The American Psychiatric Press Textbook of Psychopharmacology

The American Psychiatric Press Textbook of Psychopharmacology

Edited by

**Alan F. Schatzberg, M.D., and
Charles B. Nemeroff, M.D., Ph.D.**

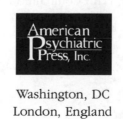

Washington, DC
London, England

Copyright © 1995 American Psychiatric Press, Inc.
ALL RIGHTS RESERVED
Manufactured in the United States of America on acid-free paper
98 97 96 95   4 3 2 1
First Edition
American Psychiatric Press, Inc.
1400 K Street, N.W., Washington, DC 20005

Library of Congress Cataloging-in-Publication Data
The American Psychiatric Press textbook of psychopharmacology / edited
  by Alan F. Schatzberg and Charles B. Nemeroff.
     p. cm.
   Includes bibliographical references and index.
   ISBN 0-88048-389-X
   1. Mental illness—Chemotherapy. 2. Psychotropic drugs.
3. Psychopharmacology. 4. Biological psychiatry. I. Schatzberg,
Alan F. II. Nemeroff, Charles B. III. American Psychiatric Press.
IV. Title: Textbook of psychopharmacology.
   [DNLM: 1. Psychotropic Drugs—pharmacology. 2. Psychotropic
Drugs—therapeutic use. 3. Mental Disorders—drug therapy. QV
77.2 A512 1995]
RC483.A515 1995
615'.78—dc20
DNLM/DLC
for Library of Congress   94-49235
                                                                      CIP

British Library Cataloguing in Publication Data
A CIP record is available from the British Library.

Cover designed by David Ryner, Echo Communications, Bethesda, Maryland

Dedicated to
Nancy, Melissa, and Lindsey;
Melissa, Matthew, Amanda, and Sarah-Frances;
and the memory of our parents.

Also dedicated to
Roland D. Ciaranello, M.D.,
who died suddenly on
December 15, 1994.

Contents

Contributors xi

Introduction xix
    Alan F. Schatzberg, M.D., and Charles B. Nemeroff, M.D., Ph.D.

Section I: Principles of Psychopharmacology
Roland D. Ciaranello, M.D., Section Editor

1 Introduction to Neurotransmitters, Receptors, Signal Transduction,
and Second Messengers 3
    Richard E. Wilcox, Ph.D., and Rueben A. Gonzales, Ph.D.

2 Molecular Neurobiology 31
    Allison C. Chin, Ph.D., Karen A. Shaw, Ph.D., and Roland D. Ciaranello, M.D.

3 Biochemical Anatomy: Insights Into the Cell Biology and Pharmacology
of Neurotransmitter Systems in the Brain 45
    Alfred Mansour, Ph.D., Derek T. Chalmers, Ph.D., Charles A. Fox, Ph.D.,
    James H. Meador-Woodruff, M.D., and Stanley J. Watson, M.D., Ph.D.

4 Electrophysiology 65
    Anthony A. Grace, Ph.D., and Benjamin S. Bunney, M.D.

5 Animal Models of Depression and Schizophrenia 81
    Jay M. Weiss, Ph.D., and Clinton D. Kilts, Ph.D.

6 Principles of Pharmacokinetics and Pharmacodynamics 125
    David J. Greenblatt, M.D.

Section II: Classes of Psychiatric Drugs: Animal and Human Pharmacology
Herbert Y. Meltzer, M.D., Section Editor

Anxiolytics and Antidepressants

7 Tricyclics and Tetracyclics 141
    William Z. Potter, M.D., Ph.D., Husseini K. Manji, M.D., F.R.C.P.C., and
    Matthew V. Rudorfer, M.D.

8   Selective Serotonin Reuptake Inhibitors 161
      Gary D. Tollefson, M.D., Ph.D.

9   Monoamine Oxidase Inhibitors 183
      K. Ranga Rama Krishnan, M.D.

10   Trazodone and Other Antidepressants 195
      Robert N. Golden, M.D., Joseph M. Bebchuk, M.D., F.R.C.P.C., and
      Martha E. Leatherman, M.D.

11   Benzodiazepines 215
      James C. Ballenger, M.D.

12   Nonbenzodiazepine Anxiolytics 231
      Jonathan O. Cole, M.D., and Kimberly A. Yonkers, M.D.

Antipsychotics

13   Antipsychotic Medications 247
      Stephen R. Marder, M.D., and Theodore Van Putten, M.D.

14   Atypical Antipsychotics 263
      Michael J. Owens, Ph.D., and S. Craig Risch, M.D.

15   Drugs to Treat Extrapyramidal Side Effects 281
      Joseph K. Stanilla, M.D., and George M. Simpson, M.D.

Drugs for Treatment of Bipolar Disorder

16   Lithium 303
      Robert H. Lenox, M.D., and Husseini K. Manji, M.D., F.R.C.P.C.

17   Antiepileptic Drugs 351
      Susan L. McElroy, M.D., and Paul E. Keck, Jr., M.D.

18   Calcium Channel Antagonists as Novel Agents for Manic-Depressive Disorder 377
      Steven L. Dubovsky, M.D.

Other Agents

19   Cognitive Enhancers 391
      Deborah B. Marin, M.D., Kenneth L. Davis, M.D., and Albert J. Speranza, Jr., M.D.

20   Sedative-Hypnotics 405
      Seiji Nishino, M.D., Ph.D., Emmanuel Mignot, M.D., Ph.D., and
      William C. Dement, M.D., Ph.D.

21   Stimulants in Psychiatry 417
      Jan Fawcett, M.D., and Katie A. Busch, M.D.

Section III: Clinical Psychobiology and Psychiatric Syndromes
David J. Kupfer, M.D., Section Editor

22 Biology of Mood Disorders 439
  Kalpana I. Nathan, M.D., Dominique L. Musselman, M.D.,
  Alan F. Schatzberg, M.D., and Charles B. Nemeroff, M.D., Ph.D.

23 Neurobiology of Schizophrenia 479
  Michael B. Knable, D.O., Joel E. Kleinman, M.D., Ph.D., and
  Daniel R. Weinberger, M.D.

24 Biology of Anxiety Disorders 501
  Murray B. Stein, M.D., and Thomas W. Uhde, M.D.

25 Biology of Alzheimer's Disease and Animal Models 523
  Donald L. Price, M.D., Lary C. Walker, Ph.D., Lee J. Martin, Ph.D.,
  David R. Borchelt, Ph.D., Philip C. Wong, Ph.D., and
  Sangram S. Sisodia, Ph.D.

26 Biology of Psychoactive Substance Dependence Disorders:
  Opiates, Cocaine, and Ethanol 537
  Roger E. Meyer, M.D.

27 Biology of Eating Disorders 557
  Regina C. Casper, M.D.

Section IV: Psychopharmacological Treatment
Donald F. Klein, M.D., Section Editor

28 Treatment of Depression 575
  Dennis S. Charney, M.D., Helen L. Miller, M.D.,
  Julio Licinio, M.D., and Ronald Salomon, M.D.

29 Treatment of Bipolar Disorder 603
  Charles L. Bowden, M.D.

30 Treatment of Schizophrenia 615
  Peter F. Buckley, M.D., and Herbert Y. Meltzer, M.D.

31 Treatment of Anxiety Disorders 641
  C. Barr Taylor, M.D.

32 Treatment of Alzheimer's Disease and Other Dementias 657
  Murray A. Raskind, M.D.

33 Treatment of Childhood and Adolescent Disorders 669
  Mina K. Dulcan, M.D., Joel D. Bregman, M.D.,
  Elizabeth B. Weller, M.D., and Ronald A. Weller, M.D.

34 Treatment of Substance-Related Disorders 707
    James W. Cornish, M.D., Laura F. McNicholas, M.D., Ph.D., and
    Charles P. O'Brien, M.D., Ph.D.

35 Treatment of Eating Disorders 725
    W. Stewart Agras, M.D.

36 Treatment of Aggressive Disorders 735
    Stuart C. Yudofsky, M.D., Jonathan M. Silver, M.D., and
    Robert E. Hales, M.D.

37 Treatment of Personality Disorders 753
    Robert L. Trestman, Ph.D., M.D., Marie deVegvar, M.D., and
    Larry J. Siever, M.D.

38 Treatment of Psychiatric Emergencies 769
    Michael J. Tueth, M.D., C. Lindsay DeVane, Pharm.D., and
    Dwight L. Evans, M.D.

39 Psychopharmacology in the Medically Ill Patient 783
    Alan Stoudemire, M.D., Michael G. Moran, M.D., and
    Barry S. Fogel, M.D.

40 Geriatric Psychopharmacology 803
    Carl Salzman, M.D., Andrew Satlin, M.D., and
    Adam B. Burrows, M.D.

41 Psychopharmacology During Pregnancy and Lactation 823
    Zachary N. Stowe, M.D., and Charles B. Nemeroff, M.D., Ph.D.

    Appendix 1: Promising Psychopharmacological Agents Available in Europe 839
    Ira D. Glick, M.D., Yves Lecrubier, M.D., Stuart A. Montgomery, M.D.,
    Oldrich Vinar, M.D., D.Sc., and Donald F. Klein, M.D.

    Index 847

Contributors

W. Stewart Agras, M.D.
Professor of Psychiatry and Director, Behavioral
Medicine Program, Stanford University School of
Medicine, Stanford, California

James C. Ballenger, M.D.
Director, Institute of Psychiatry; Director, Clinical
Research Division; and Chairman and Professor,
Department of Psychiatry and Behavioral Sciences,
Medical University of South Carolina, Charleston,
South Carolina

Joseph M. Bebchuk, M.D., F.R.C.P.C.
Clinical Instructor and Clinical
Psychopharmacology Research Fellow, Department
of Psychiatry, University of North Carolina at
Chapel Hill School of Medicine, Chapel Hill, North
Carolina

David R. Borchelt, Ph.D.
Instructor, Department of Pathology, The Johns
Hopkins University School of Medicine, Baltimore,
Maryland

Charles L. Bowden, M.D.
Nancy U. Karren Professor and Deputy Chairman,
Department of Psychiatry, and Chief, Division of
Biological Psychiatry, University of Texas Health
Science Center, San Antonio, Texas

Joel D. Bregman, M.D.
Medical Director, Emory Autism Resource Center,
Associate Professor of Psychiatry and Behavioral
Sciences and Assistant Professor of Pediatrics,
Emory University School of Medicine, Atlanta,
Georgia

Peter F. Buckley, M.D.
Assistant Professor of Psychiatry, Case Western
Reserve University School of Medicine, Cleveland,
Ohio

Benjamin S. Bunney, M.D.
Professor of Psychiatry and Pharmacology, Yale
University School of Medicine; Chief of Psychiatric
Services, Yale-New Haven Hospital; Chairman of
the Board, Yale Psychiatric Institute, New Haven,
Connecticut

Adam B. Burrows, M.D.
Instructor in Medicine, Harvard Medical School;
Staff Geriatrician and Research Fellow, Hebrew
Rehabilitation Center for Aged, Boston,
Massachusetts

Katie A. Busch, M.D.
Assistant Professor, Department of Psychiatry,
Rush-Presbyterian-St. Luke's Medical Center,
Chicago, Illinois

Regina C. Casper, M.D.
Professor, Department of Psychiatry and Behavioral
Sciences, Stanford University School of Medicine,
Stanford, California

Derek T. Chalmers, Ph.D.
Scientist, Neuroscience Section, Neurocrine
Biosciences, Inc., San Diego, California

Dennis S. Charney, M.D.
Professor of Psychiatry, Yale University School
of Medicine, New Haven, Connecticut; Chief,
Psychiatry Service, West Haven Veterans
Administration Medical Center, West Haven,
Connecticut

Allison C. Chin, Ph.D.
Research Associate, Department of Psychiatry and Behavioral Sciences, Stanford University School of Medicine, Stanford, California

Roland D. Ciaranello, M.D.
Nancy Friend Pritzker Professor of Psychiatry and Behavioral Sciences, Stanford University School of Medicine, Stanford, California

Jonathan O. Cole, M.D.
Professor of Psychiatry, Harvard Medical School, Boston, Massachusetts; Senior Staff Consultant, McLean Hospital, Affective Disorders Program, Belmont, Massachusetts

James W. Cornish, M.D.
Research Assistant Professor, Department of Psychiatry, and Director of Pharmacotherapy, Treatment Research Center, University of Pennsylvania, Philadelphia, Pennsylvania

Kenneth L. Davis, M.D.
Professor and Chairman, Department of Psychiatry, Mount Sinai Medical Center, New York, New York

William C. Dement, M.D., Ph.D.
Lowell W. and Josephine Q. Berry Professor, Department of Psychiatry and Behavioral Sciences, Stanford University School of Medicine, Stanford, California; Director, Stanford Sleep Disorders Center, Palo Alto, California

C. Lindsay DeVane, Pharm.D.
Professor of Psychiatry and Behavioral Sciences, Medical University of South Carolina, Charleston, South Carolina

Marie deVegvar, M.D.
Clinical Instructor, Mount Sinai School of Medicine, New York, New York; Clinical Director, Psychiatry Outpatient Services, Bronx Veterans Administration Medical Center, Bronx, New York

Steven L. Dubovsky, M.D.
Professor of Psychiatry and Medicine and Vice Chairman for Clinical Affairs, Department of Psychiatry, University of Colorado School of Medicine, Denver, Colorado

Mina K. Dulcan, M.D.
Osterman Professor of Child Psychiatry, Northwestern University Medical School, Evanston, Illinois; Head, Department of Child Psychiatry, Children's Memorial Medical Center, Chicago, Illinois

Dwight L. Evans, M.D.
Professor of Psychiatry, Medicine, and Neuroscience, and Chairman, Department of Psychiatry, University of Florida College of Medicine, Gainesville, Florida

Jan Fawcett, M.D.
Professor and Chairman, Department of Psychiatry, Rush-Presbyterian-St. Luke's Medical Center; Director, Rush Institute for Mental Well-Being, Chicago, Illinois

Barry S. Fogel, M.D.
Professor of Psychiatry and Human Behavior, Brown University School of Medicine, Providence, Rhode Island

Charles A. Fox, Ph.D.
Postdoctoral/Research Fellow, Mental Health Research Institute, University of Michigan, Ann Arbor, Michigan

Ira D. Glick, M.D.
Professor of Psychiatry and Director of Inpatient and Partial Hospitalization Services, Department of Psychiatry and Behavioral Sciences, Stanford University School of Medicine, Stanford, California

Robert N. Golden, M.D.
Professor and Chair of Psychiatry and Director, Clinical Psychopharmacology Research Training Program, University of North Carolina at Chapel Hill School of Medicine, Chapel Hill, North Carolina

Rueben A. Gonzales, Ph.D.
Associate Professor, Department of Pharmacology, College of Pharmacy, University of Texas, Austin, Texas

Anthony A. Grace, Ph.D.
Associate Professor of Neuroscience and Psychiatry, Center for Neuroscience, University of Pittsburgh, Pittsburgh, Pennsylvania

David J. Greenblatt, M.D.
Professor of Pharmacology and Experimental
Therapeutics, Psychiatry, and Medicine, Tufts
University School of Medicine; Division of Clinical
Pharmacology, New England Medical Center
Hospital, Boston, Massachusetts

Robert E. Hales, M.D.
Chairman, Department of Psychiatry, California
Pacific Medical Center; Clinical Professor of
Psychiatry, University of California, San Francisco,
School of Medicine, San Francisco, California

Paul E. Keck, Jr., M.D.
Associate Professor of Psychiatry and Co-Director,
Biological Psychiatry Program, University of
Cincinnati College of Medicine, Cincinnati, Ohio

Clinton D. Kilts, Ph.D.
Associate Professor of Psychiatry and Assistant
Professor of Pathology, Department of Psychiatry
and Behavioral Sciences, Emory University School
of Medicine, Atlanta, Georgia

Donald F. Klein, M.D.
Professor of Psychiatry, Columbia University
College of Physicians and Surgeons, New York,
New York; Director of Research, New York State
Psychiatric Institute, New York, New York

Joel E. Kleinman, M.D., Ph.D.
Chief, Neuropathology Section, and Deputy Chief,
Clinical Brain Disorders Branch, Division of
Intramural Research Programs, National Institute
of Mental Health, Bethesda, Maryland; NIMH
Neuroscience Center at St. Elizabeths, Washington,
DC

Michael B. Knable, D.O.
Clinical Research Associate, Division of Intramural
Research Programs, National Institute of Mental
Health, Bethesda, Maryland; NIMH Neuroscience
Center at St. Elizabeths, Washington, DC

K. Ranga Rama Krishnan, M.D.
Associate Professor of Psychiatry, Duke University
School of Medicine; Head, Division of Biological
Psychiatry, and Director, Affective Disorders
Program, Duke University Medical Center, Durham,
North Carolina

David J. Kupfer, M.D.
Thomas Detre Professor and Chairman,
Department of Psychiatry, University of Pittsburgh
School of Medicine, Western Psychiatric Institute
and Clinic, Pittsburgh, Pennsylvania

Martha E. Leatherman, M.D.
Assistant Professor of Psychiatry, University of
Texas Health Science Center at San Antonio, San
Antonio, Texas

Yves Lecrubier, M.D.
Director of Research INSERM, Hôpital de la
Salpêtrière, Paris, France

Robert H. Lenox, M.D.
Professor of Psychiatry, Pharmacology, and
Neuroscience, and Director, Molecular
Neuropsychopharmacology Program, University of
Florida College of Medicine, Gainesville, Florida

Julio Licinio, M.D.
Visiting Scientist, Intramural Research Program, and
Chief, Unit on Clinical Research, Clinical
Neuroendocrinology Branch, National Institute of
Mental Health, Bethesda, Maryland

Husseini K. Manji, M.D., F.R.C.P.C.
Visiting Scientist, Section on Clinical Pharmacology,
National Institute of Mental Health, and Molecular
Pathophysiology Branch, NIDDK, Bethesda,
Maryland

Alfred Mansour, Ph.D.
Research Investigator, Mental Health Research
Institute, University of Michigan, Ann Arbor,
Michigan

Stephen R. Marder, M.D.
Professor of Psychiatry, University of California–
Los Angeles School of Medicine; Chief, Psychiatry
Service, West Los Angeles Veterans Administration
Medical Center, Los Angeles, California

Deborah B. Marin, M.D.
Assistant Professor, Department of Psychiatry, and
Director, Division of Geropsychiatry, Mount Sinai
Medical Center, New York, New York

Lee J. Martin, Ph.D.
Assistant Professor, Departments of Pathology and
Neuroscience, The Johns Hopkins University
School of Medicine, Baltimore, Maryland

Susan L. McElroy, M.D.
Associate Professor of Psychiatry and Co-Director,
Biological Psychiatry Program, University of
Cincinnati College of Medicine, Cincinnati, Ohio

Laura F. McNicholas, M.D., Ph.D.
Assistant Professor of Psychiatry, University of
Pennsylvania School of Medicine, Philadelphia,
Pennsylvania

James H. Meador-Woodruff, M.D.
Assistant Research Scientist, Mental Health
Research Institute, University of Michigan, Ann
Arbor, Michigan

Herbert Y. Meltzer, M.D.
Douglas Bond Professor of Psychiatry, Case
Western Reserve University School of Medicine,
Cleveland, Ohio

Roger E. Meyer, M.D.
Vice President for Medical Affairs/Executive Dean
and Professor of Psychiatry, George Washington
University Medical Center, Washington, DC

Emmanuel Mignot, M.D., Ph.D.
Assistant Professor of Psychiatry and Behavioral
Sciences, Stanford University School of Medicine,
Stanford, California; Director, Center for
Narcolepsy, Stanford Sleep Research Center, Palo
Alto, California

Helen L. Miller, M.D.
Assistant Professor of Psychiatry, Yale University
School of Medicine, New Haven, Connecticut;
Director, Affective Disorders Program, West Haven
Veterans Administration Medical Center, West
Haven, Connecticut

Stuart A. Montgomery, M.D.
Professor of Psychiatry, St. Mary's Hospital Medical
School, London, England

Michael G. Moran, M.D.
Associate Professor of Psychiatry, University of
Colorado School of Medicine, Denver, Colorado

Dominique L. Musselman, M.D.
Research Fellow in Neuroendocrinology,
Department of Psychiatry and Behavioral Sciences,
Emory University School of Medicine, Atlanta,
Georgia

Kalpana I. Nathan, M.D.
Attending Psychiatrist, Department of Psychiatry,
Veterans Affairs Medical Center, Palo Alto,
California; Consulting Psychiatrist, Emergency
Psychiatric Services, Valley Medical Center, San
Jose, California

Charles B. Nemeroff, M.D., Ph.D.
Reunette W. Harris Professor and Chairman,
Department of Psychiatry and Behavioral Sciences,
Emory University School of Medicine, Atlanta,
Georgia

Seiji Nishino, M.D., Ph.D.
Visiting Assistant Professor of Psychiatry and
Behavioral Sciences, Stanford University School
of Medicine, Stanford, California; Lecturer,
Department of Neuropsychiatry, Osaka Medical
College, Osaka, Japan

Charles P. O'Brien, M.D., Ph.D.
Professor and Vice Chairman, Department of
Psychiatry, University of Pennsylvania; Chief of
Psychiatry, Veterans Administration Medical Center,
Philadelphia, Pennsylvania

Michael J. Owens, Ph.D.
Associate Director, Laboratory of
Neuropsychopharmacology, and Assistant
Professor, Department of Psychiatry and Behavioral
Sciences, Emory University School of Medicine,
Atlanta, Georgia

William Z. Potter, M.D., Ph.D.
Chief, Section on Clinical Pharmacology, National
Institute of Mental Health, Bethesda, Maryland

Donald L. Price, M.D.
Professor, Departments of Pathology, Neurology, and Neuroscience, and Director, Neuropathology Laboratory, The Johns Hopkins University School of Medicine, Baltimore, Maryland

Murray A. Raskind, M.D.
Professor and Vice Chairman for Research Development, Department of Psychiatry and Behavioral Sciences, University of Washington School of Medicine, Seattle, Washington

S. Craig Risch, M.D.
Professor of Psychiatry and Behavioral Sciences; Director, Clinical Neuropharmacology Research Program; and Director, Affective Disorders and Schizophrenia Research and Treatment Program, Institute of Psychiatry and Behavioral Sciences, Medical University of South Carolina, Charleston

Matthew V. Rudorfer, M.D.
Assistant Chief, Clinical Treatment Research Branch, Division of Clinical and Treatment Research, National Institute of Mental Health, Bethesda, Maryland

Ronald Salomon, M.D.
Assistant Professor of Psychiatry, Yale University School of Medicine, New Haven, Connecticut; Director, ECT Service, West Haven Veterans Administration Medical Center, West Haven, Connecticut

Carl Salzman, M.D.
Professor of Psychiatry, Harvard Medical School, Boston, Massachusetts; Director of Psychopharmacology, Massachusetts Mental Health Center, Boston, Massachusetts

Andrew Satlin, M.D.
Assistant Professor of Psychiatry, Harvard Medical School, Boston, Massachusetts; Director of Geriatric Psychiatry, McLean Hospital, Belmont, Massachusetts

Alan F. Schatzberg, M.D.
Kenneth T. Norris, Jr. Professor and Chairman, Department of Psychiatry and Behavioral Sciences, Stanford University Medical Center, Stanford, California

Karen A. Shaw, Ph.D.
Lecturer, Department of Biochemistry and Physiology, University of Reading, Reading, Berkshire, United Kingdom

Larry J. Siever, M.D.
Professor of Psychiatry, Mount Sinai School of Medicine, New York, New York; Director of Outpatient Department, Bronx Veterans Administration Medical Center, Bronx, New York

Jonathan M. Silver, M.D.
Director of Neuropsychiatry, Columbia Presbyterian Medical Center, and Associate Professor of Clinical Psychiatry, Columbia University, New York, New York

George M. Simpson, M.D.
Professor of Psychiatry and Pharmacology, and Director of Clinical Psychopharmacology, Medical College of Pennsylvania/Eastern Pennsylvania Psychiatric Institute, Philadelphia, Pennsylvania

Sangram S. Sisodia, Ph.D.
Assistant Professor, Department of Pathology, The Johns Hopkins University School of Medicine, Baltimore, Maryland

Albert J. Speranza, Jr., M.D.
Psychiatrist, Veterans Affairs Medical Center, New York, New York

Joseph K. Stanilla, M.D.
Clinical Instructor in Psychiatry, Medical College of Pennsylvania, Philadelphia, Pennsylvania; Clinical Director, Clinical Research Unit, Norristown State Hospital, Norristown, Pennsylvania

Murray B. Stein, M.D.
Associate Professor; Director, Anxiety & Traumatic Stress Disorders Research Program, Department of Psychiatry, University of California, San Diego

Alan Stoudemire, M.D.
Professor of Psychiatry and Behavioral Sciences, Emory University School of Medicine, Atlanta, Georgia

Zachary N. Stowe, M.D.
Assistant Professor, Department of Psychiatry and Behavioral Science; Assistant Professor, Department of Obstetrics and Gynecology; and Director, Pregnancy and Postpartum Mood Disorders Program, Emory University School of Medicine, Atlanta, Georgia

C. Barr Taylor, M.D.
Professor of Psychiatry and Associate Director, Laboratory for the Study of Behavioral Medicine, Stanford University School of Medicine, Stanford, California

Gary D. Tollefson, M.D., Ph.D.
Associate Professor of Psychiatry, University of Minnesota, Minneapolis, Minnesota; Executive Director, CNS-GI-GU Medical Division, Lilly Research Laboratories, Eli Lilly and Company, Indianapolis, Indiana

Robert L. Trestman, Ph.D., M.D.
Assistant Professor of Psychiatry and Director, Research Fellowship Training, Department of Psychiatry, Mount Sinai School of Medicine, New York, New York; Research Director, Outpatient Psychiatry, Bronx Veterans Administration Medical Center, Bronx, New York

Michael J. Tueth, M.D.
Assistant Professor of Psychiatry and Director, Geropsychiatry Outpatient Services, Department of Psychiatry, University of Florida College of Medicine, Gainesville, Florida

Thomas W. Uhde, M.D.
Professor and Chairperson, Department of Psychiatry and Behavioral Neurosciences, Wayne State University; Psychiatrist-in-Chief, Detroit Medical Center; Chairman, Department of Psychiatry, and Director, Mood and Anxiety Disorders Clinical Research Division, Detroit Receiving Hospital, Detroit, Michigan

Theodore Van Putten, M.D.*
Professor of Psychiatry, University of California–Los Angeles School of Medicine; Staff Psychiatrist, West Los Angeles Veterans Administration Medical Center, Los Angeles, California

Oldrich Vinar, M.D., D.Sc.
Associate Professor, Institute of Organic Chemistry and Biochemistry; Head, Joint Laboratory, Czech Academy of Science and State Institute for Drug Control, Prague, Czech Republic

Lary C. Walker, Ph.D.
Assistant Professor, Departments of Pathology and Psychology, The Johns Hopkins University School of Medicine, Baltimore, Maryland

Stanley J. Watson, M.D., Ph.D.
Research Scientist, Mental Health Research Institute, University of Michigan, Ann Arbor, Michigan

Daniel R. Weinberger, M.D.
Chief, Clinical Brain Disorders Branch, Division of Intramural Research Programs, National Institute of Mental Health, Bethesda, Maryland; NIMH Neuroscience Center at St. Elizabeths, Washington, DC

Jay M. Weiss, Ph.D.
Professor of Psychiatry, Department of Psychiatry and Behavioral Sciences, Emory University School of Medicine, Atlanta, Georgia; Director of Research, Georgia Mental Health Institute, Atlanta, Georgia

Elizabeth B. Weller, M.D.
Professor of Psychiatry, Pediatrics, and Neuroscience, Vice Chair of Psychiatry, and Director of Training, Child and Adolescent Psychiatry, Ohio State University School of Medicine, Columbus, Ohio

Ronald A. Weller, M.D.
Professor of Psychiatry, Director of Training, Department of Psychiatry, Ohio State University School of Medicine, Columbus, Ohio

*Deceased

Richard E. Wilcox, Ph.D.
Professor and Doluisio Fellow,
Neuropharmacology Program Head, Institute for
Neuroscience and College of Pharmacy, University
of Texas, Austin, Texas

Philip C. Wong, Ph.D.
Instructor, Department of Pathology, The Johns
Hopkins University School of Medicine, Baltimore,
Maryland

Kimberly A. Yonkers, M.D.
Assistant Professor, Department of Psychiatry and
Department of Obstetrics and Gynecology,
University of Texas Southwestern Medical Center,
Dallas, Texas

Stuart C. Yudofsky, M.D.
D.C. and Irene Ellwood Professor and Chairman,
Department of Psychiatry, Baylor College of
Medicine; Chief of Psychiatry Service, The
Methodist Hospital, Houston, Texas

Introduction

Psychopharmacology has developed as a medical discipline over approximately the past four decades. The development and early introduction of effective antidepressants, antipsychotics, and mood stabilizers were frequently based on serendipitous observations. The repeated demonstration of efficacy of these agents served as an impetus for considerable research into the neurobiological bases of emotion and cognition as well as the biological basis of the major psychiatric disorders. Moreover, the emergence of an entire new multidisciplinary field, neuropsychopharmacology, which in turn has led to newer, specific agents to alter maladaptive central neurons system processes or activity, was another by-product of these early endeavors. The remarkable proliferation of information in this area—coupled with the absence of any comparable, currently available text—led us to edit this *Textbook of Psychopharmacology*.

In order to present the rich amount of information, we have attempted to develop a context for the reader. The Textbook consists of four major sections. The first section, "Principles of Psychopharmacology," includes chapters on neurotransmitters, neuroanatomy, electrophysiology, molecular neurobiology, animal models, and pharmacokinetics. This section provides a theoretical background for the reader.

The second section, "Classes of Psychiatric Drugs: Animal and Human Pharmacology," presents information by classes of drugs. For each drug within a class, data are reviewed on preclinical and clinical pharmacology, pharmacokinetics, indications, dosages, and the like. This section is pharmacopoeia-like. We have attempted to include data on currently available drugs in the United States as well as medications that will almost certainly become available in the near future.

The third section, "Clinical Psychobiology and Psychiatric Syndromes," reviews data on the biological underpinnings of specific disorders—for example, major depression, bipolar disorder, panic disorder. The authors in this section comprehensively review the biological alterations described for each of the major psychiatric disorders, allowing the reader to better understand current psychopharmacological approaches as well as to anticipate future novel developments.

The fourth section, "Psychopharmacological Treatment," reviews state-of-the-art therapeutic approaches to patients with major psychiatric disorders as well as to those in specific age groups or circumstances: childhood disorders, emergency psychiatry, pregnancy and postpartum, the medically ill, and so forth. This section provides the reader with specific information about drug selection and their prescription. In addition, there is an Appendix on promising new agents in Europe and Canada.

This Textbook would not have been possible without the superb editorial work of the section editors—Roland Ciaranello, Herbert Meltzer, David Kupfer, and Donald Klein—as well as, of course, the authors of the chapters who so generously gave of their time. In addition, we wish to thank Claire Reinburg of the American Psychiatric Press and her staff for their editorial efforts. Finally, we extend our thanks to Marsha D. Wallace at Stanford University and Maryfrances Porter at Emory University for their invaluable assistance.

Alan F. Schatzberg, M.D.
Charles B. Nemeroff, M.D., Ph.D.

Principles of Psychopharmacology

Roland D. Ciaranello, M.D., Section Editor

Introduction to Neurotransmitters, Receptors, Signal Transduction, and Second Messengers

Richard E. Wilcox, Ph.D., and
Rueben A. Gonzales, Ph.D.

Psychopharmacology is the study of the mediation and modulation of behavior through the actions of endogenous signaling substances and drugs. A psychopharmacological mechanism is the molecular means by which behavioral change is brought about by an endogenous or exogenous chemical. Signaling molecules in the brain are small molecular weight transmitters (hormones, neurotransmitters, and neuromodulators) and cellular second messengers (e.g., cyclic adenosine monophosphate [cAMP], inositol trisphosphate [IP_3], diacylglycerol [DAG], and arachidonic acid [AA] metabolites) as well as proteins (receptors, signal-transducing guanine nucleotide-binding proteins [G proteins], enzymes, uptake carriers, etc.).

In this chapter, we consider four classes of signaling molecule: neurotransmitters, receptors, signal transducing proteins, and second messengers. Together, all of these elements participate in the integration of information within the central nervous system (CNS). There are numerous levels at which this integration can occur (e.g., the molecular, cellular, circuit [tissue], and whole brain [system] levels). The reader is probably quite familiar with examples of CNS integration that occur at the cellular and circuit levels. In this chapter, we provide a set of models for the molecular and cellular levels of integration to use throughout the remainder of this textbook. We discuss each of the four classes of signaling molecules separately throughout much of this chapter. Each class is discussed "horizontally" (see Figure 1–1) to facilitate comparison among other signaling molecules at the same level. Although this approach is necessary to allow ready comparisons within a class of signaling molecule, it is also artificial. This is because the CNS functions across classes of signaling molecule, sending information from transmitter to receptor to signal transducing protein to cellular second messenger in a "vertical" pattern of information flow within a transmitter system.

It is essential to realize that each of the biochemical information transfer pathways that exists in our brains has a primary function—to alter cellular activity, information flow, and ultimately, behavior. Fundamentally, each biochemical pathway within each of the transmitter systems of brain alters some cellular function directly. In addition, the changes in cellular activity that are produced by one biochemical pathway act to alter the functions of other pathways throughout the cell and at multiple points within the direct pathway. Thus, each biochemical pathway inside the cell also has many branch points where other pathways are activated or inhibited in their functions. Integration can occur at the level of transmitters modulating the same or different subtypes of receptors, at the level of receptors activating the same or different signal transducer proteins, and at the level of signal transducers altering the same or different second messengers inside the cell.

A presynaptic neuron's release of a transmitter activates a postsynaptic receptor that transduces a signal to the inside of the target cell and ultimately produces a postsynaptic response. For example, receptor-gated ion channels mediate fast on-off signals in the form of ion fluxes. Other information transfer processes rely on slower mechanisms, including the transduction of information from a cell surface receptor to intracellular enzymes. Activation of an ion channel may alter the activation of a cellular enzyme and may also result in attenuation of the channel's ability to respond to its transmitter for a short time.

In this chapter, we consider prototypes of each class of signaling molecule and then discuss other key members of the class comparatively—the horizontal approach of Figure 1–1. This should provide the reader with a solid core of information with which to approach the more detailed discussions in later chapters of this book, which focus on the vertical approach of transmitter systems. To achieve the status accorded a signaling molecule within its class, a putative signal substance must meet certain criteria. To highlight this concept, the sections on neurotransmitters and second messengers begin with a brief overview of the criteria that potential signal molecules within these classes have met for inclusion. The discussion within each section focuses on a few fundamental principles by which the reader can compare signaling molecules within and between functional classes.

■ NEUROTRANSMITTERS

■ Core Transmitters and the Prototype for Discussion

We will consider acetylcholine, dopamine, norepinephrine, serotonin, glutamate, and γ-aminobutyric acid (GABA) as key transmitters implicated in psychiatric disease and its pharmacological therapy.

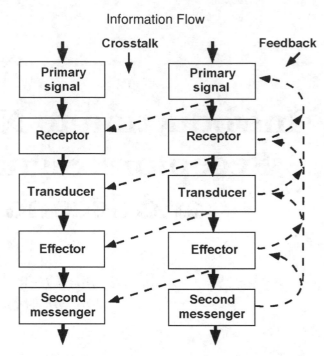

Figure 1–1. Schematic representation of the elements that mediate information processing in the central nervous system. Boldface arrows indicate "vertical" or direct transfer of information across classes of signaling molecule. Dashed arrows indicate examples of some of the potential points of integration that involve interactions between and within classes of signaling molecules. For simplicity, only a few of the numerous possible types of integration have been shown in this figure. These processes involve regulation, modulation, or fine-tuning of direct signals. Emphasized in the figure are feedback processes, in which information can flow from distal to proximal portions of a biochemical information pathway (i.e., from effector to receptor); and crosstalk, in which information can be transferred between parallel biochemical pathways through common linkages.

Dopamine, which plays a major role in schizophrenia and its pharmacotherapy (Seeman 1987), will be considered as the prototype, and other core transmitters will be compared with it.

■ Criteria for a Neurotransmitter

It is useful to follow the format of McGeer and colleagues (1987) in stating the criteria for a transmitter within anatomical, chemical, physiological, and pharmacological domains. Dopamine fulfills the anatomical criterion by being unevenly distributed within the brain, where it is especially enriched in nerve terminals. Indeed, it was the difference in the brain distributions of dopamine and norepinephrine that first gave a clue to an independent transmitter role for dopamine. The chemical criteria for dopamine are also fulfilled by the presence of the enzymes necessary for dopamine synthesis (tyrosine hydroxylase and aromatic amino acid decarboxylase; Nagatsu 1991) in terminals of dopamine neurons and by the calcium-dependent and potassium-stimulated release of endogenous dopamine from pinched-off nerve endings (synaptosomes) from the corpus striatum of basal ganglia (Leslie et al. 1985).

Local microinjections of dopamine by needle-guide cannula (chemitrode), iontophoresis, pulse pressure, and microdialysis tube infusion mimic the actions produced by stimulation of the nigrostriatal dopamine tract and other dopamine-containing pathways, such as the ventral tegmental dopaminergic projection to mesolimbic and mesocortical brain regions. This fulfills the basic physiological criterion for transmitter status. Finally, the effects of drugs on the several possible sites of action within the dopaminergic synapse (discussed in the next section) should alter behavior in ways predictable from stimulating or lesioning tracts containing dopamine in the brain. This is indeed the case and fulfills the pharmacological criterion for dopamine's transmitter status.

■ Major Sites of Drug Action—
Steps in Chemical Transmission

Tyrosine from dietary sources is taken up into dopaminergic nerve terminals through a facilitated diffusion, where it is acted upon by the cytoplasmic enzyme tyrosine hydroxylase to yield L-dopa (Figure 1–2). Subsequently, the L-dopa is taken into presynaptic vesicles where the conversion to dopamine takes place through the action of an L-aromatic amino acid decarboxylase enzyme (also termed dopa-decarboxylase). The dopamine is protected from degradation within the presynaptic terminal by storage in membranous vesicles until arrival of an action potential at the synaptic region induces a voltage-dependent calcium ion entry coupled to transmitter release (stimulus-secretion coupling). As a result of calcium entry, the vesicular contents are extruded into the immediately adjacent synaptic cleft, where dopamine diffuses to stimulate dopamine receptors. These receptors may be on the nerve terminal (axon terminal autoreceptors, because they respond to the neuron's own transmitter) or on the nondopa-

minergic target cell (postsynaptic heteroceptors, because these neurons do not secrete dopamine; Wolf and Roth 1987). Similarly, dopamine release from the dendrites or cell body can stimulate another class of impulse flow–regulating receptors (dendritic or somal autoreceptors, respectively; Roth 1984).

Clearly, dopamine cannot be released unless it is synthesized and stored properly; thus, complete inhibition of either of the above enzymatic reactions can prevent dopamine production. Such inhibition will reduce dopamine release into the synaptic cleft. This illustrates the principle of *synaptic effect*: effects of a drug or a disease on dopamine synthesis become relevant to behavior only if such changes also somehow alter the amount of dopamine released into the synaptic cleft and available to stimulate its receptors.

The hydroxylation of tyrosine is the rate-limiting step in dopamine synthesis; its inhibition by α-methyl-*p*-tyrosine (AMPT) reduces the active pool of dopamine and can serve as an index of the rate at which dopamine is "turned over" within a particular brain region. A marked behavioral activation is induced by enhancing synaptic dopamine levels through the actions of cocaine or dextroamphetamine (see next section). Conversely, inhibition of dopamine synthesis produces a behavioral quieting in humans. In animals, dopamine synthesis can reasonably be estimated either from the decline in dopamine levels after tyrosine hydroxylase inhibition or from the increases in L-dopa accumulation after inhibition of the dopa-decarboxylase enzyme (by agents such as NSD 1015; Vaughn et al. 1990). In humans, dopamine synthesis and the functional integrity of the nigrostriatal dopamine nerve terminals may be estimated from changes in the specific radioactivity of ^{18}F-fluorodopa following administration of an intravenous tracer dose using the method of positron-emission tomography (PET; Hall et al. 1992; Laihinen et al. 1992).

Newly synthesized dopamine is stored in a functional "pool" that is preferentially released on nerve stimulation. This pool is especially sensitive to inhibition by the actions of AMPT. Other dopamine, which makes up the great majority of the transmitter content of a dopamine nerve terminal, is stored in a less labile pool that is sensitive to the drug reserpine (see below). There has been some suggestion that the proximity of various synaptic vesicles to likely sites of transmitter release within the terminal may help to define these two pools anatomically. Yet a third pool of dopamine consists of the cytoplasmic transmitter (McMillen 1983).

Physiological dopamine release is dependent on the concentration of external calcium ion, because it is calcium influx down its steep concentration gradient into the nerve terminal that couples the voltage changes associated with axon potentials to the secretion of transmitter. It is convenient to study release processes in vitro using either pinched-off nerve endings (synaptosomes) or tissue slices. Biophysical properties of the respective preparations dictate that synaptosomes are typically depolarized using potassium stimulation, whereas slices are depolarized using electrical stimulation. In either instance, increasing the amount of depolarization increases the net calcium influx and dopamine release from the nerve terminal (Leslie et al. 1985; Woodward et al. 1986). In contrast to the physiological release process, certain psychostimulant drugs, such as dextro-amphetamine and methamphetamine, can enhance the release of dopamine and some other transmitters through a calcium-independent release mechanism (Robinson and Becker 1986). Such noncalcium-dependent release is thought to occur through an

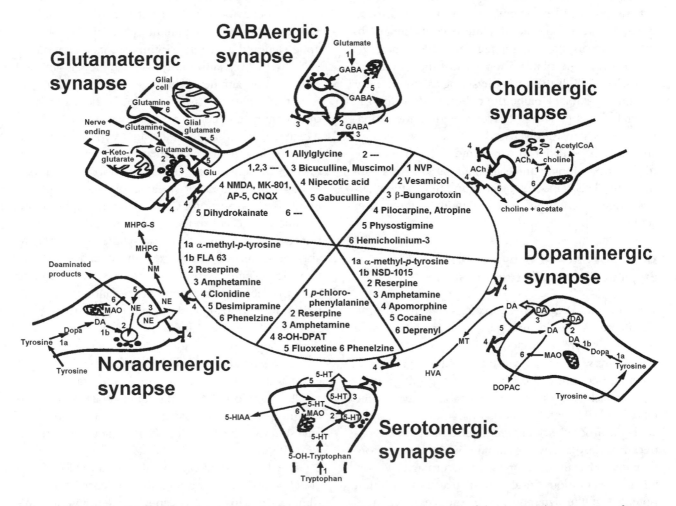

Figure 1–2. Sites of drug action for several neurotransmitter systems. The six panels of the rosette show synapses for GABA (γ-aminobutyric acid), acetylcholine (ACh), dopamine (DA), serotonin (5-HT), norepinephrine (NE), and glutamate (Glu). In general, each of the steps in synaptic transmission offers a potential target for therapeutic intervention by a drug. These steps (sites) include synthesis, vesicular uptake, transmitter release, receptor binding, cellular uptake, and transmitter metabolism. For each synapse, drugs are shown that act at the sites indicated by the numbers on the scheme. AP-5 = 2-amino-5-phosphonopentanoic acid; CNQX = 6-cyano-7-nitroquinoxaline-2,3-dione; NMDA = N-methyl-D-aspartate; NVP = naphthyl vinyl pyridinium ion; MAO = monoamine oxidase; NM = normetanephrine; MHPG = 3-methoxy-4-hydroxyphenylglycol; MHPG-S = MHPG sulfate; 5-HIAA = 5-hydroxyindoleacetic acid; MT = 3-methoxytyramine; HVA = homovanillic acid; DOPAC = 3,4-dihydroxyphenylacetic acid; 8-OH-DPAT = 8-hydroxydipropylaminotetralin. MK-801, FLA 63, and NSD 1015 are chemical code names designated by pharmaceutical companies.

exchange-diffusion process (McMillen 1983). According to this hypothesis, the amphetamine molecules are transported into the nerve terminal by the dopamine uptake carrier, exchange places with endogenous dopamine within one of the storage pools of the transmitter, and diffuse out of the terminal into the synaptic cleft, leading to an increased dopamine release.

Released dopamine can stimulate autoreceptors, which appear to be of the D_2 subfamily, located on dopamine nerve terminals. Such stimulation initiates a negative feedback effect on dopamine synthesis to reduce further release of dopamine. The consequences of dopamine stimulation are thought to involve a change in the kinetics of tyrosine hydroxylase (Saller and Salama 1986; Strait and Kuczenski 1986). This regulatory process illustrates the principle of *self-regulation* (synaptic homeostasis), whereby release of dopamine, elevating synaptic levels above baseline, initiates a set of events that tends to restore dopamine levels to their baseline. Some dopamine agonists, such as the prototype agent apomorphine or its congener *N*-n-propylnorapomorphine (NPA), can stimulate autoreceptors somewhat selectively in low doses, reducing synaptic dopamine levels without stimulating postsynaptic dopamine receptors. NPA has been used in open studies to reduce the enhanced levels of limbic system dopamine thought to be associated with the delusions and hallucinations of psychosis. Released dopamine from dendritic or somal sites can similarly exert a negative feedback action to inhibit firing of dopaminergic neurons (Chiodo 1992; Grace and Onn 1989).

In the nigrostriatal and mesolimbic dopamine systems of brain, increases in impulse flow lead to increases in dopamine synthesis, turnover, and levels of dopamine metabolites. This is a finding common to most other major transmitter systems. In contrast to most other systems, decreases in impulse flow in these two dopamine pathways, which lead to increases in dopamine content within the terminal, also lead to dramatic increases in dopamine synthesis (Bannon and Roth 1983; Deutch and Roth 1990). Although this at first seems paradoxical, there is a potential explanation. The increases in dopamine synthesis following decreases in neural firing appear to occur through an induced change in the kinetics of tyrosine hydroxylase, perhaps through a change in available intracellular calcium. These increases thus occur by a mechanism that is different from the in-

creases that follow increases in impulse flow.

Released dopamine can also stimulate postsynaptic receptors in target neurons to cause a variety of changes, depending on the type of dopamine receptor that is activated. Drugs that mimic dopamine by stimulating its receptors—agonist drugs, such as some of the agents used to treat parkinsonism—can reduce dopamine synthesis and release in the corpus striatum through negative feedback (Severson et al. 1990; Wilcox et al. 1990). At least part of this action appears to be through the stimulation of axon terminal autoreceptors. Antipsychotic drugs that block dopamine receptors, thereby acting as antagonists, prevent the actions of dopamine at these receptor sites. Thus, acute administration of antipsychotics typically halts the negative feedback action of dopamine on its synthesis and release, leading to marked increases in both actions in corpus striatum (Bartholini et al. 1989). Very low doses of antipsychotic agents appear able to block autoreceptors selectively, leading to elevations in synaptic dopamine concentrations in the absence of significant postsynaptic blockade (Bannon et al. 1986). As such, these low antipsychotic doses would not be expected to benefit psychotic symptoms such as delusions and hallucinations.

Stimulation of postsynaptic receptors by dopamine is a key event in the synaptic transmission process. Dopamine can activate at least five subtypes of dopamine receptors, which are discussed in detail below (Bunzow et al. 1988; Civelli et al. 1991; Dearry et al. 1990; Sibley and Monsma 1992; Sunahara et al. 1991; Zhou et al. 1990). Here, it is important to note that the amount of receptor stimulation is directly proportional to the concentration of dopamine. Furthermore, the cellular actions of dopamine increase to their maximum as a nonlinear, monotonic function of increasing amounts of the dopamine-receptor complex (Randall 1988). This illustrates the dose dependence of biological responses. Furthermore, because dopamine's stimulation of its receptors produces a specific sequence of cellular events, it is also important to realize that the peak time for the biological effects of a transmitter (or drug) depends on the agent's ability to get to its sites of action.

Of great relevance to the clinician is the adaptation shown by receptor systems with previous exposure to drugs. For example, chronic blockade of D_2 dopamine receptors leads to an approximate 30% increase in receptor density and to changes in postreceptor events. These changes make the system more sensitive to endogenous dopamine and to the actions of dopamine agonists (sensitization) while less sensitive to some of the biological consequences of receptor blockade.

The converse situation occurs with repeated stimulation of dopamine receptors by dopamine or dopamine agonists, resulting in a reduction of dopamine receptor numbers (downregulation) or an uncoupling of the receptors from their signal-transducing proteins (desensitization) as well as an enhanced effect of receptor blockers (Riffee et al. 1982; Severson et al. 1990; Vaughn et al. 1990). It is important to understand that sensitization or desensitization need not only follow chronic exposure to exogenous agents. Both can occur with a single exposure to a drug or hormone; indeed, they probably play a significant role in allowing adaptation of motor, emotional, and cognitive systems to changing stimuli, as has been so ably demonstrated for sensory systems. Understanding the therapeutic actions of psychoactive agents requires knowledge of the adaptations that the CNS brings into play with repeated exposure to the drug. The operational phenomenon of *tolerance,* whereby exposure to an agonist induces a smaller response to subsequent agonist doses partially through the process of desensitization, reflects the actions of the CNS to maintain relatively constant degrees of cellular activation despite marked changes in receptor stimulation (Sibley and Lefkowitz 1985).

These adaptive changes with drug exposure illustrate the principle of *synaptic resilience,* which is a form of homeostasis. Here, the CNS attempts to maintain a balanced level of receptor activation and cellular responsiveness despite marked changes in formation of drug-receptor complexes. This is accomplished by altering receptor densities (through changes in gene expression), coupling of receptor to signal transduction pathways (discussed later in this section), and transmitter release. Faulty feedback among components of a biochemical pathway extending from a cell surface receptor through second messengers and associated genes may contribute to disease symptoms (Montmayeur and Borrelli 1991). Similarly, altered balances between presynaptic and postsynaptic elements of a synapse may also contribute to manifestations of psychiatric disorder (Cole et al. 1992). In both instances, the mechanism is a disruption of synaptic resilience.

Dopamine binds to and dissociates from its receptors fairly rapidly. Subsequently, the synaptic dopamine concentration falls because of an active uptake process mediated by means of a sodium-dependent uptake carrier protein that has recently been cloned and sequenced (Kilty et al. 1991). Uptake into the nerve terminal represents the major means by which the released dopamine is removed from the synapse. A small amount of extracellular dopamine appears to be broken down by the enzyme catechol-O-methyltransferase (COMT). However, under normal circumstances this is not a clinically significant action. Drugs that inhibit the neuronal uptake carrier include the widely abused stimulant cocaine and the therapeutically used stimulant methylphenidate (Nestler 1992). Note that although both cocaine and dextroamphetamine have similar abilities to enhance the synaptic content of dopamine, which leads to increased dopamine receptor stimulation, they do so by different molecular mechanisms.

Once inside the nerve terminal, cytoplasmic dopamine is subject to metabolism by monoamine oxidase (MAO), located in the outer mitochondrial membrane. Thus, dopamine levels available for further release would tend to decline, because of catabolism by MAO, were no other processes operative. However, a second uptake carrier located in synaptic vesicle membranes (representing a gene product that appears to be distinct from that in the neuronal membrane) removes the dopamine from the cytoplasm to the protected vesicular environment. Reserpine is an inhibitor of the vesicular uptake of dopamine and certain other transmitters. Administration of this drug causes all dopamine removed from the synapse to be subject to degradation by MAO. This, in turn, leads to a profound reduction in stores of the transmitter. Note that although cocaine and reserpine have somewhat similar mechanisms ("uptake" inhibition), they actually have opposite effects on synaptic dopamine levels: cocaine increases these levels, whereas reserpine decreases them. This is because the two uptake carrier proteins are distinct not only in amino acid sequence but also in location.

Normally, metabolism by COMT and MAO does not play a major role in the functions of dopamine neurons. However, complete inhibition of the B form of MAO by deprenyl (selegiline) can significantly potentiate the actions of dopamine. Furthermore, inhibition of the A form of MAO, which preferentially acts on serotonin-like substrates, can provide an important action in the treatment of depression refractory to standard agents (Racagni et al. 1992).

Agents that depend on an intact neuron for their action are defined as indirect acting, in contrast to those drugs that bypass the neuron and directly activate or block receptors, which are defined as direct acting. These two agents respond in dramatically different ways to alterations in neuronal function or integrity. For example, loss of the nigrostriatal dopamine tract projecting to the basal ganglia (as occurs in parkinsonism) leads to a loss of effectiveness of indirect-acting agonists such as dextroamphetamine, cocaine, and methylphenidate. In contrast, the actions of direct agonists may actually be enhanced because of sensitization of receptor and postreceptor elements, as discussed previously (synaptic resilience).

■ Comparison of Dopamine and Serotonin Systems in the Brain

It is important to appreciate similarities and differences among the key transmitters most relevant to biological psychiatry. In this section, we briefly review the serotonin system, which plays a major role in affective disorders, suicide, impulsive behavior, and aggression. Serotonin (5-hydroxytryptamine [5-HT]) synthesis depends on an active uptake process for tryptophan that competes with other large neutral amino acids for entry into the brain. Serotonin synthesis also depends on a rate-limiting synthetic step, hydroxylation of tryptophan by tryptophan hydroxylase. This enzyme has a K_m for tryptophan (a kinetic measure of the affinity of the enzyme for its substrate) that is greater than the normal biological concentrations of the amino acid. Under these conditions, the availability of the substrate (tryptophan) becomes rate-limiting. These conditions allow changes in dietary tryptophan composition to alter the synthesis of brain serotonin by altering precursor availability. Serotonin is produced from 5-hydroxytryptophan (5-HTP) through the action of 5-HTP decarboxylase, which is somewhat similar to dopa-decarboxylase. In contrast to what is observed within the dopamine system, 5-HTP administration does not inhibit tryptophan hydroxylase activity, indicating that end product (serotonin) inhibition of serotonin synthesis is not normally an important controlling factor in regulation of this transmitter. However, impulse flow in

serotonin (as in dopamine) neurons may initiate changes in the kinetic properties of tryptophan hydroxylase.

Whereas all major transmitters may to some extent exhibit some circadian rhythm, there is a well-established daily rhythm of serotonin and the hormone melatonin in pineal gland. Both substances appear to be regulated by environmental light, and both are potentially involved in seasonal affective disorder (SAD; Cooper et al. 1992). Furthermore, serotonergic neurons appear to have a pacemaker role that is relevant for behavior and that may impinge on their regulation. As with the dopamine system, there appears to be some subtype specificity in serotonin autoreceptors such that these are composed primarily of the 5-HT_{1A} receptor subtype. Thus, serotonin neurons can self-regulate synaptic transmitter concentrations and receptor stimulation through negative feedback. Termination of serotonergic receptor stimulation is achieved by neuronal uptake. For example, inhibition of serotonin uptake into the nerve terminal by fluoxetine increases synaptic transmitter levels to exert a clinically significant antidepressant action (Siever et al. 1991). Similarly, serotonin degradation by MAO can be inhibited by enzyme inhibitors such as iproniazid, which also exerts an important antidepressant action in treating patients who are refractory to other types of agents.

■ Sites of Clinically Important Actions of Other Major Transmitters in the Brain

More detailed discussions of the therapeutically significant actions of the major transmitters are provided in subsequent chapters. It is important here to highlight some of the more significant differences between those transmitters not yet discussed versus dopamine and serotonin. Dopamine's status as the immediate precursor of norepinephrine suggests that most aspects of noradrenergic neuronal regulation should be similar to those observed for dopamine systems. This is indeed the case. However, all known noradrenergic systems and some brain dopamine systems (such as the mesoprefrontal tract) lack autoreceptors modulating transmitter synthesis. This lack differentiates these pathways from the nigrostriatal and mesolimbic dopamine pathways, which do have synthesis-modulating autoreceptors. Thus, the former (autoreceptor deficient) systems do *not* increase transmitter synthesis when impulse flow is interrupted, whereas the latter (autoreceptor containing) systems do (Bannon and Roth 1983).

Acetylcholine (ACh) synthesis, like that of serotonin, is regulated primarily by availability of the precursor, choline, and the action of the sodium-dependent, high-affinity choline uptake carrier. A second salient characteristic of cholinergic neurons is the extremely rapid termination of ACh action, which occurs by enzymatic degradation. This degradation occurs through the activity of the acetylcholinesterase enzyme. Thus, inhibition of ACh metabolism—in contrast to that of dopamine, serotonin, and norepinephrine—is clinically significant and has been used in attempts to treat symptoms of Alzheimer's disease and in standard therapy for myasthenia gravis (Summers et al. 1986; Taylor 1990).

The major amino acid transmitters include glutamate, the prototype excitatory substance, and GABA, the prototype inhibitory mediator. These signaling molecules offer several major contrasts to other key transmitters considered in this chapter. First, the number of synapses using these transmitters is much greater than those using all other types of monoamines and peptide transmitters combined. Second, both glutamate- and GABA-containing neurons are widely distributed within the brain, in contrast to the more restricted distribution of dopamine, serotonin, and noradrenergic neurons. Third, both glutamate and GABA have other biochemical and metabolic actions in the body in addition to their transmitter functions. These three characteristics of brain glutamate and GABA systems have major implications for biological psychiatry. The first implication is that the ubiquity of these transmitters makes it likely that some of their pathways will be dysfunctional in most diseases affecting behavior. The second implication is that this same feature renders difficult the standard pharmacotherapeutic approaches that increase or decrease synaptic levels of either transmitter. The third implication is that successful pharmacotherapy to alter either glutamate or GABA functions in the brain must take advantage of advances in receptor pharmacology derived from the cloning of the genes for glutamate and GABA receptors. In this instance, new drugs that can selectively stimulate or block subtypes of these amino acid transmitter receptors at restricted sites could thereby yield a therapeutically useful balance between symptomatic relief and side effects.

■ RECEPTORS

A receptor is one of the key elements in normal synaptic transmission and in the action of psychopharmacological agents. In fact, this site is the most likely target for most of the clinically available psychoactive agents. By interacting with receptors, drugs can alter cellular function and may thus bring a dysfunctional system back toward normal. The existence of a number of receptors was originally theorized from examination of pharmacological data. However, with the advent of modern biochemical techniques including molecular cloning, receptors are now known to exist in bewildering diversity.

■ Definition of a Receptor

The basic function of any receptor is molecular recognition of a signaling molecule, resulting in signal transduction. This statement of the operational basis of a receptor explicitly distinguishes a receptor from a binding site. The study of binding sites associated with a receptor may give us important information about the pharmacological characteristics or location of the receptor. However, it is important to keep in mind that the existence of a binding site does not necessitate the existence of a receptor. Recognition of the appropriate signal by the receptor causes its activation, which begins the process of signal transduction. The transduction process (discussed in more detail later in this section) involves another set of proteins or may be intrinsic to the receptor's structure. On a molecular level, receptor activation is accomplished by a change in the three-dimensional structure of the receptor protein.

The first basic characteristic of a receptor we will consider is the ability of the receptor to recognize specific molecules. The body in general and the brain in particular have evolved a large number of signaling molecules. Each signaling molecule, or primary messenger, has evolved as a member of a complex of transmitter, receptor, signal transducer, and effector to carry a specific type of information. This information is then used in the process of integration to lead eventually to a response, such as behavior. Receptors have evolved in turn to recognize specific signals to begin the process of integration of neuronal information. The initial event in this process is molecular recognition, which occurs through the chemical interaction between the primary messenger and the receptor protein. In the process of synaptic transmission, the molecular recognition occurs in the extracellular space, although there are other receptors that may exist within the cell, such as hormone receptors.

For all receptors, the recognition site is intrinsic to the three-dimensional structure of the receptor protein. Therefore, the primary amino acid sequence of the protein determines the nature of the recognition site and the type of receptor. Receptor polypeptides are generally transmembrane molecules with the amino acid chain looping through the membrane several times, offering a good membrane anchor. Although we know the primary amino acid sequence of a large number of receptors, we are only beginning to understand how various amino acids participate in the binding of the primary messenger molecule and, hence, the molecular recognition process in receptors such as the dopaminergic, β-adrenergic, and nicotinic cholinergic receptor proteins (Bunzow et al. 1988; Changeux et al. 1992; Hollenberg 1991). The agonist-binding site in the β-adrenergic receptor is composed of several amino acids that reside on several interacting transmembrane domains located on a single polypeptide chain. In contrast, the agonist-binding site in the nicotinic receptor has been localized primarily to amino acid residues near the N-terminal extracellular portion of a single subunit in a heteromeric complex. Models of receptors of classical neurotransmitters that are being proposed on the basis of primary amino acid structure share this feature: the amino acids that form the binding site are located at or near the extracellular face of the protein. This location is consistent with the function of the receptors in synaptic transmission.

■ Classification

Receptors can be classified based on their primary amino acid sequence or through differences in pharmacology (i.e., their ability to interact with specific drugs). Before the initial determination of the amino acid sequence of a receptor, the nicotinic cholinergic receptor (Noda et al. 1983), the only classification scheme available was pharmacological. With the knowledge of the primary amino acid sequences of a large number of neurotransmitter receptors, it has become clear that some receptors are more closely related than was previously indicated from the pharmacological classification schemes (Andersen et al.

1990; Civelli et al. 1991; Sibley and Monsma 1992). In addition, in most cases there are more receptor subtypes known from differences in primary amino acid structure than can be determined from pharmacological studies alone. For example, drugs are available that can readily distinguish between two types of dopamine receptors previously known as D_1 and D_2 (Andersen et al. 1990). However, to date there are five separate dopamine receptor subtypes with distinct primary amino acid sequences that form two receptor subfamilies: D_1-like and D_2-like.

The discordance between the number of receptor subtypes from molecular biological analysis and pharmacological studies has been found for most of the neurotransmitter receptors covered in this textbook. The lack of correspondence between pharmacology and molecular biology with regard to receptor classification points out the need for newer and more selective pharmacological agents. As these newer agents are developed, the hope is that the additional selectivity achieved will translate into better therapeutic agents with fewer side effects. Until we reach this point, however, we must rely on classic pharmacological methods for receptor classification in animal and clinical experiments, with the knowledge that a number of receptor subtypes may contribute to the overall clinical response (Albert et al. 1990; Neve et al. 1989). To this end, we discuss some general aspects of receptor pharmacology for purposes of receptor classification.

■ Drug Efficacy and Affinity

The binding of a neurotransmitter or drug (generally referred to as a ligand) to a receptor involves the interaction between the electronic forces associated with the ligand molecule and those associated with some of the projecting amino acid residues of the receptor protein. The affinity of a ligand for a particular receptor refers to the strength of interaction between it and the protein. Thus, the affinity of a ligand-receptor interaction depends only on the chemical characteristics of the drug and the receptor and may be derived solely through information obtained from binding experiments. A common measure of the affinity of a ligand for a receptor is the concentration of the ligand that is necessary to occupy one-half of the total number of receptors available (K_d, similar to the K_m from enzyme kinetics, is the reciprocal of the affinity). This parameter can be determined experimentally from radioligand-binding experiments conducted on tissue homogenates or whole cells (Limbird 1986).

Different drugs have different affinities for a particular receptor because of the varying strengths of interactions of their respective electronic fields. When the affinities of a series of drugs for various receptors are compared, the affinities of the drugs may be ranked from highest to lowest. The drugs with highest affinity will bind to the receptor at lower concentrations (i.e., it takes a lower concentration of the drug to occupy half of the receptor sites). Each receptor will be pharmacologically characterized by a series of drugs with a range of affinities from high to low. This information can then be used to define and identify particular receptors. The ability of a receptor to distinguish different drugs by their affinities is the basis of molecular recognition (Taylor and Insel 1990). Hormones and transmitters tend to have lower overall affinity for their receptors than do many drugs. This appears to serve the purpose of allowing the transmitter-receptor complex to dissociate ("reset") rapidly and thus adapt quickly to a changing environment.

Drug affinity depends only on the chemical interaction between the drug and the receptor. Therefore, knowing the affinity of a drug does not reveal anything about its activity (i.e., what the drug does to the cell, tissue, organ, or behavior of the organism). To determine the activity of a drug, an experiment must be performed in which some response is measured. This may be a biochemical response or a behavioral response. The ability of a drug to elicit a response per unit of receptors occupied is referred to as the drug's efficacy (McGonigle and Molinoff 1989; Ruffalo 1982). Strong full agonists produce the maximum response of which the tissue is capable when occupying a small fraction of the total receptors. In contrast, weaker full agonists may need to occupy a substantial fraction of the total receptors to produce the tissue maximum response. Partial agonists are not capable of producing a tissue maximum response, even when occupying all receptors. Like competitive antagonists, partial agonists can reverse or prevent the effects of high concentrations of the transmitter. Thus, this pharmacological definition of efficacy differs from the clinical use of the term that refers to the ability of a drug to elicit a therapeutic response.

In this latter instance, both agonists and antagonists may have clinical efficacy, as in the use of dopamine agonists to treat Parkinson's disease symptoms and the use of dopamine antagonists to treat schizophrenic symptoms. The pharmacological efficacy of a drug may also be used to a limited degree for receptor classification, but drug affinity is a more reliable measure for this purpose. However, the clinical efficacy of a drug depends on both pharmacological efficacy and affinity. Because drug efficacy depends on the ability of a drug to induce a conformational change in the receptor that activates it and leads to a cellular response, efficacy may depend on other proteins besides the receptor (e.g., G proteins).

■ Molecular Structure of Receptors

As we have indicated, until the mid-1980s, the only means of classifying and identifying receptors was pharmacological. In 1983, Noda and colleagues reported the initial deduction of the primary amino acid sequence of a receptor subunit—the nicotinic ACh receptor. Since then, several additional subunits of this receptor have been identified and their primary amino acid sequences reported (Changeux et al. 1992). Many other receptor proteins have been isolated and purified, their deoxyribonucleic acid (DNA) sequenced, and their amino acid sequences deduced (Figure 1–3). This new information from biochemical and molecular biological analyses of receptor structure has led to new ways of thinking about receptor structure and classification. Several general patterns are now apparent from this type of analysis that will influence the future pharmacological analysis of receptors. For example, in virtually every case where subtypes of receptors were inferred from pharmacological analysis, we now know that there are even more separate and distinct gene products than were once suspected from the pharmacological analysis. Other unsuspected general patterns have emerged and are outlined in the next section.

■ Superfamilies

The large number of receptor proteins whose sequences have been deduced have structural similarities that cut across the traditional pharmacologically identified receptor types. Five general types of receptors, which are referred to as superfamilies, can be identified from primary amino acid sequence similarities. A superfamily of receptors encompasses several

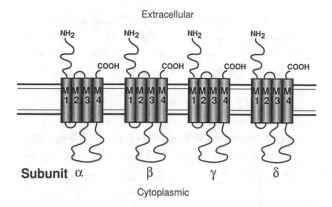

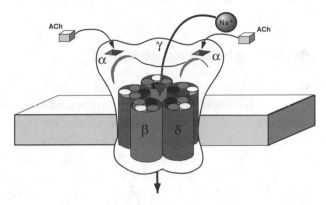

Figure 1–3. Proposed structure of the nicotinic acetylcholine receptor located at the neuromuscular junction.

Panel A: Four distinct but homologous subunits are shown that are proposed to have similar tertiary structures. Each polypeptide contains highly conserved regions, including four putative transmembrane regions.

Panel B: The proposed pentameric structure of the nicotinic acetylcholine receptor includes an ion pore that is lined by the M2 transmembrane region (black cylinder) from each of the five subunits. The acetylcholine (ACh) binding site is thought to be located primarily on the α subunits.

Source. Modified from Kandel et al. 1991, Chapter 10.

pharmacological types of these proteins. As the primary amino acid sequences of new receptors are discovered, additional superfamilies may be proposed. The major receptor superfamilies are ligand-gated ion channels, G protein–linked receptors, tyrosine kinase receptors, growth factor receptors, and hormone-like receptors. Some of these superfamilies may overlap (e.g., growth factor receptors may have tyrosine kinase activity). We will focus on the ligand-gated ion channel and G protein–linked receptor superfamilies; more is known about these superfamilies, and they have more immediate relevance to currently available psychotherapeutic agents.

■ Ligand-Gated Ion Channel Receptors

The superfamily of ligand-gated ion channel receptors is an example of a receptor type with its signal transduction mechanism contained within the structure of the receptor (i.e., an intrinsic mechanism). The most studied ligand-gated ion channel receptor is the nicotinic ACh receptor. This receptor was first isolated and purified because quantities large enough for biochemical analysis could be obtained from the electric organ of marine animals. The model for the structure of the nicotinic receptor is based on electron microscopy and functional analysis by electrophysiological recording after expression of the individual receptor subunits using molecular biological techniques (Sakmann 1992). Proof of the subunit structure or stoichiometry of other ligand-gated ion channel receptors is still lacking, but it may be inferred from the subunit sequence similarities observed by comparing primary amino acid sequences with that of the nicotinic cholinergic protein.

Four distinct subunits are required to form the functional nicotinic receptor that is located at the neuromuscular junction (motor end plate): α, β, γ, and δ. Two copies of the α subunit are present in the molecular complex to give a pentameric structure. The five subunits are arranged in a circular manner to form a central pore. Thus, each of the five subunits contributes to forming the ion channel. The α subunit has been identified to contain the ligand-binding site for the neurotransmitter ACh. Analysis of the amino acids in each subunit reveals that each contains four characteristic stretches of amino acids with a high degree of lipophilicity and that will tend to form a helical structure known as an α helix. These four domains are believed to traverse the cell membrane and are designated M1–M4. Moreover, one of the transmembrane domains, the M2, has the unique characteristic of regularly spaced amino acids containing hydroxyl groups. These hydroxyl-containing amino acids may actually form the edge of the ion pore, with the hydroxyls participating in the conduction of ions through the pore.

The primary amino acid sequences of subunits of many other ligand-gated ion channels have now been reported (e.g., certain subtypes of glutamate and GABA receptors; Burt and Kamatchi 1991; Gasic and Hollmann 1992). It is now proposed that this superfamily of receptors has used the motifs of a pentameric structure, with each subunit containing four transmembrane domains. Differences in the channel conductance properties of various receptors have been found to be due to specific amino acid residues that are at or near the M2 domain. This finding is consistent with the model that postulates that this domain forms the lining of the ion pore. For most ligand-gated ion channel receptors, we also now know that there are several forms of the different subunits, encoded by separate genes, which make up the pentameric structure. For example, at least seven distinct α subunits of the nicotinic cholinergic receptor have been discovered through molecular cloning studies (Changeux et al. 1992). It is clear that different combinations of α, β, γ, and δ subunits that make up the pentameric structure of the nicotinic receptor may lead to channels with different pharmacological and channel conductance characteristics.

Interestingly, we now know that neuronal nicotinic receptors do not need either the δ or γ subunits to form functional ion channels; that is, they can form viable receptors using only components assembled from α and β subunits. The neuronal nicotinic receptors clearly have a different pharmacology than that exhibited by the nicotinic receptors located at the neuromuscular junction. With the recent evidence that alterations in nicotinic receptors occur in Alzheimer's disease, the diversity of nicotinic receptor subtypes and differences in pharmacology among these subtypes suggest that therapeutic advantages may eventually be obtained from this knowledge.

Glutamate and GABA-A receptors represent other ligand-gated ion channel families with multiple subunit compositions. Glutamate receptors control cation flux across the membrane and mediate excitation throughout the CNS. In contrast, GABA-A receptors control anion flux across the membrane and mediate neuronal inhibition. Expression of individual subunits for both glutamate and GABA-A receptors can give rise to functional, homomeric ion channels, although the properties of these differ from those of the endogenous receptor channels. Both glutamate and GABA-A receptors exhibit a complex pharmacology, with a large number of allosteric sites associated with the receptor complex that have both positive and negative modulatory effects on channel function. Benzodiazepines and barbiturates act on the GABA-A receptors to increase channel activation, thereby leading to increased neuronal inhibition. This mechanism may play a role in the anxiolytic properties of these important neuropharmacological agents. Drugs

acting at various modulatory sites on the glutamate receptor complex are currently in development as potential agents for treatment of stroke or dementias.

The discovery of the heteromeric structure of ligand-gated ion channels has contributed to our understanding of the fundamental nature of these important molecules. However, challenges still remain. These include determining the precise subunit composition of distinct receptor proteins (receptor subtypes) that exist in the intact brain, designing drugs that interact with these different proteins selectively, and using such drugs in therapeutically valuable ways.

■ G Protein–Linked Receptors

G protein–linked receptors represent another superfamily of receptors that has been discovered as a result of deducing their primary amino acid structures from a knowledge of the DNA sequences encoding the proteins. This superfamily uses a unique signal transduction mechanism, requiring the presence of a separate membrane bound protein (called a G protein because it binds guanine nucleotides), which then interacts with another effector protein (see below). The first receptor in this superfamily to be sequenced was the β_2-adrenergic receptor (Dixon et al. 1986; Figure 1–4). Other receptors in this superfamily include subtypes of muscarinic cholinergic, dopamine, glutamate, GABA, and serotonin receptors. As with the superfamily of ligand-gated ion channels, the similarity in structure among many of the members of the G protein–linked superfamily was not discovered until a number of amino acid sequences were deduced.

Analysis of their primary amino acid sequences has led to a general model of the G protein–linked receptors (Savarese and Fraser 1992; Schwinn et al. 1991). Definitive proof that G protein–linked receptors conform to this model awaits the crystallization of the receptor proteins and analysis by X-ray crystallography. However, this evidence has been obtained for a closely related protein, bacteriorhodopsin from the purple membrane of *Halobacterium halobium,* where it acts as a proton pump (Figure 1–4; Probst et al. 1992; Smith 1989). This model G protein–linked receptor is a single polypeptide containing seven transmembrane domains that consist of stretches of hydrophobic amino acids arranged in a helical structure. The α helices are arranged with the N-terminal extending into the extracellular fluid and the C-terminal extending into the cytoplasm of the neuron. Knowledge of the amino acid sequences of many G protein–linked receptors has allowed the methods of site-directed mutagenesis and construction of chimeric proteins to be applied to their study. This has led, in turn, to a greater increase in the understanding of the functions of specific portions of these proteins.

The site-directed mutagenesis method allows the deletion, insertion, or alteration of one or more amino acids within particular domains of the protein (Cox et al. 1992; Mansour et al. 1992; Neve et al. 1991). The chimeric receptor method involves combining large portions of one receptor having a hypothesized function (e.g., ligand binding) with a portion from another receptor potentially associated with another function (e.g., G protein coupling; Kozell et al. 1992). Expression of the mutated receptors, measurement of their ligand-binding characteristics and coupling to signal transduction molecules and effectors has helped to identify sites on the proteins that play important functional roles. For example, the ligand-binding site is thought to lie within a pocket formed by the seven transmembrane domains (Probst et al. 1992). Interaction of the receptor with the G protein depends in part on a chain of amino acids that are part of the third cytoplasmic loop between the 5th and 6th transmembrane domain and, in some instances, several amino acids in the C-terminal region (Probst et al. 1992). Many of these details are summarized in panel A of Figure 1–4; further discussion of these details may be found in the figure caption.

Differences in the structural features discussed above among receptors or receptor subtypes may be important functionally and behaviorally. Thus, the long and short forms for the D_{2A} dopamine receptor differ only by 29 amino acids within the third cytoplasmic loop as a result of alternative messenger ribonucleic acid (mRNA) splicing (Chio et al. 1990). As a result, the long D_{2A} receptor produces almost double the inhibition of cAMP production stimulated by calcitonin gene-related peptide than observed with the short D_{2A} receptor (Hayes et al. 1992). Furthermore, Van Tol and colleagues (1992) have shown that a 48-base pair sequence in the third loop of the D_4 dopamine receptor exists in at least three polymorphic variants, with two repeats, four repeats, or seven repeats being the most common. The receptor forms bearing these repeats differ from one another

with respect to their ability to bind classic (spiperone) and atypical (clozapine) antipsychotic drugs.

■ Other Superfamilies

We have briefly described some of the structural and functional characteristics of the two major superfamilies of receptors that are targets for traditional psychotherapeutic agents. However, other receptor superfamilies may become important targets as new knowledge of their roles in neuronal function is forthcoming. For example, hormones that act as general homeostatic and metabolic regulators throughout the body may have unique roles to play in control of neuronal excitability. Hormone receptors are located intracellularly but generally act through molecular recognition and separate signal transduction mechanisms that involve changes in gene expression (McEwen et al. 1986). In addition, growth factors may be important not only in development of the brain but may also play a role in the maintenance of synaptic connections throughout adult life. Receptors for a number of growth factors have been cloned. Their sequence analysis has revealed structural similarities, such as the presence of a tyrosine kinase motif (i.e., these receptors have the ability to phosphorylate other proteins including themselves; Aaronson 1991).

As additional sequences for receptors become available, it seems clear that new classes of receptors will be recognized. For example, receptors for immunomodulators such as interleukins have been cloned and found to have unique structural motifs that can be combined in a variety of ways. Many of these mediators and their receptors are also found in the brain and are potential targets for therapeutic intervention. In some cases, the receptor molecule has been identified and sequenced, but sequences that code for sites that couple to known signal transduction mechanisms have not been identified. This suggests that additional transduction mechanisms are yet to be discovered.

■ SIGNAL TRANSDUCTION

Cellular information processing begins at the most basic level with a signal transduction mechanism. Signals are constantly being initiated, transduced, and integrated throughout every cell in the body. In the

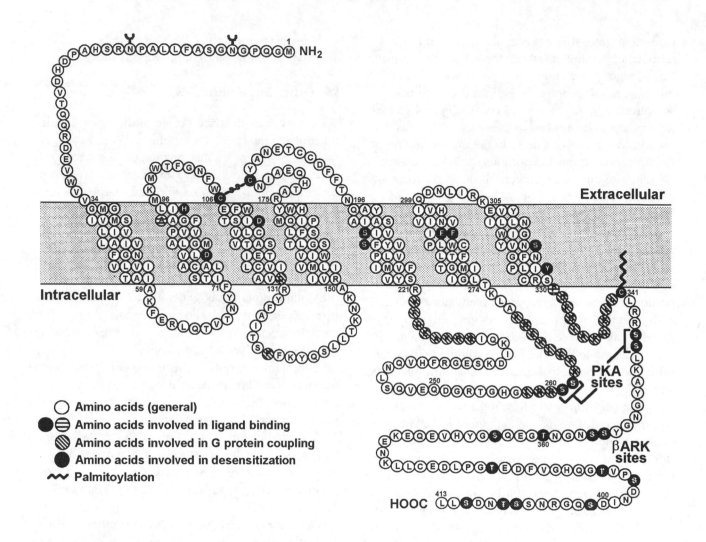

Figure 1–4. Amino acid sequence of the β₂-adrenergic receptor.

Top panel: The deduced amino acid sequence of the human β₂-adrenergic receptor. Also shown are amino acid residues thought to be involved in binding of adrenergic ligands to the active site, in coupling with the stimulatory G protein, Gₛ, in desensitization following exposure to agonist, and in anchoring the receptor to the membrane through palmitoylation. Regulatory regions of the receptor are also highlighted in the figure as consensus sequences that are phosphorylated by the enzymes protein kinase A (PKA) and β-adrenergic receptor kinase (βARK) during cAMP-dependent and cAMP-independent desensitization, respectively.
Source. Schwinn et al. 1992, p. 1666.

Right panel: A model of the possible alignment of the seven transmembrane regions of the β₂-adrenergic receptor based on a similarity to that observed for the purple membrane of *Halobacterium halobium.*
Source. Redrawn from Henderson and Unwin 1975.

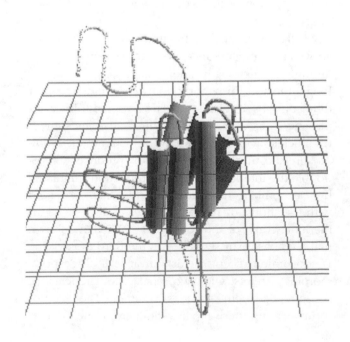

CNS, information processing and integration are clearly major functions. Therefore, understanding how signals are carried through a cell membrane is of fundamental importance. In the neuron, signals consist of changes in voltage across a membrane or changes in concentration of specific molecules or ions. Our discussion focuses on biochemical signal transduction systems that serve to convert an extracellular primary signal into an intracellular second messenger.

■ Ion-Based Signaling

The excitable nature of neurons is due to the formation of ionic gradients from outside compared with the inside of the cell (Kandel et al. 1991; Kuffler et al. 1984). These gradients are initiated and maintained by the energy-dependent ion pumps located on the plasma membrane (e.g., sodium is present in a higher concentration outside the cell, whereas potassium is in a higher concentration inside). Once the ionic gradient is formed, the difference in ion concentration across the membrane (in conjunction with the selective permeability of the membrane to certain ions) contributes to the resting membrane potential of the neuron. Under resting conditions, these properties of the neuron create a measurable voltage across the membrane, and the neuron is polarized. A polarized neuron can be excited by an appropriate stimulus. Excitation is often the result of the change in permeability of the plasma membrane toward ions such as sodium, potassium, chloride, or calcium. These permeability changes are often sudden and result from the opening of ion channels that are embedded in the neuron's plasma membrane.

A sudden change in the concentration of an ion across the membrane changes the membrane potential, and the neuron may become depolarized or hyperpolarized. Ligand-gated ion channels are a common signal transduction mechanism for altering neuronal excitability as a part of normal synaptic transmission. In this case, the primary signal is the concentration of neurotransmitter stimulating the receptor on the cell surface. The transduction mechanism involves a single molecule—the ligand-gated ion channel. The second messenger for a ligand-gated ion channel is the ion that passes into the cell. The nicotinic cholinergic receptor discussed previously is an example of this type of transduction mechanism. Ultimately, the increase in sodium within the neuron causes a depolarization that may cause the cell to fire an action potential.

■ G Protein–Linked Signaling

In contrast to the change in intracellular ion concentration mediated by ligand-gated ion channels, specific molecules are known to play a second messenger role inside cells. These molecules are generally formed through the action of an effector enzyme that is controlled through receptor activation. In contrast to standard enzyme catalytic mechanisms, one advantage of the G protein–linked pathways is the potential for amplification at several steps. In addition, this pathway is a point at which integration of neurotransmitter signals can occur because different transmitters can activate or inhibit the same enzyme. The best known second messenger molecules are probably cAMP, IP_3, and DAG, although many others have been proposed (e.g., metabolites of AA and, more recently, nitric oxide). The actions of second messengers are discussed in more detail in the following section.

It is now clear that, among the large number of diverse receptors that use second messengers as part of the signal transduction mechanism, the actual transduction process involves a set of transducing proteins called G proteins (Lamb and Pugh 1992; Spiegel 1992) that show preferential interactions with certain receptors (Senogles et al. 1990). Molecular biological analysis of these and related proteins has revealed that the family of G proteins involved in signal transduction is part of a larger superfamily of enzymes that contain GTPase activity (the ability to hydrolyze guanosine triphosphate [GTP]; Figure 1–5; Bourne et al. 1991; Gilman 1987). Figure 1–5 highlights some of the features of a model GTPase that are involved in its functions, including the extent to which the conformation of the protein can be altered during the exchange of GTP for guanosine diphosphate (GDP) on its binding site. From detailed studies of the coupling of receptors to effectors such as adenylate cyclase and phospholipase C, a general mechanism has emerged that may be applicable to the formation of other second messenger molecules. Furthermore, the psychiatric implications of altered G protein regulation are now becoming evident (Manji 1992). For example, there is evidence that supports the idea that there are changes in G proteins in schizophrenia (Okada et al. 1991).

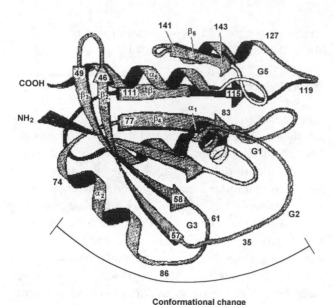

Conformational change

Figure 1–5. Model of a guanine nucleotide-binding signal transducing protein (G protein). Shown is a schematic version of the initial 166 amino acid residues of the proto-oncogene (p21^{ras}), a paradigm of the GTPase family of enzymes of which G proteins are a part. Overall, the core of the protein consists of six β sheets, which are connected to one another by α helices and hydrophilic loops. Five regions of the protein, encoded G1–G5, are critical in the reactions of this protein. The nucleotide exchange reaction (in which guanosine diphosphate [GDP] is exchanged for guanosine triphosphate [GTP] as a consequence of transmitter binding to a receptor on the cell surface), the conformational change in the G protein that results, and the hydrolysis of GTP that inactivates the G protein are all associated with various combinations of the G1–G5 regions. Also shown in the figure is the approximate magnitude of the conformational change in the protein that occurs with nucleotide exchange. *Source.* Bourne et al. 1991, p. 118.

■ **Adenylate Cyclase**

Hormone-sensitive adenylate cyclase activity has been shown to require three proteins: receptor, the heterotrimeric G protein, and the catalytic unit of the adenylate cyclase enzyme itself. Thus, these three proteins constitute a basic pathway for transmitter stimulation of cAMP synthesis (Figure 1–6; Bates et al. 1991; Strulovici et al. 1984). Activation or inhibition of the cyclase by agonist depends on the formation of an intermediate complex of agonist, receptor, and guanine nucleotide–regulated coupling protein (G$_s$ or G$_i$, respectively). The hypothesis of a ternary complex of agonist, receptor, and G protein as a regulator of second messenger function and high-affinity agonist binding to the receptor was first sug-

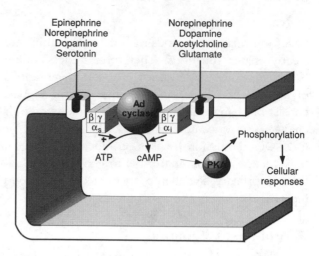

Figure 1–6. Adenylate cyclase–linked signal transduction. Agonists can stimulate or inhibit adenylate cyclase activity through separate receptors and G proteins. Activation of a receptor linked to a stimulatory G protein, G$_s$, increases the intracellular concentration of cyclic AMP (cAMP). Conversely, activation of a receptor linked to an inhibitory G protein, G$_i$, lowers the cAMP concentration inside the cell. Ad cyclase = adenylate cyclase; ATP = adenosine triphosphate; cAMP = cyclic adenosine monophosphate; PKA = protein kinase A.

gested for the hepatic glucagon receptor and, subsequently, for the β-adrenergic receptors. More generally, all hormones and neurotransmitters that act at the cell surface to stimulate or inhibit adenylate cyclase appear to function through this ternary complex (Iyengar and Birnbaumer 1987). A similar approach to the pituitary D$_2$ receptor and the striatal D$_1$ and D$_2$ receptors supports the ternary complex hypothesis for these systems. Furthermore, it is now well established that at least some D$_1$ receptors stimulate the cyclase in striatum, whereas at least some D$_2$ receptors inhibit it (Hess and Creese 1987).

At the molecular level, the best characterized of all ternary complex systems is the β$_2$-adrenergic receptor associated with adenylate cyclase through a stimulatory G protein (G$_s$; Collins et al. 1991; Schwinn et al. 1991). Reconstitution studies of the β$_2$ receptor and G$_s$ have established that agonist binding to the receptor is sensitive to guanine nucleotides. The low-affinity agonist receptor conformation reflects the receptor dissociated from G$_s$, whereas the high-affinity state reflects the agonist-receptor-G$_s$ complex (Gilman 1987). The agonist-receptor-G$_s$ complex is considered to be a relatively stable intermediate. However, its half-life is short in the presence of physiological concentrations of GTP. In the β$_2$-adrenergic receptor system, agonist binding stimulates dissociation of GDP from the G_s protein and stimulates the binding of GTP to G_s. A guanine nucleotide-binding site has been described to function as if "closed" in the absence of agonist-receptor complex and "open" (allowing nucleotide exchange) in its presence (Gilman 1987). Thus, high-affinity agonist binding is GTP sensitive in this system. Binding of GTP causes dissociation of the ternary complex and of G_s into its α and $\beta\gamma$ subunits. Concomitantly, GTP binding also shifts the receptor from a high- to a low-affinity agonist-binding conformation, thus resetting the system.

Once the β subunit of G_s is activated, it can then move in the plane of the membrane by diffusion until it interacts with adenylate cyclase. Adenylate cyclase, an integral membrane-bound protein with a channel- or transporter-like structure, is activated by $G_s\alpha$-GTP (Krupinski 1992; Krupinski et al. 1989). The substrate for this reaction is adenosine triphosphate ([ATP] in the presence of magnesium), which will normally be present in sufficient concentrations through energy-producing reactions in the cell. Thus, the major process for production of cAMP is through the receptor-activated pathway.

A receptor-activated inhibitory pathway also exists for control of cAMP levels. This pathway also requires ternary complex formation and involvement of a different G protein, G_i. Receptors that mediate this action include the α_2-adrenergic, the D_2 dopamine, and the 5-HT_{1A} serotonin receptors. The transduction mechanism may not be identical in this inhibitory pathway to that described for stimulation of adenylate cyclase. Here, it is thought that dissociation of the G_i into $G_{i\alpha}$ and $G_{i\beta\gamma}$ subunits causes the accumulation of $G_{\beta\gamma}$ subunits. These $\beta\gamma$ subunits may induce reassociation of the G_s (stimulatory) heterotrimer (α-β-γ). This is because $\beta\gamma$ subunits from one G protein appear able to substitute to some extent for $\beta\gamma$ subunits from another G protein (Spiegel et al. 1992).

A general principle of signal transduction through second messenger formation is the concept of amplification of the primary signal. In G protein–linked signaling, amplification may occur at several levels (Alousi et al. 1991). Molecular recognition may be one source of amplification whereby the transmitter may activate several receptors before it diffuses away from the receptor to its sites for uptake or catabolism. The activation of G protein through formation of the GTP-bound $G_{s\alpha}$ is another step where amplification may occur, because a single $G_{s\alpha}$ may stimulate many effector enzyme molecules before GTP hydrolysis renders the G protein α subunit unable to do so. Finally, the activated adenylate cyclase may produce many molecules of cAMP before it returns to its resting state. In pharmacological terms, signal transduction activated by the drug-receptor interaction determines the ability of the drug to produce a response for a given receptor occupancy (the drug's efficacy).

To date, the evidence suggests that dopaminergic, muscarinic, and some serotonergic receptor–G protein–adenylate cyclase systems in the brain behave similarly to the β-adrenergic receptor–cyclase systems (Savarese and Fraser 1992). Because many neurotransmitter-receptor systems use common signal transduction mechanisms, the transduction mechanism may not be expected to be a good target for therapeutic intervention in a dysfunctional brain because of the lack of specificity of a given drug acting on transducer proteins. However, there is a newly recognized diversity in these signal transduction pathways. This appears to be because of differences in the subtypes of G proteins that are required for stimulation by specific receptors and differential activation of second messenger pathways by separate G proteins. These recent findings suggest that selectivity of psychotherapeutic drugs targeted toward signal transduction may be achieved some day. Recent evidence suggests that some psychiatric drugs, such as lithium, may target the transduction systems associated with G proteins (Avissar and Schreiber 1989). This finding is consonant with the potential changes in G proteins that may be associated with other psychiatric disorders, such as schizophrenia (Manji 1992; Okada et al. 1991).

■ Phospholipase C

Another major G protein–linked signal transduction mechanism is the phosphoinositide (PI) hydrolysis pathway (Figure 1–7; Berridge 1989). Less is known about the details of this transduction mechanism. However, emerging evidence suggests that the general steps described previously for the adenylate cyclase system also operate for the PI pathway. Thus, only the major differences between this pathway and the adenylate cyclase system are covered here. Within the PI hydrolysis pathway, receptor, G protein, and effector are required and may be sufficient for the process to operate. The effector enzyme is a

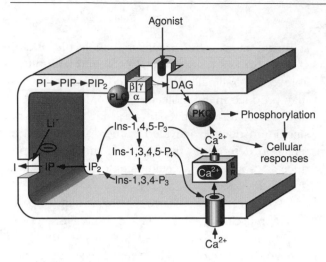

Figure 1–7. Phosphoinositide (PI)-linked signal transduction. An agonist binds to its receptor and initiates the G protein–linked signal pathway. The effector enzyme is a phosphoinositide-specific phospholipase C (PLC) that hydrolyzes membrane phosphatidylinositol-4,5-bisphosphate (PIP_2) into inositol-1,4,5-trisphosphate (Ins-1,4,5-P_3; IP_3) and diacylglycerol (DAG). Ins-1,4,5-P_3 then acts to release calcium from an endoplasmic reticulum–like store, and calcium can then activate a variety of calcium-dependent enzymes. DAG, which stays associated with the membrane, activates protein kinase C (PKC), causing phosphorylation of specific proteins leading to cellular responses. Ins-1,4,5-P_3 can be phosphorylated to Ins-1,3,4,5-P_4, which has been proposed to control influx of extracellular calcium. A series of dephosphorylation reactions controls the levels of inositol phosphates. The inositol monophosphatase is inhibited by therapeutic concentrations of lithium and can disrupt the normal function of the phosphoinositide cycle.
Source. Modified from Berridge 1989.

PI-specific phospholipase C (Berridge 1989; Fisher et al. 1992).

It is now clear that several classes of G proteins serve as transducers for the PI system, and these are distinct from those that couple receptors to adenylate cyclase. For example, new G proteins, G_q and G_{11}, have been shown to be active in coupling receptors to phospholipase C. The phospholipase C involved in the receptor-activated transduction pathway exists in several different forms that may play unique roles in specific pathways (Rhee 1991). This enzyme uses phosphatidylinositol-4,5-bisphosphate (PIP_2) as substrate. PIP_2 is a phospholipid that makes up a small portion of the plasma membrane. The phospholipase C breaks down PIP_2 into two second messengers: DAG and IP_3. In this way, the PI pathway results in a bifurcating signaling system inside the cell (Fowler and Tiger 1991).

Other Signal Transduction Systems

It is now clear that additional signal transduction systems are operative in the CNS and that the molecular diversity that has been shown within a single pathway may soon be matched by a variety of separate pathways. In most cases, the exact receptor-coupling mechanisms or roles that these novel pathways play in the control of neuronal function and ultimate behaviors are not known. Guanylate cyclase is an enzyme found in the brain in several different forms, some of which may be membrane bound and some of which appear to be cytoplasmic (Schulz et al. 1991). Stimulation of this enzyme, which results in the formation of cyclic guanosine monophosphate (GMP), may occur through direct activation of a receptor (membrane-bound form) or through intervening steps that may involve additional signaling molecules. Phospholipase A_2 is a well-established enzyme involved in signal transduction in lymphocytes, but it may also play a role in neuronal function. Receptor-activated phospholipase A_2 produces AA that can then be metabolized to several potential intracellular messenger molecules (Shimizu and Wolfe 1990; see next section).

Several growth factors that are known to have activity on neuron growth and maintenance transduce their signals through tyrosine phosphorylation that then participates in the activation of an isozyme (γ form) of PI-specific phospholipase C (Rhee 1991). The latest addition to the growing list of signal transduction systems is the pathway leading to the novel signaling molecule, nitric oxide. Recent studies have shown that pathways that lead to an increase in intracellular calcium cause activation of nitric oxide synthase, which in turn leads to the production of nitric oxide. Nitric oxide then stimulates guanylate cyclase activity, ultimately leading to increased levels of cyclic GMP. This pathway may play a role in strengthening certain synapses in an activity-dependent manner, such as with learning (Snyder 1992).

CELLULAR SECOND MESSENGERS

Our discussion in this section focuses on two types of cellular second messengers, cAMP and three second messengers derived from membrane phospholipids: IP_3, DAG, and AA metabolites. We present the criteria for considering a substance a second messenger and then discuss the prototype. Each second messenger system is described from the perspective of a few basic organizing principles to allow each of them (and other such systems that the reader will encounter) to be compared.

■ Criteria for Second Messenger Function

Specific enzymes for the production of the substance constitute the initial criterion for establishing second messenger function (Northup 1989). For example, cytosolic adenylate cyclase converts ATP to cAMP in the presence of magnesium ion. *A specific degradative-removal pathway* is the second criterion. cAMP breakdown is catalyzed by a specific cyclic nucleotide phosphodiesterase that has high activity in the CNS (Conti et al. 1992). Together, these two criteria allow a cellular substance to be present in controlled amounts in response to specific signals. This provides an optimum set of conditions for the second messenger to regulate cellular enzymatic functions and to alter gene expression (through acting on a cAMP-response element within the DNA of certain genes).

The third criterion for classifying a substance as a second messenger is that of *transmitter responsiveness*. In this instance, stimulation of a receptor (such as a D_1 dopamine receptor) by the transmitter should yield a predictable change in cellular content of the substance. *Mimicry-potentiation* is a fourth criterion. In essence, application of analogues of the substance (e.g., cAMP analogues that are resistant to hydrolysis, such as dibutyryl-cAMP or 8-bromo-cAMP) should yield cellular actions that mimic those of the transmitter (stimulation of cAMP-dependent protein kinase activity). Similarly, inhibitors of breakdown of the substance (by using phosphodiesterase inhibitors, such as theophylline or caffeine) should potentiate the cellular actions of the transmitter. Finally, *the existence of a specific output,* such as the cAMP-dependent protein kinase, is the last major criterion that a substance must fulfill to be considered a second messenger. In this context, it is interesting that blockade of dopamine receptors with antipsychotic drugs also changes cAMP levels (Kaneko et al. 1992).

■ Cyclic AMP and Adenylate Cyclase

The cAMP pathway is the prototype of an intracellular signaling system using a soluble substance that exerts its primary actions within the cytosol on a tetrameric protein kinase enzyme: cAMP-dependent protein kinase (Gao and Gilman 1991). Following production of cAMP by adenylate cyclase, four cAMP molecules bind to the two regulatory subunits of the cAMP-dependent protein kinase to initiate one of the major actions of the second messenger. The cAMP binding causes the two catalytic subunits of the protein kinase A (PKA) holoenzyme to be freed to phosphorylate various target proteins. Among the target proteins for PKA action is the cell surface receptor itself (e.g., β_2-adrenergic; Hausdorff et al. 1990; Sibley and Lefkowitz 1988). Thus, stimulation of a β-adrenergic receptor by agonist activates both a productive pathway and a regulatory pathway inside the cell. The productive pathway activates adenylate cyclase, which stimulates cAMP production. The regulatory pathway(s) will include the feedback influences that activation of the cAMP-dependent protein kinase may have on the β-adrenergic receptor by virtue of phosphorylating it, thus changing its ability to be activated by agonist. Together, this view of the β-adrenergic receptor–G protein–adenylate cyclase–PKA system provides a further example of the homeostatic consequences of activation of a second messenger pathway.

There are several isoforms of the regulatory PKA subunits that have three functional domains in common: two cAMP-binding sites per subunit near the C-terminal region, one portion of the N-terminal region to which the other regulatory subunit binds, and another portion of the N-terminal region that normally inhibits the attached catalytic subunit (Taylor et al. 1990). Each of the catalytic subunits contains an ATP-binding site and a substrate protein-binding site. This arrangement potentially allows the catalytic subunit to interact with specific amino acid sequences in several proteins. The receptor can amplify the agonist signal by interacting with several of the more numerous G protein molecules within the membrane. So, too, further signal amplification occurs inside the cell, as each catalytic subunit of the PKA transfers the γ-phosphoryl group of ATP to the hydroxyl groups of specific serine and threonine residues of many target protein molecules.

Regulation of cAMP levels occurs through the action of two basic kinds of enzymes. Several phosphodiesterases convert active cAMP to the inactive AMP to terminate the second messenger action. Also, various protein phosphatases remove phosphate groups from the target proteins to terminate the cellular responses that are mediated by the phosphorylated proteins.

It is important to note that phosphorylation may cause some proteins to be activated, whereas others (such as β_2-adrenergic receptors) become less active when phosphorylated. An autophosphorylation reaction, found with many protein kinases, causes at least some isoforms of the regulatory domain of the PKA molecule to be phosphorylated by its own catalytic subunits. This autophosphorylation causes a slower rate of interaction between regulatory and catalytic subunits than would otherwise occur (Walaas and Greengard 1991).

Significantly, multiple transmitters produce at least some of their cellular actions through increasing or decreasing cAMP levels inside the cell. This action illustrates the principle of *convergent processing* of information in the CNS. Furthermore, as we have discussed, there are several steps in the cAMP second messenger pathway—formation of a bimolecular complex of agonist and receptor, ternary complex formation, G protein activation, ternary complex and G protein heterotrimer dissociation, and activation of the catalytic unit of the cyclase enzyme. Because of the various chemical reactions involved in cAMP production, a significantly greater time is required for changes in cAMP levels than for changes in conductances of an ion channel intrinsic to the nicotinic cholinergic receptors. However, the cellular consequences of adenylate cyclase activation or inhibition often outlast those associated with altered ion fluxes through membrane channels. Together, these observations illustrate the principle of *latency-duration of action* (i.e., second messenger activity determines the temporal nature of the target cellular response).

Second messenger formation is not an end point for the cell but an intermediate reaction. The cellular response to a change in second messenger level changes the activity of other cellular proteins, often through changes in their phosphorylation state (Garattini 1992). As we discussed, increases in cAMP accumulation inside the cell activates the cAMP-dependent protein kinase by releasing its regulatory subunits. In fact, the known actions of cAMP result from activation of PKA, illustrating the principle of *protein kinase output*.

Finally, *regulation pathway participation* is a principle that refers to the observation that second messenger pathways consist of two kinds of loops: a productive pathway and one or more regulatory pathways. As was described for cAMP, activation of the productive loop in the β-adrenergic receptor system increases cAMP inside the cell. However, the increases in cAMP activate PKA that phosphorylates the receptor and thereby limits its ability to respond to further agonist stimulation. Stimulation of PKA by cAMP causes phosphorylation of residues within the cytoplasmic portion of the β-adrenergic receptor protein, making it less able to couple to the G_s transducer (desensitization). Another consequence of agonist stimulation of the β_2 receptor that is not cAMP dependent (but is dependent on agonist occupancy) is activation of the β-adrenergic receptor kinase that phosphorylates different residues on the receptor and induces modulation of the receptor by another protein, β-arrestin (Arriza et al. 1992; Attramadal et al. 1992; Benovic et al. 1986; Lohse et al. 1990). This example demonstrates one means by which activation of the pathway not only produces a cellular response (increased cAMP) but also reduces the response to further activation (desensitization; Sibley and Lefkowitz 1985, 1988).

■ Inositol Lipid-Based Second Messengers

As we discussed, the hydrolysis of PIP_2 forms both a membrane associated (diacylglycerol, DAG) and a cytosolic (IP_3) second messenger (Berridge 1989). DAG is the primary lipid regulator of a phospholipid-dependent enzyme, protein kinase C (PKC), which it activates. PKC actually is an enzyme family that phosphorylates serine and threonine residues in a variety of target protein substrates, both membranous and cytosolic (Kikkawa et al. 1989). Of the 10 known isozymes of PKC, the four major forms contain both lipid- and calcium-binding sites within the N-terminal region, whereas the catalytic domain of the molecule resides in the C-terminal region. The four so-called minor forms of the enzyme are structurally similar but lack the calcium-binding site. In the presence of ATP, the activated PKC phosphorylates substrate proteins, producing phosphoproteins that alter cellular responsiveness. To be activated by DAG, PKC must shift from a cytosolic location to a membrane position, because phospholipid is needed for the activation process.

IP_3 is a soluble product of PIP_2 cleavage and is a messenger with a short half-life (< 10 sec, although its duration of action is longer than that of many ion channel openings). IP$_3$ acts by binding to a specific IP$_3$ receptor on membrane organelles, such as endoplasmic or sarcoplasmic reticulum. The IP$_3$ receptor protein contains both an IP$_3$-binding site and a calcium channel. The IP$_3$ receptor is a tetramer consisting of similar subunits with four membrane spanning regions constituting the calcium channel. Increases in IP$_3$ levels release calcium from intracellular stores. The released calcium subsequently interacts with various cellular components such as calmodulin. This calcium-binding protein then can activate calcium- and calmodulin-dependent protein kinase to phosphorylate target proteins (Miller 1991).

Central to the regulatory roles of IP$_3$ and DAG is their recycling, which is under the control of specific enzymes (Berridge 1989). DAG may be phosphorylated to phosphatidic acid, which combines with cytidine triphosphate (CTP) to form cytidine diphosphate (CDP)-DAG. The CDP-DAG then reacts with inositol to regenerate PIs. The phosphatidylinositol, in turn, can then be phosphorylated to PIP$_2$. An alternative degradative pathway for DAG involves its hydrolysis to glycerol and constituent fatty acids. One of these is often AA, which is itself a precursor to another important lipid-derived second messenger (see Figure 1–8). IP$_3$ breakdown is catalyzed by the sequential action of phosphatases (or further phosphorylated to IP$_4$). The last of these dephosphorylations, catalyzed by an inositol monophosphatase, is inhibited by millimolar lithium concentrations (Berridge 1989). This action of lithium disrupts the entire cascade of reactions, because the production of DAG and IP$_3$ is dependent on the regeneration of PIP$_2$. This is because only locally available inositol can be used for PIP$_2$ production—inositol cannot cross the blood-brain barrier. It has been speculated that at least a part of the antimanic action of lithium ion may be mediated by its action on the regeneration of inositol phospholipids (Berridge 1989).

The principle of convergent processing is demonstrated for DAG and IP$_3$, because a large number of transmitters act through the phospholipase C pathway. The latency and duration of action of DAG and IP$_3$ are also greater than those typically observed for ionic conductance changes. Protein kinase output is obvious for DAG because of its direct action on PKC; that for IP$_3$ is less direct, but also significant, because of the activation of the calcium-calmodulin–dependent protein kinases. Finally, regulatory pathway participation is shown for both lipid-derived

second messengers. This is because these products of phospholipid hydrolysis can feed back to regulate both their own production and that of other cytosolic messengers, including cAMP. Haloperidol, a prototypic antipsychotic drug, appears to alter both cAMP and IP$_3$ accumulation (Kaneko et al. 1992). This suggests interactions between adenylate cyclase and phospholipase C pathways in the brain.

■ Arachidonic Acid Pathway

AA is typically the fatty acid that exists in the ester form at position 2 in brain phospholipid molecules. Thus, stimulation of receptors that activate the en-

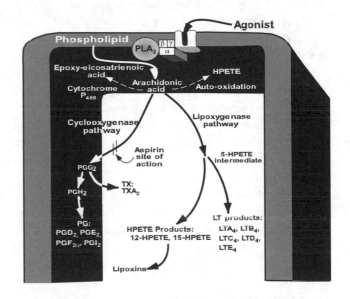

Figure 1–8. Signal transduction linked to arachidonic acid. An agonist binds to a cell surface receptor and activates a G protein, in a manner that is similar to that shown earlier for the adenylate cyclase and phosphoinositide systems. The effector enzyme is phospholipase A$_2$ (PLA$_2$), which converts membrane phospholipids to arachidonic acid (AA). The AA is then rapidly converted to several active metabolites, including prostaglandins (PG), thromboxanes (TX), leukotrienes (LT), hydroperoxy acid (HPETE) products, and lipoxins. Two major pathways are shown, reflecting the actions of cyclooxygenase and lipoxygenase. Information in the figure is not intended to be complete, but rather to illustrate some of the major known active products resulting from the actions of cyclooxygenase and lipoxygenase on AA to produce second messengers upon demand. Note the important roles of PGG$_2$ and PGH$_2$ as intermediates in the cyclooxygenase pathway and of 5-HPETE in the lipoxygenase pathway. Note also that aspirin acts to inhibit the cyclooxygenase pathway.

zyme phospholipase A_2 releases AA from the membrane, where it is quickly converted to several active eicosanoid metabolites. The term *eicosanoid* refers to one of a class of compounds, including the prostaglandins, thromboxanes, and leukotrienes, all of which are derived from AA (also called eicosatetraenoic acid; Figure 1–8). Cyclooxygenase metabolism of AA produces the prostaglandins and thromboxanes, whereas the actions of several lipoxygenases on AA yield the leukotrienes and several other metabolites (Shimizu and Wolfe 1990). A significant aspect of AA pathway function is that each of the active metabolic products must be created upon demand to function both inside and outside the target cells, because there is no storage of these substances. It is tantalizing that levels of prostaglandins and thromboxanes are increased during electroconvulsive therapy, acute cerebral ischemia, and trauma, whereas levels of a lipoxygenase product (HPETE, hydroperoxyeicosatrienoic acid) are elevated after depolarization of brain slices with potassium, glutamate, or N-methyl-D-aspartate (NMDA; Schwartz and Kandel 1991). Because drugs acting upon the AA metabolite systems of the brain are not currently used in psychiatry, they are not discussed in detail here. However, these drugs do appear to fulfill the criteria required for second messengers. Their actions also appear consonant with the principles of convergent processing, latency-duration of action, and regulation pathway participation.

■ CHAPTER SUMMARY

■ General Summary

Our focus in this chapter was on the use of model systems to provide the reader with an overview of transmitters, receptors, signal transducing proteins, and cellular second messengers.

■ Neurotransmitters— First Messengers

In this brief review of brain signaling, we have seen that certain key principles may be applied to each of the four fundamental steps in the chemical signaling process—neurotransmission, receptor binding, signal transduction, and second messenger activation. Thus, we examined several principles of neurotransmission in the brain. The first principle of neurotransmission was that of synaptic effect. Each of the steps in synaptic transmission is relevant to psychopharmacology only to the extent that it alters the synaptic transmitter content (and, hence, the amount of transmitter available to bind to receptors). Any effect of disease or drug that does not change the synaptic content of a transmitter does not alter behavior. The second principle of neurotransmission examined was that of self-regulation (synaptic homeostasis), in which each pulse of released transmitter tends to reduce its subsequent release by initiating feedback processes within its neuron.

The third principle of neurotransmission was that of dose dependence, whereby the stimulation of their receptors by all hormones, neurotransmitters, and drugs are proportional to their concentration or dose. The fourth principle of neurotransmission was that the biological effects of any chemical mediator have a characteristic latency and duration of action. The fifth principle of neurotransmission covered in this introduction was that of synaptic resilience, in which partial damage to one portion of a nerve terminal or to one aspect of a neuron's functions tends to be associated with compensatory changes in neuronal activity. These principles were considered briefly in relation to the several sites of drug action—synthesis, storage, release, binding, reuptake, and metabolism. Just as each of these sites of drug action applies in principle to any transmitter or modulator system, so do the five fundamental principles of neurotransmission. It is the task of the psychopharmacologist to discover how best to employ these principles with respect to the sites of drug action when dealing with symptoms of various diseases, as will be discussed in subsequent chapters.

■ Receptors

Receptor proteins represent the initial component of a signal transduction system for transferring the message of the neurotransmitter across the neuronal membrane into the cell. Molecular recognition of receptors for drugs or neurotransmitters is the basis of pharmacological selectivity. Receptors can be classified based on pharmacological, structural, and functional criteria. Elucidation of the primary amino acid sequences for a growing number of receptors has revealed that a few general features are used by most of these proteins, which can be separated into superfamilies on this basis. The G protein–linked superfamily contains seven transmembrane domains in a single polypeptide. The ligand-gated ion channel superfamily exists as a complex of five subunits, each of which contains four transmembrane domains.

■ Signal Transduction

Activation of the receptor by an agonist initiates the process of signal transduction. G protein–linked receptors utilize a guanine nucleotide-binding protein (G protein) to couple to the effector enzyme. The transduction process involves dissociation of the heterotrimeric G protein into α and $\beta\gamma$ subunits and exchange of bound GDP for cytosolic GTP. The activated, GTP-bound α subunit may then stimulate the activity of enzymes such as adenylate cyclase or PI-specific phospholipase C to produce second messengers (cAMP or IP_3 and DAG) inside the cell. Signal transduction through ligand-gated ion channels involves the movement of ions into or out of the cell, which alters the membrane potential, and thus the excitability of the neuron.

■ Second Messengers

The first fundamental principle of second messengers discussed was that of convergent processing, in which information conveyed by many neurotransmitters is funneled and integrated into the action of a few second messengers. Latency-duration of action was shown to distinguish the rapid mediation of biological activity by ligand-gated ion channels from the slower but more lasting actions of cellular second messengers such as cAMP. Protein kinase output is an action shared by cellular second messengers that leads, through phosphorylation of target proteins to phosphoproteins, to a variety of direct and indirect actions. These actions include effects at some distance from the site of second messenger production. Finally, regulation pathway participation is the principle whereby second messengers play a significant role in altering the ability of hormones, neurotransmitters, and drugs to change cellular second messenger levels (i.e., to change their own levels). This is accomplished by feedback actions to desensitize the receptor-signal transducer system and by feedforward actions to alter gene expression.

■ REFERENCES

Aaronson SA: Growth factors and cancer. Science 254:1146–1153, 1991

Albert PR, Neve KA, Bunzow JR, et al: Coupling of a cloned rat dopamine-D2 receptor to inhibition of adenylyl cyclase and prolactin secretion. J Biol Chem 265:2098–2104, 1990

Alousi AA, Jasper JR, Insel PA, et al: Stoichiometry of receptor-G_s-adenylate cyclase interactions. FASEB J 5:2300–2303, 1991

Andersen PH, Gingrich JA, Bates MD, et al: Dopamine receptor subtypes: beyond the D1/D2 classification. Trends Pharmacol Sci 11:231–236, 1990

Arriza JL, Dawson TM, Simerly RB, et al: The G-protein-coupled receptor kinases βARK1 and βARK2 are widely distributed at synapses in rat brain. J Neurosci 12:4045–4055, 1992

Attramadal H, Arriza JL, Aoki C, et al: β-Arrestin2, a novel member of the arrestin/β-arrestin gene family. J Biol Chem 267:17882–17890, 1992

Avissar S, Schreiber G: Muscarinic receptor subclassification and G-proteins: significance for lithium action in affective disorders and for the treatment of the extrapyramidal side effects of neuroleptics. Biol Psychiatry 26:113–130, 1989

Bannon MJ, Roth R: Pharmacology of mesocortical dopamine neurons. Pharmacol Rev 35:53, 1983

Bannon MJ, Freeman AS, Chiodo LA, et al: The pharmacology and electrophysiology of mesolimbic dopamine neurons. Handbook of Psychopharmacology 19:329–374, 1986

Bartholini G, Zivkovic B, Scatton B: Dopaminergic neurons: basic aspects, in Handbook of Experimental Pharmacology, Vol 90/11. Edited by Trendelenburg U, Weiner N. Berlin, Springer-Verlag, 1989, pp 277–317

Bates MD, Senogles SE, Bunzow JR, et al: Regulation of responsiveness at D2 dopamine receptors by receptor desensitization and adenylyl cyclase sensitization. Mol Pharmacol 35:55–63, 1991

Benovic JL, Strasser RH, Caron MG, et al: β-Adrenergic receptor kinase: identification of a novel protein kinase that phosphorylates the agonist-occupied form of the receptor. Proc Natl Acad Sci U S A 83:2797–2801, 1986

Berridge MJ: Inositol trisphosphate and diacylglycerol: two interacting second messengers. Ann Rev Biochem 56:159–193, 1989

Bourne HR, Sanders DA, McCormick F: The GTPase superfamily: conserved structure and molecular mechanism. Nature 349:117–127, 1991

Bunzow JR, Van Tol HHM, Grandy DK, et al: Cloning and expression of a rat D2 dopamine receptor cDNA. Nature 336:783–787, 1988

Burt DR, Kamatchi GL: GABA$_A$ receptor subtypes: from pharmacology to molecular biology. FASEB J 5:2916–2923, 1991

Changeux J-P, Devillers-Thiery A, Galzi J-L, et al: New mutants to explore nicotinic receptor functions. Trends Pharmacol Sci 13:299–301, 1992

Chio CL, Hess GF, Graham RS, et al: A second molecular form of D2 dopamine receptor in rat and bovine caudate nucleus. Nature 343:266–269, 1990

Chiodo LA: Dopamine autoreceptor signal transduction in the DA cell body: a "current view." Neurochem Int 20:815–845, 1992

Civelli O, Bunzow JR, Grandy DK, et al: Molecular biology of the dopamine receptors. Eur J Pharmacol—Mol Pharmacol Sec 207:277–286, 1991

Cole AJ, Bhat RV, Patt C, et al: D1 dopamine receptor activation of multiple transcription factor genes in rat striatum. J Neurochem 58:1420–1426, 1992

Collins S, Caron MG, Lefkowitz RJ: Regulation of adrenergic receptor responsiveness through modulation of receptor gene expression. Ann Rev Physiol 53:497–508, 1991

Conti M, Swinnen JV, Tsikalas KE, et al: Structure and regulation of the rat high-affinity cyclic AMP phosphodiesterases: a family of closely related enzymes. Adv Second Messenger Phosphoprotein Res 25:87–99, 1992

Cooper JR, Bloom FE, Roth RH: The Biochemical Basis of Neuropharmacology, 6th Edition. New York, Oxford University Press, 1992

Cox BA, Henningsen RA, Spanoyannis A, et al: Contributions of conserved serine residues to the interactions of ligands with dopamine D2 receptors. J Neurochem 59:627–635, 1992

Dearry A, Gingrich JA, Falardeau P, et al: Molecular cloning and expression of the gene for a human D1 dopamine receptor. Nature 347:72–76, 1990

Deutch AY, Roth RH: The determinants of stress-induced activation of the prefrontal cortical dopamine system. Prog Brain Res 85:367–403, 1990

Dixon RAF, Kobilka BK, Strader DJ, et al: Cloning of the gene and cDNA for mammalian β-adrenergic receptor and homology and rhodopsin. Nature 321:75–79, 1986

Fisher SK, Heacock AM, Agranoff BW: Inositol lipids and signal transduction in the nervous system: an update. J Neurochem 58:18–38, 1992

Fowler CJ, Tiger G: Modulation of receptor-mediated inositol phospholipid breakdown in the brain. Neurochem Int 19:171–206, 1991

Gao B, Gilman AG: Cloning and expression of a widely distributed (type IV) adenylyl cyclase. Proc Natl Acad Sci U S A 88:10178–10182, 1991

Garattini S: Pharmacology of second messengers: a critical appraisal. Drug Metab Rev 24:125–194, 1992

Gasic GP, Hollmann M: Molecular neurobiology of glutamate receptors. Annu Rev Physiol 54:507–536, 1992

Gilman AG: G proteins: transducers of receptor-generated signals. Ann Rev Biochem 56:615–649, 1987

Grace AA, Onn SP: Morphology and electrophysiological properties of immunocytochemically identified rat dopamine neurons recorded in vitro. J Neurosci 9:3463–3481, 1989

Hall H, Farde L, Halldin C, et al: Imaging of dopamine receptors using PET and SPECT. Neurochem Int 20:329S–333S, 1992

Hausdorff WP, Caron MG, Lefkowitz RJ: Turning off the signal: desensitization of β-adrenergic receptor function. FASEB J 4:2881–2889, 1990

Hayes G, Bident TJ, Selbie LA, et al: Structural subtypes of the dopamine D2 receptor are functionally distinct: expression of the cloned D2$_A$ and D2$_B$ subtypes in a heterologous cell line. Mol Endocrinol 6:920–926, 1992

Henderson R, Unwin PN: Three dimensional model of purple membrane obtained by electron microscopy. Nature 257:28–32, 1975

Hess EJ, Creese I: Biochemical characterization of dopamine receptors, in Dopamine Receptors. Edited by Creese I, Graser CM. New York, Alan R Liss, 1987, pp 1–28

Hollenberg MD: Structure-activity relationships for transmembrane signaling: the receptor's turn. FASEB J 5:178–186, 1991

Iyengar R, Birnbaumer L: Signal transduction by G-proteins. ISI Atlas of Science: Pharmacology 1:213–221, 1987

Kandel E, Schwartz J, Jessell T (eds): Principles of Neuroscience, 3rd Edition. New York, Elsevier, 1991

Kaneko M, Sato K, Horikoshi R, et al: Effect of haloperidol on cyclic AMP and inositol trisphosphate in rat striatum in vivo. Prostaglandins Leukot Essent Fatty Acids 46:53–57, 1992

Kikkawa U, Kishimoto A, Nishizuka Y: The protein kinase C family: heterogeneity and its implications. Annu Rev Biochem 58:31–44, 1989

Kilty JE, Lorang D, Amara SG: Cloning and expression of a cocaine-sensitive rat dopamine transporter. Science 254:578–579, 1991

Kozell L, Starr S, Machida C, et al: Agonist induced changes in density of D1, D2, and chimeric D1/D2 receptors. Society for Neuroscience Abstracts 18:276, 1992

Krupinski J: The adenylyl cyclase family. Mol Cell Biochem 104:73–79, 1992

Krupinski J, Coussen F, Bakalyar HA, et al: Adenylyl cyclase amino acid sequence: possible channel- or transporter-like structure. Science 244:1558–1564, 1989

Kuffler SW, Nicholls JG, Martin AR: From Neuron to Brain: A Cellular Approach to the Function of the Nervous System, 2nd Edition. Sunderland, MA, Sinauer Associates, 1984

Laihinen A, Rinne JO, Rinne UK, et al: (^{18}F)-6-Fluorodopa PET scanning in Parkinson's disease after selective COMT inhibition with nitecapone (OR-462). Neurology 42:199–203, 1992

Lamb TD, Pugh EN Jr: G-protein cascades: gain and kinetics. Trends Neurosci 15:291–298, 1992

Leslie S, Woodward J, Wilcox R.: Correlation of rates of calcium entry and endogenous dopamine release in mouse striatal synaptosomes. Brain Res 325:99–105, 1985

Limbird LE: Cell Surface Receptors: A Short Course on the Theory and Methods. Boston, MA, Martinus Nijhoff Publishing, 1986

Lohse MJ, Benovic JL, Codina J, et al: β-Arrestin: a protein that regulates β-adrenergic receptor function. Science 248:1547–1550, 1990

Manji HK: G proteins: implications for psychiatry. Am J Psychiatry 149:746–760, 1992

Mansour A, Meng F, Meador-Woodruff JH, et al: Site-directed mutagenesis of the human dopamine D2 receptor. Eur J Pharmacol—Mol Pharmacol Sec 227:205–214, 1992

McEwen BS, DeKloet ER, Rostene W: Adrenal steroid receptors and actions in the nervous system. Physiol Rev 66:1121–1188, 1986

McGeer PL, Eccles JC, McGeer EG: Molecular Neurobiology of the Mammalian Brain, 2nd Edition. New York, Plenum, 1987

McGonigle P, Molinoff P: Quantitative aspects of drug-receptor interactions, in Basic Neurochemistry, 4th Edition. Edited by Siegel G, Agranoff B, Albers RW, et al. New York, Raven, 1989, pp 183–202

McMillen BA: CNS stimulants: two distinct mechanisms of action for amphetamine-like drugs. Trends Pharmacol Sci 4:429–432, 1983

Miller RJ: The control of neuronal Ca^{2+} homeostasis. Prog Neurobiol 37:225–285, 1991

Montmayeur JP, Borrelli E: Transcription mediated by a cAMP-responsive promoter element is reduced upon activation of dopamine D_2 receptors. Proc Natl Acad Sci U S A 88:3135–3139, 1991

Nagatsu T: Genes for human catecholamine-synthesizing enzymes. Neurosci Res 12:315–345, 1991

Nestler EJ: Molecular mechanisms of drug addiction. J Neurosci 12:2439–2450, 1992

Neve KA, Henningsen RA, Bunzow JR, et al: Functional characterization of a rat dopamine D2 receptor cDNA expressed in a mammalian cell line. Mol Pharmacol 36:446–451, 1989

Neve KA, Cox BA, Henningsen RA, et al: Pivotal role of aspartate-80 in the regulation of dopamine D2 receptor affinity for drugs and inhibition of adenylyl cyclase. Mol Pharmacol 39:733–739, 1991

Noda M, Takahashi H, Tanabe T, et al: Structural homology of *Torpedo californica* acetylcholine receptor subunits. Nature 302:528–532, 1983

Northup JK: Regulation of cyclic nucleotides in the nervous system, in Basic Neurochemistry, 4th Edition. Edited by Siegel G, Agranoff B, Albers RW, et al. New York, Raven, 1989, pp 349–364

Okada F, Crow T, Roberts GW: G proteins (G_i, G_o) in the medial temporal lobe in schizophrenia: preliminary report of a neurochemical correlate of structural change. J Neural Transm Gen Sect 84:147–153, 1991

Probst WC, Snyder LA, Schuster DI, et al: Sequence alignment of the G-protein coupled receptor superfamily. DNA Cell Biol 11:1–20, 1992

Racagni G, Brunello N, Tinelli D, et al: New biochemical hypotheses on the mechanism of action of antidepressant drugs: cAMP-dependent phosphorylation system. Pharmacopsychiatry 25:51–55, 1992

Randall PK: Quantitative analysis of behavioral pharmacological data. Ann N Y Acad Sci 515:124–139,

1988

Rhee SG: Inositol phospholipid-specific phospholipase C: interaction of the γ_1 isoform with tyrosine kinase. Trends Biochem Sci 16:297–301, 1991

Riffee WH, Wilcox RE, Vaughn DM, et al: Dopamine receptor sensitivity after chronic dopamine agonists: striatal (H)-spiroperidol binding in mice after chronic administration of high doses of apomorphine, N-n-propylnorapomorphine, and dextroamphetamine. Psychopharmacology 77:146–149, 1982

Robinson TE, Becker JB: Enduring changes in brain and behavior produced by chronic amphetamine administration: a review and evaluation of animal models of amphetamine psychosis. Brain Res Rev 11:157–198, 1986

Roth R: CNS dopamine autoreceptors: distribution, pharmacology, and function. Ann N Y Acad Sci 430:27–55, 1984

Ruffalo RR Jr: Important concepts of receptor theory. J Auton Pharmacol 2:277–295, 1982

Sakmann B: Elementary steps in synaptic transmission revealed by currents through single ion channels. Science 256:503–512, 1992

Saller CF, Salama AI: Apomorphine enantiomers' effects on dopamine metabolism: receptor and non-receptor related actions. Eur J Pharmacol 121:181–188, 1986

Savarese TM, Fraser CM: In vitro mutagenesis and the search for structure-function relationships among G protein-coupled receptors. Biochem J 283:1–19, 1992

Schulz S, Yuen PST, Garbers DL: The expanding family of guanylyl cyclases. Trends Pharmacol Sci 12:116–120, 1991

Schwartz JH, Kandel ER: Synaptic transmission mediated by second messengers, in Principles of Neural Science, 3rd Edition. Edited by Kandel ER, Schwartz JA, Jessell TM. New York, Elsevier, 1991, pp 173–193

Schwinn DA, Caron MG, Lefkowitz RJ: The beta-adrenergic receptor as a model for molecular structure-function relationships in G-protein-coupled receptors, in The Heart and Cardiovascular System, 2nd Edition. Edited by Fozzard HA, et al. New York, Raven, 1991, pp 1657–1684

Seeman P: Dopamine receptors in human brain diseases, in Dopamine Receptors. Edited by Creese I, Fraser CM. New York, Alan R Liss, 1987, pp 233–245

Senogles SE, Spiegel AM, Padrell E, et al: Specificity of receptor-G protein interactions. J Biol Chem 265:4507–4514, 1990

Severson J, Randall P, Wilcox RE: Single apomorphine pretreatment results in a rapid decline in high-affinity dopamine binding to the striatal D2 receptor. Eur J Pharmacol 188:283–286, 1990

Shimizu T, Wolfe LS: Arachidonic acid cascade and signal transduction. J Neurochem 55:1–15, 1990

Sibley DR, Lefkowitz RJ: Molecular mechanisms of receptor desensitization using the β-adrenergic receptor-coupled adenylate cyclase system as a model. Nature 317:124–129, 1985

Sibley DR, Lefkowitz RJ: Biochemical mechanisms of β-adrenergic receptor regulation. ISI Atlas of Science: Pharmacology 2:66–70, 1988

Sibley DR, Monsma FJ Jr: Molecular biology of dopamine receptors. TIPS 13:61–69, 1992

Siever LJ, Kahn RS, Lawlor BA, et al: Critical issues in defining the role of serotonin in psychiatric disorders. Pharmacol Rev 43:509–525, 1991

Smith CUM: Elements of Molecular Neurobiology. New York, Wiley, 1989

Snyder SH: Nitric oxide: first in a new class of neurotransmitters? Science 257:494–496, 1992

Spiegel AM: Heterotrimeric GTP-binding proteins: an expanding family of signal transducers. Med Res Rev 12:55–71, 1992

Spiegel A, Shenker A, Weinstein L: Receptor-effector coupling by G proteins: implications for normal and abnormal signal transduction. Endocr Rev 13:536–565, 1992

Strait K, Kuczenski R: Dopamine autoreceptor regulation of the kinetic state of striatal tyrosine hydroxylase. J Pharmacol Exp Ther 29:561–569, 1986

Strulovici B, Cerione RA, Kilpatrick BF, et al: Direct demonstration of impaired functionality of a purified desensitized β-adrenergic receptor in a reconstituted system. Science 225:837–840, 1984

Summers WK, Majovski V, Marsh GM, et al: Oral tetrahydroaminoacridine in long-term treatment of senile dementia, Alzheimer type. N Engl J Med 315:1241–1245, 1986

Sunahara R, Guan HC, O'Dowd BF, et al: Cloning of the gene for a human dopamine D5 receptor with higher affinity for dopamine than D1. Nature 350:614–619, 1991

Taylor P: Anticholinesterase agents, in Goodman and Gilman's The Pharmacological Basis of Therapeutics, 8th Edition. Edited by Gilman AG, Rall TW, Nies AS, et al. New York, Pergamon, 1990, pp 131–150

Taylor P, Insel PA: Molecular basis of pharmacologic selectivity, in Principles of Drug Action, 3rd Edition. Edited by Pratt WB, Taylor P. New York, Churchill Livingstone, 1990, pp 1–102

Taylor S, Buechler J, Yonemoto W: cAMP-dependent protein kinase: framework for a diverse family of regulatory enzymes. Ann Rev Biochem 59:971–1005, 1990

Van Tol HHM, Wu CM, Guan HC, et al: Multiple dopamine D4 receptor variants in the human population. Nature 358:149–152, 1992

Vaughn D, Severson J, Woodward J, et al: Behavioral sensitization following subchronic apomorphine treatment—possible neurochemical basis. Brain Res 526:37–44, 1990

Walaas SI, Greengard P: Protein phosphorylation and neuronal function. Pharmacol Rev 43:299–350, 1991

Wilcox RE, Severson J, Woodward J, et al: Behavioral sensitization following a single apomorphine treatment—selective effects on the dopamine release process. Brain Res 528:109–113, 1990

Wolf ME, Roth RH: Dopamine autoreceptors, in Dopamine Receptors. Edited by Creese I, Fraser DM. New York, Alan R Liss, 1987, pp 45–96

Woodward JJ, Wilcox RE, Leslie SW, et al: Dopamine uptake during fast-phase endogenous dopamine release from mouse striatal synaptosomes. Neurosci Lett 71:106–112, 1986

Zhou QY, Grandy DK, Thambi L, et al: Cloning and expression of human and rat D1 dopamine receptors. Nature 347:76–80, 1990

2

Molecular Neurobiology

Allison C. Chin, Ph.D., Karen A. Shaw, Ph.D., and
Roland D. Ciaranello, M.D.

The nervous system is the most heterogeneous tissue in an organism. This heterogeneity is evident in its diverse cellular population, in the complex morphological differences between individual neurons, and in the varying array of gene products expressed by distinct cell types. Molecular neurobiology has emerged as a discipline from the confluence of molecular genetics and neuroscience. Neuroscientists have integrated a multidisciplinary approach to understanding the nervous system anatomically, electrophysiologically, and biochemically in terms of its neurochemical constituents. Molecular geneticists are concerned with understanding the biophysical structure of proteins and nucleic acids in relation to the genetic process and the nature of heredity. Recombinant deoxyribonucleic acid (DNA) technology, including genetic engineering, has accelerated the development of powerful tools and methodologies that make it feasible to manipulate the nervous system so as to facilitate an understanding of the genetic regulation underlying its development and maintenance.

The techniques of molecular biology have transformed neurobiological research and promise to have a comparable impact on clinical practice. Cloning of the molecular components involved in hearing, sight, and smell have demonstrated that different mechanisms are employed to transduce these sensory signals. The ability to generate antibodies to cloned genes or segments of genes, to "tag" or mark

progenitor cells and follow their progressive path during development, and to genetically engineer the expression of specific genes in animals has been crucial to an elucidation of the numbers and types of cells produced during the development of the nervous system. Once the requisite cell numbers and types are present, the cells will undergo axonal growth and targeting, synapse formation, regulation of neurotransmitter release, and dynamic receptor-effector coupling. The mechanisms underlying each of these processes are undergoing intensive molecular genetic scrutiny.

In this chapter, we focus on some of the basic aspects of molecular neurobiology. In the first part of this chapter, we review the molecular components of gene expression and the mechanisms underlying its regulation. In the second part, we describe methods for manipulating gene expression both in vitro and in vivo. Finally, we take a brief look at how molecular neurobiology has contributed to our understanding of a number of neurological disorders.

■ MOLECULAR COMPONENTS OF GENE EXPRESSION

■ Structural Organization of DNA

The genome is the blueprint of a cell and contains the information necessary for it to carry out its biological activity. The genome is composed of chromosomes that contain genes, the units of heredity. The total number of chromosomes per cell for any given species is unique. Humans have 23 pairs of chromosomes—1 pair of sex chromosomes and 22 pairs of autosomes. In contrast, rats have 26 pairs of chromosomes, fruit flies have 4, and maize has 10. Each chromosome contains hundreds of genes that are themselves made up of DNA. The major flow of genetic information progresses from DNA to ribonucleic acid (RNA) to protein.

The structure of DNA was discovered by Watson and Crick in 1953. The classic Watson-Crick double helix consists of two right-handed helical polynucleotide chains coiled around a central axis, such that the purine (adenine [A] and guanine [G]) and pyrimidine (cytosine [C] and thymidine [T]) bases are in parallel planes on the inside of the helix. The bases of each chain are precisely paired (i.e., the principle of complementation) through hydrogen bonds to form the most stable duplexes: A to T and C to G. In addition, each DNA strand is polarized, or oriented so that the free 5′-phosphate and 3′-hydroxyl groups are at opposite ends. These principles of polarity and complementarity also govern nucleic acid synthesis, where one strand serves as the template for the synthesis of the complementary strand.

The genetic information contained in the DNA is deciphered according to the genetic code. There are several interesting features of the code that are worth noting. First, DNA is read continuously from the 5′ to the 3′ direction. Second, groups of three nucleotides, or triplets, encode the 20 different amino acids. Thus, the four nucleotides can account for $4^3 = 64$ triplets. Third, the code is degenerate (redundant) in that each amino acid may be specified by one or more triplets. Finally, the genetic code also includes signals for the initiation and termination of messages.

The mammalian genome consists of approximately 3×10^9 nucleotides and contains the coding capacity for approximately 10^5 genes. Most of these genes share common structural features that include the site of transcription initiation (DNA to RNA) and upstream (in the 5′ direction) sequences that contain the putative promoter region. The promoter region is necessary for proper regulation of gene expression and is often identified by the presence of a sequence of TA repeats (a TATA box) that lies about 30 nucleotides upstream of the transcription initiation site. Often farther upstream reside consensus sequences

of 8–12 nucleotides that are collectively called upstream regulatory elements (UREs). Examples of UREs include consensus sequences for binding cyclic adenosine monophosphate (cAMP), hormone receptors, and a host of transcription factors.

UREs may augment transcription, as in the case of the "CAAT" box, or lead to attenuation of transcription; they serve to modulate the basal promoter activity of any given gene. Genes are organized into sequences that will appear in the messenger RNA ([mRNA] exons) and intervening noncoding sequences (introns). Although introns show no homology to one another, consensus sequences at the exon/intron junctions, or splice junctions, lead to the precise excision of noncoding intronic sequences. Regulatory elements located at the 3′ end of the gene include the polyadenylation consensus sequence, AATAAA, which signals an endonucleolytic cleavage of the mRNA 10–15 nucleotides further downstream and the subsequent addition of 100–200 adenylate groups to the mRNA. Transcriptional enhancer elements may also be found 3′ to the coding region.

■ RNA Synthesis

RNA is synthesized from a DNA template as a single-stranded polymer of ribonucleotides. Like DNA, RNA exhibits a 5′ to 3′ polarity and is composed of four nucleotides: adenosine (A), cytosine (C), guanine (G), and uridine (U). Uridine differs from thymidine in the absence of a methyl group at the 5-carbon position. An additional distinction between DNA and RNA is that the sugar moiety in the latter is ribose, which contains a hydroxyl group at the 2′ position of the pentose ring. RNA also tends to exhibit a high degree of secondary structure as the result of intrastrand hybridization (i.e., complementary sequences within a single RNA molecule may self-hybridize). The consummate example of this is the cloverleaf structure of transfer RNA (tRNA).

Three classes of RNA molecules are synthesized in the cell: mRNA, ribosomal RNA (rRNA), and tRNA. Messenger RNA carries the genetic information encoded in the gene. Ribosomal RNA is transcribed from its gene as a large precursor molecule (45S) that is cleaved to generate three smaller fragments (28S, 18S, and 5.8S). A second gene gives rise to a 5S rRNA. All the rRNA molecules are assembled with a large array of proteins to form the ribosomal subunits that are involved in protein synthesis. The tRNA molecules interface between the nucleic acids and the proteins. They are complex molecules containing "anticodons" that recognize the genetic message in the mRNA at one end and the corresponding amino acid at the other.

In the nucleus, genes undergo transcription by RNA polymerase II from the initiation site through the site of termination to generate primary transcripts. Because most genes contain introns and exons, the primary transcripts require further processing before mature mRNAs are obtained. The initial modification is the addition of a cap (usually a guanine nucleotide in a 5'-5' phosphate linkage) to the 5' end of the transcript, followed by polyadenylation at the 3' terminus. Finally, introns are removed by a process termed splicing. Mature transcripts vary greatly in length, from hundreds to several thousands of nucleotides. All three forms of RNA are involved in protein synthesis.

◼ Protein Synthesis

Mature transcripts are transported from the nucleus to the cytoplasm where they serve as templates for ribosomes and are translated into proteins. Multiple ribosomes may translate a single mRNA template simultaneously. The start codon AUG is located toward the 5' end of the transcript and signals the beginning of translation. Sequential bases of the transcript are read as nonoverlapping triplets and define the amino acids that are incorporated into the protein. At least 20 tRNA molecules serve as carriers for the different amino acids that are attached to the growing polypeptide by aminoacyl tRNA transferases. UAA, UAG, and UGA serve as signals for the termination of protein synthesis and lead to release of the polypeptide from the ribosome. The nascent polypeptide chain will then interact with itself and its environment to assume its final tertiary conformation. The genetic information only specifies the primary structure of the protein.

◼ Regulation of Gene Expression

The mammalian genome encodes an estimated 100,000 different genes in a given cell, and only 20%–30% of these are expressed in a tissue-specific manner (Milner and Sutcliffe 1983). Thus, it follows that the regulation of individual mRNA sequences plays a critical role in the abundance of specific proteins that

ultimately define the phenotype of a particular cell. Control of temporal (i.e., when during development) and spatial (i.e., where in the organism) gene expression may be exerted at multiple levels during the flow of information from DNA to protein (Figure 2–1).

One level of control is at the level of the genome. The amount of gene products could vary by loss or amplification of DNA. Most α-thalassemias occur as a result of the deletion of one or more of the adult α-globin genes. The best known example of gene amplification occurs in the frog *Xenopus,* in which the rRNA genes—already present in an abundant 500 copies—are amplified an additional 4,000-fold during oogenesis to accommodate the level of protein synthesis characteristic of early embryogenesis.

Diversity of gene products may also be arrived at by combinatorial strategies. As exemplified by the immunoglobulin gene family, multiple exon segments may be joined to produce $> 10^7$ antibody molecules. Superimposed on the diversity arising from combinatorial mechanisms is additional variability contributed

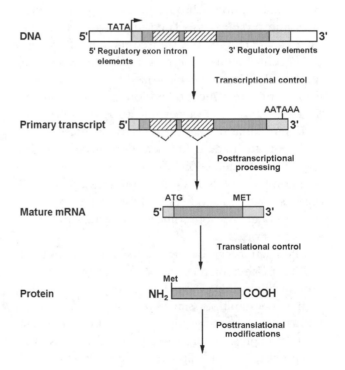

Figure 2–1. Levels of regulation on gene expression. Schematic diagram of a gene with the shaded boxes representing exons that encode the untranslated (light boxes) and coding (dark boxes) portion of the mature mRNA. The arrow denotes the transcription initiation site. The relative positions of the TATA box and 5'- and 3'-regulatory elements are as indicated.

by somatic mutation of the immunoglobulin genes. Multigene families often contain members that are expressed in distinct temporal or spatial patterns such as the hemoglobin genes and transducins, respectively. Van Tol and colleagues (1992) discovered the existence of different polymorphic forms of the dopamine D_4 receptors that contain variable repeats of a 48-base pair sequence. Moreover, the different forms of the D_4 receptors exhibit pharmacological differences in vitro. Whether or not these differences in vitro translate into meaningful distinctions in vivo remains to be seen. Nevertheless, it is intriguing to consider that one or more of these genomic controls might underlie the complexity of other receptor-effector signaling systems such as the odorant receptors (Buck 1992).

Transcriptional control has long been considered a primary form of tissue-specific gene regulation. Subtractive hybridization methods have clearly demonstrated that different cells within an organism may express overlapping but distinct populations of mRNA. A number of mechanisms exist that may affect gene transcription. Chromosomes are composed of DNA and proteins associated in a highly condensed state called chromatin. Transcription is affected by chromatin structure such that transcriptionally active regions of DNA are characterized by a "looser" chromatin structure. Decondensation of chromatin renders the DNA more accessible to RNA polymerase and transcription factors. RNA polymerase is not sufficient to initiate transcription accurately but requires the interaction of auxiliary proteins (transcription factors). Some transcription factors are ubiquitous, whereas others exhibit more restricted patterns of expression; some are activators and others are repressors.

Regulation can be envisioned not only in terms of DNA-protein interactions but also through protein-protein interactions. Some genes express transcripts with either multiple start sites; however, it is not known if all these transcripts are actually utilized. Differential expression of N-methyl-D-aspartate (NMDA) receptor subunits results in different subunit combinations in the cerebellum versus the forebrain (Kutsuwada et al. 1992). Alternative promoters may be used to direct the expression of related proteins from a single gene in different tissues, as is the case with brain-derived neurotrophic factor (Timmusk et al. 1993).

Posttranscriptional mechanisms of gene regulation are particularly relevant to molecular neurobiology. Alternative selection of splice junctions in a gene may generate transcripts that change the translational capacity of the mRNA by altering the reading frame or removing entire portions of the coding region. Multiple potassium channel components result from alternative splicing at the Shaker locus in Drosophila (Schwarz et al. 1988). Differential polyadenylation of the calcitonin/calcium gene-related peptide (CGRP) gene in the thyroid and pituitary tissues leads to the expression of two different prepeptides that are further processed to yield calcitonin or CGRP (Amara et al. 1982). The amount of accumulation of a particular mRNA could also be regulated within the nucleus by splicing or the extent of polyadenylation or transport into the cytoplasm. Additionally, the stability of individual transcripts could vary considerably to allow for differential accumulation of specific mRNAs. Finally, an increasing body of evidence is accumulating to support the regulation of gene expression by way of subcellular localization of transcripts (Kleiman et al. 1990).

Translational control of gene expression is best exemplified in systems such as sea urchins and Drosophila. Eggs of both these invertebrates contain all the maternal transcripts required for early embryogenesis; however, very little translation occurs until after fertilization. Globin synthesis requires the inactivation of an initiation factor by phosphorylation. Phosphorylation as a mechanism of activation or repression of translation initiation factors may be particularly relevant to the nervous system, where second messenger systems often regulate protein kinases that, in turn, have regulatory effects on downstream products.

Posttranslational processing of mature or precursor proteins plays a key role in regulating gene expression. Numerous neuroactive substances are derived from larger prepeptides or prohormones by endoproteolytic cleavage(s). One such example is the pro-opiomelanocortin (POMC) gene. Tissue-specific processing of POMC results in a wide array of end products, including endorphins, as well as several pituitary hormones exhibiting very different biological activity (Nakanishi et al. 1979). Peptidergic neurosecretory cells also produce neuropeptides by posttranslational cleavage of a larger precursor. The egg-laying hormone (ELH) of the mollusk Aplysia is one of three peptides that govern the egg-laying behavior. Pulse-chase labeling combined with immunoelectron microscopy studies have revealed that the ELH prohormone undergoes an ordered series of eight proteolytic cleavages to generate a set of nine bioactive peptides (Jung and Scheller 1991). Furthermore, intricate trafficking of the prohormone results in the specific and localized packaging of peptides into distinct classes of secretory vesicles. Other posttranslational modifications of gene products include glycosylation and phosphorylation. The modifications may be permanent or, as is often the case with phosphorylation, a means of dynamic regulation of a protein between its active and inactive states.

■ Gene Expression and Antipsychotic Drugs

Many drugs that interact with receptors are used therapeutically and exert profound effects on mental states (reviewed in Levy and Van de Kar 1992; Richelson 1991). Very often the drugs have a broad spectrum of activity and interact with more than one receptor subtype. In addition, the clinical use of several of the antipsychotic drugs is complicated by acute and chronic motor side effects. The serotonin-2 (5-HT$_2$) receptor is a site of action for hallucinogenic drugs that induce a state of psychosis (Pierce and Peroutka 1988). Consistent with the role of hallucinogens as agonists is the therapeutic use of 5-HT$_2$ antagonists (5-HT$_2$ blockers) as antipsychotics. Although chlorpromazine and spiperone are potent antipsychotic agents that function as 5-HT$_2$ antagonists, they are not specific for only this receptor (Glennon 1990). Haloperidol is a typical antipsychotic drug that also induces dystonia, presumably mediated by extrapyramidal motor systems in the basal ganglia. Clozapine is one of the atypical antipsychotic drugs that does not cause extrapyramidal side effects (EPS) and displays clinical efficacy equal to or greater than that of haloperidol (Baldessarini and Frankenburg 1991). However, treatment with clozapine can lead to agranulocytosis.

The isolation of cloned sequences for many receptors has facilitated a molecular understanding of the specific residues necessary for ligand binding. Site-directed mutagenesis of specific amino acids within the receptor protein can be analyzed for the consequences on ligand binding and receptor activation. For example, mutagenesis of a single serine residue in the fifth transmembrane region of the 5-HT$_2$ receptor alters the binding properties from a human pharmacology to that of a rat (Kao et al. 1992). Similar mutagenesis studies demonstrated that ketanserin, mianserin, mesulergine, and spiperone share overlapping but distinct binding domains (Choudhary et al. 1993; Wang et al. 1993). The structural information will be extremely useful in drug design to create more highly specific ligands.

Much less information is available on the effects of antipsychotic drugs on gene expression. Two groups have recently demonstrated that treatment of rats with antipsychotic drugs induces changes in receptor mRNA levels in the brain. Chronic administration of rats with sulpiride, haloperidol, loxapine, and clozapine differentially increased the expression of dopamine receptor mRNA levels. Loxapine elicited a 1.5- to 4.5-fold increase in mRNA levels for the D$_1$, D$_2$, and D$_3$ dopamine receptors, whereas haloperidol only affected the dopamine D$_3$ mRNA levels (Buckland et al. 1992). Clozapine caused a fivefold increase in D$_3$ receptor mRNA after 4 days of treatment, whereas sulpiride elicited a similar increase after 32 days (Buckland et al. 1993).

Merchant and Dorsa (1993) have demonstrated that a number of typical and atypical antipsychotic drugs differentially regulate the expression of neurotensin (NT), a peptidergic transmitter that interacts with the nigrostriatal and mesolimbic dopamine systems. Acute administration of either typical or atypical antipsychotics (e.g., haloperidol, fluphenazine, clozapine, remoxipride, and thioridazine) selectively increased NT mRNA expression in the nucleus accumbens. In contrast, only typical antipsychotics such as haloperidol and fluphenazine affected an increase in NT mRNA in the dorsal striatum. These differences may reflect a functional significance of the therapeutic effects of these drugs. The effects of antipsychotic drugs on the regulation of gene expression adds another dimension to their role as therapeutic agents.

■ MANIPULATION OF GENE EXPRESSION

The genetic engineering revolution is universally regarded as having originated with the discovery of the structure of DNA by Watson and Crick in 1953. For more detailed understanding about the organization of DNA, methods had to be developed to reveal the exact nucleotides of selected DNA (and, ultimately, gene) sequences. The stage was set in the 1960s and 1970s for the isolation of the enzyme DNA ligase that can join DNA chains together, the discovery of sequence-specific methylase enzymes that modified DNA by methylation, and the identification of restriction enzymes that generated site-specific endonucleolytic cleavages. In particular, a restriction enzyme digest of DNA generates a restriction map, or a series of DNA fragments that are characteristic of that particular piece of DNA. Restriction fragments led the way to the rapid development of powerful methods of DNA sequencing. In 1973, Boyer and Cohen developed the first practical method for systematically cloning specific DNA fragments, regardless of their origin (Cohen et al. 1973). They mixed plasmid DNA fragments that had been digested by the same restriction enzyme together in the presence of DNA ligase to generate the first hybrid plasmid DNAs. The recombinant DNA molecules were subsequently propagated in bacteria. By the mid-1970s, the ability to exploit recombinant DNA methodology was at its full potential.

The ability to clone DNA has emerged as one of the most powerful tools of molecular biology. This technology has accelerated analysis of gene structure, generation of protein sequence information, production of antibodies to specific epitopes of a particular antigen, and studies of functional aspects of proteins by gene transfer. It is possible to clone genes directly from genomic DNA, or to clone DNA from mRNA transcripts and thereby clone only the expressed gene products.

■ cDNA Cloning

Nearly every mRNA molecule has a stretch of adenine nucleotides called a poly A tail at its 3′-end. When short chains of poly T are mixed with the mRNA, they hybridize with the poly A tail to form an mRNA molecule with a double-stranded poly dA–poly dT tail. An enzyme called reverse transcriptase, isolated from RNA tumor viruses, can use this oligo dT as a primer and the mRNA as a template to synthesize DNA (Figure 2–2). This enzyme reverses the first step of gene expression—hence its name. If the mRNA and DNA strands are separated, the DNA strand can be used as a template for the synthesis of the complementary DNA strand by DNA polymerase I. Because the end result is a double-stranded DNA molecule that is

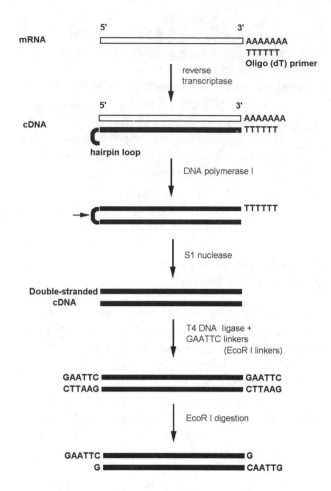

Figure 2–2.   Complementary DNA (cDNA) synthesis.

complementary to the mRNA, it is called cDNA.

The cDNA molecule can be inserted into a cloning vector after further processing and propagated as recombinant DNA in bacteria (Figure 2–3). The ends of the cDNA molecules can be modified by methylation, restriction enzyme digestion, or the addition of nucleotide tails or artificial linkers in order to make them compatible with the cloning vector. A variety of vectors are available for cloning, including bacterial plasmids, bacteriophages, and recombinant phagemids. The choice of vectors is determined by the sizes of the DNA fragments to be cloned and the strategy to be employed in identifying the relevant cDNA clones. Because the original mRNA used as template represents a mixed population of transcripts, the cDNA will also be heterogeneous in size and sequence. Furthermore, the more abundant a particular transcript, the easier it will be to identify its corresponding cDNA. This pool of cDNAs is called a "cDNA library."

The cDNA library may be screened to identify the

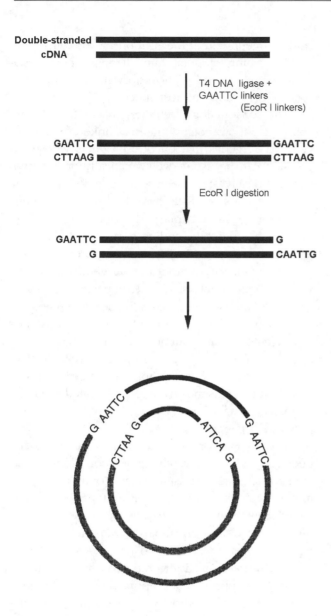

Figure 2–3. cDNA cloning.

cDNA clones may be sequenced to determine the primary structure of the protein, expressed in a suitable host cell (transfection) to carry out functional studies, or used to screen genomic DNA for the gene encoding the target protein.

■ Genomic Cloning

Analysis of the structure and organization of chromosomal genes requires a genomic DNA library. The principles of constructing a genomic library are similar to those involved in the generation of cDNA libraries. Genomic DNA is digested with a restriction enzyme and (because the average size of the genomic fragments is around 20 kb) cloned into bacteriophage vectors that are capable of stably carrying these large pieces of foreign DNA. A genomic library is readily screened with radiolabeled cDNA plasmid probes. Often, several genomic clones need to be isolated and characterized in order to recover all the sequences that encode a given gene. Recombinant clones containing these longer chromosomal fragments also facilitate examination of regions flanking the coding sequences of a gene at both the 5'- and 3'- ends that may be involved in the regulation of its expression.

■ Restriction Fragment Length Polymorphisms

Cloned cDNAs and genomic DNA fragments have served as extremely important diagnostic tools in molecular medicine. Restriction fragment length polymorphism (RFLP) analysis takes advantage of the fact that restriction enzyme digestion of DNA generates specific restriction maps (Figure 2–4). Naturally occurring or mutationally induced variations in particular gene sequences result in differences in the restriction maps, or polymorphisms. In this type of analysis, genomic DNA is digested with one or more restriction enzymes and size-fractionated on agarose gels, and the DNA is then immobilized on filter membranes. The DNA-containing filters are hybridized with radiolabeled recombinant DNA probes for particular target genes and the hybridized products visualized by autoradiography. The distinct polymorphisms known as RFLPs have been useful in the chromosomal mapping of genes using somatic cell hybrids, following patterns of inheritance of disease-related genes and in forensic medicine.

clones of interest by a number of different methods. If amino acid sequence for the protein is available, short synthetic nucleic acids (oligonucleotides) may be constructed based on the genetic code and codon usage. Alternatively, antibodies directed against the protein might exist in the absence of any sequence information. In this case, the cDNAs would be cloned in vectors that would allow expression of the foreign DNA in bacterial hosts. Recombinants would be screened using the antibody. Positive clones may be propagated in bacterial hosts to generate large homogeneous cultures from which the recombinant DNA may be extracted for more extensive analysis. The

A

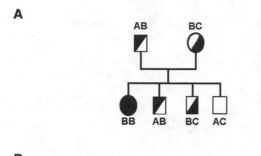

B

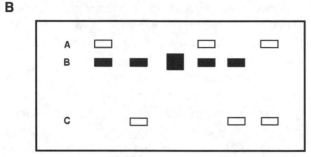

Figure 2–4. RFLP analysis of an inherited disorder. Open, hatched, and black boxes or circles indicate wild type, carriers, and affected individuals, respectively.

Panel A: Pedigree of a male (box) and female (circle) who are both carriers for a particular genetic trait. They have four offspring: one affected child and three non-affected children (two are carriers and one is wild type for the gene).

Panel B: Restriction fragment length polymorphism analysis of DNA isolated from each of the individuals. The parents are polymorphic for the gene and have "genotypes" of AB and BC. The "genotypes" of the children are BB, AB, BC, and AC. Because the affected child's genotype is BB, the RFLP analysis demonstrates that the B fragment segregates with the disease and would be useful in diagnostic tests.

■ Expression of Recombinant Genes

The ability to express cloned genes epitomizes the power of the recombinant DNA technology. Introduction of recombinant cDNAs in host cells (i.e., through transfection) that endogenously express the target gene have allowed a functional examination of the protein at a subcellular level. A number of methods have been developed to transfect foreign DNA into mammalian cells, including calcium phosphate precipitation, lipofection, and electroporation. Once the DNA has been transfected, it is selectively retained by virtue of selectable markers (normally conferring resistance to a specific antibiotic). The use of recombinant plasmids harboring site-directed mutations has revealed amino acid sequences necessary for a variety of normal cellular functions. These include targeting and localization of proteins, ion-specific gating of potassium channels, posttranslational modification by phosphorylation, and agonist specificity in different host species.

The construction of chimeric plasmids that contain putative promoter sequences linked to reporter genes (i.e., genes that encode products whose expression can be assayed enzymatically or immunohistochemically) have been seminal in understanding the interactions of *cis-* and *trans-*regulation of gene expression. Chimeric plasmids usually contain sequences that flank the coding portion of a gene. Deletions that systematically remove portions of the putative regulatory region may be generated with a variety of endonucleases and exonucleases and subsequently transfected into cell lines. Such experiments have led to the identification of consensus DNA elements (*cis* sequences) that bind *trans-*acting factors such as hormone receptors, cyclic nucleotides, and transcription factors. Transfection assays with chimeric plasmids have also delimited promoter regions necessary for mediating cell-type specific expression of genes.

The expression of recombinant plasmids has been assayed in vivo by the generation of transgenic animals. The use of constitutive and/or inducible promoters such as the heat shock and viral promoters have been used to overexpress specific cDNAs in flies, worms, and mammals. Chimeric promoter-reporter constructs similar to those described here have been introduced into the germ line of animals to assay for appropriate temporal and spatial regulation of gene expression. More recently, the site-specific recombination of a target gene in mice has been used to generate null mutations ("knockouts"). The knockout transgenic mice serve as in vivo "test tubes" to determine whether a gene is essential for survival and to gain insight into the contributions of a particular gene to an organism's normal development.

■ MOLECULAR GENETIC APPROACHES TO NEURODEGENERATIVE DISORDERS

In the last two decades, coupling of the explosive developments in molecular genetics and neuroscience has had a profound impact on basic science and clinical medicine. Several different strategies have been employed in the hope of finding a cure for a variety of neurodegenerative disorders. One approach is to screen cDNA libraries generated from "normal" and affected individuals. This strategy is particularly useful if the target gene is known, because oligonucleotide or antibody probes might be readily obtained. In this manner, human liver cDNA libraries were screened to identify clones encoding mutant phenylalanine hydroxylase (PH) cDNAs. A second strategy is to systematically hone in on the target gene using RFLP analysis to screen pedigrees of the families of afflicted individuals and look for the cosegregation of DNA markers with the inheritance of the disease. The recent isolation of the gene for Huntington's disease (HD) exemplifies this approach (Huntington's Disease Collaborative Research Group 1993). This cloning effort required the concerted cooperation of eight different research groups and would have been impossible without the availability of extensive family histories across multiple generations. Animal models of different neurodegenerative disorders have also been used to elucidate the mechanisms underlying the disease process. In 1990, the first implants of fetal tissues into individuals with Parkinson's disease (PD) were described (Freed et al. 1990; Lindvall et al. 1990). The ultimate goal of all these strategies is to find a cure for the disorder in question.

■ Cloning Target Genes: Sequence Analysis and RFLP Diagnosis

Phenylketonuria (PKU) was one of the first inherited diseases in which mental retardation was linked to a metabolic disorder (reviewed in Eisensmith and Woo 1991). PKU is an autosomal recessive disorder in which the level of serum phenylalanine is considerably elevated as a result of a liver PH deficiency. Several mutant PH cDNAs, identified by RFLP assays, have been cloned and characterized by sequence analysis (Okano et al. 1991; Woo et al. 1983). In one case, the mutation gives rise to an alternatively spliced transcript that generates a truncated protein product that is enzymatically inactive. The second mutant gene contains a single base change ($C \rightarrow T$) that results in an amino acid substitution (arg $\rightarrow$ trp). Although this protein is of normal length, it is also enzymatically inactive.

The availability of the PH cDNA has been useful in prenatal diagnosis for PKU and shows the most promise for identification of maternal PKU. In maternal PKU, afflicted mothers whose phenylalanine levels are not controlled by dietary restriction give birth to infants with symptoms of classic PKU, including mental retardation. This fetal pathology is a direct result of the elevated phenylalanine in the maternal circulation and can be prevented by placing phenylketonuric females on dietary phenylalanine restriction during pregnancy. Identification of the gene mutation allows direct testing for the inheritance of the defective gene.

The isolation of the HD gene was a triumphant feat in molecular genetic medicine. The genetic defect causing HD was mapped to chromosome 4 in 1983, but 10 years would go by before the Huntington's gene would be cloned (Gusella et al. 1983; Huntington's Disease Collaborative Research Group 1993). HD is a progressive neurodegenerative disorder that is inherited in an autosomal dominant fashion; homozygotes for the disease do not differ clinically from heterozygotes. Typically, the disease is manifested in middle-aged adults, but juvenile onset of HD occurs occasionally. The symptoms of HD include characteristic motor disturbances and dementia, culminating in a vegetative state within 10 to 20 years of onset.

Analyses of the HD gene have revealed that the mutation is an expanded, unstable trinucleotide repeat, $(CAG)_n$, which may be in the coding sequence. The repeat is considered unstable, because its length tends to expand with successive generations but contracts on occasion. It is not yet clear whether the trinucleotide repeat is translated so its effect may be exerted either at the mRNA or protein level. Another curiosity is why the effects of this mutation are so pronounced in the brain when the gene is expressed in cells throughout the body. Thus, the next challenge facing the HD research community is to determine the normal function of the "huntingtin" protein, as the product of this gene has been named, and to elucidate the mechanism whereby the trinucleotide repeat leads to the neuropathology of HD.

The repeat expansion in HD may prove to be a common mutational mechanism in human genetic disease. The presence of trinucleotide repeats have been described in three other disorders, the fragile X syndrome, myotonic dystrophy (MD), and Kennedy's disease (KD). Symptoms of the fragile X syndrome include a form of X-linked mental retardation and a fragile chromosome site localized to Xq27.3. The expression of this disease is directly associated with transcriptional suppression, or inactivation, of the *FMR1* gene, presumably by the expansion of a $(CGG)_n$ repeat in the 5'-untranslated region of the gene (Fu et al. 1992; Kremer et al. 1991; Verkerk et al. 1991).

FMRP, the *FMR1* gene product, has been shown to be an RNA binding protein that interacts with a selective but substantial fraction of human brain mRNA (Ashley et al. 1993). MD is an autosomal dominant neuromuscular disorder and the most common form of muscular dystrophy. The unstable trinucleotide repeat, $(CTG)_n$, resides in the 3'-untranslated region of the MD gene that encodes a myotonin protein kinase (Aslanidis et al. 1992; Brook et al. 1992; Buxton et al. 1992; Fu et al. 1992; Harley et al. 1992; Mahadevan et al. 1992). KD, a rare X-linked recessive disorder typified by spinal and bulbar muscular atrophy, is caused by expansion of the trinucleotide $(CAG)_n$ in the coding sequence of the androgen receptor gene (Biancalana et al. 1992; LaSpada et al. 1991). As in the case of HD, the repeat length in the fragile X syndrome and myotonic dystrophy tends to increase with transmission to the next generation. The parallels between HD and MD are particularly striking, as there appears to be a correlation with repeat length and age at disease onset. Although the ability to clone genes has provided an understanding of how the mutations give rise to their respective gene defects, the mechanisms underlying these disease processes remain unknown.

Many other examples of neurodegenerative diseases exist for which the genetics have outpaced a cellular and molecular understanding of the genes' products. Identification of the gene products for the different diseases could provide target proteins for possible drug therapy. Genes for Alzheimer's disease (AD), neurofibromatosis type 1 (NF1), and neurofibromatosis type 2 (NF2) have been cloned, but how the defective gene products underlie their respective diseases is unclear. Associations have been made for monoamine oxidase A (MAO-A) and dopamine D_4 receptors to abnormal behavior (Brunner et al. 1993; Seeman et al. 1993).

The pathogenesis of AD is correlated with the 40-amino acid peptide derived from the β-amyloid precursor protein (APP) (Koo et al. 1993; Selkoe 1991). Hypotheses for the molecular basis of the disease process revolve around the direct or indirect neurotoxicity of this peptide. The search is on for inhibitors of peptide production. Demonstration that APP can interact with heterotrimeric guanosine triphosphate (GTP)-binding proteins, important components of the intracellular signal transduction machinery, provides additional targets for investigation (Nishimoto et al. 1993).

The neurofibromatoses are characterized by a predisposition to peripheral tumors (NF1; reviewed in Gutmann and Collins 1993) or schwannomas and meningiomas of the cranial nerves and the spinal nerve roots (NF2) (Rouleau et al. 1993; Trofatter et al. 1993). The gene for NF1 resides on chromosome 17 and encodes neurofibromin, a protein related to a family of GTPase-activating proteins. Recent evidence suggests that neurofibromin is essential for inhibition of cell proliferation by negative regulation of the *ras* proto-oncogene, which is already a target for cancer therapeutics (Basu et al. 1992). The NF2 gene, on chromosome 22, gives rise to a gene product that is structurally related to a family of proteins involved in the association of integral membrane proteins with the cytoskeleton (Rouleau et al. 1993; Trofatter et al. 1993). Monoamine oxidase A and B (MAO-A and MAO-B) metabolize serotonin, dopamine, and noradrenaline. A point mutation in the *MAOA* gene, which results in a complete deficiency of the MAO-A enzyme, segregates with an X-linked borderline mental retardation and prominent aggressive behavior (Brunner et al. 1993). In each of these cases, an understanding of the "normal" function of the gene products provides insight into the mechanisms that go awry in the disease state.

■ Animal Models

Animal models for neurodegenerative diseases are invaluable resources. Whether they represent natural or genetically engineered resources, they are useful tools for analyzing the normal functions of genes and their products and the consequences of harboring the defective gene. The nematode *Caenorhabditis elegans* has proved to be an excellent system for investigating the mechanisms underlying programmed cell death (Driscoll 1992). In this organism, the lineage of all 959 cells of the adult is known, as well as the lineage of the 131 cells that die during development (Sulston et al. 1983). Invertebrates such as the fruit fly and the grasshopper have been used to dissect the genes involved in the axonal growth cone and pathway finding of motor neurons in developing organisms (Thomas et al. 1984).

Preliminary studies have correlated elevated levels of dopamine D_4 receptors in the schizophrenia striatum (Seeman et al. 1993). Dopamine D_4 receptors were six times higher in tissues from subjects with schizophrenia compared with brains of control subjects or subjects with AD or HD. It will be interesting to see what the phenotype of rats expressing elevated levels of the dopamine D_4 receptors will be. A progressive neuropathy that resembles amyotrophic lateral sclerosis has been generated in transgenic mice by overexpression of the human neurofilament heavy chain (Cöte et al. 1993). Several mouse models exist for human motor neuron disease, including trembler (*tr*) and progressive motor neuropathy (*pmn*). The trembler mutation, an autosomal dominant disorder, is considered a model for both Charcot-Marie-Tooth disease type 1 (CMT1) and hereditary neuropathy with liability to pressure palsies (HNPP) (Chance et al. 1993). The clinical manifestations of all three diseases are characterized by hypomyelination of peripheral neurons.

CMT1 is an autosomal dominant disorder that has been mapped to several loci, including chromosomes 1 (CMT1B) and 17 (CMT1A). HNPP has also been mapped to chromosome 17. CMT1A is associated with a duplication of a region 17p11, which includes the gene for peripheral myelin protein 22 (PMP-22). HNPP is correlated with a deletion of this same DNA region. *Tr* has been mapped to a syntenic region on mouse chromosome 11. Although the genetic region of 17p11 contains enough DNA to encode an estimated 20–30 genes, it is possible that HNPP and CMT1A are phenotypic consequences of the aberrant expression of the same gene.

The motor neuron degeneration in *pmn* mice progresses rapidly (Sendtner et al. 1992). The phenotype of mutant mice treated with ciliary neurotrophic factor (CNTF) included significantly longer life spans, exhibition of improved motor behavior, and increased myelination in axons of the phrenic nerve. CNTF is a polypeptide that has been purified from chick ocular tissue and rat sciatic nerve. Interestingly, *pmn* mice express normal levels of CNTF mRNA and protein. The mechanism(s) by which CNTF mediates motor neuron survival have yet to be elucidated. Biotechnology companies have reportedly begun clinical trials of CNTF with individuals who have amyotrophic lateral sclerosis (Oppenheim 1992). Several other proteins such as growth-promoting activity factor, fibroblast growth factor 5, leukemia-inhibitory factor, and insulin-like growth factor support the survival of motor neurons in vitro and can be tested for their therapeutic value in treating degenerating motor neurons (Mudge 1993). The first fetal implants in rat models of PD described anatomical and functional repair (Björklund and Stenevi 1979).

■ Gene Therapy via Fetal Implants

Implantation of human fetal tissue is fraught with biological, clinical, and ethical considerations (Gage 1993). A review of studies conducted by three different groups who implanted fetal tissue into PD patients raises the concern that basic questions regarding what tissue should be used and where still need to be addressed. Although it is generally agreed that the appropriate tissue is fetal mesencephalon, the age of the fetuses and the treatment of the tissue (i.e., time between abortion and transplantation) that would yield optimal cell survival but an adequate window of time for testing the tissue quality (i.e., absence or presence of viral, fungal, and bacterial contamination) are points of dispute. It is also agreed that the transplantation site should be the caudate and putamen, where dopaminergic neurons project (and the target areas in PD that are depleted of dopamine). Differences in experimental protocol concern whether or not bilateral implants should be carried out and how many dopamine neurons should be implanted (from one or more fetuses). Hope remains that therapeutic benefits can be gained by grafts, but further clinical investigations await methodological advances.

■ Summary

Molecular biology has had a profound impact on the neurosciences. The availability of recombinant DNA technology has led to considerable progress in identifying products encoded by genes that segregate with a particular neurodegenerative disorder. The cloned genes represent valuable tools for prenatal diagnosis, investigation of normal cellular functions of the gene products and the molecular basis underlying the defects, design of therapeutic agents, and—perhaps one day—therapy by gene replacement.

■ REFERENCES

Amara SG, Jonas V, Rosenfeld MG, et al: Alternative RNA processing in calcitonin gene expression generates mRNAs encoding different polypeptide products. Nature 298:240–244, 1982

Ashley CT Jr, Wilkinson KD, Reines D, et al: *FMR1* protein: conserved RNP family domains and selective RNA binding. Science 262:563–566, 1993

Aslanidis C, Jansen G, Amemiya C, et al: Cloning of the essential myotonic dystrophy region and mapping of the putative defect. Nature 355:548–551, 1992

Baldessarini RJ, Frankenburg FR: Clozapine, a novel antipsychotic agent. N Engl J Med 324:746–754, 1991

Basu TN, Gutmann DH, Fletcher JA, et al: Aberrant regulation of *ras* proteins in malignant tumour cells from type 1 neurofibromatosis patients. Nature 356:713–715, 1992

Biancalana V, Serville F, Pommier J, et al: Moderate instability of the trinucleotide repeat in spinobulbar muscular atrophy. Human Molecular Genetics 1:255–258, 1992

Björklund A, Stenevi U: Reconstruction of the nigrostriatal dopamine pathway by intracerebral nigral transplants. Brain Res 177:555–560, 1979

Brook JD, McCurrach ME, Harley HG, et al: Molecular basis of muscular dystrophy: expansion of a trinucleotide (CTG) repeat at the 3′ end of a transcript encoding a protein kinase family member. Cell 68:799–808, 1992

Brunner HG, Nelen M, Breakfield XO, et al: Abnormal behavior associated with a point mutation in the structural gene for monoamine oxidase A. Science 262:578–580, 1993

Buck L: The olfactory multigene family. Curr Opin Genet Dev 2:467–473, 1992

Buckland PR, O'Donovan MC, McGuffin P: Changes in dopamine D1, D2, and D3 receptor mRNA levels in rat brain following antipsychotic treatment. Psychopharmacology (Berl) 106:479–483, 1992

Buckland PR, O'Donovan MC, McGuffin P: Clozapine and sulpiride up-regulate dopamine D3 receptor mRNA levels. Neuropharmacology 32:901–907, 1993

Buxton J, Shelbourne P, Davies J, et al: Detection of an unstable fragment of DNA specific to individuals with myotonic dystrophy. Nature 355:547–548, 1992

Chance PF, Alderson MK, Leppig KA, et al: DNA deletion associated with hereditary neuropathy with liability to pressure palsies. Cell 72:143–151, 1993

Choudhary MS, Craigo S, Roth BL: A single point mutation (Phe^{340} [→] Leu^{340}) of a conserved phenylalanine abolishes 4-[^{125}I]iodo-(2,5-dimethoxy)-phenylisopropylamine and [^{3}H]mesulergine but not [^{3}H]ketanserin binding to 5-hydroxytryptamine$_2$ receptors. Mol Pharmacol 43:755–761, 1993

Cohen S, Chang A, Boyer H, et al: Construction of biologically functional bacterial plasmids in vitro. Proc Natl Acad Sci U S A 70:3240–3244, 1973

Côte F, Collard JF, Julien JP: Progressive neuronopathy in transgenic mice expressing the human neurofilament heavy gene: a mouse model of amyotrophic lateral sclerosis. Cell 73:35–46, 1993

Driscoll M: Molecular genetics of cell death in the nematode *Caenorhabditis elegans*. J Neurobiol 23:1327–1351, 1992

Eisensmith RC, Woo SL: Phenylketonuria and the phenylalanine hydroxylase gene. Molecular Biology and Medicine 8:3–18, 1991

Freed CR, Breeze RE, Rosenberg NL, et al: Transplantation of human fetal dopamine cells for Parkinson's disease. Arch Neurol 47:505–512, 1990

Fu YH, Pizzuti A, Fenwick RG, et al: An unstable triplet repeat in a gene related to myotonic muscular dystrophy. Science 255:1256–1259, 1992

Gage FH: Fetal implants put to the test. Nature 361:405–406, 1993

Glennon RA: Serotonin receptors: clinical implications. Neurosci Biobehav Rev 14:35–47, 1990

Gusella JF, Wexler NS, Conneally PM, et al: A polymorphic DNA marker genetically linked to Huntington's disease. Nature 306:234–238, 1983

Gutmann DH, Collins FS: The neurofibromatosis type I gene and its protein product, neurofibromin. Neuron 10:335–343, 1993

Harley HG, Brook JD, Floyd J, et al: Expansion of an unstable DNA region and phenotypic variation in myotonic dystrophy. Nature 355:545–546, 1992

Huntington's Disease Collaborative Research Group: A novel gene containing a trinucleotide repeat that is expanded and unstable on Huntington's disease chromosomes. Cell 72:971–983, 1993

Jung LJ, Scheller RH: Peptide processing and targeting in the neuronal secretory pathway. Science

251:1330–1335, 1991

Kao HT, Adham N, Olsen MA, et al: Site-directed mutagenesis of a single residue changes the binding properties of the serotonin 5-HT$_2$ receptor from a human to a rat pharmacology. FEBS Lett 307:324–328, 1992

Kleiman R, Banker G, Steward O: Differential subcellular localization of particular mRNAs in hippocampal neurons in culture. Neuron 5:821–830, 1990

Koo EH, Park L, Selkoe D: Amyloid beta-protein as a substrate interacts with extracellular matrix to promote neurite outgrowth. Proc Natl Acad Sci U S A 90:4748–4752, 1993

Kremer EJ, Pritchard M, Lynch M, et al: Mapping of DNA instability at the fragile X to an trinucleotide repeat sequence p(CGG)$_n$. Science 252:1711–1714, 1991

Kutsuwada T, Kashiwabuchi N, Mori H, et al: Molecular diversity of the NMDA receptor channel. Nature 358:36–41, 1992

LaSpada AR, Wilson EM, Lubahn DB, et al: Androgen receptor gene mutations in X-linked spinal and bulbar muscular atrophy. Nature 352:77–79, 1991

Levy AD, Van de Kar LD: Endocrine and receptor pharmacology of serotonergic anxiolytics, antipsychotics and antidepressants. Life Sci 51:83–94, 1992

Lindvall O, Brundin P, Widner H, et al: Grafts of fetal dopamine neurons survive and improve motor function in Parkinson's disease. Science 247:574–577, 1990

Mahadevan M, Tsilfidis C, Sabourin L, et al: Myotonic dystrophy mutation: an unstable CTG repeat in the 3' untranslated region of the gene. Science 255:1253–1255, 1992

Merchant KM, Dorsa DM: Differential induction of neurotensin and c-fox gene expression by typical versus atypical antipsychotics. Proc Natl Acad Sci U S A 90:3447–3451, 1993

Milner RJ, Sutcliffe JG: Gene expression in rat brain. Nucleic Acids Res 11:5497–5520, 1983

Mudge AW: Motor neurons find their factors. Nature 363:213–214, 1993

Nakanishi S, Inoue A, Kita T, et al: Nucleotide sequence of cloned cDNA for bovine corticotropin β-lipotropin precursor. Nature 278:423–428, 1979

Nishimoto I, Okamoto T, Matsuura Y, et al: Alzheimer amyloid protein precursor complexes with brain GTP-binding protein G$_o$. Nature 362:75–79, 1993

Okano Y, Wang T, Eisensmith RC, et al: Phenylketonuria missense mutations in the Mediterranean. Genomics 9:96–103, 1991

Oppenheim RW: High hopes of a trophic factor. Nature 35:451–452, 1992

Pierce PA, Peroutka SJ: Antagonism of 5-hydroxytryptamine$_2$ receptor mediated phosphatidylinositol turnover by D-lysergic acid diethylamide. J Pharmacol Exp Ther 247:918–925, 1988

Richelson E: Psychopharmacology of classical and atypical antipsychotics. Yakubutsu Seishin Kodo 11:71–74, 1991

Rouleau GA, Merel P, Lutchman M, et al: Alteration in a new gene encoding a putative membrane-organizing protein causes neuro-fibromatosis type 2. Nature 363:515–521, 1993

Schwarz TL, Tempel BL, Papazian DM, et al: Multiple potassium-channel components are produced by alternative splicing at the *Shaker* locus in *Drosophila*. Nature 331:137–142, 1988

Seeman P, Gun HC, Van Tol HHM: Dopamine D4 receptors elevated in schizophrenia. Nature 365:441–445, 1993

Selkoe DJ: The molecular pathology of Alzheimer's disease. Neuron 6:487–498, 1991

Sendtner M, Schmalbruch H, Stickli KA, et al: Ciliary neurotrophic factor prevents degeneration of motor neurons in mouse mutant progressive neuronopathy. Nature 358:502–504, 1992

Sulston JE, Schierenberg E, White JG, et al: The embryonic cell lineage of the nematode *Caenorhabditis elegans*. Dev Biol 100:64–119, 1983

Thomas JB, Bastiani MJ, Bate M, et al: From grasshopper to *Drosophila:* a common plan for neuronal development. Nature 310:203–206, 1984

Timmusk T, Palm K, Metsis M, et al: Multiple promoters direct tissue-specific expression of the rat BDNF gene. Neuron 10:475–489, 1993

Trofatter JA, MacCollin MM, Rutter JL, et al: A novel moesin-, ezrin-, radixin-like gene is a candidate for the neurofibromatosis 2 tumor suppressor. Cell 72:791–800, 1993

Van Tol HHM, Wu CM, Guan HC, et al: Multiple dopamine D4 receptor variants in the human population. Nature 358:149–152, 1992

Verkerk AJM, Pieretti M, Sutcliffe JS, et al: Identification of a gene (*FMR-1*) containing a CGG repeat coincident with a breakpoint cluster region exhibiting length variation in fragile X syndrome. Cell 65:905–914, 1991

Wang CD, Gallaher TK, Shih JC: Site-directed mutagenesis of the serotonin 5-hydroxytryptamine$_2$ receptor: identification of amino acids necessary for ligand binding and receptor activation. Mol Pharmacol 43:931–940, 1993

Watson JD, Crick FHC: A structure for deoxyribonucleic acid. Nature 171:737–738, 1953

Woo SL, Lidsky AS, Guttler R, et al: Cloned human phenylalanine hydroxylase gene allows prenatal diagnosis and carrier detection of classical phenylketonuria. Nature 306:151–155, 1983

■ SELECTED READINGS

Alberts B, Bray D, Lewis J, et al: Molecular Biology of the Cell, 2nd Edition. New York, Garland Publishing, 1989

Davidson EH: Gene Activity in Early Development, 3rd Edition. Orlando, FL, Academic Press, 1986

Lewin B: Genes IV, 4th Edition. Cambridge, England, Oxford University Press, 1990

Smith CUM: Elements of Molecular Neurobiology. New York, Wiley, 1989

3

Biochemical Anatomy: Insights Into the Cell Biology and Pharmacology of Neurotransmitter Systems in the Brain

Alfred Mansour, Ph.D., Derek T. Chalmers, Ph.D., Charles A. Fox, Ph.D., James H. Meador-Woodruff, M.D., and Stanley J. Watson, M.D., Ph.D.

In this chapter, we cannot possibly describe all of the relevant cellular biology and anatomy for each and every clinical condition affecting the central nervous system (CNS) and the therapeutic compounds relevant to each condition's treatment. Ideally, we could provide an overview of the 30 to 50 most relevant neurotransmitter systems and their associated cell biology and anatomy. But such an undertaking would require several volumes in its own right and is obviously impractical here. We have opted to focus instead on two major neurotransmitter systems, dopamine (DA) and serotonin (5-HT), each of which is central to the current theories of certain psychiatric illnesses and the drugs used to treat them.

Our primary aim in this chapter, then, is to provide the conceptual links between the neurotransmitter systems in the brain and the modes of action of psychotherapeutic drugs using the DA and 5-HT systems as prototypical examples. These links occur at several different levels of neuronal organization and require a knowledge of gross neuroanatomy, neuronal circuitry, synaptic regulation, and cellular biol-

ogy. We discuss each of these levels, with a particular emphasis on neuronal circuits, as they are fundamental to our understanding the biological basis of drug action.

Early anatomists recognized that the brain is a complex organ. Based on gross anatomical criteria, the brain could be divided into several regions, including the brain stem, cerebellum, midbrain, hypothalamus, thalamus, and cerebral cortex. In addition to gross anatomical divisions, differences were noted in cell morphology. For example, pyramidal neurons in the cerebral cortex were observed to be structurally different from the small round neurons in the suprachiasmatic nucleus of the hypothalamus and the large pigmented neurons of the substantia nigra. More recently, neuroscientists demonstrated that neurons can be classified by biochemical as well as structural criteria, thus revolutionizing anatomy and heralding the era of biochemical neuroanatomy. Investigators can now clearly demonstrate that neurons in the CNS have specific complements of neurotransmitters, transporters, receptors, guanine nucleotide-binding proteins (G proteins), and other signal trans-duction molecules. Identification of neurons in the CNS in terms of their biochemical constituents and examination of how they may form functional networks or circuits is in fact one of the major tasks of present-day neuroanatomists, and one of the main focuses of this chapter.

■ DOPAMINE SYNTHESIZING CELL GROUPS

Brain DA projections are organized into four major circuits—the nigrostriatal, mesolimbic, tuberoinfundibular, and incertohypothalamic systems. Each system has specific anatomical and biochemical characteristics, and their activity regulates specific components of brain function.

The nigrostriatal circuit is one of the most extensive DA systems in the brain (Figure 3–1). Its importance in brain functioning is evidenced by the dramatic deficits in motor function observed in individuals with Parkinson's disease, a disorder that results in the destruction of most of the dopaminergic neurons in this circuit. Two groups of dopaminergic neurons, A8 and A9, form the presynaptic components of the circuit. The A8 cells are located in the mesencephalic reticular formation and are closely associated with the A9 dopaminergic neurons, whereas

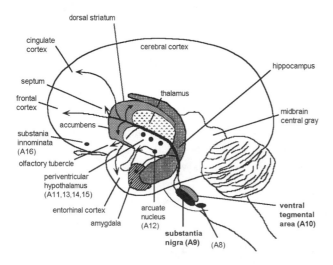

Figure 3–1. Dopaminergic cell groups and their projections. Presynaptic receptors are found on dopamine producing cells and postsynaptic receptors are found in their projection fields. See the text and Table 3–2 for details on dopamine binding and mRNA distributions.

A9 dopaminergic neurons are located in the pars compacta region of the substantia nigra. The A8 and A9 neurons give rise to axons that travel to the forebrain through the medial forebrain bundle. These axons terminate mainly in the caudate nucleus and putamen, with a small group of axons also providing DA to the central amygdaloid nucleus (Anden et al. 1964; Ungerstedt 1971).

Neurons in the A10 cell group are the point of origin for the mesolimbic system; A10 dopaminergic neurons are located in the midbrain, medial to the A9 cells and in the ventral tegmental area. This system runs parallel to the nigrostriatal system, with its axons ascending through the lateral hypothalamus in the medial forebrain bundle (Figure 3–1). Unlike the nigrostriatal system, the mesolimbic dopaminergic projection has a more diverse group of targets, including the nucleus accumbens; olfactory tubercle; bed nucleus of the stria terminalis; lateral septum; and the frontal, cingulate, and entorhinal regions of the cerebral cortex (Lindvall 1975; Lindvall et al. 1974; Moore 1978; Nauta et al. 1978; Ungerstedt 1971).

The tuberoinfundibular system consists of the dopaminergic cells in the arcuate nucleus of the hypothalamus and their projections. These A12 neurons send axons from their ventromedial location in the caudal hypothalamus to the external layer of the median eminence, where they terminate in the region of the hypothalamo-hypophyseal portal vessels (Hökfelt 1967; Hökfelt et al. 1976). This dopaminergic cell group is in a strategic position to influence the output of endocrine cells in the pituitary gland.

Cells in the A11, A13, A14, and A15 groups make up the incertohypothalamic dopaminergic system of the diencephalon. A11 cells are located in the caudal periventricular hypothalamus dorsal to the A12 cells that are found in the infundibular region of the hypothalamus. The zona incerta, a region of the dorsolateral caudal hypothalamus, contains the A13 dopaminergic cells. The A14 cells are in the periventricular hypothalamus rostral to the A11 periventricular dopaminergic cells. Finally, the A15 dopaminergic neurons of the hypothalamus are found rostral, dorsal, and lateral to the A14 cells in the region of the paraventricular and supraoptic hypothalamic nuclei (Pearson et al. 1990). This diffuse DA system modulates many aspects of hypothalamic function.

In rats, the olfactory bulbs contain the only group of dopaminergic cells in the telencephalon. This group of cells is referred to as A16. Unlike other dopaminergic cells that in some cases have quite extensive projections, A16 cells are interneurons and only participate in local olfactory bulb circuitry. However, a vestige of this olfactory DA system is observed in humans. These A16 cells are located in the substantia innominata region of the rostral forebrain (Pearson et al. 1990).

■ Dopamine Receptor Types and Their Neuroanatomical Distributions

Most of what we know concerning the distribution of DA in the CNS was well established in the 1970s using what are now considered conventional histochemical techniques. With development of selective ligands and binding conditions for the DA systems, we have been able to examine the other side of the synapse and selectively label the receptors to which DA can bind. However, it was not until the application of molecular biological techniques to the CNS in the 1980s that we had a real appreciation of the complexity and diversity of the DA and 5-HT receptors in the brain and the way drugs may interact to produce their physiological and behavior effects. This technology has allowed the identification of many families and types of receptors, including the DA and 5-HT receptors, in addition to other neurotransmitters, receptors, transporters, and G proteins that were previously unappreciated with conventional techniques.

Numerous behavioral and pharmacological studies initially identified two types of DA receptors, D_1 and D_2. Each receptor type has a distinct anatomical distribution (Bouthenet et al. 1987; Boyson et al. 1986; Charuchinda et al. 1987; Dawson et al. 1988; Mansour et al. 1990; Wamsley et al. 1989) and pharmacology and has been associated with different behavioral effects (Clark and White 1987; Stoof and Kebabian 1984). But with the advent of molecular biological approaches, the number of proteins that can bind DA has increased to five and is likely to expand further. The five DA receptor types (D_1–D_5) can be divided into D_1 and D_2 receptor families and appear to be part of the superfamily of seven transmembrane, G protein–coupled receptors. The D_2 family consists of D_2, D_3, and D_4 (Bunzow et al. 1988; Sokoloff et al. 1991; Van Tol et al. 1991), whereas the D_1 family consists presently of the D_1 and D_5 receptors (Dearry et al. 1990; Monsma et al. 1990; Sunahara et al. 1990, 1991; Zhou et al. 1990).

The D_2 receptor family has a high affinity for antipsychotic drugs such as haloperidol, chlorpromazine, and clozapine and has been shown to be negatively coupled (D_2, D_3, D_4) to the second messenger adenylate cyclase. Within the D_2 family, each receptor has its own pharmacologically distinct profile (Table 3–1). For example, D_3 receptors have a high affinity for DA and quinpirole as compared to D_2, and D_4 receptors show a 10-fold higher affinity for clozapine as compared to D_2 and D_3. Similarly, raclopride has a far greater affinity for D_2 and D_3 compared to D_4. Many of the clinically used antipsychotic drugs (particularly at higher doses) clearly affect all three of these DA receptors, and further research is necessary to develop truly selective DA antagonists that may be used therapeutically. This is particularly important given the extrapyramidal and other undesired side effects often observed with chronic administration of antipsychotic medication.

The D_1 family, consisting of D_1 and D_5, can be differentiated from the D_2 family in its affinity for experimental drugs SCH23390 (antagonist) and SKF39383 (agonist) that do not bind to the D_2 family of receptors. The D_1 and D_5 subtypes can be differentiated from each other in terms of their anatomical

Table 3–1.   Drug dissociation constants (K_i values [nM])

Agonists	D_2	D_3	D_4
Bromocriptine	5.3	7.4	340.0
Apomorphine	24.0	20.0	4.1
Dopamine	474.0	25.0	28.0
Quinpirole	576.0	5.1	46.0

Antagonists	D_2	D_3	D_4
Haloperidol	0.45	9.8	5.1
Spiperone	0.07	0.6	0.05
(−) Sulpiride	9.2	25.0	52.0
Raclopride	1.8	3.5	237.0
Clozapine	56.0	180.0	9.0
Chlorpromazine	2.8	6.1	37.0
Pimozide	2.4	3.7	43.0

Note. The K_i values were derived from Bunzow et al. 1988 and Van Tol et al. 1991. The lower the numerical value, the higher the affinity a drug has for a receptor subtype. Relative selectivities may be estimated from ratios of K_i values across receptor subtype. The minus sign before sulpiride refers to the negative enantiomer of sulpiride.

distribution (Fremeau et al. 1991; Mansour et al. 1991; Meador-Woodruff et al. 1991, 1992; Mengod et al. 1991) and their affinity for DA, with the D_5 receptor having a higher affinity for the endogenous ligand (Sunahara et al. 1991). Although the D_2 receptor family may be of greater importance for psychiatry given the large number of therapeutic compounds that bind to these sites, the D_1 family of receptors should not be ignored. A great deal of pharmacological and electrophysiological evidence suggests an interaction between D_1-like and D_2-like receptors, with D_1 sites having enabling or modulating effects on D_2 (Clark and White 1987).

The D_1 and D_2 families of receptors can be further differentiated with respect to their gene structures. Members of the D_2 receptor family have multiple introns in the coding regions of their genes allowing the production of multiple messenger RNA (mRNA) variants by alternate DNA splicing. Two functional forms of the D_2 receptor that differ by 29 amino acids have been identified (Dal Toso et al. 1989; Giros et al. 1989; Monsma et al. 1989), and two additional variants of the D_3 have been described (Giros et al. 1991). Multiple forms of the D_4 receptor have also been described that vary in the number of insertions within the putative third intracellular loop (Van Tol et al. 1992). On the other hand, the D_1 and D_5 receptor genes contain no introns in their coding regions resulting in single D_1 and D_5 receptor proteins. Pseudogenes of the D_5 receptor that encode truncated forms of the D_5 receptor have been described in humans (Weinshank et al. 1991) but do not appear to be functional.

Anatomically, the DA receptor subtypes have five distinct distributions (Bouthenet et al. 1991; Mansour et al. 1990, 1991; Meador-Woodruff et al. 1989, 1991, 1992; Mengod et al. 1991; O'Malley et al. 1992; Weiner et al. 1991) supporting the notion that they may play functionally different roles in the CNS. However, before we review their anatomy, a brief discussion of the methods used in identifying these receptors is necessary to put these data into perspective. Brain receptors can be anatomically characterized in one of three ways: 1) with in situ hybridization techniques, to localize their mRNA; 2) with receptor autoradiograph techniques, to localize the binding sites; and 3) with immunohistochemical techniques, to localize the receptor proteins themselves.

In situ hybridization allows the selective identifi-

cation of the mRNAs of each receptor and, therefore, the cell bodies that synthesize these receptors. Receptor autoradiographic techniques, on the other hand, rely on the pharmacological identification of binding sites that may be present on both cell bodies and fibers in the CNS. Immunohistochemical techniques directly label the receptor proteins, which may be localized in cell bodies and fibers, but they also use antibodies generated to selective amino acid stretches of the receptors. In situ hybridization provides excellent cellular resolution and mRNA quantitation but little information concerning cellular projections when used alone. Receptor autoradiography provides a measure of receptor quantitation and allows the mapping of possible brain projections when used in combination with in situ hybridization. However, it is dependent on the development of selective ligands that currently do not exist for the D_4 and D_5 receptors. Immunohistochemical identification of receptors provides excellent cellular resolution of the receptor protein and can be applied to any known amino acid sequence, but it is not quantitative, and certain antibodies may often be difficult to develop. To date, only antibodies to the D_1 and D_2 receptors have been described. Clearly, then, each method has its limitations and advantages. It is only with an integration of mRNA, binding site, and protein distributions that we can achieve an accurate understanding of the anatomy of these receptors.

It should be recognized that we do not have the same amount of information for each of the DA receptors and that much of the distribution information is derived from studies using rats as animal models. The distributions of D_1 and D_2 have been studied the most, partly because of their relatively high levels of mRNA and protein expression in the brain. The mRNA distributions for D_3, D_4, and D_5 have been described in the CNS of the rat. However, their levels are low, and we are probably detecting signals only in those regions of highest mRNA abundance. Also, antibodies have not been developed for the D_3, D_4, and D_5 receptors, and only one selective ligand (7-hydroxydipropylaminotetralin [7-OH-DPAT]) has been developed for D_3. Further research is necessary to develop more selective and sensitive means of measuring these receptors and extending these findings to humans.

Despite these limitations, there is a great deal of evidence to indicate that the five DA receptors have different and often complementary distributions in the CNS (Table 3–2). We will limit our description of the DA receptors to rats and note if it differs from what is presently known of that of humans. As the D_2 receptor was cloned first, we have the best appreciation of its distribution in the brain. High levels of D_2 mRNA, binding, and immunohistochemical staining can be observed in numerous dopaminergic projection fields, including the caudate-putamen, nucleus accumbens, olfactory tubercle, and lateral septum, in addition to being localized in the DA-producing cells of the substantia nigra, ventral tegmental area, olfactory bulb, and zona incerta. Such a distribution would suggest both a postsynaptic and presynaptic, or autoreceptor, function (Nagy et al. 1978).

The term *presynaptic* is often confusing, but we use it to refer to receptors on both presynaptic nerve terminals and cell bodies. Presynaptic receptors located on DA-producing cells are also often referred to as autoreceptors, because they are thought to regulate DA release. Autoreceptors have also been described for the serotonergic system and are discussed later in this chapter. It should be kept in mind that the distribution of these receptors is often not homogeneous throughout an anatomical region. For example, in the caudate-putamen, mediolateral, rostral-caudal, and dorsoventral regions, gradients have been observed. D_2 receptor binding and mRNA are most concentrated dorsolaterally and in the more rostral portion of the caudate-putamen. These differences, as well as a wealth of other anatomical data, suggest that the striatum may be subdivided further into anatomically and biochemically defined compartments that may be functionally distinct. The core of the nucleus accumbens and the dorsal caudate-

putamen have been implicated, for example, in motor control and integration, whereas the shell of the nucleus accumbens and the ventral caudate-putamen are associated with limbic functions (Heimer et al. 1991). Other regions in which D_2 receptor mRNA and binding have been demonstrated include the hippocampus, lateral and medial hypothalamus, lateral mammillary nuclei, interpeduncular nucleus, and periaqueductal gray.

Despite the related pharmacology of the D_3 receptor, the distribution of this receptor varies markedly from that of D_2 and D_4. Like the D_2 receptor, D_3 receptor mRNA and binding have been localized to both dopaminoceptive (or postsynaptic) and DA-containing (presynaptic) cells. The two distributions differ in that the D_3 DA receptors appear to be more concentrated in dopaminoceptive fields associated with limbic function, such as the islands of Calleja, stria terminalis, ventral caudate-putamen, and nucleus accumbens. These regions receive dopaminergic projections from the ventral tegmental area and are part of the mesolimbic DA system. These regions also receive nondopaminergic projections from other limbic structures, including the prefrontal cortex and amygdala. The localization of D_3 receptors in the ventral tegmental area suggests that, like the D_2 receptor, they may serve an autoreceptor function. But given their more "limbic" distribution, drugs selective for D_3 may be less apt to produce the extrapyramidal side effects (EPS) often seen with D_2 antagonists. Other areas containing D_3 receptors include the septum, hippocampus, medial mammillary nuclei of the hypothalamus, and lobules 9 and 10 of the cerebellum. The D_3 receptor clearly needs to be

Table 3–2.   Dopamine receptor messenger ribonucleic acid (mRNA) distribution

	D_1	D_5	D_2	D_3	D_4
Anatomical distribution	Highest mRNA levels in caudate-putamen, olfactory tubercle, nucleus accumbens, amygdala, and cortex. No detectable mRNA in substantia nigra and pituitary.	mRNA localized in the parafascicular nucleus of the thalamus, hippocampus, and dentate gyrus.	Highest mRNA levels in basal ganglia including the caudate-putamen, nucleus accumbens, olfactory tubercle, substantia nigra, and ventral tegmental area. D_2 mRNA levels also high in pituitary.	D_3 mRNA shows a more "limbic" distribution with high levels in olfactory tubercle and nucleus accumbens. Only low levels observed in caudate-putamen and no D_3 detected in pituitary.	mRNA localized in cortex, hypothalamus, hippocampus, and olfactory bulb. Comparatively little in nigrostriatal system. Overall mRNA levels at least 10-fold lower compared with D_2.

considered as a possible site of action when evaluating the effects of antipsychotic drugs previously thought to function by antagonizing D_2 receptors.

The D_4 receptor has a similar pharmacology to the D_2 and D_3 receptors, differing in affinities for only a few compounds such as clozapine (Van Tol et al. 1991). However, the anatomical distribution of D_4 has been difficult to determine, but is probably different from the typical receptor autoradiographic distributions described with D_2-like ligands. D_4 mRNA is difficult to detect in the basal ganglia and pituitary but appears to be present in the islands of Calleja, hypothalamus, hippocampus, neocortex, and allocortex. Of the D_2-like family, D_4 has been the most difficult to characterize because of its relatively low levels in the CNS, but it may be the most interesting from a psychiatric point of view. Several polymorphic variants of the D_4 receptor have been described in humans (Van Tol et al. 1992). Each consists of 16 amino acid repeats in the putative third cytosolic loop of the D_4 receptor. One-, four-, and sevenfold repeats have been described that appear to differ in their affinity for clozapine and [^{3}H]-spiperone and their ability to couple to G proteins. Perhaps with the development of selective D_4 antibodies for immunohistochemistry and ligands for receptor binding, the distribution and function of this receptor will be better understood.

The D_1 receptor distribution partially overlaps with that of the D_2-like family of receptors, especially in the basal forebrain, but represents a fourth dopaminergic receptor distribution. One distinguishing feature of the D_1 receptor is that it is not an autoreceptor (Table 3–2) and therefore not localized in DA-producing cells of the substantia nigra, ventral tegmental area, hypothalamus, and olfactory bulb. D_1 receptor mRNA and binding are more widespread in the CNS as compared to the D_2-like family of receptors, with detectable levels of mRNA in the caudate-putamen, nucleus accumbens, olfactory tubercle, neo- and allocortex, ventral dentate gyrus, amygdala (basolateral, lateral, central, basomedial, and cortical nuclei), suprachiasmatic nucleus of the hypothalamus, and cerebellum. Marked discrepancies between high levels of D_1 receptor binding and no receptor mRNA can be observed in a number of structures, including the globus pallidus, entopeduncular and subthalamic nuclei, and the substantia nigra (pars reticulata) that likely reflect receptor transport from its cell of origin to the terminal areas. Other regions

containing D_1 receptor binding and no detectable mRNA include the medial septum, stratum moleculare of the hippocampus, superior and inferior colliculi, periaquaductal gray, and medial geniculate body.

As is the case with the D_2 receptor family, D_1 receptor mRNA and binding is differentially distributed within specific brain nuclei. For example, higher levels of D_1 mRNA are observed in the dorsomedial and ventrolateral caudate-putamen and in the deeper layers (V, VI) of neocortex. Similarly, differences in D_1 mRNA levels can be observed between the core and shell of the nucleus accumbens, which have been associated with limbic and motor functions, respectively. As seen with D_2, there is a rostral-caudal gradient in D_1 mRNA and binding in the nucleus accumbens, with highest levels observed rostrally.

In contrast to the D_1 receptor, the distribution of the D_5 is far more restricted. In situ hybridization studies suggest that this receptor is restricted in rats to the hippocampus and parafascicular nucleus of the thalamus (Meador-Woodruff et al. 1992). Despite the 10-fold greater sensitivity of the D_5 receptor for DA compared with D_1, it does not appear to be localized in traditional dopaminergic projection regions. Rather, the D_5 receptor localization in the parafascicular nucleus suggests an integrative role, because it receives afferent projections from the substantia nigra and has efferent projection to the striatum.

Dopamine receptor colocalization. As is apparent from the preceding discussion, although each DA receptor has a distinct distribution, there are regions of overlap, particularly in forebrain and midbrain structures such as the caudate-putamen, nucleus accumbens, olfactory tubercle, hippocampus, and substantia nigra. This suggests that there may be a colocalization of multiple DA receptors within the same cells. This has been an area of controversy, and the true extent of colocalization is unclear. Behavioral, electrophysiological, and pharmacological evidence suggest extensive colocalization of D_1, D_2 (for review, see Clark and White 1987), and possibly D_3 receptors within the caudate-putamen and nucleus accumbens. Unfortunately, the anatomical data are currently divided, with extreme points of view of little or no colocalization of D_1 and D_2 in the striatum (Gerfen et al. 1991), to complete colocalization of D_1, D_2, and D_3 in striatonigral projecting neurons (Surmeier et al. 1992). More research is necessary to determine how regional differences may contribute to the extent of colocalization and the relative colocalization with D_3 and D_4 receptors. This is of critical functional significance in understanding the role of the DA receptors in the nigrostriatal and mesolimbic systems and in the cellular regulation of the striatum by psychotropic drugs.

■ Serotonin-Synthesizing Cell Groups

The 5-HT–synthesizing neurons consist of a heterogeneous population of cells in the brain stem (Figure 3–2). Based on the original description by Dahlstrom and Fuxe (1964) in rat brain stem, serotonergic cell groups were coded B1–B9 with respect to their rostral-caudal location (B9 being the most rostral supralemniscal region). It is apparent that these serotonergic nuclei can be further divided into rostral and caudal subdivisions with respect to target projection areas. The rostral division, localized in the midbrain and pons, provides ascending projections to the forebrain; the caudal division, located in the medulla oblongata, sends descending projections to the spinal cord. In this chapter, we focus on the ascending serotonergic system.

Most ascending serotonergic projections originate in the dorsal (B_6 and B_7) and median (B_5 and B_8) raphe nuclei of the brain stem. However, both the caudal linear nucleus (B_8) of the midbrain and the more ventral supralemniscal (B_9) cell group contribute to rostral serotonergic afferents (for a review, see Tork 1985). The dorsal raphe nucleus, located in the ventral portion of the periaqueductal gray matter, contains the greatest number of 5-HT neurons in the brain (estimated at ~ 165,000 in humans). Based on cell densities and morphology, several subregions are identifiable within the nucleus: interfascicular, ventral, ventrolateral, dorsal (lateral and medial), and caudal (Steinbusch and Nieuwenhuys 1983; Tork 1985). The dorsal subnucleus, which extends into the periaqueductal gray matter, contains the largest number of serotonergic neurons in this region. The median raphe nucleus is located in the central portion of the pons, ventral to the dorsal raphe nucleus. The morphology of cells in this nucleus is similar to that found in the dorsal raphe. Here, however, 5-HT cells are found along the midline and are only one-third of those found in the dorsal raphe (Tork 1990).

Unlike the distinct subsystems involved in dopaminergic circuitry, virtually every area of the brain receives projections from the raphe nuclei described above (Figure 3–2). This provides a clear anatomical basis for the involvement of 5-HT in a diverse array of cognitive and behavioral functions. Ascending projections travel initially in the medial forebrain bundle before branching to innervate specific target regions, including the hippocampus, hypothalamus, cerebral cortex, septal nuclei, caudate-putamen, and thalamus. The ascending serotonergic system can be thought of as a dual projection system, with projection areas receiving input that originates in both the dorsal and median raphe nuclei. However, the proportion of projection fibers arising from each nucleus varies considerably in different brain structures. For example, the vast majority of fibers innervating the dentate gyrus originate within the median raphe nucleus, with little apparent input from the dorsal raphe cells. On the other hand, striatal innervation arises predominantly from dorsal raphe cells, with minimal input from the median raphe (Tork 1990). Thus, the median raphe-hippocampal system may be considered important in relation to serotonergic influence of limbic hippocampal function, whereas dorsal raphe-striatal projections relate to basal ganglia function.

In each projection area, serotonergic input exhibits a distinct innervation pattern. Thus, within the hippocampal formation, 5-HT fibers are particularly concentrated within stratum laconosum moleculare and stratum oriens of cornu ammonis (CA) subfields,

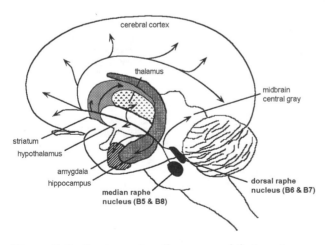

Figure 3–2. Serotonergic cell groups and their projections. Presynaptic receptors are found on serotonin-producing cells, and postsynaptic receptors are located in their projection fields. See the text and Table 3–4 for details on serotonin receptor binding and mRNA distributions.

but sparse across the pyramidal cell layer of the CA subfields and the granule cell layer of dentate gyrus (Tork 1985). In a similar fashion, raphe input to the cerebral cortex in the rat is concentrated in superficial lamina, with fewer axons found in deeper layers (Lidov et al. 1980). Comparison of 5-HT fiber distributions with specific 5-HT receptor distributions in anatomical subregions (see next section) provides valuable insight into the role of 5-HT receptor subtypes within specific 5-HT circuits. This information is useful in considering the action of 5-HT drugs in the brain.

■ Serotonin Receptors and Their Distributions

Like DA, the actions of 5-HT are mediated by multiple receptors. Serotonin receptors were originally divided into two subtypes, 5-HT$_1$ and 5-HT$_2$, on the basis of pharmacological profile (Peroutka and Snyder 1979). However, more recent pharmacological and biochemical data indicate the presence of at least four major 5-HT receptor families—5-HT$_1$, 5-HT$_2$, 5-HT$_3$, and 5-HT$_4$—with some families containing multiple subtypes. Thus, the 5-HT$_1$ receptor family, defined as exhibiting high affinity for 5-HT, has been subdivided into six receptor subtypes, 5-HT$_{1A-1F}$. This complex pharmacology has been confirmed and extended with molecular cloning techniques (Adham et

al. 1993; Albert et al. 1990; Hamblin and Metcalf 1991; Julius et al. 1988; McAllister et al. 1992; Voigt et al. 1991). Indeed, the speed at which nucleic acid sequences for serotonin-like receptors have become available has far outpaced the availability of specific serotonergic pharmacological tools, similar to what has occurred with the DA receptors. Based on sequence information and pharmacological profiles, at least 12 5-HT receptors have been identified in the brain to date (Table 3–3), with the proposed "5-HT$_6$" and "5-HT$_7$" receptors being the most novel (Amlaiky et al. 1992; Ruat et al. 1993). In a similar fashion to DA receptors, most cloned 5-HT receptors belong to the superfamily of G protein–coupled receptors that appear to span the plasma membrane seven times. A notable exception is the 5-HT$_3$ receptor that belongs to the ligand-gated ion channel family.

A detailed description of the anatomical distribution for all of the presently known 5-HT receptors is beyond the scope of our discussion in this chapter. Therefore, only their cellular mRNA distribution (where available) is presented in Table 3–4. The distribution of the 5-HT$_1$ and 5-HT$_2$ receptors follows, as they are particularly relevant in understanding the actions of psychotherapeutic drugs with serotonergic properties. For purposes of clarity, the 5-HT receptors have been divided into their pre- and postsynaptic localization. Although most available distribution data are derived from rat brain studies, it is apparent

Table 3–3. Pharmacological characteristics of 5-HT receptors

| | 5-HT$_1$ receptor subtypes | | | | | |
	5-HT$_{1A}$	5-HT$_{1B}$	*5-HT$_{1C(2C)}$	5-HT$_{1D}$	5-HT$_{1E}$	5-HT$_{1F}$
Selective pharmacological agents	Azaperones (8-OH-DPAT, ipsapirone)	None	None	None	None	None
Nonselective agents	5-HT 5-CT (–) Pindolol	5-HT 5-CT (–) Pindolol	5-HT Mesulergine Metergoline	5-HT 5-CT Metergoline	5-HT Methiothepin Methysergide	5-HT Sumatriptan Methysergide

| | Non–5-HT$_1$ receptor subtypes | | | | | |
	5-HT$_2$	5-HT$_3$	5-HT$_4$	5-HT$_5$	5-HT$_6$	5-HT$_7$
Selective pharmacological agents	DOB DOI	Zacopride ICS 205-930	None	None	None	None
Nonselective agents	Mesulergine Ketanserin Spiperone	—	5-HT 5-MeOT Zacopride	Ergotamine Methiothepin 5-CT	Methysergide Bufotenine Ergotamine	5-HT 5-CT 5-MeOT

Note. 8-OH-DPAT = 8-hydroxydipropylaminotetralin; 5-CT = 5-carboxyamidotryptamine; DOB = 4-bromo-2,5-dimethoxyamphetamine; DOI = 4-iodo-2,5-dimethoxyamphetamine; 5-MeOT = 5-methoxytryptamine.
* Based on nucleotide sequence homology and second messenger linkage, the 5-HT$_{1C}$ receptor has been reclassified as the 5-HT$_{2C}$ receptor.

Table 3–4. Serotonin receptor messenger ribonucleic acid (mRNA) distribution

	5-HT_{1A}	5-HT_{1B}	5-HT_1 receptor subtypes			
			5-HT_{1C}	5-HT_{1D}	5-HT_{1E}	5-HT_{1F}
Anatomical distribution	mRNA localized in limbic brain areas; hippocampus, septum, amygdala, and raphe nuclei (somatodendritic)	mRNA expression in raphe neurons and hippocampus (CA_1) striatum and cortex	High level of mRNA expression in choroid plexus, also expressed in subiculum, hypothalamus, and dorsal raphe	mRNA found in hippocampus striatum and amygdala	Binding in human neocortex	mRNA found in neocortex, hippocampus, and dorsal raphe
Pre- versus postsynaptic	Pre- and postsynaptic	Pre- and postsynaptic	Postsynaptic/presynaptic?	Pre- and postsynaptic?	Pre- and postsynaptic ?	Pre- and postsynaptic

	5-HT_2	$^*5\text{-HT}_3$	Non-5-HT_1 receptor subtypes			
			5-HT_4	5-HT_5	5-HT_6	5-HT_7
Anatomical distribution	mRNA localized in neocortex (1.V), claustrum, pontine nuclei, and hippocampus	mRNA expression in cortex, hippocampus (CA_1), amygdala, and dorsal raphe	Binding in hippocampus and midbrain	mRNA expression in cortex, hippocampus, and cerebellum	mRNA found in hippocampus	mRNA expression in hippocampus, amygdala, and raphe nuclei
Pre- versus postsynaptic	Postsynaptic	Pre- and postsynaptic	Postsynaptic?	Postsynaptic	Postsynaptic	Pre- and postsynaptic

*Ligand-gated channel.

from human mapping studies that 5-HT receptor binding sites display a similar distribution in both species.

5-HT receptors (5-HT_{1B} and 5-HT_{1D}) located presynaptically are responsible for negative feedback control of 5-HT release from serotonergic terminals. Consistent with this, 5-HT_{1B} and 5-HT_{1D} receptor mRNAs have been detected within both dorsal and median raphe nuclei of mouse and rat brain, whereas 5-HT_{1B} binding sites are found predominantly in raphe projection areas such as the neocortex (Maroteaux et al. 1992; Voigt et al. 1991). Until recently, the 5-HT_{1D} receptor was thought to represent a variant of the 5-HT_{1B} receptor that was present in the human brain, but not in that of the mouse or rat. However, it is now clear that this proposed species dichotomy is inaccurate—a 5-HT_{1B} receptor has been cloned from human brain (Jin ct al. 1992), and a gene encoding a 5-HT_{1D}-like receptor has been found in rat brain (Hamblin et al. 1992). Thus, *both* of these receptors may act to control presynaptic 5-HT release within 5-HT circuits.

Presynaptic serotonergic activity is also controlled by 5-HT autoreceptors located on the soma and/or dendrites of 5-HT cells. Electrophysiological data indicate that activation of 5-HT_{1A} receptors on raphe neurons results in decreased firing of 5-HT cells (Sprousc and Aghajanian 1987). In keeping with these findings, 5-HT_{1A} receptor mRNA and 5-HT_{1A} receptors are both found in raphe neurons (Chalmers and Watson 1991), suggesting a local synthesis of these sites. These receptors represent important sites for presynaptic regulation of serotonergic circuitry, as they may act to modulate serotonergic "tone" within brain systems. Consequently, these somatodendritic 5-HT_{1A} receptors may be important sites for serotonergic drug action (see next section). In addition to 5-HT_{1A} receptors, 5-HT_{1B}, 5-HT_{1C}, 5-HT_{1F}, 5-HT_3, and 5-HT_7 receptors may also be present on serotonergic cells in raphe nuclei (Adham et al. 1993; Hoffman and Mezey 1989; Ruat et al. 1993; Voigt et al. 1991). However, the functional role of these sites in this region remains to be clarified.

In situ hybridization histochemistry indicates that 5-HT_{1A} receptor mRNA is present in great abundance within the hippocampus, septal nuclei, amygdaloid nuclei, and entorhinal cortex (Chalmers and Watson 1991), key anatomical structures related to limbic function. The presence of 5-HT_{1A} receptors in each of these anatomical regions confirms a local postsynaptic localization for these sites. It is therefore evident that any drugs acting at 5-HT$_{1A}$ sites may alter function within multiple anatomical components of circuitry associated with emotional control. In addition to the 5-HT$_{1A}$ receptor, the 5-HT$_{1C/2C}$ receptor is also expressed within limbic areas, particularly the ventral hippocampus, septum, amygdala, and cingulate cortex (Hoffman and Mezey 1989). Again, such an anatomical distribution raises the possibility that this receptor may play a role in serotonergic regulation of affect. However, the extremely high level (10× above limbic structures) of 5-HT$_{1C/2C}$ mRNA expression in epithelial cells of the choroid plexus indicates that the primary role of this receptor may relate to cerebrospinal fluid production.

Early receptor binding experiments using [^{3}H]-spiperone indicated a high level of 5-HT$_2$ receptors in neocortex. Autoradiographic studies using the selective 5-HT$_2$ antagonist ketanserin indicated high levels of receptor binding within laminae I and V of neocortex and within the claustrum and other parts of the basal ganglia. Other in situ hybridization studies have confirmed the synthesis of 5-HT$_2$ receptors within neocortical cells (Mengod et al. 1990), indicating that these sites are indeed present on intrinsic cortical cells. The morphology of 5-HT$_2$-immunoreactive cells in this region (Morilak et al. 1992) indicates that 5-HT$_2$ receptors are most likely localized on γ-aminobutyric acid (GABA)ergic interneurons or cholinergic cells within the neocortex.

In addition to their role as autoreceptors, it is likely that the 5-HT$_{1B}$ and 5-HT$_{1D}$ receptors also act as postsynaptic 5-HT receptors in some brain regions. 5-HT$_{1B}$ receptor transcripts are found in cells within CA$_1$ and subicular subfields of hippocampus and layer IV of neocortex and entorhinal cortex (Voigt et al. 1991). Thus, these sites may not only regulate presynaptic serotonergic input to limbic areas but may also participate in mediating postsynaptic serotonergic effects.

■ Synaptic Regulation

The number of DA and 5-HT receptor subtypes and the lack of selective ligands has made it more difficult to determine exactly which receptors and circuits may be activated following pharmacological treatments. As can be seen from Table 3–1, many drugs previously thought to bind to D$_2$ receptors actually bind to D$_2$, D$_3$, and D$_4$ sites at different levels of oc-

cupancy depending on the drug concentration. Similarly, all drugs examined thus far that bind D$_1$ with high affinity also bind D$_5$ receptors (Sunahara et al. 1991; Weinshank et al. 1991). The absence of receptor-specific compounds is also evident within the serotonergic system where, to date, most 5-HT receptor subtypes are characterized in terms of agonist profiles, and few receptor specific ligands are available (Table 3–3).

Despite these kinds of limitations, the issues of synaptic regulation may be examined on a more conceptual level. When a physician administers a drug, this should not be viewed as activating a specific receptor or family of receptors, but rather as activating or inhibiting specific cell groups or circuits. The smallest functional units of such circuits are synapses, and one mode of drug action is the modulation of neurotransmission across synapses. The DA and 5-HT receptor distributions that we have presented here may be thought of as potential sites of synaptic transmission that need to be kept in mind in understanding psychotropic drug action. Selective D$_3$ or D$_4$ agonists, if they existed, would activate entirely different sets of synapses than D$_2$ agonists, given the differences in their distributions. Similarly, D$_5$ agonists would have markedly different sites of action compared to D$_1$ drugs, because the receptors are differentially distributed.

Presynaptic mechanisms. Presynaptic mechanisms control the level of neurotransmitter released into the synapse and can be modulated by drugs that affect neurotransmitter synthesis, breakdown, release, and reuptake. Figures 3–3 and 3–4 illustrate pre- and postsynaptic mechanisms of regulation.

Neurotransmitter synthesis. In the case of dopaminergic neurons, the conversion of tyrosine to dihydroxyphenylalanine (dopa) by tyrosine hydroxylase is the rate-limiting step in DA production. The amount of DA in the synapse can be affected through drugs such as α-methyl-p-tyrosine, an effective tyrosine hydroxylase inhibitor used to reduce catecholamine levels. In an analogous fashion, inhibition of tryptophan hydroxylase by $para$-chlorophenylalanine blocks the conversion of tryptophan to 5-hydroxytryptophan, the rate-limiting step for 5-HT synthesis. These drugs are not given clinically but have been used in animal research paradigms.

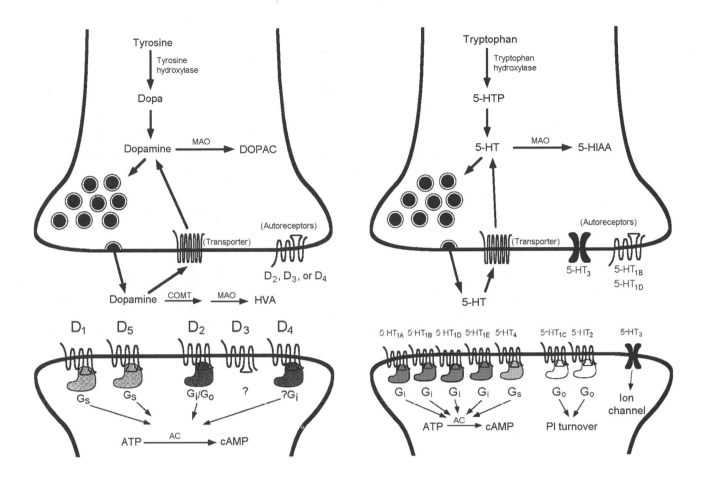

Figure 3–3. Schematic representation of a dopaminergic synapse. Dopaminergic cells synthesize dopamine from dihydroxyphenylalanine (dopa), which in turn is synthesized from tyrosine. The conversion of tyrosine to dopa by tyrosine hydroxylase is the rate-limiting step in the synthesis of dopamine. Once dopamine is synthesized, it is packaged into secretory granules until it is released into the synapse. Once released, dopamine can interact with postsynaptic receptors (D_1–D_5) or presynaptically located autoreceptors (D_2, D_3, or D_4); these receptors appear to be members of the seven transmembrane domain, G protein–coupled superfamily of receptors. The D_1 and D_5 receptors appear to be coupled to adenylate cyclase (AC) via G_s. D_2 appears to be coupled to AC through either G_i or G_o, whereas D_4 may be coupled via G_i. Dopamine can also undergo reuptake into the synthesizing cell for repackaging into granules via a transporter molecule that appears to be contained in the presynaptic cell membrane, spanning this membrane 12 times. Dopamine catabolism can occur both intracellularly as well as extracellularly: monoamine oxidase (MAO) degrades dopamine to 3,4-dihyroxyphenylacetic acid (DOPAC) in the intracellular route. Extraneuronally, dopamine is converted to homovanillic acid (HVA) by the sequential activities of catechol-O-methyltransferase (COMT) and MAO. ATP = adenosine triphosphate; cAMP = cyclic adenosine monophosphate.

Figure 3–4. Schematic representation of a serotonergic synapse. Serotonin (5-HT) and dopamine synthesizing cells have many similarities: 5-HT is synthesized from 5-hydroxytryptophan (5-HTP), which in turn is synthesized from tryptophan. This conversion of tryptophan to 5-hydroxytryptophan by tryptophan hydroxylase is the rate limiting step in 5-HT synthesis. Like dopamine, 5-HT is packaged into secretory granules following synthesis. Following release, 5-HT can interact with a complement of postsynaptic receptors as well as autoreceptors, or undergo reuptake by a transporter with many similarities to the dopamine transporter. Most of the 5-HT receptors are also members of the superfamily of seven transmembrane domain, G protein–coupled receptors. Most of the $5-HT_1$ receptors and the $5-HT_4$ site are coupled to adenylate cyclase (AC) through G_i. $5-HT_{1C/2C}$ and $5-HT_2$, however, are linked to phosphoinositide (PI) turnover via G_o. The $5-HT_3$ receptor is structurally and functionally distinct, acting as an ion channel. The $5-HT_{1B}$, $5-HT_{1D}$, and $5-HT_3$ receptors have also been shown to serve as autoreceptors. $5-HT_{1A}$ may also serve as an autoreceptor in somatodendritic synapses. Serotonin can serve as a substrate for monoamine oxidase (MAO), resulting in the formation of the metabolite 5-hydroxyindoleacetic acid (5-HIAA). ATP = adenosine triphosphate; cAMP = cyclic adenosine monophosphate.

Neurotransmitter breakdown. Drugs that inhibit the oxidative breakdown of catecholamines and indoleamines, such as monoamine oxidase inhibitors (MAOIs), can be used clinically to elevate monoamine levels, as in the drug treatment of depression. The antidepressant drugs pargyline, phenelzine, and tranylcypromine act to inhibit the action of MAO, thereby blocking the catabolism of DA and 5-HT. This acts to increase monoamine content within the brain that presumably leads to augmentation of monoaminergic tone.

Release. Release of neurotransmitter is controlled by a number of factors. The more proximal determinant of release is intracellular Ca^{2+} levels. As Ca^{2+} increases, the levels of neurotransmitter release are increased. However, in the long term, release of neurotransmitters is dependent on the presence of autoreceptors. Autoreceptors are specific receptors found on neurotransmitter-producing cell bodies or presynaptic terminals that, when stimulated, inhibit transmitter release. Members of the D_2 and $5-HT_1$ families of receptors would be examples of autoreceptors.

A feature of DA neurons is that they can release DA not only from presynaptic terminals, but also from their cell bodies and dendrites (Geffen et al. 1976). Consistent with this, D_2 and D_3 receptors have been identified in several dopaminergic cell groups. D_2 receptors are perhaps the best documented in this regard and have been identified in the midbrain DA cell groups (A8–A10), zona incerta, and olfactory bulb. It is unclear at present whether specific members of the D_2 family may predominate in particular DA-producing cell groups. For example, D_2 may be the dominant DA receptor subtype in the ventral tegmental area and zona incerta, whereas in the substantia nigra D_2 and D_3 may act as autoreceptors.

The actions of the DA autoreceptors have been best explored in the substantia nigra and ventral tegmental area, where DA agonists have been shown to inhibit DA release and cell firing (Aghajanian and Bunney 1977; Skirboll et al. 1979; White and Wang 1984). Numerous antipsychotics have in fact been specifically designed to selectively activate the autoreceptors, thereby reducing DA activity without producing EPS. To some extent these drugs have been successful, but there are not enough clinical data to know whether they are superior to conventional pharmacological therapies. It was hoped with the

original cloning of the D_2 receptor and the subsequent identification of a longer isoform that one form of the D_2 might be the postsynaptic D_2, whereas the other might represent the D_2 autoreceptor. However, the multiple forms of the D_2 receptor appear to have identical anatomical distributions in the brain (Meador-Woodruff and Mansour 1991; Snyder et al. 1991).

In a similar fashion, $5-HT_{1A}$, $5-HT_{1B}$, and $5-HT_{1C/2C}$ receptors are localized on the 5-HT–containing cells of the brain stem. As we have indicated, these sites most probably act to regulate presynaptic serotonergic activity.

Reuptake. Specific proteins have recently been identified that selectively remove neurotransmitters from the synapse back into the cell cytosol and subsequently to storage granules. To date, specific transporter molecules have been described for DA, 5-HT, norepinephrine, GABA, glycine, and glutamate (see Amara 1992). Two types of DA transporters have been identified. One is localized in storage vesicles and is important in the relatively nonspecific reuptake into catecholamine storage granules. A second is localized in the presynaptic membrane and is responsible for the selective reuptake of neurotransmitter released into the synaptic cleft. For the DA and 5-HT transporters, neurotransmitter influx is linked to cotransport of sodium and chloride ions across the cell plasma membrane.

A number of drugs can affect levels of transmitter by binding to the uptake sites and effectively controlling synaptic levels of neurotransmitter. Cocaine, for example, binds to the DA and norepinephrine transporters in the presynaptic membrane, inhibiting reuptake and thereby increasing the levels of catecholamines in the synaptic cleft. There is some evidence to suggest that this may in fact represent the underlying mechanism related to cocaine-reinforced behavior (Ritz et al. 1987). Similarly, the tricyclic antidepressants (TCAs), such as imipramine, fluoxetine, and amitriptyline, can act to block the action of the 5-HT transporter, preventing the reuptake of 5-HT from the synapse and prolonging the action of 5-HT at synaptic receptors.

Postsynaptic mechanisms. Unlike presynaptic regulation mechanisms, where the emphasis is on the amount of neurotransmitter released into the synapse, postsynaptic mechanisms of regulation involve the ability of a neurotransmitter to produce biophysical changes in the postsynaptic membrane. As is the case for the presynaptic cell, transduction of information in the postsynaptic cells can be modulated at a number of different levels.

DA antagonists have been prescribed in the treatment of psychotic disorders for nearly 40 years. Many of the antipsychotic drugs used today are believed to derive their therapeutic efficacy at least partly from their ability to block dopaminergic transmission by acting as antagonists at postsynaptic DA receptor sites. Typical antipsychotics are likely to have their effects at predominantly D_2 and D_3 and (to a lesser extent) D_4 receptors. Patients resistant to typical antipsychotics are often treated with atypical antipsychotics such as clozapine, which may be acting predominantly at the D_4 receptor (Seeman 1992). Antipsychotic drugs clearly also have potent effects on other nondopaminergic receptors, such as muscarinic, adrenergic, and serotonergic receptors that should not be ignored in understanding their mechanism of action. For example, although clozapine has a high affinity for D_4, it also has a good affinity for D_2 and a number of non-DA receptors, including serotonergic and muscarinic receptors (Fitton and Heel 1990).

■ REGULATION

Acute administration of a DA receptor agonist or antagonist has little or no effect on receptor number. With repeated administration, however, DA antagonists such as haloperidol produce long-lasting increases in D_2 receptor number in rats (Boyson et al. 1988; Hess et al. 1988) that may be associated with the EPS sometimes observed in humans. However, it is unclear whether this represents a change at the gene transcription level, because changes in mRNA following chronic haloperidol treatment are inconsistent. Some investigators suggest that the D_2 receptor protein may become more stabilized following chronic antagonist treatment rather than undergoing increased biosynthesis (Srivastava et al. 1990; Van Tol et al. 1990). Of the studies reporting an increase in D_2 mRNA following chronic haloperidol treatment (Buckland et al. 1992; Kopp et al. 1992), one study suggests that the shorter isoform of D_2 mRNA is particularly increased (Arnauld et al. 1991). D_1 receptor binding has also been reported to increase with chronic D_1 antagonist treatment (Creese and Chen 1985), but it is unclear whether this represents a transcriptional change. Only one study is presently available concerning D_3 (Buckland et al. 1992) that shows an increase in D_3 mRNA levels following chronic antagonist treatment; but there are no reports on the regulation of D_4 or D_5 receptors by DA agonists or antagonists. The tools to measure these receptors, however, are inadequate or have only recently became available.

With regard to the 5-HT system, although the acute effects of both MAOIs and reuptake blockers is to increase the concentration of 5-HT within the brain, the therapeutic effects of these drugs occur only after subchronic treatment (2–3 weeks). The mechanism for this delayed response is unclear. However, there is some evidence to support the longstanding theory that drug action is related to slowly developing adaptive changes in postsynaptic serotonergic parameters in response to alterations in presynaptic input. For example, cortical 5-HT_2 receptors have been reported to be downregulated after chronic antidepressant treatment (Goodwin et al. 1984), and the number of hippocampal 5-HT_{1A} receptors is specifically increased after chronic treatment with a TCA (Welner et al. 1989).

Interestingly, the increase in hippocampal 5-HT_{1A} receptors after tricyclic treatment appears to have a functional correlate, because tricyclic drugs also enhance the suppressant effect of 5-HT_{1A} activation on hippocampal pyramidal cells (deMontigny and Aghajanian 1978). Bearing in mind the importance of the hippocampus in limbic circuitry, it is possible that alterations in 5-HT_{1A} receptors in this anatomical region contribute to the beneficial effects of selective antidepressants (i.e., enhancing serotonergic input to hippocampal cells). Somatodendritic 5-HT_{1A} receptors located *presynaptically* on serotonergic cell bodies also appear to be sensitive to regulation by specific antidepressants. Both MAOIs and specific 5-HT reuptake inhibitors have been found to desensitize 5-HT_{1A} autoreceptors in raphe nuclei after chronic treatment (Blier and deMontigny 1983, 1985). Such a receptor response may act to disinhibit serotonergic cells and consequently enhance serotonergic input to projection areas. Desensitization of somatodendritic 5-HT_{1A} receptors may also be the mode of action by which 5-HT_{1A} agonists such as buspirone and gepirone produce anxiolytic and antidepressant effects (Welner et al. 1989). However, it remains possible that these drugs may produce their effects by regulating postsynaptic $5-HT_{1A}$ receptors in regions expressing high levels of these sites (i.e., the hippocampus and other limbic structures).

The high levels of $5-HT_2$ receptors within neocortical regions, particularly the claustrum, may underlie the hallucinogenic effects of $5-HT_2$ agonists. Some $5-HT_2$ antagonists, such as ritanserin, have been shown to have therapeutic effects in generalized anxiety and to improve negative symptoms in schizophrenia (Leysen and Pauwels 1990). The mechanism of action for these effects is unclear but may be related to transynaptic effects of the drugs or serotonergic-dopaminergic interactions in selective circuits. $5-HT_3$ receptor antagonists possess potent antiemetic properties that relate to the high concentration of these receptors in both the nucleus tractus solitarius and the area postrema (Tyers 1990). There is some evidence to suggest that some $5-HT_3$ antagonists may be anxiolytic (Briley and Chopin 1991).

■ RECEPTOR COUPLING

Regulation of receptor number is not the only means a cell has to control the level of signal transmission. Many of the DA and 5-HT receptors, as we have indicated earlier, are coupled to G proteins. It is thought that when agonists bind to these receptors they undergo a conformational change, allowing G proteins to tightly bind to the receptor, initiating a cascade of events including the activation of a host of second messengers of which adenylate cyclase is one (Vallar and Meldolesi 1989). Effectiveness of signal transduction is not only dependent on the number of receptors and their affinity for the ligand, but also on the efficiency of coupling to G proteins and the ability to activate second messenger systems. For example, with lesions of DA cells in the substantia nigra, as occurs with Parkinson's disease, there is no change in D_1 receptor number or affinity but an uncoupling of the receptor from adenylate cyclase in striatal cells (Ariano 1989). It is also apparent that a variety of antidepressants regulate the expression of G proteins in various brain regions following chronic administration (Lesch and Manji 1992).

The best information we have to date is that D_2 is coupled to a subset of G proteins referred to as G_i and G_o, whereas D_1 and D_5 are coupled to G_s (Figure 3–3). However, with the family of G proteins growing, this is clearly too simplistic a description and may well depend on the cell type in which these receptors are found. In the future, drugs may not only be targeted to specific receptor subtypes but also to particular G proteins to which they are coupled.

It should be kept in mind that adenylate cyclase is not the only second messenger found in the brain. DA D_2 receptor activation has also been linked to decreases in phospholipase C and changes in K^+ and Ca^{2+} currents, as well as to increases in arachidonic acid (Freedman and Weight 1988; Lledo et al. 1992; Pionelli et al. 1991). Similarly, in addition to adenylate cyclase inhibition, $5-HT_{1A}$ receptors are also linked to K^+ and Ca^{2+} channels (probably through a G protein) in specific anatomical regions. $5-HT_{1B}$, $5-HT_{1D}$, and $5-HT_{1E}$ receptors are linked to inhibition of adenylate cyclase, whereas $5-HT_{1C}$ and $5-HT_2$ receptors may couple to inositol phosphate production (Figure 3–4).

■ CONCLUSION

In emphasizing receptor selectivities and pre- and postsynaptic mechanisms, it is often easy to forget that these receptors and cells are part of complicated circuits. Despite their importance, we know only a small fraction of the potential circuits in the CNS. Neuronal circuits can be identified with traditional anterograde and retrograde anatomical tracing techniques. A more recent way of measuring functional circuits has been the visualization and quantification of what are known as immediate early genes, of which c-fos and c-jun are examples. Under basal conditions, the mRNA and protein levels of these molecules are low and thus difficult (if not impossible) to detect. Within minutes following cellular activation or inhibition that would occur after drug administration or behavioral treatment, the expression levels of these immediate early genes increase dramatically. By examining the cellular expression of these genes before and after experimental treatments, one can produce maps of the cells and circuits that are transcriptionally active. For example, investigators have used these techniques to examine the effects of amphetamine. They have demonstrated the activation of specific subpopulations of cells in a number of brain areas including the caudate-putamen, nucleus accumbens, and specific cortical areas (Graybiel et al. 1990). By colocalizing these immediate early gene products and specific receptor subtypes, we can begin to develop an appreciation of which circuits are activated during a pharmacological treatment.

Perhaps the most important lesson to be learned from the preceding analysis of the DA and 5-HT systems is the prevalence of—if not the necessity for—diversity in the nervous system. This is manifest in the number of receptor families, receptor subtypes, coupling mechanisms, and possible second messenger systems that can be stimulated under normal physiological conditions or through the administration of drugs. This diversity is further amplified when complex anatomical and biochemical circuitry and the colocalization of multiple receptors and neurotransmitters occur within the same cells. The obvious question is: why have mammals evolved such a complicated means of neuronal communication? It may well be an adaptive mechanism to maximize the processing and integration of information. This is the primary function of the CNS and is what differentiates humans from invertebrates.

Although this analysis has been restricted to the DA and 5-HT systems, it could easily have focused on a number of other neurotransmitter or neuropeptide systems. The concepts would have been the same. An emphasis on neuronal circuitry, synaptic regulation, and cellular and molecular biology would similarly apply to many other neurotransmitter systems. Research on the organization of the DA and 5-HT receptor systems has made great strides in the last 5 years and promises to further our understanding of the nervous system and the physiological basis of mental disorders.

◼ REFERENCES

Adham N, Kao HT, Schechter LE, et al: Cloning of another human serotonin receptor (5-HT$_{1F}$): a fifth 5-HT$_1$ receptor subtype coupled to the inhibition of adenylate cyclase. Proc Natl Acad Sci U S A 90:408–412, 1993

Aghajanian GK, Bunney BS: Dopamine autoreceptors: pharmacological characterization by microintophoretic single cell recording studies. Naunyn Schmiedebergs Arch Pharmacol 297:1–7, 1977

Albert PR, Zhou QY, Van Tol HHM, et al: Cloning, functional expression and mRNA tissue distribution of the rat 5-hydroxytryptamine$_{1A}$ receptor gene. J Biol Chem 265:5825–5832, 1990

Amara SG: A tale of two families. Nature 360:420–421, 1992

Amlaiky N, Plassat JL, Ramboz S, et al: The mouse 5-HT$_5$ and 5-HT$_6$ receptors—two new "5-HT$_{1D}$-like" serotonin receptors: cloning and expression. Society for Neuroscience Abstracts 18:212, 1992

Anden NE, Dahlstrom A, Fuxe K, et al: Demonstration and mapping out of nigroneostriatal dopamine neurons. Life Sci 3:523–530, 1964

Ariano MA: Long term changes in striatal D$_1$ dopamine receptor distribution after dopaminergic deafferentation. J Neurosci 32:203–212, 1989

Arnauld E, Arsaut J, Demotes-Mainard J: Differential plasticity of the dopaminergic D2 receptor mRNA isoforms under haloperidol treatment, as evidenced by in situ hybridization in rat anterior pituitary. Neurosci Lett 130:12–16, 1991

Blier P, deMontigny C: Electrophysiological investigations on the effect of repeated zimelidine administration on serotonergic transmission in the rat. J Neurosci 3:1270–1278, 1983

Blier P, deMontigny C: Serotonergic but not noradrenergic neurons in rat central nervous system adapt to long term treatment with monoamine oxidase inhibitors. Neuroscience 16:949–955, 1985

Bouthenet M-L, Martres MP, Sales N, et al: A detailed mapping of dopamine D$_2$ receptors in rat central nervous system by autoradiography with [^{125}I]Iodosulpride. Neuroscience 20:117–155, 1987

Bouthenet M-L, Souil E, Matres M-P, et al: Localization of dopamine D$_3$ receptor mRNA in the rat brain using in situ hybridization histochemistry: comparison with D$_2$ receptor mRNA. Brain Res 564:203–219, 1991

Boyson SJ, McGonigle P, Molinoff PB: Quantitative autoradiographic localization of the D$_1$ and D$_2$ subtypes of dopamine receptors in rat brain. J Neurosci 6:3177–3188, 1986

Boyson SJ, McGonigle P, Luthin GR, et al: Effects of chronic administration of neuroleptic and anticholinergic agents on the densities of D$_2$ dopamine and muscarinic cholinergic receptors in rat striatum. J Pharmacol Exp Ther 244:987–993, 1988

Briley M, Chopin P: Serotonin in anxiety: evidence from animal models, in 5-Hydroxytryptamine in Psychiatry. Edited by Sandler M, Coppen A, Harnett S. New York, Oxford Medical Publications, 1991, pp 177–197

Buckland PR, O'Donovan MC, McGuffin P: Changes

in D_1, D_2, and D_3 receptor mRNA levels in rat brain following antipsychotic treatment. Psychopharmacology (Berl) 106:479–483, 1992

Bunzow JR, Van Tol HHM, Grandy DK, et al: Cloning and expression of a rat D_2 dopamine receptor cDNA. Nature 336:783–787, 1988

Chalmers DT, Watson SJ: Comparative anatomical distribution of 5-HT_{1A} receptor mRNA and 5-HT_{1A} binding in rat brain—a combined in situ hybridization/in vitro receptor autoradiographic study. Brain Res 561:51–60, 1991

Charuchinda C, Supavilai P, Karobath M, et al: Dopamine D_2 receptors in the rat brain: autoradiographic visualization using a high affinity selective agonist ligand. J Neurosci 7:1352–1360, 1987

Clark D, White FJ: Review: D_1 dopamine receptor—the search for a function: a critical evaluation of the D_1/D_2 dopamine classification and its functional implications. Synapse 1:345–388, 1987

Creese I, Chen A: Selective D_1 dopamine receptor increase following chronic treatment with SCH23390. Eur J Pharmacology 109:127–128, 1985

Dahlstrom A, Fuxe K: Evidence for the existence of monoamine-containing neurons in the central nervous system, I: demonstration of monoamines in cell bodies of brain stem neurons. Acta Physiol Scand Suppl 232:1–55, 1964

Dal Toso R, Sommer B, Ewert M, et al: The dopamine D_2 receptor: two molecular forms generated by alternative splicing. EMBO J 8:4025–4034, 1989

Dawson TM, Barone P, Sidhu A, et al: The D_1 dopamine receptor in the rat brain: quantitative autoradiographic localization using an iodinated ligand. Neuroscience 26:83–100, 1988

Dearry A, Gingrich JA, Falardeau P, et al: Molecular cloning and expression of the gene for a human D_1 dopamine receptor. Nature 347:72–76, 1990

deMontigny C, Aghajanian GK: Tricyclic antidepressants: long term treatment increases responsivity of rat forebrain neurons to serotonin. Science 202:1303–1306, 1978

Fitton A, Heel RC: Clozapine—a review of pharmacological properties, and therapeutic use in schizophrenia. Drugs 40:722–747, 1990

Freedman JE, Weight FF: Simple K^+ channels activated by D_2 dopamine receptors in acutely dissociated neurons from rat corpus striatum. Proc Natl Acad Sci U S A 85:3618–3622, 1988

Fremeau RT, Duncan GE, Fornaretto M-G, et al: Localization of D_1 dopamine receptor mRNA in brain

supports a role in cognitive, affective, and neuroendocrine aspects of dopaminergic neurotransmission. Proc Natl Acad Sci U S A 88:3772–3776, 1991

Geffen LB, Jessell TM, Cuello AC, et al: Release of dopamine from dendrites in rat substantia nigra. Nature 260:258–261, 1976

Gerfen CR, McGinty JF, Young WS: Dopamine differentially regulates dynorphin, substance P, and enkephalin expression in striatal neurons: in situ hybridization histochemical analysis. J Neurosci 11:1016–1031, 1991

Giros B, Sokoloff P, Martes M-P, et al: Alternative splicing directs the expression of two D_2 dopamine receptor isoforms. Nature 342:923–926, 1989

Giros B, Martes M-P, Pilon C, et al: Shorter variants of the D_3 dopamine receptor produced through various patterns of alternative splicing. Biochem Biophys Res Commun 176:1584–1592, 1991

Goodwin GM, Green AR, Johnson P: 5-HT_2 receptor characteristics in frontal cortex and 5-HT_2 receptor-mediated head twitch behaviour following antidepressant treatment to mice. Br J Pharmacol 83:235–242, 1984

Graybiel AM, Moratalla R, Robertson HA: Amphetamine and cocaine induce drug specific activation of the c-fos gene in striosome-matrix compartments and limbic subdivisions of the striatum. Proc Natl Acad Sci U S A 87:6912–6919, 1990

Hamblin MW, Metcalf MA: Primary structure and functional characterization of a human 5-HT_{1D} serotonin receptor. Mol Pharmacol 40:143–148, 1991

Hamblin MW, McGuffin RW, Metcalf MA, et al: Distinct 5-HT_{1B} and 5-HT_{1D} serotonin receptors in rat: structural and pharmacological comparison of the two cloned receptors. Molecular and Cellular Neurosciences 3:578–587, 1992

Heimer L, Zahm DS, Churchill L, et al: Specificity in the projection patterns of accumbal core and shell in the rat. Neuroscience 41:89–125, 1991

Hess EJ, Norman AB, Cresse I: Chronic treatment with dopamine receptor antagonists: behavioral and pharmacologic effects of D_1 and D_2 dopamine receptors. J Neurosci 8:2361–2370, 1988

Hoffman BJ, Mezey E: Distribution of serotonin 5-HT_{1C} receptor mRNA in adult rat brain. FEBS Lett 247:453–462, 1989

Hökfelt T: The possible ultrastructural identification of tubero-infundibular dopamine containing nerve endings in the median eminence of the rat. Brain

Res 5:121–3, 1967

Hökfelt T, Johansson O, Fuxe K, et al: Immuno-histochemical studies on the localization and distribution of monoamine neuron systems in the rat brain, I: tyrosine hydroxylase in the mes- and diencephalon. Medical Biology 54:427–453, 1976

Jin H, Oksenberg D, Ashkenazi A, et al: Characterization of the human 5-hydroxytryptamine$_{1B}$ receptor. J Biol Chem 267:5735–5738, 1992

Julius D, McDermott R, Axel R, et al: Molecular characterization of a functional cDNA encoding the serotonin$_{1C}$ receptor. Science 241:558–564, 1988

Kopp J, Lindefors N, Brene S, et al: Effect of raclopride on dopamine D_2 receptor mRNA expression in rat brain. Neuroscience 47:771–779, 1992

Lesch KP, Manji HK: Signal-transducing G proteins and antidepressant drugs: evidence for modulation of alpha subunit gene expression in rat brain. Biol Psychiatry 32:549–579, 1992

Leysen JE, Pauwels PJ: 5-HT$_2$ receptors, roles and regulation, in The Neuropharmacology of Serotonin. Edited by Whitaker-Azmitia PM, Peroutka S. Ann N Y Acad Sci 600:183–193, 1990

Lidov HGW, Grzanna R, Molliver ME: The serotonin innervation of the cerebral cortex in the rat—an immunohistochemical analysis. Neuroscience 5:207–227, 1980

Lindvall O. Mesencephalic dopamine afferents to the lateral septal nucleus of the rat. Brain Res 87:89–95, 1975

Lindvall O, Bjorkland A, Moore A, et al: Mesencephalic dopamine neurons projecting to the neocortex. Brain Res 81:325–331, 1974

Lledo PM, Hornburger V, Bockaert J, et al: Differential G-protein-mediated coupling of D_2 dopamine receptors to K$^+$ and Ca^{2+} currents in rat anterior pituitary cells. Neuron 8:455–463, 1992

Mansour A, Meador-Woodruff JH, Bunzow JR, et al: Localization of dopamine D_2 receptor mRNA and D_1 and D_2 receptor binding in the rat brain and pituitary: an in situ hybridization-receptor autoradiographic analysis. J Neurosci 10:2587–2600, 1990

Mansour A, Meador-Woodruff JH, Zhou Q-Y, et al: A comparison of D_1 receptor binding and mRNA in rat brain using receptor autoradiographic and in situ hybridization techniques. Neuroscience 45:359–371, 1991

Maroteaux L, Saudou F, Amlaiky N, et al: Mouse 5-HT$_{1B}$ serotonin receptor: cloning, functional expression and localization in motor control centers. Proc Natl Acad Sci U S A 89:3020–3024, 1992

McAllister G, Charlesworth A, Snodin C, et al: Molecular cloning of a serotonin receptor from human brain (5-HT$_{1E}$): a fifth 5-HT$_1$-like subtype. Proc Natl Acad Sci U S A 89:5517–5521, 1992

Meador-Woodruff JH, Mansour A: Expression of the dopamine D_2 receptor gene in brain. Biol Psychiatry 30:985–1007, 1991

Meador-Woodruff JH, Mansour A, Bunzow JR, et al: Distribution of D_2 dopamine receptor mRNA in rat brain. Proc Natl Acad Sci U S A 86:7625–7628, 1989

Meador-Woodruff JH, Mansour A, Healy DJ, et al: Comparison of the distributions of D_1 and D_2 dopamine receptor mRNAs in the rat brain. Neuropsychopharmacology 5:231–242, 1991

Meador-Woodruff JH, Mansour A, Grandy DK, et al: Distribution of D_5 dopamine receptor mRNA in rat brain. Neurosci Lett 145:209–212, 1992

Mengod G, Pompeiano M, Inocencia M, et al: Localization of the mRNA for the 5-HT$_2$ receptor by in situ hybridization histochemistry: correlation with the distribution of receptor sites. Brain Res 524:139–143, 1990

Mengod G, Vilaro, MT, Niznik HB, et al: Visualization of a dopamine D_1 receptor mRNA in human and rat brain. Molecular Brain Research 10:185–191, 1991

Monsma FJ, McVittie LD, Gerten CR, et al: Multiple D_2 dopamine receptors produced by alternative RNA splicing. Nature 342:926, 1989

Monsma FJ, Mahan LC, McVittie LD, et al: Molecular cloning and expression of a D_1 dopamine receptor linked to adenylyl cyclase activation. Proc Natl Acad Sci U S A 87:6723–6727, 1990

Moore RY: Catecholamine innervation of the basal forebrain, I: the septal area. J Comp Neurol 177:665–684, 1978

Morilak DA, Garlow SJ, Ciaranello RD: Localization and description of 5-HT$_2$ immunoreactive neurons in the rat brain. Soc Neurosci Abstract 18:212, 1992

Nagy JI, Lee T, Seeman P, et al: Direct evidence for presynaptic and postsynaptic dopamine receptors in brain. Nature 274:278–281, 1978

Nauta WJH, Smith GP, Faull RLM, et al: Efferent connections and nigral afferents of the nucleus accumbens septi in the rat. Neuroscience 3:385–401, 1978

O'Malley KL, Harmon S, Tang L, et al: The rat dopamine D_4 receptor: sequence, gene structure, and demonstration of expression in the cardiovascular system. New Biol 4:137–146, 1992

Pearson J, Halliday G, Sakamoto N, et al: Catecholeminergic neurons, in The Human Nervous System. Edited by Paxinos G. Sydney, Australia, Academic Press, 1990, pp 1023–1050

Peroutka SJ, Snyder SH: Multiple serotonin receptors: differential binding of [3H]-5-hydroxytryptamine, [3H]-lysergic acid diethylamide and [3H]-spiperidol. Mol Pharmacol 16:687–699, 1979

Pionelli D, Pilon C, Giros B, et al: Dopamine activation of the arachidonic acid cascade via a modulatory mechanism as a basis of D_1/D_2 receptor synergism. Nature 353:164–167, 1991

Ritz MC, Lamb RJ, Goldberg SR, et al: Cocaine receptors on dopamine transporters are related to self administration of cocaine. Science 237:1219–1223, 1987

Ruat M, Traiffort E, Leurs R, et al: Molecular cloning, characterization, and localization of a high-affinity serotonin receptor ($5-HT_7$) activating cAMP formation. Proc Natl Acad Sci U S A 90:8547–8551, 1993

Seeman P: Dopamine receptor sequences—therapeutic levels of neuroleptics occupy D_2 receptors, clozapine occupies D_4. Neuropsychopharmacology 7:261–284, 1992

Skirboll LR, Grace AA, Bunney BS: Dopamine auto- and postsynaptic receptors: electrophysiological evidence for differential sensitivity to dopamine agonists. Science 206:80–82, 1979

Snyder LA, Roberts JL, Sealfon SC: Distribution of dopamine D_2 receptor mRNA splice variants in the rat by solution hybridization/protection assay. Neurosci Lett 122:37–40, 1991

Sokoloff P, Giros B, Martes M-P, et al: Molecular cloning and characterization of a novel dopamine receptor (D_3) as a target for neuroleptics. Nature 347:146–151, 1991

Sprouse JS, Aghajanian GK: Electrophysiological responses of serotonergic dorsal raphe neurons to $5-HT_{1A}$ and $5-HT_{1B}$ agonists. Synapse 1:3–9, 1987

Srivastava LK, Morency MA, Bajwa SB, et al: Effect of haloperidol on expression of dopamine D_2 receptor mRNAs in rat brain. J Mol Neurosci 2:155–161, 1990

Steinbusch HWM, Nieuwenhuys R: The raphe nuclei of the rat brainstem: a cytoarchitectonic and immunohistochemical study, in Chemical Neuroanatomy. Edited by Emson PC. New York, Raven, 1983, pp 131–207

Stoof JC, Kebabian JW: Two dopamine receptors: biochemistry, physiology and pharmacology. Life Sci 35:2281–2296, 1984

Sunahara RK, Niznik HB, Weiner DM, et al: Human dopamine D_1 receptor encoded by an intronless gene on chromosome 5. Nature 347:80–83, 1990

Sunahara RK, Guan H-C, O'Dowd BF, et al: Cloning of the gene for a human dopamine D5 receptor with higher affinity for dopamine than D1. Nature 350:614–619, 1991

Surmeier DJ, Eberwine J, Wilson CJ, et al: Dopamine receptor subtypes co-localize in rat striatonigral neurons. Proc Natl Acad Sci U S A 89:10178–10182, 1992

Tork I: Raphe nuclei and serotonin containing systems, in The Rat Nervous System, Vol 2. Edited by Paxinos G. Sydney, Australia, Academic Press, 1985, pp 43–78

Tork I: Anatomy of the serotonergic system, in The Neuropharmacology of Serotonin. Edited by Whitaker-Azmitia P, Peroutka S. Ann N Y Acad Sci 600:9–35, 1990

Tyers MB: $5-HT_3$ receptors, in The Neuropharmacology of Serotonin. Edited by Whitaker-Azmitia PM, Peroutka S. Ann N Y Acad Sci 600:194–205, 1990

Ungerstedt U: Stereotaxic mapping of the monoamine pathways in the rat brain. Acta Physiol Scand Suppl 367:1–49, 1971

Vallar L, Meldolesi J: Mechanisms of signal transduction at the dopamine D_2 receptor. Trends Pharmacol Sci 10:74–77, 1989

Van Tol HHM, Riva M, Civelli O, et al: Lack of effect of chronic dopamine receptor mRNA level. Neurosci Lett 111:303–308, 1990

Van Tol HHM, Bunzow JR, Guan H-C, et al: Cloning of the gene for a human dopamine D_4 receptor with high affinity for the antipsychotic clozapine. Nature 350:610–614, 1991

Van Tol HHM, Wu CM, Guan H-C, et al: Multiple dopamine D_4 receptor variants in the human population. Nature 358:149–152, 1992

Voigt MM, Laurie DJ, Seeburg PH, et al: Molecular cloning and characterization of a rat brain cDNA encoding a 5-hydroxytryptamine$_{1B}$ receptor. EMBO J 10:4017–4023, 1991

Wamsley JK, Gehlert DR, Filloux FM, et al: Comparison of the distribution of D_1 and D_2 dopamine receptors in the rat brain. J Comp Neurol 2:119–137, 1989

Weiner DM, Levey AI, Sunahara RK, et al: D_1 and D_2 dopamine receptor mRNA in rat brain. Proc Natl Acad Sci U S A 88:1859–1863, 1991

Weinshank RL, Adham N, Macchi M, et al: Molecular cloning and characterization of a high affinity dopamine receptor (D_{1B}) and its pseudogene. J Biol Chem 266:22427–22435, 1991

Welner SA, deMontigny C, Desroches J, et al: Autoradiographic quantification of serotonin$_{1A}$ receptors in rat brain following antidepressant drug treatment. Synapse 4:347–352, 1989

White FJ, Wang RY: Pharmacological characterization of dopamine autoreceptors in the rat ventral tegmental area: microiontophoretic studies. J Pharmacol Exp Ther 231:275–280, 1984

Zhou QY, Grandy DK, Thambi L, et al: Cloning and expression of human and rat D_1 dopamine receptors. Nature 347:76–80, 1990

4

Electrophysiology

Anthony A. Grace, Ph.D., and Benjamin S. Bunney, M.D.

There are a number of approaches that can be used to analyze the structure and function of the nervous system in health and disease. Many of these techniques—for example, the biochemical analysis of neurotransmitter and metabolite levels, anatomical studies of axonal projection sites or neurotransmitter enzymes, or molecular biological studies of messenger levels and turnover—examine the nervous system at the level of groups or populations of neurons. In contrast, electrophysiology by its very nature is oriented toward the physiological analysis of individual neurons. In this chapter, we present descriptions of preparations and techniques that are in a general sense applicable to many systems, with specific examples drawn from the dopaminergic system to draw upon our field of expertise.

The employment of electrophysiological techniques for the analysis of neuronal physiology is dependent on the unique properties of the neuronal membrane. Like many other cell types, the neuron possesses an electrochemical gradient across its membrane. The electrochemical gradient itself is a product of two forces: an electrical potential force that is derived from the voltage difference between the inside and the outside of the cell, and a chemical potential force that results from the unequal distribution of ions across the membrane. Cells set up and maintain this electrochemical gradient as a result of the selective permeability of their membranes to particular ionic species. Thus, the membrane exhibits a rather high degree of permeability to ions such as

potassium but is relatively impermeable to other ions such as sodium and calcium.

In the resting state, cells have a very low internal concentration of sodium and calcium. To achieve this state, the cell must expend energy (in the form of adenosine triphosphate [ATP] hydrolysis) to extrude sodium from the intracellular space in exchange for potassium ions. The extrusion of sodium sets up both a chemical gradient (because sodium attempts to exist in equal concentrations across the membrane) as well as an electrical gradient (because sodium is positively charged and is not freely permeable across the membrane; thus, net positive charges are being removed from inside of the cell). To partially counter this electrical gradient, potassium—which is more permeable—flows down the electrical gradient to become concentrated inside the cell. However, as it is doing this, it is also setting up an opposing chemical gradient, because it is achieving higher concentrations within the cell than outside of the cell. When the electrical force drawing potassium into the cell balances the chemical force of the concentration gradient forcing potassium out of the cell, the membrane is at equilibrium—with high extracellular sodium concentration, relatively high intracellular potassium concentrations, and with a transmembrane potential causing the inside of the cell to be negatively charged with respect to its environment.

A typical resting membrane potential for a neuron is rather small, being on the order of −70 mV with respect to the extracellular fluid. In actuality, potassium itself is not freely permeable. A small electrochemical gradient exists in most neurons that attempts to force potassium out of the cell and draw the membrane potential to more negative values. Although the scenario is somewhat more complicated than this (e.g., involving charged proteins and other ionic species with selective permeabilities), this is a rough approximation as to how a cell gains an electrochemical gradient via the energy-dependent extrusion of sodium.

It should be noted that neurons are not the only cells that have transmembrane potentials. In fact, all living cells have an electrochemical gradient across their membranes that they use for transporting glucose and other essential materials and accumulating them against a concentration gradient. Such energy-dependent processes are usually coupled to other gradients from which they derive this energy. For example, a compound may be taken up and concentrated by linking its transport to sodium, which itself has a large electrochemical gradient in the opposite direction. What makes the neuron unique is its ability to rapidly change the permeability of its membrane to one or more ion species in a regenerative manner. It is this process that underlies the generation of an action potential, sets up active propagation of an action potential down an axon, and triggers the process that ultimately results in neurotransmitter release. It also provides the electrophysiologist with a measure of neuronal activity that can be assayed by recording the electrical activity generated by the neuron.

The action potential is a regenerative phenomenon, meaning that the events that initiate the action potential also serve as the force that drives this event to completion. Normally, a given neuron receives information in the form of synaptic potentials. For example, an axon terminal synapsing on the neuron releases a neurotransmitter, which binds to the neuron and selectively alters the permeability of its membrane by opening ion channels linked to its binding site. An ion channel that opens in response to a neurotransmitter is referred to as a ligand-gated channel. If the neurotransmitter causes activation of a channel that increases the permeability of the membrane to a negatively charged ion that exists in high concentrations in the extracellular fluid (e.g., chloride), the influx of chloride down its electrochemical gradient causes a negative shift in the membrane potential of the cell, thereby increasing the potential difference across the membrane, or a hyperpolarization of the

cell. If activation of this channel causes a positively charged ion such as sodium to flow down its electrochemical gradient and into the cell, it will cause a brief decrease in the membrane potential (i.e., a depolarization) of the neuron.

Because a change in the membrane potential alters the electrochemical gradient of potassium across the membrane, potassium ions will flow through their respective channels to restore the membrane to its resting level. Thus, if a neurotransmitter depolarizes the membrane, it causes an efflux of potassium ions and a return of the membrane potential to resting levels. However, if the depolarization is sufficiently large, another type of channel is activated—the voltage-gated or voltage-dependent sodium channel. In response to a given level of depolarization, this channel increases its permeability to sodium to allow more of this ion to enter the cell. The result is a further depolarization of the membrane and consequently increased activation of this voltage-dependent channel. Because of the positive feedback nature of this event, it is referred to as regenerative, as the depolarization augments the very factor that causes the cell to be depolarized. The membrane potential at which this regenerative process is initiated is thus the threshold potential for action potential generation, with a hyperpolarization of the cell causing a decrease in its excitability and a depolarization increasing the likelihood that it will generate an action potential.

The regenerative depolarization of the membrane has limits, however. One limit is the equilibrium potential for sodium. The equilibrium potential is the membrane potential at which the electrochemical gradient for a particular ion is zero, with no net flux of the ion across a membrane. This would occur when the membrane potential is sufficiently positive to oppose the further influx of the positively charged sodium ion down its concentration gradient. Although this potential is usually about +40 mV in many cells, the action potential does not actually reach this value. Instead, another voltage-activated channel that is selectively permeable to potassium is activated. The resultant massive increase in potassium permeability starts to return the membrane potential to its original state, thereby inactivating the regenerative sodium conductance. The increase in potassium permeability is actually sufficient to drive the membrane potential negative to the resting potential and toward the equilibrium potential for potassium (i.e., approximately −80 to −90 mV), before the subsequent decrease in voltage-dependent potassium conductance returns the membrane to its original resting state.

The equilibrium potential of an ion determines the net effect that opening its associated ion channels will have on the neuron. The equilibrium potential occurs when the membrane is depolarized or hyperpolarized sufficiently to exactly offset the effects of the concentration gradient on the ion, with the result that there is no net flux of this ion across the membrane. For example, because of the very high concentration of sodium outside of the neuron compared with inside the cell, the large concentration gradient for sodium across the membrane attempts to force sodium into the neuron. Therefore, to oppose this concentration gradient, the membrane potential of the neuron would have to be highly positive to provide an electrical gradient of equivalent force. This occurs at approximately +40 mV for sodium. Potassium, on the other hand, has an equilibrium potential that is about 10–20 mV more negative than the resting potential, due in part to the fact that the ATP hydrolysis used to extrude sodium exchanges it for potassium. As a result, increasing potassium permeability causes a hyperpolarization of the neuron because of an efflux of potassium down its concentration gradient.

Another common ionic species is chloride. This ion is negatively charged and therefore has an electrical gradient that would act against it entering the cell. However, the concentration of chloride is so much higher in the extracellular fluid that the chemical gradient predominates. As a consequence, opening chloride ion channels causes chloride to flow into the cell, hyperpolarizing the membrane (Figure 4–1). In fact, the opening of chloride ion channels is the mechanism through which the primary inhibitory neurotransmitter in the brain (i.e., γ-aminobutyric acid [GABA]) decreases neuronal activity.

Neurons within the vertebrate nervous system have additional conductances that provide them with unique functions. One of these conductances is the voltage-gated calcium conductance. Like sodium, calcium also exists in higher concentrations outside of the neuron compared to inside the cell. However, the gradient is even more extreme than it is for sodium. Even though there is much less calcium in the extracellular fluid than sodium, the equilibrium potential for calcium is close to +240 mV because of the extremely low intracellular concentration of this ion. The neuron maintains this low intracellular concentration so as to use this ion for specialized purposes. Thus, calcium influx is known to cause neurotransmitter release, activate calcium-gated ion channels, and trigger second messenger systems (e.g., the calcium-regulated protein kinase). Calcium channels, like their sodium counterparts, are also voltage gated and are known to cause calcium influx into the neuron during the action potential. Furthermore, the calcium can also influence the excitability of the cell by activating the calcium-activated potassium current, which then causes a large membrane hyperpolarization following the spike, known as an afterhyperpolarization, that delays the occurrence of a subsequent spike in that neuron. After entering the neuron, calcium is rapidly sequestered into intracellular organelles to terminate its action and reset the neuron before the next event. Therefore, calcium can alter the physiological activity and the biochemical properties of the neuron it affects (Llinás 1988).

■ ELECTROPHYSIOLOGICAL TECHNIQUES

By employing electrophysiological techniques to assess information about a neuron, such as that described previously, experiments can be designed to investigate differences in the physiological properties of neurons of interest, the interaction between neurotransmitter systems that are known to be involved in behavioral or pathological conditions, and the mode of action of pathomimetic or psychotherapeutic agents. Furthermore, this can be done using a broad range of electrophysiological techniques and preparations. In attempting to gain such information, it is important to note that there is no technique that is "best." Each approach has its relative strengths and weaknesses, and only through integrating information gained at these various levels will a more complete comprehension of neuronal function be achieved.

■ Electroencephalographic Recordings

There are a number of parameters of neuronal activity that can be assessed electrophysiologically. These parameters can be selectively assessed depending on the method of recording used. Five recording meth-

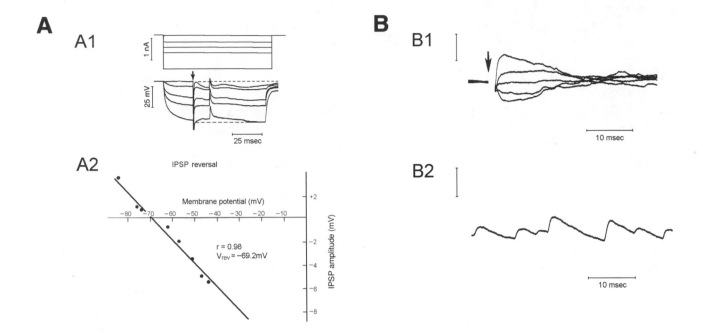

Figure 4–1. At least three techniques can be used to determine the ionic species that mediates a synaptic response: determining the reversal potential of the ion, reversing the membrane potential deflection produced by changing the concentration gradient of the ion across the membrane, and determining the reversal potential (or blocking the synaptic response) after applying a specific ion channel blocker.

In this example, three techniques are used to illustrate the involvement of a chloride ion conductance increase evoked in dopamine-containing neurons by stimulation of the striatonigral gamma-aminobutyric acid (GABA)-ergic projection.

Panel A: The reversal potential of a response may be determined by examining the amplitude of the response as the membrane potential of the neuron is varied. In this example, we have superimposed several responses of the neuron evoked at increasingly hyperpolarized membrane potentials (top traces), with the membrane potential altered by injecting current through the electrode and into the neuron (bottom traces = current injection). *Panel A1:* A synaptic response in the form of an inhibitory postsynaptic potential (IPSP) is evoked in a dopamine neuron by stimulating the GABAergic striatonigral pathway (arrow). When increasing amplitudes of hyperpolarizing current (lower traces) are injected into the neuron through the electrode, there is a progressive hyperpolarization of the membrane (top traces). As the membrane is made to be more negative, the IPSP diminishes in amplitude, eventually being replaced by a depolarizing response. *Panel A2:* Plotting the amplitude of the evoked response (y-axis) versus the membrane potential at which it was evoked (x-axis) illustrates how the synaptic response changes with membrane potential. The membrane voltage at which the synaptic response is equal to zero (i.e., −69.2 mV in this case) is the reversal potential of the ion

mediating the synaptic response (i.e., the potential at which the electrochemical forces working on the ion are zero). Therefore, there is no net flux of ion across the membrane. At more negative membrane potentials, the flow of the ion is reversed, causing the chloride ion (in this case) to exit the cell and result in a depolarization of the membrane.

Panel B: The flow of an ion across a membrane may also be altered by changing the concentration gradient of the ion across the membrane. Normally, chloride ions flow from the outside of the neuron (where they are present at a higher concentration) to the inside of the neuron (where their concentration is lower), causing the membrane potential to become more negative. In this case, the concentration of chloride ion across the membrane of the dopamine neuron is reversed by using potassium chloride as the electrolyte in the intracellular recording electrode. *Panel B1:* Soon after the neuron is impaled with the potassium chloride-containing electrode, stimulation of the striatonigral pathway (arrow) evokes an IPSP (bottom trace). However, as the recording is maintained, chloride is diffusing from the electrode into the neuron, causing the electrochemical gradient to progressively decrease over time. As a result, each subsequent stimulation pulse evokes a smaller IPSP, eventually causing the IPSP to reverse to a depolarization (top trace). The depolarization is caused by an efflux of chloride out of the neuron and down its new electrochemical gradient. This has caused the reversal potential of the chloride-mediated response to change from a potential that was negative to the resting potential to one that is now positive to the resting potential. *Panel B2:* After injecting chloride ions into the neuron, spontaneously occurring IPSPs that were not readily observed in the control case are now readily seen as reversed IPSPs (i.e., depolarizations) occurring in this dopamine neuron recorded in vivo.

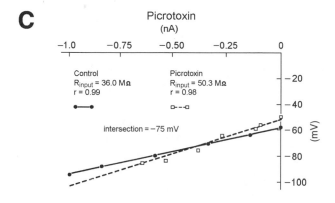

C

Picrotoxin
(nA)

Control
R_{input} = 36.0 MΩ
r = 0.99

Picrotoxin
R_{input} = 50.3 MΩ
r = 0.98

intersection = −75 mV

Figure 4–1. *(continued) Panel C:* Another means for determining the ionic conductance involved in a response is by using a specific ion channel blocker. This can be done in two ways: by using the drug to block an evoked response, or (as shown in this example) by examining the effects of administering the drug on the neuron to determine if the cell is receiving synaptic events that alter the conductance of the membrane to this ion. To do this, the current/voltage relationship of the cell is first established. This is done by injecting hyperpolarizing current pulses into the neuron (x-axis) and recording the membrane potential that is present during the current injection (y-axis). These values are then plotted on the graph (filled circles), with the resting membrane potential being the membrane potential at which no current is being injected into the neuron (y-intercept). The slope of the resultant regression line (solid line) is equal to the input resistance of the neuron (R_{input} = 36 megohms). After administration of the chloride ion channel blocker picrotoxin, a new current/voltage relationship is established in a similar manner. Picrotoxin caused a depolarization of the membrane (y-intercept of dashed line is more positive) and an increase in the neuron input resistance (the slope of the dashed line is larger). The intersection of the membrane current/voltage plots obtained before and after picrotoxin administration is then calculated. By definition, this point of intersection (i.e., −75 mV) is the reversal potential of the response to picrotoxin, because a neuron at this membrane potential would show no net change in membrane potential on drug administration.

Source. Adapted from Grace and Bunney 1985 with permission of the publisher.

ods are reviewed here: electroencephalographic (EEG) recordings, field potential recordings, single unit extracellular recordings, intracellular recordings, and patch clamp recordings. Which of these parameters are being measured is essentially a function of the type of electrode used. In recording EEGs, the desired signal is very small in amplitude, and as a consequence a large electrode that sums activity over large regions of the brain surface is used. Although

this is less invasive than other techniques, the information it can yield is comparatively narrow, in that simultaneous activation of a large array of neurons must occur for the potentials to be recorded at the scalp. As a consequence, stimulus presentation and EEG averaging are typically required to separate the signal desired from the background noise.

■ Field Potential Recordings

The next level of analysis is the recording of field potentials. This method uses a recording electrode with a smaller tip and a higher resistance, with the electrophysiological measures confined to a small population of neurons surrounding the electrode tip. This technique is still dependent on the simultaneous activation of a number of cells; but because the electrode is inserted into the brain, the cells do not have to be at the surface of the skull as in the EEG recordings. Furthermore, the activation can consist of stimulation of an afferent pathway. Nonetheless, the array of neurons sampled must have a common orientation for the massed activity to be measurable. Therefore, such measures are typically restricted to cortical structures such as the neocortex and hippocampus. Using this method, the current resulting from the parallel activation of excitatory and inhibitory afferents can be measured, as well as the electrophysiological response of a population of neurons to such stimulation. However, as with EEG recordings, such an approach is of limited value in psychopharmacological research.

■ Single Unit Extracellular Recordings

The next level of recording involves examining the electrophysiology of individual neurons using extracellular single unit recording techniques. This involves placing an electrode in close proximity to a single neuron for the purpose of recording its spike discharge. This is achieved by using an electrode with a smaller tip and a higher resistance, resulting in the sampling of a smaller volume of tissue (i.e., the somata of individual neurons). Because the region sampled by the electrode is smaller, the signal is larger in amplitude and the background noise is less. This enables easy recording of the spontaneous spike discharge of a single neuron within the brain of a living (but typically anesthetized) animal. The cells examined are located through the use of an atlas and a stereotaxic apparatus. By using the stereotaxic apparatus to hold the head of the animal in a precise orientation, a brain atlas may be used to accurately place the recording electrodes within the region of the brain desired. Furthermore, if a dye is dissolved in the electrolyte within the recording pipette, the dye may be ejected into the recording site for subsequent histological verification of the region recorded.

Because the recording electrode is placed near the outside surface of the neuron, there is less of a concern that the activity recorded is a result of damage to the neuron itself, as may be the case with intracellular recording techniques. Furthermore, a large number of neurons may be sampled in a given animal. However, as a consequence, the amount of information that can be obtained from a neuron is limited. Typically, the research is relegated to recording information related to action potential firing (e.g., the firing rate of the neuron, its pattern of spike discharge, and how these states of activity may be affected by stimulation of an afferent pathway or administration of a drug [Figure 4–2]). Nonetheless, when combined with the appropriate pharmacological techniques, extracellular recording has yielded a substantial amount of valuable information related to drug action or neuronal interconnections of physiologically important neuronal types. For example, by using a series of coordinated pharmacological and physiological techniques, it was possible to define a unique extracellular waveform as that associated with the discharge of a dopamine-containing neuron (Bunney et al. 1973; Grace and Bunney 1983). This provided the basis for studies that yielded information defining the mode of action of antipsychotic drugs (Bunney and Grace 1978; Grace 1992).

Extracellular recordings from neurons measure the current flow generated around a neuron as it generates spikes. For this reason, extracellular action potentials generally are composed of two components: a positive-going component followed by a negative-going component. The positive-going component is a reflection of the ion flux across the neuronal membrane surrounding the electrode that occurs during the depolarizing phase of the action potential, with the negative phase reflecting the repolarization. Because the extracellular recording electrode is measuring current across the membrane occurring in concert with changes in intracellular membrane potential, and because current is defined in terms of the first

derivative (i.e., rate of change) of voltage, the extracellularly recorded action potential (or "spike") waveform is typically a first derivative of the action potential voltage with respect to time (Terzuolo and Araki 1961). This phenomenon underlies the biphasic nature of the extracellularly recorded event (Figure 4–3). Furthermore, the recorded spike is largest when the recording electrode is placed near the active site of spike generation, because the current density is greatest (and thus the voltage drop induced across the electrode largest) at this site.

■ Intracellular Recordings

With intracellular recording, an electrode with a much smaller tip and a much higher electrical resistance is inserted into the membrane of the neuron. Although the tip of the electrode is smaller, the signal measured is much larger than with extracellular recording, because it is measuring the potential difference across the membrane directly rather than relying on transmembrane current density changes outside of the neuron. As a result, electrical activity occurring within the neuron can be measured that would be nearly impossible to measure extracellularly, such as spontaneously occurring or evoked (via afferent pathway stimulation) electrical potentials generated by neurotransmitter release (or postsynaptic potentials). Furthermore, because the membrane potential of the neuron may be altered by injecting depolarizing or hyperpolarizing current into the cell through the electrode, the equilibrium potential (also known as the reversal potential) of the response may be determined. In addition, the overall conductance of the membrane may be measured by injecting known levels of current and measuring the membrane voltage deflection produced. By applying this information using Ohm's law, the input resistance of the cell can be determined. This could be important in assessing drug effects. A drug could increase the input resistance of the membrane, making it more responsive to current generated by afferent synapses, without changing the membrane potential of the neuron. Indeed, such a condition has been proposed to underlie the mechanism through which norepinephrine increase the amplitude of the response of a neuron to a stimulus without affecting its basal firing rate (i.e., increasing its "signal-to-noise" ratio; Freedman et al. 1977; Woodward et al. 1979).

Using the intracellular recording electrode, it is

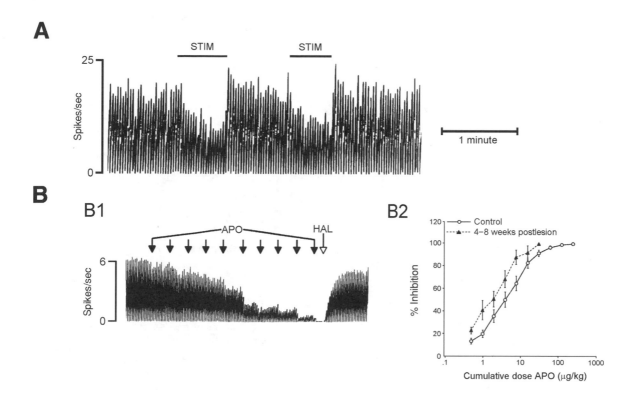

Figure 4–2. Extracellular recording techniques are an effective means of assessing the effects of afferent pathway stimulation or drug administration on neuron activity. On the other hand, the measures that can be performed are typically restricted to changes in firing rates or in the pattern of spike discharge.

Panel A: This firing rate histogram illustrates the response of a substantia nigra–zona reticulata neuron to stimulation of the γ-aminobutyric acid (GABA)ergic striatonigral pathway. A common method for illustrating how a manipulation affects the firing rate of a neuron is by constructing a firing rate histogram. This is typically done by using some type of electronic discriminator and counter to count the number of spikes that a cell fires in a given period of time. In this example, the counter counts spikes over a 10-second interval, and converts this number to a voltage, which is then plotted out on a chart recorder. The counter then resets to zero, and begins counting spikes over the next 10-second interval. Therefore, in the firing rate histogram illustrated, the height of each vertical line is proportional to the number of spikes that the cell fires during each 10-second interval, with the calibration bar on the left showing the equivalent firing frequency in spikes per second. During the period at which the striatonigral pathway is stimulated (horizontal bars above trace marked "STIM"), the cell is inhibited, as reflected by the decrease in the height of the vertical lines. When the stimulation is terminated, a rebound activation of cell firing is observed. *Source.* Adapted from Grace and Bunney 1985 with permission of the publisher.

Panel B: In this example, a similar histogram is used to illustrate the effects of a drug on the firing of a neuron.

Panel B1: This figure shows the well-known inhibition of dopamine neuron firing rate upon administration of the dopamine agonist apomorphine (APO). Each of the filled arrows represents the intravenous administration of a dose of apomorphine. After the cell is completely inhibited, the specificity of the response is tested by examining the ability of the dopamine antagonist haloperidol (HAL [open arrow]) to reverse this response. Typically, drug sensitivity is determined by administering the drug in a dose-response fashion. This is done by giving an initial drug dose that is subthreshold for altering the firing rate of the cell. The first dose is then repeated, with each subsequent dose given being twice that of the previous dose. This is continued until a plateau response is achieved (in this case, a complete inhibition of cell discharge). *Panel B2:* The drug is administered in a dose-response manner in order to facilitate the plotting of a *cumulative* dose-response curve, with drug doses plotted on a logarithmic scale (i.e., a log dose-response curve). In order to compare the potency of two drugs or the sensitivity of two cells to the same drug, a point on the curve is chosen during which the fastest rate-of-change of the response is obtained. The point usually chosen is that at which the drug dose administered causes 50% of the maximal change obtained (i.e., the ED_{50}). As can be observed in this example, the dopamine neurons recorded after a partial dopamine depletion (dashed line) are substantially more sensitive to inhibition by apomorphine than the dopamine neurons recorded in control (solid line) rats. *Source.* Adapted from Pucak and Grace 1991 with permission of the publisher.

C

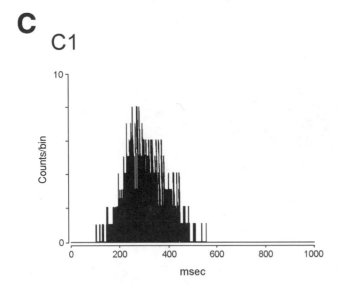

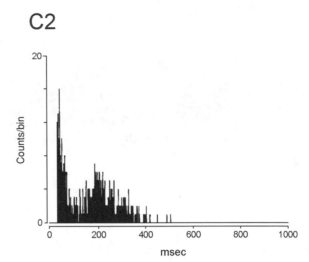

Figure 4–2. *(continued) Panel C:* In addition to determining the firing rate of a neuron, extracellular recording techniques may be used to assess the effects of drugs on the pattern of spike discharge. This is typically done by plotting an interspike interval histogram. In this paradigm, a computer is connected to a spike discriminator, and a train of 500 or so spikes is analyzed. The computer is used to time the delay between subsequent spikes in the train (i.e., the time interval between spikes), and plots this in the form of a histogram, in which the x-axis represents time between subsequent spikes, and the y-axis shows the number of interspike intervals that exhibited a specific delay (bin = range of time; e.g., for 1 msec bins, all intervals between 200.0 msec and 200.99 msec).

Panel C1: The cell is firing irregularly (as shown by the primarily normal distribution of intervals around 200 msec) with some spikes occurring after longer-than-average delays (i.e., bins above 400 msec, probably due to spontaneous IPSPs delaying spike occurrence). *Panel C2:* In contrast, this cell is firing in bursts, which consists of a series of 3–10 spikes with comparatively short interspike intervals (i.e., approximately 70 msec) separated by long delays between bursts (i.e., events occurring above 150-msec intervals). The computer determined that, in this case, the cell was discharging 79% of its spikes in bursts, compared with 0% in *Panel C1*.
Source. Adapted from Grace and Bunney 1984a with permission of the publisher.

also possible to inject specific substances into the neuron. For example, second messengers or calcium chelators may be introduced into the neuron to examine how they alter neuronal physiology or the neuron's response to drugs. Furthermore, by injecting the neuron with a fluorescent dye or enzymatic marker, the morphology of the specific cell impaled may be recovered and examined (Figure 4–4). This technique can be combined with immunocytochemistry to examine the neurotransmitter synthesized by the cell under study (e.g., Grace and Onn 1989).

Inserting an electrode into the membrane of a cell to measure transmembrane voltage and manipulating its membrane by injecting current is commonly known as "current clamp," because the amount and direction of ionic current crossing the membrane of the cell can be controlled by the experimenter, such as when determining the reversal potential of a response. Another technique that is effective in neuro-

physiological research involves the use of "voltage clamp" techniques. With voltage clamping, the membrane potential of the neuron is maintained at a set voltage level by injecting current into the cell. This is achieved by rapid feedback electronics that adjusts the current injected to accurately offset any factors that may act to change this potential. Thus, when the neuron is exposed to a drug that opens ion channels, the effects of the ionic influx are precisely counterbalanced by altering the current injected into the neuron by the voltage clamp device. The amount of additional current that must be injected into the neuron to maintain the membrane potential at its set point is therefore the inverse of the transmembrane current generated by the drug. By using specific ion channel blockers or by altering the extracellular ionic environment of the neuron, the precise ionic mechanism and conductance changes induced in a neuron by a drug or neurotransmitter may be determined.

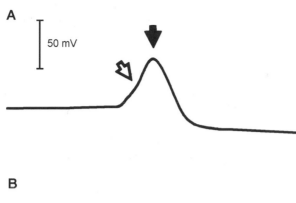

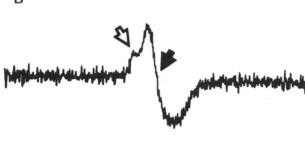

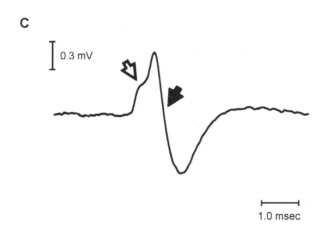

Figure 4–3. Relationship between action potentials recorded intracellularly and those recorded extracellularly from dopamine-containing neurons.

Panel A: During intracellular recordings, an action potential is initiated from a negative resting membrane potential (e.g., –55 mV), reaches a peak membrane potential (solid arrow), and is followed by a repolarization of the membrane and usually an afterhyperpolarization. An inflection in the rising phase of the spike (open arrow) is often observed. This is known to reflect the delay between the initial segment spike that initiates the action potential (occurring prior to the open arrow) and the somatodendritic action potential that it triggers (occurring after the open arrow).

Panel B: Using a computer, the membrane voltage deflection occurring during the action potential in *Panel A* is differentiated with respect to time, resulting in a pattern that shows the rate of change of membrane voltage. Note that the inflection is exaggerated (open arrow) and the peak of the action potential crosses zero (solid arrow), since at the peak of a spike the rate of change reaches zero before reversing to a negative direction.

Panel C: A trace showing a typical action potential in a dopamine neuron recorded extracellularly. The extracellular action potential resembles the differentiated intracellular action potential *Panel B*. This is because the extracellular electrode is actually measuring the current crossing the membrane during the action potential, and is therefore by definition equivalent to the absolute value of the first derivative of the voltage trace *Panel A*. The amplitude of the extracellular spike is indicated in volts, since the parameter measured is actually the voltage drop produced across the electrode tip by the current flux, and is therefore much smaller than the actual membrane voltage change that occurs in *Panel A*.

Source. Adapted from Grace and Bunney 1983 with permission of the publisher.

■ Patch Clamp Recordings

A final level of analysis to be discussed is one directed at assessing the response of individual ionic channels in the membrane of a neuron. Actually, this technique may be described more as a type of high-resolution extracellular recording. In this method, a glass pipette with a comparatively large tip is drawn, and the tip is fire-polished to make it very smooth. The electrode tip is then placed against the membrane surface of a neuron under visual control. Typically, the neuronal membrane is first cleaned of debris with a jet of fluid to permit a tight seal between the electrode and the membrane. A small suction is then applied to the pipette to tighten its seal with the membrane. Because such an attachment provides a high resistance junction with the membrane, the minute transmembrane currents that are generated as a result of the opening and closing of individual ionic channels may be monitored. The biophysical characteristics (e.g., open time, inactivation rate) of specific ion channels and how they may be modified by drugs applied via the pipette lumen or to other regions of the neuron being studied can be determined.

■ PREPARATIONS USED IN ELECTROPHYSIOLOGICAL RESEARCH

As with the various types of recordings that can be performed, so, too, there are several preparations

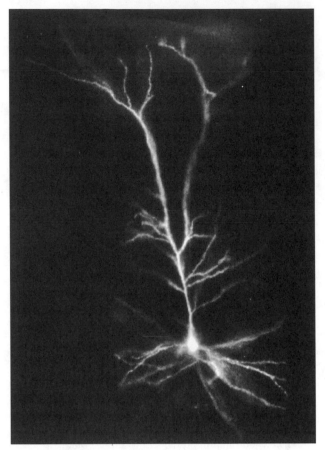

Figure 4–4. During intracellular recordings, the recording pipette is filled with an electrolyte to enable the transmission of membrane voltage deflections to the preamplifier. The electrode may also be filled with substances for injection into the neuron impaled, such as a morphological stain. In this example, the electrode was filled with the highly fluorescent dye Lucifer yellow. Because this dye has a negative charge at neutral pH, it may be ejected from the electrode by applying a negative current across the electrode, with the result that the Lucifer yellow carries the negative current flow from the electrode and into the neuron. Because this dye diffuses rapidly in water, it quickly fills the entire neuron impaled. The tissue is then fixed in a formaldehyde compound, the lipids clarified by dehydration-defatting or by using dimethylsulfoxide (Grace and Llinás 1985) and the tissue examined under a fluorescence microscope. In this case, a brightly fluorescing pyramidal neuron in layer 3 of the neocortex of a guinea pig is recovered.

that can be employed in this analysis. No single preparation is "best"; instead, each is associated with specific advantages and shortcomings. As usual, a more complete picture of the functioning of a system can be gained by taking advantage of the unique perspective provided by each preparation and designing the experiments accordingly. Except for the first cat-

egory listed, all preparations pertain to the mammalian vertebrate preparation.

■ Simpler Nervous Systems— Invertebrates and Lower Vertebrate Preparations

We include a reference to this preparation for completeness; more comprehensive reviews regarding the use of nonmammalian model systems can be found elsewhere (Kandel 1978). However, depending on the application, use of these preparations may yield varying degrees of relevance. With respect to the use of phylogenetically lower species as models for psychopharmacological studies in humans, much of the data related to anatomy, cellular physiology, and behavior would be of limited value. Nonetheless, there are several unique advantages associated with the study of the nervous systems of these organisms: the nervous system is more accessible, the small number of neurons allows for simple and replicable identification of specific neurons, the large neuronal size enables more stable impalement and more complex procedures, and so on. On the other hand, these advantages are often more than counterbalanced by the fact that the nervous system of these organisms are substantially different from those of vertebrates and humans, even at the single neuronal level. As a result, information derived from these systems is likely to be substantially less applicable to behavioral control in the mammalian class.

In contrast, information provided regarding the study of some second messenger systems or receptor transduction mechanisms appear to be more directly transferable to the vertebrate. Thus, it appears that nature is more likely to conserve the most basic functional units of neurotransmitter actions throughout phylogeny, with decreasing levels of homology as the functional units are assembled into more complex systems of neurons and networks.

■ In Vivo Electrophysiological Recordings

Protocols that employ the in vivo preparation focus on the living, intact, anesthetized animal as the subject of the study. Recording the activity of neurons in the intact animal has a number of advantages over studies performed in isolated tissues. For example, the health of the tissue or neuron under study is more easily maintained and monitored. Furthermore, the neuron can be examined in its normal ionic and cellular microenvironment, with its normal complement of afferent connections intact. In addition, neurons recorded in vivo are more likely to be spontaneously active, facilitating the use of extracellular recordings and investigations into the actions of inhibitory neurotransmitters.

With respect to psychopharmacological research, the in vivo preparation provides the most direct link between neurophysiology and behavior. A drug that is known to elicit a characteristic behavioral response can be administered systemically to examine how the drug affects neurons that are likely to participate in the behavioral response. For similar reasons, this preparation is also the most effective for investigating the mode of action of psychotherapeutic drugs on specific neuronal systems. Although the precise locus of action through which the systemically administered drugs act to achieve these effects may be difficult to determine directly, it can nonetheless be determined whether a given drug ultimately influences the activity of a neuronal system of interest.

There are also experimental parameters that present difficulties that, although not insurmountable, add complexity to the experimental paradigm. For example, the researcher cannot visually identify the nucleus or the cell to be recorded and must often rely on indirect techniques for cell identification. However, there are ways to enhance the ability to identify cell types. Thus, unlike the in vitro preparations, cells may be identified with respect to the projection sites of their axons by employing antidromic activation: stimulation of the axon terminal region to evoke an action potential that is conducted back down the axon and subsequently recorded at the soma. Furthermore, by using in vivo intracellular recording, the neuron in question may be stained with dye and its location, morphology, and neurotransmitter content identified post hoc by a variety of histochemical and immunocytochemical techniques (e.g., Grace and Bunney 1983; Onn et al. 1994). In addition, although the precise locus of action of systemically administered drugs cannot be determined, the drug effects obtained can be compared with those produced by directly applying the drug to the neuron through microiontophoresis (Figure 4–5 [Bloom 1974]).

On the other hand, the properties that confer distinct advantages on the in vivo preparation with respect to examining how drugs act in the intact organism also limit the type of data that may be collected. Regarding drug administration, there are some drugs that do not readily cross the blood-brain barrier or that exert their actions on neurons via an effect on peripheral organs. Thus, although dopamine cells can be excited by microiontophoretic administration of cholecystokinin (Skirboll et al. 1981), the excitation produced by systemic administration of this peptide has been shown to be mediated peripherally and affects the brain via the vagus (Hommer et al. 1985). In addition, the inability to control the microenvironment of the neuron restricts the analysis of the ionic mechanisms underlying cell firing or drug action, because the researcher is unable to administer ion channel blockers to the entire neuron surface or change the ionic composition of the extracellular fluid. Therefore, whereas the in vivo preparation affords many advantages with respect to examining how behaviorally or therapeutically effective drugs may exert their actions through defined neuronal systems, examination of the site of action or the membrane mechanisms underlying these responses is more readily accessible using in vitro systems.

■ In Vitro Electrophysiological Recordings From Brain Slices

Recordings of neurons maintained in vitro have led to significant advances in our understanding of the ionic mechanisms underlying neurotransmitter and drug action. This preparation consists of slices 300–400 μm thick cut from the brain of an animal soon after decapitation. If this procedure is done carefully and the brain slices rapidly placed into oxygenated physiological saline, the neurons within the slices will remain alive and healthy, often for 10 hours or more. Because the neurons are recorded in a chamber with oxygenated media superfused over the slice, several advantages may be realized:

1. Both intracellular and extracellular recordings are more stable owing to the absence of blood and breathing pulsations.
2. Visual control over electrode placement is achieved.
3. The ionic composition of the microenvironment may be controlled precisely.
4. There is little interference from the activity of long-loop afferents, and the near-absence of spontaneous spike discharge limits the contribution of local circuit neurons to the responses.

A

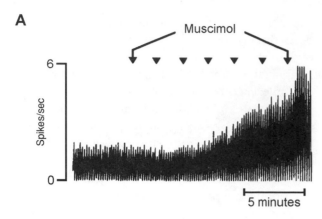

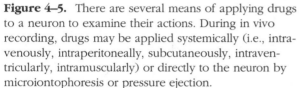

B

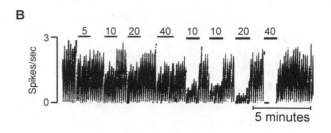

Figure 4–5. There are several means of applying drugs to a neuron to examine their actions. During in vivo recording, drugs may be applied systemically (i.e., intravenously, intraperitoneally, subcutaneously, intraventricularly, intramuscularly) or directly to the neuron by microiontophoresis or pressure ejection.

Panel A: Administration of a drug systemically is useful for determining how a drug affects neurons in the intact organism, irrespective of whether the action is direct or indirect. In this case, intravenous administration of the GABA agonist muscimol (solid arrows) causes a dose-dependent increase in the firing rate of this dopamine-containing neuron.

Panel B: In contrast, administering a drug directly to a neuron will provide information about the site of action of the drug, at least as it concerns the discharge of the neuron under study. In this case, γ-aminobutyric acid (GABA) is administered directly to a dopamine neuron by microiontophoresis. In this technique, several drug-containing pipettes are attached to the recording electrode. The pH of the drug solutions are adjusted to ensure that the drug molecules are in a charged state

(e.g., GABA is used at pH = 4.0 to give it a positive charge), and the drug is ejected from the pipette tip by applying very small currents to the drug-containing pipette. Because the total diameter of the microiontophoretic pipette tip is only about 5 μm, the drugs ejected typically only affect the cell being recorded. In this case, GABA is applied to a dopamine neuron by microiontophoresis; the horizontal bars show the time during which the current is applied to the drug-containing pipette, and the amplitude of the current (indicated in nA) is listed above each bar. Note that, unlike the excitatory effects produced by a systemically administered GABA agonist in *Panel A,* direct application of GABA will *inhibit* dopamine neurons. This has been shown to be due to inhibition of a much more GABA-sensitive inhibitory interneuron by the systemically administered drug, and illustrates the need to compare direct drug administration and systemic drug administration to ascertain the site of action of the drug of interest.

Source. Adapted from Grace and Bunney 1985 with permission of the publisher.

Furthermore, in contrast to microiontophoresis, the concentration of drug in the solution can be controlled precisely. This is also the most complex preparation that can be used for patch clamp recordings, because it is possible to remove debris and place the patch pipette on selected neurons under visual control using a high-resolution optics system (Edwards et al. 1989).

Nonetheless, because of the isolated nature of this system, the results obtained may not precisely reflect the physiology of the intact system. For example, dopamine neurons recorded in vivo have been characterized by their burst-firing discharge pattern (Grace and Bunney 1984b), which appears to be important in regulating neurotransmitter release (Gonon 1988). However, dopamine neurons recorded in vitro do not fire in bursting patterns (Grace

and Onn 1989 [Figure 4–6]). On the other hand, this distinction provides what may be an ideal system for examining the factors enabling burst firing to occur in vivo. Therefore, the most complete model of the functioning of a system or of its response to drug application can be derived by comparing the results obtained in vitro with those in the intact organism.

■ Recordings From Dissociated Neurons and Neuronal Cell Cultures

Recordings from isolated neurons are in actuality a subset of in vitro recording methods, with many of the same advantages in terms of accessibility and stability. Furthermore, because the neurons can be completely visualized, performing advanced techniques such as patch clamping is more easily done. A unique

A

B

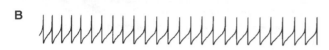

Figure 4–6. Variation (sometimes substantial) in patterns of activity of a neuron type, depending on the preparation in which it is recorded.

Panel A: Extracellular recordings of a dopamine neuron in an intact, anesthetized rat (i.e., in vivo) illustrates the typical irregular firing pattern of the cell, with single spikes occurring intermixed with bursts of action potentials.

Panel B: In contrast, intracellular recordings of a dopamine neuron recorded in an isolated brain slice preparation (i.e., in vitro) illustrate the pacemaker pattern that has been found to occur exclusively in identified dopamine neurons in this preparation. For dopamine neurons, a pacemaker firing pattern is rarely observed in vivo, and burst firing has never been observed in the in vitro preparation. However, although the activity recorded in vitro is obviously an abstraction compared to the firing pattern of this neuron in vivo, a comparative study in each preparation does provide the opportunity to examine what factors may underlie the modulation of firing pattern in this neuronal type.

Source. Adapted from Grace 1987 and Grace and Bunney 1983 with permission of the publishers.

advantage of this system can also be obtained via coculturing different neuronal populations. For example, defining the effects of a noradrenergic synapse on a hippocampal pyramidal neuron more precisely may be possible by coculturing these cell types and allowing them to make synapses. In this way, the researcher has visual control over impaling neurons that comprise a presynaptic and postsynaptic pairing. On the other hand, the synapses formed are not necessarily limited to those that occur naturally in the intact organism, both in terms of the location of the synapse on the neuron and the classes of neurons that are interconnected. Furthermore, the altered neuronal morphology present in these preparations may alter the response of the neurons to drugs. Nonetheless, when the analysis is limited to well-defined responses, such as second messenger actions or ion channel measures, this system affords an unparalleled level of accessibility.

▩ RELATIONSHIP BETWEEN BIOCHEMICAL AND ELECTROPHYSIOLOGICAL MEASURES OF NEURONAL ACTIVITY

The methods outlined here are directed at analyzing the activity of individual neurons as a means of assessing their role in pharmacological responses or behavioral actions. This is based on the premise that the discharge of a neuron in some manner reflects its release of transmitter onto a postsynaptically located target neuron. As such, biochemical measures of neurotransmitter levels would be predicted to correspond to the activity changes occurring during electrophysiological recordings from neurons (Roth 1987). In several cases, such approaches have been fruitful in defining the physiological relevance of recorded neuron activity. One case in which this has proven valuable is in the analysis of firing pattern. For example, dopamine neurons, like many other cell types in the central nervous system, are capable of discharging trains of action potentials in two patterns of activity: single spiking and burst firing. However, their range of firing rates is comparatively restricted, with most cells firing only between 2–8 Hz. Nonetheless, using information on the temporal relationship between spikes in bursts (Grace and Bunney 1984b), studies using in vivo voltammetry to measure dopamine levels have shown that dopamine cells firing in bursts will release 2–3 times more neurotransmitter per spike from their terminals than those discharging at similar frequencies but in a steady firing pattern (Gonon 1988). Therefore, in this case knowledge of the physiological firing pattern provided information to the electrochemist that resulted in the elucidation of the physiological consequence of burst firing in this system.

However, the extrapolation between biochemical and electrophysiological measures may not always be valid. Thus, recordings from single neurons may not necessarily reflect the activity across the population of neurons of interest. Therefore, a drug that exerts an action via activation of the nonfiring population of neurons may be missed if its actions are assessed on single spontaneously discharging neurons (Bunney and Grace 1978; Grace and Bunney 1984a). Furthermore, the response may be confined to a topographically defined subset of neurons mediating a particular response (e.g., one would not predict a change in the activity of neurons regulating movement of the leg if the response involves a reaching movement of the arm). With respect to biochemical measurements, there may be actions of transmitters at presynaptic terminals that could dramatically alter the amount of neurotransmitter they release independent of neuronal discharge (e.g., Grace 1991). On the other hand, electrophysiological measures enable researchers to examine responses that occur very rapidly. Indeed, a massive but transient activation of spike discharge in a neuronal system may evoke a substantial behavioral response, whereas biochemical measures of neurotransmitter release performed over a long time course may dilute the impact of the transient event. Therefore, although the results obtained from each measure may not be directly comparable, the electrophysiological measures are better optimized for detecting transient events.

■ SUMMARY

In this chapter, we reviewed a number of electrophysiological techniques and preparations used in the analysis of nervous system function. Each approach is characterized by a set of unique advantages and potential shortcomings inherent in the method. Nonetheless, it should be apparent that no single technique has an overwhelming advantage in psychopharmacological research. Instead, by fitting the preparation to the question at hand, and through the judicious comparison of data obtained from intact versus isolated preparations, the various limitations may be systematically overcome to yield a more broadly applicable model of psychopharmacological action.

■ REFERENCES

Bloom FE: To spritz or not to spritz: the doubtful value of aimless iontophoresis. Life Sci 14:1819–1834, 1974

Bunney BS, Grace AA: Acute and chronic haloperidol treatment: comparison of effects on nigral dopaminergic cell activity. Life Sci 23:1715–1728, 1978

Bunney BS, Walters JR, Roth RH, et al: Dopaminergic neurons: effect of antipsychotic drugs and amphetamine on single cell activity. J Pharmacol Exp Ther 185:560–571, 1973

Edwards FA, Konnerth A, Sakmann B, et al: A thin slice preparation for patch clamp recordings from neurones of the mammalian central nervous system. Pflugers Arch 414:600–612, 1989

Freedman R, Hoffer BJ, Woodward DJ, et al: Interaction of norepinephrine with cerebellar activity evoked by mossy and climbing fibers. Exp Neurol 55:269–288, 1977

Gonon FG: Nonlinear relationship between impulse flow and dopamine released by rat midbrain dopaminergic neurons as studied by in vivo electrochemistry. Neuroscience 24:19–28, 1988

Grace AA: The regulation of dopamine neuron activity as determined by in vivo and in vitro intracellular recordings, in The Neurophysiology of Dopamine Systems. Edited by Chiodo LA, Freeman AS. Detroit, MI, Lake Shore Publications, 1987, pp 1–67

Grace AA: Phasic versus tonic dopamine release and the modulation of dopamine system responsivity: a hypothesis for the etiology of schizophrenia. Neuroscience 41:1–24, 1991

Grace AA: The depolarization block hypothesis of neuroleptic action: implications for the etiology and treatment of schizophrenia. J Neural Transm 36 (suppl):91–131, 1992

Grace AA, Bunney BS: Intracellular and extracellular electrophysiology of nigral dopaminergic neurons, I: identification and characterization. Neuroscience 10:301–315, 1983

Grace AA, Bunney BS: The control of firing pattern in nigral dopamine neurons: single spike firing. J Neurosci 4:2866–2876, 1984a

Grace AA, Bunney BS: The control of firing pattern in nigral dopamine neurons: burst firing. J Neurosci 4:2877–2890, 1984b

Grace AA, Bunney BS: Opposing effects of striatonigral feedback pathways on midbrain dopamine cell activity. Brain Res 333:271–284, 1985

Grace AA, Llinás R: Dehydration-induced morphological artifacts in intracellularly stained neurons: circumvention using rapid DMSO clearing. Neuroscience 16:461–475, 1985

Grace AA, Onn SP: Morphology and electrophysiological properties of immunocytochemically identified rat dopamine neurons recorded in vitro. J Neurosci 9:3463–3481, 1989

Hommer DW, Palkovits M, Crawley JN, et al: Cholecystokinin-induced excitation in the substantia nigra: evidence for peripheral and central components. J Neurosci 5:1387–1392, 1985

Kandel ER: A Cell-Biological Approach to Learning (Grass Lecture Monograph 1). Bethesda, MD, Society for Neuroscience, 1978, pp 1–90

Llinás RR: The intrinsic electrophysiological properties of mammalian neurons: a new insight into CNS function. Science 242:1654–1664, 1988

Onn SP, Berger TW, Grace AA: Identification and characterization of striatal cell subtypes using in vivo intracellular recording and dye-labelling in rats, III: morphological correlates and compartmental localization. Synapse 16:231–254, 1994

Pucak ML, Grace AA: Partial dopamine depletions result in an enhanced sensitivity of residual dopamine neurons to apomorphine. Synapse 9:144–155, 1991

Roth RH: Biochemical correlates of the electrophysiological activity of dopaminergic neurons: reflections on two decades of collaboration with electrophysiologists, in Neurophysiology of Dopaminergic Systems—Current Status and Clinical Perspectives. Edited by Chiodo LA, Freeman AS. Detroit, MI, Lake Shore Publications, 1987, pp 187–203

Skirboll LR, Grace AA, Hommer DW, et al: Peptide-monoamine coexistence: studies of the actions of a cholecystokinin-like peptide on the electrical activity of midbrain dopamine neurons. Neuroscience 6:2111–2124, 1981

Terzuolo CA, Araki T: An analysis of intra- versus extracellular potential changes associated with activity of single spinal motoneurons. Ann N Y Acad Sci 94:547–558, 1961

Woodward DJ, Moises HC, Waterhouse BD, et al: Modulatory actions of norepinephrine in the central nervous system. Federation Proceedings 38:2109–2116, 1979

Animal Models of
Depression and Schizophrenia

Jay M. Weiss, Ph.D., and Clinton D. Kilts, Ph.D.

Animal models of both depression and schizophrenia have played a significant role in the development of current treatments for these disorders. Despite this, animal models of these disorders have yet to achieve more than a small percentage of their ultimate promise because existing models remain imperfect approximations of their target pathologies. However, the ability to study physiological and environmental processes under experimental control that is not possible when human patients are the subject population makes animal models of such value for development of effective treatments that efforts to improve animal models are continuously ongoing. In this chapter, we summarize the development of such models to date.

■ TYPES OF ANIMAL MODELS

Animal models can be divided into two categories. The first category can be called *animal assay* models. Models in this category use behavioral and/or physiological responses of animals to assess processes, usually physiological processes, that already-

existing evidence indicates are important in a disorder. For example, evidence from drug and other studies indicates that alteration in the activity of dopamine, a neurotransmitter in the brain, is important in schizophrenia and Parkinson's disease. Rats show turning (rotational) behavior when receptors for dopamine in the brain are stimulated. The sensitivity of receptors and activity of the dopaminergic system in the brain can be assessed in animals by measuring such turning behavior; thus, this response in the animal serves as an assay for a physiological function of importance in behavioral pathology. The second category consists of models that can be called ***homologous*** models. These models endeavor to recreate the human disorder in animals. In these models, treatments are administered to animals in the hope of causing the animals to resemble individuals who are afflicted with the disorder.

Both the animal assay and homologous models are very useful. The first type finds its major use in drug screening and development of new drugs. By permitting researchers to determine how various compounds affect physiological processes that are important in pathology, animal assay models make it

---

The authors express their sincere appreciation to Lorna Clarke and Barbara House, without whose dedicated efforts this chapter would not have been possible.

possible to rapidly assess the potential usefulness of drug compounds and, in some cases, to discover new drugs that unexpectedly affect an important physiological process. Of course, a limitation of this type of model is that it assumes a priori that a particular physiological process is important in a disorder, and the usefulness of the model rests on this assumption.

The second type of animal model is also valuable, perhaps even more so than the first. Once perfected, a homologous model reproduces a disorder (as closely as can be done) in an animal. Unlike the animal assay type, a homologous model is not designed with the assumption that a particular physiological abnormality underlies a disorder. Consequently, because the perfected homologous model reproduces a disorder, it is then possible to study the model as a means to discover the underlying cause (i.e., the physiological defect) in the disorder. In addition, such a model can be used to test for *totally novel treatments* for the disorder; that is, because a perfected homologous model reproduces the disorder without making any assumptions regarding its physiological basis, researchers can test any potential treatment on the animal model to see if it can reverse the disorder. Because the physiological basis of a disorder can be discovered if a disorder is produced in animals, and because completely new treatments may be tested as well, major advances in the understanding and treatment of a disorder will rapidly follow the development of an adequate homologous model.

CRITERIA FOR EVALUATING ANIMAL MODELS

Soon after animal models of behavioral disorders, particularly depression, came into use, criteria were proposed by which such models could be evaluated. Although these criteria have been constructed primarily for evaluation of homologous models, animal assays can also be evaluated by applying those aspects of the criteria applicable to such models. Interestingly, a considerable degree of consensus has developed with regard to one particular set of criteria, which has been widely accepted in the field despite the occasional recommendations for some modifications.

Criteria Proposed by McKinney and Bunney

The criteria that have been widely accepted are those proposed by McKinney and Bunney (1969). They proposed that the usefulness and/or validity of an animal model of any behavioral disorder could be determined on the basis of the similarity of the animal model to the human disorder with respect to four criteria:

1. Etiology
2. Symptomatology
3. Biochemistry
4. Response to treatment

In other words, the "goodness" or validity of an animal model of any behavioral, psychological, or psychiatric disorder can be determined by the extent to which the animal model 1) is produced by etiological factors similar to those that produce the human disorder, 2) resembles the human disorder in manifestations or symptomatology, 3) has an underlying pathophysiological basis similar to that of the human disorder, and 4) responds as does the human disorder to appropriate therapeutic treatments. Before commenting further on these particular criteria, we will examine other suggestions and/or amplifications.

Criteria Proposed by Abramson and Seligman

In a book that reviewed a wide variety of animal models, Abramson and Seligman (1977) proposed a different set of criteria:

1. Is the analysis of the laboratory phenomenon (model) thorough in describing the essential features of its cause, prevention, and cure?
2. Is the similarity of symptoms convincingly demonstrated?
3. To what extent are physiology, cause, cure, and prevention similar to the human disorder?
4. Does the model describe in all instances a naturally occurring psychopathology or only a subgroup?

In actuality, these criteria do not suggest anything markedly different from those proposed by McKinney and Bunney (1969) but appear to address issues such as the quality of the research that is carried out to establish the model (i.e., is the analysis thorough enough? are symptoms convincingly demonstrated?). The third criterion seems to repeat those proposed by McKinney and Bunney, with the exception that etiology is omitted from this particular list. Finally, the last criterion simply asks for judgment regarding whether the model reproduces a particular subgroup of a disorder. However, once this issue is settled, the same criteria would be used to evaluate the model, whether it represented some global disorder or a subgroup.

■ Criteria Proposed by Willner

The most significant attempt to improve upon the simple schema of McKinney and Bunney (1969) was offered by Willner (1984). This investigator suggested that animal models should be evaluated for different types of validity—predictive validity, face validity, and construct validity. Each of these categories was said to possess five characteristics. Predictive validity is determined by whether a model correctly identifies 1) pharmacological antidepressant treatments of 2) different types 3) without showing false positives or 4) negatives, and 5) by whether drug dosages that are effective in the model correlate in potency with those found to be effective in the clinic. Face validity is said to be determined by whether 1) antidepressant effects are present only on chronic administration, and whether the symptoms of the model 2) resemble a number of the symptoms of depression that are 3) specific to depression 4) found in a particular subtype of depression, and 5) the model should not show characteristics that are not seen clinically. Finally, construct validity requires that 1) the behavioral features of the model and 2) the features of depression that the model seeks to reproduce can be unambiguously interpreted, 3) are homologous, and stand in an established 4) empirical and 5) theoretical relationship to depression.

Although these criteria are long and detailed, it is unclear how they add constructively to those proposed by McKinney and Bunney (1969). For example, predictive validity, which Willner (1984) applies only to antidepressant medications, would seem to be subsumed under the McKinney and Bunney criterion of response to treatment. Moreover, the first characteristic listed by Willner under face validity—that antidepressant medication has therapeutic effects only on chronic administration—would seem to be

an aspect of this criterion rather than of another. Thus, what Willner describes as predictive validity as well as the chronicity requirement for the effects of drugs could well be seen simply as a more elaborate description of McKinney and Bunney's last general criterion. (It should also be noted that Willner's schema omits any mention of nonpharmacological treatments, which not only are effective in ameliorating depression but also could conceivably be modeled in an animal.) A similar judgment could be made regarding face validity, which would seem to be subsumed under McKinney and Bunney's requirement of symptom similarity. Moreover, the specific requirements proposed by Willner for this category may be excessively restrictive. In particular, it is unclear why a model that includes all salient clinical features of depression (which presumably are also reversible by antidepressant treatment) would be of lesser value if the model showed additional changes as well; depression in humans is rarely uncontaminated by other changes or disturbances.

Potentially the most significant contribution embodied in Willner's (1984) suggestions is the addition of construct validity. By pointing out the need to define characteristics clearly and unambiguously, Willner draws attention to the fact that attributes of the human disorder are often poorly described, which makes modeling exceedingly difficult. However, the need for construct validity could be said to apply to every aspect of both the animal response being generated (and measured) and the human behavior that researchers attempt to match in an animal model, all of these characteristics falling within the criteria of McKinney and Bunney (1969). In other words, these aspects of construct validity, like many of the Abramson and Seligman (1977) criteria, appear to set requirements for how any criterion, including those proposed by McKinney and Bunney, should be established and/or evaluated, but such requirements do not themselves expand the actual list of criteria proposed by McKinney and Bunney.

There is, however, one exception to this in Willner's (1984) criteria. It is that aspect of construct validity stipulating that responses seen in the animal model should "stand in theoretical relationship to depression." This stipulation could be regarded as trivial—one that might be fulfilled by, for example, conceptually linking reduced motor activity in rats to psychomotor retardation in humans. However, defining a theoretical basis for a model would ordinarily be understood to require more than this. What would be expected by this requirement is *to establish a link across different levels of analysis,* such as linking a syndrome of different behaviors to an underlying generalized cognitive deficit or physiological defect. Thus, this criterion potentially expands the scope of homologous models by promoting modeling not only of responses and/or syndromes of responses but also of *processes* involved in abnormal behavior. For example, researchers might model deficits in the appreciation of pleasure (for depression) or the inability to properly exclude irrelevant stimuli (for schizophrenia). Moreover, it can be argued that ultimately the most satisfactory and appropriate models for behavioral disorders reflect critical processes.

But despite potential positive attributes of this suggestion, it is also important to consider the appreciable dangers in using the criterion described above. To model a critical process, two major assumptions must be made: 1) that the particular process one addresses is affected (disturbed) in the disorder, and 2) that the behavioral change measured in the animal validly represents that process rather than being caused by some other unrelated influence. In short, adopting this approach means that researchers are no longer strictly bound by symptom similarity of the behavior seen in the model to that seen in the disorder; the link to the disorder is accomplished through a series of theoretical formulations. In considering this course, it should be recalled that the field of abnormal psychology is emerging from a long period during which disorders were defined by hypothetical underlying processes; these were usually psychodynamic in nature. Today, proponents of theoretically based models are likely to replace psychodynamic processes with physiological ones as the appropriate basis for abnormal psychology. For example, in the case of depression, "anger turned inward" is likely to be replaced by "deficits in brain dopaminergic transmission mediating pleasure." However, although aspects of the latter formulation may be easier (and more fashionable) to measure than the former, the underlying concerns with respect to modeling are similar. This is because even a physiologically based formulation of an underlying deficit is presently a conjecture. It needs to be emphasized that little is actually known at present about the pathophysiology underlying abnormal psychology. No reliable physiological abnormalities denote any diagnostic group. The wealth of information available in the physiolog-

ical realm relates largely to drug action that describes processes involved in counteracting or ameliorating abnormal responses, which ultimately may relate only indirectly to what is physiologically disturbed in the affected patient. As a result, although theoretically based models are likely to provide interesting and valuable information about the relationship of certain behaviors to physiological changes, they face no fewer fundamental problems in establishing their validity as models of diagnostic categories than did the psychodynamic formulations they have replaced.

The thrust of DSM-III, DSM-III-R, and DSM-IV (American Psychiatric Association 1980, 1987, 1994) has been to move away from diagnosis related to theoretical constructs and toward diagnosis based on directly observable markers. This trend is accentuated in the call for basing the diagnosis of depression on behavioral "signs" rather than even on reported symptoms (Mitchell and Potter 1993; Parker et al. 1990). Consequently, reproducing the symptoms or "signs" of abnormal psychological conditions in animal models, and finding these symptoms to be ameliorated by effective treatments, must continue to be the goal of current models, or researchers risk slipping back to pre–DSM-III diagnosis. *The appropriate goal for models is to achieve empirical validity, regardless of theoretical validity.* For depression, this pursuit is aided by the considerable repertoire of motor and vegetative symptoms found in this disorder. For schizophrenia, on the other hand, symptoms and signs in the human disorder are predominantly evidence of cognitive disturbance, so that reproducing these specific symptoms in an animal model is much more difficult. As is seen in the discussion of models for schizophrenia, attempting to duplicate disturbed processes appears to be the most productive avenue at present, despite the conceptual risks.

In conclusion, the concise, straightforward schema proposed by McKinney and Bunney (1969) appears to be the most adequate set of criteria yet suggested for evaluating animal models. As Sir Martin Roth (1976) commented in addressing diagnosis of affective disorders, "good classifications are simple and parsimonious" (p. 86).

◼ MODELS OF DEPRESSION

In this section, a description of each model is given. These descriptions begin by focusing on procedural aspects by which the model is produced and then summarize attributes of the model, particularly those that permit evaluation according to the criteria of McKinney and Bunney (1969). The allocation of models to either the animal assay category or the homologous model category can occasionally be somewhat arbitrary, but heavy emphasis is placed here on face validity with respect to symptomatology. For example, in accord with the view that a fundamental aspect of depression is a slowing, or retardation, of function (e.g., Cohen et al. 1982; Nelson and Charney 1981; Parker et al. 1990), models are classified here as homologous when reduced motor activity is the primary symptom shown by the animal, though the model may be deficient in other ways. Conversely, models of depression are not classified as homologous when hyperactivity is a significant feature, except in those cases where the model shows evidence that functioning is otherwise generally retarded and/or that the hyperactivity seen in the model is because of agitation.

■ Animal Assay Models

Muricide. Some rats will spontaneously kill mice when the mice are presented to them. Horovitz and colleagues (1965) noted that administration of imipramine, iproniazid (a monoamine oxidase inhibitor [MAOI]), and dextroamphetamine blocked the tendency of such rats to kill mice, and that this effect could not be attributed to drug-induced debilitation or sedation. Subsequent studies confirmed that tricyclic antidepressants (TCAs; i.e., desipramine [DMI], imipramine), MAOIs, and amphetamines have this effect, but antihistamines did also (Sofia 1969a, 1969b). It should be noted that antidepressants accomplished this effect with acute administration.

Yohimbine lethality. The drug yohimbine can be administered to mice in dosages that are lethal; administration of sublethal doses was found to be lethal when accompanied by the administration of TCAs and MAOIs (Quinton 1963). Malick (1981) reported that atypical antidepressants (i.e., bupropion, nomifensine, mianserin, iprindole) also produced this effect, whereas antipsychotics and most tranquilizers did not. An important exception is that electroconvulsive therapy (ECT) does not potentiate lethality; also, anticholinergics and antihistaminics do. The drugs have these effects when administered acutely.

Amphetamine potentiation. Amphetamine produces a number of effects in rats, including hyperthermia, increased locomotor activity, and improved shuttle box avoidance performance. Antidepressants, both TCAs and MAOIs, have been found to potentiate these responses (Carlton 1961; Halliwell et al. 1964; Morpurgo and Theobald 1965). As with the models previously described, these effects are observed after acute administration of drug. It can be noted that the various effects measured in conjunction with this test derive from the catecholamimetic action of amphetamine; consequently, the ability of a drug or treatment to potentiate these effects of amphetamine primarily detects ability to potentiate catecholaminergic neurotransmission.

Kindling. Electrical stimulation of certain brain regions (e.g., amygdala, cortex) apparently sensitizes the brain region to initiate seizure activity so that, following such stimulation, considerably less electrical stimulation delivered to the brain region is required to initiate seizure activity than is the case when electrical stimulation of that brain region has not been given previously. Babington and Wedeking (1973) reported that TCAs reduced the likelihood of development of seizures in "kindled" animals. Other drugs such as tranquilizers and sedatives also blocked kindled seizures. However, only the antidepressants that were tested (i.e., amitriptyline, nortriptyline, imipramine) blocked seizures initiated in the amygdala at considerably lower doses than were needed to block seizures kindled in the neocortex; all other drugs tested were equipotent against seizures initiated at both sites. Subsequently, ECT was found to produce the same effect (Babington 1975), but MAOIs did not. Drugs are effective in this model when given acutely.

Circadian rhythm readjustment. Rats are normally active during the dark period of the day and are quiet (less active) during the light period. If the light-dark periods are switched, the animals must readjust their activity to this shift in the light-dark cycle. The rapidity with which animals will shift their activity to the new dark period and decrease their activity to the new light period is facilitated by administration of the TCA imipramine or the MAOI pargyline (Baltzer and Weiskrantz 1975). A stimulant (amphetamine) and a tranquilizing agent (chlordiazepoxide) were not effective. In treatments reported to be effective, drugs were administered repeatedly (i.e., for 10 days before the light-dark shift, and for approximately 2 weeks thereafter).

Lesioning of the olfactory bulbs. Bilateral lesions of the olfactory bulbs produce a number of behavioral effects. This procedure generally results in hyperactivity in novel situations such as the open field (Janscar and Leonard 1980) and exaggerated responses to excitatory stimuli (Cairncross et al. 1977). Perhaps related to the hyperactivity, animals with olfactory bulb lesions also show deficits in passive avoidance performance (Archer et al. 1984; Rigter et al. 1977) as well as superior performance in the two-way shuttle avoidance task (Archer et al. 1984), which is highly dependent on high levels of motor activity for good acquisition (e.g., Weiss et al. 1968). However, olfactory bulb lesions also produce poor performance in one-way avoidance (King and Cairncross 1974), suggesting that decreased fearfulness may contribute to both poor passive avoidance and enhanced shuttle avoidance (i.e., shuttle avoidance is performed better in animals whose fear level is low). Activity in the Porsolt swim test has been reported to be unaffected by bulbectomy (Gorka et al. 1985), but bulbectomy was found to increase activity in a swim task that emphasized escape attempts (Stockert et al. 1988). Lesioning of the olfactory bulbs was initially reported to produce a sustained elevation of circulating corticosterone in the rat, thus mimicking the hypocortisolemia seen in severe depression, but this response may have been generated as an acute reaction to the measurement procedures (see discussion in van Reizen and Leonard 1991).

Regarding pharmacological tests, deficits in avoidance behavior, particularly passive avoidance, produced by bulbectomy were found to be reversed by TCAs (i.e., amitriptyline, imipramine, clomipramine), atypical antidepressants (i.e., mianserin, viloxazine), and a serotonin (5-HT) uptake inhibitor, while this deficit was exaggerated by tranquilizers and neuroleptics (Cairncross et al. 1975b, 1977; Rigter et al. 1977; van Riezen et al. 1977). Drugs were effective in such tests when administered chronically. Increased open-field activity of bulbectomized animals was found to be diminished by selective serotonin reuptake inhibitors (SSRIs), which were effective when given acutely as well as chronically (Earley and Leonard 1985).

Differential operant responding for low reinforcement (DRL). Seiden, O'Donnell, and colleagues screened a wide variety of drugs for their effects on rats when the animals are reinforced for a low rate of responding. In this task, an animal is taught to press a lever to receive a food reward. After the response is acquired, the animal is placed on a "differential reinforcement of low rate 72 second" (or DRL72) schedule, which requires the animal to wait 72 seconds after making a response before making another response in order to obtain the food reward; making a second response in less than 72 seconds after the first causes no reinforcement and simply resets the timing sequence so that the animal must wait an additional 72 seconds before responding to receive a reward.

In several studies (McGuire and Seiden 1980a, 1980b; O'Donnell and Seiden 1982, 1983, 1985), these investigators found that ECT and a variety of antidepressant drugs including TCAs (i.e., DMI, imipramine, nortriptyline, clomipramine), MAOIs (i.e., tranylcypromine, iproniazid, phenelzine), atypical antidepressants (i.e., iprindole, mianserin, trazodone), and SSRIs (i.e., zimeldine, fluoxetine) all improved the ability of animals to inhibit responding and then obtain reward. Danysz and colleagues (1988) found similar detection of antidepressants. This effect was usually seen with acute administration of drug, but further improvements in performance were seen when the drug was administered repeatedly. Antipsychotic, psychomotor stimulant, narcotic analgesic, anxiolytic, antihistaminic, and anticholinergic agents did not improve performance.

Seiden and O'Donnell (1985) described findings indicating that the improved ability to obtain rewards on a DRL schedule could not be explained simply by the possibility that antidepressant treatment decreased response rate. This was because anxiolytics and phenothiazines also decreased response rate but did so to such an extent that the number of reinforcements decreased dramatically. However, Pollard and Howard (1986) found in two studies that non-antidepressant drugs (i.e., chlorpromazine, haloperidol, buspirone) could reduce response rate moderately to produce an increase in reinforcements similar to that of antidepressants, and they argue that this test is not specific for antidepressant drugs. (It can be noted that the absolute magnitude of an effect seen in this test situation is often small—for example, reinforcements may increase from an average of 15 under "no-drug" conditions to 20–25 under "drug conditions"—so that the results are quite sensitive to small changes in response rate. On the other hand, the lever-press response that is used permits investigators to test the same animals repeatedly and under all conditions, so that small effects can be discerned and become statistically significant.)

Seiden and colleagues (1985) have done testing to determine whether a specific monoamine neurotransmitter might be responsible for the increase in reinforced responding on a DRL72 schedule that is seen when antidepressants are given. Lesions of the dorsal bundle noradrenergic system that innervates the forebrain (i.e., lesioning the axons originating from the locus ceruleus [LC]) did not block the ability of DMI to increase the number of rewards obtained, but partial lesioning of brain dopamine did reduce this effect somewhat. Such results point to dopamine as the important catecholamine neurotransmitter (O'Donnell and Seiden 1984); however, 1) partial lesions of brain dopamine are of uncertain functional effect and can even result in enhancement of dopaminergic neurotransmission, and 2) bupropion, which preferentially potentiates dopamine by blocking its reuptake, was found to be ineffective in increasing reinforced responding in the test (Seiden et al. 1985). Consequently, the neurotransmitter basis of the phenomenon has not yet been clarified.

Isolation-induced hyperactivity. When rats were housed individually as soon as they were weaned, they were found to be hyperactive as adults when tested in a novel environment. Garzon and Del Rio (1981; Garzon et al. 1979) found this hyperactivity (i.e., increased activity of isolated rats relative to nonisolated rats) to be attenuated or abolished by TCAs (i.e., amitriptyline, clomipramine, DMI), MAOIs (i.e., phenelzine, clorgiline), and atypical antidepressants (i.e., iprindole, mianserin, trazodone). The hyperactivity of isolated rats was not affected by antipsychotic medication (i.e., chlorpromazine, haloperidol), anxiolytics (i.e., chlordiazepoxide, diazepam), and amphetamine.

These investigators have tested several drugs in an attempt to elucidate the neurotransmitter mechanism underlying the hyperactivity. The activity difference between isolated and nonisolated rats is abolished by the postsynaptic dopamine receptor agonist apomorphine and also by higher doses of nomifensine, which blocks dopamine as well as nor-

epinephrine reuptake. Interestingly, the lowest dose of nomifensine used (5 mg/kg intraperitoneally) markedly increased the difference between isolated and nonisolated animals. Hyperactivity of isolated animals was also blocked by cyproheptadine, a serotonin receptor antagonist, as well as by salbutamol, a β-adrenergic receptor stimulant. Based on this array of pharmacological results, the nature of isolation-induced hyperactivity does not appear easily explained in relation to any one particular monoamine. All of the drug effects described here were seen with acute administration. One potential concern in the use of this testing procedure, which was emphasized by the investigators and considered throughout their studies, is that many of the drugs used will affect motor activity of normal (i.e., nonisolated) animals, so that drugs can eliminate differences between isolated and nonisolated animals by either markedly increasing or decreasing activity in general. Care must therefore be taken to use drug doses that do not considerably change normal motor patterns when this model is employed.

■ Summary Observations Regarding Animal Assay Models

Animal assays are, almost by definition, useful (or not useful) depending on their ability to screen for drugs or other potential treatments for depression. As is observed from the preceding descriptions, many of these models detect antidepressant medication when the drug is administered acutely. The first observation that can be made is that, although this might at first appear to be a deficiency because antidepressant medication is effective in patients only after repeated administration, it may not be so in an animal assay model. A drug screen can be viewed as most useful if it specifically detects effective antidepressant medication when the drug is given only once, and is therefore highly efficient. In evaluating animal assays, it should be kept in mind that such assays use responses of animals, whether behavioral or physiological, in a manner that is not different from an in vitro assay; that is, the response of the animal, even if it is a behavioral one, is no more than a "readout" of drug action. As researchers increasingly require that the drug mimic the effects observed in human patients (i.e., effectiveness only when administered chronically), they are effectively moving toward criteria that are applicable to homologous models, and requiring the behavioral response of the animal to resemble the behavioral response of the depressed patient. Consequently, an animal assay that responds to acute administration of a treatment is as useful, and perhaps more useful, than one that requires chronic administration of the treatment.

Lesioning of the olfactory bulbs produces one of the more interesting models described under the category of animal assays. This model has one of the best profiles for detection of known antidepressants, responding to TCAs and atypical antidepressants as well as to 5-HT uptake blockers, whereas stimulants (amphetamine) as well as the anticholinergic atropine were ineffective; however, the single MAOI that was tested, tranylcypromine, was ineffective. The ability of olfactory bulbectomy to act as a screen for antidepressant medication may appear anomalous at first given the nature of the manipulation, but studies have determined that neurotransmitter changes resulting from lesions of the olfactory bulbs may account for the ability of this seemingly unusual procedure to generate a model relevant to depression. For instance, all effective TCAs potentiate the effects of released norepinephrine by blocking reuptake (e.g., Richelson and Pfenning 1984), which was a key observation that led to the catecholamine hypothesis of depression (Bunney and Davis 1965; Schildkraut and Kety 1967). This hypothesis originally proposed that a deficit in brain norepinephrine, which noradrenergic reuptake blockers and MAOIs corrected, was responsible for depression. Lesioning of the olfactory bulbs produces a marked depletion of norepinephrine in the forebrain, possibly by interruption of noradrenergic axons as they course by the olfactory bulbs in projecting to the neocortex (Cairncross et al. 1973, 1975a). Moreover, Shipley and colleagues (1985) reported that 40% of neurons of the LC project to the rat olfactory bulb, which is 10 times as many LC cells as project to any other part of the cerebral cortex; consequently, altered activity of a significant number of the noradrenergic cells that innervate the forebrain is likely to follow a lesion of the olfactory bulbs.

But, as could be expected, the consequences of bulbectomy are not simple. Lesions of the olfactory bulbs affect not only norepinephrine but also serotonergic, cholinergic, and γ-aminobutyric acid (GABA)-ergic systems (see review by Leonard and Tuite 1981). Moreover, the behavioral effects of bulbectomy cannot be reproduced simply by reducing forebrain norepinephrine. This last point was made in a particularly illuminating series of experiments by Archer and colleagues (1984), who used the drug DSP-4 to destroy forebrain noradrenergic terminals on axons of LC cells and found that this procedure did not mimic effects seen after olfactory bulbectomy. In contrast to manipulating noradrenergic systems, Cairncross and colleagues administered neurotoxins that destroy serotonergic neurons (i.e., 5,6- and 5,7-dihydroxytrytamine) and produced behavioral effects similar to those seen with bulbectomy (reviewed in Cairncross et al. 1979), which suggests that the deficit induced by bulbectomy might be serotonergic in nature. However, Leonard and Tuite (1981) have argued that the effects of these neurotoxins are notably smaller in magnitude than those produced by bulbectomy. When we also consider that these effects of serotonergic neurotoxins can be reversed by treatment with mianserin (Wren 1976, reported in Leonard and Tuite 1981), a drug that blocks α_2-adrenergic receptors (Robson et al. 1978), it appears that, at the least, both norepinephrine and serotonin need to be considered in the eventual resolution of how the bulbectomy model is generated.

■ Homologous Models

As was stated previously, the models discussed in this section represent those in which the animal shows responses similar to those seen in clinical depression. Inclusion of the model in this section does not require the symptom profile to be extensive—the animal may manifest only one particular response that appears similar to what is seen in clinical depression—although animal models included here may also reproduce a number of changes, behavioral or physiological, that can be related to depressive responses.

Reserpine-induced reduction of motor activity. Reserpine and reserpine-like compounds, such as tetrabenazine, inactivate the ability of synaptic vesicles to retain monoamines; as a consequence of this action, release of monoamines follows administration of these drugs, and there is then a long-term reduction in monoamine stores, resulting in depletion of dopamine norepinephrine, epinephrine, and serotonin in the brain and periphery. The depletion of amines produces a variety of physiological and behavioral effects, and antidepressants have been shown to counteract a number of these. Domenjoz and Theobald (1959) first reported that imipramine could block the ability of reserpine to potentiate hypnotic effects. Costa and colleagues (1960) then reported that reserpine-induced decreases in rectal temperature and heart rate and increases in diarrhea and ptosis were blocked by imipramine. These effects would ordinarily cause this model to be classified as an animal assay, but reserpine will also decrease motor activity, and antidepressants will counteract this effect as well. Vernier and colleagues (1962) reported that imipramine would antagonize reserpine-induced sedation, which was quantified largely by decreased motor activity. In addition to imipramine, other TCAs also antagonize reserpine-induced (or tetrabenazine-induced) depression of motor activity. MAOIs have a similar effect (Howard et al. 1981). The "reserpinized rodent" constitutes one of the earliest animal models of depression. The observation that reserpine suppresses motor activity was apparently a key factor in suggesting the catecholamine hypothesis of depression.

Given the ability of TCAs and MAOIs to potentiate the action of monoamines, in retrospect it is not surprising that these substances antagonize the effects of reserpine on a variety of responses, including reserpine's ability to depress motor activity. On the other hand, a variety of compounds that do not appear to be effective antidepressant medications, such as amphetamine and cocaine, also yield positive results in antagonizing reserpine-induced reduction of motor activity. Thus, this test apparently detects the ability of a treatment or drug to potentiate central aminergic transmission rather than its specificity for antidepressant action. The effects described here are also seen with acute administration of drug, rather than requiring chronic administration. Finally, the test is not known to detect non-TCAs such as iprindole.

Depression of active responding induced by 5-hydroxtryptophan. Based on early studies suggesting that lysergic acid diethylamide (LSD) produced psychoactive effects by interacting with serotonergic receptors, Aprison hypothesized that serotonin might be importantly involved in behavioral states. Consequently, Aprison and colleagues injected the serotonin precursor 5-hydroxytryptophan (5-HTP) into pigeons, and subsequently rats, and observed that the treatment produced marked suppression of active responding for food reinforcement (summa-

rized in Aprison et al. 1978). This reduction in active behavior seen following increased 5-HT release due to administration of 5-HTP was blocked by TCAs (i.e., amitriptyline, imipramine) as well as non-TCAs (i.e., mianserin, iprindole) (Nagayama et al. 1981). Two features of the model do not reproduce what is seen in depression: 1) acute administration of the antidepressants was effective in blocking the behavioral depression, and 2) drugs that block 5-HT reuptake (e.g., fluoxetine) increased 5-HTP–induced behavioral depression markedly (Nagayama et al. 1980), so that this class of antidepressants exacerbates rather than prevents depression in this model.

Swim test immobility. A test proposed by Porsolt and colleagues involves placing a rodent (a rat or mouse) into a beaker of water and determining the amount of time that the animal remains immobile. The typical procedure that has been used is to place the animal in the tank for 15 minutes on day 1; as a result of this exposure, active coping attempts are extinguished so that the animal ceases movement by the end of the session. The following day, the animal is returned to the water tank for 5 minutes where immobility is timed. Between the first and second exposure to the swim tank, the drug (or other treatment) is given, often a single drug administration shortly before the immobility test, or 2–3 drug administrations during the 24 hours between the first and second exposures to the swim tank. Effective antidepressants cause animals to show less immobility on the second (test) exposure than is shown by vehicle-treated or untreated animals. The test situation with an animal showing the immobile response is illustrated in Figure 5–1.

This test detects a wide range of antidepressant treatments, including all TCAs tested (i.e., imipramine, DMI, amitriptyline, nortriptyline), MAOIs (i.e., nialamide, iproniazid), atypical antidepressants (i.e., iprindole, mianserin, nomifensine), and ECT (Porsolt et al. 1978; see also review by Borsini and Meli 1988). Deprivation of REM (rapid eye movement) sleep, which is therapeutic in depression, is also detected by this test (Hawkins et al. 1980). The test does not respond to anxiolytics or phenothiazines. However, it will show false positives to a variety of different substances (for a complete list, see De Pablo et al. 1989), particularly stimulants (i.e., amphetamine and caffeine). Also, a significant weakness of this test, given the current preference for antidepressant med-

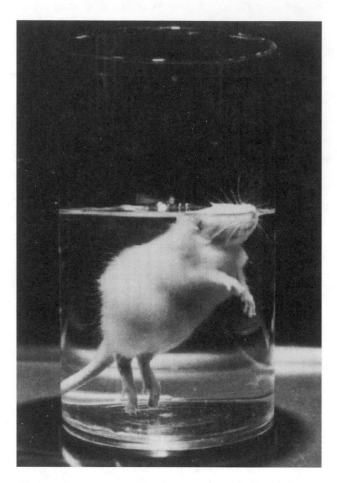

Figure 5–1. Rat showing characteristic posture of immobility.
Source. Reproduced with permission of Raven Press from Porsolt RD: Behavioral despair, in *Antidepressants: Neurochemical, Behavioral, and Clinical Perspectives.* Edited by Enna SJ, Malick JB, Richardson E. New York, Raven, 1981, p 121.

ication, is its poor detection of SSRIs, which was noted early on by Porsolt and colleagues (1979; Satoh et al. 1984).

Perhaps because of its ease of use and ability to detect drugs of antidepressant potential, the Porsolt swim test is currently the most widely used pharmacological test for antidepressants. A number of interesting and significant characteristics have been discovered regarding this model. First, drugs work when given acutely, which does not reproduce the clinical efficacy of antidepressant drugs that require repeated administration. However, larger effects are often seen when drugs have been given repeatedly before testing. (In this regard, the effects of SSRIs need to be assessed after chronic administration of drug.) Second, although the test was initially de-

scribed as "behavioral despair," there is little evidence that exposure of animals to this test situation produces a significant degree of anything that might be called despair. Rather, immobility in the standard test situation appears to be explained, at least in part, by the animal's learning to adopt an immobile posture with the rear feet or tail balanced on the bottom of the swim tank, thereby supporting the head above the top of the water (see Figure 5–1; also see De Pablo et al. 1989; Hawkins et al. 1978). Thus, effective drugs appear to cause the animal on the test day to attempt active behavior instead of continuing to practice a previously learned immobile posture. Modifications of the original test situation using deeper water to prevent the animal from standing on the bottom of the tank have been employed in several situations (e.g., Abel 1991; De Pablo et al. 1989; Weiss et al. 1981); under these conditions, the immobility that is measured represents more unambiguously a loss of motivation to engage in active coping attempts than is the case when the animal can partially resolve its dilemma by standing on the floor of the tank. Third, although "despair" has not been shown to characterize the model, stress may well be involved in the model's ability to detect antidepressant effects. Borsini and colleagues (1989) showed that the initial exposure of the rat to the swim tank, although typically done to extinguish active behavior, produces consequences similar to those produced by known stressors (i.e., cold, restraint, footshock), and that exposing the rat to the swim tank on the day before the test considerably enhances the capacity of the test to detect antidepressants. Thus, the swim test, as usually conducted, appears to determine how treatments counteract "stress-induced" immobility. Fourth, antidepressant medication particularly increases "escape-like" motor activity that occurs early in the swim test, which can be discriminated from general increases in motor activity that can be detected late in swim tests of long duration (Armario et al. 1988; Kitada et al. 1981). This establishes a way to discriminate between antidepressant action and nonspecific stimulation of motor activity in the swim test.

Various investigators have examined the neurochemical basis of swim test immobility, studying antidepressant-treated animals to try to uncover mechanisms of drug action as well as nondrugged animals to obtain possible clues to neurophysiological pathology underlying depression. In non–drug-treated rodents, depression-like behavior (i.e., swim test immobility) was increased by potentiating cholinergic transmission (Hasey and Hanin 1991) and blocking catecholamine synthesis with α-methyl-*p*-tyrosine (Gil et al. 1992). To decrease swim test immobility, several investigators have focused, not surprisingly, on brain dopamine, prominently related to motor activity. Activity in the swim test has been increased by 1) blocking dopamine reuptake and stimulating D_2 receptors (Borsini et al. 1988), 2) stimulating the ventral tegmental cell bodies projecting to forebrain dopaminergic regions (Plaznik et al. 1985a), and 3) infusing into the nucleus accumbens norepinephrine, phenylephrine ($α_1$ receptor stimulant), isoproterenol (β-adrenergic receptor stimulant), and apomorphine (dopamine receptor stimulant) (Plaznik et al. 1985b). Plaznik and colleagues (1985a) have argued that only the noradrenergic manipulations specifically affect activity in the swim test that represents escape-like responses, whereas stimulation of dopamine directly decreases swim test immobility by increasing motor activity in general. Finally, Murua and Molina (1990) suggest that opiate mechanisms may be involved in producing immobility, having found that naloxone reduced immobility in stressed rats.

Regarding the mechanism of action of antidepressant drugs, studies using the swim test have focused on analyzing DMI's mode of action. The therapeutic (anti-immobility) effect of DMI in the swim test can be blocked by the dopamine receptor (D_2) antagonist sulpiride (Cervo and Samanin 1987) and lesions of the LC (by the neurotoxin 6-hydroxydopamine) (Plaznik et al. 1985a). The latter finding indicates that norepinephrine is essential for the therapeutic effect of DMI, perhaps not surprising given the extreme potency with which DMI blocks norepinephrine reuptake (Richelson and Pfenning 1984). Kitada and colleagues (1986) showed that pharmacological stimulation of adrenergic β receptors attenuated the anti-immobility effects of DMI, therefore suggesting that the essential function of norepinephrine in DMI's therapeutic effect is to downregulate β receptors, a long-held theory regarding why certain antidepressants are effective (Sulser 1979; Vetulani et al. 1976).

Clonidine withdrawal. Whereas acute administration of the drug clonidine causes rats to be inactive in the swim test, it is also possible to produce long-lasting inactivity in this test in drug-free animals. A procedure to accomplish this was reported by Hoffman and Weiss (1986). When clonidine was administered to rats for 2 weeks and was then abruptly withdrawn, the animals, which were now drug-free, showed a depression of activity in the swim test that lasted for several weeks. The long-lasting nature of this reduction in motor activity permits examination of the effects of long-term treatment regimens. Only DMI has been tested to date. When given daily for 2 weeks, DMI reversed the depression of swim test activity seen in this model; when chronic DMI administration was halted, activity in the swim test again became depressed. It was also observed that DMI did not increase swim test activity after being given for only 1 day. Further studies of this model have not been conducted.

Tail suspension test. When a mouse is suspended in the air by its tail, it will struggle to free itself. Steru and colleagues (1985) reported that antidepressant drugs increase the amount of time spent in such struggling. Struggling is increased by TCAs, MAOIs, and atypical antidepressants but is not increased by neuroleptics, anxiolytics, or anticholinergics. However, struggling time is also increased by psychostimulants (dextroamphetamine). Drugs work in this test when given acutely, and consequently this model has been proposed to be, and has been used exclusively as, a screening technique for pharmacological treatments. However, because effective treatments counteract a form of immobility (i.e., cessation of struggling), the test is thought to be related to the Porsolt swim test and is therefore listed here as a homologous model.

Neonatal clomipramine. In this model, rat pups are injected with clomipramine (15 mg/kg) twice daily on postnatal days 8 through 21. When tested at 90+ days of age, these animals show decreased sexual activity, intracranial self-stimulation, aggressive behavior, and motor hyperactivity in a novel situation (Hartley et al. 1990; Neill et al. 1990; Vogel et al. 1990a). Relative to control animals that had been injected neonatally with saline, clomipramine-injected rats also show changes in sleep behavior that have been associated with depression, including reduced latency to enter REM sleep following sleep onset and frequent onset of REM periods (Vogel et al. 1988, 1990b). Based on these behavioral effects, the investigators who developed the procedure proposed it as a means to model endogenous, as opposed to reactive, depression (Vogel et al. 1990c). One drawback to this model appears to be the hyperactivity evidenced by the animals in that patients manifesting "endogenous" depression are likely to be the most seriously affected who will show psychomotor retardation rather than hyperactivity. Testing of treatment efficacy on this model has been very limited; preliminary data were given (Vogel et al. 1990c) showing that imipramine treatment for 4 days reduced locomotor hyperactivity of the animals treated neonatally with clomipramine. Although this treatment uses an inducing stimulus that seems to have little relation to whatever normal physiological conditions may give rise to susceptibility to depression, the hypothesis offered by the investigators is that a physiological defect is present in endogenous depression, and administering clomipramine neonatally somehow reproduces this defect.

Lesioning of the dorsomedial amygdala in dogs.
When the dorsomedial amygdala is lesioned electrolytically in dogs, one of the most dramatic syndromes resembling severe depression is produced. Fonberg has reported that these animals display lethargy, negativism, reluctance to eat, and, to the extent that this can be judged in a dog, saddened facial expression (Fonberg 1969a, 1969b; summarized in Fonberg 1972). In terms of symptom profile, the appearance of these animals ranks with the "monkey separation" model (see next section) as producing the most similarity to what is observed in severe retarded depression (see Figure 5–2). The effect of antidepressant medication on this syndrome has not yet been reported. Despite its dramatic appearance, the model has been little studied, and perhaps is likely to remain so given the problems of using dogs as subjects. Also, some questions can be raised as to its relevance. Fonberg has reported that lesioning of the lateral hypothalamus, which is now well known to disturb dopaminergic axons ascending to the striatum and frontal brain, produces in the dog a similar phenomenon, which raises the question of whether the dorsolateral amygdala lesions simply produce a variant of the "lateral hypothalamic syndrome" that is produced by lesioning of dopamine inputs of the basal ganglia. If this is the case, it would mean that either the model is unrelated to clinical depression, or the resemblance of these dogs' symptoms to those seen in very severe retarded depression indicates that

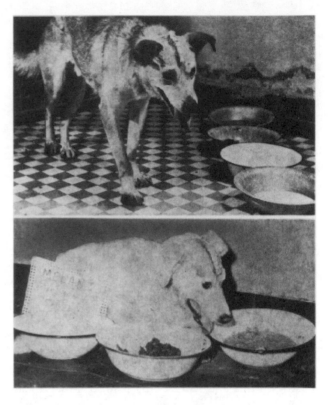

Figure 5–2. Two dogs (upper and lower) after bilateral dorsomedial amygdala damage. Note the animals' lack of interest in the various kinds of food presented, and their sad appearance.

Source. Reproduced with permission of the Ciba Foundation from Fonberg E: Control of emotional behaviour through the hypothalamus and amygdaloid complex. *Ciba Found Symp* 8:132, 1972.

clinical depression involves disturbance of these dopaminergic systems, which is simply seen in extreme form when the brain lesions are made in the dogs.

Isolation/separation-induced depression in monkeys. Behavioral responses that appear similar to those seen in severe depression have been elicited by separating young monkeys from their mothers and normal social setting or from their juvenile peers. Following separation, animals initially display high activity accompanied by much vocalization; this is labeled as the stage of "agitation" or "protest" and usually lasts 24–36 hours. Following this, the behavior pattern changes markedly, with the animal then showing decreased activity, huddling and self-clasping, dejected and saddened facial expression, and generally decreased activity and exploration

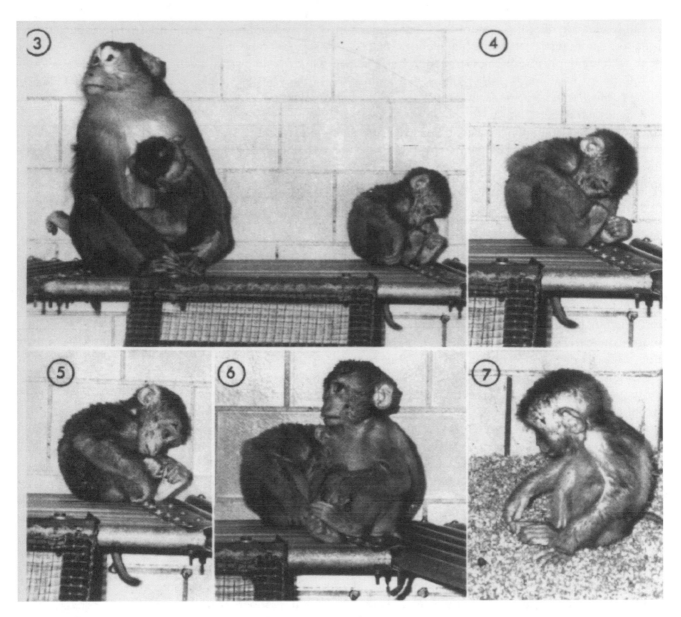

Figure 5–3. Depressed pigtail infant showing characteristic hunched-over posture with flexion throughout. He is completely disengaged from the mother and infant nearby who are in ventral-ventral contact.

Figure 5–4. Depressed pigtail infant showing characteristic posture including head between legs. Note slightly opened eyes as he sucks his penis.

Figure 5–5. Depressed pigtail infant showing characteristic posture and dejected facies.

Figure 5–6. Two depressed pigtail infants. The one in rear shows characteristic hunched-over posture. The one in front has lifted his head to look across pen. Despite their passive contact, they are quite disengaged from each other.

Figure 5–7. Depressed infant showing aimless, tentative exploration of bedding during early stages of recovery.

Source. Reproduced with permission of Williams & Wilkins from Kaufman IC, Rosenblum LA: The reaction to separation in infant monkeys: anaclitic depression and conservation-withdrawal. *Psychosom Med* 29:655, 1967.

(e.g., Kaufman and Rosenblum 1967; McKinney et al. 1971) (see Figures 5–3 through 5–7). This constellation of depressive-type behaviors can persist for 5 or 6 days before gradually remitting; however, in some cases, it lasts even longer. Depression-related behaviors are diminished by long-term administration of imipramine, and symptoms reappear if the drug is withheld (Suomi et al. 1978). Also, the drug appears not to work soon after it is administered but requires long-term administration, thus paralleling what is seen with antidepressant administration in humans.

Studies exploring underlying biochemical changes in this model are of interest. Kraemer and colleagues (Kraemer 1986) have shown that animals that are isolated for long periods of time have norepinephrine levels in the cerebrospinal fluid (CSF) that are approximately half the levels seen in normal animals. These investigators have also reported that animals having low CSF levels of norepinephrine are more susceptible to depressive-like symptoms when separated than are animals with higher levels of norepinephrine. Porsolt and colleagues (1984) also reported that acute administration of imipramine, which blocks norepinephrine reuptake, increased both motor activity and vocalizations during the protest stage, making responses during this initial stage more extreme. These data suggest that norepinephrine and adrenergic receptors in the brain are importantly involved in this type of depression, suggesting such hypotheses as 1) decreased CSF norepinephrine in susceptible animals is indicative of low norepinephrine release and, consequently, supersensitive adrenergic receptors in these animals, or 2) animals prone to depression, having low CSF norepinephrine, are vulnerable to norepinephrine depletion in the brain when subjected to stress, which results in depression.

Separation of Siberian hamsters. Siberian dwarf hamsters (*phodopus sungorus pallas*) form stable male-female mating pairs that ordinarily remain together even after pups are born, with the male participating in rearing activities. Crawley (1984) developed a model in which Siberian hamster pairs, maintained in the laboratory, were separated 3–4 weeks after they had formed mating pairs, and thereafter the animals were housed in individual cages. During the period after separation (3–4 weeks was generally monitored), the male hamsters showed decreased daily running-wheel activity, decreased activity when tested in an open field, increased body weight, and decreased social interaction when an unfamiliar animal of the opposite sex was introduced into the cage. Separated females showed a smaller decrease in running-wheel activity but no change in the other measures. All of these changes could be reversed by reuniting the separated pair. The changes in behavior described here could not be attributed to

the isolation (i.e., single housing) of animals after separation because similar changes were not seen in animals that had been maintained in single-sex groups and were then individually housed. Effects of one antidepressant, imipramine, were tested in this model. Administration of imipramine (10 mg/kg) daily for 2 weeks following separation eliminated a number of activity-related changes shown by male hamsters in the open field (but not total distance traversed in the open field). Imipramine administration also did not eliminate the increase in body weight or the decrease in social interaction with an unfamiliar animal of the other sex. Regarding neurochemical differences, males were found to show evidence of decreased 5-HT turnover (possibly decreased release), as indicated by lower 5-hydroxyindoleacetic acid (5-HIAA)/5-HT ratios in cortex, diencephalon, and mesencephalon (Crawley 1983). Further studies of this model have not been reported.

Exhaustion stress. Hatotani and colleagues (1982) exposed female rats to forced running in an activity wheel until the animals were exhausted, as indicated by rectal temperature reaching 33° C or less. After exposure to three sessions of forced running, each separated by a 24-hour rest period, spontaneous motor activity in the rats was markedly depressed for several weeks. This depression of motor activity was marked by complete suppression of the diurnal peaks in spontaneous motor activity seen in nonstressed animals. Motor activity was returned to normal by daily injections of imipramine; a therapeutic response was seen only after the drug was administered for longer than 10 days. The other characteristic described for this model is that a marked increase in intensity of histochemical fluorescence of noradrenergic cell bodies in the brain accompanies the exhaustion-induced decrease in motor activity, thereby indicating that activation of noradrenergic neurons in the brain appears to be increased by the exhaustion-stress procedure. Conversely, fluorescence of dopamine neurons of the tuberoinfundibular system in the hypothalamus was much weaker in stressed animals, which was thought to indicate decreased activity in these dopaminergic neurons.

Chronic mild stress model. First introduced by Katz, Roth, and Carroll, this model is generated by exposing rats to a succession of different stressful conditions over a period of either 2 weeks (Roth and

Katz 1981) or 3 weeks (Katz et al. 1981a), stressful conditions consisting of mild uncontrollable foot-shock, cold swim, changing of housing conditions, reversal of light and dark periods, and food and water deprivation. The sequence of stressors is concluded with exposure to noise at 95 decibels and bright light for 1 hour, followed by testing of spontaneous motor activity in an open field; the effect measured in these studies is a decrease in open-field activity seen in chronically stressed animals relative to animals that have not been exposed to the chronic stress regimen. Although changes were sometimes of small magnitude (20%–30% relative to nonstressed animals), a reduction in open-field activity nevertheless reliably characterized chronically stressed animals in a number of studies. Katz and colleagues principally analyzed effects of treatment (Katz 1981; Katz and Baldrighi 1982; Katz and Hersh 1981; Katz and Sibel 1982a, 1982b; Katz et al. 1981b). They showed that the decrease in activity in the open field could be reduced by TCAs (i.e., imipramine, amitriptyline), an MAOI (i.e., tranylcypromine), atypical antidepressants (i.e., mianserin, bupropion, iprindole), and ECT, and was not consistently reversed by an anticholinergic, antihistaminic, anxiolytic, or neuroleptic drug. This profile indicated that the decreased activity in the open field produced by "chronic stress" is selectively responsive to antidepressant medications. Katz and colleagues also reported that stress-induced elevations in corticosteroids were antagonized by antidepressant medication.

An interesting effect reported in one paper of the series has been followed up by a considerable amount of research because of its hypothesized relevance to depression. Katz (1982) reported that the chronic stress regimen decreased the hedonic value of a stimulus, and that this change could be reversed by treatment with imipramine. It was found in this study that normal rats would ingest increasingly larger amounts of fluid that contained progressively larger concentrations of sucrose or saccharin, but that greater consumption of more palatable solutions was not seen when consumption was measured within 24–48 hours after conclusion of the 3-week chronic stress regimen. When chronically stressed rats were treated with imipramine during the 3-week stress procedure, the amount of sucrose solution they ingested was equivalent to that ingested by unstressed animals, although the interpretation of this therapeutic effect is complicated by the fact that the imipra-

mine treatment decreased saccharin consumption in the control animals that were exposed to no stress at all. Nevertheless, these results indicate that the tendency of rats to take in larger than normal amounts of a palatable solution was reduced by the chronic stress regimen.

Subsequent studies have followed up on this result on the assumption that it may model what Klein (1975) has termed the principal characteristic of depression: the inability to experience pleasurable events. Reward and hedonic effects have been related to the dopaminergic system of the brain (e.g., Wise and Rompre 1989). Tekes and colleagues (1986) showed that the chronic stress regimen decreased indicants of dopamine turnover in the brain, and that these changes in dopamine turnover were antagonized by chronic treatment with a TCA (amitriptyline) and an MAOI (deprenyl). Moreau and colleagues (1992) found that a similar stress regimen increased the threshold for electrical self-stimulation through electrodes in the ventral tegmental area of the brain (dopamine cell body region), and that this reduction in self-stimulation was countered by DMI. Willner and colleagues (Muscat et al. 1988, 1990, 1992; Sampson et al. 1991; Willner et al. 1992) have published a number of studies showing that chronic mild stress decreases intake of palatable solutions, that these effects can be counteracted by treatment with antidepressants, and that chronic stress alters dopamine turnover and dopamine receptors in the brain. Although these studies make clear that the chronic stress regimen does alter various aspects of dopaminergic systems in the brain, the interpretation of changes in intake that were observed is more ambiguous. For example, studies do not appear to demonstrate that animals exposed to the chronic stress regimen ever lose their preference for palatable substances (e.g., sucrose, saccharin) in comparison with tap water; but, rather, only the degree to which they will overconsume these palatable substances in comparison with tap water decreases in animals exposed to chronic stress. Thus, it is not evident that the chronic stress regimen has not simply decreased total consumption rather than affecting preference. It is well known that stressful conditions will decrease consumption of both food and liquid (e.g., Pare 1965; Weiss 1968). From the clinical perspective, the emphasis of these studies on the dopaminergic system raises the question of why antidepressants that preferentially potentiate dopaminergic transmission (e.g., bupropion) appear to be no faster acting or better (and perhaps less so) than classic TCAs that block norepinephrine uptake or SSRIs.

Uncontrollable shock (or the "learned helplessness") model. In the late 1960s, several studies showed that exposing animals, both rats as well as dogs, to electric shocks that they could not control resulted in quite different responses than were seen in animals that received the same shocks while having control over them. Seligman, Maier, and Solomon found that exposing dogs to uncontrollable shock made the animals unable to acquire an active (shuttle) avoidance-escape response (Overmier and Seligman 1967; Seligman and Maier 1967; Seligman et al. 1971). At the same time, Weiss (1968) observed that exposure of rats to uncontrollable shock decreased subsequent food and water intake in the home cage and caused body weight loss, these changes being virtually absent in animals that received the same shocks while exerting control over them. In these studies, the rats also became more fearful after receiving uncontrollable shock than they did after receiving controllable shock. In the mid-1970s, both Seligman and Maier found that the avoidance-escape deficit resulting from uncontrollable shock could be produced in rats and dogs (Maier et al. 1973; Seligman and Beagley 1975). In 1974, Seligman hypothesized that exposure to uncontrollable events produces a depression-like response, and that exposure of animals to uncontrollable shock therefore constituted a model for the study of depression. Subsequently, Weiss and colleagues (1981) showed that uncontrollable shock, but not controllable shock, decreased active behavior and increased immobility in a swim test. Figure 5–8 shows an experimental setting that generates this model.

Perhaps because it has been studied more widely than any other, the uncontrollable shock model has been found to reproduce the largest list of symptoms found in human depression. In 1982, Weiss and colleagues listed the various effects of uncontrollable shock and showed that these symptoms correspond closely with those listed in DSM-III, which was then the standard for diagnosis of depression in humans. The symptoms produced by uncontrollable shock now include 1) decreases in food and water consumption, 2) loss of body weight, 3) loss of ability to initiate normal active behavior, 4) loss of normal grooming activity, 5) loss of normal competitiveness

and play-like activities, 6) alteration of sleep patterns, particularly marked by early morning awakening, 7) loss of responding for rewarding brain stimulation, and 8) increased errors in discrimination tasks (for references, see Weiss 1991).

Responsivity to antidepressant treatment of animals exposed to uncontrollable shock has been examined by various investigators. All studies concerned with this issue have measured the ability of antidepressant treatment to reverse the deficit in avoidance-escape performance produced by uncontrollable shock. Poor performance of active avoidance-escape responses following uncontrollable shock was first reported to be reversed by DMI (Leshner et al. 1979) and then by nortriptyline (Telner and Singhal 1981). Sherman and colleagues (1982) then conducted a large study in which the avoidance-escape deficit was reversed by a wide variety of antidepressant medications—including TCAs, atypical antidepressants, and MAOIs—and ECT, whereas it was not corrected by stimulants or antipsychotic medications. Martin and colleagues have also found deficits to be reversed by SSRIs (P. Martin et al. 1990) as well as TCAs and MAOIs (P. Martin et al. 1987). In these studies, drugs have generally been given for only 1–3 days between the uncontrollable shock and testing, although Leshner and colleagues tested effects after 7 days of drug administration. Although this might suggest beneficial effects of acute drug administration, Telner and Singhal (1981) reported no effects early in drug administration but positive effects later. A difficulty with establishing efficacy after long-term (i.e., 2 weeks) drug administration is that the symptoms in this model tend to dissipate (see last paragraph in this section).

Regarding the pathophysiology that underlies the behavioral symptoms produced by uncontrollable shock, investigations have again focused on reduced motor activity produced by uncontrollable shock. Studies of the physiological mechanism underlying this deficit have been extensive, with disturbance of central noradrenergic, serotonergic, cholinergic, GABAergic systems and endorphins and enkephalins hypothesized by different investigators to be responsible for the deficit. Of these various formulations, the most well-developed hypotheses are those emphasizing disturbance of norepinephrine and 5-HT; these hypotheses not only are based on data showing that pharmacological manipulation of these systems can produce and/or reverse the behavioral deficit, but,

**Avoidance/Escape
(Controlling Stressor)**   **Yoked
(No Control Over Stressor)**   **Box Condition
(No Stressor)**

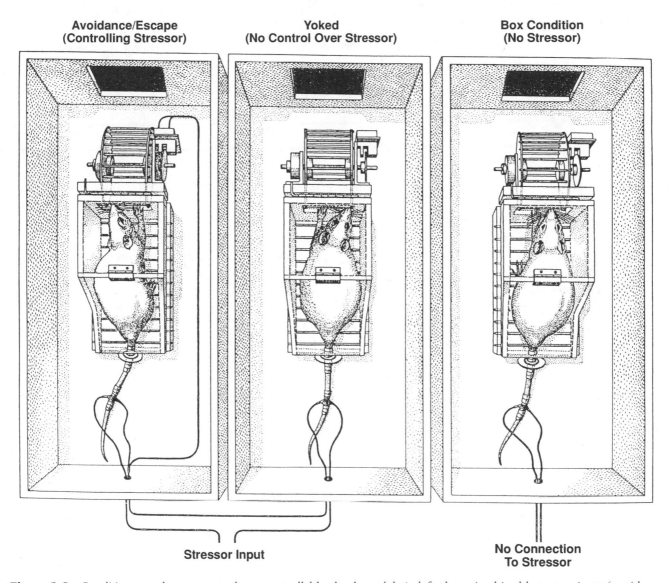

Stressor Input   **No Connection
To Stressor**

Figure 5–8. Conditions used to generate the uncontrollable-shock model. At left, the animal is able to terminate (avoid and/or escape) the stressor (electric shock to the tail) by turning the wheel at the front of its box enclosure, while at center the "yoked" animal receives exactly the same shocks (through fixed tail electrodes wired in series with the avoidance-escape animal), but none of its wheel-turn responses have any effect on shock. At the right, the "no-stressor" animal simply remains in the box apparatus with no tail-shock stressor being received throughout the procedure. Subsequent to this procedure, the yoked animal at center shows depression-related behavioral changes, while the avoidance-escape and box-condition animals do not show these behavioral changes.

Source. Reprinted with permission of Elsevier Science Publishers B.V. from Weiss JM, Goodman PA, Losito BG, et al: Behavioral depression produced by an uncontrollable stressor: relationship to norepinephrine, dopamine, and serotonin levels in various regions of the rat brain. *Brain Research Reviews* 3:173, 1981.

most importantly, also include studies showing that uncontrollable shock alters the implicated neurotransmitter system to produce changes potentially able to mediate the behavioral deficit observed after shock.

The hypothesis relating effects of uncontrollable shock to noradrenergic changes is the most detailed and specific one offered at present. It states that strong uncontrollable shock depletes norepinephrine in terminals of the LC region, which causes increased burst firing of LC cells by reducing transmitter available to stimulate inhibitory somatodendritic α_2 receptors on LC cell bodies (summarized in Weiss 1991). Thus, this formulation attributes depression produced by uncontrollable shock to disinhibition (which results in increased activity) of LC neurons.

These findings in turn suggest that depressive symptomatology in the uncontrollable shock model results from an excess of norepinephrine released in the terminal regions to which the LC neurons project (e.g., hippocampus, cortex, forebrain), which would be the presumed consequence of hyperactivity of LC neurons. It can also be noted that this formulation appears to complement the findings of Henn and colleagues, who reported that β-adrenergic receptors are upregulated in animals that are susceptible to the behavior-depressing effects of uncontrollable shock (Henn et al. 1985; J. V. Martin et al. 1990). Both higher-than-normal release of norepinephrine from LC terminals and upregulated β receptors would potentiate postsynaptic noradrenergic activity.

The data relating 5-HT to deficits produced by uncontrollable shock are currently less clear than those supporting the noradrenergic hypothesis. Although serotonergic receptors are altered by uncontrollable shock (J. V. Martin et al. 1990), the investigators who have studied these changes point out they do not appear well correlated with the behavioral deficit. Also, the data are contradictory regarding whether 5-HT release in the brain is increased (Edwards et al. 1992; Petty et al. 1990) or decreased (Petty and Sherman 1983) as a consequence of uncontrollable shock. Thus, 5-HT seems affected, but the nature of the change is unclear.

Finally, it should be mentioned that deficits in responding for electrical (rewarding) brain stimulation that occur after uncontrollable shock seem related to changes in dopaminergic mesocorticolimbic regions (e.g., Zacharko and Anisman 1991).

A significant drawback to the uncontrollable shock model is that most of the depression-like symptoms produced in the model (described previously in this section) do not last beyond 48–72 hours after exposure to uncontrollable shock; in some instances, the loss of symptoms at about this time is rather abrupt (e.g., Desan et al. 1988; Overmier and Seligman 1967; Weiss et al. 1981; Zacharko et al. 1983). Although the lack of persistence of the symptoms appears to be a deficiency in this model, it may be a clue to the model's underlying pathophysiology. Weiss and colleagues (1981) noted that the disappearance of behavioral depression at 2–3 days postshock corresponds to the time at which the enzyme tyrosine hydroxylase, whose activity is the primary determinant of norepinephrine synthesis, shows a marked increase specifically in the LC. Thus,

salient behavioral symptoms disappear at the same time as a rise in norepinephrine synthesis capacity occurs in the LC, based on a well-known biochemical correlate of the habituation (i.e., induction of tyrosine hydroxylase) in that brain region. Although induction of tyrosine hydroxylase in the LC is surely only one of many neurophysiological changes occurring at the time when behavior normalizes in animals subjected to uncontrollable shock, the correspondence of these events points to the possibility that specific compensatory changes in noradrenergic systems participate in the cessation of depressive symptomatology. With respect to habituation, the chronic stress model described previously may be an extension of the uncontrollable shock model, which avoids habituation and its therapeutic consequences by continually exposing animals to mild and varied stressors. In this event, the two models would be based on the same fundamental mechanisms.

A final point relevant to this model concerns the controversial issue of interpretation. The model produced by exposure of animals to uncontrollable shock is often called the *learned helplessness* model, a term derived from the original interpretation offered by Seligman, Maier, and colleagues (e.g., Seligman and Maier 1967; Seligman et al. 1971). These investigators hypothesized that the poor avoidance responding following exposure to uncontrollable shock occurred because the animals learned that they were helpless during exposure to the shock, that "nothing I do matters." This cognition was said to cause the various consequences that followed uncontrollable shock; in fact, Seligman's (1974) original hypothesis linking the consequences of uncontrollable shock to depression argued that as evidence of this, depressed individuals made many comments indicative of their feelings of helplessness. In contrast, Weiss (1980; Weiss et al. 1970) and others (e.g., Anisman and Bignami 1978; Anisman et al. 1991) argued that the inference of the "I am helpless" cognition to nonhuman animals was extremely difficult, if not impossible, to test, and that a simpler explanation was available—that exposure to uncontrollable shock (as opposed to shock that can be controlled) is extremely stressful, and the depression-like symptoms observed are produced by this high degree of stress. According to this view, the depression-like symptoms resulting from uncontrollable shock are stress induced. Shortly after this controversy crystallized, the last symptom listed in the second paragraph of this section—that uncontrollable shock causes increased errors in discrimination tasks—was reported. When first described, this finding was thought to demonstrate that exposure to uncontrollable shock diminished an animal's ability to make associations as would be predicted if uncontrollable shock indeed led to a "learned helplessness" cognition (Jackson et al. 1978). However, Minor and colleagues (1984, 1988) carefully analyzed the phenomenon in further studies and found that the deficits in learning ability seen in these experiments could be accounted for by increased emotionality and/or fearfulness produced by uncontrollable shock. These studies linked the effects to changes in the concentration of norepinephrine in the forebrain, thus suggesting that deficits in discrimination learning were produced by a stress-induced change (Minor et al. 1984, 1988). Despite the durability of the "learned helplessness" label for the model discussed here, there is as yet no substantial evidence that the consequences of uncontrollable shock in animals involve a "learned helplessness" cognition.

■ Models Using Selective Breeding (Genetic Selection)

Despite the ability of homologous models to approximate symptoms seen in depression and respond to treatments effective in combating human clinical depression, each of the various models described here nevertheless lacks elements found in the human disorder. For example, the uncontrollable shock model, which appears to reproduce the most complete symptom profile of any animal model of depression, does not generate symptoms that last long enough to model the longevity of human clinical depression; that is, certain significant depression-like features in this animal model disappear within 48–72 hours (see previous discussion). Attempts to correct this and other shortcomings of existing animal models have given rise to a salient new development in this area— the use of selective breeding procedures to attempt to produce populations of animals that either 1) have a higher likelihood of showing the appropriate characteristics than is the case in a normal population of animals, or 2) display characteristics of the disorder to a more pronounced extent than is seen in normal populations. Thus, investigators are now attempting to incorporate into their models the clinical observation that not all individuals appear to be equally

likely to become depressed in that there is often a genetic component to the expression of behavioral disorders.

It should be noted that the models described in this section often use standard procedures described previously for various models (e.g., uncontrollable shock, swim test) and therefore the models included here could have been described under previously defined models. However, because genetic selection procedures constitute recent, and perhaps the most promising, developments now being conducted in the construction of animal models of depression, these models are addressed here in a separate section.

The first model considered is one in which animals were selectively bred for susceptibility and resistance to a behavioral deficit produced by uncontrollable shock (Henn et al. 1985). Henn, Edwards, and colleagues exposed animals to uncontrollable grid shock and then tested animals for their ability to depress a lever to escape from grid shock. In a normal population of Sprague Dawley rats used by these investigators, only 5%–20% of the animals showed impaired escape behavior (i.e., long latencies of more than 20 seconds to escape) after receiving uncontrollable shock. Long latencies, which the investigators termed "failure to escape," can be attributed to decreased motor activity, and hence constitute a depression-like symptom generated in the uncontrollable shock model. These investigators repeatedly tested for, and then bred, animals that showed failure to escape after uncontrollable shock, and they also bred animals that performed the escape response quite well (i.e., showed short escape latencies). After four generations of selective breeding, the proportion of animals showing failure to escape had increased to 45% among offspring bred for this characteristic, whereas 0% of animals bred for rapid escape showed poor escape performance. The authors also reported that, among animals bred for susceptibility to poor escape performance, uncontrollable shock also reduced appetite and caused weight loss.

Effects of antidepressant treatment have been assessed on animals selectively bred for poor escape performance. Henn et al. (1985) reported that when such animals were given placebo (or vehicle), they showed normal escape performance after 3–5 weeks of repeated escape training. In contrast, antidepressant treatment was reported to produce normal escape responding after 5 days. Effective antidepressants were said to include TCAs, MAOIs, and atypical antidepressants, although details were not given.

These investigators have also sought to uncover brain mechanisms that might underlie the poor escape performance of animals selectively bred for this characteristic. They reported that poor performance after uncontrollable shock was accompanied by upregulation of β-adrenergic receptors in the hippocampal region as well as exaggerated cyclic adenosine monophosphate (cAMP) responses to norepinephrinc. This physiological characteristic of animals selectively bred for depression-related symptomatology appears consistent with a well-known action of antidepressants, which is to downregulate β receptors. However, a significant question remains concerning all of these studies (as well as a number of others by this group) in which physiological differences have been examined in animals that show escape deficits following uncontrollable shock in contrast with those that do not show such deficits (Edwards et al. 1991a, 1991b, 1992; Lachman et al. 1993; J. V. Martin et al. 1990; Papolos et al. 1993). When animals fail to escape in the lever-press test, these particular animals always receive considerably more grid shock than do animals that do not fail to escape, so that a difference observed in any particular physiological parameter might result from the fact that these animals received a large amount of grid shock during the test rather than this difference having predisposed these animals to perform poorly. This issue needs to be clarified in order to determine whether the various differences reported in these studies are produced by differential amounts of shock received during testing, or whether they are inherent in the animals before the shock experience and are somehow involved in mediating the poor performance.

Another model derives from rats initially selected as highly responsive to cholinergic agonists (reviewed in Overstreet 1993). In this model, animals were originally differentiated by the extent to which various responses (i.e., decreased body temperature, body weight, drinking behavior) were affected by potentiation of acetylcholine (by use of the anticholinesterase drug diisopropylfluorophosphate). Selective breeding was then undertaken for animals that were sensitive or resistant to pharmacological manipulation of cholinergic activity. Two lines have been developed—the Flinders sensitive line (FSL) and the Flinders resistant line (FRL). Based on the hypothesis that depressed individuals are hypersensitive to cholinergic agonists, it was suspected that the "sensitive" (FSL) rats might show an increased propensity to exhibit depressive symptomatology. Consistent with this hypothesis, the FSL rats showed reduced motor activity (measured in the open field and the swim test) relative to FRL rats, and this difference was exaggerated by exposure to uncontrollable footshock (Overstreet 1986). FSL rats also show increased REM sleep (Shiromani et al. 1988), which may relate to differences in REM shown by depressed patients. This model also has been reported to respond to several different antidepressant drugs, including SSRIs (Overstreet 1993). Of considerable interest regarding underlying pathophysiology, recent studies indicate that despite the initial selection of these animals because of sensitivity to cholinergic agonists, affecting cholinergic receptors pharmacologically does not alter the reduced motor activity shown in the model, whereas intervening with drugs that affect norepinephrine (imipramine, DMI) does counteract this symptom (Schiller et al. 1992). Thus, the hypoactivity in the model appears related to classic catecholaminergic systems that had been previously linked to depression.

These investigators have also begun to explore the possibility that the fawn-hooded rat might be used as an animal model of depression (Overstreet et al. 1992) and have compared fawn-hooded animals with rats of the Flinders lines. The fawn-hooded rat shows reduced sensitivity to serotonergic drugs and consequently has been characterized as showing deficient serotonergic neurotransmission (Aulakh et al. 1988; Wang et al. 1988). In view of the antidepressant effects of SSRIs, it has been suggested that the fawn-hooded animal might constitute a depression-susceptible rat. Overstreet and colleagues (1992) found that the fawn-hooded rat showed decreased motor activity following exposure to uncontrollable shock, although the extent of this deficiency was not as great as that found in the Flinders sensitive line. The researchers observed that the fawn-hooded rat as opposed to its normal progenitor (the Wistar rat) showed a marked preference for alcohol. Consequently, the investigators argued that the fawn-hooded rat may also be used as an animal model for alcoholism. Antidepressant drugs have not yet been tested in this model.

Finally, in a series of brief reports, Golda and Petr proposed that the spontaneous hypertensive rat (derived from the Wistar line) can be used as an animal model of depression. They have demonstrated that exposure of the hypertensive rats to grid shock results in a decrease in motor activity that can be seen up to 9 weeks after exposure to the shock (Golda and Petr 1986). The stress-induced suppression of motor activity has been dissociated from changes in spontaneous exploratory activity (Golda and Petr 1987a) and threshold for reaction to shock (Golda and Petr 1987b). The effects of a variety of drugs in reversing this shock-induced decrease in motor activity have been reported by these investigators (Golda and Petr 1987a, 1987c); however, only one drug related to classic antidepressants (an MAOI) was tested (and showed positive results). A significant question that remains regarding this model is whether the depression in motor activity described in these studies represents a response other than that produced by conditioned fear (i.e., freezing behavior by the rats). The brief reports that present the findings do not make clear whether motor activity was tested in a location different from the one in which the animals initially received inescapable grid shock. If the location was the same, the phenomenon being investigated (i.e., long-term suppression of motor activity) could simply reflect the durability of conditioned fear, and consequently could be unrelated to reduced motor activity that is analogous to a depression-like symptom.

■ Summary Observations Regarding Homologous Models of Depression

Neither an overall summary of depression models nor an evaluation of the strengths and weaknesses of such models is undertaken here; this endeavor should be the prerogative of the reader based on the preceding material. As an aid to this process, the attributes of the various homologous models are summarized in Table 5–1, with the characteristics of each described according to the criteria of McKinney and Bunney (1969).

We offer one additional point, an observation that arises from surveying the various animal models of depression. One of the most useful functions of animal models is to explore potential pathophysiology underlying depression as well as neurochemical mechanisms underlying antidepressant drug action. In addressing these issues, investigators have almost always focused on single neurotransmitter systems to explain changes seen in any model. This is good science in the reductionist tradition because such theories have led to clear, specific hypotheses that could then be tested. This having been said, the message we can now glean from the considerable number of relevant studies employing animal models is that explaining depression-related behavior as well as the action of drugs appears to require reference to multiple transmitter systems interacting with one another.

As a specific example of how interacting neurochemical systems must be considered, we can examine what research has told us about the mechanism by which DMI exerts antidepressant action as revealed in the swim test. Studies show that DMI potently reduces immobility in the swim test through noradrenergic mechanisms. Although this conclusion might be conjectured from the dominant norepinephrine reuptake blocking action of the drug, it is further indicated by the ability of neurotoxic lesions of the LC to completely block the therapeutic (i.e., antiimmobility) effect of DMI (Plaznik et al. 1985a), as well as by the attenuation of this effect by stimulation of β-adrenergic receptors (Kitada et al. 1986) that norepinephrine presumably downregulates. In addition, Platt and Stone (1982) showed that repeated exposure to a stressor produces the therapeutic (antiimmobility) effect in the swim test, which further implicates norepinephrine because this amine system shows by far the most distinct habituational changes of the various monoamines in the brain. But despite compelling evidence that changes in norepinephrine and adrenergic receptors are involved in how DMI decreases immobility in the swim test, it is not evident how norepinephrine acting independently anywhere in the brain could accomplish this effect because this transmitter has little claim to direct action on motor systems (see discussion in Weiss et al. 1980). When we add to this the several studies showing that stimulation of dopamine and dopaminergic receptors, particularly in the nucleus accumbens, can initiate motor activity (Plaznik et al. 1985b), and, most importantly, that blockade of D_2 receptors will block the effects of DMI (Cervo and Samanin 1987), we are led to conclude that limbic dopamine is needed to produce DMI's therapeutic effects. On the other hand, increasing dopamine release did not counteract immobility in the swim test (Borsini et al. 1988), so that simply potentiating dopaminergic transmission in any manner is not sufficient for a therapeutic effect; in contrast, infusing norepinephrine

Table 5–1. Homologous animal models of depression

	Etiology	Symptomatology	Responsiveness to treatment	Biochemistry
Reserpine-induced depression	?	Decreased motor activity	* Responds to TCAs and MAOIs ** Responds to acute drug administration; also responds to stimulants, α-adrenergic agonists, β-blockers, and antihistamines	Disruption of monoaminergic neurotransmission
5-HTP-induced depression	?	Decreased active responding (for food reward)	* Responds to various antidepressants (amitriptyline, imipramine, iprindole, mianserin, trazodone) ** Responds to acute drug pretreatment; also responds to methysergide; responds negatively to fluoxetine	Augmentation of serotonergic neurotransmission
Swim-test immobility	"Behavioral despair," but more evidence points to learned inactivity and/or stress-induced inactivity	Decreased motor activity	* Responds to TCAs, MAOIs, atypical antidepressants, ECT, and REM sleep deprivation; weak response to 5-HT reuptake inhibitors; responds to chronic drug administration, but ** Responds to acute drug administration; also responds to stimulants, anticholinergics, and antihistamines	Decreased motor activity produced by potentiating cholinergic transmission or blocking catecholamines; decreased activity counteracted by increased catecholaminergic transmission and (in stressed animals) blocking opiate receptors
Clonidine withdrawal	?	Decreased motor activity	* Responds to chronic but not acute DMI administration	(?) Subsensitivity of α2 receptors
Tail suspension	?	Decreased escape-related motor activity	* Responds to TCAs, MAOIs, and atypical antidepressants ** Responds to acute administration of drug; also responds to stimulants (D-amphetamine)	
Neonatal clomipramine	?	Decreased sexual activity, aggression, responding for brain stimulation; decreased REM latency; motor hyperactivity	** Responds to imipramine (decreases motor hyperactivity)	
Dorsomedial amygdala lesion in dogs	?	Decreased appetite (feeding and drinking); decreased grooming; animals show lethargy and "negativism"		(?) Decreased DA in forebrain

			Responsiveness to treatment	
Separation-induced depression in primates	Separation	Agitation, sleeplessness, "protest" followed by decreased activity, social activity, appetite, play; self-clasping, hunched posture, and "sad" facial expression	* Chronic imipramine decreases some symptoms (self-clasping, vocalizations); acute imipramine has opposite effect (i.e., exacerbates "protest" reactions)	Decreased NE in CSF; i.e., (?) decreased noradrenergic activity in brain
Separation of Siberian hamsters	Separation	Decreased social interaction and exploratory activity, increase in body weight of males	* Responds (some symptoms) to repeated administration of imipramine	Decreased 5-HT turnover in males
Exhaustion stress	Exposure to a highly stressful, uncontrollable situation (i.e., forced exercise)	Decreased spontaneous motor activity, loss of body weight, hypothermia, loss of normal estrous cycling	* Responds (i.e., more rapid recovery of motor activity) to imipramine	Elevation of NE in brain stem noradrenergic cell body regions in animals showing reduced spontaneous activity; also decreased hypothalamic DA
Chronic, mild stress	Exposure to series of stressful, uncontrollable conditions during 2- to 3-week period	Decreased active behavior (in open field), failure to respond to pleasurable stimuli (but possibly decreased consumption?), elevated steroids	* Responds to TCAs, MAOIs, atypical antidepressants, and ECT; does not respond to stimulants, antihistamines, or anxiolytics	Decreased mesocorticolimbic dopaminergic activity linked to deficit in responding for brain stimulation and (?) decreased response to pleasurable stimuli
Uncontrollable shock-induced depression	Exposure to a highly stressful, uncontrollable situation	Decreased appetite (feeding and drinking), weight loss; decreased motor activity in a variety of tests; decreased grooming, play, competitiveness; decreased sleep marked by early morning waking; also, decreased responding for electrical brain stimulation	* Responds (deficit in active responding) to TCAs, MAOIs, atypical antidepressants, ECT, but not to antipsychotics or stimulants (amphetamine and caffeine) or antihistamines; does not respond to anxiolytics except when given during exposure to uncontrollable shock	Deficit in active behavior linked to 1) decreased NE release in the region of the LC leading to (?) increased NE release in projection regions of the LC; 2) increased concentration of β-adrenergic receptors in the hippocampal region; and 3) altered serotonergic release in forebrain (cortex and septum). Decreased responding for brain stimulation linked to deficit in mesocorticolimbic dopaminergic activity

Note. ? = relationship to depression is unclear, uncertain, or conjectural. (?) = statement that follows is an extrapolation or derivation from other results, has not been directly observed or measured, or is a theoretical hypothesis Under "Responsiveness to treatment," effects listed after * are consistent with changes seen in human clinical depression; effects listed after ** are not consistent. CSF = cerebrospinal fluid; DA = dopamine; DMI = desipramine; ECT = electroconvulsive therapy; 5-HT = serotonin; 5-HTP = 5-hydroxytryptophan; LC = locus ceruleus; MAOI = monoamine oxidase inhibitor; NE = norepinephrine; REM = rapid eye movement; TCA = tricyclic antidepressant.

and adrenergic receptor agonists into the nucleus accumbens did accomplish this effect (Plaznik et al. 1985b). All of this leads to the conclusion that neither norepinephrine nor dopamine alone can currently explain the action of DMI; rather, the therapeutic effect of DMI requires norepinephrine to influence limbic dopamine. Both elements appear necessary to orchestrate the antidepressant response that animals show to DMI. In conclusion, also note that when other models responsive to diverse pharmacological agents that affect different neurochemical systems are examined, there is no instance in which a manipulation restricted to only one neurotransmitter system is able to reproduce pathophysiology or drug action (e.g., Danysz et al. 1988; Plaznik et al. 1988).

To summarize, the value of animal models is to permit, relative to examining the human patient, rapid and detailed physiological studies. A considerable body of work of this nature has been carried out, and these studies suggest that we will not solve the problem of treating depression without paying attention to the interaction of neurotransmitter systems. The metaphor of Parkinson's disease, with its specific pathophysiological defect related to dopamine in the basal ganglia, appears inadequate for addressing the problem of depression.

■ MODELS OF SCHIZOPHRENIA

The disruption of normal cognitive operations is the hallmark of schizophrenia. As such, it can be argued that schizophrenia is a uniquely human disorder that cannot be modeled in animals. At the very least, it can be asserted that the inability of animal models to incorporate elements of language that are invaluable to the expression and examination of schizophrenia creates an enormous barrier to model development. Nevertheless, the potential benefits for understanding the neurobiology and improving treatment that would accrue from the study of valid models of a disorder as prevalent and debilitating as schizophrenia have resulted in the proposal of a variety of related animal models (for reviews see Dunn et al. 1990; Lyon 1990). Animal assay models exist for screening of antipsychotic drugs. In addition, a variety of animal models of schizophrenia that can be classified as homologous have been generated based on hypotheses that describe underlying deficits in schizophrenia in both physiological and psychological terms.

■ Animal Assay Models

Animal behavioral models stressing their predictive pharmacology represent by far the greatest effort expended in the development and use of animal models of schizophrenia. The demonstrated efficacy of neuroleptics, both phenothiazine and nonphenothiazine drugs, in the treatment of psychosis (e.g., Cott and Kurtz 1987; Kane 1987) established the basis for testing the effects of these drugs on responses of animals, and then screening for potentially new antipsychotic medications by assessing the ability to produce similar effects. As with animal assays for depression, such models reflect pharmacological similarity of the responses that are measured to the pharmacology of schizophrenia; these responses observed in the animal may bear little or no relevance to the symptoms of schizophrenia.

Conditioned avoidance responding. Perhaps the most studied pharmacological model has been the inhibitory effects of neuroleptic antipsychotics on conditioned avoidance responding (CAR) to aversive stimuli (Cook and Catania 1964; Worms et al. 1983). In this test, subjects (usually rodents) are conditioned to make an active response (e.g., locomotion in a shuttle box, pole climbing) to avoid or escape footshock. Neuroleptic administration results in a deficit in avoidance responding, with escape behavior impaired only by greater drug doses. The differential effect of neuroleptics on avoidance and escape behavior distinguishes neuroleptics from other avoidance-disrupting drugs such as barbiturates, MAOIs, and benzodiazepines that exhibit overlapping dose-effect relationships for avoidance and escape behavior (Arnt 1982). In addition to drug specificity, CAR paradigms exhibit significant positive correlations between the potency of neuroleptic antipsychotics to inhibit avoidance responding (ED_{50} values) and their clinical potency as reflected in their average administered daily dose (Kuribara and Tadokoro 1981). However, the model has several features that limit its relationship to the pharmacology of schizophrenia. First, inhibition of avoidance responding by neuroleptic antipsychotics exhibits tolerance with repeated drug administration (Fregnan and Chieli 1980; Nielsen et al. 1974; Sanger 1985). Second, the atypical antipsychotic drug clozapine is not effective in the CAR test (Sanger 1985). Although CAR paradigms have use as a screening technique for neuroleptic antipsychotics, they appear to be of limited value in identifying mechanistically novel antipsychotics.

Catalepsy test. The induction of catalepsy (the inability to correct an externally imposed body posture) (Sanberg et al. 1988) represents an additional animal behavioral screen for neuroleptic antipsychotics (Worms et al. 1983). However, drug-induced catalepsy is neither specific nor sensitive for antipsychotic drugs, exhibits tolerance with repeated neuroleptic administration, and demonstrates a poor correlation with the therapeutic potency of antipsychotics (Dunn et al. 1990). Despite having virtually no strength as an animal behavioral model of antipsychotics, catalepsy tests do have value in the study of the neuropharmacology of extrapyramidal function (Sanberg et al. 1988) and as a rapid behavioral screen for predicting the motor side effects of potential antipsychotic drugs.

Paw test. The paw test (Ellenbroek et al. 1987) is a recent addition to pharmacological behavioral models related to schizophrenia. The test reflects the effect of drug administration to rats on the spontaneous retraction of their extended forelimbs and hindlimbs (Ellenbroek and Cools 1988). Neuroleptic antipsychotics increase the time to retraction of the hindlimb and forelimb with equipotent effects for both limbs, whereas atypical antipsychotics increase hindlimb retraction time (HRT) at lower doses than those required to increase forelimb retraction time (FRT). From these observations, it was proposed that drug effects on HRT and FRT are separate measures of the antipsychotic potential and liability for extrapyramidal side effects (EPS), respectively, of tested drugs. The paw test appears superior to previously developed screening techniques in that it distinguishes neuroleptics from atypical antipsychotics, with members of the latter class exhibiting positive effects rather than being false negatives in the test.

As a pharmacological model of schizophrenia, the paw test shows antipsychotic drug specificity and lack of effect of anticholinergics on the HRT. Another positive aspect of the model is that drug-induced increases in the HRT do not develop tolerance with repeated administration of antipsychotic drugs (Ellenbroek and Cools 1988). Although additional tests of antipsychotic drug sensitivity and specificity are needed to establish the predictive strength of this model, the paw test appears to represent a unique behavioral screen for the distinct clinical pharmacology of neuroleptic and atypical antipsychotics (Kane et al. 1988).

Self-stimulation paradigms. Neuroleptic administration produces an inhibition of operantly conditioned lever-pressing for intracranial electrical stimulation (Worms et al. 1983) or intravenous doses of cocaine (Roberts and Vickers 1984). Both paradigms appear to be models of the dopaminergic pharmacology of brain reward mechanisms, and drug effects are typically interpreted as an induction of an anhedonic state (Ettenberg et al. 1981). Intracranial electric self-stimulation (ICSS) paradigms may also (or alternatively) model the effects of neuroleptics on motor function, as the inhibitory effects of flupentixol on ICSS obtained when ICSS is delivered after lever-pressing are not observed in rats that obtain ICSS by nose-poking, a motorically simple task (Ettenberg et al. 1981). An inhibition of ICSS and an increase in cocaine self-administration is exhibited by many neuroleptic and atypical antipsychotics (Worms et al. 1983; Roberts and Vickers 1984). A notable exception is clozapine, which actually decreases cocaine self-administration (Roberts and Vickers 1984). These authors also reported an excellent correlation (for a limited number of antipsychotics other than clozapine) between potency for increasing cocaine intake by self-administration and daily clinical dose for antipsychotic effects. Antipsychotic drug specificity and tolerance development represent unresolved issues for both self-stimulation paradigms. Collectively, these self-stimulation paradigms would seem better able to predict the negative effect of a drug on dopamine-mediated reward mechanisms than its antipsychotic potential.

■ Homologous Models

These models aspire to a direct relevance between the behavior shown in the animal model and behavioral responses seen in schizophrenia and/or underlying processes that are thought to define schizophrenia. Homologous animal models of schizophrenia can be subdivided into three types. The first type reflects the previously made point that the signs and symptoms of schizophrenia express disturbances in cognitive operations, and these can only be represented in nonhuman animals by theoretically based constructs. Modeling of psychophysiological processes that are believed to be disturbed in schizophrenia has largely focused on deficits in information processing and stimulus filtering (Braff and Geyer 1990; Freedman et al. 1991; Nuechterlein and Dawson 1984). As might be expected, such animal models do not necessarily reproduce observable consequences (i.e., symptoms) seen in the disorder. Moreover, it has been shown that deficits in these processes and the diagnostic symptoms of schizophrenia in patients may not covary over time (Penn et al. 1993). A second type of homologous model reproduces a salient symptom seen in schizophrenia, the disturbance of social behavior. Finally, the third type of model reproduces physiological disturbances linked theoretically to the etiology of schizophrenia.

With respect to these latter models, it should be noted that progression from knowledge of etiology to development of models represents the most rational approach to establishing models, but that pharmacological models of schizophrenia are an excellent example of the reverse progression (Iversen 1987). A defect of brain dopamine function (i.e., overactivity), which neuroleptic medication presumably counteracts, has been taken as an etiological fact of schizophrenia, and models then reproduce the "hyperdopaminergic" state in animals to study the consequences of this state.

Latent inhibition paradigms. The latent inhibition (LI) of conditioned responses by preexposure to a to-be-conditioned stimulus is a well-studied model of selective attention (Lubow et al. 1982). Operationally, it is proposed that the neutral presentation of a stimulus retards the subsequent learning of conditioned associations to the stimulus (Lubow 1973). Conceptually, LI paradigms are models of the ability to accurately categorize a stimulus based on its changing salience. The phenomenon of LI attempts to reproduce attentional deficits in schizophrenia that are expressed as the use of inefficient and inflexible processing strategies to filter stimuli. LI also contains parallels with nonattentional constructs of schizophrenia such as deficits in the control of behavior by context (Lubow 1989) and the influence of prior experience on the perception of current events (Hemsley 1987).

The empirical strength of LI paradigms as models

of brain functions affected by schizophrenia is derived from animal behavioral pharmacology and human behavioral studies. Initial interest in LI paradigms stemmed from their being affected by amphetamine (Solomon et al. 1981; Weiner et al. 1984), a drug thought to induce psychosis (see subsection on chronic amphetamine intoxication). More recent studies of LI have emphasized the response of these paradigms to antipsychotic drugs (Christison et al. 1988; Dunn et al. 1993; Feldon and Weiner 1991; Weiner and Feldon 1987). For example, administering haloperidol to rats facilitates the LI of conditioned response suppression by stimulus preexposure (Christison et al. 1988; Weiner and Feldon 1987). The facilitation of LI by haloperidol exhibits a potency similar to the clinical potency of haloperidol, is self-limiting at higher doses, and does not exhibit tolerance with repeated drug administration (Dunn et al. 1993). Also, LI is enhanced by structurally diverse neuroleptic antipsychotics (see Figure 5–9) as well as being affected by atypical antipsychotics, although clozapine, fluperlapine, amperozide, and olanzapine *decrease* LI.

Significantly, the effects of neuroleptic and atypical antipsychotics on LI, though distinct, are confined to the effect of stimulus preexposure on conditioned suppression. Conditioned responses in the absence of stimulus preexposures were found to be unaffected by drug administration (Dunn et al. 1993). This pattern of effect is not mimicked by anxiolytics, sedative hypnotics, antidepressants, a nonantipsychotic phenothiazine, or morphine (Dunn et al. 1993). A challenge for this model will be to define conditions (e.g., a deficit in LI) that produce a convergence for all efficacious antipsychotic drugs on a common behavioral effect, or an appreciation of the mechanisms (e.g., 5-HT–dopamine actions) underlying the distinct effects on LI of neuroleptic versus atypical antipsychotics as a key to understanding their distinct clinical pharmacology (Kane et al. 1988).

Human behavioral studies lend further support to LI phenomena as animal models of symptoms or psychopathological constructs of schizophrenia. Using a variation of LI paradigms used in animals, Baruch and colleagues (1988a) demonstrated that LI of a learned stimulus association by stimulus preexposure was absent in patients with acute schizophrenia; control subjects without schizophrenia and a group of subjects with chronic schizophrenia exhibited clear LI. These results led to the proposal that LI paradigms represent a model of the positive symptoms and causal mechanisms (i.e., hyperdopaminergia) of acute but not chronic schizophrenia (Baruch et al. 1988a). However, a more plausible and testable hypothesis based on the animal pharmacology of LI is that differences in antipsychotic medication underlie the group differences in LI performance. It is worth noting that all three groups readily learned the stimulus association in the absence of stimulus preexposure. Dopamine receptors negatively modulate LI in both animal and human paradigms. The administration of apomorphine, amphetamine, and D_1 or D_2/D_3 dopamine receptor agonists inhibits LI in rats (C. D. Kilts, L. Dunn, R. J. Scibilia, unpublished data, 1994), whereas amphetamine administration inhibits

LI in nonschizophrenic human subjects (Gray et al. 1992). Latent inhibition paradigms appear to be promising models of brain functions sensitive to schizophrenia, antipsychotic drugs, and dopamine receptor activation.

Blocking paradigms. Blocking paradigms, like LI tasks, represent models of selective attention and the influence of context and prior experience on current perception and learning (Gray et al. 1991). Blocking tasks also involve a stimulus preexposure, conditioning, and behavioral testing component (Kamin 1969). Stimulus preexposure, unlike LI paradigms, involves the conditioned association of the stimulus (CS-A) with an unconditioned stimulus (UCS). In conditioning, a compound stimulus (CS-A plus CS-B) is pre-

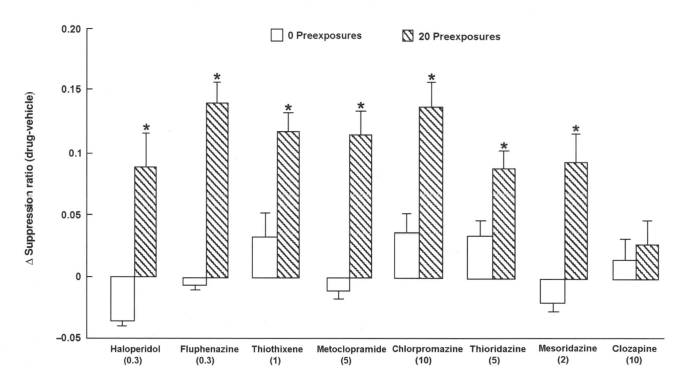

Figure 5–9. Effect of structurally diverse neuroleptic antipsychotics and clozapine on the latent inhibition (LI) of conditioned response suppression by 20 stimulus preexposures. (See Dunn et al. 1993 for details of the LI paradigm.) Preexposure to the to-be-conditioned stimulus (house light) weakens its ability to serve as a conditioned stimulus (CS) in classical conditioning with the unconditioned stimulus (footshock), so that stimulus-preexposed animals exhibit a decreased conditioned response (suppression of spout licking) to the CS relative to nonpreexposed subjects. The amount of suppression that occurs is expressed as a ratio that is calculated by A/A + B, where A represents the time to complete licks 81–90 prior to the onset of the CS, and B represents the time to complete licks 91–100 following onset of the CS. Results above present the difference (or delta) in ratio that was measured in drug-treated groups relative to control animals that were given vehicle (i.e., vehicle-treated ratio subtracted from drug-treated ratio). All neuroleptic antipsychotics tested enhanced the LI effect, as reflected in a significantly greater delta suppression ratio. Numbers in parentheses represent the mg/kg dose administered daily for 7 consecutive days prior to stimulus preexposures. Asterisk (*) denotes statistical significance ($P < .05$) compared with delta suppression ratios calculated in the absence of stimulus preexposure.

sented, followed by the same UCS. In testing, the conditioned response to CS-B is measured; preexposure (prior association of CS-A and the UCS) weakens (or "blocks") the response to CS-B. As models of the differential processing of stimuli of different relevance, LI and blocking tasks differ in the simultaneous presentation of different stimuli (blocking) versus sequential processing of the same stimulus (LI).

Blocking tasks were used initially as models of amphetamine-induced or -exacerbated psychosis (Crider et al. 1982). The negative effect of amphetamine on the blocking effect was antagonized by haloperidol administration (Crider et al. 1982). However, the ability of blocking tasks to detect a range of antipsychotic drugs has not yet been tested. It can be noted that testing of humans indicates the presence of a deficit in the stimulus blocking effect in schizophrenia (Jones et al. 1992). Acutely ill schizophrenic patients fail to exhibit blocking of conditioned associations to CS-B by CS-A; nonschizophrenic control subjects and patients with anxiety disorder or chronic schizophrenia exhibit a clear blocking effect. The validation of blocking behavior as an animal model (distinct from LI) of brain functions relevant to schizophrenia must await the study of the sensitivity, specificity, and potency of the effects of antipsychotic drugs and the assessment of tolerance development with repeated drug administration.

Prepulse inhibition of the startle reflex. An additional animal model of the information processing–stimulus filtering deficits of schizophrenia is represented by the inhibition of the startle reaction to an acoustic or tactile stimulus when the startling stimulus is preceded by a weak prestimulus (hence, prepulse inhibition, or PPI) (Braff et al. 1978). The PPI effect is often proposed to represent an animal behavior model of sensorimotor gating functions. The model is postulated to reproduce gating deficits found in schizophrenia. Based on this hypothesis, it has been used to probe the neural and pharmacological substrates of schizophrenia (Braff and Geyer 1990; Swerdlow et al. 1986, 1990, 1994). Parallels between rats and humans in the graded response and threshold for PPI defined by a range of prepulse intensities and in the startle stimuli (Swerdlow et al. 1994) support the contention that similar operations underlie PPI in both species. Like LI and blocking paradigms, PPI (of an eye blink reflex) is absent or

dramatically reduced in patients with schizophrenia compared with nonschizophrenic control subjects (Braff and Geyer 1990; Braff et al. 1978, 1992). Like LI (Baruch et al. 1988b), PPI is also diminished in psychosis-prone individuals (Simmons 1990). However, deficits in PPI are not unique to schizophrenia but are also observed in patients with Huntington's disease or obsessive-compulsive disorder (Swerdlow et al. 1993, 1994).

As behavioral models of stimulus-filtering functions that are disrupted by schizophrenia, PPI paradigms differ from LI paradigms with respect to modulation by dopamine receptors and effects of antipsychotic drugs. PPI is inhibited by the administration of D_2 but not D_1 receptor agonists, although D_1 receptor agonists potentiate the disruptive effects of D_2 receptor activation on PPI (Peng et al. 1990). In contrast, the LI of a conditioned response suppression by stimulus preexposure is inhibited by the activation of either D_1 or D_2/D_3 dopamine receptors in the absence of apparent interactive effects between receptor subtypes (C. D. Kilts, L. Dunn, R. J. Scibilia, unpublished data, 1994). The specific dopamine projections involved in modulating PPI and LI also appear to differ. The selective activation of dopamine receptors in the nucleus accumbens inhibits PPI of the startle reflex (Swerdlow et al. 1990, 1991) but does not affect the LI of conditioned suppression (Killcross and Robbins 1993). These differences suggest that LI and PPI of the startle reflex represent distinct aspects of stimulus filtering with different neural mechanisms. These paradigms would therefore have distinct strengths and applications as models of the psychobiological "symptom" of information processing deficits in schizophrenia.

Differences between LI and PPI are also seen in response to antipsychotic drugs. LI in normally functioning animals is significantly affected by antipsychotic drug administration; neuroleptic antipsychotics enhance the negative impact of stimulus preexposure on associative learning. In contrast, sensorimotor gating measured by PPI is not affected by the administration of antipsychotic drugs to normally functioning animals (Swerdlow et al. 1994). Antipsychotic drugs do antagonize decreases in PPI of the startle reflex produced by apomorphine (Swerdlow and Geyer 1993; Swerdlow et al. 1991, 1994) or isolation rearing (Geyer et al. 1993). That a deficit in PPI is needed to reveal an effect of antipsychotic drugs may represent a source of strength for the PPI model as the substrates of drug action in schizophrenia are those brain functions that are degraded by the genetic and psychosocial factors unique to this disorder. In other words, a "defect state" may be a requirement of valid animal models of antipsychotic drug effects in schizophrenia.

However, the contention that antipsychotic drug effects on induced deficits in PPI in animals represent a model of the pharmacology of sensorimotor gating abnormalities in schizophrenia (Swerdlow et al. 1991, 1994) is undermined by the apparently negligible effect of antipsychotic medication on PPI deficits in schizophrenic patients (Braff and Geyer 1990). This inconsistency highlights a means for validating animal models—the testing of predictions from the model in human behavioral studies. Are the modeled behaviors (e.g., PPI, LI) affected differently in distinct symptom subtypes of schizophrenia, by different classes of antipsychotic drugs in a within-subject crossover design, or by the patients' gender? The attempt to correlate results of clinical behavioral research with animal behavioral models represents both the best effort in model testing and the ultimate goal of animal modeling—to learn about the clinical condition. The study of PPI phenomena in humans may reveal highly useful information concerning the neurobiology of stimulus processing deficits in schizophrenia, but not concerning the mode of action of antipsychotic drugs. Perhaps Carlton's (1978) assessment of the restricted relevance of animal behavioral models is partly correct in that a *complete* relationship between an animal model and schizophrenia is not a necessary requirement and places too much strain on the model.

Rodent interaction. The degradation of social skills in schizophrenia is a hallmark of this disorder (Mueser et al. 1991) and the distinguishing feature of subgroups of schizophrenia (Carpenter et al. 1988; Kibel et al. 1993). Deterioration of social skills is associated with the chronic phase of schizophrenia and its deficit form (Carpenter et al. 1988) or negative syndrome (Kibel et al. 1993). A modification of the rat social interaction (SI) paradigm, developed and tested as an animal behavioral model of anxiolytic drug activity (Gardner and Guy 1984), has been proposed as an animal model of the effects of antipsychotic drugs on social behaviors affected by schizophrenia (Corbett et al. 1993). Active, nonaggressive behavioral interactions between pairs of familiar or unfamiliar rats were timed following the acute administration of antipsychotic or nonantipsychotic drugs. Antipsychotic drug administration significantly altered SI behaviors between unfamiliar, but not familiar, pairs compared with vehicle-injected control pairs; neuroleptic antipsychotics decreased SI, whereas atypical antipsychotics increased SI. As a comparison, diazepam administration enhanced SI in both familiar and unfamiliar pairs of rats. SI paradigms thus have possible use as behavioral screens for drugs of potential value in the treatment of the deficits in social skills observed in schizophrenia. Several considerations support a cautious use of these models. The effectiveness of clozapine in this test may be explained in part by the anxiolytic properties of this drug (Spealman et al. 1982). Also, the negative influence of neuroleptic antipsychotics on SI is difficult to reconcile with their beneficial (i.e., ameliorative) effects on negative symptoms (Labarca et al. 1993; Meltzer et al. 1986). A critical test of the model strength of SI will be the determination of antipsychotic drug effects following chronic drug administration.

Social behavior in monkeys. An obvious limitation of the use of SI models is the conceptual distance between interactive behavior in rodent pairs and deficits in social skills and social withdrawal exhibited by schizophrenic patients in complex human social contexts. These deficiencies have been addressed by an ethological analysis of monkeys in the context of their complex, well-organized social structure (Ellenbroek 1991). Observed SIs are compiled into a behavioral ethogram. Monkeys exhibit a wide and rich repertoire of social behaviors; as a result, they approximate better the social setting of humans. For instance, drug effects on the interactive behavior of the alpha and beta males and the females of a social group can be described and changes analyzed in terms of group social structure or individual social bonds (Ellenbroek et al. 1989). Monkey social behavior in models of schizophrenia has largely been studied in conjunction with amphetamine-induced social isolation (Arnett et al. 1989; Ellenbroek et al. 1989; Miczek and Yoshimura 1982), which is thought to be analogous to social withdrawal symptoms seen in the negative (or deficit) forms of schizophrenia.

Amphetamine administration to monkeys markedly reduces the duration and number of both active and passive social behaviors, with a resulting increase in spatial distance between socially living monkeys (Arnett et al. 1989; Ellenbroek 1991; Ellenbroek et al. 1989). Amphetamine-induced social isolation is observed following either chronic or acute drug administration, and different social behaviors are differentially affected. For instance, acute amphetamine administration 1) decreased behavioral items of the ethogram, such as grooming and huddling, 2) had no significant effect on looking at other animals, and 3) increased submissive behaviors (Ellenbroek et al. 1989; Miczek and Yoshimura 1982). The social withdrawal observed in monkeys following amphetamine administration and the complex pattern (compared with that of rodents) of drug-induced stereotyped behaviors have been proposed as models of both negative and positive symptoms, respectively, of schizophrenia in a single paradigm (Ellenbroek 1991). The amphetamine-induced social isolation in monkeys has characteristics of a deficient ability to interpret communicative signals and/or a hyperdopaminergic state.

The validity of this model has not been demonstrated beyond a shared lack of effect of noradrenergic and opiate receptor antagonists, benzodiazepines, and neuroleptic antipsychotics on deficits in social function in schizophrenia and this animal behavioral model (Ellenbroek 1991). However, the assertion that neuroleptics lack effect is dubious for both the clinical symptoms and the animal behaviors. The needed test of efficacy for the atypical antipsychotics on amphetamine-induced social isolation in monkeys has apparently not been conducted. The fact that this model is produced by a dopaminomimetic drug limits its application as a screen for novel antipsychotics and as a tool for studying the mechanism of schizophrenia. However, this animal model is unique in reproducing the degraded complex social behaviors of the negative, or deficit, form of schizophrenia. A more systematic analysis of the monkey behaviors associated with social withdrawal induced by other nonpharmacological means, and a more thorough analysis of the behavioral pharmacology of antipsychotic drugs, would seem worthwhile in the development and testing of such a model.

Chronic amphetamine intoxication. Animal behavioral models based on an induced hyperdopaminergic state derive from the long-held belief in the involvement of the neurotransmitter dopamine

in the neurochemical pathology of schizophrenia (Carlson 1988; Davis et al. 1991). Indirect evidence for a hyperactivity of dopamine neurons innervating the subcortical limbic system in schizophrenia is inferred from the behavioral symptoms of patients, their exacerbation by dopaminomimetics (Angrist et al. 1985; Davidson et al. 1987), and their therapeutic response to antidopaminergic treatment (Creese et al. 1976). More recent reformulations of the dopamine hypothesis of schizophrenia include postulating a hypoactivity of dopamine neurons innervating the prefrontal cortex as the neural basis of the negative/deficit symptom complex in schizophrenia (Davis et al. 1991). The behavioral effects of the drug-induced activation of brain dopamine receptors have long been proposed as an animal model of psychotic symptoms (Ellinwood and Kilbey 1977; Ellinwood et al. 1972; Ellison et al. 1978).

Chronic amphetamine intoxication models in cats and monkeys have focused on elicited behaviors that are interpreted as parallels of motor and cognitive symptoms of schizophrenia (Ellinwood and Kilbey 1977; Nielsen et al. 1983). Motor disturbances observed in the end stage of chronic amphetamine administration in animals include restless shifting and awkward postures; behavioral effects include fragmented, perseverative, or abortive behaviors with situationally irrelevant responses and reduced or inappropriate social behaviors. Nielsen and associates (1983) also described apparent amphetamine-induced hallucinatory behavior in monkeys consisting of behavioral sequences oriented toward nonexistent stimuli. Not surprisingly, treatment with neuroleptic antipsychotics resulted in a rapid cessation of these effects of chronic amphetamine administration. Chronic amphetamine intoxication models thus produce animal behavioral analogues of even the most human of the positive and negative symptoms of schizophrenia. Historically, these models have added considerable momentum to the purported role of dopamine in the neurochemical pathology of schizophrenia. However, a caution in interpreting these models is worth noting because of the possibility that effects of amphetamine and other dopaminomimetics may reflect actions on neural mechanisms related to treatment but not to etiology. The use of in vivo functional brain imaging techniques (e.g., positron-emission tomography) may demonstrate parallels between the functional neuroanatomy of schizophrenia (Liddle et al. 1992; Tamminga et al. 1992) and that of chronic amphetamine intoxication, and thus may strengthen the model beyond its behavioral parallels.

Hippocampal damage. Models in which the hippocampus of animals is damaged have gained added significance with the demonstration that changes in the volume of the hippocampus (and amygdala) currently represent the most consistently observed component of the neuropathology of schizophrenia (Bogerts et al. 1993; Shenton et al. 1992). Bilateral lesioning of the hippocampus in animals affects specific behaviors (e.g., attention, arousal, habituation), cognitive operations (e.g., learning, memory), and physiological reactions (e.g., skin conductance) that parallel a constellation of deficits associated with schizophrenia (Schmajuk 1987). Behavioral deficits following hippocampal lesioning can be reversed by administration of clinically efficacious antipsychotics (Schmajuk 1987).

More recent formulations of the hippocampal lesion model have shown the model to reproduce diverse phenomenological aspects of schizophrenia. Bilateral lesions of the ventral hippocampus of young adult (42-day-old) rats produced by intracerebral microinjection of the excitatory amino acid neurotoxin ibotenic acid resulted in changes in postoperative behavior as well as pharmacological and biochemical estimates of brain dopamine systems (Lipska et al. 1992). Specifically, hippocampal damage increased spontaneous exploratory behavior and amphetamine-induced locomotion while inducing an increase in the estimated activity of dopamine neurons innervating the limbic (ventral) striatum and a decrease in the activity of dopamine neurons of the medial prefrontal cortex. Hippocampal damage in these studies was not associated with an altered behavioral responsivity to environmental stimuli (i.e., stressors).

The hippocampal damage paradigm has also been strengthened by the addition of developmental features. Schizophrenia represents a disorder with a defined developmental latency. The index episode typically occurs at postpubertal ages in late adolescence or early adulthood (Kendler et al. 1987). Moreover, the neuroanatomical alterations associated with schizophrenia (e.g., decreased volume of the amygdaloid-hippocampal complexes of the temporal lobes) are thought to represent early developmental pathology that remains functionally quiescent until adolescence or adulthood (Crow 1990; Weinberger

1987). In the animal model described here, ibotenic acid–induced hippocampal damage of rats at postnatal day 7 results in a delayed emergence of an enhanced (relative to sham-operated controls) locomotor response to a novel environment, an intraperitoneal injection of saline or amphetamine, or a swim stressor (Lipska et al. 1993). Behavioral effects of lesions were noted at postpubertal postnatal day 56, but not prepubertal day 35, following lesion on postnatal day 7. Behavioral effects were interpreted as being suggestive of an enhanced response of mesolimbic dopamine neurons to stressful environmental and pharmacological stimuli. The neonatal hippocampal damage model thus possesses analogues of the postpubertal onset and stress vulnerability of schizophrenia and of the neurochemical construct of limbic dopamine dysregulation (Lipska et al. 1993).

It should be noted that, despite the similarities described here, the observed changes in hippocampal volume (Bogerts et al. 1993; Shenton et al. 1992) or cytoarchitecture (Conrad et al. 1991) in adult schizophrenic patients represent subtle, asymmetric changes, in contrast with the robust loss of neuropil, gliosis, and cavitation observed in the hippocampus of lesioned animals. Also, changes in neuroanatomy associated with schizophrenia are not confined to the hippocampal formation.

High ambient pressure. The psychotogenic effects of exposure to high ambient pressure (Stoudemire et al. 1984) has led to the conclusion that high pressure–induced changes in neurotransmission and behavior represent a method by which schizophreniform psychosis can be produced (Abraini et al. 1993). In addition to neurological and other psychiatric symptoms, deep-sea divers experiencing very high pressure exhibit neuroleptic-reversible delusions, hallucinations, paranoid thoughts, and agitation (Stoudemire et al. 1984). The exposure of rats to environments of high ambient pressure results in neuroleptic-reversible increases in spontaneous locomotor activity and correlated increases in the dopamine content of the nucleus accumbens and caudate putamen (Abraini et al. 1993). The high pressure–induced behavioral-neurochemical model has its strength in parallels with a key component of the dopamine hypothesis of schizophrenia—the hypothetical overactivity of mesolimbic dopamine neurons. An additional strength of the model is that the inducing condition (i.e., high pressure) does not involve a presumption of underlying causes of schizophrenia, and consequently makes possible studies of the mechanistic bases and pharmacology of schizophrenia's consequences in an attempt to understand these aspects of psychotic disorders. An obvious weakness of the model is its lack of relevance to inducing conditions of schizophrenia.

■ Models Using Selective Breeding (Genetic Selection)

Even those animal models of schizophrenia that are arguably best able to reproduce symptoms or psychophysiological constructs of schizophrenia (e.g., LI, blocking, PPI) have multiple shortcomings. An example is the apomorphine-induced deficit in PPI of the startle reflex, in which an induced behavioral deficit is a prerequisite for demonstrating antipsychotic drug effects (Swerdlow et al. 1994). This manipulation produces a short-lived behavioral deficit that differs from the enduring deficiency that characterizes schizophrenia. As with animal models of depression, behavioral genetic techniques offer a promising approach by which models may be improved. However, the technique has yet to be used extensively.

The one area in which genetic selection techniques have been applied has been drug response. As explained earlier, drug-produced interference with CAR has been used as a screening technique for antipsychotic medication. Genetically distinct strains of mice differ greatly in the effect of neuroleptic antipsychotics on CAR (Fuller 1970) and induction of catalepsy (Fink et al. 1982), and these observations constituted the impetus for developing pharmacogenetic models of response to neuroleptic antipsychotics. A significant proportion (7%–30%) of newly admitted patients with schizophrenia exhibit little or no therapeutic response to neuroleptic therapy (Kane et al. 1988; Kolakowska et al. 1985), whereas a smaller subgroup of patients demonstrate a rapid and robust response to neuroleptic antipsychotics (Garver et al. 1984). Selective breeding programs have been used to develop genetic animal models of neuroleptic response and nonresponse in gerbils (Upchurch and Schallert 1983) and in mice (Hitzeman et al. 1991). Using the cataleptic response to haloperidol administration as the selected behavior, a significant bidirectional response to selection has been demonstrated in mice. By the seventh generation, the hal-

operidol-nonresponsive (HNR) line exhibited no catalepsy following haloperidol (2 mg/kg) administration, whereas the haloperidol-responsive (HR) line exhibited a robust cataleptic response of long duration to 1 mg/kg haloperidol (Hitzeman et al. 1991). Behavioral differences in drug response to haloperidol were not attributable to differences between lines in the pharmacokinetics of haloperidol. The response to selection generalized to D_2 dopamine receptor antagonists other than haloperidol, suggesting that alterations in brain D_2 receptor density or function may underlie the difference in response.

It should also be noted that selective breeding techniques for good and poor CAR learning have long been known to result in the generation of distinct lines of rats (Bignami 1965; Brush 1991; Brush et al. 1979). The three major strains of rats resulting from successful bidirectional selection for CAR acquisition include the Roman, Syracuse, and Australian High and Low Avoidance strains (Brush 1991). Although these breeding programs have convincingly demonstrated the hereditary influences on CAR, the effect of genetic selection on the response of CAR to antipsychotic drug administration has not been systematically examined. Finally, genetic selection programs with respect to the LI model are currently under development.

■ Summary Observations Regarding Models of Schizophrenia

The signs and symptoms of schizophrenia reflect cognitive disturbances that have no prima facie duplication in animal behavior. As such, animal behavioral models of schizophrenia have sought validation in pharmacological parallels, as well as parallels with psychophysiological and neurochemical constructs of schizophrenia. The utility of such models in elucidating the neurobiology of schizophrenia and/or as targets for the development of mechanistically novel antipsychotics with improved efficacy and decreased side effects is dependent on an increased number of facts of schizophrenia that may be modeled. Noninvasive, in vivo imaging techniques will play a major role in the discovery of the neurobiological facts of schizophrenia. The application of improved techniques of magnetic resonance imaging has identified a neuropathology of schizophrenia (Breier et al. 1992; Shenton et al. 1992) that suggests a disorder in neocortical-limbic communication. Similarly, the application of functional brain imaging techniques to schizophrenia has demonstrated that schizophrenia has a functional neuroanatomy represented by alterations in functional neural circuits (Liddle et al. 1992; Tamminga et al. 1992). In solving the mysteries of schizophrenia, these findings provide important clues as to the "what" and "where" of the effects of schizophrenia on the brain and offer leads in defining why such effects occur and how they affect cognitive processes. These findings also furnish needed facts concerning the neurobiology of schizophrenia for use as targets for animal modeling and model validation.

Finally, future animal behavioral models related to schizophrenia should manifest "appropriate" deficits in psychophysiology before using models to probe the neurochemistry, neuroanatomy, and pharmacology of schizophrenia. The reverse order has typically been pursued. In particular, it should be recognized that the psychopharmacology of schizophrenia is often unique, because drugs interact with the abnormalities in neurochemistry and neuroanatomy that underlie the disorder. The dependency of pharmacology on a "defect state" for accurate assessment suggests that the search for novel treatments for schizophrenia using animal models needs to proceed from the development of valid symptom models.

■ REFERENCES

Abel EL: Alarm substance emitted by rats in the forced-swim test is a low volatile pheromone. Physiol Behav 50:723–727, 1991

Abraini JH, Ansseau M, Fechati T: Pressure-induced disorders in neurotransmission and spontaneous behavior in rats: an animal model of psychosis. Biol Psychiatry 34:622–629, 1993

Abramson LY, Seligman MEP: Modeling psychopathology in the laboratory: history and rationale, in Psychopathology: Experimental Models. Edited by Maser JD, Seligman MEP. San Francisco, CA, WH Freeman & Company, 1977, pp 1–26

American Psychiatric Association: Diagnostic and Statistical Manual of Mental Disorders, 3rd Edition. Washington, DC, American Psychiatric Association, 1980

American Psychiatric Association: Diagnostic and Statistical Manual of Mental Disorders, 3rd Edition, Revised. Washington, DC, American Psychiatric Association, 1987

American Psychiatric Association: Diagnostic and Statistical Manual of Mental Disorders, 4th Edition. Washington, DC, American Psychiatric Association, 1994

Angrist B, Pedselow E, Rubinstein M, et al: Amphetamine response and relapse risk after depot neuroleptic discontinuation. Psychopharmacology (Berl) 85:277–301, 1985

Anisman H, Bignami G: A comparative neurochemical, pharmacological, and functional analysis of aversively motivated behaviors: caveats and general consideration, in Psychopharmacology of Aversively Motivated Behavior. Edited by Anisman H, Bignami G. New York, Plenum, 1978, pp 487–512

Anisman H, Shanks N, Zakman S, ct al: Multisystem regulation of performance deficits induced by stressors: an animal model of depression, in Animal Models in Psychiatry, Vol 2. Edited by Iverson MTM. Clifton, NJ, Humana Press, 1991, pp 1–55

Aprison MH, Takahashi R, Tachiki K: Hypersensitive serotonergic receptors involved in clinical depression—a theory, in Neuropharmacology and Behavior. Edited by Haber B, Aprison MH. New York, Plenum, 1978, pp 23–53

Archer T, Soderberg U, Ross SB, ct al: Role of olfactory bulbectomy and DSP4 treatment in avoidance learning in the rat. Behav Neurosci 98:496–505, 1984

Armario A, Gavalda A, Marti O: Forced swimming test in rats: effect of desipramine administration and the period of exposure to the test on struggling behavior, swimming, immobility and defecation rate. Eur J Pharmacol 158:207–212, 1988

Arnett L, Ridley R, Gamble S, et al: Social withdrawal following amphetamine administration to marmosets. Psychopharmacology (Berl) 99:222–229, 1989

Arnt J: Pharmacology specificity of conditioned avoidance response inhibition in rats: inhibition by neuroleptics and correlation to dopamine receptor blockade. Acta Pharmacologica et Toxicologica 51:321–329, 1982

Aulakh CS, Wozniak KM, Hill JL, et al: Differential neuroendocrine responses to the 5-HT agonist m-chlorophenylpiperazine in fawn-hooded rats relative to Wistar and Sprague-Dawley rats. Neuroendocrinology 48:401–406, 1988

Babington RG: Antidepressives and the kindling effect, in Antidepressants. Edited by Fielding S, Lal H. Mount Kisco, NY, Futura Publishing, 1975, pp 113–124

Babington RG, Wedeking PW: The pharmacology of seizures induced by sensitization with low intensity brain stimulation. Pharmacol Biochem Behav 1:461–467, 1973

Baltzer V, Weiskrantz L: Antidepressant agents and reversal of diurnal activity cycles in the rat. Biol Psychiatry 10:199–209, 1975

Baruch I, Hemsley DR, Gray JA: Differential performance of acute and chronic schizophrenics in a latent inhibition task. J Nerv Ment Dis 176:598–606, 1988a

Baruch I, Hemsley DR, Gray JA: Latent inhibition and "psychotic proneness" in normal subjects. Personality and Individual Differences 9:777–783, 1988b

Bignami G: Selection for high rates and low rates of avoidance conditioning in rat. Animal Behavior 13:221–227, 1965

Bogerts B, Lieberman JA, Ashtari M, et al: Hippocampus-amygdala volumes and psychopathology in chronic schizophrenia. Biol Psychiatry 33:236, 1993

Borsini F, Meli A: Is the forced swimming test a suitable model for revealing antidepressant activity? Psychopharmacology (Berl) 94:147–160, 1988

Borsini F, Lecci A, Mancinelli A, et al: Stimulation of dopamine D_2 but not D_1 receptors reduces immobility time of rats in the forced swimming test: implication for antidepressant activity. Eur J Pharmacol 148:301–307, 1988

Borsini F, Lecci A, Sessarego A, et al: Discovery of antidepressant activity by forced swimming test may depend on pre-exposure of rats to a stressful situation. Psychopharmacology (Berl) 97:183–188, 1989

Braff D, Stone C, Callaway E, et al: Prestimulus effects on human startle reflex in normals and schizophrenics. Psychophysiology 15:339, 1978

Braff DL, Geyer MA: Sensorimotor gating and schizophrenia: human and animal model studies. Arch Gen Psychiatry 47:181–188, 1990

Braff DL, Grisson C, Geyer MA: Gating and habituation of the startle reflex in schizophrenic patients. Arch Gen Psychiatry 49:206, 1992

Breier A, Buchanan RW, Elkashef A, et al: Brain morphology and schizophrenia. Arch Gen Psychiatry 49:921–926, 1992

Brush FR: Genetic determination of individual differences in avoidance learning: behavioral and endocrine characteristics [review]. Experientia 47:1039–1050, 1991

Brush FR, Froehlich JC, Sakellaris PC: Genetic selection for avoidance behavior in the rat. Behav Genet 9:309–316, 1979

Bunney WE Jr, Davis JM: Norepinephrine in depressive reactions: a review. Arch Gen Psychiatry 13:483–494, 1965

Cairncross KD, Schofield S, King HG: The implication of noradrenaline in avoidance learning in the rat. Prog Brain Res 39:481–485, 1973

Cairncross KD, Schofield SPM, Bassett JR: Endogenous brain norepinephrine levels following bilateral olfactory bulb ablation. Pharmacol Biochem Behav 3:425–427, 1975a

Cairncross KD, King MG, Schofield SPM: Effect of amitriptyline on avoidance learning in rats following olfactory bulb ablation. Pharmacol Biochem Behav 3:1063–1067, 1975b

Cairncross KD, Cox B, Forster C, et al: The olfactory bulbectomized rat: a simple model for detecting drugs with antidepressant potential. Br J Pharmacol 61:497P, 1977

Cairncross KD, Cox B, Forster C, et al: Olfactory projection systems, drugs and behaviour: a review. Psychoneuroendocrinology 4:253–272, 1979

Carlson A: The current status of the dopamine hypothesis of schizophrenia. Neuropsychopharmacology 1:179–186, 1988

Carlton PL: Potentiation of the behavioral effects of amphetamine by imipramine. Psychopharmacologia 2:364–376, 1961

Carlton PL: Theories and models in psychopharmacology, in Psychopharmacology: A Generation of Progress. Edited by Lipton MA, DiMascio A, Killam KF. New York, Raven, 1978, pp 553–561

Carpenter WT, Heinrichs DW, Wagman AMI: Deficit and nondeficit forms of schizophrenia: the concept. Am J Psychiatry 145:578–601, 1988

Cervo L, Samanin R: Evidence that dopamine mechanisms in the nucleus accumbens are selectively involved in the effect of desipramine in the forced swimming test. Neuropharmacology 26:1469–1472, 1987

Christison GW, Atwater GE, Dunn LA, et al: Haloperidol enhancement of latent inhibition: relation to therapeutic action? Biol Psychiatry 23:746–749, 1988

Cohen RM, Weingartner H, Smallberg SA, et al: Effort

and cognition in depression. Arch Gen Psychiatry 39:593–597, 1982

Conrad AJ, Abebe T, Austin R, et al: Hippocampal pyramidal cell disarray in schizophrenia as a bilateral phenomenon. Arch Gen Psychiatry 48:431, 1991

Cook L, Catania AC: Effects of drugs on avoidance and escape behavior. Federation Proceedings 23:818–835, 1964

Corbett R, Hartman H, Kerman LL, et al: Effects of atypical antipsychotic agents on social behavior in rodents. Pharmacol Biochem Behav 45:9–17, 1993

Costa E, Garattini S, Valzelli L: Interactions between reserpine, chlorpromazine, and imipramine. Experientia 16:461–463, 1960

Cott JM, Kurtz NM: New pharmacological treatments for schizophrenia, in Handbook of Schizophrenia, Vol 2: Neurochemistry and Neuropharmacology of Schizophrenia. Edited by Henn FA, DeLisi LE. New York, Elsevier, 1987, pp 203–207

Crawley JN: Preliminary report of a new rodent separation model of depression. Psychopharmacol Bull 19:537–541, 1983

Crawley JN: Evaluation of a proposed hamster separation model of depression. Psychiatry Res 11:35–47, 1984

Creese I, Burt DR, Snyder SH: Dopamine receptor binding predicts clinical and pharmacological potencies of antipsychophrenic drugs. Nature 261:717, 1976

Crider A, Solomon PR, McMahon MA: Disruption of selective attention in the rat following chronic d-amphetamine administration: relationship to schizophrenic attention disorder. Biol Psychiatry 17:351–360, 1982

Crow TJ: Temporal lobe asymmetries as the key to the etiology of schizophrenia. Schizophr Bull 16:433–443, 1990

Danysz W, Plaznik A, Kostowski W, et al: Comparison of desipramine, amitriptyline, zimeldine and alaproclate in six animal models used to investigate antidepressant drugs. Pharmacol Toxicol 62:42–50, 1988

Davidson MK, Lindsey JR, Davis JK: Requirements and selection of an animal model. Isr J Med Sci 23:551–555, 1987

Davis KL, Kahn RS, Ko G, et al: Dopamine in schizophrenia: a review and reconceptualization. Am J Psychiatry 148:1474–1486, 1991

De Pablo JM, Parra A, Segovia S, et al: Learned im-mobility explains the behavior of rats in the forced swimming test. Physiol Behav 46:229–237, 1989

Desan PH, Silbert LH, Maier SF: Long-term effects of inescapable stress on daily running activity and antagonism by desipramine. Pharmacol Biochem Behav 30:21–29, 1988

Domenjoz R, Theobald W: Zur pharmakologie des Tofranil ®(N-(3-dimethylaminopropyl)-iminodi-benzylhydrochlorid). Archives Internationales de Pharmacodynamie et de Therapie 120:450–489, 1959

Dunn LA, Kilts CD, Nemeroff CB: Animal behavioral models for drug development in psychopharmacology, in Modern Drug Discovery Technology. Edited by Moos WH, Clark JS. Chichester, England, VCH & Ellis Horwood, 1990, pp 259–280

Dunn LA, Atwater GE, Kilts CD: Effects of antipsychotic drugs on latent inhibition: sensitivity and specificity of an animal behavioral model of clinical drug action. Psychopharmacology (Berl) 112:315–323, 1993

Earley B, Leonard BE: Effect of two specific-serotonin re-uptake inhibitors on the behaviour of the olfactory bulbectomized rat in the "open field" apparatus, in Clinical and Pharmacological Studies in Psychiatric Disorders. Edited by Burrows GD, Norman TR, Dennerstein L. London, John Libby, 1985, pp 234–240

Edwards E, Harkins K, Wright G, et al: Modulation of [3H]paroxetine binding to the 5-hydroxytryptamine uptake site in an animal model of depression. J Neurochem 56:1581–1586, 1991a

Edwards E, Harkins K, Wright G, Henn FA: 5-HT$_{1b}$ receptors in an animal model of depression. Neuropharmacology 30:101–105, 1991b

Edwards E, Kornrich W, Van Houtten P, et al: In vitro neurotransmitter release in an animal model of depression. Neurochem Int 21:29–35, 1992

Ellenbroek BA: The ethological analysis of monkeys in a social setting as an animal model for schizophrenia, in Animal Models in Psychopharmacology (Advances in Pharmacological Sciences Series). Edited by Olivier B, et al. Basel, Switzerland, Birkhauser Verlag, 1991, pp 265–284

Ellenbroek B, Cools AR: The paw test: an animal model for neuroleptic drugs which fulfills the criteria for pharmacological isomorphism. Life Sci 42:1205–1213, 1988

Ellenbroek BA, Peeters BW, Honig WM, et al: The paw test: a behavioural paradigm for differentiating between classical and atypical neuroleptic drugs. Psychopharmacology (Berl) 93:343–348, 1987

Ellenbroek BA, Willemen APM, Cools AR: Are antagonists of dopamine D_1 receptors drugs that attenuate both positive and negative symptoms of schizophrenia? Neuropsychopharmacology 2:191–199, 1989

Ellinwood EH Jr, Kilbey MM: Chronic stimulant intoxication models of psychosis, in Animal Models in Psychiatry and Neurology, Vol I. Edited by Hanin I, Usdin E. Oxford, England, Pergamon, 1977, pp 61–74

Ellinwood EH Jr, Sudilovsky A, Nelson LM: Behavioral analysis of chronic amphetamine intoxication. Biol Psychiatry 4:215–225, 1972

Ellison G, Eison MS, Huberman HS: Stages of constant amphetamine intoxication: delayed appearance of paranoid-like behaviors in rat colonies. Psychopharmacology (Berl) 56:293–299, 1978

Ettenberg A, Koob ZGF, Bloom FE: Response artifact in the measurement of neuroleptic induced anhedonia. Science 213:357, 1981

Feldon J, Weiner I: The latent inhibition model of schizophrenic attention disorder: haloperidol and sulpiride enhance rats' ability to ignore irrelevant stimuli. Biol Psychiatry 29:635–646, 1991

Fink JS, Swerdloff A, Reis DJ: Genetic control of dopamine receptors in mouse caudate nucleus: relationship of cataleptic response to neuroleptic drugs. Neurosci Lett 32:301–306, 1982

Fonberg E: Effects of small dorsomedial amygdala lesions on food intake and acquisition of instrumental alimentary reactions in dogs. Physiol Behav 4:739–743, 1969a

Fonberg E: The role of the hypothalamus and amygdala in food intake, alimentary motivation and emotional reaction. Acta Biologiae Experimentalis 29:335–358, 1969b

Fonberg E: Control of emotional behaviour through the hypothalamus and amygdaloid complex. Ciba Found Symp 8:131–161, 1972

Freedman R, Waldo MR, Bickford-Wimer P, et al: Elementary neuronal dysfunctions in schizophrenia. Schizophr Res 4:233–243, 1991

Fregnan GB, Chieli T: Classical neuroleptics and deconditioning activity after single or repeated treatments. Arzneimittelforschung 30:1865–1870, 1980

Fuller JL: Strain differences in the effects of chlorpromazine and chlordiazepoxide upon active and passive avoidance in mice. Psychopharmacologia 16:261–271, 1970

Garzon J, Del Rio J: Hyperactivity induced in rats by long-term isolation: further studies on a new model for the detection of antidepressants. Eur J Pharmacol 74:287–294, 1981

Garzon J, Fuentes JA, Del Rio J: Antidepressants selectively antagonize the hyperactivity induced in rats by long-term isolation. Eur J Pharmacol 59:293–296, 1979

Gardner C, Guy A: A social interaction model of anxiety sensitive to acutely administered benzodiazepines. Drug Development Research 4:207–216, 1984

Garver DL, Zemlan F, Hirschowitz J, et al: Dopamine and non-dopamine psychoses. Psychopharmacology (Berl) 84:138–145, 1984

Geyer MA, Wilkinson LS, Humby T, et al: Isolation rearing of rats produces a deficit in prepulse inhibition of acoustic startle similar to that in schizophrenia. Biol Psychiatry 34:361–372, 1993

Gil M, Marti J, Armario A: Inhibition of catecholamine synthesis depresses behavior of rats in the holeboard and forced swim tests: influence of previous chronic stress. Pharmacol Biochem Behav 43:597–601, 1992

Golda V, Petr R: Behaviour of genetically hypertensive rats in an animal model of depression and in an animal model of anxiety. Activitas Nervosa Superior 28:274–275, 1986

Golda V, Petr R: Animal model of depression: drug induced changes independent of changes in exploratory activity. Activitas Nervosa Superior 29:114–115, 1987a

Golda V, Petr R: Animal model of depression: retention of motor depression not predictable from the threshold of reaction to the inescapable shock. Activitas Nervosa Superior 29:113–114, 1987b

Golda V, Petr R: Animal model of depression: effect of nicotergoline and metergoline. Activitas Nervosa Superior 29:115–117, 1987c

Gorka Z, Earley B, Leonard BE: Effect of bilateral olfactory bulbectomy in the rat, alone or in combination with antidepressants, on the learned immobility model of depression. Neuropsychobiology 13:26–30, 1985

Gray JA, Feldon J, Rawlins JNP, et al: The neuropsychology of schizophrenia. Behavior and Brain Sciences 14:1–35, 1991

Gray NS, Pickering AD, Hemsley DR, et al: Abolition of latent inhibition by a single 5 mg dose of d-amphetamine in man. Psychopharmacology (Berl) 307:425–430, 1992

Halliwell G, Quinton RM, Williams FE: A comparison of imipramine, chlorpromazine and related drugs in various tests involving autonomic functions and antagonism of reserpine. Br J Pharmacol 23:330–350, 1964

Hartley P, Neill D, Hagler M, et al: Procedure- and age-dependent hyperactivity in a new animal model of endogenous depression. Neurosci Biobehav Rev 14:69–72, 1990

Hasey G, Hanin I: The cholinergic-adrenergic hypothesis of depression reexamined using clonidine, metoprolol, and physostigmine in an animal model. Biol Psychiatry 29:127–138, 1991

Hatotani N, Nomura J, Kitayama I: Changes in brain monoamines in the animal model for depression, in New Vistas in Depression, Advances in the Biosciences, Vol 40. Edited by Langer SZ, Takahashi R, Segawa T, et al. Oxford, England, Pergamon, 1982, pp 65–72

Hawkins J, Hicks RA, Phillips N, et al: Swimming rats and human depression. Nature 274:512, 1978

Hawkins J, Phillips N, Moore JD, et al: Emotionality and REMD: a rat swimming model. Physiol Behav 25:167–171, 1980

Hemsley DR: An experimental psychological model for schizophrenia, in Search for the Causes of Schizophrenia. Edited by Hafner H, Gattaz WF, Janzarik W. Berlin, Springer-Verlag, 1987, pp 179–188

Henn FA, Johnson J, Edwards E, et al: Melancholia in rodents: neurobiology and pharmacology. Psychopharmacol Bull 21:443–446, 1985

Hitzemann R, Daines K, Bier-Langing CM, et al: On the selection of mice for haloperidol response and non-response. Psychopharmacology (Berl) 103:244–250, 1991

Hoffman LJ, Weiss JM: Behavioral depression following clonidine withdrawal: a new animal model of long-lasting depression? Psychopharmacol Bull 22:943–949, 1986

Horovitz ZP, Ragozzino PW, Leaf RC: Selective block of rat mouse-killing by antidepressants. Life Sci 4:1909–1912, 1965

Howard JL, Soroko FE, Cooper BR: Empirical behavioral models of depression, with emphasis on tetrabenazine antagonism, in Antidepressants: Neurochemical, Behavioral, and Clinical Perspectives. Edited by Enna SJ, Malick JB, Richardson E. New York, Raven, 1981, pp 107–120

Iversen SD: Is it possible to model psychotic state in animals? Journal of Psychopharmacology 1:154–156, 1987

Jackson RL, Maier SF, Rapaport PM: Exposure to inescapable shock produces both activity and associative deficits in the rat. Learning and Motivation 9:69–98, 1978

Janscar S, Leonard BE: The effects of olfactory bulbectomy on the behaviour of rats in the open field. Isr J Med Sci 149:80–81, 1980

Jones SH, Gray JA, Hemsley DR: Loss of the Kamin blocking effect in acute but not chronic schizophrenics. Biol Psychiatry 32:739–755, 1992

Kamin LJ: Predictability, surprise, attention and conditioning, in Punishment and Aversive Behaviour. Edited by Campbell BA, Church RM. New York, Appleton-Century-Crofts, 1969, pp 279–296

Kane JM: Neuroleptic treatment of schizophrenia, in Handbook of Schizophrenia, Vol 2: Neurochemistry and Neuropharmacology of Schizophrenia. Edited by Henn FA, DeLisi LE. New York, Elsevier, 1987, pp 179–226

Kane J, Honigfeld G, Singer J, et al: Clozapine for the treatment resistant schizophrenic. Arch Gen Psychiatry 45:789–796, 1988

Katz RJ: Animal model of depression: effects of electroconvulsive shock therapy. Neurosci Biobehav Rev 5:273–277, 1981

Katz RJ: Animal model of depression: pharmacological sensitivity of a hedonic deficit. Pharmacol Biochem Behav 16:965–968, 1982

Katz RJ, Baldrighi G: A further parametric study of imipramine in an animal model of depression. Pharmacol Biochem Behav 16:969–972, 1982

Katz RJ, Hersh S: Amitriptyline and scopolamine in an animal model of depression. Neurosci Biobehav Rev 5:265–271, 1981

Katz RJ, Sibel M: Animal model of depression: tests of three structurally and pharmacologically novel antidepressant compounds. Pharmacol Biochem Behav 16:973–977, 1982a

Katz RJ, Sibel M: Further analysis of the specificity of a novel animal model of depression—effects of an antihistaminic, antipsychotic and anxiolytic compound. Pharmacol Biochem Behav 16:979–982, 1982b

Katz RJ, Roth KA, Carroll BJ: Acute and chronic stress effects on open field activity in the rat: implications for a model of depression. Neurosci Biobehav Rev 5:247–251, 1981a

Katz RJ, Roth KA, Schmaltz K: Amphetamine and

tranylcypromine in an animal model of depression: pharmacological specificity of the reversal effect. Neurosci Biobehav Rev 5:259–264, 1981b

Kaufman IC, Rosenblum LA: The reaction to separation in infant monkeys: anaclitic depression and conservation-withdrawal. Psychosom Med 29:648–675, 1967

Kendler KS, Tsuang MT, Hays P: Age at onset in schizophrenia. Arch Gen Psychiatry 44:881, 1987

Kibel DA, Lafont I, Liddle PF: The composition of the negative syndrome of chronic schizophrenia. Br J Psychiatry 162:744, 1993

Killcross AS, Robbins TW: Differential effects of intra-accumbens and systemic amphetamine on latent inhibition using an on-baseline, within-subject conditioned suppression paradigm. Psychopharmacology (Berl) 110:479–489, 1993

King MG, Cairncross KD: Effects of olfactory bulb section on brain noradrenaline, corticosterone and conditioning in the rat. Pharmacol Biochem Behav 2:347–353, 1974

Kitada Y, Miyauchi T, Satoh A, et al: Effects of antidepressants in the rat forced swimming test. Eur J Pharmacol 72:145–152, 1981

Kitada Y, Miyauchi T, Kosasa T, et al: The significance of b-adrenoceptor down regulation in the desipramine action in the forced swimming test. Naunyn Schmiedebergs Arch Pharmacol 333:31–35, 1986

Klein DF: Differential diagnosis and treatment of the dysphorias, in Depression: Behavioral, Biochemical, Clinical and Treatment Concepts. Edited by Simpson GM, Gallant DM. New York, Spectrum, 1975, pp 127–154

Kolakowska T, Williams AO, Arden M, et al: Schizophrenia with good and poor outcome, I: early clinical features, response to neuroleptics and signs of organic dysfunction. Br J Psychiatry 146:229–239, 1985

Kraemer GW: Causes of changes in brain noradrenaline systems and later effects on responses to social stressors in rhesus monkeys: the cascade hypothesis. Ciba Found Symp 123:216–233, 1986

Kuribara H, Tadokoro S: Correlation between anti-avoidance activities of antipsychotic drugs in rats and daily clinical doses. Pharmacol Biochem Behav 14:181–192, 1981

Labarca R, Silva H, Jerez S, et al: Differential effects of haloperidol on negative symptoms in drug-naive schizophrenic patients: effects on plasma homovanillic acid. Schizophr Bull 9:29, 1993

Lachman HM, Papolos DF, Boyle A, et al: Alterations in glucocorticoid inducible RNAs in the limbic system of learned helpless rats. Brain Res 609:110–116, 1993

Leonard BE, Tuite M: Anatomical, physiological, and behavioral aspects of olfactory bulbectomy in the rat. Int Rev Neurobiol 22:251–286, 1981

Leshner AI, Remler H, Biegon A, et al: Desmethylimipramine (DMI) counteracts learned helplessness in rats. Psychopharmacology (Berl) 66:207–208, 1979

Liddle PF, Firston KJ, Frith CD, et al: Patterns of cerebral blood flow in schizophrenia. Br J Psychiatry 160:179–186, 1992

Lipska BK, Jaskiw GE, Chrapusta S, et al: Ibotenic acid lesion of the ventral hippocampus differentially affects dopamine and its metabolites in the nucleus accumbens and prefrontal cortex in the rat. Brain Res 585:1–6, 1992

Lipska BK, Jaskiw GE, Weinberger DR: Postpubertal emergence of hyperresponsiveness to stress and amphetamine after neonatal excitotoxic hippocampal damage: a potential animal model of schizophrenia. Neuropsychopharmacology 9:67–75, 1993

Lubow RE: Latent inhibition. Psychol Bull 79:398–407, 1973

Lubow RE: Latent Inhibition and Conditioned Attention Theory. New York, Cambridge University Press, 1989

Lubow RE, Weiner I, Feldon J: An animal model of attention, in Behavioral Models and the Analysis of Drug Action. Edited by Spiegelstein MY, Levy A. Amsterdam, Elsevier, 1982, pp 89–107

Lyon M: Animal models of mania and schizophrenia, in Behavioral Models in Psychopharmacology: Theoretical, Industrial and Clinical Perspectives. Edited by Wilner P. Cambridge, England, Cambridge University Press, 1990, pp 253–310

Maier SF, Albin RW, Testa TJ: Failure to learn to escape in rats previously exposed to inescapable shock depends on nature of escape response. Journal of Comparative and Physiological Psychology 85:581–592, 1973

Malick JB: Yohimbine potentiation as a predictor of antidepressant action, in Antidepressants: Neurochemical, Behavioral, and Clinical Perspectives. Edited by Enna SJ, Malick JB, Richardson E. New York, Raven, 1981, pp 141–155

Martin JV, Edwards E, Johnson JO, et al: Monoamine

receptors in an animal model of affective disorder. J Neurochem 55:1142–1148, 1990

Martin P, Soubrie P, Simon P: The effect of monoamine oxidase inhibitors compared with classical tricyclic antidepressants on learned helplessness paradigm. Prog Neuropsychopharmacol Biol Psychiatry 11:1–7, 1987

Martin P, Soubrie P, Puech AJ: Reversal of helpless behavior by serotonin uptake blockers in rats. Psychopharmacology (Berl) 101:403–407, 1990

McGuire PS, Seiden LS: Differential effects of imipramine in rats as a function of DRL schedule value. Pharmacol Biochem Behav 13:691–694, 1980a

McGuire PS, Seiden LS: The effects of tricyclic antidepressants on performance under a differential-reinforcement-of-low-rates schedule in rats. J Pharmacol Exp Ther 214:635–641, 1980b

McKinney WT, Bunney WE: Animal model of depression. Arch Gen Psychiatry 21:240–248, 1969

McKinney WT, Suomi SJ, Harlow HF: Depression in primates. Am J Psychiatry 127:49–56, 1971

Meltzer HY, Sommers AA, Luchins DJ: The effect of neuroleptics and other psychotropic drugs on negative symptoms in schizophrenia. J Clin Psychopharmacol 6:329, 1986

Miczek K, Yoshimura H: Disruption of primate social behavior by d-amphetamine and cocaine: differential antagonism by antipsychotics. Psychopharmacology (Berl) 76:163, 1982

Minor TR, Jackson RL, Maier SF: Effects of task-irrelevant cues and reinforcement delay on choice-escape learning following inescapable shock: evidence for a deficit in selective attention. J Exp Psychol Anim Behav Process 10:543–556, 1984

Minor TR, Pelleymounter MA, Maier SF: Uncontrollable shock, forebrain norepinephrine, and stimulus selection during choice-escape learning. Psychobiology 16:135–145, 1988

Mitchell PB, Potter WZ: Major depression: the validity of a diagnosis. Depression 1:180, 1993

Moreau JL, Jenck F, Martin JR, et al: Antidepressant treatment prevents chronic unpredictable mild stress-induced anhedonia as assessed by ventral tegmentum self-stimulation behavior in rats. Eur J Pharmacol 2:43–49, 1992

Morpurgo C, Theobald W: Influence of imipramine-like compounds and chlorpromazine on the reserpine-hypothermia in mice and the amphetamine-hyperthermia in rats. Medicina et Pharmacologia Experimentalis 12:226–232, 1965

Mueser KT, Bellack AS, Douglas MS, et al: Prevalence and stability of social skill deficits in schizophrenia. Schizophr Res 5:167–176, 1991

Murua VS, Molina VA: An opiate mechanism involved in conditioned analgesia influences forced swim-induced immobility. Physiol Behav 48:641–645, 1990

Muscat R, Towell A, Willner P: Changes in dopamine autoreceptor sensitivity in an animal model of depression. Psychopharmacology (Berl) 94:545–550, 1988

Muscat R, Sampson D, Willner P: Dopaminergic mechanism of imipramine action in an animal model of depression. Biol Psychiatry 28:223–230, 1990

Muscat R, Papp M, Willner P: Antidepressant-like effects of dopamine agonists in an animal model of depression. Biol Psychiatry 31:937–946, 1992

Nagayama H, Hingtgen JN, Aprison MH: Pre- and postsynaptic serotonergic manipulations in an animal model of depression. Pharmacol Biochem Behav 13:575–579, 1980

Nagayama H, Hingtgen JN, Aprison MH: Postsynaptic action by four antidepressive drugs in an animal model of depression. Pharmacol Biochem Behav 15:125–130, 1981

Neill D, Vogel G, Hagler M, et al: Diminished sexual activity in a new animal model of endogenous depression. Neurosci Biobehav Rev 14:73–76, 1990

Nelson JC, Charney DS: The symptoms of major depressive illness. Am J Psychiatry 138:1–13, 1981

Nielsen M, Fjalland B, Pedersen V, et al: Pharmacology of neuroleptics upon repeated administration. Psychopharmacology (Berl) 34:95, 1974

Nielsen EB, Lyon M, Ellison G: Apparent hallucinations in monkeys during around-the-clock amphetamine for seven to fourteen days: possible relevance to amphetamine psychosis. J Nerv Ment Dis 171:222–233, 1983

Nuechterlein KH, Dawson ME: Information processing and attentional functioning in the developmental course of schizophrenic disorders. Schizophr Bull 10:160–203, 1984

O'Donnell JM, Seiden LS: Effects of monoamine oxidase inhibitors on performance during differential reinforcement of low response rate. Psychopharmacology (Berl) 78:214–218, 1982

O'Donnell JM, Seiden LS: Differential-reinforcement-of-low-rate 72-second schedule: selective effects of antidepressant drugs. J Pharmacol Exp Ther 224:80–88, 1983

O'Donnell JM, Seiden LS: Altered effects of desipramine on operant performance after 6-hydroxy-dopamine-induced depletion of brain dopamine or norepinephrine. J Pharmacol Exp Ther 229:629–635, 1984

O'Donnell JM, Seiden LS: Effect of the experimental antidepressant AHR-9377 on performance during differential reinforcement of low response rate. Psychopharmacology (Berl) 87:283–285, 1985

Overmier JB, Seligman MEP: Effects of inescapable shock upon subsequent escape and avoidance learning. Journal of Comparative and Physiological Psychology 63:28–33, 1967

Overstreet DH: Selective breeding for increased cholinergic function: development of a new animal model of depression. Biol Psychiatry 21:49–58, 1986

Overstreet DH: The Flinders sensitive line rats: A genetic animal model of depression. Neurosci Biobehav Rev 17:51-68, 1993

Overstreet DH, Rezvani AH, Janowsky DS: Genetic animal models of depression and ethanol preference provide support for cholinergic and serotonergic involvement in depression and alcoholism. Biol Psychiatry 31:919–936, 1992

Papolos DF, Edwards E, Marmur R, et al: Effects of the antiglucocorticoid RU 38486 on the induction of learned helpless behavior in Sprague-Dawley rats. Brain Res 615:304–309, 1993

Pare WP: Stress and consummatory behavior in the albino rat. Psychol Rep 16:399–405, 1965

Parker G, Hadzi-Pavlovic D, Boyce P, et al: Classifying depression by mental state signs. Br J Psychiatry 157:55–65, 1990

Peng RY, Mansbach RS, Braff DL, et al: A D_2 dopamine receptor agonist disrupts sensorimotor gating in rats: implications for dopaminergic abnormalities in schizophrenia. Neuropsychopharmacology 3:211–217, 1990

Penn DL, Van Der Dose AJW, Spaulding WD, et al: Information processing and social cognitive problem solving in schizophrenia. J Nerv Ment Dis 181:13–20, 1993

Petty F, Sherman AD: Learned helplessness induction decreases in vivo cortical serotonin release. Pharmacol Biochem Behav 18:649–650, 1983

Petty F, Kramer GL, Phillips TR, et al: Learned helplessness and serotonin: in vivo microdialysis. Society for Neuroscience Abstracts 16:752, 1990

Platt JE, Stone EA: Chronic restraint stress elicits a positive antidepressant response on the forced swim test. Eur J Pharmacol 82:179–181, 1982

Plaznik A, Danysz W, Kostowski W: Mesolimbic noradrenaline but not dopamine is responsible for organization of rat behavior in the forced swim test and an anti-immobilizing effect of desipramine. Pol J Pharmacol Pharm 37:347–357, 1985a

Plaznik A, Danysz W, Kostowski W: A stimulatory effect of intraaccumbens injections of noradrenaline on the behavior of rats in the forced swim test. Psychopharmacology (Berl) 87:119–123, 1985b

Plaznik A, Tamborska E, Hauptmann M, et al: Brain neurotransmitter systems mediating behavioral deficits produced by inescapable shock treatment in rats. Brain Res 447:122–132, 1988

Pollard GT, Howard JL: Similar effects of antidepressant and non-antidepressant drugs on behavior under an interresponse-time > 72-s schedule. Psychopharmacology (Berl) 89:253–258, 1986

Porsolt RD: Behavioral despair, in Antidepressants: Neurochemical, Behavioral, and Clinical Perspectives. Edited by Enna SJ, Malick JB, Richardson E. New York, Raven, 1981, pp 121–139

Porsolt RD, Anton G, Blavet N, et al: Behavioural despair in rats: a new model sensitive to antidepressant treatments. Eur J Pharmacol 47:379–391, 1978

Porsolt RD, Bertin A, Blavet N, et al: Immobility induced by forced swimming in rats: effects of agents which modify central catecholamine and serotonin activity. Eur J Pharmacol 57:201–210, 1979

Porsolt RD, Roux S, Jalfre M: Effects of imipramine on separation-induced vocalizations in young rhesus monkeys. Pharmacol Biochem Behav 20:979–981, 1984

Quinton RM: The increase in the toxicity of yohimbine induced by imipramine and other drugs in mice. Br J Pharmacol 21:51–66, 1963

Richelson E, Pfenning M: Blockade by antidepressants and related compounds of biogenic amine uptake into rat brain synaptosomes: most antidepressants selectively block norepinephrine uptake. Eur J Pharmacol 104:277–286, 1984

Rigter H, van Riezen H, Wren A: Pharmacological validation of a new test for the detection of antidepressant activity of drugs. Br J Pharmacol 59:451–452, 1977

Roberts DCS, Vickers G: Atypical neuroleptics increase self-administration of cocaine: an evaluation of a behavioural screen for antipsychotic activity. Psychopharmacology (Berl) 82:135–139, 1984

Robson RD, Antonaccio MJ, Saelens JK, et al: Antagonism by mianserin and classical a-adrenoceptor blocking drugs of some cardiovascular and behavioral effects of clonidine. Eur J Pharmacol 47:431–442, 1978

Roth M: A classification of affective disorders based on a synthesis of new and old concepts, in Research in the Psychobiology of Human Behavior. Edited by Meyer E, Brady JV. Baltimore, MD, Johns Hopkins University Press, 1976, pp 75–114

Roth KA, Katz RJ: Further studies on a novel animal model of depression: therapeutic effects of a tricyclic antidepressant. Neurosci Biobehav Rev 5:253–258, 1981

Sampson D, Willner P, Muscat R: Reversal of antidepressant action by dopamine antagonists in an animal model of depression. Psychopharmacology (Berl) 104:491–495, 1991

Sanberg PR, Bunsey MD, Giordano M, et al: The catalepsy test: its ups and down. Behav Neurosci 102:748–759, 1988

Sanger DJ: The effect of clozapine on shuttle box avoidance responding in rats: comparison with haloperidol and chlordiazepoxide. Pharmacol Biochem Behav 23:231, 1985

Satoh H, Mori J, Shimomura K, et al: Effect of zimelidine, a new antidepressant, on the forced swimming test in rats. Jpn J Pharmacol 35:471–473, 1984

Schildkraut JJ, Kety SS: Biogenic amines and emotion. Science 156:23–33, 1967

Schiller GD, Pucilowski O, Wienicke C, et al: Immobility-reducing effects of antidepressants in a genetic animal model of depression. Brain Res Bull 28:821–823, 1992

Schmajuk NA: Animal models of schizophrenia: the hippocampally lesioned animal. Schizophr Bull 13:317–327, 1987

Seiden LS, O'Donnell JM: Effects of antidepressant drugs on DRL behavior, in Behavioral Pharmacology: The Current Status. New York, Alan R. Liss, 1985, pp 323–338

Seiden LS, Dahms JL, Shaughnessy RA: Behavioral screen for antidepressants: the effects of drugs and electroconvulsive shock on performance under a differential-reinforcement-of-low-rate schedule. Psychopharmacology (Berl) 86:55–60, 1985

Seligman MEP: Depression and learned helplessness, in The Psychology of Depression: Contemporary Theory and Research. Edited by Friedman RJ, Katz MM. Washington, DC, VH Winston, 1974, pp 83–125

Seligman MEP, Beagley G: Learned helplessness in the rat. Journal of Comparative and Physiological Psychology 88:534–541, 1975

Seligman MEP, Maier SF: Failure to escape traumatic shock. Journal of Experimental Psychology 74:1–9, 1967

Seligman MEP, Maier SF, Solomon RL: Unpredictable and uncontrollable aversive events, in Aversive Conditioning and Learning. Edited by Brush FR. New York, Academic Press, 1971, pp 347–400

Shenton ME, Kikinis R, Jolesz FA, et al: Abnormalities of the left temporal lobe and thought disorder in schizophrenia. N Engl J Med 327:604–612, 1992

Sherman AD, Sacquitne JL, Petty F: Specificity of the learned helplessness model of depression. Pharmacol Biochem Behav 16:449–454, 1982

Shipley MT, Halloran FJ, De La Torre J: Surprisingly rich projection from locus coeruleus to the olfactory bulb in the rat. Brain Res 329:294–299, 1985

Shiromani PJ, Overstreet D, Levy D, et al: Increased REM sleep in rats selectively bred for cholinergic hyperactivity. Neuropsychopharmacology 1:127–133, 1988

Simons RF: Schizotypy and startle prepulse inhibition. Psychophysiology 27 (suppl):S6, 1990

Sofia RD: Effects of centrally active drugs on four models of experimentally-induced aggression in rodents. Life Sci 8:705–716, 1969a

Sofia RD: Structural relationship and potency of agents which selectively block mouse killing (muricide) behavior in rats. Life Sci 8:1201–1210, 1969b

Solomon CR, Crider A, Winkleman JW, et al: Disrupted latent inhibition in the rat with chronic amphetamine or haloperidol-induced supersensitivity: relationship to schizophrenic attention disorder. Biol Psychiatry 16:519, 1981

Spealman RD, Kelleher RT, Goldberg SR, et al: Behavioral effects of clozapine: comparison with thioridazine, chlorpromazine, haloperidol and chlordiazepoxide in squirrel monkeys. J Pharmacol Exp Ther 224:127, 1982

Steru L, Chermat R, Thierry B, et al: The tail suspension test: a new method for screening antidepressants in mice. Psychopharmacology (Berl) 85:367–370, 1985

Stockert M, Serra J, DeRobertis E: Effect of olfactory bulbectomy and chronic amitriptyline treatment in rats ^{3}H-imipramine binding and behavioral analysis by swimming and open field tests. Pharmacol Biochem Behav 29:681–686, 1988

Stoudemire A, Miller J, Schmitt F, et al: Development of an organic affective syndrome during a hyperbaric diving experiment. Am J Psychiatry 141:1251–1254, 1984

Sulser F: New perspectives on the mode of action of antidepressant drugs. Trends Pharmacol Sci 1:92–94, 1979

Suomi SJ, Seaman SF, Lewis JK, et al: Effects of imipramine treatment of separation-induced social disorders in rhesus monkeys. Arch Gen Psychiatry 35:321–325, 1978

Swerdlow NR, Geyer MA: Clozapine and haloperidol in an animal model of sensorimotor gating deficits in schizophrenia. Pharmacol Biochem Behav 44:741–744, 1993

Swerdlow NR, Geyer M, Braff D, et al: Central dopamine hyperactivity in rats mimics abnormal acoustic startle in schizophrenics. Biol Psychiatry 21:23, 1986

Swerdlow NR, Braff DL, Masten VL, et al: Schizophrenic-like sensorimotor gating abnormalities in rats following dopamine infusion into the nucleus accumbens. Psychopharmacology (Berl) 101:414–420, 1990

Swerdlow NR, Keith VA, Braff DL, et al: The effects of spiperone, raclopride, SCH 23390 and clozapine on apomorphine-inhibition of sensorimotor gating of the startle response in the rat. J Pharmacol Exp Ther 256:530, 1991

Swerdlow NR, Benbow CH, Zisook S, et al: A preliminary assessment of sensorimotor gating in patients with obsessive compulsive disorder. Biol Psychiatry 33:298, 1993

Swerdlow NR, Braff DL, Taaid N, et al: Assessing the validity of an animal model of deficient sensorimotor gating in schizophrenic patients. Arch Gen Psychiatry 51:139–154, 1994

Tamminga CA, Thaker GK, Buchanan R, et al: Limbic system abnormalities identified in schizophrenia using position emission tomography with fluorodeoxyglucose and neocortical alteration with deficit syndrome. Arch Gen Psychiatry 49:522–530, 1992

Tekes K, Tothfalusi T, Magyar K: Irregular chronic stress related selective presynaptic adaptation of dopaminergic system in rat striatum: effects of (−) deprenyl and amitriptyline. Acta Physiol Pharmacol Bulg 12:21–28, 1986

Telner JI, Singhal RL: Effects of nortriptyline treatment on learned helplessness in the rat. Pharmacol Biochem Behav 14:823–826, 1981

Upchurch M, Schallert T: A behavioral analysis of the offspring of "haloperidol-sensitive" and "haloperidol-resistant" gerbils. Behav Neural Biol 39:221–228, 1983

van Riezen H, Leonard BE: Effects of psychotropic drugs on the behavior and neurochemistry of olfactory bulbectomized rats, in Psychopharmacology of Anxiolytics and Antidepressants. Edited by File SE. New York, Pergamon, 1991, pp 231–250

van Riezen H, Schnieden H, Wren AF: Olfactory bulb ablation in the rat: behavioural changes and their reversal by antidepressant drugs. Br J Pharmacol 60:521–528, 1977

Vernier VG, Hanson HM, Stone CA: The pharmacodynamics of amitriptyline, in Psychosomatic Medicine: the First Hahnemann Symposium. Edited by Nodine JH, Moyer JH. Philadelphia, PA, Lea & Febiger, 1962, pp 683–690

Vetulani J, Stawarz RJ, Dingell JV, et al: A possible mechanism of action of antidepressant treatments. Naunyn Schmiedebergs Arch Pharmacol 293:109–114, 1976

Vogel G, Hartley P, Neill D, et al: Animal depression model by neonatal clomipramine: reduction of shock induced aggression. Pharmacol Biochem Behav 31:103–106, 1988

Vogel G, Neill D, Hagler M, et al: Decreased intracranial self-stimulation in a new animal model of endogenous depression. Neurosci Biobehav Rev 14:65–68, 1990a

Vogel G, Neill D, Kors D, et al: REM sleep abnormalities in a new animal model of endogenous depression. Neurosci Biobehav Rev 14:77–83, 1990b

Vogel G, Neill D, Hagler M, et al: A new animal model of endogenous depression: a summary of present findings. Neurosci Biobehav Rev 14:85–91, 1990c

Wang P, Aulakh CS, Hill JL, et al: Fawn-hooded rats are subsensitive to the food intake suppressant effects of 5-HT agonists. Psychopharmacology (Berl) 94:558–562, 1988

Weinberger DR: Implications of normal brain development for the pathogenesis of schizophrenia.

Arch Gen Psychiatry 44:660, 1987

Weiner I, Feldon J: Facilitation of latent inhibition by haloperidol in rats. Psychopharmacology (Berl) 91:248–253, 1987

Weiner I, Lubow RE, Feldon J: Abolition of expression but not acquisition of latent inhibition by chronic amphetamine in rats. Psychopharmacology (Berl) 83:194, 1984

Weiss JM: Effects of coping responses on stress. Journal of Comparative and Physiological Psychology 65:251–260, 1968

Weiss JM: Coping behavior: explaining behavioral depression following uncontrollable stressful events. Behav Res Ther 18:485–504, 1980

Weiss JM: Stress-induced depression: critical neurochemical and electrophysiological changes, in Neurobiology of Learning, Emotion and Affect. Edited by Madden J IV. New York, Raven, 1991, pp 123–154

Weiss JM, Krieckhaus EE, Conte R: Effects of fear conditioning on subsequent avoidance and movement. Journal of Comparative and Physiological Psychology 65:413–421, 1968

Weiss JM, Stone EA, Harrell N: Coping behavior and brain norepinephrine level in rats. Journal of Comparative and Physiological Psychology 72:153–160, 1970

Weiss JM, Bailey WH, Pohorecky LA, et al: Stress-induced depression of motor activity correlates with regional changes in brain norepinephrine but not in dopamine. Neurochem Res 5:9–22, 1980

Weiss JM, Goodman PA, Losito BG, et al: Behavioral depression produced by an uncontrollable stressor: relationship to norepinephrine, dopamine, and serotonin levels in various regions of the rat brain. Brain Research Reviews 3:167–205, 1981

Weiss JM, Bailey WH, Goodman PA, et al: A model for neurochemical study of depression, in Behavioral Models and the Analysis of Drug Action. Edited by Spiegelstein MY, Levy A. Amsterdam, Elsevier, 1982, pp 195–223

Willner P: The validity of animal models of depression. Psychopharmacology (Berl) 83:1–16, 1984

Willner P, Muscat R, Papp M: Chronic mild stress-induced anhedonia: a realistic animal model of depression. Neurosci Biobehav Rev 16:525–534, 1992

Wise RA, Rompre PP: Brain dopamine and reward. Annu Rev Psychol 40:191–225, 1989

Worms P, Broekkamp CLE, Lloyd KG: Behavioral effects of neuroleptics, in Neuroleptics: Neurochemical, Behavioral, and Clinical Perspectives. Edited by Coyle JT, Enna SJ. New York, Raven, 1983, pp 93–117

Wren AF: Master's thesis, Manchester University, United Kingdom, 1976 (reported in Leonard and Tuite 1981)

Zacharko RM, Anisman H: Stressor-induced anhedonia in the mesocorticolimbic system. Neurosci Biobehav Rev 15:391–405, 1991

Zacharko RM, Bowers WJ, Kokkinidis L, et al: Region-specific reductions of intracranial self-stimulation after uncontrollable stress: possible effects of reward processes. Behav Brain Res 9:129–141, 1983

6

Principles of Pharmacokinetics and Pharmacodynamics

David J. Greenblatt, M.D.

The discipline of pharmacokinetics uses mathematical models to describe and predict the time-course of drug concentrations and amounts in various body fluids. The application of pharmacokinetic principles to clinical psychiatry and psychopharmacology has undergone major advances during the last 30 years. One reason for this progress is the availability of improved techniques for quantitation of drug concentrations in plasma and tissues, using methods such as gas chromatography, liquid chromatography, and mass spectroscopy (Friedman and Greenblatt 1986). For essentially all drugs used to treat mental illness, reliable methods are now available to quantitate serum or plasma concentrations of these compounds and their metabolites after single doses or during chronic therapy. The second reason for progress in pharmacokinetics is the general availability of computer methods for nonlinear regression analyses, which are essential for fitting of data to theoretical models (Harmatz and Greenblatt 1987; Motulsky and Ransnas 1987).

Pharmacodynamics refers to the study of the time-course and intensity of drug effects on the organism, whether human or experimental animal. Again, major progress in this field is attributable to technological advances in the capacity to measure drug effects. The newest discipline of kinetic-dynamic modeling uses similar mathematical methods to link drug concentrations directly to clinical effects. Successful kinetic-dynamic modeling ultimately validates the clinical value of both pharmacokinetics and pharmacodynamics.

In this chapter, I review some current advances in our understanding of pharmacokinetic and pharmacodynamic methodologies and their application to kinetic-dynamic modeling.

■ PHARMACOKINETICS

■ Implications of the Two-Compartment Model

Lipophilic psychotropic drugs generally do not behave as if the body were a single homogeneous space. The two-compartment model, which resolves

Supported in part by Grant MH-34223 from the Department of Health and Human Services.
The author is grateful for the collaboration and assistance of Richard I. Shader, Jerold S. Harmatz, Lisa L. von Moltke, Bruce L. Ehrenberg, and Lawrence G. Miller.

the living organism into two distinct mathematical spaces, enhances the precision of describing and predicting drug behavior but also increases mathematical complexity (Figure 6–1). The characteristics of this model have been described in detail in many previous publications (Gibaldi and Perrier 1975; Greenblatt and Koch-Weser 1975; Greenblatt and Shader 1985; Wagner 1975). The model assumes that intravenously administered medications are introduced directly into the "central" compartment, which consists of the circulating blood as well as other high-flow tissues such as brain, heart, lung, liver, and endocrine organs. Irreversible drug elimination, either by hepatic biotransformation or renal excretion, takes place only via the central compartment. Reversible distribution occurs between central and "peripheral" compartments, with a finite period of time (usually between 30 minutes and 6 hours after intravenous drug dosage) required for distribution equilibrium to be attained. The peripheral compartment is usually considered to be inaccessible to direct measurement and is not a site of drug elimination or clearance.

This model predicts that rapid intravenous drug administration will yield a biphasic serum or plasma drug concentration curve (Figure 6–2). The initial rapid phase of drug disappearance is due largely to distribution, followed thereafter by a slower phase of disappearance attributable mainly to elimination or clearance. The interdependency of distribution, elim-

ination, and duration of action is increasing recognized. A drug's elimination half-life refers to the apparent half-life of disappearance in the postdistributive elimination phase. This does not necessarily correspond to its duration of action, which actually depends on the absolute plasma concentration relative to a hypothetical minimum effective concentration (MEC). Drug action may be terminated during the distribution phase and may have little to do with elimination half-life following a single dose (Figure 6–2). The absolute size of the dose also is of critical importance, because a proportional change in dose will produce corresponding changes in all plasma concentrations. This may change duration of action in a nonproportional manner, depending on the MEC for the particular drug action in question (Figure 6–3).

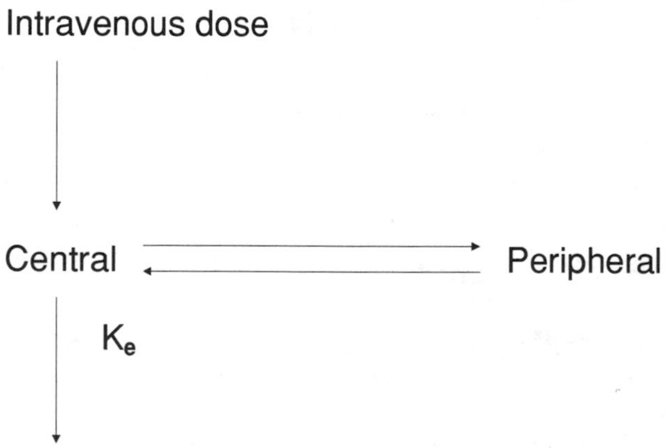

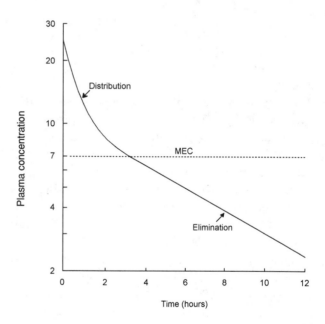

Figure 6–2. Predicted plasma concentration curve following a rapid intravenous injection (at time zero) of a drug whose behavior is consistent with a two-compartment model. The curve is biphasic: there is a rapid disappearance phase due mainly to distribution, followed by a slower phase of disappearance attributable mainly to elimination. The elimination half-life of this drug is 6 hours; note that this refers to the slower rate of disappearance during the elimination phase, after distribution equilibrium is complete. Also assume that this drug has a minimum effective concentration (MEC) of 7 units. At plasma levels above the MEC, the drug is clinically effective; below this, the drug has no activity. Note that the duration of action of this drug is short (approximately 3 hours), despite its elimination half-life of 6 hours. This is because the plasma level falls below the MEC during the distribution phase.

Intravenous dose

Central ⟷ Peripheral

K_e

Figure 6–1. Schematic representation of the two-compartment open model. It is assumed that intravenously administered medications are given directly into the central compartment. Irreversible elimination (via hepatic biotransformation or renal excretion) only occurs via the central compartment; K_e is the first-order elimination rate constant. Reversible distribution occurs between central and peripheral compartments.

These principles are equally applicable following oral drug administration (Greenblatt 1991). The mathematics become more complex, because the drug is actually administered into an extravascular site such as the gastrointestinal tract. It is then absorbed into the systemic circulation, followed by the previously described processes of distribution and elimination (Figure 6–4). If the absorption rate is rapid, the plasma concentration curve will begin at zero, rapidly reach a peak, and decline thereafter in biphasic fashion. The duration of drug action depends on dosage, plasma concentrations during the distribution and elimination phases, and location of the particular MEC in question (Figure 6–5). Thus, with oral as well as intravenous dosage, elimination half-life does not necessarily predict the duration of drug action after a single dose.

The Steady-State Condition

Continuous drug administration with a regular dosage schedule will eventually lead to the steady-state condition, at which time the mean plasma drug concentration remains constant as long as the dosing rate remains the same and there is no change in drug clearance. The mean steady-state concentration is

often of considerable importance, because it may predict the likelihood of therapeutic efficacy or side effects (Friedman and Greenblatt 1986). However, the relationship may be complicated by interdose fluctuation unless the drug is given by continuous intravenous infusion. Under usual circumstances, drugs are administered by multiple discrete doses. There is not really one unique steady-state plasma concentration; it rises and falls above the mean value during each dosage interval (Figure 6–6). Drugs with short half-life values tend to undergo greater interdose fluctuation. Clinicians may observe phenomena such as transient toxicity when plasma levels are at maximum just following a dose, or "breakthrough" symptoms when levels fall toward the end of a dose interval (Figure 6–6). To cope with this problem, clinicians may need to subdivide the daily dosage and give it more frequently. For some drugs, "sustained release" formulations are available that reduce interdose fluctuation by providing a slow absorption profile.

Many psychotropic drugs have pharmacologically active metabolites (Caccia and Garattini 1990, 1992; Greenblatt and Shader 1987). This pharmacokinetic feature has both benefits and drawbacks. The presence of an active metabolite tends to "cushion" the effect of interdose fluctuation at steady state, because plasma levels of metabolites usually undergo less up-and-down fluctuation than do levels of the

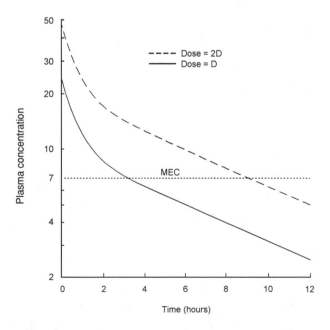

Figure 6–3. For the same drug discussed in Figure 6–2, a doubling of the dose (from D to 2D) disproportionately increases the duration of action, which is determined by the length of time that the plasma level exceeds the minimum effective concentration (MEC).

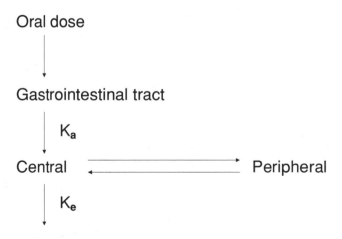

Figure 6–4. Modification of the two-compartment model (from Figure 6–1) to include oral administration. It is assumed that drug absorption from the gastrointestinal tract is a first-order process, having a rate constant K_a. As the drug reaches the central compartment, the processes of distribution and elimination take place as in Figure 6–1. K_e = first-order elimination rate constant.

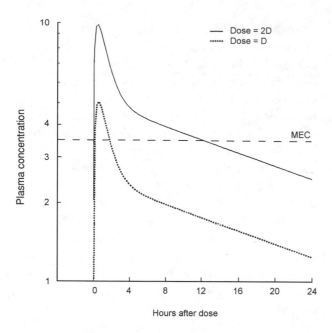

Figure 6–5. The duration of drug action after oral dosage may be determined mainly by distribution rather than elimination, as with intravenous dosage (Figure 6–3). Doubling of the dose (from D to 2D) may disproportionately increase the duration of action. MEC = minimum effective concentration.

parent drug (Figure 6–7). However, the relation between plasma drug concentration and clinical outcome is more complex, because levels of the parent drug and any active metabolites that are present must be considered simultaneously. Some metabolites have half-life values much longer than those of the parent drug. Discontinuation of a medication of this type can lead to drug effects that persist well beyond the disappearance of the parent drug, owing to sustained levels of the long half-life metabolite. The pharmacokinetic behavior of fluoxetine and its metabolite, norfluoxetine, is an example of this situation (Greenblatt et al. 1992; Pato et al. 1991; Schenker et al. 1988).

Differences among drugs in the time-course and severity of discontinuation syndromes usually are explained by pharmacokinetic properties (Greenblatt et al. 1990). This relationship is most convincingly supported by studies of the class of benzodiazepines. Abrupt discontinuation of chronic therapy with short half-life benzodiazepines (such as alprazolam and lorazepam) is much more likely to produce discontinuation syndromes of rapid onset than is termination of treatment with a long half-life benzodiazepine such as diazepam, desmethyldiazepam, or any pre-

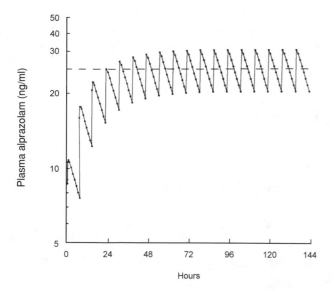

Figure 6–6. Predicted plasma alprazolam concentrations if an oral dosing regimen of 1.0 mg every 8 hours is started at time zero. It is assumed that the elimination half-life of alprazolam is 12 hours. At steady state, the plasma level rises and falls after each dose; this is termed *interdose fluctuation*. If the horizontal dashed line (corresponding to 25 ng/ml) is the minimum effective concentration (as defined in Figure 6–2), there will be "breakthrough" of symptoms toward the end of each dose interval.

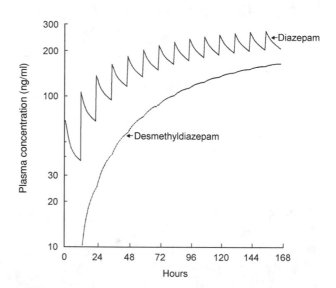

Figure 6–7. Predicted plasma concentrations of diazepam (DZ) and its major metabolite, desmethyldiazepam (DMDZ), if an oral dosing regimen of 5 mg every 12 hours is started at time zero. Kinetic behavior of DZ and DMDZ were based on previous study (Greenblatt et al. 1989c). Note that interdose fluctuation of DZ plasma levels at steady state is considerably less than that of alprazolam (see Figure 6–6). There is almost no interdose fluctuation of DMDZ plasma levels.

cursor of desmethyldiazepam (Busto et al. 1986; Noyes et al. 1991; Rickels et al. 1988, 1990). The difference is attributable to rapid elimination of active substances from blood and brain following discontinuation of the short half-life compounds. When short half-life benzodiazepines are tapered rather than abruptly discontinued, the discontinuation profile becomes largely indistinguishable from that of a long half-life derivative (Schweizer et al. 1990).

There is little tenable support for the hypothesis that benzodiazepines with high receptor affinity (such as alprazolam) are more likely to produce discontinuation syndromes than "low-affinity" benzodiazepines. The most obvious counterexample comes from a comparison of alprazolam and clonazepam. Both of these compounds have high benzodiazepine receptor affinity, but the half-life of alprazolam is considerably shorter than that of clonazepam (Greenblatt and Shader 1987; Greenblatt et al. 1987). Clinical differences between these two compounds after drug discontinuation are explained by the difference in half-life and have little to do with receptor affinity as such.

■ The Predictability of Drug Interactions

The increasing popularity of the selective serotonin reuptake inhibitor (SSRI) antidepressants, of which fluoxetine is the prototype (Table 6–1), has brought pharmacokinetic drug interactions back to the consciousness of psychopharmacologists contemplating combined drug therapy. The class of SSRIs appears to have the secondary pharmacological property of reversibly inhibiting the activity of hepatic drug-metabolizing enzymes. The introduction of fluoxetine into clinical practice was followed by experimental and clinical reports of drug interactions, in which coadministration of fluoxetine caused decreased clearance and elevated plasma drug concentrations of certain other coadministered medications (Table 6–2; Ciraulo and Shader 1990). In some cases, these interactions were of clinical importance (Preskorn et al. 1990). The various SSRIs (and their metabolites) that are already available, as well as those under investigation, are not equivalent in their capacity to inhibit drug metabolism. Nor is the metabolism of every drug equally affected by SSRI coadministration.

A simple count of the number of medications that may be coadministered with SSRIs raises the discour-

Table 6–1. Selective serotonin reuptake inhibitor antidepressants and their metabolites

Parent drug	Clinically important metabolite
Fluoxetine	Norfluoxetine
Sertraline	Desmethylsertraline
Paroxetine	
Fluvoxamine[*]	

[*] Under investigation through mid-1994.

Table 6–2. Representative drugs whose metabolism is reportedly impaired by fluoxetine or norfluoxetine

Drug	Reference
Valproate	Sovner and Davis 1991
Desipramine	Preskorn et al. 1990, 1994; Wilens et al. 1992
Haloperidol	Goff et al. 1991
Imipramine	Bergstrom et al. 1992
Alprazolam	Greenblatt et al. 1992; Lasher et al. 1991
Diazepam	Lemberger et al. 1988

aging necessity for literally hundreds of clinical pharmacokinetics studies that must be done to delineate which drugs will interact, the extent of their interaction, and whether they can be coadministered safely. However, recent advances in the field of cytochrome biochemistry fortunately have revealed some logical consistencies. A pattern of predictability has emerged that may render at least some of the clinical pharmacokinetic studies unnecessary (Brosen 1990; Gonzalez 1992a; Guengerich 1992, 1993; Murray 1992). Of many biochemically distinct human liver cytochromes that have been identified, the P_{450}-2D6 subfamily, together with the P_{450}-3A subfamily (3A3 and 3A4), collectively account for the metabolism of many drugs used in clinical practice (Table 6–3). The 2D6 subfamily is notorious for its genetic polymorphism. The human population can be divided into a majority of "normal metabolizers" and a smaller group of "slow metabolizers." The latter group will have relatively low clearance and increased plasma levels of any drug metabolized by cytochrome P_{450}-2D6; the "at-risk" group can be identified by administering a test substance such as sparteine, debrisoquin, or dextromethorphan. SSRIs are important inhibitors of the 2D6 subfamily at clinically relevant concentrations.

Table 6–3. Partial list of drugs metabolized by cytochromes P_{450}-3A (3A3 and 3A4) and by P_{450}-2D6

Metabolized by 3A (3A3 or 3A4)	Metabolized by 2D6
Cyclosporine	Propranolol
Nifedipine	Propafenone
Midazolam	Timolol
Quinidine	Metoprolol
Lidocaine	Desipramine
Triazolam	Nortriptyline
Alprazolam	Codeine
Terfenadine	
Diltiazem	

Again, not all SSRIs are equal in their capacity to inhibit. Paroxetine is the most potent inhibitor, followed by fluoxetine and norfluoxetine, and then by sertraline and desmethylsertraline (Crewe et al. 1992; Otton et al. 1993; Skjelbo and Brøsen 1992; von Moltke et al. 1994a). The cytochrome P_{450}-3A subfamily, on the other hand, is not subject to genetic polymorphism; that is, the distribution of enzyme activity in the population is not bimodal or polymodal, as it is with 2D6. SSRIs also inhibit the activity of 3A cytochromes, but as a class the SSRIs are less potent against 3A than against 2D6. Again, not all SSRIs are equal, and the order of activity is not the same as for inhibition of 2D6. Although data on this subject are much more limited, it appears that norfluoxetine is a more potent inhibitor than either sertraline or desmethylsertraline, which in turn are more potent than fluoxetine itself (von Moltke et al. 1992). Data on paroxetine are incomplete. The potential problems of combining SSRIs with other medications can be approached more logically if the specific cytochrome subfamily responsible for metabolism of the other medications has been identified. This knowledge will increase the accuracy of predicting whether a pharmacokinetic interaction is likely and which specific SSRI can be chosen to minimize the likelihood of interference (Gonzalez 1992b; Peck et al. 1993; von Moltke et al. 1994b).

■ PHARMACODYNAMICS

Following a single oral dose of a psychotropic medication, its clinical effect will increase, reach a maximum, and then decline with time. The time-course and intensity of drug action or response comprises the discipline of pharmacodynamics. The capacity to understand and predict individual differences in drug response is, in a sense, the ultimate task in psychopharmacology, because the objective of therapy is to produce therapeutic benefit without side effects or toxicity.

Recent advances in the understanding of pharmacodynamics are partly attributable to enhanced precision and objectivity in the measurement of human drug response. The emergence of the discipline of kinetic-dynamic modeling, whereby drug concentration is used as a direct predictor of response, is also significant.

■ Methods of Measurement

Each class of psychotropic drugs produces unique pharmacodynamic effects, and a correspondingly unique set of problems with measurement. The methodological problems facing investigators studying antidepressant drugs, antipsychotic agents, and sedative-anxiolytics vary widely and may in fact differ for various medication subgroups within the larger category. Some of the lessons learned from pharmacodynamic studies of sedative-anxiolytic drugs serve to illustrate available approaches to quantitation and the limitations associated with each.

Benzodiazepine derivatives and other compounds acting via the γ-aminobutyric acid (GABA)–benzodiazepine complex apparently act by interaction with this receptor site, enhancement of the action of GABA, opening of the chloride channel, entry of chloride ion into the cell, and cell hyperpolarization (Figure 6–8) (Haefely 1990; Zorumski and Isenberg 1991). The final common pathway is the benzodiazepine agonist effect of "sedation." However, this action has many clinical facets, depending on the therapeutic objective and clinical setting of drug administration. For example, the "primary therapeutic actions" consist of antianxiety-antipanic effects, sleep enhancement, or reduction of seizure activity. Commonly accompanying these therapeutic actions are typical side effects such as excessive or persistent sedation, drowsiness, ataxia, incoordination, slowed reaction time, or slowed psychomotor performance. Some effects may be ambiguous; for example, impaired memory may be a desired therapeutic effect in the context of premedication before

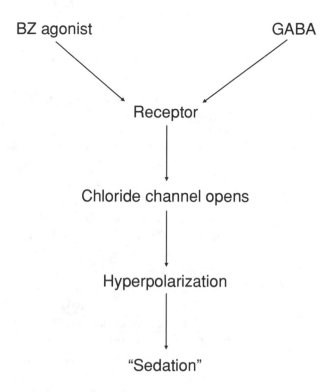

BZ agonist   GABA

Receptor

Chloride channel opens

Hyperpolarization

"Sedation"

Figure 6–8. Schematic representation of the mechanism of action of benzodiazepine (BZ) agonists via the γ-aminobutyric acid (GABA)–benzodiazepine receptor complex.

general anesthesia, or sedation prior to endoscopy or cardioversion. In other circumstances, it might be an undesired side effect. Finally, benzodiazepines produce some effects whose direct link to clinical efficacy or side effects are not directly established. These include increased beta activity on the electroencephalogram (EEG), reduced saccadic eye movement velocity, elevated concentrations of plasma growth hormone, and reduced plasma concentrations of cortisol and adrenocorticotropic hormone (ACTH; Hommer et al. 1986; Mandema and Danhof 1992; Roy-Byrne et al. 1990).

Ironically, the accuracy, reliability, and objectivity of methods for measuring the pharmacodynamic effects of benzodiazepines become greater as the effects become more removed from the primary therapeutic action (Greenblatt et al. 1991a). What we really want to know is the time-course and intensity of primary therapeutic effects, but these are the most difficult to measure. Clinical anxiolytic or sedative properties can be quantitated via global assessments by patients or by a trained observer. Alternatively,

rating instruments can be targeted to specific symptoms or symptom groups. These measurement approaches have historically been extremely useful in clinical psychopharmacology, but they have important limitations. Because they are subjective, ratings will be influenced by the outlook, expectation, and experience of the patient or observer. Drug effects usually must be evaluated as change scores relative to both the pretreatment baseline condition and to inactive placebo. Special populations (e.g., elderly patients) may have a unique frame of reference for interpreting rating scale items or perceived drug effects, which creates additional methodological complications.

Quantitation of secondary effects of benzodiazepine agonists has also provided important data on the pharmacodynamic properties of these drugs. These testing procedures generally focus on the broad category of psychomotor performance, including measures of reaction time, speed and accuracy of task performance, and capacity for information acquisition and recall. These procedures are partly objective, in that a given test provides a specific numeric result. Again, change scores are the most meaningful; drug effects must be compared to baseline performance and to effects of placebo. A principal drawback of the psychomotor performance procedures is that they are influenced by practice. Subjects' performance will progressively improve if they undertake a test repeatedly in the absence of medication. This can greatly complicate interpretation of drug-related changes and must be carefully accounted for in the experimental design. The study of special populations (such as elderly patients) may also be complicated, because their baseline performance may be different from that of a "control" population (Greenblatt et al. 1991b). There is no well-established method for normalizing or controlling for differences in baseline performance capacity when comparing drug effects between populations. Finally, the extent to which drug effects on laboratory performance tests apply to real-life tasks is not clearly established. This is of particular concern for complex laboratory tests, such as simulated automobile operation, for which the consequences of error are negligible in the laboratory but potentially lethal on the road.

Increasing attention has focused on the fully objective measures of pharmacodynamic effects of benzodiazepines. Of particular interest is the computerized analysis of the EEG, which can directly quantitate benzodiazepine effects either by evaluation of the "beta" frequency band by fast-Fourier transform, or by aperiodic analysis (Mandema and Danhof 1992; Stanski 1992; Swerdlow and Holley 1987). These methods are fully objective, unresponsive to placebo, and not altered by practice or experience. There is no theoretical basis to allow direct linkage of EEG changes to clinical assessment either of therapeutic effects or psychomotor side effects. Nonetheless, empirical evidence shows that the pharmacodynamic profile of EEG changes in response to benzodiazepine administration closely intercorrelates with other measures of drug activity (Friedman et al. 1992).

■ Kinetic-Dynamic Modeling

Kinetic-dynamic modeling procedures subsume time and look directly at the relation of drug concentrations to drug effect (Dingemanse et al. 1988; Holford and Sheiner 1982; Stanski 1992). The objective is to determine precisely how much variably in drug effect is attributable to measurable drug concentrations (Greenblatt and Harmatz 1993).

The application of a specific model reflects theoretical and empirical considerations. The model should fit the data but should not extract from the data more information than is actually available. The

Sigmoid-E_{max} model is of considerable importance. When it fits the data, investigators are reassured about the concentration-effect relationship, because many drug-receptor interactions fit the same model (Figure 6–9). The linkage is characterized by three features: 1) E_{max}, which is the maximum drug effect (relative to baseline) and cannot be exceeded no matter how high the drug concentration; 2) EC_{50}, a concentration at which the drug effect is 50% of E_{max}; and 3) A, an exponent of unknown biological significance related to the "steepness" of the curve in its linear phase. When applicable, this model allows quantitation of individual differences in sensitivity to a given drug, relative "potencies" of drugs having the same mechanism of action, and the quantitative and qualitative effects of pharmacologic potentiators or antagonists. However, not all data sets are consistent with this model. Many are consistent with simpler relationships, such as linear or exponential equations (Friedman et al. 1992; Greenblatt and Harmatz 1993; Greenblatt et al. 1991b).

The assumption that plasma drug concentrations are proportional to drug concentrations at the site of action may need to be modified for purposes of kinetic-dynamic modeling. Intravenous administration of diazepam to healthy volunteer subjects produced

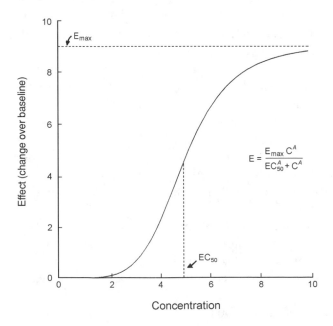

Figure 6–9. Schematic representation of the Sigmoid-E_{max} model, relating concentration (C, on the x-axis) to effect (E, on the y-axis). See text for explanation of E_{max}, EC_{50}, and the exponent A.

$$E = \frac{E_{max}\, C^A}{EC_{50}^A + C^A}$$

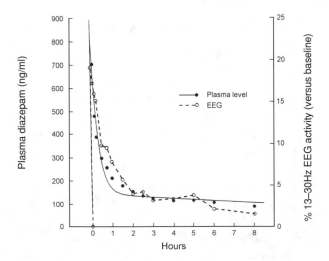

Figure 6–10. A series of healthy volunteer subjects received 0.15 mg/kg of diazepam by 1-minute intravenous infusion. Mean plasma diazepam concentrations and mean changes over baseline in the fraction of electroencephalogram (EEG) activity falling in the "beta" range (13–30 cycles per second) during the first 8 hours after dosage are shown on the graph. Note that the time-course of plasma concentrations closely parallels the pharmacodynamic effect on the EEG (Greenblatt et al. 1989a).

changes in the EEG that closely paralleled plasma drug concentrations (Figure 6–10; Greenblatt et al. 1989a). The effect-concentration relationship was well described by the Sigmoid-E_{max} model (Figure 6–11). However, after intravenous administration of lorazepam, maximum pharmacodynamic effect was delayed by some 30 minutes following drug injection

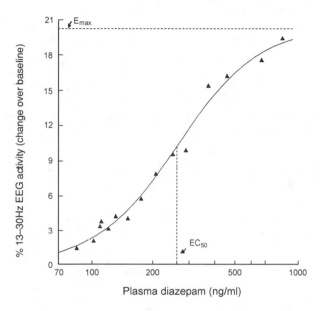

Figure 6–11. The concentration-effect relationship from Figure 6–10 is consistent with a Sigmoid-E_{max} model, with E_{max} = + 20.2% and EC_{50} = 269 ng/ml (Greenblatt et al. 1989a).

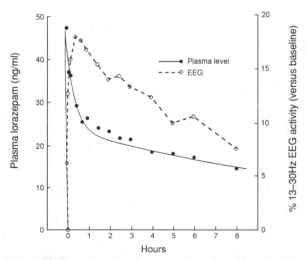

Figure 6–12. After intravenous administration of 0.046 mg/kg of lorazepam by 1-minute intravenous infusion, maximum effects on the electroencephalogram do not occur until about 30 minutes after the infusion (Greenblatt et al. 1989b).

(Figure 6–12; Greenblatt et al. 1989b). This is attributable to a delay in drug entry into the brain (Greenblatt and Sethy 1990). The relationship of plasma concentration to pharmacodynamic effect was not consistent with any physiological model, because plasma concentrations immediately after drug injection are not proportional to drug concentrations at the site of action (Figure 6–13). To account for this complication, the pharmacokinetic model is modified to include an "effect site," which equilibrates with plasma after a finite delay that itself can be assigned a half-life (Colburn 1981; Sheiner et al. 1979). The relation of drug effect to effect-site concentrations, as opposed to plasma concentrations, allows the application of reasonable models to the kinetic-dynamic relationship (Figure 6–14).

■ CONCLUSION

The clinical response to a given dose of a given psychotropic medication varies considerably among individuals in a given population of patients. One component of this variance is pharmacokinetic: the

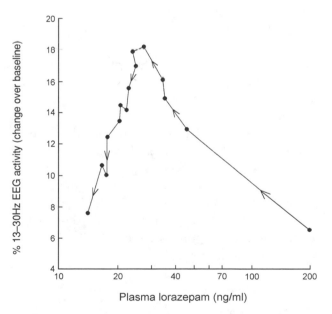

Figure 6–13. In the case of lorazepam (Figure 6–12), a plot of plasma concentration versus effect yields a "hook," because the time of maximum plasma level does not correspond to the time of maximum effect. This is termed *counterclockwise hysteresis* and is explained by the finite time necessary for lorazepam in plasma to equilibrate with brain tissue. The arrows are in the direction of increasing time (Greenblatt et al. 1989b).

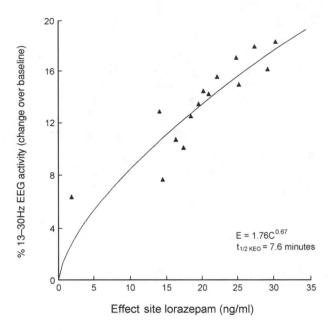

Figure 6–14. To undertake kinetic-dynamic modeling, it is necessary to postulate that equilibration of plasma lorazepam with lorazepam at the "effect site" occurs with a half-life of 7.6 minutes ($t_{1/2KEO}$). Using this assumption, effect-site lorazepam is related to pharmacodynamic effect (E) via an exponential model.

same dose will produce different plasma concentration in different individuals. The other component is pharmacodynamic: the same concentration will produce different responses in different individuals. We are moving toward greater understanding and increased predictability of these two components of variance. Advances in pharmacokinetics have increased the predictability of individual variations of distribution, elimination, and clearance. Advances in pharmacodynamic techniques and in kinetic-dynamic modeling have narrowed down the variance component attributable to intrinsic differences and drug sensitivity. Our capacity to achieve desired therapeutic efficacy without side effects will continue to improve as the data base expands.

■ REFERENCES

Bergstrom RF, Peyton AL, Lemberger L: Quantification and mechanism of the fluoxetine and tricyclic antidepressant interaction. Clin Pharmacol Ther 51:239–248, 1992

Brosen K: Recent developments in hepatic drug oxidation: implications for clinical pharmacokinetics. Clin Pharmacokinet 18:220–239, 1990

Busto U, Sellers EM, Naranjo CA, et al: Withdrawal reaction after long-term therapeutic use of benzodiazepines. N Engl J Med 315:854–859, 1986

Caccia S, Garattini S: Formation of active metabolites of psychotropic drugs: an updated review of their significance. Clin Pharmacokinet 18:434–459, 1990

Caccia S, Garattini S: Pharmacokinetic and pharmacodynamic significance of antidepressant drug metabolites. Pharmacol Res 26:317–329, 1992

Ciraulo DA, Shader RI: Fluoxetine drug-drug interactions. J Clin Psychopharmacol 10:48–50, 213–217, 1990

Colburn WA: Simultaneous pharmacokinetic and pharmacodynamic modeling. J Pharmacokinet Biopharm 9:367–388, 1981

Crewe HK, Lennard MS, Tucker GT, et al: The effect of selective serotonin re-uptake inhibitors on cytochrome $P_{450}2D6$ (CYP2D6) activity in human liver microsomes. Br J Clin Pharmacol 34:262–265, 1992

Dingemanse J, Danhof M, Breimer DD: Pharmacokinetic-pharmacodynamic modeling of CNS drug effects: an overview. Pharmacol Ther 38:1–52, 1988

Friedman H, Greenblatt DJ: Rational therapeutic drug monitoring. JAMA 256:2227–2233, 1986

Friedman H, Greenblatt DJ, Peters GR, et al: Pharmacokinetics and pharmacodynamics of oral diazepam: effect of dose, plasma concentration, and time. Clin Pharmacol Ther 52:139–150, 1992

Gibaldi M, Perrier D: Pharmacokinetics. New York, Marcel Dekker, 1975

Goff DC, Midha KK, Brotman AW, et al: Elevation of plasma concentrations of haloperidol after the addition of fluoxetine. Am J Psychiatry 148:790–792, 1991

Gonzalez FJ: Human cytochromes P_{450}: problems and prospects. Trends Pharmacol Sci 13:346–352, 1992a

Gonzalez FJ: In vitro systems for prediction of rates of drug clearance and drug interactions. Anesthesiology 77:413–415, 1992b

Greenblatt DJ: Benzodiazepine hypnotics: sorting the pharmacokinetic facts. J Clin Psychiatry 52 (suppl 9):4–10, 1991

Greenblatt DJ, Harmatz JS: Kinetic-dynamic modeling in clinical psychopharmacology. J Clin Psychopharmacol 13:231–234, 1993

Greenblatt DJ, Koch-Weser J: Clinical pharmacokinetics. N Engl J Med 293:702–705, 964–970, 1975

Greenblatt DJ, Sethy VH: Benzodiazepine concentrations in brain directly reflect receptor occupancy: studies of diazepam, lorazepam, and oxazepam. Psychopharmacology 102:373–378, 1990

Greenblatt DJ, Shader RI: Pharmacokinetics in Clinical Practice. Philadelphia, PA, WB Saunders, 1985

Greenblatt DJ, Shader RI: Pharmacokinetics of antianxiety agents, in Psychopharmacology: The Third Generation of Progress. Edited by Meltzer HY. New York, Raven, 1987, pp 1377–1386

Greenblatt DJ, Miller LG, Shader RI: Clonazepam pharmacokinetics, brain uptake, and receptor interactions. J Clin Psychiatry 48 (suppl 10):4–9, 1987

Greenblatt DJ, Ehrenberg BL, Gunderman J, et al: Pharmacokinetic and electroencephalographic study of intravenous diazepam, midazolam, and placebo. Clin Pharmacol Ther 45:356–365, 1989a

Greenblatt DJ, Ehrenberg BL, Gunderman J, et al: Kinetic and dynamic study of intravenous lorazepam: comparison with intravenous diazepam. J Pharmacol Exp Ther 250:134–140, 1989b

Greenblatt DJ, Harmatz JS, Friedman H, et al: A large-sample study of diazepam pharmacokinetics. Ther Drug Monit 11:652–657, 1989c

Greenblatt DJ, Miller LG, Shader RI: Benzodiazepine discontinuation syndromes. J Psychiatr Res 24 (suppl 2):73–79, 1990

Greenblatt DJ, Harmatz JS, Shader RI: Clinical pharmacokinetics of anxiolytics and hypnotics in the elderly: therapeutic considerations. Clin Pharmacokinet 21:165–177, 262–273, 1991a

Greenblatt DJ, Harmatz JS, Shapiro L, et al: Sensitivity to triazolam in the elderly. N Engl J Med 324:1691–1698, 1991b

Greenblatt DJ, Preskorn SH, Cotreau MM, et al: Fluoxetine impairs clearance of alprazolam but not of clonazepam. Clin Pharmacol Ther 52:479–486, 1992

Guengerich FP: Human cytochrome P-450 enzymes. Life Sci 50:1471–1478, 1992

Guengerich FP: Bioactivation and detoxication of toxic and carcinogenic chemicals. Drug Metab Dispos Biol Fate Chem 21:1–6, 1993

Haefely WE: The $GABA_A$-benzodiazepine receptor: biology and pharmacology, in Handbook of Anxiety, Vol 3, The Neurobiology of Anxiety. Edited by Burrows GD, Roth M, Noyes R Jr. Amsterdam, Netherlands, Elsevier, 1990, pp 165–188

Harmatz JS, Greenblatt DJ: A SIMPLEX procedure for fitting nonlinear pharmacokinetic models. Comput Biol Med 17:199–208, 1987

Holford NHG, Sheiner LB: Kinetics of pharmacologic response. Pharmacol Ther 16:143–166, 1982

Hommer DW, Matsuo V, Wolkowitz O, et al: Benzodiazepine sensitivity in normal human subjects. Arch Gen Psychiatry 43:542–551, 1986

Lasher TA, Fleishaker JC, Steenwyk RC, et al: Pharmacokinetic-pharmacodynamic evaluation of the combined administration of alprazolam and fluoxetine. Psychopharmacology 104:323–327, 1991

Lemberger L, Rowe H, Bosomworth JC, et al: The effect of fluoxetine on the pharmacokinetics and psychomotor responses of diazepam. Clin Pharmacol Ther 43:412–419, 1988

Mandema JW, Danhof M: Electroencephalogram effect measures and relationships between pharmacokinetics and pharmacodynamics of centrally acting drugs. Clin Pharmacokinet 23:191–195, 1992

Motulsky HJ, Ransnas LA: Fitting curves to data using nonlinear regression: a practical and nonmathematical review. FASEB J 1:365–374, 1987

Murray M: P_{450} enzymes: inhibition mechanisms, genetic regulation and effects of liver disease. Clin Pharmacokinet 23:132–146, 1992

Noyes R, Garvey MJ, Cook B, et al: Controlled discontinuation of benzodiazepine treatment for patients with panic disorder. Am J Psychiatry 148:517–523, 1991

Otton SV, Wu D, Joffe RT, et al: Inhibition by fluoxetine of cytochrome P_{450} 2D6 activity. Clin Pharmacol Ther 53:401–409, 1993

Pato MT, Murphy DL, DeVane CL: Sustained plasma concentrations of fluoxetine and/or norfluoxetine four and eight weeks after fluoxetine discontinuation. J Clin Psychopharmacol 11:224–225, 1991

Peck CC, Temple R, Collins JM: Understanding consequences of concurrent therapies. JAMA 269:1550–1552, 1993

Preskorn SH, Beber JH, Faul JC, et al: Serious adverse effects of combining fluoxetine and tricyclic antidepressants. Am J Psychiatry 147:532, 1990

Preskorn SH, Alderman J, Chung M, et al: Pharmacokinetics of desipramine coadministered with sertraline or fluoxetine. J Clin Psychopharmacol 14:90–98, 1994

Rickels K, Fox IL, Greenblatt DJ, et al: Clorazepate and lorazepam: clinical improvement and rebound anxiety. Am J Psychiatry 145:312–317, 1988

Rickels K, Schweizer E, Case WG, et al: Long-term therapeutic use of benzodiazepines, I: effects of abrupt discontinuation. Arch Gen Psychiatry 47:899–907, 1990

Roy-Byrne PP, Cowley DS, Greenblatt DJ, et al: Reduced benzodiazepine sensitivity in panic disorder. Arch Gen Psychiatry 47:534–540, 1990

Schenker S, Bergstrom RF, Wolen RL, et al: Fluoxetine disposition and elimination in cirrhosis. Clin Pharmacol Ther 44:353–359, 1988

Schweizer E, Rickels K, Case WG, et al: Long-term therapeutic use of benzodiazepines, II: effects of gradual taper. Arch Gen Psychiatry 47:908–916, 1990

Sheiner LB, Stanski DR, Vozeh S, et al: Simultaneous modeling of pharmacokinetics and pharmacodynamics: application to d-tubocurarine. Clin Pharmacol Ther 25:358–371, 1979

Skjelbo E, Brøsen K: Inhibitors of imipramine metabolism by human liver microsomes. Br J Clin Pharmacol 34:256–261, 1992

Sovner R, Davis JM: A potential drug interaction between fluoxetine and valproic acid. J Clin Psychopharmacol 11:889, 1991

Stanski DR: Pharmacodynamic modeling of anesthetic EEG drug effects. Annu Rev Pharmacol Toxicol 32:423–447, 1992

Swerdlow BN, Holley FO: Intravenous anaesthetic agents: pharmacokinetic-pharmacodynamic relationships. Clin Pharmacokinet 12:79–110, 1987

von Moltke LL, Greenblatt DJ, Shader RI: In vitro inhibition of alprazolam oxidation by fluoxetine and norfluoxetine. J Clin Pharmacol 32:764, 1992

von Moltke LL, Greenblatt DJ, Cotreau-Bibbo MM, et al: Inhibition of desipramine hydroxylation in vitro by serotonin-reuptake-inhibitor antidepressants, and by quinidine and ketoconazole: a model system to predict drug interactions in vivo. J Pharmacol Exp Ther 268:1278–1283, 1994a

von Moltke LL, Greenblatt DJ, Harmatz JS, et al: Cytochromes in psychopharmacology. J Clin Psychopharmacol 14:1–4, 1994b

Wagner JG: Fundamentals of Clinical Pharmacokinetics. Hamilton, IL, Drug Intelligence Publications, 1975

Wilens TE, Biederman J, Baldessarini RJ, et al: Fluoxetine inhibits desipramine metabolism. Arch Gen Psychiatry 49:752, 1992

Zorumski CF, Isenberg KE: Insights into the structure and function of GABA-benzodiazepine receptors: ion channels and psychiatry. Am J Psychiatry 148:162–173, 1991

Classes of Psychiatric Drugs: Animal and Human Pharmacology

Herbert Y. Meltzer, M.D., Section Editor

Anxiolytics and Antidepressants

7

Tricyclics and Tetracyclics

William Z. Potter, M.D., Ph.D., Husseini K. Manji, M.D., F.R.C.P.C., and Matthew V. Rudorfer, M.D.

From the 1960s until the late 1980s, tricyclic antidepressants (TCAs) represented the major pharmacological treatment for depression in the United States. They still provide the surest antidepressant response for moderately to severely nondelusionally depressed patients, especially those with a primary depression of the endogenous or melancholic type who may be candidates for hospitalization (Potter et al. 1991). Furthermore, the original tertiary amine tricyclics—first imipramine, then amitriptyline and clomipramine (in Europe)—all included in their biochemical spectrum of effects at least a moderate degree of serotonin reuptake inhibition at therapeutic doses. It was the recognition of this fact that led to the development of the selective serotonin reuptake inhibitors (SSRIs). Thus, the clinical pharmacology of the tricyclics forms the basis of our current understanding of how to best use most antidepressants and of theories on mechanisms of action.

In this chapter, we selectively review what has been learned about tricyclics and the subsequently introduced heterocyclic in both clinical and preclinical studies over the past three decades. Our emphasis will be on their comparative pharmacology and on those findings most relevant to deciding when to treat a patient with any of these compounds.

■ HISTORY AND DISCOVERY

The synthesis of iminodibenzyl, the "tricyclic" core of imipramine, and the description of its chemical characteristics dates to 1889 (Baldessarini 1985). As Baldessarini noted, it was only after 1948, when Hafliger and Schindler synthesized a series of more than 40 derivatives of iminodibenzyl to be screened as possible antihistamines, sedatives, analgesics, and antiparkinsonian drugs, that the pharmacological properties were investigated. Out of this effort emerged imipramine, a dibenzapine compound, which was distinguished from the phenothiazines only by replacement of the sulfur with an ethylene linkage. Interestingly, the best known phenothiazine, chlorpromazine, was not synthesized until 1952, although attempts to use promethazine (which had been available for some time) to reduce motor agitation had been carried out for more than a decade (Laborit et al. 1952). Following their screening in animals, a few iminodibenzyl derivatives, including imipramine, were selected on the basis of their sedative or hypnotic properties for therapeutic trials as agents to calm agitated and/or psychotic patients.

In the meantime, and starting with reports in 1952 and 1953, a wide variety of clinical effects of

The authors thank Penny Nolton for her editorial assistance in preparing this chapter.

chlorpromazine were described, including an ameliorative effect on psychosis. It was thus with a view toward imipramine as a phenothiazine analogue that a few years later Kuhn (1958) assessed its ability to quiet agitated psychotic patients but found it relatively ineffective. On the other hand, he noticed that imipramine seemed to produce remarkable improvement in a subset of patients who were identified as depressed. Kuhn followed up on this chance observation with subsequent administration of imipramine to patients with a variety of depressive syndromes. He suggested that imipramine was most useful in "endogenous" depressions characterized by regression and inactivity, an impression not that different from what is held by most clinicians today after more than three decades of controlled trials (see next section).

■ STRUCTURE-ACTIVITY RELATIONSHIPS

As shown in Figure 7–1, there are nine drugs marketed in the United States as antidepressants that may be classified as tricyclic and one (maprotiline) as tetracyclic. (In the case of the tricyclic clomipramine, it has been approved only for treatment of obsessive-compulsive disorder.) This simplistic and loose classification is a product of convention and implies somewhat greater similarity of structure and function than actually exists. In most instances, it is the nature of the side chain, not the cyclic structure, which is most easily related to function.

To clarify this point, the first two compounds, imipramine and desipramine, are distinguished only by a methyl group on the propylamine side chain. As we discuss in detail in both the "Pharmacology" and "Side Effects" sections, this simple alteration from a tertiary amine (3°; e.g., imipramine) to a secondary amine (2°; e.g., desipramine) side chain has widespread effects. This is the case in terms of both monoamine uptake inhibition—3° amines are more potent as inhibitors of serotonin (5-HT) and 2° amines more potent as inhibitors of norepinephrine (NE) uptake— as well as interaction with α_1-adrenergic, histaminergic, and muscarinic receptors—3° amines being more than an order of magnitude more potent. Interestingly, the core dibenzapine (tricyclic) structure—the same iminodibenzyl synthesized a century ago,

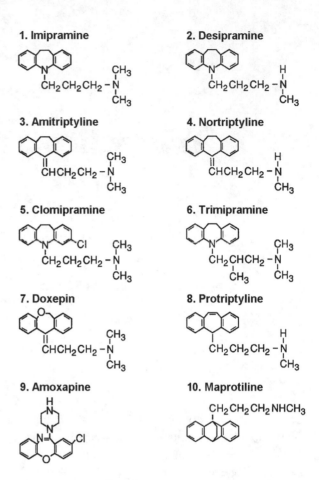

Figure 7–1. Drugs marketed in the United States as tricyclics (1–9) and tetracyclic (10).

which is common to both imipramine and desipramine—has no significant pharmacological activity in concentrations similar to those required for imipramine to produce effects in preclinical "antidepressant" models (Bickel and Brodie 1964).

Consideration of the next two compounds, amitriptyline and nortriptyline, makes these concepts about the structure-activity relationship even clearer. The core tricyclic structure is a dibenzocycloheptadiene that must be presumed to occupy more or less the same molecular space as iminodibenzyl. Given the same propylamine side chains, the profile of pharmacological effects is qualitatively the same for the respective 3° and 2° amine forms, amitriptyline and nortriptyline, as for imipramine and desipramine. However, absolute potencies in terms of monoamine reuptake and receptor inhibitions are affected by modification of the tricyclic structure. For instance, amitriptyline is more potent than imipramine in terms of cholinergic, α_1-adrenergic, and histaminergic receptor blockade, as well as 5-HT uptake inhibition (but less potent in terms of NE uptake inhibition).

The fifth compound, clomipramine, differs from imipramine only in the addition of a chloride atom to one of the tricyclic benzene rings. This confers an increase in potency as an inhibitor of 5-HT reuptake as well as an inhibitor of histaminergic receptors and some loss of potency as an inhibitor of NE uptake (Hall and Ogren 1981). Clomipramine's demethylated 2° amine metabolite, however, is a potent NE uptake inhibitor and is extensively formed in humans (see below).

Trimipramine, the sixth compound, is also closely related to imipramine, but here in terms of the addition of a methyl group to the second carbon of the propylamine side chain. Precise comparisons of the pharmacodynamics of trimipramine with other tricyclics are limited, but available data show that in its parent form it is somewhat less potent than imipramine as a NE uptake inhibitor (Randrup and Braestrup 1977) but more potent as an antihistamine (Psychoyos 1981). In some preparations it has been claimed to have significant potency as a dopamine uptake inhibitor, although this property is not established in humans (Randrup and Braestrup 1977).

Doxepin, the seventh compound, is most closely related to amitriptyline; the only difference involves an oxygen in place of a carbon, such that the central cycloheptadene ring is converted to a oxepinylidene. Consistent with the principles previously described, this modification has effects only on the potency of the 3° amine's actions. Here, 5-HT uptake inhibition is decreased in comparison to that produced by amitriptyline, and NE uptake inhibition is somewhat increased (Pinder et al. 1977). In other words, doxepin's biochemical profile most closely resembles that of imipramine, consistent with the retention of the 3° amine side chain.

The eighth compound, protriptyline, is closely related to nortriptyline, from which it is distinguished by desaturation of two saturated central ring carbons. This change further enhances this 2° amine's potency as a NE uptake inhibitor. Through some unknown mechanism, it also greatly reduces the metabolism, such that it has a three- to fourfold longer half-life (Moody et al. 1977; Ziegler et al. 1978) and achieves steady-state concentrations similar to those achieved on nortriptyline at one-third of the dose.

The last tricyclic on the list, amoxapine, deviates the most, because it is derived more directly from an active neuroleptic, loxapine, which has a very different middle ring. Although there are two benzene rings (one with a chlorine as for clomipramine), the central ring and side chain have little similarity to the other tricyclics. Nonetheless, amoxapine does share the property of potent NE uptake inhibition (Richelson and Pfenning 1984), which could not be predicted from its structure. What could be expected more, given its close relationship to loxapine, is that amoxapine and its metabolite, 7-hydroxyamoxapine, produce dopamine receptor blockade at therapeutic doses (Coupet et al. 1979).

The last compound shown in Figure 7–1, maprotiline, has been called a heterocyclic, although this appellation is ultimately misleading, given the abundance of "hetero"-cyclic drugs not included. Even the term *tetracyclic* is confusing and is used only to relate maprotiline to the "classic" tricyclics (compounds 1–8 in Figure 7–1). In the case of maprotiline, an ethylene-type bridge between the two central carbons of a six-member middle ring produces a more rigid core structure but a compound similar in biochemical properties to desipramine and nortriptyline, given the presence of the identical 2° amine side chain (Wells and Gelenberg 1981). Maprotiline may achieve somewhat greater *selectivity* (but not potency) as a NE uptake inhibitor, because it has apparently negligible effects as a 5-HT uptake inhibitor following its chronic administration in humans (Turner and Ehsanullah 1977).

■ PHARMACOLOGICAL PROFILE

■ Primary Biochemical Effects

As we have defined them, the classic TCAs are imipramine, amitriptyline, and their close structural analogues. Observations of their ability to block the reuptake of the neurotransmitters 5-HT and NE into their respective nerve terminals formed the basis of the monoamine hypothesis of depression (Bunney and Davis 1965; Prange 1965; Schildkraut 1965). These biochemical activities are still considered the pharmacological essence of their therapeutic effect. Both are metabolized to the 2° amines (on the side chain), nortriptyline and desipramine, which are themselves marketed as antidepressants (Figure 7–1).

Of these four compounds, desipramine is the most biochemically selective with respect to both neurotransmitter uptake inhibition and relative lack of interaction with other systems for a given plasma concentration. In actual clinical use, nortriptyline is almost as specific. It is effective at substantially lower plasma concentrations (see below); and, as we noted in the discussion of structure-activity relationships, the so-called heterocyclic maprotiline is also relatively specific for NE uptake inhibition. Compared with most other tricyclic compounds, desipramine and maprotiline block the reuptake of NE at low concentrations unlikely to affect the uptake of 5-HT. Morcover, desipramine has little affinity for muscarinic-cholinergic, histaminergic, and α-adrenergic receptors (Table 7–1), although its potency in these cases is still considerably higher than that seen with the SSRIs and bupropion.

The availability of TCAs that showed relative specificity and/or potency with regard to inhibition of NE or 5-HT uptake, together with the clinical impression that different compounds were effective in different patients, led to the theory that there were noradrenergic and serotonergic forms of depression (Beckmann and Goodwin 1975; Maas et al. 1972). Convincing evidence to support this hypothesis has not been forthcoming. Comparisons of treatment responses to desipramine (the most selective NE inhibitor) with those of an early selective 5-HT inhibitor, zimeldine, and later with fluoxetine and other SSRIs, have produced no consistent differences (Potter 1984). Another study in which patients who did not respond to desipramine were to be treated with clomipramine, the most potent tricyclic 5-HT uptake inhibitor, could not be completed, because the failure rate of endogenomorphically depressed patients to desipramine was extremely low (Stewart et al. 1980). Thus, specific pharmacology has not translated into specific antidepressant effects.

The rationale for selecting a tricyclic on the basis of its specific biochemical pharmacology is weakened further by findings that even drugs with *acute* biochemical specificity have common effects on multiple biochemical systems with *chronic* administration in humans. For example, both NE and 5-HT uptake inhibitors reduce the production of the neurotransmitters' respective metabolites, 3-methoxy-4-hydroxyphenylglycol (MHPG) and 5-hydroxyindoleacetic acid (5-HIAA) in cerebrospinal fluid (Aberg-Wistedt et al. 1982; Potter et al. 1985). Moreover, other antidepressants, such as monoamine oxidase inhibitors (MAOIs) and bupropion (which has no clearly defined mechanism of action), can at least reduce output of NE (Golden et al. 1988). Finally, recent experiments in animals have demonstrated that antidepressant drugs and electroconvulsive shock alter the density and function of receptors for both NE and 5-HT in the brain after 1–2 weeks of administration (see below under "Mechanism of Action"). Therefore, the administration of any currently available drug as a test for biochemical specificity of effect in depression is not warranted.

Table 7–1. In vitro acute biochemical activity of tricyclic antidepressants[a]

	Reuptake inhibition			Receptor affinity				
	NE	5-HT	DA	α_1	α_2	H_1	MUSC	D_2
Imipramine	+	+	0	++	0	+	++	0
Desipramine	+++	0	0	+	0	0	+	0
Amitriptyline	±	++	0	+++	±	++++	++++	0
Nortriptyline	++	±	0	+	0	+	++	0
Clomipramine	+	+++	0	++	0	+	++	0
Trimipramine	+	0	0	++	±	+++	++	+
Doxepin	++	+	0	++	0	+++	++	0
Protriptyline	++	0	0	+	0	+	++	0
Amoxapine	++	0	0	++	±	±	0	++
Maprotiline	++	0	0	+	0	++	+	0

Note. NE = norepinephrine; 5-HT = serotonin; DA = dopamine; α_1 = α_1-adrenergic receptor; α_2 = α_2-adrenergic receptor; H_1 = histamine-1 receptor; MUSC = muscarinic cholinergic receptor; D_2 = dopamine$_2$ receptor.
[a] Relative potencies from earlier reviews (i.e., Potter 1984; Potter et al. 1991; Richelson and Nelson 1984; Richelson and Pfenning 1984).

This brings us to a consideration of the diverse biochemical effects associated with use of tricyclic compounds, most of which have at least some physiological relevance if no direct relationship to antidepressant outcome. These medications are considered pharmacologically "dirty drugs." That is, in addition to exertion of their presumed desired mode of action (i.e., inhibition of monoamine neurotransmitter uptake), they bind to a host of receptors in the brain and periphery (Table 7–1), with consequent unwanted actions. The relationships of these diverse biochemical actions to side effects and toxicity are discussed in the next section.

■ Pharmacokinetics

From a clinical point of view, the most important advances from studying the pharmacology of TCAs have emerged from studies of their pharmacokinetics (Amsterdam et al. 1981; Rudorfer and Potter 1987). TCAs are well absorbed following oral administration, although peak plasma levels occur over the relatively wide range of 2–6 hours. Most TCAs have a half-life of approximately 24 hours, which allows for once-a-day dosing (Table 7–2). Less than 5% of a dose is excreted unchanged, with metabolism occurring primarily in the liver through the mixed function oxidases. The tricyclics undergo demethylation, aromatic hydroxylation, and glucuronide conjugation of the hydroxy metabolite (Figure 7–2). The demethylated metabolites of 3° amines are pharmacologically active, as are the hydroxy metabolites of both 3° and 2° amines (Bertilsson et al. 1979; Potter et al. 1979). Conjugation contributes the most to rendering the lipophilic tricyclics water soluble and easier to excrete by the kidneys. The glucuronide metabolites are considered inactive, both because they have no identified effects on biological systems in the concentrations achieved and because they do not cross the blood-brain barrier (reviewed in detail in Potter et al. 1980).

The rates of metabolism of TCAs are determined by individual genetics, varying 30- to 40-fold with 7%–9% of a Caucasian population classifiable as "slow hydroxylators" (Brosen et al. 1985; Evans et al. 1980). Great progress has recently been made in understanding the exact source of slow hydroxylation. Individuals can be so classified on the basis of the urinary ratio of debrisoquin/4-hydroxydebrisoquin in an 8-hour collection following an oral dose of 10 mg

debrisoquin (an antihypertensive). A high ratio means that a person is a "slow hydroxylator." It was recognized that metabolism of another test compound, sparteine, correlated with that of debrisoquin and what was termed the sparteine-debrisoquin oxidation polymorphism is now known to be determined by P_{450}-2D6 (CYP-2D6), a specific isozyme of

Table 7–2. Elimination half-life ($t_{1/2}$) of tricyclic antidepressants

	$t_{1/2}$ (hours)	
	Mean	**Range**
Imipramine	12	7–22
	28	18–34
Desipramine	18	10–31
Amitriptyline	24	20–30
	36	31–46
Nortriptyline	28	22–39
	33	18–58
Clomipramine	24	20–39
Trimipramine	24	16–38
Doxepin	16	8–24
	17	10–47
Protriptyline	74	54–92
Amoxapine	10	8–18
Maprotiline	43	27–58

Source. Modified from Rudorfer and Potter 1987 with values from one or more studies using more sensitive high-performance liquid chromatography (HPLC) and/or gas chromatography/mass spectrometry (GC/MS) assays, with added information on trimipramine and amoxapine from Abernethy et al. 1984 and Calvo et al. 1985, respectively.

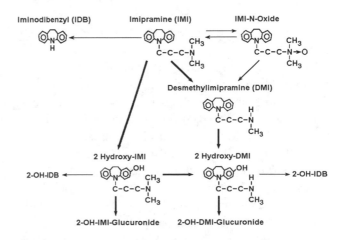

Figure 7–2. Known metabolic pathways for the major tricyclic antidepressant (TCA) imipramine in humans. Similar pathways apply to other TCAs.

the P_{450} microsomal enzymes. Furthermore, it has been explicitly shown that P_{450}-2D6 is responsible for the 2-hydroxylation of imipramine and desipramine and that mutations of the P_{450}-2D6 gene are responsible for slow metabolism through these pathways (Brosen et al. 1991; Dahl et al. 1992). The P_{450} isozyme(s) responsible for TCA demethylation reactions have not yet been identified. It is assumed, however, that most TCAs will depend on the P_{450}-2D6 enzyme for major hydroxylation reactions, which are a necessary prelude to glucuronidation. Of particular relevance to current therapeutics are the SSRI fluoxetine and its metabolite norfluoxetine. They are particularly potent inhibitors of P_{450}-2D6 (Brosen and Skjelbo 1991), which explains why parent TCA concentrations are dramatically elevated in patients taking fluoxetine. Of course, there are other medications (including the SSRI paroxetine) that can induce or inhibit hepatic P_{450} enzymes that will decrease or increase plasma TCA levels (see "Drug Interactions").

Some of the demethylated metabolites of TCAs that show differential pharmacodynamics as discussed here actually exceed concentrations of the parent compound. For example, the 3° amine and potent 5-HT uptake inhibitor clomipramine is metabolized to desmethylclomipramine concentrations that exceed those of the parent compound at steady state (Traskman et al. 1979). Because desmethylclomipramine (as would be expected for a 2° amine) is a potent NE uptake inhibitor, the in vitro selectivity of clomipramine as a 5-HT uptake inhibitor is lost upon its administration to patients.

Other metabolic pathways may also be relevant to clinical effects. Based on both animal and clinical studies, it has been suggested that hydroxy-TCA metabolites, which are rarely assayed, may be more cardiotoxic than their parent precursors (Jandhyala et al. 1977; Young et al. 1984), although the most recent evidence shows that no such generalization is possible. For instance, the clinically predominant E enantiomer of 10-hydroxy-nortriptyline is considerably *less* toxic than nortriptyline itself, whereas the minor Z-10-OH enantiomer has cardiotoxicity similar to the parent 3° amine (Pollock et al. 1992a). On the other hand, elevated plasma concentrations of E-10-hydroxynortriptyline have been associated with poorer antidepressant response (Young et al. 1988).

Although TCA pharmacokinetics may also be influenced by age, changes in pharmacodynamic responses as a function of aging are more important.

Elderly patients are more sensitive to at least the anticholinergic and α_1-antagonistic effects of tricyclics, as reflected in drug-induced delirium (Sunderland et al. 1987) and orthostatic hypotension (Glassman et al. 1979, 1987), respectively, independent of any processes that might elevate plasma concentrations. Increased concentrations must of course be considered, because it is more probable that secondary decreases of P_{450} activity and hepatic blood flow will occur in elderly patients, either from concomitant medical illness and/or medication. Thus, in earlier more naturalistic studies, elevated concentrations of TCAs were sometimes reported as a function of age (Linnoila et al. 1981; Nies et al. 1977; Ziegler and Biggs 1977). However, in more controlled prospective studies, concentrations of parent TCAs or rates of hydroxylation activity do not differ between otherwise healthy old versus young subjects (Asberg et al. 1971; Cutler et al. 1981; Pollock et al. 1992b; Young et al. 1984).

With regard to active metabolites, however, the known decline of renal clearance with age predictably reduces the urinary excretion of unconjugated hydroxy metabolites, resulting in substantial increases of their steady-state concentrations in elderly patients (Kitanaka et al. 1982; Pollock and Perel 1989; Young et al. 1984). This makes for elevations, especially in the case of nortriptyline, to a toxic or countertherapeutic range of hydroxynortriptyline (Young et al. 1988; see previous discussion). At the other end of the spectrum, in many studies of prepubescent children, TCA clearance is higher than in adults; a lower plasma concentration is often achieved at the same mg/kg dose (Geller 1991; Rapoport and Potter 1981).

Controlling for plasma concentration is, of course, essential to any evaluation of pharmacodynamics. This is particularly important in longer-term studies of clinical response in which there is a high likelihood of problems with compliance. To show compliance, concentrations must be stable over time. This is also necessary information for establishing nonresponse to a TCA, defined as lack of clinical improvement when therapeutic concentrations are present for 4–6 weeks. However, there are uncertainties concerning what is "therapeutic."

Despite a current appreciation for the great variability in metabolism of tricyclic drugs and a consequent need to individualize treatment, definitive therapeutic concentrations are not well established for all TCAs. Most critical analyses agree that therapeutic levels have been defined for only nortriptyline, imipramine, and desipramine (American Psychiatric Association Task Force 1985; Perry et al. 1987; Rudorfer and Potter 1987). Nonetheless, attempts have been made to provide estimates of reasonable therapeutic ranges for all marketed TCAs based on cumulative experience with therapeutic monitoring rather than on prospective controlled studies (Orsulak 1989). Lack of response, toxicity, minimizing adverse effects by using the minimal effective dose, or suspected pharmacokinetic interactions (e.g., with neuroleptics or fluoxetine) are indications for measurement of plasma drug levels. Even without such measurements, daily doses of tricyclic drugs other than nortriptyline or protriptyline can be increased to 300–350 mg of imipramine or the equivalent if side effects allow. With nortriptyline, dose increases require monitoring, because plasma levels > 150 ng/ml are as ineffective as those yielding a subtherapeutic (< 50 ng/ml) level.

TCAs also have a narrow therapeutic index with considerable risk of significant toxicity when blood concentrations are 2–6 times therapeutic ones, such that a 1-week supply may be fatal if taken all at once (Gram 1990; Rudorfer and Robins 1982). In general, concentrations > 1000 ng/ml are associated with prolongation of the QRS interval, an effect that may even be seen at 500 ng/ml (Preskorn and Irwin 1982; Rudorfer and Young 1980a; Spiker et al. 1975). This relatively narrow therapeutic index is of special concern for depressed patients with suicide potential who may intentionally take an overdose, although specific pharmacodynamic properties that might contribute to fatal arrhythmia, for instance, are not clearly established in humans with regard to a concentration-response relationship. Nonetheless, TCA blood concentrations may remain elevated for several days after overdose, presenting a cardiac risk even after apparent clinical improvement (Jarvis 1991). Furthermore, central nervous system toxicity in terms of coma, shock, respiratory depression, delirium, seizures, and hyperpyrexia may well contribute as much to fatalities as the quinidine-like effects on cardiac conduction of the TCAs.

■ MECHANISM OF ACTION

Our discussion on pharmacology so far has been in terms primarily of clomipramine and the four most closely related TCAs marketed in the United States. Despite the 10 examples of this class in Figure 7–1 (if the tetracyclic maprotiline is included) that acutely affect NE and 5-HT uptake to varying extents, the bulk of data on biochemical effects in humans is provided by studies with imipramine, desipramine, nortriptyline, and clomipramine. Because (as we have noted) all of these reduce indices of NE and 5-HT turnover (i.e., total synthesis and metabolism in humans), it is assumed that all other TCAs will too. Given what has been learned from preclinical studies about chronic "adaptive" changes following TCAs (which we describe below), the commonality of biochemical findings is not so surprising.

Several major flaws in the original hypothesis about the mechanism of action of TCAs as simply enhancing intrasynaptic NE and/or 5-HT began to appear in the mid-1970s and are briefly outlined here. First, antidepressant drugs such as iprindole and bupropion are weak inhibitors of monoamine uptake at best (Ferris et al. 1981; Zis and Goodwin 1979). Similarly, several potent reuptake inhibitors, most notably cocaine and amphetamine, do not produce convincing evidence of antidepressant effects in controlled trials. Finally, the most compelling objection—and the one raised most frequently—is the large temporal discrepancy between the rapid drug-induced biochemical effects on monoamine uptake, which occur within hours, and the antidepressant response, which generally occurs after at least 7–14 days.

At this point, we should note that our knowledge about the complex cascade of events that translate *any* biochemical event into long-term changes in mood and affect is limited. Thus, the temporal discordance discussed here need not prima facie represent evidence against the "classical monoamine hypotheses" of antidepressant drug action. Nevertheless, this has led to extensive research and the formulation of the "receptor sensitivity hypothesis of antidepressant drug action." This postulates that alterations in the sensitivity of various receptors observed only after chronic drug administration is directly related to the mechanism of antidepressant drug action. It is beyond the scope of this chapter to review the extensive literature regarding alterations in various receptor systems, and only a few major ones are highlighted here. Several excellent reviews are available (Charney et al. 1991; Heninger and Charney 1987; Sugrue 1983; Sulser 1984).

Vetulani and Sulser (1975) were the first to demonstrate that chronic (but not acute) administration of various antidepressants to rats reduces the activity of the NE-stimulated adenylate cyclase in the limbic forebrain. Activation of adenylate cyclase results in an increase in intracellular cyclic adenosine monophosphate (cAMP). cAMP has been shown to be an important "second messenger" mediating the physiological effects of various hormones and neurotransmitters. The stimulation of brain adenylate cyclase by NE is at least partially mediated by β-adrenoceptors (Sulser et al. 1978). Several researchers have since showed that the actual number of forebrain β-adrenoceptors is also reduced following chronic administration of many (but not all) TCAs. Moreover, a reduction in β-adrenoceptors was observed not only with imipramine and desipramine, but also with MAOIs and the atypical antidepressants iprindole and mianserin (Sulser et al. 1978).

Chemically diverse and unrelated antidepressants were thus all found to be capable of decreasing the density of β-adrenoceptors and/or the responsiveness of the β-adrenoceptor–coupled adenylate cyclase system following chronic administration. By contrast, other drugs that share common pharmacological properties with the TCAs, such as various anticholinergic and antihistaminergic agents, all fail to produce similar changes in β-adrenoceptor function. Finally, other neurotransmitter receptors including muscarinic-cholinergic, histaminergic, and dopaminergic receptors are not consistently altered during chronic administration of antidepressants to animals (Hauger and Paul 1983).

The time course of the antidepressant-induced decrease in β-adrenoceptors in animals is in keeping with the delayed therapeutic effects of these drugs in humans. Interestingly, both electroconvulsive therapy (ECT) and rapid eye movement (REM) sleep deprivation (which are both clinically effective antidepressants) decrease cerebral β-adrenoceptors in animals somewhat faster than the chemical antidepressants do (Mogilnicka et al. 1980; Sulser et al. 1978), a finding that may be related to their relatively rapid antidepressant effects in patients. The most intuitively obvious explanation for the decrease in brain β-adrenoceptors following chronic antidepressant administration is that all of these drugs somehow increase the intrasynaptic concentration of NE.

In addition to reducing the number of central β-adrenoceptors, TCAs (as well as SSRIs and MAOIs) also appear to alter the number and/or function of serotonin receptors in various forebrain regions (Charney et al. 1991; Heninger and Charney 1987). Single-unit electrophysiological investigations have consistently shown enhanced serotonergic transmission in various postsynaptic brain regions following chronic antidepressant administration. In particular, evidence suggests that there is increased throughput at the 5-HT$_{1A}$ receptor in the hippocampus in the absence of consistent alterations in the density of the receptors themselves, suggesting an enhancement of the coupling to second messenger generating systems.

Because many receptor systems are known to homeostatically downregulate and desensitize in response to increased transmitter availability, the antidepressant-induced downregulation of β-receptors has generally been regarded as an "adaptive phenomenon." However, there are several problems with this seemingly parsimonious explanation, including the lack of β-receptor downregulation in several areas of the brain receiving dense noradrenergic innervation. The ascending serotonergic projections from the midbrain therefore represent another monoaminergic neurotransmitter system that is affected by antidepressants.

There are multiple subtypes of serotonin receptors, among them the broadly inclusive 5-HT$_2$ class as well as the 5-HT$_{1A}$ class referred to previously. Chronic administration of antidepressants to rats decreases the number of 5-HT$_2$ receptors in the brain, and with some drugs this reduction is quite dramatic (Peroutka and Snyder 1980). Because acute administration of antidepressants fails to alter 5-HT$_2$ receptors (Lerer 1987; Vetulani et al. 1981), it is unlikely that this decrease is the result of residual drug present in the membrane preparation. Indeed, many antidepressants are far more potent in reducing 5-HT$_2$ receptors than β-adrenoceptors (with the possible exception of desipramine, which is more effective in reducing β-adrenoceptors). However, because the most effective treatment, electroconvulsive shock, increases the density of rat cortical 5-HT$_2$ receptors, direct antidepressant properties clearly cannot be ascribed to a reduction in 5-HT$_2$ numbers.

Evidence also suggests that a functional linkage exists between the noradrenergic and serotonergic neurotransmitter systems, although how this relates to receptor regulation remains to be defined. For instance, destruction of the noradrenergic system (with

6-hydroxydopamine) markedly reduces the ability of several antidepressants (including ECT) to enhance serotonin-mediated behaviors in rats (Green and Deakin 1980). Monoamine neurotransmitter system interactions may provide a basis for unifying several major hypotheses of depression and the mechanism of action of antidepressants (Hsiao et al. 1987; Potter et al. 1985). These interactions also highlight the difficulty in isolating a drug effect to a specific neurotransmitter system; with chronic administration, subtle and permissive interactions between systems are to be expected.

The potential clinical relevance of these studies designed to explore the mechanisms of action of TCAs in comparison with those of other antidepressants lies in their highlighting two phenomena. First, whatever the balance of acute biochemical effects, all TCAs produce qualitatively similar chronic changes and hence would not be expected to show major differences in degree or type of antidepressant efficacy. Second, biochemical changes occur over a period of 1–2 weeks and may take even longer to stabilize with extended escalation of dose—a phenomenon that argues against any therapeutic advantage of one compound over another in speed of response.

The preceding notwithstanding, the possibility remains that NE (and 5-HT) uptake inhibition may not be necessary or a sufficient condition to initiate and sustain the chain of biochemical events leading to therapeutic response. Although the most obvious explanation for the decrease in brain β-adrenoceptors following chronic administration remains that these drugs somehow increase the intrasynaptic concentration of NE and/or 5-HT, we return our discussion to the ability of other atypical antidepressants, like iprindole, to downregulate β-adrenoceptors, which requires that other mechanism(s) be evoked (Manier et al. 1989). Indeed, several investigators (including us) have shown that chronic in vitro treatment in systems lacking presynaptic input (e.g., human fibroblasts or cultured C6 glioma cells) results in a similar downregulation and desensitization of the β-adrenergic receptor (Manji et al. 1991a). We are currently investigating the mechanisms(s) by which antidepressants downregulate β-adrenergic receptors, focusing on possible effects of crosstalk with protein kinase C (Manji et al. 1991b).

Another point to emphasize is that in terms of presumed core biochemical effects, TCAs are best distinguished from SSRIs by their universal ability to potently inhibit NE uptake and more variably inhibit 5-HT uptake. Thus, a third phenomenon can be highlighted: TCAs are more "broad-spectrum" in their effects on neurotransmitter systems than SSRIs and hence may ultimately prove to have a different spectrum of clinical effects.

In keeping with this suggestion, researchers in a series of Danish studies have concluded that SSRIs may not be as effective in treatment of severely depressed inpatients as is clomipramine, although the latter clearly has more severe side effects (Bech 1988; Danish University Antidepressant Group 1990). Indeed, there is a paucity of studies of SSRIs on inpatients; and even in outpatients, it is often difficult to distinguish SSRIs from placebo. It is appropriate to wonder if the "classic" patients who participated in studies of TCAs in the 1960s and early 1970s differ substantially from the outpatient groups studied today. If so, generalizations about response to all depressions from studies done 20 years apart are not valid. There remain, however, a number of clinical predictors that help to identify the most appropriate patients to receive TCAs, and some of these are highlighted here.

■ INDICATIONS

■ Major Depression and Melancholia

It is now generally accepted that patients with melancholic depression require pharmacotherapy or ECT (Potter et al. 1991). Earlier studies suggested that melancholic depression responded better to TCAs than did depression not meeting the criteria for melancholia (Paykel 1972; Raskin and Crook 1976). But most recent data fail to support such selectivity of response, perhaps reflecting the changing population available for studies (Paykel 1989). A review concluded that, allowing for the limitations of the research base, a good premorbid personality, psychomotor retardation, and intermediate severity with melancholia predict good response to tricyclic drug therapy (Joyce and Paykel 1989). Severity has long been identified as a predictor of response to TCAs (Stewart et al. 1989), whereas good premorbid personality is consistent with observations that primary depression (i.e., depression not preceded by other psychiatric diagnoses or medical illness) responds best to drugs (Coryell and Turner 1985; Fairchild et al. 1986). Identification of symptoms that most consistently change following treatment with desipramine has been used to develop a scale for measuring response to TCAs that may prove useful in future studies (Nelson and Mazure 1990).

Overall, TCAs produce an antidepressant response rate of 80% in nonpsychotic patients with unipolar depression who show melancholic features, have an illness duration of less than 1 year, and are maintained at plasma levels in selected ranges for 4–6 weeks. Estimates of lower response rates in these patients most likely result from inadequate dosage over too short a time. The critical importance of adjusting for wide interindividual differences in the pharmacokinetics of the TCAs has already been described.

■ "Atypical" Depression

Although they are not formally considered in DSM-III-R (American Psychiatric Association 1987), atypical forms of depression are often encountered. The term "atypical" previously referred simply to the absence of melancholic features. However, in the United States, atypical depression is more and more used as a label for combinations of mood reactivity (i.e., inability to experience a positive response to favorable events), overeating, oversleeping, and chronic oversensitivity to rejection (Liebowitz et al. 1988). Patients with atypical depression show a lower response rate to TCAs versus MAOIs (Paykel et al. 1982; Quitkin et al. 1991; Ravaris et al. 1980). However, the concept of atypical depression is imprecise, and one recent report suggests that SSRIs may be as effective as MAOIs in its treatment. Given the probability of shifts in patient populations under study, it seems premature to conclude that TCAs should be avoided in treating patients with atypical features.

■ Delusional (With Psychotic Features) Depression

Patients who both meet the criteria for major depression and have delusions show a very poor response rate to monotherapy with traditional TCAs (Glassman et al. 1977; Perry et al. 1982). Successful pharmacotherapy of such delusional or psychotic depressions requires a combination of a neuroleptic and a TCA (Spiker et al. 1985). Because amoxapine, the tricyclic

metabolite of loxapine, possesses dopamine blocking as well as monoamine uptake inhibitory properties, it may be effective by itself in treating delusional depression (Anton et al. 1985; Coupet et al. 1979). However, the opportunity to independently adjust the neuroleptic and antidepressant components is lost. A potentially important detail regarding combination therapy concerns the ability of some neuroleptic drugs to block the metabolism of TCAs, which necessitates special attention to doses and possibly to blood level monitoring (Gram et al. 1974). Alternatively, the response rates to ECT among patients with delusional depressions are excellent (86% in the aggregate from a dozen studies [Kroessler 1985]).

■ Obsessive-Compulsive Disorder (OCD)

Only one TCA, clomipramine, has been shown to produce significant therapeutic benefit in OCD patients, despite attempts to treat this disorder with other members of the drug class, such as desipramine for adults and children (Ananth et al. 1981; Insel et al. 1985; Leonard et al. 1989; Thoren et al. 1980). This is believed to be a function of the potent 5-HT reuptake-inhibiting properties of clomipramine, because most SSRIs tested to date also produce benefit in OCD. It is significant that the specified upper dose of clomipramine in U.S. product labeling is 250 mg, because there is an increased incidence of seizures at higher doses. Unfortunately, studies reporting seizures did not include data on blood levels, and it is almost certain that those patients who are rapid metabolizers of clomipramine will require higher doses. These higher doses may well be safe in such rapid metabolizers. The experience of European research teams with clomipramine treatment indicates that many patients tolerate doses up to 450 mg/day, experiencing only those side effects that would be expected from a 3° amine TCA at therapeutic doses (Collins 1973).

■ Enuresis

Nocturnal enuresis in children can clearly benefit from TCAs, with imipramine being the one member of the class that has received U.S. product labeling for this indication. Recommended doses are low (i.e., 25–50 mg at bedtime in children under 12 and up to 75 mg in those 12 or over). No other TCAs are specifically "approved" for treatment of enuresis, although others with a 3° amine profile of action may be assumed to share similar effects (see earlier section on "Structure Activity Relationships"). The mechanism of action is not known. The beneficial effect may be related to the anticholinergic effect or to modifications of sleep processes. Controlled trials with plasma blood level monitoring provide strong evidence of an antienuretic effect of imipramine (Rapoport et al. 1980). Earlier studies support the use of amitriptyline and nortriptyline for the treatment of nocturnal enuresis in children (Forsythe and Merrett 1969; Lake 1968). Suggested amitriptyline doses are 10–20 mg at bedtime for children ages 6 to 10 years and 25–50 mg at bedtime for children age 11 years or older.

■ Panic Disorder

Although we have referred to tricyclic *antidepressants* in this chapter, it is clear that at least some members of this class are effective treatments for panic disorder, even in the absence of depression. It should be noted that use of TCAs in treatment of panic disorder is not included in U.S. product labeling. Nonetheless, such use has played a considerable role in the treatment of panic disorder (including that with agoraphobia), with controlled studies supporting the use of both the 3° amine imipramine and the 2° amine nortriptyline (Jobson et al. 1978; Munjack et al. 1988; Uhde and Nemiah 1989; Zitrin et al. 1980). Ultimate doses and presumably plasma levels are the same as those used in the treatment of depression.

One special consideration in the treatment of panic disorder with TCAs is that, particularly with the 2° amines, too rapid escalation of dose may increase anxiety and even precipitate a panic attack. It is therefore recommended that patients be started with low doses (e.g., 10–20 mg) building up to typical therapeutic doses (100–250 mg) over weeks rather than days.

■ Other Uses

A surprisingly diverse number of uses for TCAs are recorded not only in the clinical literature but also in a current authoritative American reference such as the USPDI (1993) and an international pharmacopoeia, *Therapeutic Drugs* (Dollery 1991, 1992). Listed in alphabetical order are those uses referred to in one

or the other sources with the associated TCAs (Table 7–3). This list is important for two reasons: 1) in terms of appreciating that many prescriptions of TCAs have nothing to do with the presence of depression or other psychiatric disorders, and 2) in understanding how TCAs are useful in any single condition, which may clarify why it is useful for others and ultimately contribute to knowledge on their pathophysiologies.

■ SIDE EFFECTS AND TOXICOLOGY

As indicated in Table 7–4, there are distinctions among properties of specific TCAs in the expected frequency and severity of adverse effects. Thus, as predicted from the variety of greater receptor affinities of the 3° amine tricyclics for a variety of receptors (Table 7–1), in general they produce more pronounced anticholinergic, antihistaminic (H_1 and H_2), sedative, and hypotensive actions than their 2° amine counterparts. We have recently reviewed the possible relationships between the various side effects observed in human subjects and the specific biochemical actions of the full range of antidepressants

Table 7–3. Uses of one or more tricyclic antidepressants (TCAs) not included in product labeling

Use	Specified TCAs[*]
Anxiety/panic	Clomipramine, desipramine, doxepin, imipramine
Bulimia	Amitriptyline, desipramine, imipramine
Cataplexy/narcolepsy	Clomipramine, desipramine, imipramine, protriptyline
Enuresis	Amitriptyline, clomipramine, nortriptyline
Migraine (prophylaxis)	Amitriptyline
Nausea with chemotherapy	Nortriptyline
Neuralgia (chronic pain)	Amitriptyline, desipramine, doxepin, imipramine, nortriptyline
Peptic ulcer	Amitriptyline, doxepin, imipramine
Urticaria/pruritis	Doxepin, nortriptyline

[*] At least one mention in USPDI (1993) or *Therapeutic Drugs* (Dollery 1991, 1992).

Table 7–4. Possible clinical side effects of blocking various receptors

Property	Possible clinical consequences
Blockade of muscarinic receptors	Blurred vision Dry mouth Sinus tachycardia Constipation Urinary retention Cognitive dysfunction
Blockade of α_1-adrenergic receptors	Potentiation of the antihypertensive effect of prazosin and terazosin Postural hypotension, dizziness, drowsiness Reflex tachycardia
Blockade of α_2-adrenergic receptors	Blockade of the antihypertensive effects of clonidine and α-methyldopa
Blockade of dopamine D_2 receptors	Extrapyramidal movement disorders
Blockade of histamine (H_1) receptors	Sedation Weight gain

(Rudorfer et al. 1994). The salient details concerning TCAs are presented below.

■ Cardiovascular Effects

TCAs commonly produce a benign rise in heart rate, often on the order of 15–20 beats per minute. Although this is sometimes ascribed to vagal inhibition, the rise in heart rate appears most consistently after use of 2° amine tricyclics, such as desipramine, for which NE reuptake blockade clearly plays a role (Ross et al. 1983). α_1-Adrenergic antagonism is more marked after 3° amine TCAs and is now the most likely basis of any orthostatic hypotension observed with use of those drugs. Such orthostatic hypertension usually produces only transient benign dizziness upon standing in young physically healthy patients but can lead to falls and injury in older individuals (Ray 1992). Some experts prefer nortriptyline among the TCAs in terms of minimizing orthostatic hypotension in elderly patients, both because of relatively less potency at α_1 receptors and obtaining therapeutic effects at low blood levels.

The most potentially dangerous TCA cardiac effect (i.e., of a quinidine-like membrane stabilization resulting in slowed impulse conduction) was discussed in the subsection "Pharmacokinetics." Although such slowed impulse conduction produces only an innocuous prolongation of electrocardiogram (ECG) parameters during routine TCA dosing in physically healthy individuals (Laird et al. 1993; Rudorfer and Young 1980a)—and can suppress preexisting premature atrial or ventricular contractions—it may precipitate frank bundle branch or complete heart block in cardiac patients (Glassman et al. 1987), with consequent morbidity or mortality. This property may relate to cases of sudden death in patients taking therapeutic doses of TCAs, most recently reported in several children taking desipramine (Riddle et al. 1993). Widening of the QRS complex on the ECG, which has been correlated with red blood cell concentrations of tricyclic desmethyl metabolites (Amitai et al. 1993), has become a standard index of serious TCA poisoning, especially in overdose situations (Jarvis 1991). Preskorn and Fast (1991) have speculated that the association of serious cardiac conduction slowing with supratherapeutic TCA plasma concentrations may explain some cases of sudden death during tricyclic therapy in presumed slow metabolizers of these drugs. Recent data have raised concern that the risk of sudden death during TCA treatment among patients with ventricular arrhythmias or ischemic heart disease may be greater than previously appreciated (Glassman et al. 1993). And, as we have noted, there continue to be disturbing reports of sudden death in children treated with TCAs (Riddle et al. 1993).

The possibility of TCA-induced impaired left ventricular function may have been overestimated in the past (Glassman et al. 1987) but is reported occasionally in patients with severe underlying heart disease (Dalack et al. 1991). An earlier suggestion of greater cardiac safety of doxepin has been refuted by Roose and associates (1991), who demonstrated the usual TCA adverse effects (and consequent poor tolerability) of doxepin in cardiac patients with depression.

■ Anticholinergic Effects

Especially with 3° amine TCAs, antimuscarinic actions of TCAs are universal, presenting minor annoyances to most young, healthy patients but posing major hazards to those who are physically compromised. Even the commonly experienced side effect of dry mouth has been associated with serious dental pathology. Reduced tear flow and impaired visual accommodation, with resultant blurred vision, may impair daily function and pose a hazard to contact lens wearers (reviewed by Nierenberg and Cole 1991). Constipation may be a minor discomfort, responsive to increased fluids and bulk laxatives; or it could progress to life-threatening paralytic ileus in medically vulnerable patients. A similar spectrum exists for urinary retention, a major risk of TCA use in older men with prostatic hypertrophy. Narrow-angle glaucoma may constitute a contraindication to the use of medications with any anticholinergic effects.

Tertiary amine TCAs are particularly prone to produce cognitive toxicity, ranging from confusion and memory impairment to frank delirium in elderly patients who show increased sensitivity to anticholinergics (Sunderland et al. 1987). Although some cases of TCA-related sexual dysfunction have been ascribed to anticholinergic effects, such a correlation was not observed in a recent survey (Balon et al. 1993). Indeed, sexual dysfunction has emerged as a more prominent adverse effect associated with the use of SSRIs. Thus, this potent 5-HT uptake–inhibiting property of clomipramine, rather than its strong anticholinergic effects, may explain the high incidence of sexual dysfunction observed with this TCA (Aizenberg et al. 1991).

Although correlations between TCA plasma levels and anticholinergic effects have been identified (Rudorfer and Young 1980b), these side effects are maximal at subtherapeutic plasma concentrations of 3° amine forms (Preskorn and Fast 1991), rendering dosage adjustment inefficient in combating them. Although counteracting cholinergic agents, such as bethanechol, are sometimes used in the treatment of peripheral antimuscarinic actions of TCAs (Rosen et al. 1993), and symptomatic relief can be obtained with use of artificial saliva or tears, most clinically significant problems require change of medication. Thus, the 3° amine TCAs should to be avoided in standard antidepressant doses, or used judiciously (Rahman et al. 1991), in geriatric patients. It should be noted that even desipramine, which has the lowest anticholinergic activity among the classical tricyclics, still produces appreciable muscarinic blockade at therapeutic blood levels (Ross et al. 1983; Rudorfer and Young 1980b).

■ Sedation

This action of the tricyclics, reflecting antihistaminic and α-blocking as well as anticholinergic activity—particularly the 3° amines (Table 7–2)—is one of the few side effects that can be used therapeutically in drug selection. Thus, the 3° amine TCAs are commonly used in a once-daily nighttime dose to symptomatically address sleep disturbance in depressed patients with insomnia (Potter et al. 1991). An incidental benefit of antihistaminic potency of the TCAs has been the antiallergic and antiulcer activities noted in Table 7–3, especially for amitriptyline, doxepin, and trimipramine.

■ Weight Gain

Use of TCAs is often associated with a degree of weight gain, which more than compensates for any prior weight loss associated with depression-related anorexia. This is believed to result from the antihistaminic and possibly α-receptor blocking actions of the TCAs, as well as a TCA-induced carbohydrate craving and slowing of metabolism that is still not well understood. In one survey of clinical practice (Berken et al. 1984), outpatients treated with amitriptyline—possibly the worst offender among the TCAs—gained an average of > 7 kg (with craving for sweets) during 6 months of treatment. Weight gain was related to dose with subsequent loss of weight following drug discontinuation. This side effect does appear to vary among the TCAs (Fernstrom et al. 1986) and is minimal or absent with the most stimulatory members of the class (e.g., protriptyline and desipramine).

■ DRUG-DRUG INTERACTIONS

TCAs interact, pharmacodynamically and/or pharmacokinetically, with a variety of other compounds. The well-established adverse cognitive and psychomotor consequences of combining 3° amine tricyclics with alcohol (Shoaf and Linnoila 1991) are primarily of a pharmacodynamic nature, although pharmacokinetics may be relevant. As reviewed by Shoaf and Linnoila (1991), tricyclic clearance is generally decreased by acute dosing with ethanol but increased by chronic alcohol use (in the absence of cirrhotic liver damage). Most adverse TCA pharmacodynamic interactions with other medications involve additive sedative or anticholinergic effects (e.g., with hypnotics or neuroleptics).

The dependence of tricyclics on hepatic metabolism is the basis of pharmacokinetic interactions with drugs that induce or impair the liver cytochrome P_{450} microsomal enzyme system (Rudorfer and Potter 1987). The most dramatic, frequent, and clinically relevant of such interactions is that between the SSRI fluoxetine and TCAs (Brosen and Skjelbo 1991; Nelson et al. 1991; Otton et al. 1993). Several weeks' treatment with fluoxetine markedly reduces TCA clearance and raises TCA blood levels two- to fourfold. In vitro studies with human liver microsomes suggest that sertraline may also decrease TCA clearance, but not to the same extent as fluoxetine (Lydiard et al. 1993; Otton et al. 1993). In such cases, plasma drug concentration monitoring is of obvious use in accounting for and correcting kinetically based interactions.

■ Potentially Hazardous Interactions

The following listing is a distillation of warnings provided in the USPDI (1993) and/or *Therapeutic Drugs* (Dollery 1991, 1992).

MAOIs. As discussed in most sources, giving TCAs to individuals on MAOIs may produce stroke, hyperpyrexia, convulsions, and death through a variety of mechanisms. It is nonetheless possible to safely combine most TCAs with MAOIs, especially if treatment begins with a 3° amine compound. The one exception is clomipramine, which (because of its potent 5-HT uptake inhibiting action) can produce a potentially fatal "serotonin syndrome" when combined with MAOIs.

Norepinephrine and epinephrine. Following administration of the biogenic amines NE and epinephrine for other medical conditions, unexpectedly large increases in blood pressure and a greater incidence of arrhythmias may occur in individuals on TCAs.

Phenothiazines. Additive anticholinergic effects may occur with phenothiazines, which may be manifested apace of psychosis and/or agitation, especially in elderly subjects. Nonetheless, combinations of phenothiazines with TCAs are appropriate and necessary for the treatment of delusional depression, as we have noted (Spiker et al. 1985).

■ Other Significant Reactions

Barbiturates. These drugs can increase the metabolism of TCAs, requiring higher than usual doses of the antidepressant to achieve a therapeutic effect.

Cimetidine. The use of cimetidine can block the metabolism of both 3° and 2° amine TCAs. Lower doses may therefore be appropriate in patients on this H_2-receptor antagonist. Other H_2-receptor antagonists are not reported to decrease the metabolism of TCAs.

Clonidine. The effects of clonidine are reduced or blocked by desipramine, presumably secondary to its ability to increase noradrenaline in the synapse. Other TCAs can be expected to have a similar effect.

Guanethidine. All TCAs can be expected to block the antihypertensive effects of guanethidine by inhibiting its uptake into nerve endings, although this effect should be most marked with the most potent NE uptake inhibitors.

Haloperidol. Haloperidol can block the metabolism of TCAs, depending on the dose and sequence of administration, thereby potentially raising their plasma concentrations into a toxic or nontherapeutic range.

Methylphenidate. The use of methylphenidate has been reported to block the metabolism of TCAs, but not to the same extent as antipsychotic drugs.

Phenothiazines. The phenothiazines, in particular, can block the metabolism of TCAs, depending on dose and sequence of administration.

Phenytoin. The concentrations of phenytoin may be elevated into a toxic range by administration of TCAs.

Warfarin. The activity of this anticoagulant may be increased by administration of TCAs, which are competitive inhibitors of warfarin metabolism.

■ REFERENCES

Abernethy DR, Greenblatt DJ, Shader RI: Trimipramine kinetics and absolute bioavailability: use of gas-liquid chromatography with nitrogen-phosphorus detection. Clin Pharmacol Ther 35: 348–353, 1984

Aberg-Wistedt A, Ross SB, Jostell KG, et al: A double-blind study of zimelidine, a serotonin uptake inhibitor, and desipramine, a noradrenaline uptake inhibitor, in endogenous depression, II: biochemical findings. Acta Psychiatr Scand 66:66–82, 1982

Aizenberg D, Zemishlany Z, Hermesh H, et al: Painful ejaculation associated with antidepressants in four patients. J Clin Psychiatry 52:461–463, 1991

American Psychiatric Association Task Force: Task Force on the Use of Laboratory Tests in Psychiatry: tricyclic antidepressants—blood level measurements and clinical outcome. Am J Psychiatry 142:155–162, 1985

American Psychiatric Association: Diagnostic and Statistical Manual of Mental Disorders, 3rd Edition, Revised. Washington, DC, American Psychiatric Association, 1987

Amitai Y, Erikson T, Kennedy EJ, et al: Tricyclic antidepressants in red cells and plasma: correlation with impaired intraventricular conduction in acute overdose. Clin Pharmacol Ther 54:219–227, 1993

Amsterdam J, Brunswick D, Mendels J: The clinical application of tricyclic antidepressant pharmacokinetics and plasma levels. Am J Psychiatry 137:653–662, 1981

Ananth J, Pecknold JC, Van der Steen N: Double blind comparable study of clomipramine and amitriptyline in obsessive neurosis. Prog Neuropsychopharmacol Biol Psychiatry 5:257–262, 1981

Anton RF, Ressner EL, Hitri A, et al: Efficacy of amoxapine in psychotic depression: relationship to serum prolactin and neuroleptic activity. J Clin Psychiatry Monograph 3:8–13, 1985

Asberg M, Cronholm B, Sjoqvist F, et al: Relationship between plasma levels and therapeutic effect of nortriptyline. British Medical Journal 3:331–334, 1971

Baldessarini RJ: Drugs and the treatment of psychiatric disorders, in The Pharmacological Basis of Therapeutics, 4th Edition. Edited by Gilman AG, Goodman IS, Rall TW, et al. New York, Macmillan, 1985, pp 387–445

Balon R, Yeragani VK, Pohl R, et al: Sexual dysfunction during antidepressant treatment. J Clin Psychiatry 54:209–212, 1993

Bech P: A review of the antidepressant properties of serotonin reuptake inhibitors. Adv Biol Psychiatry 17:58–69, 1988

Beckmann H, Goodwin FK: Antidepressant response to tricyclics and urinary MHPG in unipolar patients. Arch Gen Psychiatry 32:17–22, 1975

Berken GN, Weinstein DO, Stern WC: Weight gain: a side effect of tricyclic antidepressants. J Affect Disord 7:133–138, 1984

Bertilsson L, Mellstrom B, Sjoqvist F: Pronounced inhibition of noradrenaline uptake by 10-hydroxy-metabolites of nortriptyline. Life Sci 25:1285–1291, 1979

Bickel MN, Brodie, BB: Structure and antidepressant activity of imipramine analogues. Int J Neuropharmacology 3:611–621, 1964

Brosen K, Skjelbo E: Fluoxetine and norfluoxetine are potent inhibitors of $P_{450}IID6$—the source of the sparteine/debrisoquine oxidation polymorphism. Br J Clin Pharmacol 31:136–137, 1991

Brosen K, Otton SV, Gram LF: Sparteine oxidation polymorphism in Denmark. Acta Pharmacol Toxicol 57:357–360, 1985

Brosen K, Zeugin T, Myer UA: Role of $P_{450}IID6$, the target of the sparteine/debrisoquin oxidation polymorphism, in the metabolism of imipramine. Clin Pharmacol Ther 49:609–617, 1991

Bunney WE, Davis JM: Norepinephrine in depressive reactions: a review. Arch Gen Psychiatry 13:483–494, 1965

Calvo B, Garcia MJ, Pedraz JL, et al: Pharmacokinetics of amoxapine and its active metabolites. Int J Clin Pharmacol Ther Toxicol 23:180–185, 1985

Charney DS, Delgado PL, Southwick SM, et al: Current hypotheses of the mechanism of antidepressant treatments: implications for the treatment of refractory depression, in Advances in Neuropsychiatry and Psychopharmacology, Vol 2. Edited by Amsterdam JD. New York, Raven, 1991, pp 23–41

Collins GH: The use of parenteral and oral clomipramine (Anafranil) in the treatment of depressive states. Br J Psychiatry 122:189–190, 1973

Coryell W, Turner R: Outcome with desipramine therapy in subtypes of nonpsychotic major depression. J Affect Disord 9:149–154, 1985

Coupet I, Rauh CE, Szucs-Myers VA, et al: 2-chloro-11(piperazinyl)[b,f][1,4]oxazepine (amoxepine), an antidepressant with antipsychotic properties—a possible role for 7-hydroxyamoxapine. Biochem Pharmacol 28:2514–2515, 1979

Cutler NR, Zavadil AP III, Eisdorfer C, et al: Concentration of desipramine in elderly women. Am J

Psychiatry 138:1235–1237, 1981

Dahl ML, Johansson I, Palmertz MP, et al: Analysis of the CYP2D6 gene in relation to debrisoquin and desipramine hydroxylation in a Swedish population. Clin Pharmacol Ther 51:12–17, 1992

Dalack GW, Roose SP, Glassman AH: Tricyclics and heart failure. Am J Psychiatry 148:1601, 1991

Danish University Antidepressant Group: Paroxetine: a selective serotonin reuptake inhibitor showing better tolerance, but weaker antidepressant effect than clomipramine in a controlled multicenter study. J Affect Disord 18:289–299, 1990

Dollery C (ed): Therapeutic Drugs. Edinburgh, Churchill Livingstone, 1991, 1992

Evans DAP, Mahgoub A, Sloan TP, et al: A family and population study of the genetic polymorphism of debrisoquine oxidation in a white British population. J Med Genet 17:102–105, 1980

Fairchild CJ, Rush AJ, Vasavada N, et al: Which depressions respond to placebo? Psychiatry Res 18:217–226, 1986

Fernstrom MD, Krowinski RL, Kupfer DJ: Chronic imipramine treatment and weight gain. Psychiatry Res 17:269–273, 1986

Ferris RM, White HL, Cooper BR, et al: Some neurochemical properties of a new antidepressant, bupropion hydrochloride (Wellbutrin). Drug Development Research 1:21–35, 1981

Forsythe WI, Merrett JD: A controlled trial of imipramine and nortriptyline in the treatment of enuresis. Br J Clin Pract 23:210–215, 1969

Geller B: Psychopharmacology of children and adolescents: pharmacokinetics and relationships of plasma/serum levels to response. Psychopharmacol Bull 27:401–409, 1991

Glassman A, Perel J, Shostak M, et al: Clinical implication of imipramine plasma levels for depressive illness. Arch Gen Psychiatry, 34:197–204, 1977

Glassman AH, Bigger JT Jr, Giardina EV, et al: Clinical characteristics of imipramine induced orthostatic hypotension. Lancet 1:468–472, 1979

Glassman AH, Roose SP, Giardina EGV, et al: Cardiovascular effects of tricyclic antidepressants, in Psychopharmacology: The Third Generation of Progress. Edited by Meltzer HY. New York, Raven, 1987, pp 1437–1442

Glassman AH, Roose SP, Bigger JT Jr: The safety of tricyclic antidepressants in cardiac patients: risk-benefit reconsidered. JAMA 269:2673–2675, 1993

Golden RN, Markey SP, Risby ED, et al: Antidepres-sants reduce whole-body norepinephrine turnover while maintaining 6-hydroxymelatonin output. Arch Gen Psychiatry 45:144–149, 1988

Gram LF: Inadequate dosing and pharmacokinetic variability as confounding factors in assessment of efficacy of antidepressants. Clin Neuropharmacol 13 (suppl 1):S35–S44, 1990

Gram LF, Overo KF, Kirk L: Influence of neuroleptics and benzodiazepines on metabolism of tricyclic antidepressants in man. Am J Psychiatry 131:863–866, 1974

Green AR, Deakin JFW: Brain noradrenaline depletion prevents ECS-induced enhancement of serotonin and dopamine-mediated behavior. Nature 285:232–233, 1980

Hall H, Ogren SO: Effects of antidepressant drugs on different receptors in the brain. Eur J Pharmacol 70:393–407, 1981

Hauger RL, Paul SM: Neurotransmitter receptor plasticity: alterations by antidepressants and antipsychotics. Psychiatric Annals 13:399–407, 1983

Heninger GR, Charney DS: Mechanism of action of antidepressant treatments: implications for the etiology and treatment of depressive disorders, in Psychopharmacology: The Third Generation of Progress. Edited by Meltzer HY. New York, Raven, 1987, pp 535–545

Hsiao JK, Agren H, Rudorfer MV, et al: Monoamine neurotransmitter interactions and the prediction of antidepressant response. Arch Gen Psychiatry 44:1078–1083, 1987

Insel TR, Mueller EA, Alterman I, et al: Obsessive-compulsive disorder and serotonin: is there a connection? Biol Psychiatry 20:1174–1188, 1985

Jandhyala B, Steenberg M, Perel JM, et al: Effects of several tricyclic antidepressants on the hemodynamics and myocardial contractility of anesthetized dogs. Eur J Pharmacol 42:403–410, 1977

Jarvis MR: Clinical pharmacokinetics of tricyclic antidepressant overdose. Psychopharmacol Bull 27:541–550, 1991

Jobson K, Linnoila M, Gillam J, et al: Successful treatment of severe anxiety attacks with tricyclic antidepressants: a possible mechanism of action. Am J Psychiatry 135:863–864, 1978

Joyce PR, Paykel ES: Predictors of drug response in depression. Arch Gen Psychiatry 46:89–99, 1989

Kitanaka I, Ross RI, Cutler NR, et al: Altered hydroxy-desipramine concentrations in elderly depressed patients. Clin Pharmacol Ther 31:51–55, 1982

Kroessler D: Relative efficacy rates for therapies of delusional depression. Convulsive Therapy 1:173–182, 1985

Kuhn R: The treatment of depressive states with G22355 (imipramine hydrochloride). Am J Psychiatry 115:459–464, 1958

Laborit H, Huguenard P, Alluaume R: Un nouveau stabilisateur végétatif: le 4560 RP [A new vegetative stabilizer: 4560 RP]. Presse Méd 60:206–208, 1952

Laird LK, Lydiard RB, Morton WA, et al: Cardiovascular effects of imipramine, fluvoxamine and placebo in depressed outpatients. J Clin Psychiatry 54:224–228, 1993

Lake B: Controlled trial of nortriptyline in childhood enuresis. Med J Aust 5(2) (suppl 14):582–585, 1968

Leonard HL, Swedo S, Rapoport JL, et al: Treatment of obsessive compulsive disorder in children and adolescents with clomipramine and desipramine: a double-blind crossover comparison. Arch Gen Psychiatry 46:1088–1092, 1989

Lerer B: Neurochemical and other neurobiological consequences of ECT: implications for the pathogenesis and treatment of affective disorders, in Psychopharmacology: The Third Generation of Progress. Edited by Meltzer HY. New York, Raven, 1987, pp 577–588

Liebowitz MR, Quitkin FM, Stewart JW, et al: Antidepressant specificity in atypical depression. Arch Gen Psychiatry 45:129–137, 1988

Linnoila M, George L, Guthrie S, et al: Effect of alcohol consumption and cigarette smoking on antidepressant levels of depressed patients. Am J Psychiatry 138:841–842, 1981

Lydiard RB, Anton RF, Cunningham T: Interactions between sertraline and tricyclic antidepressants [letter]. Am J Psychiatry 150:1125–1126, 1993

Maas JW, Fawcett JA, Dekirmenjian H: Catecholamine metabolism, depressive illness, and drug response. Arch Gen Psychiatry 26:353–363, 1972

Manier DH, Gillespie DD, Sulser F: Dual aminergic regulation of central beta adrenoreceptors: effect of "atypical" antidepressants and 5-hydroxy-tryptophan. Neuropsychopharmacology 2:89–95, 1989

Manji HK, Chen G, Bitran JA, et al: Chronic exposure of C6 glioma cells to desipramine desensitizes β-adrenoceptors, but increases K_I/K_H ratio. Eur J Pharmacol 206:159–162, 1991a

Manji HK, Chen G, Bitran JA, et al: Down-regulation of beta receptors by desipramine in vitro involves PKC/phospholipase A_2. Psychopharm Bull 27:247–253, 1991b

Mogilnicka E, Arbilla S, Depoortere H, et al: Rapid-eye-movement sleep deprivation decreases the density of ^{3}H-dihydroalprenolol and ^{3}H-imipramine binding sites in the rat cerebral cortex. Eur J Pharmacol 65:289–292, 1980

Moody JP, Whyte SF, MacDonald AJ, et al: Pharmacokinetic aspects of protriptyline plasma levels. Eur J Clin Pharmacol 11:51–56, 1977

Munjack DJ, Isigli R, Zulueta A, et al: Nortriptyline in the treatment of panic disorder and agoraphobia with panic attacks. J Clin Psychopharmacol 8:204, 1988

Nelson JC, Mazure CM: A scale for rating tricyclic response in major depression: the TRIM. J Clin Psychopharmacol 10:252–260, 1990

Nelson JC, Mazure CM, Bowers MB Jr, et al: A preliminary open study of the combination of fluoxetine and desipramine for rapid treatment of major depression. Arch Gen Psychiatry 48:303–307, 1991

Nierenberg AA, Cole JO: Antidepressant adverse drug reactions. J Clin Psychiatry 52 (suppl):40–47, 1991

Nies A, Robinson DS, Friedman DS, et al: Relationship between age and tricyclic antidepressant plasma levels. Am J Psychiatry 134:790–793, 1977

Orsulak PJ: Therapeutic monitoring of antidepressant drugs: guidelines updated. Ther Drug Monit 11:497–507, 1989

Otton SV, Wu D, Joffe RT, et al: Inhibition by fluoxetine of cytochrome P_{450} 2D6 activity. Clin Pharmacol Ther 53:401–409, 1993

Paykel ES: Depressive typologies and response to amitriptyline. Br J Psychiatry 120:147–156, 1972

Paykel ES: Treatment of depression: the relevance of research for clinical practice. Br J Psychiatry 155:754–763, 1989

Paykel ES, Rowan PR, Parker RR, et al: Response to phenelzine and amitriptyline in subtypes of outpatient depression. Arch Gen Psychiatry 39:1041–1049, 1982

Perry PJ, Morgan DE, Smith RE, et al: Treatment of unipolar depression accompanied by delusions. J Affect Disord 4:195–200, 1982

Perry PJ, Pfohl BM, Holstad SG: The relationship between antidepressant response and tricyclic antidepressant plasma concentrations. Clin Pharmacokinet 13:381–392, 1987

Peroutka SJ, Snyder SH: Long term antidepressant

treatment decreases spiroperidol-labeled serotonin receptor binding. Science 210:88–90, 1980

Pinder RM, Brogden RN, Speight TM, et al: Doxepin up-to-date: a review of its pharmacological properties and therapeutic efficacy with particular reference to depression. Drugs 13:161–218, 1977

Pollock BG, Perel JM: Tricyclic antidepressants: contemporary issues for therapeutic practice. Can J Psychiatry 34:609–617, 1989

Pollock BG, Everett G, Perel JM: Comparative cardiotoxicity of nortriptyline and its isomeric 10-hydroxymetabolites. Neuropsychopharmacology 6:1–10, 1992a

Pollock BG, Perel JM, Altieri LP, et al: Debrisoquine hydroxylation phenotyping in geriatric psychopharmacology. Psychopharmacol Bull 28:163–168, 1992b

Potter WZ: Psychotherapeutic drugs and biogenic amines: current concepts and therapeutic implications. Drugs 28:127–143, 1984

Potter WZ, Calil NM, Manian AA, et al: Hydroxylated metabolites of tricyclic antidepressants: preclinical assessment of activity. Biol Psychiatry 14:601–613, 1979

Potter WZ, Bertilsson L, Sjoqvist F: Clinical pharmacokinetics of psychotropic drugs fundamental and practical aspects, in The Handbook of Biological Psychiatry. Edited by Van Praag NM, Rafaelson O, Lader O, et al. New York, Marcel Dekker, 1980, pp 71–134

Potter WZ, Scheinin M, Golden RN, et al: Selective antidepressants and cerebrospinal fluid: lack of specificity on norepinephrine and serotonin metabolites. Arch Gen Psychiatry 42:1171–1177, 1985

Potter WZ, Rudorfer MV, Manji HK: The pharmacologic treatment of depression: an update. N Engl J Med 523:633–642, 1991

Prange AI: The pharmacology and biochemistry of depression. Diseases of the Nervous System 25:217–221, 1965

Preskorn SH, Fast GA: Therapeutic drug monitoring for antidepressants: efficacy, safety, and cost effectiveness. J Clin Psychiatry 52 (suppl):23–22, 1991

Preskorn SH, Irwin HA: Toxicity of tricyclic antidepressants: kinetics, mechanism, intervention: a review. J Clin Psychiatry 43:151–156, 1982

Psychoyos S: Antidepressant inhibition of H_1-H_2-histamine-receptor-mediated adenylate cyclase in [2-^{3}H]adenine-prelabeled vesicular preparations from guinea pig brain. Biochem Pharmacol 30:2182–2185, 1981

Quitkin FM, Harrison W, Stewart JW, et al: Response to phenelzine and imipramine in placebo nonresponders with atypical depression. Arch Gen Psychiatry 48:319–323, 1991

Rahman MK, Akhtar MJ, Savla NC, et al: A double-blind randomized comparison of fluvoxamine with dothiepin in the treatment of depression in elderly patients. Br J Clin Pract 45:255–258, 1991

Randrup A, Braestrup C: Uptake inhibition of biogenic amines by newer antidepressant drugs: relevance to the dopamine hypothesis of depression. Psychopharmacol 53:309–314, 1977

Rapoport J, Potter WZ: Tricyclic antidepressants: use in pediatric psychopharmacology, in Pharmacokinetics: Youth and Age. Edited by Raskin A, Robinson D. Amsterdam, Elsevier, 1981, pp 105–123

Rapoport JL, Mikkelson EJ, Zavadil AP, et al: Childhood enuresis II: psychopathology, tricyclic concentration in plasma and anti-enuretic effect. Arch Gen Psychiatry 37:1146–1152, 1980

Raskin A, Crook TA: The endogenous-neurotic distinction as a predictor of response to antidepressant drugs. Psychol Med 6:59–70, 1976

Ravaris CL, Robinson DS, Ives JO, et al: Phenelzine and amitriptyline in the treatment of depression: a comparison of present and past studies. Arch Gen Psychiatry 37:1075–1080, 1980

Ray WA: Psychotropic drugs and injuries among the elderly: a review. J Clin Psychopharmacol 12:386–396, 1992

Richelson E, Nelson A: Antagonism by antidepressants of neurotransmitter receptors of normal human brain in vitro. J Pharmacol Exp Ther 230:94–102, 1984

Richelson E, Pfenning M: Blockade by antidepressants and related compounds of biogenic amine uptake into rat brain synaptosomes: most antidepressants selectively block norepinephrine uptake. Eur J Pharmacol 130:277–286, 1984

Riddle MA, Geller B, Ryan N: Another sudden death in a child treated with desipramine. J Am Acad Child Adolesc Psychiatry 32:792–797, 1993

Roose SP, Dalack GW, Glassman AH, et al: Is doxepin a safer tricyclic for the heart? J Clin Psychiatry 52:338–341, 1991

Rosen J, Pollock BG, Altieri LP, et al: Treatment of nortriptyline's side effects in elderly patients: a double-blind study of bethanechol. Am J Psychiatry 150:1249–1251, 1993

Ross RI, Zavadil AP, Calil NM, et al: The effects of desmethylimipramine on plasma norepinephrine, pulse and blood pressure in volunteers. Clin Pharmacol Ther 33:429–437, 1983

Rudorfer MV, Potter WZ: Pharmacokinetics of antidepressants, in Psychopharmacology: The Third Generation of Progress. Edited by Meltzer HY. New York, Raven, 1987, pp 1353–1364

Rudorfer MV, Robins E: Amitriptyline overdose: clinical effects of tricyclic antidepressant plasma levels. J Clin Psychiatry 43:457–460, 1982

Rudorfer MV, Young RC: Desipramine: cardiovascular effects and plasma levels. Am J Psychiatry 137:984–986, 1980a

Rudorfer MV, Young RC: Anticholinergic effects and plasma desipramine levels. Clin Pharmacol Ther 28:703–706, 1980b

Rudorfer MV, Manji HK, Potter WZ: Comparative tolerability profiles of the newer versus older antidepressants. Drug Saf 10:18–46, 1994

Schildkraut JJ: The catecholamine hypothesis of affective disorders: a review of supporting evidence. Am J Psychiatry 122:509–522, 1965

Shoaf SE, Linnoila M: Interaction of ethanol and smoking on the pharmacokinetics and pharmacodynamics of psychotropic medications. Psychopharmacol Bull 27:577–594, 1991

Spiker D, Weiss A, Chang S, et al: Tricyclic antidepressant overdose: clinical presentation and plasma levels. Clin Pharmacol Ther 18:539–546, 1975

Spiker DG, Weiss JC, Dealy RS, et al: The pharmacologic treatment of delusional depression. Am J Psychiatry 142:430–436, 1985

Stewart JW, Quitkin F, Fyer A, et al: Efficacy of desmethylimipramine in endogenomorphically depressed patients. Psychopharmacol Bull 16:52–54, 1980

Stewart JW, Quitkin FM, Liebowitz MR, et al: Efficacy of desipramine in depressed outpatients: response according to Research Diagnostic Criteria and severity of illness. Arch Gen Psychiatry 40:202–207, 1989

Sugrue MF: Chronic antidepressant therapy and associated changes in central monoaminergic function. Pharmacol Ther 21:1–37, 1983

Sulser F: Antidepressant treatments and regulation of norepinephrine-receptor-coupled adenylate cyclase systems in brain. Adv Biochem Psychopharmacol 39:249–261, 1984

Sulser F, Vetulani J, Mobley PL: Mode of action of antidepressant drugs. Biochem Pharmacol 27:257–261, 1978

Sunderland T, Tariot PN, Cohen RM, et al: Anticholinergic sensitivity in patients with dementia of the Alzheimer type and age-matched controls: a dose-response study. Arch Gen Psychiatry 44:418–426, 1987

Thoren P, Asberg M, Cronholm B, et al: Clomipramine treatment of obsessive compulsive disorder: a controlled clinical trial. Arch Gen Psychiatry 37:1281–1289, 1980

Traskman L, Asberg M, Bertilsson L, et al: Plasma levels of chlorimipramine and its dimethyl metabolite during treatment of depression. Clin Pharmacol Ther 26:600–610, 1979

Turner P, Ehsanullah RSB: Clomipramine and maprotiline on human platelet uptake of 5-hydroxytryptamine and dopamine in vitro: relevance to their antidepressive and other central actions? Postgrad Med J 53 (suppl 4):14–18, 1977

Uhde TW, Nemiah JC: Panic and generalized anxiety disorders, in Comprehensive Textbook of Psychiatry, 5th Edition. Edited by Sadock BJ. Baltimore, MD, Williams & Wilkins, 1989, pp 952–972

USPDI: Drug Information For the Health Care Professional, 13th Edition. Rockville, MD, United States Pharmacopeial Convention, Inc., 1993

Vetulani J, Sulser F: Action of various antidepressant treatments reduces reactivity of noradrenergic cyclic AMP generating systems in limbic forebrain. Nature 257:495–496, 1975

Vetulani J, Lebrecht U, Pilc A: Enhancement of responsiveness of the central system and serotonin-2-receptor density in rat frontal cortex by electroconvulsive treatments. Eur J Pharmacol 76:81–85, 1981

Wells BG, Gelenberg AJ: Chemistry, pharmacology, pharmacokinetics, adverse effects and efficacy of the antidepressant maprotiline hydrochloride. Pharmacotherapy 1:121–139, 1981

Young RC, Alexopoulos GS, Shamoian CA, et al: Plasma 10-hydroxynortriptyline in elderly depressed patients. Clin Pharmacol Ther 35:540–544, 1984

Young RC, Alexopoulos GS, Shindledeker R, et al: Plasma 10-hydroxynortriptyline and therapeutic response in geriatric depression. Neuropsychopharmacology 1(3):213–215, 1988

Ziegler VE, Biggs JT: Tricyclic plasma levels: effect of age, race, sex, and smoking. JAMA 238:2167–2169,

1977

Ziegler VE, Biggs IT, Wylie LT, et al: Protriptyline kinetics. Clin Pharmacol Ther 23:580–584, 1978

Zis AP, Goodwin FK: Novel antidepressants and the biogenic amine hypothesis of depression: the case of iprindole and mianserin. Arch Gen Psychiatry 36:1097–1107, 1979

Zitrin CM, Klein DF, Woerner MG: Treatment of agoraphobia with group exposure in vivo and imipramine. Arch Gen Psychiatry 37:63–72, 1980

8

Selective Serotonin Reuptake Inhibitors

Gary D. Tollefson, M.D., Ph.D.

The class of selective serotonin reuptake inhibitors (SSRIs) represents an important advance in pharmacotherapy and has been the catalyst for substantial serotonin-oriented basic and clinical research. Increasing evidence suggests that this drug class has a broad spectrum of potential indications. In general, a more advantageous safety profile has propelled these agents to their current level of popularity. Although the members of this category share a number of common features, this discussion also highlights some of their unique differences.

■ HISTORY AND DISCOVERY

Serotonin (5-HT) is an indoleamine with wide distribution in plants, animals, and humans. Pioneering histochemistry by Falck and colleagues (1962) demonstrated that 5-HT was localized within specific neuronal pathways and cell bodies. These originate principally from two discrete nuclei, the medial and dorsal raphe. Across animal species, 5-HT innervation is widespread. Although regional variations exist, several limbic structures manifest especially high levels of 5-HT (Amin et al. 1954).

However, 5-HT levels in the central nervous system (CNS) represent only a small fraction of that found in the body (Bradley 1989). Because 5-HT does not cross the blood-brain barrier, it must be synthesized locally. Release into the synapse may occur from two reservoirs, cytoplasmic and vesicular (Elks et al. 1979). Following release, 5-HT is principally inactivated by uptake into nerve terminals through a Na^+/K^+ adenosine triphosphatase (ATPase)-dependent carrier (Shaskan and Snyder 1970). The transmitter is subsequently subject to either degradation by monoamine oxidase (MAO) or vesicular restorage. Abnormalities in central 5-HT function have been hypothesized to underlie disturbances in mood, anxiety, satiety, cognition, aggression, and sexual drive to highlight a few. As described by Fuller (1985), there are several loci at which therapeutic drugs might alter 5-HT neurotransmission (see Figure 8–1). The 5-HT uptake site is the focus of this chapter. The recent explosion of knowledge regarding the 5-HT system can largely be traced to the development of compounds that block this uptake site.

■ STRUCTURE-ACTIVITY RELATIONSHIPS

Drugs that inhibit 5-HT uptake vary in their selectivity (see Table 8–1). Despite the tendency to lump the contemporary SSRIs into the same class designation, significant structural and activity differences exist. Their structural formulae help illustrate this diversity (see Figure 8–2). Both paroxetine and sertraline exist as single isomers; in contrast, fluoxetine and citalopram are racemic. Fluvoxamine has no optically active forms. Structural differences bestow both pharmacokinetic and pharmacodynamic heterogeneity.

The family of SSRIs manifests diverse structural and activity relationships. Such data are in vitro and thus subject to methodologic variability (Thomas et al. 1987). Paroxetine appears to be the most potent in vitro SSRI, whereas citalopram may be the most selective. However, it is noteworthy that in vitro potency does not necessarily equate with in vivo dosing experience, clinical efficacy, profile of adverse events, and so on. Of the SSRIs, sertraline is the only class member that is a more potent inhibitor of dopamine (DA) than noradrenaline (NA) uptake. Only

clomipramine (through its metabolite) appears to have potential for a higher NA-to-5-HT uptake ratio.

The tricyclic antidepressants (TCAs) have been characterized by their inhibitory activity at a number of other receptor targets mediating their adverse event profile (Hall and Ogren 1981; Snyder and Yamamura 1977; U'Prichard et al. 1978). These include histaminergic, α_1-adrenergic, and muscarinic receptors. For most of the SSRIs, inhibitory activity

Table 8–1. Inhibition of [^{3}H]-monoamine uptake into rat brain synaptosomes in vitro

Compound	K_1(nM)		
	[^{3}H]-5-HT	[^{3}H]-NE	[^{3}H]-DA
Paroxetine	1.1	350	2,000
Citalopram	1.8	8,800	> 10,000
Fluvoxamine	6.2	1,100	> 10,000
Sertraline	7.3	1,400	230
Clomipramine	7.4	96	9,100
Fluoxetine	25	500	4,200
Amitriptyline	87	79	4,300

Source. Relative values from a series of related trials from Boyer and Feighner 1991.

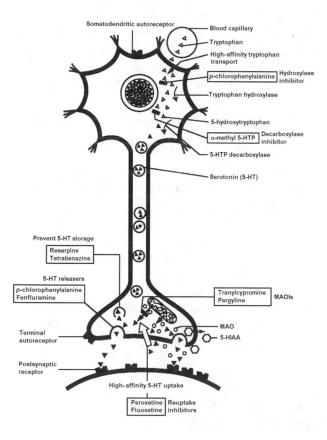

Figure 8–1. Serotonin neuron showing the main steps in the life cycle of serotonin and the sites at which drugs act. For clarity, drugs acting at 5-HT receptors have been omitted.
Source. Marsden 1991. Used with permission.

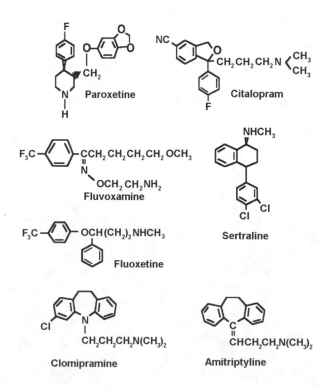

Figure 8–2. Structural formulae of the SSRIs and some TCAs.

(IC_{50}) at histaminergic or adrenergic sites is in the micromolar range and thus unlikely to be of clinical significance. Sertraline is an exception with an IC_{50} of 245 nM based on displacement of ^{3}H-prazosin from rat cortical membrane binding (Stockmeier et al. 1987). This affinity is approximately one-fourth that exhibited by imipramine. SSRI activity at the muscarinic receptor is negligible for fluoxetine, fluvoxamine, citalopram, and sertraline; however, paroxetine has an IC_{50} of 89 nM, which suggests some increased chance for anticholinergic events. Although of uncertain clinical relevance, sertraline also demonstrates a high affinity for the sigma binding site in vitro. In contrast, neither paroxetine nor fluoxetine is significantly active there (Schmidt et al. 1989). The sigma binding site is of theoretical interest in schizophrenia and related psychoses. Stauderman and colleagues (1992) demonstrated that fluoxetine and paroxetine inhibited the binding of ^{3}H-nitrendipine to L-type calcium channels. However, this was at concentrations that were probably in excess of those achieved during in vivo treatment of depression.

In summary, in vitro radioligand-binding techniques demonstrate that SSRIs have a lower probability of many of the troublesome side effects associated with TCAs and are relatively selective in their 5-HT uptake inhibition, yet retain an individual variability in their receptor pharmacology. (For a general review of radioligand binding of several SSRIs versus conventional TCAs, see Thomas et al. 1987.)

PHARMACOLOGICAL PROFILE

Serotonin (5-HT)

The action of an SSRI extends beyond the inhibition of 5-HT uptake. As evidenced in Figure 8–3, there is a family of at least nine 5-HT receptor subtypes residing at pre- and/or postsynaptic locations. 5-HT$_{1A}$ binding sites include both somatodendritic and presynaptic autoreceptors (which inhibit 5-HT firing) and postsynaptic receptors. The latter are predominantly hippocampal and demonstrate an increased sensitivity after chronic antidepressant exposure (Aghajanian et al. 1988). Antidepressant-induced changes at the 5-HT$_{1B}$ binding site are not definitive (Sleight et al. 1988). Reduced sensitivity of 5-HT$_{1B}$ sites may uniquely characterize the SSRIs. The R

enantiomer of fluoxetine antagonizes the 5-HT$_{1C}$ receptor at near-micromolar concentrations (Wong et al. 1991) in vitro; however, the relevance of this observation to other models and the extent to which other SSRIs share this interaction are unknown.

5-HT$_2$ receptors are located postsynaptically throughout the hippocampus, cortex, and spinal cord. Functionally, they inhibit postsynaptic propagation of a nerve impulse. The upregulation of 5-HT$_2$ binding sites has been implicated in major depression (Pandey et al. 1990). Although receptor studies are not conclusive, 5-HT$_2$ behavioral models (e.g., 5-HTP head twitch response) reveal that potentiation diminishes after chronic SSRI exposure consistent with 5-HT$_2$ receptor adaptation (Marshall et al. 1988). After chronic administration, many contemporary antidepressants downregulate or reduce the density of 5-HT$_2$ binding sites in rat frontal cortex (Peroutka and Snyder 1980). Some but not all SSRIs have been associated with this effect (Fraser et al. 1988). These adaptive changes have been cited as essential for an antidepressant response (Cowen 1991). However, the apparent absence of such activity in several of the SSRIs calls into question how essential this effect is.

These factors may not be exclusionary. An interaction between 5-HT$_{1A}$- and 5-HT$_2$-binding sites seems quite plausible. 5-HT$_2$ antagonists attenuate a 5-HT$_{1A}$ agonist's (8-hydroxydipropylaminotetralin [8-OH-DPAT]) ability to release 5-HT (Backus et al. 1990). SSRIs, as a drug class, have been reported to normalize both 5-HT$_{1A}$ and 5-HT$_2$ receptor density among depressed patients (Leonard 1992).

Studies of fluoxetine (Blier et al. 1988), citalopram (Chaput et al. 1986), paroxetine (deMontigny et al. 1989), fluvoxamine (Dresse and Scuvee-Moreau 1984), and sertraline (Heym and Koe 1988) have re-

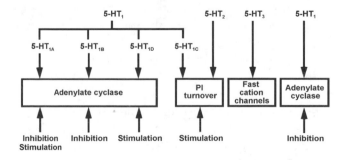

Figure 8–3. Main effector links between 5-HT binding sites and neuronal responses.

vealed that SSRIs transiently inhibit dorsal raphe firing, decrease terminal autoreceptor function, and ultimately increase net 5-HT synaptic transmission within CA_3 pyramidal cells in the hippocampus. Blier and colleagues (1990) concluded that electrophysiologic studies suggest that most antidepressants enhance net 5-HT after chronic administration, albeit at different loci—the TCAs through enhanced sensitivity of postsynaptic 5-HT$_{1A}$ receptors and the SSRIs (and MAO inhibitors [MAOIs]) through a reduced sensitivity among somatodendritic (5-HT$_{1A}$) and terminal autoreceptors (5-HT$_{1D}$). This intriguing set of observations may help explain why certain depressed patients fail to respond to one category of antidepressant but will respond to another, as well as why there is a reported TCA-SSRI synergy among some nonresponders.

■ Noradrenaline

Chronic administration of most somatic treatments for depression downregulates or reduces the density of β-NA binding sites in the brain (Bergstrom and Kellar 1979). This includes traditional NA-specific and mixed uptake inhibitors (Charney et al. 1981). However, results with the SSRIs have been less consistent (Johnson 1991). Despite their in vitro 5-HT selectivity, several of these agents (e.g., fluoxetine by autoradiography and sertraline by autoradiography or membrane binding) induce β-NA receptor downregulation.

Most studies with the SSRIs have not shown a consistent change in β-NA binding or β-NA stimulated cyclic adenosine monophosphate (cAMP) production. However, Baron and colleagues (1988) reported that fluoxetine coadministered with desipramine augmented the expected desipramine reduction in cortical β-NA receptors. Asakura and colleagues (1987) noted that coadministration with mianserin or maprotiline also increased the duration of downregulation. Sertraline induces downregulation and reduced production at the β-receptor second messenger cAMP (Koe et al. 1987). In contrast, investigations with fluvoxamine, paroxetine, and citalopram have failed to yield consistent results. In general, the greater the 5-HT selectivity of a compound, the less in vitro evidence for β-NA downregulation has been seen. Thus, β-NA downregulation may not be an essential feature for clinical efficacy. However, indirect effects are impossible to exclude.

Current data do not support a significant effect on α-NA receptor affinity or density by the SSRIs. Studies employing several different radiolabels to investigate paroxetine (Nelson et al. 1989), fluoxetine (Wong et al. 1985), and citalopram (Nowak 1989) have shown a relative inactivity at this site. Studies with sertraline or fluvoxamine are limited; however, a weak α$_1$ affinity (2–4 times less than imipramine) has been reported with sertraline (Stockmeier et al. 1987). Fluoxetine has been reported to reduce desipramine-induced growth hormone release after 4 weeks of treatment (O'Flynn et al. 1991). This effect suggests a possible indirect activity at the α$_2$-NA receptor.

In summary, the majority of SSRIs do not manifest significant NA activity. However, relative differences in adrenoceptor affinity exist across the class; the clinical significance of these differences is negligible based on present information.

■ Dopamine

Animal studies provide evidence that the 5-HT system may exert tonic inhibition on the central dopaminergic system. Thus, hypothetically SSRIs might diminish dopaminergic transmission. An anecdotal increase in extrapyramidal side effects (EPS) during fluoxetine therapy (Bouchard et al. 1989) has been attributed to this theory. 5-HT agonists also exert a facilitatory influence on DA release (Benloucif and Galloway 1991) that can be antagonized by the 5-HT$_1$ blocker pindolol. On the contrary, evidence suggests that SSRIs may actually sensitize mesolimbic DA receptors (Arnt et al. 1984a, 1984b). Many structurally diverse antidepressants are associated with a net enhancement of mesolimbic DA (Klimek and Maj 1990). The benefits of antidepressants in an animal model of depression can be antagonized by either a D$_1$ (SCH23390) or D$_2$ blocker (sulpiride) (Sampson et al. 1991). Repeated administration of several SSRIs increased the hypermotility response to several dopaminergic agents, including amphetamine, methylphenidate (Arnt et al. 1984b), quinpirole (Maj et al. 1984), or apomorphine (Plaznik and Kostowski 1987).

The induction of catalepsy or inhibition of apomorphine-induced catalepsy is not a property of the SSRIs. Clomipramine (CMI) was reported by Balsara and co-workers (1979) to augment neuroleptic effects in a rodent model. Within the family of SSRIs, citalopram reportedly downregulated rat striatolimbic D_1 receptors (Klimek and Nielsen 1987). Both citalopram and fluoxetine have been inactive in displacing D_2 blockers (Peroutka and Snyder 1980). Baldessarini and co-workers (1992) reported that fluoxetine "even at high doses or with repeated treatment" demonstrated "no significant inhibition of the DA-metabolism—increasing actions of haloperidol" (p. 191). In summary, the SSRIs do not appear to exert a significant effect on the DA system. However, in a clinical setting, a plethora of variables (e.g., pharmacokinetic interactions) make simple conclusions regarding DA-mediated events unreliable.

Gamma-Aminobutyric Acid (GABA)

A series of antidepressants (including several SSRIs) have been shown to enhance GABAergic activity. GABA receptors include both type A (GABA-A, linked to chloride ionophores and the benzodiazepine recognition site) and type B (GABA-B, comodulatory with NA and 5-HT). Upregulation of the GABA-B (i.e., baclofen-recognizing) type has been ascribed to a variety of antidepressants, including SSRIs, and electroconvulsive therapy (Lloyd et al. 1985). Presynaptic changes have been hypothesized to induce chronic postsynaptic adaptive responses (Perez et al. 1991). However, not all investigators have been able to reliably demonstrate such effects (Pratt and Bowery 1989). Thus, any GABA-based mechanism for the SSRIs remains a matter of speculation.

Miscellaneous

Neuroendocrine and neurotransmitter dysfunction in major depression have been linked to corticotropin-releasing factor (CRF) in locus ceruleus (LC) neurons. Antidepressants have been hypothesized to reverse CRF-related increases in LC discharge. Sertraline has been proposed as an acute functional CRF antagonist (Valentino and Curtis 1991). However, net 5-HT enhancement by an SSRI would be expected to promote the release of CRF (Fuller 1985). The role for SSRIs as CRF antagonists awaits further clarification; however, activity through 5-HT$_{1A}$ receptors has been proposed by Lorens and Van der Kar (1987).

In summary, the SSRIs enhance central 5-HT through increased output and/or increased postsynaptic receptor sensitivity (Blier et al. 1987). However, such changes alone do not guarantee a clinically meaningful response (Charney et al. 1984). It is likely that a prerequisite change in baseline 5-HT function and/or a "permissive" set of interactions with other colocalized neurotransmitter receptors is involved in the highly individualized responses seen in depressed patients.

PHARMACOKINETICS AND DISPOSITION

Pharmacokinetic variability within the SSRI class is seen when comparing drug half-life, percentage protein-bound, and volume of distribution (Leonard 1992). Table 8–2 summarizes several differential features. As an example, fluvoxamine exhibits a shorter half-life (16 versus 36–48 hours), less extensive binding (77% versus 95%–99%), and a smaller volume of distribution (5 versus 20–42 L/kg) than either fluoxetine or sertraline.

Any discussion of drug half-life must also include consideration of the presence or absence of active metabolites. Both fluoxetine and have metabolites that probably contribute to their therapeutic efficacy. Fluoxetine is principally metabolized to norfluoxetine, which may exceed the plasma concentration of its parent with chronic administration (Lemberger et al. 1985a). The elimination half-life of norfluoxetine is slower (7–15 days) than that of fluoxetine (3–5 days). Norfluoxetine demonstrates approximately near equal selective uptake inhibition of both 5-HT and NA (Wong et al. 1975). In contrast, CMI is metabolized (by N-demethylation) to desmethylchlomipramine, a potent inhibitor of NA uptake (Benfield et al. 1980). Thus, as plasma levels of this desmethyl metabolite rise relative to its parent, selectivity is significantly altered.

In an intermediate position, the desmethyl metabolite of sertraline manifests uptake inhibition of serotonin, albeit of a magnitude approximately one-tenth that of the parent (Heym and Koe 1988). The elimination half-life of desmethylsertraline also exceeds that of its parent (66 versus 24 hours) (Doogan and Caillard 1988). The principal desmethyl metabolite of citalopram is approximately 4 times less potent as an SSRI than its parent and 11 times more potent as a NA uptake inhibitor (Hyttel 1982). However, this metabolite's concentration is typically less than that of citalopram, and the former only weakly crosses the

Table 8–2. A comparison of several selective uptake inhibitors of serotonin

	Fluoxetine	Paroxetine	Sertraline	Citalopram	Clomipramine	Fluvoxamine
Volume of distribution (L/kg)	3–40	17	20	12–16	> 1,000	> 5
Percent protein-bound (%)	94	95	99	80	97	77
Peak plasma level (hours)	6–8	2–8	6–8	1–6	2–6	2–8
Parent half-life ($T_{1/2}$)	24–72	20	25	33	19–37	15
Major metabolite $T_{1/2}$	7–15 days	N/A	66 hours	N/A	54–77	N/A
Standard dose range (mg)	20–80	10–50	50–200	10–40	25–250	50–300
Absorption altered by a fast or fed status	No	No	Yes	No	Yes	No
Altered $T_{1/2}$ in the geriatric patient	No	Yes	Yes	Yes	Yes	No
Reduced clearance in renal patients	±	+	±	±	?	±

blood-brain barrier. Thus, an antidepressant contribution from the metabolite is likely negligible.

On the far end of the continuum, paroxetine (Haddock et al. 1989) and fluvoxamine (Claassen 1983) have metabolites with minimal or no activity. The advantages of SSRIs with a relatively longer half-life include greater protection against patient noncompliance, postdiscontinuation relapse, or abrupt "withdrawal" syndromes. Conversely, those drugs require a greater vigilance for drug-drug interaction following their discontinuation (e.g., the recommended 5-week washout from fluoxetine before initiating an MAOI; Ciraulo and Shader 1990). A key point is that variability in drug half-life does not predict or correlate with onset of antidepressant activity.

■ MECHANISM OF ACTION

The drugs discussed here represent uptake inhibitors that demonstrate a high degree of selectivity in blocking the neuronal uptake of serotonin. Based on this mechanism they can be further considered as indirect 5-HT agonists. In the absence of pharmacological manipulation, the 5-HT uptake into the presynaptic nerve terminal typically leads to its inactivation. The SSRIs, through blockade of the reuptake process, acutely enhance serotonergic neurotransmission by permitting serotonin to act for an extended time at synaptic binding sites. A net result is an acute increase in synaptic 5-HT. In this sense, the SSRIs produce a similar effect as would be seen with the direct-acting agonists (e.g., members of the aryl-piperazine family such as quipazine and MK-212).

However, one distinct difference separating the SSRIs from the direct-acting agonists is that the SSRIs are dependent on neuronal release of serotonin for their action. That is, they can be considered as augmentors of basal physiological signals. But they are neither direct stimulators of postsynaptic receptor function nor independent of presynaptic neuronal integrity. The clinical relevance of this differentiation might explain SSRI nonresponse. If this select subpopulation were characterized such that the release of 5-HT from presynaptic neuronal storage sites was substantially compromised, and in turn their net synaptic 5-HT concentration was negligible, we would not expect a clinically meaningful response to an SSRI. With minimal 5-HT in the synapse, there is little uptake to inhibit.

5-HT receptors also include a family of presynaptic autoreceptors that suppress the further release of 5-HT, thus limiting the degree of postsynaptic receptor stimulation that can be achieved. DeMontigny and colleagues (1989) have investigated the mechanism of action of several SSRIs. The authors suggest that the enhanced efficacy of serotonergic synaptic transmission is not the result of increased postsynaptic sensitivity. Rather, longer-term SSRI treatment induced a desensitization of somatodendritic and terminal 5-HT autoreceptors. Such a desensitization would permit 5-HT neurons to reestablish a normal rate of firing despite sustained reuptake blockade. These neurons in turn could release a greater amount of 5-HT per impulse into the synaptic cleft. This progressive modification reportedly occurs over a time course compatible with a delayed therapeutic efficacy observed in SSRI trials.

■ INDICATIONS

■ Depression

A plethora of placebo-controlled, double-blind trials have established the clear superiority of the SSRIs over placebo (Kasper et al. 1992). Statistically significant reductions from baseline in the Hamilton Rating Scale for Depression (HRS-D; Hamilton 1967) score have been seen as early as the second week of treatment; however, the rate and quality of response to an SSRI is highly individualized (range 10–42 days). This probably reflects the underlying biologic heterogeneity of major depression. Overall, the efficacy of the SSRIs versus conventional TCAs has been comparable or slightly better (Feighner et al. 1989; Guelfi et al. 1987; Wernicke et al. 1987). However, this has not been universal (Pcsclow ct al. 1989; vanPraag et al. 1987). Several trials have also established that the SSRIs may be effective among either TCA-resistant (Delgado et al. 1988; Tyrer et al. 1987) or MAOI-resistant (Weilburg et al. 1989) depression.

In general, the range for dose titration with most of the SSRIs is relatively narrow (see Table 8–2) (Altamura et al. 1988; Amin et al. 1989). Higher dosages are often associated with increased adverse event rates that may compromise patient management. Prescribing a conservative introductory dose—followed by patience—is recommended accordingly. In their study of fluoxetine, Schweizer and colleagues (1990) reported a delayed therapeutic benefit in 108 subjects treated with 20 mg for 3 weeks and then randomized to either 20 mg or 60 mg for another 5 weeks. Both groups did equally well after 8 weeks.

However, implementation of earlier high-dose therapy may be appropriate in some circumstances (e.g., in a patient with a history of treatment resistance). Conversion of nonresponders by prescribing at the higher end of the dose range has been described with fluoxetine and paroxetine (Fava et al. 1992; Hebenstreit et al. 1989). However, extreme dosages of sertraline (200–400 mg/day) have been associated with a reduced efficacy (Guy et al. 1986). Unfortunately, plasma level studies have contributed little toward a better understanding of these phenomena. To date, most studies have failed to confirm any relationship between clinical response and plasma concentration with paroxetine (Tasker et al. 1989), fluoxetine (Kelly et al. 1989), citalopram (Hebenstreit et al. 1989), or fluvoxamine (De-Wilde and Doogan

1982). This suggests that synaptic concentrations and/or pharmacodynamic effects are not accurately reflected by plasma levels. The issue of a linear versus curvilinear dose-response pattern with the SSRIs also remains unanswered.

Continued SSRI efficacy during maintenance therapy has been demonstrated in a number of trials (Danion 1989; Dufour 1987; Ferrey et al. 1989; Montgomery et al. 1988). One of the largest revealed a recurrence among 54 of 94 placebo subjects (57%) versus 23 of 88 fluoxetine-maintained subjects (26%; $P < .0001$) who had at least 4.5 months of recovery before their randomization (Montgomery et al. 1988). Study participants had been required to have at least two previous episodes. Similar outcomes favoring the SSRI include a smaller blinded trial ($N = 289$) with sertraline (Doogan and Caillard 1988) and open trials of fluvoxamine (Feldmann and Dunbar 1982) and citalopram (Pedersen et al. 1982) have been reported.

Although the SSRIs are often thought of as "activating," considerable evidence supports their utility in depression with anxious features. Montgomery (1989a) conducted a meta-analysis of several fluoxetine trials that indicated efficacy in depression, including the features of anxiety and psychomotor agitation. Similar findings have been reported by Jouvent and colleagues (1989) and Beasley and colleagues (1991). Dunbar (1990) demonstrated analogous benefits with paroxetine. Fluvoxamine reduced comorbid anxiety to a extent similar to that of a comparator benzodiazepine in trials conducted by Charbannes and Douge (1989) and Laws and colleagues (1990).

What has emerged from comparative blinded depression trials is that the risk-benefit profile of an SSRI is often superior to that of conventional TCAs. Boyer and Feighner (1991) reviewed this literature. A favorable comparison to the standard TCAs is particularly interesting in light of the HRS-D's emphasis on somatic and sleep symptoms. These items may improve independent of mood status secondary to the characteristic sedative and anticholinergic effects of the TCAs, while remaining unchanged or slightly accentuated by an SSRI during the first 1–2 weeks of treatment (Montgomery 1989b; Shaw and Crimmins 1989).

From a clinician's perspective, the particular advantage enjoyed by the SSRIs is their unique adverse event profile. This translates into superior patient acceptance and compliance in most cases. Within controlled clinical trials, the rate of early treatment discontinuations with a TCA comparator have been severalfold higher than those with the novel SSRIs (Jenike et al. 1989a; Shrivastava et al. 1992). Thus, the SSRIs represent a significant addition to our therapeutic armamentarium and demonstrate a favorable safety profile compared with the TCAs, and at least comparable efficacy.

■ Obsessive-Compulsive Disorder (OCD)

More than 20 years ago, the TCA clomipramine was observed to reduce OCD symptoms (Renynghe de Voxurie 1968). CMI differs from imipramine by virtue of a chloride substitution at the third carbon atom. This parachlor substitution confers a potent 5-HT inhibitory profile (Ross and Renyi 1977). The advantage of this 5-HT selectivity in the treatment of OCD has been demonstrated in comparative trials where non-SSRIs such as desipramine (Zohar et al. 1988) or clorgiline (Insel et al. 1983) exhibit a less robust effect. This differential response represents a cornerstone in the 5-HT hypothesis of OCD (Benkelfat et al. 1989). CMI plasma concentrations—unlike those of its less selective metabolite (desmethylclomipramine)—may correlate with clinical response (Insel et al. 1983) and reduced cerebrospinal fluid (CSF) 5-hydroxyindoleacetic acid (5-HIAA) (Thoren et al. 1980). Sertraline (Bick and Hackett 1989), fluvoxamine (Goodman et al. 1989), and fluoxetine (Jenike et al. 1989b) have also been shown to be effective in treatment of OCD independent of a patient's comorbid mood status. The principal difference among these agents has been their adverse event profile (e.g., a more predominant anticholinergic spectrum of adverse events with clomipramine).

A precise explanation of this selective advantage in OCD is unknown. A heightened level of metabolic activity in the orbital region and caudate dysfunction have been reported by Baxter and colleagues (1992). These features appear responsive to either somatic (fluoxetine 60–80 mg) or behavioral interventions. Hypothetically, an SSRI may selectively enhance an inhibitory or disregard signal to the orbitofrontal region and in turn, reduce resistance to these impulses (Insel 1992). Hypersensitivity of the 5-HT system has been theorized. Receptor downregulation, associated with long-term SSRI therapy, has been offered as a potential explanation (Zohar et al. 1988). This hypothetical neuroadaptation is supported by a positive correlation between symptomatic improvement from baseline in CSF 5-HIAA (Thoren 1980) or platelet 5-HT concentration (Flament et al. 1985) improvement. Chronic administration of fluoxetine attenuates ipsapirone-induced hypothermia and adrenocorticotropic hormone (ACTH) and cortisol release among primary OCD patients. Although these data support a model of drug-induced 5-HT_{1A} subsensitivity and/or dampened postreceptor signal, the magnitude of change fails to correlate with the degree of clinical improvement (Lesch et al. 1991). An SSRI-mediated decrease in 5-HT responsivity is consistent with the observed latency in symptomatic improvement.

Because OCD is a chronic disorder, prolonged SSRI therapy may be necessary. Pato and colleagues (1988) conducted a double-blind discontinuation study with clomipramine. Subjects had been treated for 5–27 months before drug discontinuation. Sixteen subjects (89%) experienced a symptomatic worsening after drug discontinuation. Thus, it would appear that an SSRI maintenance strategy should be seriously considered for OCD patients. For individuals who have experienced minimal or only moderate improvement with an SSRI, a number of augmentation strategies have been proposed (see Goodman et al. 1992). Promising candidates include tryptophan, fenfluramine, lithium, buspirone, trazodone, or a neuroleptic.

■ Panic Disorder

Preclinical, neuroanatomical, neurophysiological, and behavioral studies support a role for 5-HT in panic disorder (Kahn et al. 1988). Target candidates include 5-HT_{1A} (hippocampus), 5-HT_2 (neocortex), and 5-HT_3 (amygdala/hippocampus). A functional interaction with NA systems is plausible. With the increased number of 5-HT selective drugs available, a number of preliminary trials have been conducted. Both zimeldine and clomipramine were reported to be antipanic agents in two early placebo-controlled trials (Evans et al. 1986; Westenberg et al. 1987). In 1987, Gorman and colleagues reported a fluoxetine dose of 20 mg was effective for 7 individuals in an open-label study of 16 subjects; however, this starting dose was not well tolerated among 8 others. Schneier and colleagues (1990) treated 25 panic patients, but they employed a lower starting dose (5 mg). Of the 25 subjects, 19 improved, with only 4 demonstrating an intolerance. These two studies suggest a 5-HT role in panic disorder, and they also imply that panic patients may have a greater sensitivity to SSRIs than their nonpanic counterparts. Not unexpectedly, other SSRIs have subsequently been found to also be effective in treating panic disorder. Trials employing citalopram (Humble et al. 1989) and fluvoxamine (den-Boer et al. 1987) further confirm that 5-HT reuptake inhibition is a direct or indirect mechanism benefiting some patients with panic disorder.

■ Schizophrenia

Evidence of a 5-HT role in schizophrenia dates back to the 1950s (Woolley and Campbell 1962). The chemical similarities between 5-HT and several hallucinogenic ergot alkaloids led to the demonstration that lysergic acid diethylamide (LSD) suppressed the firing rate of 5-HT neurons in the raphe nucleus (Aghajanian et al. 1970). A number of complex interrelationships between the 5-HT and DA systems have since been described (Korsgaard et al. 1985).

Further evidence for a 5-HT contribution in schizophrenia includes elevated platelet 5-HT (Meltzer 1987), altered postmortem $5-HT_2$ binding profiles (see Murphy 1990), and diminished CSF 5-HIAA (Ninan et al. 1984). Reduced 5-HIAA levels have further been proposed to differentiate acute versus chronic schizophrenia (Bowers 1978), positive versus negative symptoms (Yesavage 1984), subclassify patients with more severe delusional and mood presentations (Lindstrom 1985), or to characterize a better prognosis (Bowers 1978). King and colleagues (1985) also reported a correlation between platelet 5-HT, CSF 5-HIAA, and autistic mannerisms and posturing. Csernansky and colleagues (1990) found that negative symptom severity, as determined from the Brief Psychiatric Rating Scale (Overall and Gorham 1962), correlated directly with CSF 5-HIAA concentrations.

The pharmacotherapy of schizophrenia with selective 5-HT agents includes trials with both agonists and antagonists. However, experience with SSRIs has been relatively limited. The mixed SSRI/releasing agent fenfluramine was reported in a study by Stahl and colleagues (1985) to reduce negative symptoms in 3 of 12 schizophrenic patients. Several preclinical observations call attention to the possible utility of $5-HT_2$ and $5-HT_3$ receptor antagonists. Improvement of negative symptoms, independent of mood or extrapyramidal improvements, was observed during a 7-week placebo-controlled trial with fluvoxamine (Silver and Nassar 1992). Similar therapeutic benefits have been reported during open-label experiences with fluoxetine in which negative symptoms, aggressive behaviors, mood, or psychosis improved (Goff et al. 1990; Goldman and Janecek 1990).

■ Eating Disorders

Manipulation of central 5-HT results in significantly altered feeding behaviors (e.g., an increased satiety response) (Carruba et al. 1986). Blundell (1986) reported that pharmacological enhancement of 5-HT reduced meal size, rate of eating, and body weight. The predominant locus of this 5-HT effect is likely within the hypothalamus. In general, an antidepressants' ability to diminish appetite and in turn reduce weight is related to its ability to block 5-HT uptake (Angel et al. 1988). One notable exception is paroxetine, a highly potent 5-HT uptake inhibitor that versus conventional TCAs in clinical trial experience was associated with a similar proportion of subjects with weight gain (Dechant and Clissold 1991). Selective $5-HT_{1A}$ activation in some patients may explain weight gain (Dourish et al. 1986).

Bulimia

5-HT involvement in bulimia nervosa (BN) has been based on several recent observations (Jimerson et al. 1989; Kaye et al. 1988). Kaye and colleagues (1988) hypothesized that variations in the ratio of tryptophan to other amino acids consequent to recurrent bingeing and vomiting mediated both satiety and mood. Some patients with BN, independent of mood status, manifest a blunted prolactin response to m-chlorophenylpiperazine (m-CPP). This has been interpreted as evidence of postsynaptic 5-HT hypersensitivity within select hypothalamic pathways (Brewerton et al. 1990).

Goldbloom and colleagues (1988) reported the V_{max} of platelet 5-HT uptake was increased among nondepressed bulimic patients. Jimerson and colleagues (1989) observed a significant inverse association between CSF 5-HIAA and symptom severity. However, much of the support for a 5-HT role in BN comes from pharmacotherapeutic experience. Agents with at least some degree of 5-HT uptake inhibition have been found to be useful in BN (see Brewerton et al. 1990). Clinical trials with fenfluramine (Russell 1985) and fluoxetine (Freeman and Hampson 1987) have revealed a positive effect on treatment of bulimic activity. In a large placebo-controlled trial, Enas and colleagues (1989) studied dosing of 20 mg versus 60 mg of fluoxetine in 382 outpatient bulimic women. A clinical benefit was observed in binge frequency, purging, mood, and carbohydrate craving. Based on an open trial by Mitchell and co-workers (1989), therapeutic benefits of the SSRIs may also be apparent among patients previously resistant to TCAs.

Anorexia

A 5-HT disturbance in anorexia was postulated by Fanelli and colleagues (1986). Coppen and colleagues (1976) reported a reduction in plasma L-tryptophan among anorexic patients. Subsequent studies have also suggested the presence of decreased platelet imipramine binding (Weizman et al. 1986); however, these have not been uniformly replicated. Brewerton and colleagues (1990) have suggested that hypothalamic 5-HT responsivity at or beyond postsynaptic sites is abnormal in subjects with anorexia nervosa.

Pharmacologic trials with SSRIs have been relatively sparse. Lacey and Crisp (1980) reported that weight-recovered anorexia nervosa patients who received clomipramine had more stable eating habits and weight maintenance. Efficacy of the SSRI has been linked to the obsessional quality demonstrated by many eating disorder patients.

■ Alcoholism

Although under a very complex regulative system, a substantial amount of evidence supports a 5-HT dysfunction in alcoholism (reviewed in Tollefson and Montague-Clouse 1989). Preclinical studies employing chemical or surgical ablation of 5-HT pathways enhance alcohol consumption, whereas 5-HT–enhancing drugs ameliorate it. For example, Murphy and colleagues (1988) reported beneficial effects with fluoxetine and fluvoxamine in reducing alcohol intake in a select rat strain. Ballenger and colleagues (1979) have eloquently proposed a 5-HT "deficiency" based on CSF 5-H1AA studies.

A series of clinical trials with SSRIs have shown a reduction in the pattern or nature of alcohol consumption (see Tollefson and Montague-Clouse 1989). This is in contrast to the non–5-HT selective TCAs, whose efficacy has been less robust. Naranjo and colleagues (1987) tested citalopram in a double-blind placebo-controlled crossover study of 39 non-

depressed alcoholic subjects. The 40-mg dose, unlike the 20-mg arm, reduced the number of drinks consumed and increased abstinent days. Similar results with zimeldine, fluoxetine, and viqualine have been reported by this group (Naranjo and Sellers 1989). Although a precise explanation for this differential is missing, the 5-HT$_{1C}$/5-HT$_2$ and 5-HT$_3$ receptors (see Murphy 1990) have been implicated in alcohol abuse. The beneficial effect of the SSRIs appear to be independent of their antidepressant activity. Among heavy abusers of alcohol, however, a reduction in benefit may emerge (Gorelick 1989).

From a risk-benefit point of view, it is reassuring that there does not appear to be an SSRI potentiation of the effects of alcohol (Allen and Lader 1989; Lemberger et al. 1985b). Any therapeutic role for the SSRIs in the treatment of alcoholism should assume that they would be part of a multifaceted treatment program.

■ Obesity

SSRIs have been extensively investigated for an impact on food consumption. This interest stems from evidence that perturbation of 5-HT receptors modifies animal feeding behavior (Garattini et al. 1986). This modification appears independent of a local gastrointestinal effect (e.g., the perception of nausea). 5-HT innervation to the hypothalamus influences satiety and may selectively affect carbohydrate consumption (Wurtman et al. 1981). Fuller and Wong (1989) have reviewed appetite-relevant mechanisms for fluoxetine. In a trial of 45 obese individuals, Darga and colleagues (1991) reported significantly greater weight loss (–8.2 kg) among fluoxetine-diet subjects than in placebo-diet subjects through 45 weeks. Peak weight loss occurred around week 29. Unfortunately, some subjects began to regain portions of their loss after 52 weeks. Long-term benefits may be better sustained when combining fluoxetine with behavior modification (Marcus et al. 1990).

Sertraline has also been associated with an inhibitory effect on food intake (Lucki et al. 1988). Among depressed subjects, mild to moderate weight loss especially characterized individuals who were overweight before treatment.

Future weight loss studies need to address the mechanism underlying weight regain among a subset of subjects, to better identify optimal long-term candidates for pharmacotherapy, and to establish therapeutic monitors that allow the clinician to assess realistic weight loss targets.

Sleep

Fluoxetine decreases rapid eye movement (REM) and increases nonrapid eye movement (NREM) sleep at dose ranges of 5–40 mg/kg in rodent models (Gao et al. 1992). Citalopram (Hilakivil et al. 1987) and fluvoxamine (Scherschlicht et al. 1982) also shorten REM sleep in laboratory animal models. This is a common property of many antidepressant medications. Interestingly, both fluoxetine and sertraline induce higher rates of sedation as dosages are increased. In contrast, paroxetine demonstrates a dose-dependent increase in arousal, wakening, reduced slow wave sleep, and REM suppression (Kleinlogel and Burki 1987).

Suicidality

Evidence implicating 5-HT in suicide or violence is compelling. Reduced CSF 5-HIAA concentrations distinguishes the suicidally versus nonsuicidally depressed patient (Edman et al. 1986; Ninan et al. 1984). In vitro binding assays have shown an increased density or B_{max} of 5-HT$_2$ receptors in depressed and suicidal individuals (Pandey et al. 1990). Both observations are consistent with a relative state of 5-HT depletion among suicidal subjects. The American College of Neuropsychopharmacology (1992) reviewed evidence that antidepressants result in substantial improvement or remission of suicidal ideation and impulses in the vast majority of patients. SSRIs were thought to potentially "carry a lower risk for suicide than older tricyclic antidepressants" (p. 181). Further, this task force stated that there was no evidence that the SSRIs triggered emergent suicidal ideation above base rates associated with depression.

Miscellaneous

A broad variety of other medical disorders may also benefit from an SSRI trial. However, most of these potential uses are based on anecdote or open-label experience and thus require confirmation. Diminished 5-HT activity has been implicated in the personality features of impulsivity, anger, hostility, and aggression (Coccaro et al. 1989). These clinical attributes best associate with DSM-III-R (American Psychiatric Association 1987) Cluster B personality

features. Clinical trials in borderline personality disorder reported by Cornelius and colleagues (1989) and Norden (1989) are encouraging. SSRIs may have an adjunctive role in the management of these challenging conditions.

Other potential uses include treatment of late luteal phase dysphoric disorder (Wood et al. 1992), premature ejaculation (R. Crenshaw, personal communication, February 1993), behavioral complications following head trauma (Cassidy 1989), migraine headache prophylaxis (Adly et al. 1992), complications accompanying Alzheimer's disease (Nyth et al. 1989), chronic pain (Gilbert-Rahola et al. 1989), diabetic neuropathy (Theesen and Marsh 1989), and fibrositis (Geller 1989). The broad involvement of 5-HT systems in modulating behavior and cognition supports the wide potential utility of the SSRIs. Further contributions from the laboratory and clinical experience should mutually enrich our knowledge about the appropriate roles for this exciting class of drugs.

SIDE EFFECTS AND TOXICOLOGY

Side effects—or the relative absence thereof—are how the SSRIs have distinguished themselves. Although not associated with the receptor heterogeneity that mediates conventional adverse events associated with the TCAs (Richelson and Nelson 1984), SSRIs possess their own unique side-effect profile (Figure 8–4).

For most patients, the SSRIs are better tolerated (e.g., the number of early trial discontinuations attributable to an adverse event is lower than with comparator TCAs; see Boyer and Feighner 1991). As a general guideline in three-arm trials, a 5%–10% incidence of early discontinuations because of an adverse event occurred for the placebo group, 10%–20% for the SSRI group, and 30%–35% for the TCA group. Not unexpectedly, agents that selectively enhance synaptic 5-HT within the CNS may induce agitation, anxiety, sleep disturbance, tremor, sexual dysfunction (primarily anorgasmia), or headache. Clinical features at baseline do not appear to predispose a patient to any one of these CNS events (Montgomery 1989b). Although CNS events may be seen with the SSRIs, it has been suggested that overall

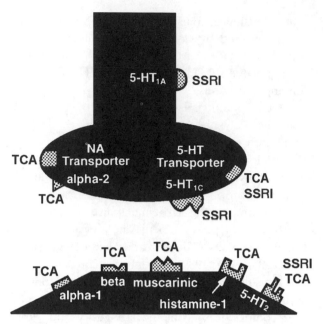

Figure 8–4. Relative specificity of TCAs versus SSRIs. Receptor heterogeneity has minimal therapeutic relevance, while increasing the risks of treatment-related adverse events.

they demonstrate a more favorable profile of behavioral toxicity than the conventional TCAs.

Certain autonomic adverse events also characterize the SSRIs. These may include dry mouth, sweating, or weight change. Because the enteric nervous system is richly innervated by 5-HT, events may also include altered gastrointestinal motility, nausea, and so on.

As was discussed previously, the SSRIs are unlikely to alter DA function. Anecdotal reports of EPS (Meltzer et al. 1979) associated with the SSRIs apparently are not any more frequent than has been reported historically with the TCAs (Fann et al. 1976; Zubenko et al. 1987), MAOIs (Teusink et al. 1984), or trazodone (Papini et al. 1982). Very rare events including arthralgia, lymphadenopathy, inappropriate antidiuretic syndrome, agranulocytosis, and hypoglycemia have been reported during clinical trials or postmarketing surveillance; however, causality typically is uncertain.

One additional rare and life-threatening idiosyncratic event associated with the SSRIs (and more prominently their interaction with MAOIs or other 5-HT enhancers) is the central serotonin syndrome (CSS). This phenomenon appears to represent an overactivation of central 5-HT receptors and may manifest with features including abdominal pain, diarrhea, sweating, fever, tachycardia, elevated blood pressure, altered mental state (e.g., delirium), myoclonus, increased motor activity, irritability, hostility, and mood change. Severe manifestations of this syndrome can induce hyperpyrexia, cardiovascular shock, or death. The rank order potency of antidepressants to inhibit the ex vivo uptake of 5-HT has been related to their potential induction of the CSS in tranylcypramine-treated rats (see Johnson 1991). Realistically, data are inadequate to rate one MAOI or SSRI as more or less likely to be associated with a CSS. The risk of the CSS seems to be increased when an SSRI is administered temporally with a second 5-HT–enhancing agent (e.g., an MAOI) (Marley and Wozniak 1984a, 1984b). The sequence with greatest risk appears to be to go from using an SSRI to an MAOI. In this scenario, drug half-life (and that of any active metabolite, where applicable) should serve as a guide. A standard recommendation would be to wait at least five times the half-life of the SSRI or its metabolite, whichever is longer.

Although some variability in adverse event frequency has been reported among the SSRIs, they all are characterized by the above-mentioned features. One notable exception is clomipramine. This tricyclic molecule is also active at muscarinic receptors and also has an adverse event profile similar to that of other TCAs. Tolerance of an adverse event may vary by dose and/or length of exposure; higher doses are typically associated with higher rates of adverse events (Bressa et al. 1989). Many events such as activation are transient, usually beginning early in the course of therapy and then remitting (Beasley et al. 1991). Comparisons between A.M. versus P.M. administration do not appear to change efficacy (Usher et al. 1991); however, the latter was associated with fewer intolerable side effects in a fluvoxamine trial (Siddiqui et al. 1985). Individual differences suggest the need for some flexibility in dosing schedules.

TCAs are known to behave like type IA antiarrhythmics and thus in a dose-dependent fashion may retard His-Purkinje conduction. SSRIs are essentially devoid of this property. In clinical trials, the incidence of increased heart rate or conduction disturbance has been extremely unusual across several of the SSRIs (Edwards et al. 1989; Fisch 1985; Guy and Silke 1990). However, very high doses of citalopram reportedly mimicked TCA-like cardiovascular effects in a feline model (Boeck et al. 1984). Klok and colleagues (1981) has also reported that 2 of 16 patients in a study of fluvoxamine experienced a rhythm disturbance. Although TCAs are relatively safer, vigilance is recommended in the predisposed patient. SSRIs are not associated with α-adrenergic antagonism and thus have been rarely associated with orthostatic hypotension. These therapeutic advantages of the SSRIs translate into a wider safety profile. Though they are not free of risk, the SSRIs appear to be better tolerated at therapeutically effective dosages for most patients when compared with the TCAs. Further refinement in SSRI dosing and schedules for administration should improve their safety record.

DRUG-DRUG INTERACTIONS

Although several significant interactions exist, the SSRIs are unlikely to be associated with many of the conventional problems seen with earlier antidepressants. These include cumulative effects with concomitant CNS depressants (e.g., alcohol), anticholinergic agents, or antihistaminic compounds. The structural differences among the SSRIs (see Figure 8–2) offer a basis for some intraclass differences. Paroxetine and fluoxetine are examples of SSRIs that are relatively free of interaction with CNS depressants such as benzodiazepines (Bannister et al. 1989; Lemberger et al. 1988). Lithium concentrations are generally unaffected; combined therapy with the SSRI fluoxetine has been associated with both synergistic (Pope et al. 1988) and negative clinical outcomes (Hadley and Cason 1989). Two notable interactions include paroxetine or fluvoxamine with warfarin (increased bleeding time), which may introduce the need to reduce the dose of a concomitant hypoglycemic agent. Secondly, cimetidine may impair first-pass SSRI metabolism and thus increase parent drug concentrations (Bannister et al. 1989).

One system that has been scrutinized and that is the basis for a series of potentially relevant clinical antidepressant drug interactions is the cytochrome P_{450} family (Brosen and Gram 1989). A genetic polymorphism exists for a number of cytochrome isoenzymes. One consequence is the significant intersubject variability in steady-state plasma levels reported with the antidepressants, including the SSRIs. Those individuals occupying the higher plasma level strata typically have been identified as "poor metabolizers." This segment represents approximately 8% of the white population. In general, their plasma half-life and steady-state SSRI concentrations would be longer and higher, respectively, and thus may represent a higher risk for toxicity and/or drug interactions. A phenotype of "fast" or extensive versus poor metabolism can be demonstrated with test drugs such as debrisoquin.

SSRIs (e.g., paroxetine) are both substrates and potent inhibitors of sparteine or debrisoquin oxidation through cytochrome P_{450}IID6. Sindrup and colleagues (1992) demonstrated that paroxetine can convert normal or extensive metabolizers to the poor metabolizer phenotype. However, this effect rapidly reverses after drug discontinuation. Based on the inhibition of sparteine oxidation by human liver microsomal cytochrome P_{450}IID6, Crewe and colleagues (1992) put the following 5-HT antidepressants in rank order, from most potent to least: paroxetine, fluoxetine, sertraline, fluvoxamine, citalopram, clomipramine, and amitriptyline.

By inhibition of IID6 and related enzymes, the SSRIs may elevate the concentration of concomitantly administered drugs. This has its greatest clinical relevance when the second agent has a narrow therapeutic index. Examples of such agents that merit vigilance include flecainide, quinidine, carbamazepine, propafenone, TCAs, and several antipsychotics (Rudorfer and Potter 1989). The clinical consequence of such an interaction may either enhance or impair efficacy and/or heighten the adverse event profile. A relevant example is drug-induced inhibition of the 2-hydroxylation of imipramine (Skjelbo and Brosen 1992), which can lead to a severalfold increase in plasma imipramine. The inhibition of *N*-demethylation of imipramine represents yet another possible mechanism. In cases where an SSRI is coadministered with such drugs, conservative introduction of the SSRI and careful plasma level monitoring are advised.

Drug Overdosage

A major advantage of the non-TCA SSRIs relative to other antidepressants has been their superior therapeutic index (Cooper 1988; Pedersen et al. 1982). The number of deaths per 1 million prescriptions across several such SSRIs (0–6) is substantially lower than that of the conventional TCAs (8–53) or MAOIs (0–61) (Leonard 1992).

Borys and colleagues (1992) reported on 234 cases of fluoxetine overdosage (232–1390 ng/ml) obtained in a prospective multicenter study. Fluoxetine was the sole ingestant in 87 cases and taken in combination with alcohol and/or other drugs in the remaining 147 cases. Common symptoms included tachycardia, sedation, tremor, nausea, and emesis. The authors concluded that the emergent symptoms were minor and of short duration, and aggressive supportive care thus "is the only intervention necessary" (p. 115).

The SSRIs currently represent an important addition to the therapeutic armamentarium for the depressed patient at risk for a drug overdosage.

■ CONCLUSION

The SSRIs have been shown to be a safe and effective drug class. They are frequently better tolerated than conventional TCAs and exhibit a superior safety profile in overdosage for patients with comorbid medical illness. Preliminary evidence suggests a broad utilitarian role for SSRIs in the treatment of psychopathology. As our experience with these compounds broadens, we can expect a continued explosion in our scientific knowledge about the 5-HT system and its interface with human pathophysiology.

■ REFERENCES

Adly C, Straumanis J, Chesson A: Fluoxetine prophylaxis of migraine. Headache 32:101–104, 1992

Aghajanian JK, Foote WE, Sheard MH: Action of psychotogenic drugs on midbrain raphe neurons. J Pharmacol Exp Ther 171:178–187, 1970

Aghajanian JK, Sprouse JS, Rasmussen K: Electrophysiology of central serotonin receptor subtypes, in The Serotonin Receptors. Edited by Sanders-Bush C. Clifton, NJ, Humana Press, 1988, pp 225–252

Allen D, Lader M: Interactions of alcohol with amitriptyline: fluoxetine and placebo in normal subjects. Int Clin Psychopharmacol 4 (suppl 1):7–14, 1989

Altamura AC, Montgomery SA, Wernicke JF: The evidence for 20 mg a day of fluoxetine as the optimal dose in the treatment of depression. Br J Psychiatry 153:109–112, 1988

American College of Neuropsychopharmacology: Suicidal behavior and psychotropic medication (consensus statement). Neuropsychopharmacology 8(2):177–183, 1992

American Psychiatric Association: Diagnostic and Statistical Manual of Mental Disorders, 3rd Edition, Revised. Washington, DC, American Psychiatric Association, 1987

Amin AH, Crawford TBB, Gaddum JH: The distribution of substance P and 5-hydroxytryptamine in the central nervous system of the dog. J Physiol 126:596–618, 1954

Amin M, Lehmann H, Mirmiran J: A double-blind, placebo-controlled, dose-finding study with sertraline. Psychopharmacol Bull 25:164–167, 1989

Angel I, Taranger MA, Claustrey Y, et al: Anorectic activities of serotonin uptake inhibitors: correlation with their potencies at inhibiting serotonin uptake in vivo and with ^{3}H-mazindol binding in vitro. Life Sci 43:651–658, 1988

Arnt J, Hyttel J, Overo FK: Prolonged treatment with the specific 5-HT uptake inhibitor citalopram: effect on dopaminergic and serotonergic functions. Pol J Pharmacol Pharm 36:221–230, 1984a

Arnt J, Overo KF, Hyttel J, et al: Changes in rat dopamine and serotonin function in vivo after prolonged administration of the specific 5-HT uptake inhibitor citalopram. Psychopharmacology (Berl) 84:457–465, 1984b

Asakura M, Tsukamoto T, Kubota H, et al: Role of serotonin in regulation of β-adrenoceptors by antidepressants. Eur J Pharmacol 141:95–100, 1987

Backus LI, Sharp T, Grahame-Smith DJ: Behavioral evidence for a functional interaction between central 5-HT$_2$ and 5-HT$_{1A}$ receptors. J Pharmacol 100:793–799, 1990

Baldessarini RJ, Marsh ER, Kula NS: Interactions of fluoxetine with metabolism of dopamine and serotonin in rat brain regions. Brain Res 579:152–156, 1992

Ballenger J, Goodwin F, Major L, et al: Alcohol and central serotonin metabolism in man. Arch Gen Psychiatry 36:224–227, 1979

Balsara JJ, Jadhav JH, Chandorkar AG: Effect of drugs influencing central serotonergic mechanisms on haloperidol-induced catalepsy. Psychopharmacology (Berl) 62:67–69, 1979

Bannister SJ, Houser VP, Hulse JD, et al: Evaluation of the potential for interactions of paroxetine with diazepam, cimetidine, warfarin and digoxin. Acta Psychiatr Scand 80:102–106, 1989

Baron BM, Ogden AM, Siegel BW, et al: Rapid downregulation of β-adrenoceptors by co-administration of desipramine and fluoxetine. Eur J Pharmacol 154:125–134, 1988

Baxter LR, Schwartz JM, Bergman KS, et al: Caudate glucose metabolic rate changes with both drug and behavior therapy for obsessive-compulsive disorder. Arch Gen Psychiatry 49:681–689, 1992

Beasley CM, Sayler ME, Bosomworth JC, et al: High-dose fluoxetine: efficacy and activating-sedating effects in agitated and retarded depression. J Clin Psychopharmacol 11:166–174, 1991

Benfield DP, Harries CM, Luscombe DK: Some pharmacological aspects of desmethylclomipramine. Postgrad Med J 56 (suppl 1):13–18, 1980

Benkelfat C, Murphy DL, Zohar J, et al: Clomipramine in obsessive-compulsive disorder: further evidence for a serotonergic mechanism of action. Arch Gen Psychiatry 46:23–28, 1989

Benloucif S, Galloway MP: Facilitation of dopamine release in vivo by serotonin agonists: studied with microdialysis. Eur J Pharmacol 200:1–8, 1991

Bergstrom DA, Kellar JK: Adrenergic and serotonergic receptor binding in rat brain after chronic desmethylimipramine treatment. J Pharmacol Exp Ther 209:256–261, 1979

Bick PA, Hackett E: Sertraline is effective in obsessive-compulsive disorder, in Psychiatry Today: VIII World Congress of Psychiatry Abstracts. Edited by Stefanis CN, Soldatos CR, Rabavilas AD. New York, Elsevier, 1989, p 152

Blier P, deMontigny C, Chaput Y: Modifications of the serotonin system by antidepressant treatments: implications for the therapeutic response in major depression. J Clin Psychopharmacol 7:24S–35S, 1987

Blier P, Chaput Y, deMontigny C: Long-term 5-HT reuptake blockade but not monoamine oxidase inhibition, decreases the function of terminal 5-HT autoreceptors: an electrophysiological study in the rat brain. Naunyn Schmiedebergs Arch Pharmacol 337:246–254, 1988

Blier P, deMontigny C, Chaput Y: A role for the serotonin system in the mechanism of action of antidepressants. J Clin Psychiatry 51 (suppl 4):14–20, 1990

Blundell JE: Serotonin manipulations and the structure of feeding behaviour. Appetite 7 (suppl):39–56, 1986

Boeck V, Jorgensen A, Overo KF: Comparative animal studies on cardiovascular toxicity of tri- and

tetracyclic antidepressants and citalopram; relation to drug plasma levels. Psychopharmacology (Berl) 82:275–281, 1984

Borys DJ, Setzer SC, Ling LJ, et al: Acute fluoxetine overdose: A report of 234 cases. Am J Emerg Med 10:115–120, 1992

Bouchard RH, Pourcher E, Vincent P: Fluoxetine and extrapyramidal side effects. Am J Psychiatry 146:1352–1353, 1989

Bowers MB Jr: Serotonin systems in psychotic states, in Biochemistry of Mental Disorders. Edited by Usdin E, Mandell A. New York, Marcel Dekker, 1978, pp 191–204

Boyer WF, Feighner JP: The efficacy of selective serotonin uptake inhibitors in depression, in Selective Serotonin Uptake Inhibitors. Edited by Feighner JP, Boyer WF. Chichester, England, Wiley, 1991, pp 89–108

Bradley PB: Introduction to Neuropharmacology. Boston, MA, Butterworth & Company, 1989, p 351

Bressa GM, Brugnoli R, Pancheri P: A double-blind study of fluoxetine and imipramine in major depression. Int Clin Psychopharmacol 4 (suppl 1):69–73, 1989

Brewerton TD, Brandt HA, Lessem MD, et al: Serotonin in eating disorders, in Serotonin in Major Psychiatric Disorders. Edited by Coccaro EF, Murphy DL. Washington, DC, American Psychiatric Press, 1990, pp 153–184

Brosen K, Gram LF: Clinical significance of the sparteine/debrisoquine oxidation polymorphism. Eur J Clin Pharmacol 36:537–547, 1989

Carruba MO, Mantegazza P, Memo M, et al: Peripheral and central mechanisms of action of serotonergic anorectic drugs. Appetite 7 (suppl): 105–113, 1986

Cassidy JW: Fluoxetine: a new serotonergically active antidepressant [Special issue: visual system dysfunction]. Journal of Head Trauma Rehabilitation 4:67–69, 1989

Chaput Y, deMontigny C, Blier P: Effects of a selective 5-HT reuptake blocker citalopram on the sensitivity of 5-HT autoreceptors, electrophysiological studies in the rat. Naunyn Schmiedebergs Arch Pharmacol 333:342–348, 1986

Charbannes JP, Douge R: Efficacy on anxiety of fluvoxamine versus prazepam, diazepam with anxiodepressed patients, in Psychiatry Today: VIII World Congress of Psychiatry Abstracts. Edited by Stefanis CN, Soldatos CR, Rabavilas AD. New York,

Elsevier, 1989, p 282

Charney DS, Menkes DB, Heninger GR: Receptor sensitivity and the mechanism of action of antidepressant treatment. Arch Gen Psychiatry 38:1160–1180, 1981

Charney DS, Heninger GR, Sternberg DE: Serotonin function and mechanism of action of antidepressant treatment. Arch Gen Psychiatry 41:359–365, 1984

Ciraulo DA, Shader RI: Fluoxetine drug-drug interactions: I. antidepressants and antipsychotics. J Clin Psychopharmacol 10:48–50, 1990

Claassen V: Review of the animal pharmacology and pharmacokinetics of fluvoxamine. Br J Clin Pharmacol 15:349S–355S, 1983

Coccaro EF, Siever LJ, Klar HM, et al: Serotonergic studies in patients with affective and personality disorders: correlated with suicidal and impulsive aggressive behavior. Arch Gen Psychiatry 46:587–599, 1989

Cooper GL: The safety of fluoxetine—an update. Br J Psychiatry 153:77–86, 1988

Coppen AJ, Gupta RK, Eccleston EG, et al: Plasma tryptophan in anorexia nervosa. Lancet 1:961, 1976

Cornelius JR, Soloff PH, Perel JM, et al: Fluoxetine trial in borderline personality. New Research Program and Abstracts, 142nd Annual Meeting of the American Psychiatric Association, May 1989, p 192

Cowen PJ: Serotonin receptor subtypes: implications for psychopharmacology. Br J Psychiatry 159 (suppl 12):7–14, 1991

Crewe HK, Lennard MS, Tucker GT, et al: The effect of selective serotonin reuptake inhibitors on the cytochrome P_{450}IID6 activity in human liver microsomes. Br J Clin Pharmacol 34:262–265, 1992

Csernansky JG, King RJ, Faustman WO, et al: 5-HIAA in cerebrospinal fluid and deficit schizophrenic characteristics. Br J Psychiatry 156:501–507, 1990

Danion JM: The effectiveness of fluoxetine in acute studies and long-term treatment, in Psychiatry Today: VIII World Congress of Psychiatry Abstracts. Edited by Stefanis CN, Soldatos CR, Rabavilas AD. New York, Elsevier, 1989, p 334

Darga LL, Carroll-Michals L, Botsford SJ, et al: Fluoxetine's effect on weight loss in obese subjects. Am J Clin Nutr 54:321–325, 1991

Dechant KL, Clissold SP: Paroxetine. Drugs 41:225–253, 1991

Delgado PL, Price LH, Charney DS, et al: Efficacy of fluvoxamine in treatment-refractory depression. J Affect Disord 15:55–60, 1988

deMontigny C, Chaput Y, Blier P: Long term tricyclic and electroconvulsive treatment increases responsiveness of dorsal hippocampus 5-HT$_{1A}$ receptors: an electrophysiological study. Society of Neuroscience Abstracts 15:854, 1989

den-Boer JA, Westenberg HG, Kamerbeek WD, et al: Effect of serotonin uptake inhibitors in anxiety disorders; a double-blind comparison of clomipramine and fluvoxamine. Int Clin Psychopharmacol 2:21–32, 1987

De-Wilde JE, Doogan DP: Fluvoxamine and chloripramine in endogenous depression. J Affect Disord 4:249–259, 1982

Doogan DP, Caillard V: Sertraline: a new antidepressant. J Clin Psychiatry 49 (suppl):46–51, 1988

Dourish CT, Hutson PH, Kennett GA, et al: 8-OH-DPAT-induced hyperphagia: its neural basis and possible therapeutic relevance. Appetite 7 (suppl):127–140, 1986

Dresse A, Scuvee-Moreau J: The effects of various antidepressants on the spontaneous firing rates of noradrenergic and serotonergic neurones. Clin Neuropharmacol 7 (suppl 1):572–573, 1984

Dufour H: Fluoxetine: long-term treatment and prophylaxis in depression. Paper presented at the International Fluoxetine Symposium, Tyrol, Austria, October 13–17, 1987

Dunbar GC: The efficacy profile of paroxetine, a new antidepressant, compared with imipramine and placebo. 17th Collegium Internationale Neuro-Psychopharmacologicum Congress Abstracts 1:17, 1990

Edman G, Asberg M, Levander S, et al: Skin conductance habituation and cerebrospinal fluid 5-hydroxyindoleacetic acid in suicidal patients. Arch Gen Psychiatry 43:586–592, 1986

Edwards JG, Goldie A, Papayanni-Papasthatis S: Effect of paroxetine on the electrocardiogram. Psychopharmacology (Berl) 97:96–98, 1989

Elks ML, Youngblood WW, Kizer JS: Serotonin synthesis and release in brain slices, independence of tryptophan. Brain Res 172:471–486, 1979

Enas GG, Pope HJ, Vevine LR: Fluoxetine and bulimia nervosa: double-blind study. New Research Program and Abstracts, 142nd Annual Meeting of the American Psychiatric Association, 1989, p 204

Evans L, Kenardy J, Schneider P, et al: Effect of a selective serotonin uptake inhibitor in agoraphobia with panic attacks. Acta Psychiatr Scand 73:49–53, 1986

Falck B, Hillarp NA, Thieme G, et al: Fluorescence of catecholamines and related compounds condensed with formaldehyde. J Histochem Cytochem 10:348–354, 1962

Fanelli FR, Cangiano C, Cecil F, et al: Plasma tryptophan and anorexia in human cancer. European Journal of Cancer and Clinical Oncology 22:89–95, 1986

Fann WE, Sullivan JL, Richman BW: Dyskinesia's associated with tricyclic antidepressants. Br J Psychiatry 128:490–493, 1976

Fava M, Rosenbaum JF, Cohen L, et al: High dose fluoxetine in the treatment of depressed patients not responsive to a standard dose of fluoxetine. J Affect Disord 25:229–234, 1992

Feighner JP, Boyer WF, Meredith CH, et al: A placebo-controlled inpatient comparison of fluvoxamine maleate and imipramine in major depression. Int Clin Psychopharmacol 4:239–244, 1989

Feldmann HS, Dunbar HC: Long-term study of fluvoxamine: a new rapid-acting antidepressant. International Pharmacopsychiatry 17:114–122, 1982

Ferrey G, Gailledrau J, Beuzen JN: The interest of fluoxetine in prevention of depressive recurrences, in Psychiatry Today: VIII World Congress of Psychiatry Abstracts. Edited by Stefanis CN, Soldatos CR, Rabavilas AD. New York, Elsevier, 1989, p 99

Fisch C: Effect of fluoxetine on the electrocardiogram. J Clin Psychiatry 46:42–44, 1985

Flament MF, Rapoport JL, Berg CJ, et al: Clomipramine treatment of childhood obsessive-compulsive disorder: a double blind, controlled study. Arch Gen Psychiatry 42:977–983, 1985

Fraser A, Offord SJ, Lucki I: Regulation of serotonin receptors and responsiveness in the brain, in The Serotonin Receptors. Edited by Sanders-Bush C. Clifton, NJ, Humana Press, 1988, pp 319–362

Freeman CPL, Hampson M: Fluoxetine as a treatment for bulimia nervosa. Int J Obes 11:171–177, 1987

Fuller RW: Drugs altering serotonin synthesis and metabolism, in Neuropharmacology of Serotonin. Edited by Green AR. New York, Oxford University Press, 1985, pp 1–20

Fuller RW, Wong DT: Fluoxetine: a serotonergic appetite suppressant drug. Drug Development Research 17:1–15, 1989

Gao B, Duncan WC Jr, Wehr ATA: Fluoxetine decreases brain temperature and REM sleep in Syrian hamsters. Psychopharmacology (Berl) 106(3):321–329, 1992

Garattini S, Mennini T, Bendotti C, et al: Neurochemical mechanism of action of drugs which modify feeding via the serotonergic system. Appetite 7 (suppl):15–38, 1986

Geller SA: Treatment of fibrositis with fluoxetine hydrochloride (Prozac). Am J Med 87:594–595, 1989

Gilbert-Rahola J, Elorza J, Casas J: Analgesic effects of the antidepressants fluvoxamine and clovoxamine, in Psychiatry Today: VIII World Congress of Psychiatry Abstracts. Edited by Stefanis CN, Soldatos CR, Rabavilas AD. New York, Elsevier, 1989, p 269

Goff DC, Brotman AW, Waites M, et al: Trial of fluoxetine added to neuroleptics for treatment-resistant schizophrenic patients. Am J Psychiatry 147:492–494, 1990

Goldbloom DS, Hicks LK, Garfinkel PE: Platelet serotonin uptake in bulimia nervosa, in New Research: Program and Abstracts of the 141st Annual Meeting of the American Psychiatric Association, Washington, DC, May 1988, p 137

Goldman MB, Janecek HM: Adjunctive fluoxetine improves global function in chronic schizophrenia. J Neuropsychiatry Clin Neurosci 2:429–431, 1990

Goodman WK, Price LH, Rasmussen SA, et al: Efficacy of fluvoxamine in obsessive-compulsive disorder: a double-blind comparison with placebo. Arch Gen Psychiatry 46:36–44, 1989

Goodman WK, McDougle CJ, Price LH: Pharmacotherapy of obsessive compulsive disorder. J Clin Psychiatry 53 (suppl 4):29–37, 1992

Gorelick DA: Serotonin uptake blockers and the treatment of alcoholism. Recent Dev Alcohol 7:267–281, 1989

Gorman JM, Liebowitz MR, Fyer AJ, et al: An open trial of fluoxetine in the treatment of panic attacks. J Clin Psychopharmacol 7:329–332, 1987

Guelfi JD, Dreyfus JF, Pichot P: Fluvoxamine and imipramine: results of a long-term controlled trial. Int Clin Psychopharmacol 2:103–109, 1987

Guy S, Silke B: The electrocardiogram as a tool for therapeutic monitoring: a critical analysis. J Clin Psych 51 [12, suppl B]:37–39, 1990

Guy W, Manov G, Wilson WH: Double blind dose determination study of new antidepressant—sertraline. Drug Development Research 9:267–272,

1986

Haddock RE, Johnson AM, Langley PE, et al: Metabolic pathway of paroxetine in animals and man and the comparative pharmacological properties of its metabolites. Acta Psychiatr Scand 80 (suppl 350):24–26, 1989

Hadley A, Cason MP: Mania resulting from lithium-fluoxetine combination [letter]. Am J Psychiatry 146:1637–1638, 1989

Hall H, Ogren SO: Effects of antidepressant drugs on different receptors in rat brain. Eur J Pharmacol 70:393–407, 1981

Hamilton M: Development of a rating scale for primary depressive illness. British Journal of Social and Clinical Psychology 6:278–296, 1967

Hebenstreit GF, Fellerer K, Zoechling R, et al: A pharmacokinetic dose titration study in adult and elderly depressed patients. Acta Psychiatr Scand 80:81–84, 1989

Heym J, Koe BK: Pharmacology of sertraline: a review. J Clin Psychiatry 49 (suppl):40–45, 1988

Hilakivil I, Kovala T, Leppavuori, et al: Effects of serotonin and noradrenaline uptake blockers on wakefulness and sleep in cats. Pharmacol Toxicol 60:161–166, 1987

Humble M, Koczkas C, Wistedt B: Serotonin and anxiety: an open study of citalopram in panic disorder, in Psychiatry Today: VIII World Congress of Psychiatry Abstracts. Edited by Stefanis CN, Soldatos CR, Rabavilas AD. New York, Elsevier, 1989, p 151

Hyttel J: Citalopram—pharmacological profile of a specific serotonin uptake inhibitor with antidepressant activity. Prog Neuropsychopharmacol Biol Psychiatry 6:277–295, 1982

Insel TR: Toward a neuroanatomy of obsessive-compulsive disorder. Arch Gen Psychiatry 49:739–744, 1992

Insel TR, Murphy DL, Cohen RM, et al: Obsessive-compulsive disorder: a double blind trial of clomipramine and clorgiline. Arch Gen Psychiatry 40:605–612, 1983

Jenike MA, Baer L, Greist JH: Clomipramine versus fluoxetine in obsessive-compulsive disorder: a retrospective comparison of side effects and efficacy. J Clin Psychopharmacol 10:122–124, 1989a

Jenike MA, Buttolph L, Baer L, et al: Open trial of fluoxetine in obsessive-compulsive disorder. Am J Psychiatry 146:909–911, 1989b

Jimerson DC, Lesem MD, Kaye WH, et al: Serotonin and symptom severity in eating disorders. Biol Psychiatry 25 (suppl 7A):143A, 1989

Johnson AM: The comparative pharmacological properties of selective serotonin re-uptake inhibitors in animals, in Selective Serotonin Uptake Inhibitors. Edited by Feighner JP, Boyer WF. Chichester, England, Wiley, 1991, pp 37–70

Jouvent R, Baruch P, Ammar S, et al: Fluoxetine efficacy in depressives with impulsivity vs blunted affect, in Psychiatry Today: VIII World Congress of Psychiatry Abstracts. Edited by Stefanis CN, Soldatos CR, Rabavilas AD. New York, Elsevier, 1989, p 398

Kahn RS, vanPraag HM, Wetzler S, et al: Serotonin and anxiety revisited. Biol Psychiatry 23:189–208, 1988

Kasper S, Fuger J, Moller HJ: Comparative efficacy of antidepressants. Drugs 43 (suppl 2):11–23, 1992

Kaye WH, Gwirtsman HE, Brewerton TD, et al: Bingeing behavior and plasma amino acids: a possible involvement of brain serotonin in bulimia nervosa. Psychiatry Res 23:31–43, 1988

Kelly MW, Perry J, Holstad SG, et al: Serum fluoxetine and norfluoxetine concentrations and antidepressant response. Ther Drug Monit 11:165–170, 1989

King R, Faull KF, Stahl SM, et al: Serotonin and schizophrenia: correlations between serotonergic activity and schizophrenic motor behavior. Psychiatry Res 14:235–240, 1985

Kleinlogel H, Burki HR: Effects of the selective 5-hydroxytryptamine uptake inhibitors, paroxetine and zimeldine, on EEG sleep and waking changes in the rat. Neuropsychobiology 17:206–212, 1987

Klimek V, Maj J: Repeated administration of antidepressant drugs enhanced agonist affinity for mesolimbic D-2 receptors. J Pharm Pharmacol 41:555–558, 1990

Klimek V, Nielsen M: Chronic treatment with antidepressants decreases the number of [^{3}H]-SCH 23390 binding sites in rat striatum and limbic system. Eur J Pharmacol 139:163–169, 1987

Klok CJ, Brouwer GJ, vanPraag HM, et al: Fluvoxamine and clomipramine in depressed patients: a double-blind clinical study. Acta Psychiatr Scand 80:145–146, 1981

Koe BK, Koch SW, Lebel LA, et al: Sertraline, a selective inhibitor of serotonin uptake, induces subsensitivity of β-adrenoceptor of rat brain. Eur J Pharmacol 141:187–194, 1987

Korsgaard S, Gerlach J, Christensson E: Behavioral aspects of serotonin-dopamine interaction in the monkey. Eur J Pharmacol 118:245–252, 1985

Lacey JH, Crisp AH: Hunger, food intake and weight: the impact of clomipramine on a refeeding anorexia nervosa population. Postgrad Med J 56 (suppl 1):79–85, 1980

Laws D, Ashford JJ, Anstee JA: A multicentre double-blind comparative trial of fluvoxamine versus lorazepam in mixed anxiety and depression treated in general practice. Acta Psychiatr Scand 81:185–189, 1990

Lemberger L, Bergstrom RF, Wolen RL, et al: Fluoxetine: clinical pharmacology and physiological disposition. J Clin Psychiatry 46:14–19, 1985a

Lemberger L, Rowe H, Bergstrom RF, et al: Effect of fluoxetine on psychomotor performance, physiologic response and kinetics of ethanol. Clin Pharmacol Ther 37:658–664, 1985b

Lemberger L, Rowe H, Bosomworth JC, et al: The effect of fluoxetine on the pharmacokinetics and psychomotor responses of diazepam. Clin Pharmacol Ther 43:412–419, 1988

Leonard BE: Pharmacological differences of serotonin reuptake inhibitors and possible clinical relevance. Drugs 43 (suppl 2):3–10, 1992

Lesch KP, Hoh A, Schulte HM, et al: Obsessive-compulsive disorder. Psychopharmacology (Berl) 105(3):415–420, 1991

Lindstrom LA: Low HVA and normal 5-H1AA CSF levels on drug-free schizophrenic patients compared to healthy volunteers: correlations to symptomatology and family history. Psychiatry Res 14:265–273, 1985

Lloyd KG, Thuret F, Pilc A: Upregulation of γ-aminobutyric acid (GABA)B binding sites in rat frontal cortex: a common action of repeated administration of different classes of antidepressant and electroshock. J Pharmacol Exp Ther 235:191–199, 1985

Lorens SA, Van der Kar LD. Differential effects of serotonin (5-HT$_{1A}$ and 5-HT$_2$) agonists and antagonists on renin and corticosterone secretion. Neuroendocrinology 45:305–310, 1987

Lucki I, Kreider MS, Simansky KJ: Reduction of feeding behaviour by the serotonin uptake inhibitor sertraline. Psychopharmacology (Berl) 96:289–295, 1988

Maj J, Rogoz Z, Skuza G, et al: Repeated treatment with antidepressant drugs potentiates the locomotor response to (+)-amphetamine. J Pharm Pharmacol 36:127–130, 1984

Marcus MD, Wing RR, Ewing L, et al: Double-blind, placebo-controlled trial of fluoxetine plus behavior modification in the treatment of obese binge eaters and non-binge eaters. Am J Psychiatry 147:876–881, 1990

Marley E, Wozniak KM: Interactions of a non-selective monoamine oxidase inhibitor, phenelzine, with inhibitors of 5-hydroxytryptamine, dopamine or noradrenaline re-uptake. J Psychiatr Res 18:173–189, 1984a

Marley E, Wozniak KM: Interactions of non-selective monoamine oxidase inhibitors, tranylcypromine and nialamide, with inhibitors of 5-hydroxytryptamine, dopamine or noradrenaline re-uptake. J Psychiatr Res 18:191–203, 1984b

Marsden CA: The neuropharmacology of serotonin in the central nervous system, in Selective Serotonin Re-Uptake Inhibitors. Edited by Feighner JP, Boyer WF. Chichester, England, Wiley, 1991, pp 11–35

Marshall EF, Nelson DR, Johnson AM, et al: Desensitisation of central 5-HT$_2$ receptor mechanisms after repeated administration of the antidepressant paroxetine. Journal of Psychopharmacology 2:194, 1988

Meltzer HY: Biological studies in schizophrenia. Schizophr Bull 13:77–111, 1987

Meltzer HY, Young M, Metz J, et al: Extrapyramidal side effects and increased serum prolactin following fluoxetine, a new antidepressant. J Neural Transm 45:165–175, 1979

Mitchell JE, Pyle RL, Eckert ED, et al: Response to alternative antidepressants in imipramine non-responders with bulimia nervosa. J Clin Psychopharmacol 9:291–293, 1989

Montgomery SA: Fluoxetine in the treatment of anxiety, agitation and suicidal thoughts, in Psychiatry Today: VIII World Congress of Psychiatry Abstracts. Edited by Stefanis CN, Soldatos CR, Rabavilas AD. New York, Elsevier, 1989a, p 335

Montgomery SA: New antidepressants and 5-HT uptake inhibitors. Acta Psychiatr Scand 80 (suppl 350):107–116, 1989b

Montgomery SA, Dufour H, Brion S, et al: The prophylactic efficacy of fluoxetine in unipolar depression. Br J Psychiatry 153:69–76, 1988

Murphy DL: Neuropsychiatric disorders and 5-HT receptors. Neuropsychopharmacology 3:457–471, 1990

Murphy JM, Waller MB, Gatto GJ, et al: Effects of fluoxetine on the intragastric self-administration of ethanol in the alcohol preferring P line of rats. Alcohol 5:283–286, 1988

Naranjo CA, Sellers EM: Serotonin uptake inhibitors attenuate ethanol intake in problem drinkers. Recent Dev Alcohol 7:255–266, 1989

Naranjo CA, Sellers EM, Sullivan JT, et al: The serotonin uptake inhibitor citalopram attenuates ethanol intake. Clin Pharmacol Ther 41:266–274, 1987

Nelson DR, Thomas DR, Johnson AM: Pharmacological effects of paroxetine after repeated administration to animals. Acta Psychiatr Scand 80 (suppl 350):21–23, 1989

Ninan PT, van-Kammen DP, Scheinin M, et al: CSF 5-hydroxyindoleacetic acid levels in suicidal schizophrenic patients. Am J Psychiatry 141:566–569, 1984

Norden MJ: Fluoxetine in borderline personality disorder. Prog Neuropsychopharmacol Biol Psychiatry 13:885–893, 1989

Nowak G: Long term effect of antidepressant drugs and electroconvulsive shock (ECS) on cortical α_1-adrenoceptors following destruction of dopaminergic nerve terminals. Pharmacol Toxicol 64:469–470, 1989

Nyth AL, Gottfries CG, Elgen K, et al: The clinical efficacy of citalopram in treatment of emotional disturbances in dementia disorders, in Psychiatry Today: VIII World Congress of Psychiatry Abstracts. Edited by Stefanis CN, Soldatos CR, Rabavilas AD. New York, Elsevier, 1989, p 503

O'Flynn K, O'Keane V, Lucey JV, et al: Effect of fluoxetine on noradrenergic mediated growth hormone release: a double blind, placebo-controlled study. Biol Psychiatry 30:377–382, 1991

Overall JE, Gorham DR: The Brief Psychiatric Rating Scale. Psychol Rep 10:799–812, 1962

Pandey GN, Pandey SC, Janicak PG, et al: Platelet serotonin-2 receptor binding sites in depression and suicide. Biol Psychiatry 28:215–222, 1990

Papini M, Martinetti MJ, Pasquinelli A: Trazadone symptomatic extrapyramidal disorders of infancy and childhood. Ital J Neurol Sci 3:161–162, 1982

Pato MT, Zohar-Kadouch RC, Zohar J, et al: Return of symptoms after discontinuation of clomipramine in patients with obsessive-compulsive disorder. Am J Psychiatry 145:1525, 1988

Pedersen OL, Kragh-Srensen P, Bjerre M, et al: Citalopram, a selective serotonin reuptake inhibitor: clinical antidepressive and long-term effect—a phase II study. Psychopharmacology (Berl) 77:199–204, 1982

Perez J, Tinelli D, Bianchi E, et al: cAMP binding proteins in the rat cerebral cortex after administration of selective 5-HT and NE reuptake blockers with antidepressant activity. Neuropsychopharmacology 4:57–64, 1991

Peroutka SJ, Snyder SH: Long-term antidepressant treatment decreases spiroperidol-labelled serotonin receptor binding. Science 210:88–90, 1980

Peselow ED, Filippi AM, Goodnick P, et al: The short- and long-term efficacy of paroxetine HCl, B: data from a double-blind crossover study and from a year-long term trial vs. imipramine and placebo. Psychopharmacol Bull 25(2):272–276, 1989

Plaznik A, Kostowski W: The effects of antidepressants and electroconvulsive shocks on the functioning of the mesolimbic dopaminergic system: a behavioural study. Eur J Pharmacol 135:389–396, 1987

Pope HG Jr, McElroy SL, Nixon RA: Possible synergism between fluoxetine and lithium in refractory depression. Am J Psychiatry 145:1292–1294, 1988

Pratt GD, Bowery NG: Autoradiographical analysis of GABAB sites in rat frontal cortex following chronic antidepressant treatment. Presented at the 1st International GABAB Symposium, Cambridge, England, September 1989

Renynghe de Voxurie GE: Anafranil (g34586) in obsessive neurosis. Acta Neurol Belg 68:787–792, 1968

Richelson E, Nelson A: Antagonism by antidepressants of neurotransmitter receptors of normal human brain in vitro. J Pharmacol Exp Ther 230:94–102, 1984

Ross SB, Renyi AL: Inhibition of the neuronal uptake of 5-hydroxytryptamine and noradrenaline in rat brain by (Z) and (E)-3-(4-bromophenyl)-N-,N-dimethyl-3(3-pyridil)allylamines and their secondary analogues. Neuropharmacology 16:57–63, 1977

Rudorfer MV, Potter WZ: Combined fluoxetine and tricyclic antidepressants. Am J Psychiatry 146:562–564, 1989

Russell GFM: Bulimia revisited. International Journal of Eating Disorders 4:681–692, 1985

Sampson D, Willner P, Muscat R: Reversal of antidepressant action by dopamine antagonists in an animal model of depression. Psychopharmacology (Berl) 104:491–495, 1991

Scherschlicht R, Polc P, Schneeberger J, et al: Selective suppression of rapid eye movement sleep in cats by typical and atypical antidepressants. Adv Biochem Psychopharmacol 31:359–364, 1982

Schmidt A, Lebel L, Koe BK, et al: Sertraline patently displaces (+)-[^{3}H]-3-PPP binding to a sites in rat brain. Eur J Pharmacol 165:335–336, 1989

Schneier FR, Liebowitz MR, Davies SO, et al: Fluoxetine in panic disorder. J Clin Psychopharmacol 10:119–121, 1990

Schweizer E, Rickels K, Amsterdam JD, et al: What constitutes an adequate antidepressant trial for fluoxetine? J Clin Psychiatry 51:8–11, 1990

Shaskan EG, Snyder SH: Kinetics of serotonin accumulation into slices from rat brain: relationship to catecholamine uptake. J Pharmacol Exp Ther 163:425, 1970

Shaw DM, Crimmins R: A multicentre trial of citalopram and amitriptyline in major depressive illness, in Citalopram: the New Antidepressant from Lundbeck Research. Edited by Montgomery SA. Amsterdam, Excerpta Medica, 1989, pp 43–49

Shrivastava RK, Shrivastava SHP, Overweg N, et al: Depression. J Clin Psychiatry 53 (suppl 2):48–51, 1992

Siddiqui UA, Chakravarti SK, Jesinger DK: The tolerance and antidepressive activity of fluvoxamine as a single dose compared to a twice-daily dose. Curr Med Res Opin 9:681–690, 1985

Silver H, Nassar A: Fluvoxamine improves negative symptoms in treated chronic schizophrenia: an add-on double-blind, placebo-controlled study. Biol Psychiatry 31:698–704, 1992

Sindrup SH, Brosen K, Gram LF, et al: The relationship between paroxetine and sparteine oxidation polymorphism. J Clin Pharmacol Ther 51:278–287, 1992

Skjelbo E, Brosen K: Inhibitors of imipramine metabolism by human liver microsomes. Br J Clin Pharmacol 34:256–261, 1992

Sleight AJ, Marsden CA, Martin KF, et al: Relationship between extracellular 5-hydroxytryptamine and behaviour following monoamine oxidase inhibition and L-tryptophan. Br J Pharmacol 93:303–310, 1988

Snyder SH, Yamamura HI: Antidepressants and the muscarinic acetylcholine receptor. Arch Gen Psychiatry 34:236–239, 1977

Stahl SM, Uhr SB, Berger PA: Pilot study on the effects of fenfluramine on negative symptoms in twelve inpatients. Biol Psychiatry 20:1098–1102, 1985

Stauderman KA, Gandhi DC, Jones DJ: Fluoxetine-induced inhibition of synaptosomal [^{3}H] 5-HT release: possible calcium-channel inhibition. Life Sci 50:2125–2138, 1992

Stockmeier CA, McLeskey SW, Blendy JA, et al: Electroconvulsive shock but not antidepressant drugs increase α_1-adrenoceptor binding sites in rat brain. Eur J Pharmacol 139:259–266, 1987

Tasker TCG, Kaye CM, Zussman BD, et al: Paroxetine plasma levels: lack of correlation with efficacy or adverse events. Acta Psychiatr Scand 80:152–155, 1989

Teusink JP, Alexopoulos GS, Shamoian CA: Parkinsonian side effects induced by a monoamine oxidase inhibitor. Am J Psychiatry 141:118–119, 1984

Theesen KA, Marsh WR: Relief of diabetic neuropathy with fluoxetine. DICP 23:572–574, 1989

Thomas DR, Nelson DR, Johnson AM: Biochemical effects of the antidepressant paroxetine, a specific 5-hydroxytryptamine uptake inhibitor. Psychopharmacology (Berl) 93:193–200, 1987

Thoren P, Asberg M, Bertilsson L, et al: Clomipramine treatment of obsessive-compulsive disorder, II: biochemical aspects. Arch Gen Psychiatry 37:1289–1294, 1980

Tollefson GD, Montague-Clouse J: The interrelationship of anxiety and alcoholism: a serotonin hypothesis. Family Practice Recertification 11:79–88, 1989

Tyrer P, Marsden CA, Casey P, et al: Clinical efficacy of paroxetine in resistant depression. Journal of Psychopharmacology 1:251–257, 1987

U'Prichard DC, Greenberg DA, Sheehan PB, et al: Tricyclic antidepressants: therapeutic properties and affinity for α-noradrenergic receptor binding sites in the brain. Science 199:197–198, 1978

Usher RW, Beasley CM, Bosomworth JC: Efficacy and safety of morning versus evening fluoxetine administration. J Clin Psychiatry 52:134–136, 1991

Valentino RJ, Curtis AL: Pharmacology of locus coeruleus spontaneous and sensory evoked activity. Prog Brain Res 88:249–256, 1991

vanPraag HM, Kahn R, Asnis GM, et al: Therapeutic indications for serotonin-potentiating compounds: a hypothesis. Biol Psychiatry 22:205–212, 1987

Weilburg JB, Rosenbaum JF, Biederman J, et al: Fluoxetine added to non-MAOI antidepressants converts non-responders to responders: a preliminary report. J Clin Psychiatry 50:447–449, 1989

Weizman R, Carmi M, Tyano S, et al: High affinity [^{3}H]

imipramine binding and serotonin uptake to platelets of adolescent females suffering from anorexia nervosa. Life Sci 38:1235–1242, 1986

Wernicke JF, Bremner JD, Bosomworth J, et al: The efficacy and safety of fluoxetine in the long-term treatment of depression. Paper presented at the International Fluoxetine Symposium, Tyrol, Austria, October 13–17, 1987

Westenberg HGM, den Boer JA, Kahn RS: Psychopharmacology of anxiety disorders: on the role of serotonin in the treatment of anxiety states and phobic disorders. Psychopharmacol Bull 23:145–149, 1987

Wong DT, Bymaster FP, Horng JS, et al: A new selective inhibitor for uptake of serotonin into synaptosomes of rat brain: 3-(p-trifluoromethylphenoxy)-N-methyl-3-phenylpropylamine. J Pharmacol Exp Ther 193:804–811, 1975

Wong DT, Reid LR, Bymaster FP, et al: Chronic effects of fluoxetine, a selective inhibitor of serotonin uptake, on neurotransmitter receptors. J Neural Transm 64:251–269, 1985

Wong DT, Threlkeld PG, Robertson DW: Affinities of fluoxetine, its enantiomers, and other inhibitors of serotonin uptake for subtypes of serotonin receptors. Neuropsychopharmacology 5(1):43–47, 1991

Wood SH, Mortola JF, Chan Y, et al: Treatment of premenstrual syndrome with fluoxetine: a double-blind placebo-controlled crossover study. Obstet Gynecol 80:339–344, 1992

Woolley DW, Campbell NK: Exploration of the central nervous system serotonin in humans. Ann N Y Acad Sci 90:108–117, 1962

Wurtman JJ, Wurtman RJ, Growdon JH, et al: Carbohydrate craving in obese people: suppression by treatments affecting serotonergic transmission. International Journal of Eating Disorders 1:2–15, 1981

Yesavage JA: Correlates of dangerous behavior by schizophrenics in hospital. J Psychiatr Res 18:225–231, 1984

Zohar J, Insel TR, Zohar-Kadouch RC, et al: Serotonergic responsivity in obsessive-compulsive disorder: effects of chronic clomipramine treatment. Arch Gen Psychiatry 45:167–172, 1988

Zubenko GS, Cohen BM, Lipinski JF: Antidepressant-related akathisia. J Clin Psychopharmacol 7:254–257, 1987

9

Monoamine Oxidase Inhibitors

K. Ranga Rama Krishnan, M.D.

Monoamine oxidase inhibitors (MAOIs) were first identified as effective antidepressants in the late 1950s. Two reports suggested that iproniazid, an antituberculosis agent, had mood-elevating properties in patients who had been treated for tuberculosis (Bloch et al. 1954; Selikoff et al. 1952). Following these observations, two studies demonstrated that iproniazid did indeed have antidepressant properties (Crane 1957; Kline 1958). Zeller (1963) reported that iproniazid caused potent inhibition of MAO enzymes both in vivo and in vitro in the brain. He also demonstrated that the medication reversed some of the actions of reserpine. Because reserpine produced significant depression as a side effect, it was suggested that iproniazid might have mood-elevating properties.

The use of iproniazid soon fell into disfavor because of its significant hepatotoxicity. Other MAOIs, both hydrazine derivatives (e.g., isocarboxazid and phenylhydrazine) and nonhydrazine derivatives (e.g., tranylcypromine), were introduced. These MAOIs were not specific for any subtype of MAO enzyme and were irreversible inhibitors of MAO (see next section). Their use has been rather limited, because hypertensive crisis by the MAOIs may occur in some patients from potentiation of the pressor effects of amines (such as tyramine) in food (Blackwell et al. 1967).

In the last few years, there has been a resurgence of interest in the development of new MAOIs—those that are more specific subtypes of MAO enzyme and those that are reversible in nature. New MAOIs, such as deprenyl or selegiline hydrochloride, an MAO β-inhibitor, have been introduced (Table 9–1).

Reversible MAO α-inhibitors such as moclobemide are currently being evaluated. Moclobemide has been introduced in Europe and is now being tested in the United States.

■ MONOAMINE OXIDASE ISOENZYMES

MAO is widely distributed in mammals. Two isoenzymes, monoamine oxidase A (MAO-A) and monoamine oxidase B (MAO-B), are of special interest to psychiatry (Cesura and Pletscher 1992). Both are present in the central nervous system (CNS) as well as in some peripheral organs. Both MAO-A and MAO-B are present in discrete cell populations within the CNS. MAO-A is present in both dopamine and norepinephrine neurons, whereas MAO-B is present to a greater extent in serotonin-containing neurons. They are also present in nonaminergic neurons in various subcortical regions of the brain. Glial cells also express MAO-A and MAO-B (Cesura and Pletscher 1992). The physiological function of these two isoenzymes has not been fully elucidated. The main substrates for MAO-A are epinephrine, norepinephrine, and serotonin. The main substrates for MAO-B are phenylethylamine, phenylethanolamine, tyramine, and benzylamine. Dopamine and tryptamine are metabolized by both isoenzymes. It is interesting to note that the substrates are not the same as the localization of the MAO subtypes. The reason for this discrepancy is unknown. It is possible that the occurrence of the MAO-B form in serotonin neurons may actually protect these neurons from amines other than serotonin that could be toxic to them (Cesura and Pletscher 1992).

The primary structures of both MAO-A and MAO-B have been fully described. MAO-A has 527 amino acids to MAO-B's 520. About 70% of the amino acid sequence of the two forms are homologous. The genes for both are located on the short arm of the human X-chromosome. Both are linked and have been located in the XP11.23-P11 region and XP22.1 region, respectively. The genes are about 70 kilobases and consist of about 15 exons and 14 introns. MAO-A has two messenger ribonucleic acid (mRNA) transcripts of 2.1 and 5.0 kilobytes in length. MAO-B has a 3-kilobyte mRNA single transcript (Cesura and Pletscher 1992). A rare inherited disorder, Norrie's disease, is characterized by deletion of both genes. Patients with this disorder have very severe mental retardation and blindness. The pathophysiology of the presentation is unknown.

The subunit composition of MAO is unknown. The enzyme is primarily present in the outer mitochondrial membrane; flavin adenine dinucleotide (FAD) is a cofactor for both MAO-A and MAO-B enzymes.

Because the cofactor domain is the same for both MAO isoenzymes, the structural differences responsible for substrate specificity are believed to lie in regions of the protein that bind to the hydrophobic moiety of the substrate. Although dopamine is considered to be a mixed substrate for both MAO-A and MAO-B, the breakdown of dopamine in the striatal regions of the brain is preferentially by MAO-B. In other regions, MAO-A may be more important. It is possible that there may be regional differences in which isoenzyme is responsible for the metabolism of other biogenic amines that are substrates for both forms of MAO (see Cesura and Pletscher 1992).

■ ENZYME KINETICS

The kinetics of the enzyme have not been well studied for MAO-A. More information is available on the enzyme kinetics for MAO-B. It appears that the enzyme kinetics depend on the nature of the substrate. Some substrates (e.g., tyramine) go through ping-pong mechanisms characterized by first oxidation of the amine to the imine form that is subsequently released from the reduced enzyme before reoxidation of the latter occurs. For other substrates (e.g., benzylamine), a tertiary complex is formed with the enzyme and oxygen (Husain et al. 1982; Pearce and Roth 1985; Ramsay and Singer 1991).

■ MONOAMINE OXIDASE INHIBITORS

■ Mechanism of Action

The target function of MAOIs is a regulation of the monoamine content within the nervous system. Because it is bound to the outer site of plasma membrane of the mitochondria, MAO in neurons is unable to deaminate amines that are present inside stored vesicles and can metabolize only on amines that are present in the cytoplasm. As a result, MAO maintains low cytoplasmic concentration of amines within the cells. Inhibition of neuronal MAO produces an increase in the MAO content within the cytoplasm. It was initially believed that the therapeutic action of the MAOIs was due to this amine accumulation (Finberg and Youdim 1984; Murphy et al. 1984, 1987). More recently, it was suggested that secondary adaptive mechanisms may be important for their antidepressant action.

After several weeks of treatment, MAOIs produce effects such as a reduction in the number of β-adrenoceptors, α_1- and α_2-adrenoceptors, and 5-HT$_1$

Table 9–1. Classification of MAOI drugs by structure, selectivity, and reversibility

Drug	Hydrazine	Selective	Reversible
Phenelzine	Yes	No	No
Isocarboxazid	Yes	No	No
Tranylcypromine	No	No	No
Deprenyl	No	Yes[1,3]	No
Moclobemide	No	Yes[2]	Yes
Brofaromine	No	Yes[2]	Yes

[1] Selective for MAO-B at lower doses.
[2] Selective for MAO-A.
[3] Becomes nonselective at higher doses.

and 5-HT$_2$ receptors. These changes are similar to that produced by chronic tricyclic antidepressants (TCAs) and other antidepressant treatment (DaPrada et al. 1984, 1989).

MAOIs can be subdivided not only on the basis of the particular type of enzyme inhibition, but also by whether or not the inhibition they produce is reversible or irreversible. The reversible MAOIs are basically chemically inert substrate analogues. These are recognized by the enzyme as substrates and are converted into intermediates by the normal mechanism. These converted compounds react to the inactive site of the enzyme and form a stable bound enzyme. This effect occurs gradually, and there is usually a correlation between the plasma concentration of the reversible inhibitors and pharmacological action.

The classic MAOIs inhibit both forms of the enzyme and have been divided into two main subtypes: hydrazine and nonhydrazine derivatives. The hydrazine derivatives are related to iproniazid, two of which are currently available—isocarboxazid (Marplan) and phenelzine (Nardil). The nonhydrazine irreversible MAOI is tranylcypromine (Parnate). Tranylcypromine is chemically similar to amphetamine. Clorgiline is an example of an irreversible MAOI-A, whereas L-deprenyl (selegiline) is an irreversible MAOI-B. Reversible inhibitors of MAO-A that are currently available include brofaromine and moclobemide.

Three classic MAOIs (i.e., tranylcypromine, phenelzine, and isocarboxazid) are of clinical interest. It is important to recognize that these drugs, in addition to their inhibition of MAO, also exert other actions that may be clinically relevant. Thus, these compounds can block MAO uptake: tranylcypromine then isocarboxazid equals phenelzine. In addition, tranylcypromine, because of its structural similarity to amphetamine, is believed to exert stimulant-like actions in the brain. There are many issues common to all three of these MAOIs.

■ Efficacy

Many studies have been conducted examining the efficacy of these compounds in the treatment of different types of depression. MAOIs have been found to be effective in treating patients with major depression or atypical depression (Davidson et al. 1987; Himmelhoch et al. 1982, 1991; Johnstone 1975;

Johnstone and Marsh 1973; McGrath et al. 1986; Paykel et al. 1982; Quitkin et al. 1979, 1990, 1991; Rowan et al. 1981; Thase et al. 1992; Vallejo et al. 1987; White et al. 1984; Zisook et al. 1985). Although early studies of relatively low-dose regimens suggested that MAOI efficacy was lower than that of TCAs, more recent studies have documented that their efficacy is comparable (Table 9–2).

Quitkin and colleagues (1979, 1991) reviewed both phenelzine and tranylcypromine studies in patients with either atypical and neurotic depression or melancholic depression. They reported that phenelzine appeared to be effective for treatment of atypical depression.

Relatively few studies of endogenous depressive patients have been conducted. It is difficult to conclude from the limited number of patient studies initially done that phenelzine is effective in treatment of these patients. There have also been very few well-controlled studies of tranylcypromine versus placebo. Three of the four studies of tranylcypromine versus placebo showed that tranylcypromine was more effective. In one study, a nonsignificant trend was found favoring tranylcypromine. More recently, studies have documented the efficacy of tranylcypromine in treating anergic depression and in high doses for patients with treatment-resistant depression (Himmelhoch et al. 1982, 1991; Thase et al. 1992; White et al. 1984).

The heterogeneity of acetylation rate may account for some of the variance in response to phenelzine (Johnstone 1975; Johnstone and Marsh 1973; Paykel et al. 1982; Rowan et al. 1981). Half of the

Table 9–2. Indications for use of MAOIs

Definitely effective	Other possible uses
Atypical depression	Obsessive-compulsive disorder
Major depression	
Dysthymia	Narcolepsy
Melancholia	Headache
Panic disorder	Chronic pain syndrome
Bulimia	Generalized anxiety disorder
Atypical facial pain	
Anergic depression	
Treatment-resistant depression	
Parkinson's disease*	

* Selegiline is the only MAOI that is useful in the treatment of Parkinson's disease.

patients in a given population are often slow acetylators. An initial study by Johnstone and Marsh (1973) suggested that slow acetylators demonstrate greater improvement with phenelzine than fast acetylators. Other groups have been unable to confirm the relationship between acetylation, acetylator type, and response to MAOI.

MAOIs are used in a wide range of psychiatric disorders. Early studies suggested that MAOIs are particularly effective in patients who have atypical depression originally defined as depression with anxiety or chronic pain, reversed vegetative symptoms, and rejection sensitivity (Quitkin et al. 1990).

The concept of atypical depression is still a subject of considerable controversy and has not been completely validated. In general, patients with atypical depression have an earlier onset than melancholic patients and have increased prevalence of dysthymia, alcohol abuse, sociopathy, and atypical depression in their relatives. The best differentiating criterion appears to be that phenelzine and other irreversible MAOIs are more effective than TCAs in treating these patients (Cesura and Pletscher 1992; Quitkin et al. 1990; Zisook et al. 1985).

Some studies have also suggested that MAOIs are effective in treating typical major depression and melancholic depression (Davidson et al. 1987; McGrath et al. 1986; Vallejo et al. 1987).

TREATMENT OF VARIOUS PSYCHIATRIC DISORDERS

Panic Disorder

Both single-blind and double-blind studies have demonstrated that phenelzine and iproniazid are effective in treating panic disorder (Lydiard et al. 1989; Quitkin et al. 1990; Tyrer et al. 1973). About 50%–60% of patients with panic disorder respond to MAOIs. In the early stages of treatment, patients sometimes have a worsening of symptoms. This is reduced in clinical practice by combining the MAOI with a benzodiazepine for the initial phase of the study. It has also been suggested that phenelzine has an antiphobic action in addition to its antipanic effect (Kelly et al. 1971). The time-course of effect and the dose used is similar to that for major depression.

Social Phobia

Liebowitz and colleagues (1992) have demonstrated that phenelzine is effective in treating social phobia. In an open-label study, Versiani and colleagues (1988) suggested that tranylcypromine is also effective and also demonstrated the efficacy of moclobemide in a double-blind study (Versiani et al. 1992). In clinical experience, about 50% of patients respond to MAOIs. The onset of response is gradual (usually about 2–3 weeks).

Obsessive-Compulsive Disorder (OCD)

Although initial case reports suggested that MAOI may be effective in treatment of OCD (Jenike 1981), there are no double-blind studies that suggest efficacy.

Posttraumatic Stress Disorder

The classic MAOI phenelzine has been proven effective for treatment of posttraumatic stress disorder (PTSD), both in single-blind trials (Kosten et al. 1991) and in a double-blind crossover trial.

Generalized Anxiety Disorder (GAD)

MAOIs are not usually used for treating GAD because the risk-benefit ratio favors the use of azaspirones or benzodiazepines. MAOIs are used primarily in treatment-resistant GAD patients.

Bulimia Nervosa

Both isocarboxazid and phenelzine have been shown to be effective in treating some symptoms of bulimia nervosa (Kennedy et al. 1988; McElroy et al. 1989; Walsh et al. 1985, 1987).

Premenstrual Dysphoria

Preliminary studies as well as clinical experience suggest that MAOIs may be effective in treatment of premenstrual dysphoria (Glick et al. 1991).

Chronic Pain

MAOIs are believed to be effective in the treatment of atypical facial pain as well as for other chronic pain syndromes. However, only limited data on these conditions are available. The classic MAOIs have not been found to be effective for treating neurological disorders such as Parkinson's disease and Alzheimer's dementia. However, the MAO-B inhibitor L-deprenyl has been shown to be effective in slowing the progression of Parkinson's disease (Cesura and Pletscher 1992), but the mechanism underlying this effect is unknown.

■ SIDE EFFECTS OF MONOAMINE OXIDASE INHIBITORS

Side effects of MAOIs are generally more severe or frequent than for other antidepressants (Zisook 1984). The most frequent ones include dizziness, headache, dry mouth, insomnia, constipation, blurred vision, nausea, peripheral edema, forgetfulness, fainting spells, trauma, hesitancy of urination, weakness, and myoclonic jerks. Loss of weight and appetite can occur with isocarboxazid (Davidson and Turnbull 1982). Hepatotoxicity is rarer with the currently available MAOIs compared with iproniazid. However, elevation of liver enzymes such as serum glutamic-oxaloacetic transaminase (SGOT) and serum glutamic-pyruvic transaminase (SGPT) are found in 3%–5% of patients. Liver function tests must be conducted only when there are symptoms such as malaise, jaundice, or excessive fatigue.

Some side effects first emerge during maintenance treatment (Evans et al. 1982). These include weight gain (which occurs in almost half of the patients), edema, muscle cramps, carbohydrate craving, sexual dysfunction (which is usually anorgasmia), pyridoxine deficiency (Goodheart et al. 1991), hypoglycemia, hypomania, urinary retention, and disorientation. Peripheral neuropathy is a rare side effect of MAOIs (Goodheart et al. 1991). Weight gain is more of a problem with the hydrazine compounds such as phenelzine than with tranylcypromine. Edema is also more common with phenelzine than with tranylcypromine.

The management of some of these side effects can be problematic. Orthostatic hypotension is common with MAOIs. Addition of salt and of salt-retaining steroids such as flurohydrocortisol are sometimes effective in treating orthostatic hypotension. Elastic support stockings are also helpful. Small amounts of coffee or tea taken during the day also keep the blood pressure up. The dose of flurohydro-

cortisol should be carefully adjusted, because in elderly patients it could provoke cardiac failure resulting from fluid retention.

Sexual dysfunction that occurs with these compounds is also difficult to treat. Common problems include anorgasmia, decreased libido, impotence, and delayed ejaculation (Harrison et al. 1985; Jacobson 1987). Cyproheptadine is sometimes effective in treating sexual dysfunction such as anorgasmia. Bethanechol may also be effective in some patients. Weight gain because of the hydrazine derivatives is an indication to switch to tranylcypromine. Speech blockage is a rare side effect with MAOIs (Goldstein and Goldberg 1986).

Insomnia sometimes occurs as an intermediate or late side effect of these compounds. Changing the time of administration does not seem to be much help, though dosage reduction is sometimes helpful. Adding trazodone at bedtime is effective; however, this should be done with caution. Myoclonic jerks, peripheral neuropathy, and paresthesia, when present, are also difficult to treat. When a patient has paresthesia, evaluation for peripheral neuropathy and pyridoxine deficiency should be done. In general, patients on MAOIs should also take concomitant pyridoxine therapy. When myoclonic jerks are seen, patients can be treated with cyproheptadine (Periactin).

■ Dietary Interactions of Monoamine Oxidase Inhibitors

After the MAOIs were introduced, a number of reports of severe headaches in patients who were taking these compounds were published (Anonymous 1970; Cronin 1965; Hedberg et al. 1966; Simpson and Gratz 1992). It was shown that these headaches were due to a drug-food interaction. The risk of such an interaction is highest for tranylcypromine and lower for phenelzine, providing the dose of the latter is kept low. The interaction of MAOI with food has been attributed to increased tyramine levels. Tyramine, which has a pressor action, is present in a number of foodstuffs. It is normally broken down by the MAO enzymes and has both direct and indirect sympathomimetic actions. The classic explanation of this side effect may not be entirely accurate; in fact, it has been suggested that the potentiation by an MAOI of tyramine may be secondary to increased release of noradrenaline rather than MAOIs. Adrenaline would increase the indirect sympathetic activity of tyramine. The spontaneous occurrence of hypertensive crises in a few patients lends support to this hypothesis (O'Brien et al. 1992; Zajecka and Fawcett 1991).

The tyramine effect is potentiated by MAOIs 10- to 20-fold. A mild tyramine interaction can be seen with about 6 mg of tyramine; 10 mg can produce a moderate episode and 25 mg a severe one, characterized by hypertension, occipital headache, palpitations, nausea, vomiting, apprehension, occasional chills, sweating, and restlessness. On examination, neck stiffness, pallor, mild pyrexia, dilated pupils, and motor agitation may sometimes be seen. The reaction usually develops within 20 minutes to 1 hour after ingestion of the food. Occasionally, the reaction can be very severe and may lead to alteration of consciousness, hyperpyrexia, cerebral hemorrhage, and death. Death is exceedingly rare and has been calculated to be about 0.01%–0.02% for tranylcypromine.

The classic treatment of the hypertensive reaction is to give 5 mg of phentolamine intravenously (Youdim et al. 1987; Zisook 1984). More recently, nifedipine, a calcium channel blocker, has been shown to be effective. Nifedipine has an onset of action in about 5 minutes, and it lasts approximately 3–5 hours; in fact, some have suggested that patients should carry nifedipine with them for immediate use in the event of a hypertensive crisis.

Because of the drug interaction of the classic MAOIs with food, a number of dietary recommendations are usually made (see Table 9–3). These recommendations are quite varied.

Table 9–3.   Food restrictions for MAOIs

To be avoided	To be used in moderation
Cheese (except for cream cheese)	Coffee
Overripe aged fruit (banana peel)	Chocolate
	Colas
Fava beans	Tea
Sausage, salami	Soy sauce
Sherry, liquors	Beer, other wines
Sauerkraut	
Monosodium glutamate	
Pickled fish	
Brewer's yeast	
Beef and chicken liver	
Fermented products	
Red wine	

All the MAOI diets recommend restriction of cheese (except for cream and cottage cheese), wine, beer, sherry, liquors, pickled fish, overripe aged fruit, brewer's yeast, fava beans, beef and chicken liver, and fermented products. Other diets also recommend restriction of all alcoholic beverages, coffee, chocolate, colas, tea, yogurt, soy sauce, avocados, and bananas. The more restrictive the diet, the greater the risk of patient noncompliance. Further, many of the compounds (e.g., avocados, bananas) rarely cause hypertensive crisis, and only if overripe fruit is eaten—or, in the case of bananas, if the skin is eaten (which is uncommon in the United States). Similarly, unless a person ingests large amounts of caffeine, the interaction is usually not clinically significant.

In evaluating patients who have had a drug-food reaction, it is also important to evaluate the hypertensive reaction and differentiate it from histamine headache, which can occur with an MAOI. Histamine headaches are usually accompanied by hypotension, colic, loose stools, salivation, and lacrimation (Cooper 1967). When patients are placed on classic MAOIs, they should be given oral instructions as well as printed cards outlining these instructions.

In addition to the food interaction, drug interactions are extremely important (see next section). Each patient should be given a card indicating that he or she is taking an MAOI and should be instructed to carry it at all times. A med bracelet indicating that the wearer takes an MAOI is also a good idea.

■ DRUG INTERACTION

The extensive inhibition of MAO by MAOI enzymes raises the potential for a number of drug interactions. These interactions are particularly important because many over-the-counter medications can interact with the MAOIs. These include cough syrups containing sympathomimetic agents, which, in the presence of an MAOI, can precipitate a hypertensive crisis.

Another area of caution is the use of MAOIs in patients who need surgery. Interactions in this setting include those with narcotic drugs, especially meperidine. Meperidine when administered with MAOIs can produce a syndrome characterized by coma, hyperpyrexia, and hypertension. This has been reported primarily with phenelzine but also with tranylcypromine (Mendelson 1979; Stack et al. 1988). Stack and colleagues (1988) have noted that this syndrome is most likely to occur with meperidine and may be related to its serotonergic properties. Similar reactions have not been reported to any significant extent with other narcotic analgesics such as morphine or codeine. In fact, many patients probably receive these medications without problem. Only a small fraction of the patients probably have this interaction, and it could reflect an idiosyncratic effect. In general, current opinion favors the use of morphine or fentanyl when intra- or postoperative narcotics are needed in patients receiving MAOIs.

The issue of whether directly acting sympathomimetic amines interact with MAOIs is more controversial. Intravenous administration of sympathomimetic amines to patients receiving MAOIs fails to provoke hypertension. When a bolus infusion of catecholamines is given to healthy normal volunteer subjects who have been on phenelzine or tranylcypromine for a week, a potentiation of the pressor effect of phenylephrine is found, but no clinically significant potentiation of cardiovascular effects of norepinephrine, epinephrine, or isoproterenol (Wells 1989).

In general, direct sympathomimetic amine–MAOI interactions do not appear to produce significant cardiovascular problems, but rather a low incidence of hypertensive episodes in the presence of indirect sympathomimetics. Ideally, these compounds should not be used in patients receiving MAOIs. A direct-acting compound is preferable to an indirect-acting one. Other interactions that have been reported include a barbiturate-MAOI interaction. These interactions should be considered clinically insignificant.

■ MOCLOBEMIDE

Moclobemide is a reversible inhibitor of MAO-A enzyme (RIMA) (Amrein et al. 1989). The drug displays a higher potency in vivo than in vitro. Therefore, it has been suggested that moclobemide is a prodrug and is metabolized to a form with higher affinity for MAO-A than the parent compound. The recovery of MAO-A activity after single or repeated moclobemide administration is much shorter than that seen with other MAOIs including clorgiline, the irreversible MAO-A inhibitor. One of the metabolites of moclobemide does inhibit MAO-B; however, this action is minimally significant in humans. Moclobemide, when administered to rats, increases concentration of serotonin, norepinephrine, epinephrine, and dopa-

mine in rat brain (see Haefely et al. 1992). These effects are short lasting and parallel the time-course of MAO-A inhibition. In addition, unlike other irreversible inhibitors, repeated administration does not increase the inhibition.

In animals, moclobemide has been shown to only partially potentiate the blood pressor effect of oral tyramine. The reason for this is that it is a reversible inhibitor with a low affinity for the MAO isoenzymes, easily displaced by the pressor amines ingested in food. Based on these studies, moclobemide is thought to be safer than other irreversible MAOIs.

■ Pharmacokinetics

Following oral administration of moclobemide, peak plasma concentrations are reached within 1 hour. The drug is about 50% bound to plasma proteins and is extensively metabolized; only 1% of the compound is excreted in the urine, unchanged. The half-life of the compound is approximately 12 hours.

■ Efficacy

Moclobemide has been studied in all types of depression (Gabelic and Kuhn 1990; Larsen et al. 1991; Rossel and Moll 1990). Controlled trials have demonstrated its superiority to placebo. In addition, it has been found to as effective as imipramine, desipramine, clomipramine, and amitriptyline in the treatment of depression. The dose required is 300–600 mg per day.

Not unlike the classic MAOIs, moclobemide has been found to be more effective in both endogenous and nonendogenous suppression. In addition, in combination with antipsychotics, the drug appears to be effective in treating psychotic depression (Amrein et al. 1989). It has also been shown to be effective in treating bipolar endogenous depression.

■ Treatment of Other Psychiatric Disorders

Versiani and colleagues (1992) have compared the MAOI phenelzine, moclobemide, and placebo and demonstrated that both phenelzine and moclobemide are superior to placebo in treating patients with social phobia. Based on the efficacy of classic MAOIs in the treatment of other psychiatric disorders such as bulimia, panic disorder, and PTSD, it is likely that these patients would respond to the reversible MAOIs. Additional trials are required to confirm the utility in other psychiatric disorders.

■ Side Effects

Nausea was the only side effect noted to be greater in patients on moclobemide compared with those on placebo. Thus, the profile of the drug appears to be ideal in that there are few or no major side effects. Case reports have demonstrated no toxicity following overdoses of up to 20 g (Amrein et al. 1989).

■ Food and Drug Interactions

Intravenous tyramine pressor tests indicate a single dose of moclobemide increases tyramine sensitivity (Cusson et al. 1991). However, this increase is marginal compared with the increase associated with other MAOIs. Under most conditions, there appears to be limited drug-food interaction. However, to minimize even mild tyramine pressor effects, it would be preferable to administer moclobemide after a meal rather than before it. In a study where tyramine was administered in dosages up to 100 mg, inpatients pretreated with moclobemide produced no significant changes in blood pressure. The drug also has minimal effect on cognitive performance. There is no effect on body weight or hematological parameters (Wesnes et al. 1989; Youdim et al. 1987).

■ Drug Interactions

Unlike the other MAOIs, a number of studies have been undertaken to examine potential drug interaction (Amrein et al. 1992). No drug interaction with lithium or in combination with TCAs has been reported. The drug has also been combined with fluoxetine and other selective serotonin reuptake inhibitors (SSRIs) with no significant interaction. No interactions with benzodiazepines or neuroleptics have been reported (Amrein et al. 1992). Parallel data suggest that moclobemide can potentiate the effects of meperidine (pethidine); it is therefore possible that the narcotic-MAOI interaction can occur. Until proven otherwise, it would be prudent to avoid the combination of moclobemide with opiates such as meperidine. A pharmacokinetic interaction has been observed with cimetidine that requires the reduction of the moclobemide dose because cimetidine reduces the clearance of moclobemide.

■ MAO-B INHIBITOR, DEPRENYL, AND SELEGILINE HYDROCHLORIDE

Selegiline hydrochloride is an irreversible MAO-B inhibitor (Cesura and Pletscher 1992). Its primary use is in treatment of Parkinson's disease as an adjunct to L-dopa and carbidopa. The average daily dose for Parkinson's disease is 5–10 mg a day. The exact mechanism of action of MAO-B in Parkinson's disease is unknown. Selegiline is metabolized to levoamphetamine, methamphetamine, and N-desmethylselegiline.

The efficacy of selegiline in treating depression has not been well studied. The few studies that have examined its utility have been equivocal. The dose required for treating depression may be much higher than that required to treat Parkinson's disease. Clinical experience suggests that doses of 20–40 mg a day are needed. At these doses, dietary interactions could occur. Because MAO-B is not involved in the intestinal tyramine interaction, it is likely that, at low doses of 5–10 mg a day, dietary interaction with selegiline would probably be minimal; therefore, no drug interactions have been reported. An interaction between selegiline and narcotics has been reported and should be kept in mind. Selegiline has been found to have no adverse effects when combined with other antidepressants during treatment of depression in Parkinson's patients. The few side effects that have been noted with selegiline include nausea, dizziness, and light-headedness. When the drug is abruptly discontinued, nausea, hallucinations, and confusion have been reported.

■ SUMMARY

Various MAOIs have been shown to be effective in treating a wide variety of psychiatric disorders, including depression, panic disorder, social phobia, and PTSD. The classic MAOIs are currently used only rarely as first-line medication because of potential dietary interaction and other long-term side effects. With the introduction of RIMAs such as moclobemide and brofaromine, which have fewer side effects and no dietary restrictions, first-line usage should increase. In fact, the risk-benefit ratio for these compounds are highly favorable compared with other antidepressants. The MAO-B inhibitor selegiline is currently used to reduce the progression of Parkinson's disease. Its utility in treating other degenerative disorders is currently being assessed. It is possible that new applications and wider use of these compounds will be found in the near future.

■ REFERENCES

Amrein R, Allen SR, Guentert TW, et al: Pharmacology of reversible MAOI. Br J Psychiatry 144:66–71, 1989

Amrein R, Guntert TW, Dingemanse J, et al: Interactions of moclobemide with concomitantly administered medication: evidence from pharmacological and clinical studies. Psychopharmacology (Berl) 106:S24–S31, 1992

Anonymous: Cheese and tranylcypromine. British Medical Journal 3(718):354, 1970

Blackwell B, Marley E, Price J, et al: Hypertensive interactions between monoamine oxidase inhibitors and food stuffs. Br J Psychiatry 113:349–365, 1967

Bloch RG, Doonief AS, Buchberg AS, et al: The clinical effect of isoniazid and iproniazid in the treatment of pulmonary tuberculosis. Ann Intern Med 40:881–900, 1954

Cesura AM, Pletscher A: The new generation of monoamine oxidase inhibitors. Prog Drug Res 38:171–297, 1992

Cooper AJ: MAO inhibitors and headache. British Medical Journal 2:426, 1967

Crane GE: Iproniazid (Marsilid) phosphate, a therapeutic agent for mental disorders and debilitating disease. Psychiatry Research Reports 8:142–152, 1957

Cronin D: Monoamine-oxidase inhibitors and cheese. British Medical Journal 5469:1065, 1965

Cusson JR, Goldenberg E, Larochelle P: Effect of a novel monoamine oxidase inhibitor, moclobemide on the sensitivity to intravenous tyramine and norepinephrine in humans. J Clin Pharmacol 31:462–467, 1991

DaPrada M, Kettler R, Burkard WP, et al: Moclobemide, an antidepressant with short-lasting MAO-A inhibition: brain catecholamines and tyramine pressor effects in rats, in Monoamine Oxidase and Disease: Prospects for Therapy With Reversible Inhibitors. Edited by Tipton KF, Dostert P, Strolin Benedetti M. New York, Academic Press, 1984, pp 137–154

DaPrada M, Kettler R, Keller HH, et al: Neurochemical profile of moclobemide, a short-acting and reversible inhibitor of monoamine oxidase type A. J Pharmacol Exp Ther 248:400–414, 1989

Davidson J, Turnbull C: Loss of appetite and weight associated with the monoamine oxidase inhibitor isocarboxazid. J Clin Psychopharmacol 2:263–266, 1982

Davidson J, Raft D, Pelton S: An outpatient evaluation of phenelzine and imipramine. J Clin Psychiatry 48:143–146, 1987

Evans DL, Davidson J, Raft D: Early and late side effects of phenelzine. J Clin Psychopharmacol 2:208–210, 1982

Finberg JPM, Youdim MBH: Reversible monoamine oxidase inhibitors and the cheese effect, in Monoamine Oxidase and Disease: Prospects for Therapy With Reversible Inhibitors. Edited by Tipton KF, Dostert P, Strolin Benedetti M. New York, Academic Press, 1984, pp 479–485

Gabelic I, Kuhn B: Moclobemide (Ro 11-1163) versus tranylcypromine in the treatment of endogenous depression. Acta Psychiatr Scand Suppl 360:63, 1990

Glick R, Harrison W, Endicott J, et al: Treatment of premenstrual dysphoric symptoms in depressed women. J Am Med Wom Assoc 46:182–185, 1991

Goldstein DM, Goldberg RL: Monoamine oxidase inhibitor-induced speech blockage. J Clin Psychiatry 47:604, 1986

Goodheart RS, Dunne JW, Edis RH: Phenelzine associated peripheral neuropathy clinical and electrophysiologic findings. Aust N Z J Med 21:339–340, 1991

Haefely W, Burkard WP, Cesura AM, et al: Biochemistry and pharmacology of moclobemide: a prototype RIMA. Psychopharmacology (Berl) 106 (suppl):S6–S15, 1992

Harrison WM, Stewart J, Ehrhardt AA, et al: a controlled study of the effects of antidepressants on sexual function. Psychopharmacol Bull 21:85–88, 1985

Hedberg DL, Gordon MW, Glueck BC Jr: Six cases of hypertensive crisis in patients on tranylcypromine after eating chicken livers. Am J Psychiatry 122:933–937, 1966

Himmelhoch JM, Fuchs CZ, Symons BJ: A double-blind study of tranylcypromine treatment of major anergic depression. J Nerv Ment Dis 170:628–634,

1982

Himmelhoch JM, Thase ME, Mallinger AG, et al: Tranylcypromine versus imipramine in anergic bipolar depression. Am J Psychiatry 148:910–916, 1991

Husain M, Edmondson DE, Singer TP: Kinetic studies on the catalytic mechanism of liver monoamine oxidase. Biochemistry 21:595–600, 1982

Jacobson JN: Anorgasmia caused by an MAOI [letter]. Am J Psychiatry 144:527, 1987

Jenike MA: Rapid response of severe obsessive-compulsive disorder to tranylcypromine. Am J Psychiatry 138:1249–1250, 1981

Johnstone EC: Relationship between acetylator status and response to phenelzine. Mod Probl Pharmacopsychiatry 10:30–37, 1975

Johnstone EC, Marsh W: The relationship between response to phenelzine and acetylator status in depressed patients. Proc R Soc Lond [Biol] 66:947–949, 1973

Kelly D, Mitchell-Heggs N, Sherman D: Anxiety and the effects of sodium lactate assessed clinically and physiologically. Br J Psychiatry 119:129–141, 1971

Kennedy SH, Warsh JJ, Mainprize E, et al: A trial of isocarboxazid in the treatment of bulimia. J Clin Psychopharmacol 8:391–396, 1988

Kline NS: Clinical experience with iproniazid (Marsilid). Journal of Clinical and Experimental Psychopathology 19 (suppl 1):72–78, 1958

Kosten TR, Frank JB, Dan E, et al: Pharmacotherapy for posttraumatic stress disorder using phenelzine or imipramine. J Nerv Ment Dis 179:366–370, 1991

Larsen JK, Gjerris A, Holm P, et al: Moclobemide in depression: a randomized, multicentre trial against isocarboxazide and clomipramine emphasizing atypical depression. Acta Psychiatr Scand 84:564–570, 1991

Liebowitz MR, Schneier F, Campeas R, et al: Phenelzine vs atenolol in social phobia: a placebo-controlled comparison. Arch Gen Psychiatry 49:290–300, 1992

Lydiard RB, Laraia MT, Howell EF, et al: Phenelzine treatment of panic disorder: lack of effect on pyridoxal phosphate levels. J Clin Psychopharmacol 9:428–431, 1989

McElroy SL, Keck PE Jr, Pope HG Jr, et al: Pharmacological treatment of kleptomania and bulimia nervosa. J Clin Psychopharmacol 9:358–360, 1989

McGrath PJ, Stewart JW, Harrison W, et al: Phenelzine treatment of melancholia. J Clin Psychiatry 47:420–422, 1986

Mendelson G: Narcotics and monoamine oxidase-inhibitors [letter]. Med J Aust 1:400, 1979

Murphy DL, Garrick NA, Aulakh CS, et al: New contribution from basic science of understanding the effects of monoamine oxidase inhibiting antidepressants. J Clin Psychiatry 45:37–43, 1984

Murphy DL, Sunderland T, Garrick NA, et al: Selective amine oxidase inhibitors: basic to clinical studies and back, in Clinical Pharmacology in Psychiatry. Edited by Dahl SG, Gram A, Potter W. Berlin, Springer Verlag, 1987, pp 135 146

O'Brien S, McKeon P, O'Regan M, et al: Blood pressure effects of tranylcypromine when prescribed singly and in combination with amitriptyline. J Clin Psychopharmacol 12:104–109, 1992

Paykel ES, West PS, Rowan PR, et al: Influence of acetylator phenotype on antidepressant effects of phenelzine. Br J Psychiatry 141:243–248, 1982

Pearce LB, Roth JA: Human brain monoamine oxidase type B: mechanism of deamination as probed by steady-state methods. Biochemistry 24:1821–1826, 1985

Quitkin F, Rifkin A, Klein DF: Monoamine oxidase inhibitors: a review of antidepressant effectiveness. Arch Gen Psychiatry 36:749–760, 1979

Quitkin FM, McGrath PJ, Stewart JW, et al: Atypical depression, panic attacks, and response to imipramine and phenelzine: a replication. Arch Gen Psychiatry 47:935–941, 1990

Quitkin FM, Harrison W, Stewart JW, et al: Response to phenelzine and imipramine in placebo nonresponders with atypical depression: a new application of the crossover design. Arch Gen Psychiatry 48:319–323, 1991

Ramsay RR, Singer TP: The kinetic mechanisms of monoamine oxidases A and B. Biochem Soc Trans 19:219–223, 1991

Rossel L, Moll E: Moclobemide versus tranylcypromine in the treatment of depression. Acta Psychiatr Scand Suppl 360:61–62, 1990

Rowan PR, Paykel ES, West PS, et al: Effects of phenelzine and acetylator phenotype. Neuropharmacology 20(12B):1353–1354, 1981

Selikoff IJ, Robitzek EH, Ornstein GG: Toxicity of hydrazine derivatives of isonicotinic acid in the chemotherapy of human tuberculosis. Quarterly Bulletin of Sea View Hospital 13:17, 1952

Simpson GM, Gratz SS: Comparison of the pressor effect of tyramine after treatment with phenelzine and moclobemide in healthy male volunteers. J Clin Pharm Ther 52:286–291, 1992

Stack CG, Rogers P, Linter SPK: Monoamine oxidase inhibitors and anaesthesia: a review. Br J Anaesth 60:222–227, 1988

Thase ME, Mallinger AG, McKnight D, et al: Treatment of imipramine-resistant recurrent depression, IV: a double-blind crossover study of tranylcypromine for anergic bipolar depression. Am J Psychiatry 149:195–198, 1992

Tyrer PJ, Candy J, Kelly D: A study of the clinical effects of phenelzine and placebo in the treatment of phobic anxiety. Psychopharmacologia 32:237–254, 1973

Vallejo J, Gasto C, Catalan R, et al: Double-blind study of imipramine versus phenelzine in Melancholias and Dysthymic Disorders. Br J Psychiatry 151:639–642, 1987

Versiani M, Mundim FD, Nardi AE, et al: Tranylcypromine in social phobia. J Clin Psychopharmacol 8:279–283, 1988

Versiani M, Nardi AE, Mundim FD, et al: Pharmacotherapy of social phobia: a controlled study with moclobemide and phenelzine. Br J Psychiatry 161:353–360, 1992

Walsh BT, Stewart JW, Roose SP, et al: A double-blind trial of phenelzine in bulimia. J Psychiatr Res 19(2–3):485–489, 1985

Walsh BT, Gladis M, Roose SP, et al: A controlled trial of phenelzine in bulimia. Psychopharmacol Bull 23:49–51, 1987

Wells DG: MAOI revisited. Can J Anaesth 36:64–74, 1989

Wesnes KA, Simpson PM, Christmas L, et al: Acute cognitive effects of moclobemide and trazodone, alone and in combination with alcohol, in the elderly. Br J Clin Pharmacol 27:647P–648P, 1989

White K, Razani J, Cadow B, et al: Tranylcypromine vs nortriptyline vs placebo in depressed outpatients: a controlled trial. Psychopharmacology (Berl) 82:258–262, 1984

Youdim MBH, DaPrada M, Amrein R (eds): The cheese effect and new reversible MAO-A inhibitors. Proceedings of the Round Table of the International Conference on New Directions in Affective Disorders, Jerusalem, 5–9 April 1987

Zajecka J, Fawcett J: Susceptibility to spontaneous MAOI hypertensive episodes [letter]. J Clin Psychiatry 52:513–514, 1991

Zeller EA: Diamine oxidase, in The Enzymes, Vol 8, 2nd Edition. Edited by Boyer PD, Lardy H, Myrback K. London, Academic Press, 1963, pp 313–335

Zisook S: Side effects of isocarboxazid. J Clin Psychiatry 45(7 part 2):53–58, 1984

Zisook S, Braff DL, Click MA: Monoamine oxidase inhibitors in the treatment of atypical depression. J Clin Psychopharmacol 5:131–137, 1985

10

Trazodone and Other Antidepressants

Robert N. Golden, M.D., Joseph M. Bebchuk, M.D., F.R.C.P.C., and Martha E. Leatherman, M.D.

Several important antidepressants are often classified as "atypical," because they do not readily fit into the familiar categories of tricyclic antidepressants (TCAs), monoamine oxidase inhibitors (MAOIs), or selective serotonin reuptake inhibitors (SSRIs). In this chapter, we review the basic and clinical pharmacology of the five "other" antidepressants currently available for clinical use in the United States (in the order in which they became available): trazodone, amoxapine, bupropion, venlafaxine, and nefazodone. In addition, we highlight the experience with nomifensine (an antidepressant that was available for a short time in the mid-1980s), review the putative antidepressant properties of alprazolam, and briefly discuss select novel compounds that are currently in development as potential new antidepressants.

■ TRAZODONE

■ History and Discovery

Trazodone was first synthesized in Italy in the mid-1960s. Initial investigations were conducted there as well as in Germany and Czechoslovakia in the early 1970s. In 1976, the first British studies were initiated, and in 1978, studies began in the United States (Boschmans et al. 1987).

Trazodone differed from the conventional antidepressants then available in several ways. First, it was the first triazolopyridine derivative to be developed as an antidepressant. Second, it was developed as an outgrowth of a specific hypothesis (i.e., that depression is caused by an imbalance in the brain mechanisms responsible for the emotional integration of adverse, unpleasant experiences). For this reason, new animal models utilizing the response to noxious stimuli or situations (rather than the usual models) were used as screening tests for developing the drug (Silvestrini 1980). In fact, trazodone is inactive in classical antidepressant screening tests, such as the reserpine model, the potentiation of yohimbine toxicity, and the behavioral despair–forced swim paradigm (Rudorfer et al. 1984), yet it inhibits painful and conditioned emotional responses (Silvestrini and Lisciani 1973). Trazodone shares certain properties with benzodiazepines and neuroleptics, including sedation and suppression of rapid eye movement (REM) sleep (Yamatsu et al. 1974). Also, it shares with the phenothiazines the ability to suppress self-stimulation behavior and amphetamine effects, and it produces substantial blockade of α-adrenergic receptors (Cohen et al. 1983). In sharp contrast to most other antidepressants available at the time, it shows minimal effects on muscarinic cholinergic receptors (Taylor et al. 1980). Thus, when it was introduced, trazodone represented a new approach to the development of antidepressant compounds and provided a pharmacological profile that was distinct from that of conventional antidepressants.

Shortly after trazodone was introduced for clinical use in the United States in 1982 under the brand name Desyrel, it quickly became a widely prescribed medication, capturing up to one-third of the American market. More recently, with the availability of the extremely popular SSRIs, trazodone's use has declined. It is now available in generic formulation.

■ Structure-Activity Relations

Trazodone is chemically unrelated to other antidepressant drugs, although it does resemble some of the side chain components of TCAs and the phenothiazines. Its structure (Figure 10–1) includes a triazole moiety that may be critical to its antidepressant activity (Brogden et al. 1981).

■ Pharmacological Profile

Trazodone's effects on serotonergic systems are complex. Trazodone itself is a relatively weak serotonin reuptake inhibitor compared with the more potent SSRIs such as fluoxetine and sertraline (Hyttel 1982). However, it is relatively specific for serotonin (5-HT) uptake inhibition, with minimal effects on norepinephrine or dopamine reuptake (Hyttel 1982). In addition, trazodone exhibits some serotonin receptor antagonist activity (Brogden et al. 1981). Furthermore, its active metabolite, m-chlorophenylpiperazine (m-CPP), is a potent direct 5-HT agonist. Trazodone can thus be considered a mixed serotonergic agonist and antagonist, with the relative amount of m-CPP accumulation affecting the relative degree of the predominant agonist activity.

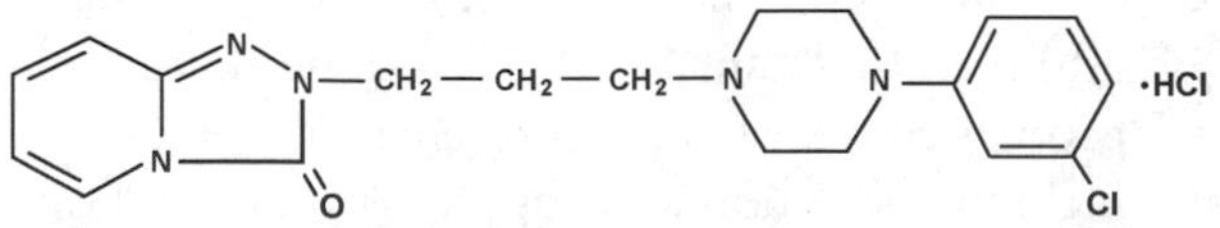

Figure 10–1. Chemical structure for trazodone.

In vivo, trazodone is virtually devoid of anticholinergic activity, and in clinical studies, the incidence of anticholinergic side effects is similar to that of placebo (Boschsmans et al. 1987; Schuckit 1987). Trazodone is a relatively weak blocker of presynaptic α_2-adrenergic receptors and a relatively potent antagonist of postsynaptic α_1-adrenergic receptors (Brogden et al. 1981). The latter property probably accounts for trazodone's propensity to cause orthostatic hypotension, as discussed in "Indications."

■ Pharmacokinetics and Disposition

Trazodone is well absorbed after oral administration, with peak blood levels occurring about 1 hour after dosing when taken on an empty stomach, and approximately 2 hours after dosing when taken with food. Its protein binding is 89%–95%. Elimination appears to be biphasic, consisting of an initial alpha phase followed by a slower beta phase, with half-lives of 3 to 6 and 5 to 9 hours, respectively.

Trazodone undergoes extensive hepatic metabolism, including hydroxylation, splitting at the pyridine ring, oxidation, and N-oxidation (Garattini 1974). Less than 1% of the drug is excreted unchanged in the feces and urine (Caccia et al. 1981). The active metabolite m-CPP is cleared more slowly than the parent compound (i.e., it has a half-life of 4–14 hours), and it reaches higher concentrations in the brain than in plasma (Caccia et al. 1981).

The relationship between steady-state blood levels and clinical response to trazodone remains unclear. In a study of geriatric patients, plasma concentrations of trazodone were lower in responders than in nonresponders (Spar 1987). However, this study was limited by the lack of a fixed-dose design (increasing the chances that patients who were destined to be nonresponders would have continued dose increases, yielding relatively higher plasma levels) and its small sample size. Another study, also conducted with geriatric patients, found a positive relationship between steady-state trazodone plasma concentrations and clinical response in a sample of 11 subjects (Monteleone and Gnocchi 1990). Well-designed studies examining the relationship between plasma m-CPP concentrations, as well as trazodone levels, have not yet been reported. Such studies could shed light on the question of trazodone's mechanism of action, in which m-CPP might play a critical role (see next subsection).

■ Mechanism of Action

Trazodone's ultimate mechanism of action remains unclear. The mixed agonist and antagonist profile for its effects on serotonin is interesting. Although the drug is often referred to as a serotonin reuptake inhibitor, such labeling overlooks the complexity of its effects on this neurotransmitter system. For example, binding studies confirm that trazodone does demonstrate relative selectivity for 5-HT reuptake sites (Hyttel 1982); yet in vivo, it blocks the head-twitch response induced by classic 5-HT agonists in animals (Brogden et al. 1981). In addition, the potent 5-HT agonist properties of trazodone's major metabolite, m-CPP, probably play a role in the mechanism of action of the parent compound. It is also interesting to note that trazodone (unlike the vast majority of antidepressants) does not produce downregulation of β-adrenergic receptors in rat cortex (Sulser 1983).

■ Indications

The primary indication for trazodone is in the treatment of major depression. In more than two dozen double-blind placebo-controlled studies in Europe and the United States, trazodone's efficacy has been consistently superior to placebo and equivalent to conventional TCAs (Golden et al. 1988a). In a review of the double-blind studies published after trazodone's release in the United States, Schatzberg (1987) found trazodone's therapeutic efficacy to be similar to that of TCAs in patients with either endogenous or nonendogenous depression. Furthermore, the accumulated data suggest that trazodone may have a more pronounced, earlier onset of anxiolytic action compared with conventional antidepressants—perhaps reflecting its potent sedative properties (Schatzberg 1987). Lader's (1987) review of the European literature yielded similar findings: data from open and double-blind trials suggest that trazodone's antidepressant efficacy is comparable to that of amitriptyline, doxepin, and mianserin. Also, trazodone demonstrated anxiolytic properties, low cardiotoxicity, and relatively mild side effects (Lader 1987).

Questions have been raised regarding trazodone's effectiveness in treating severely ill patients, especially those with prominent psychomotor retardation (Klein and Muller 1985). Shopsin and colleagues (1981) have pointed out that several unpublished, double-blind controlled studies by independent groups at different institutions found extremely low rates of response to trazodone (i.e., 10%–20%) in depressed patients. Lader (1987) acknowledged that the actual numbers of patients with severe psychomotor retarded depression reported in individual studies have been too small to resolve the ongoing impression among many clinicians that trazodone's efficacy is limited in this population.

Because trazodone has minimal anticholinergic activity, it was especially welcomed as a treatment for depressed geriatric patients when it first became available in 1982. Three double-blind studies have shown that trazodone possesses antidepressant efficacy similar to that of other antidepressants in geriatric patients (Gerner 1987). Unfortunately, orthostatic hypotension, leading to dizziness and the risk of falling, can have devastating consequences in elderly people. This side effect, along with sedation, often makes trazodone less acceptable in this population, compared with newer compounds that share its lack of anticholinergic activity but not the rest of its side-effect profile. Still, trazodone is often helpful for treatment of depressed geriatric patients with severe agitation and insomnia. In fact, there are case reports of its use in controlling agitation and hostility associated with dementia in geriatric patients (Greenwald et al. 1986; Simpson and Foster 1986). Prescribing trazodone to control aggression in nongeriatric patients with organic mental disorders has yielded mixed results in a small number of patients (Gedye 1991; Pinner and Rich 1988).

Trazodone has been reported to demonstrate antianxiety properties as well. In a study based in a general practice setting, the anxiolytic efficacy of trazodone was equal to that of chlordiazepoxide (Wheatley 1976). Another report found that trazodone has antianxiety properties in doses as low as 50 mg/day (Schwartz and Blendl 1974). Many clinicians also use low-dose trazodone as a sleep-promoting agent, especially in patients for whom benzodiazepines may be risky (e.g., patients with sleep apnea or histories of sedative hypnotic abuse). A limited number of case reports describe improvement in obsessive-compulsive disorder (OCD) and associated depression (Baxter 1985; Kim 1987; Lydiard 1986; Prasad 1984), but a double-blind placebo-controlled study found that trazodone lacked antiobsessional effects (Pigott et al. 1992). Finally, there are a handful of reports describing the use of trazodone in the treatment of bulimia nervosa, including a well-designed placebo-controlled trial in 42 women that found trazodone to be superior to placebo in reducing the frequency of episodes of binge-eating and vomiting (Hudson et al. 1989).

■ Side Effects and Toxicology

As mentioned previously, trazodone lacks the anticholinergic side effects of TCAs, making it especially useful in those situations where antimuscarinic effects would be particularly problematic (e.g., patients with prostatic hypertrophy, closed-angle glaucoma, severe constipation). Its propensity to cause sedation is a dual-edged sword. For many patients, the relief from agitation, anxiety, and insomnia can be rapid; for others, including those with considerable psychomotor retardation and with low energy, therapeutic doses of trazodone may not be tolerable because of sedation.

Trazodone elicits orthostatic hypotension in some patients, probably as a consequence of α_1-adrenergic receptor blockade. Trazodone-related syncope in elderly patients has been reported (Nambudiri et al. 1989). At therapeutic doses, it has no negative inotropic effect on the heart, and therefore no tendency to cause heart failure. However, there are case reports of cardiac arrhythmias emerging in apparent relationship to trazodone treatment, both in patients with preexisting mitral valve prolapse and in those with negative personal and family histories of cardiac disease (Janowsky et al. 1983; Lippman et al. 1983).

A relatively rare but dramatic side effect associated with trazodone is priapism. More than 200 cases have been reported (Thompson et al. 1990), and the manufacturer estimates the incidence of any abnormal erectile function to be approximately 1 in 6,000 male patients. It appears that the risk for this side effect is greatest during the first month of treatment at low doses (i.e., less than 150 mg/day). Early recognition of any abnormal erectile function, including prolonged or inappropriate erections, is important, coupled with prompt discontinuation of trazodone treatment. Also, there is a clinical report of another psychosexual side effect: three women experienced increased libido above premorbid levels in association with trazodone treatment. After resolution of their depression, two of the subjects were reluctant to discontinue the medication because of this side effect (Gatrell 1986).

As with nearly all antidepressants, mania has been observed in association with trazodone treatment. The switch to mania has been described in bipolar patients as well as in those individuals previously diagnosed as unipolar (Arana and Kaplan 1985; Knobler 1986; Lennhoff 1987; Zmitek 1987).

An important advantage that trazodone possesses in comparison with TCAs, MAOIs, and a few of the other second-generation antidepressants, is a wider therapeutic margin. It appears that trazodone is relatively safer in overdose situations, especially when it is the only agent taken. Fatalities are rare, even with large overdoses; uneventful recoveries have been reported following ingestion of doses as high as 6,000–9,200 mg (Ayd 1984). In one report, 9 of 29 overdose cases were fatal, and all 9 patients had taken other central nervous system (CNS) depressants in addition to trazodone (Gamble and Peterson 1986). When trazodone overdoses occur, clinicians should carefully monitor for hypotension, a potentially serious toxic effect.

■ Drug-Drug Interactions

Trazodone can potentiate the effects of other CNS depressants. In mice, it increases hexobarbital sleeping time (Silvestrini et al. 1968). In a single case report, phenytoin toxicity emerged with the addition of trazodone therapy (Dorn 1986). Patients should be warned about increased drowsiness and sedation when trazodone is combined with other CNS depressants, including alcohol.

In theory, the combination of trazodone with other pro-serotonergic agents could lead to the "serotonin syndrome" (Sternbach 1991). This toxic syndrome has been reported to result from the combined use of trazodone and buspirone (Goldberg and Huk 1992). Lithium potentiation of trazodone treatment has been described, however, without any mention of such toxicity (Birkhimer et al. 1983). As with other antidepressants, the combination of trazodone with an MAOI should be handled with great caution. However, there are case reports of the successful combination of trazodone with an MAOI in treatment-refractory depressed patients (Zimmer et al. 1984). As Rudorfer and Potter (1989) have pointed out, adding trazodone to ongoing MAOI treatment could enable clinicians to use it to treat MAOI-induced insomnia.

Trazodone inhibits the antihypertensive effects of

clonidine (van Zwieten 1977). For this reason, Georgotas and colleagues (1982) recommend avoiding the combined use of these two agents. On the other hand, trazodone itself can cause hypotension (especially orthostatic hypotension). In fact, the manufacturer points out in the package insert that concomitant administration of Desyrel with antihypertensive therapy may require a reduction in the dose of the antihypertensive agent.

■ AMOXAPINE

■ History and Discovery

Amoxapine (Asendin) is a dibenzoxapine tricyclic compound. It was one of the first of the second-generation antidepressants available for clinical use in the United States. Within a few years after its introduction in 1980, more than 1 million prescriptions had been filled. With the emergence of other antidepressants with different side-effect profiles, amoxapine has become less of a focus of attention.

■ Structure-Activity Relations

Amoxapine shares some structural similarities with conventional TCAs and is a dibenzoxapine derivative (see Figure 10–2). It is the N-demethylated metabolite of loxapine, a compound that was developed by the same pharmaceutical company and marketed as an antipsychotic (Loxitane). With their similar chemical structures, it is not surprising that amoxapine and

loxapine both block dopamine receptors and also share some side effects (see next subsection).

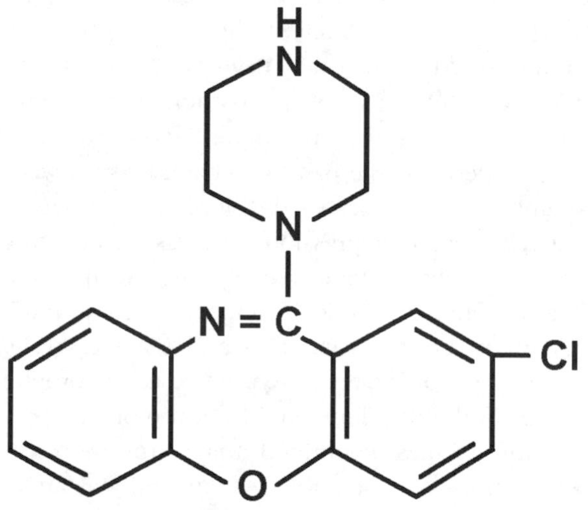

■ Pharmacological Profile

Amoxapine is a relatively potent inhibitor of norepinephrine reuptake and a weak inhibitor of serotonin reuptake. Its anticholinergic properties are similar to those of imipramine (Greenblatt et al. 1978). In addition, amoxapine (along with its active metabolites) blocks dopamine receptors, which can account for its neuroleptic-like profile.

Amoxapine demonstrates antidepressant activity in conventional animal screening tests. In addition, it also shows neuroleptic effects. Thus, it can both produce catalepsy (like conventional neuroleptics) and prevent or reverse catalepsy induced by standard neuroleptics (like conventional antidepressants) (Chermat et al. 1979).

■ Pharmacokinetics and Disposition

Amoxapine is almost completely absorbed following oral administration, with peak serum levels occurring at 1–2 hours. Its plasma half-life is approximately 8 hours. The major metabolite is 8-hydroxyamoxapine, which has a half-life of about 30 hours; 7-hydroxyamoxapine, which has a half-life of about 4 hours, is also an important metabolite because of its potent activity as a dopamine receptor blocker (Lydiard and Gelenberg 1981).

■ Mechanism of Action

Amoxapine blocks the reuptake of norepinephrine and is also a weak inhibitor of serotonin reuptake. These properties are shared by its hydroxylated metabolites (Rudorfer and Potter 1989). Both amoxapine and 7-hydroxyamoxapine block dopamine receptors, with potencies that are roughly comparable to those of the neuroleptics thioridazine and haloperidol, respectively (Rudorfer et al. 1984). This antagonism of dopaminergic neurotransmission probably accounts for amoxapine's efficacy in the treatment of psychotic depression, but it also plays a role in the various neuroleptic side effects associated with its use.

■ Indications

In double-blind controlled trials, amoxapine's efficacy in the treatment of depression is comparable to

Figure 10–2. Chemical structure for amoxapine.

that of conventional TCAs (Lydiard and Gelenberg 1981). Initial claims by the manufacturer for an earlier onset of action have failed to gain support from independent controlled trials, which show no difference in onset of clinical response with amoxapine compared with conventional TCAs (Mason et al. 1990; Prusoff et al. 1981). In fact, one study found that compared with amoxapine, amitriptyline demonstrated an earlier onset of improvement in some measures of depression and was more effective in inducing complete recovery (Mason et al. 1990). There are also reports of early relapse among amoxapine responders (Mason et al. 1990; Zetin et al. 1983).

Although dopamine receptor blockade by amoxapine and its active metabolite leads to various side effects (see next subsection), this pharmacological property can be advantageous in certain situations. For example, amoxapine is effective in the treatment of psychotic depression, which does not respond well to conventional antidepressants alone. In a double-blind study, Anton and Burch (1990) found that amoxapine was as effective as the combination of amitriptyline and perphenazine in the treatment of major depression with psychotic features. A case series described the successful treatment of psychogenic vomiting associated with depression, in which the antidopaminergic activity of amoxapine treatment probably accounted for the almost immediate cessation of vomiting (Golden et al. 1988b). However, the use of amoxapine in these clinical situations is similar to the prescription of any "fixed combination" medication, in that the physician surrenders the ability to titrate the dose or discontinue the individual components of the treatment independent of one another.

Side Effects and Toxicology

Amoxapine is associated with the usual TCA side effects, including relatively mild anticholinergic effects, mild sedation, and orthostatic hypotension. In addition, amoxapine demonstrates neuroleptic-like side effects. These include parkinsonian symptoms, akathisia, and acute dystonic reactions (Lydiard and Gelenberg 1981). Galactorrhea and amenorrhea with hyperprolactinemia have been reported (Gelenberg et al. 1979). In addition, withdrawal dyskinesia and persistent tardive dyskinesia have been reported (Huang 1986; Price and Giannini 1986; Thornton and

Stahl 1984), as has neuroleptic malignant syndrome (Taylor and Schwartz 1988).

Unfortunately, amoxapine does not appear to be any safer in overdose situations than conventional antidepressants. In a retrospective study of antidepressant overdoses, it was found to be associated with a disproportionate number of deaths and seizures (Litovitz and Troutman 1983). Another survey found that the seizure rate following amoxapine overdose was about twice that seen with maprotiline (24.5% versus 12.2%) and more than 8 times the rate following TCA overdoses (3.0%). It is striking that cardiovascular toxicity is relatively mild following amoxapine overdose. Rudorfer and Potter (1989) have pointed out that this may invalidate the usual emergency room procedure of gauging the severity of antidepressant overdose on the basis of prolongation of the QRS interval on the electrocardiogram.

Drug-Drug Interactions

Amoxapine may enhance the response to alcohol and other CNS depressants. As with other TCAs, the combined use of amoxapine with MAOIs may result in hypertensive reactions.

BUPROPION

History and Discovery

In the 1960s, a group of pharmacologists decided to search for a new antidepressant compound that was active in conventional antidepressant screening models, yet was 1) different chemically, pharmacologically, and biochemically from TCAs; 2) not an inhibitor of MAO; 3) not sympathomimetic; 4) not anticholinergic; and 5) not a cardiac depressant. It was believed that the first two characteristics would maximize the chances of developing a unique approach to treating depression, whereas the next three features would provide a compound with a side-effect profile far superior to that of existing antidepressant medications (Soroko and Maxwell 1983). The culmination of this intensive research program resulted in the development of bupropion.

Early studies confirmed that bupropion possessed efficacy comparable to conventional antidepressants but a side-effect profile that was generally viewed as milder and safer, with a notable lack of substantial anticholinergic toxicity and relatively innocuous effects on cardiovascular function. Then in 1986, just as the drug was about to be released, a small number of patients in a study of nondepressed bulimic subjects receiving bupropion were reported to have had seizures. The manufacturer voluntarily withdrew the drug pending further (and extensive) clinical investigations. Finally, in 1989, bupropion (Wellbutrin) was released for clinical use in the United States.

■ Structure-Activity Relations

Bupropion's chemical structure is unique among the antidepressants (Figure 10–3). It is a unicyclic aminoketone. The lack of complex heterocyclic fused rings, as well as the more common functional groups (e.g., N-methylpiperazine) often found in neuroleptics, is thought to contribute to bupropion's lack of the side effects usually seen in polycyclic antidepressants (Mehta 1983). Bupropion's chemical structure does resemble certain psychostimulants in some respects (including amphetamine and the diet pill diethylpropion [Tenuate]) (Mehta 1983), which may account for certain shared characteristics (Golden 1988).

■ Pharmacological Profile

Bupropion is a relative weak inhibitor of dopamine reuptake, with modest effects on norepinephrine reuptake and no effect on serotonin reuptake

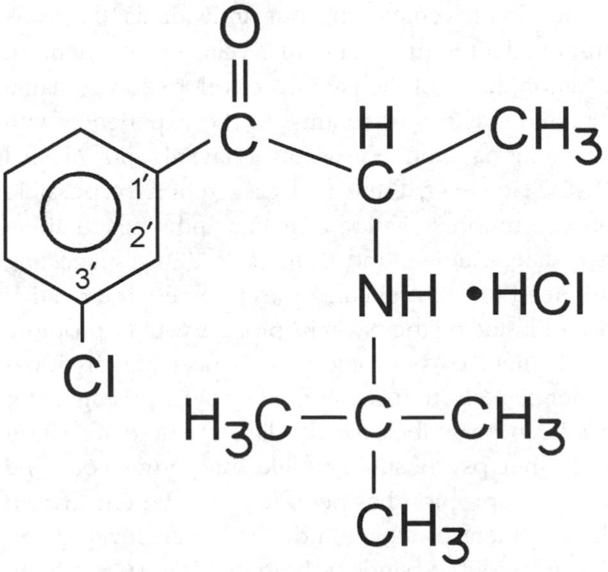

Figure 10–3. Chemical structure for bupropion.

(Richelson 1991). It does not appear to be associated with downregulation of postsynaptic β-adrenergic receptors. Also, it does not have significant effects on 5-HT$_2$, α$_2$-adrenergic, imipramine, or dopaminergic receptors in brain tissue (Ferris and Beaman 1983). It lacks anticholinergic activity and is at least 10 times weaker than TCAs in its cardiac depressant effects (Soroko and Maxwell 1983).

Bupropion is active in the classic animal models for predicting antidepressant activity (Soroko and Maxwell 1983). Furthermore, its active metabolites, especially hydroxybupropion, have been shown to possess antidepressant profiles in mice (Martin et al. 1990). This finding may be relevant to preliminary observations from human studies exploring the roles these metabolites might play in determining clinical outcome (see next subsection) (Golden 1991).

■ Pharmacokinetics and Disposition

Bupropion is rapidly absorbed following oral administration, with peak blood levels occurring within 2 hours (Lai and Schroeder 1983). Mean protein binding in healthy subjects is 85% (Findlay et al. 1981). The elimination is biphasic, with an initial phase of approximately 1.5 hours and a second phase of about 14 hours.

Bupropion undergoes extensive hepatic metabolism, including a pronounced first-pass effect. Three active metabolites—hydroxybupropion, threo-hydrobupropion, and erythro-hydrobupropion—predominate over the parent compound in both plasma and cerebrospinal fluid (CSF) at steady state and may play an important role in determining clinical response (see below) (Golden et al. 1988c).

There does not appear to be a consistent, clear relationship between steady-state bupropion plasma concentrations and clinical response (Goodnick 1991). Preskorn (1983) found a curvilinear relationship between antidepressant efficacy and trough bupropion plasma concentrations, with the greatest efficacy associated with bupropion plasma concentrations greater than 25 ng/ml but less than 100 ng/ml. On the other hand, Goodnick (1992) reported better response with trough levels less than 30 ng/ml. In another study, there was no relationship between plasma bupropion concentrations and clinical response. However, higher concentrations for each of the three active metabolites, especially hydroxybupropion, were significantly related to poor clinical outcome (Golden et al. 1988c). More clinical studies are needed to clarify the potential utility of plasma bupropion metabolite measurements in clinical care. Preskorn (1991) has proposed that bupropion be the next antidepressant to undergo aggressive study for the value of therapeutic drug monitoring.

■ Mechanism of Action

The mechanism of action for bupropion remains unclear (Ascher et al., in press). From the start, its effects on dopaminergic function have been a focus of investigation. Some of the behavioral effects of bupropion, including stimulation of locomotor activity and effects on the Porsolt forced swim test, are abolished following the destruction of dopaminergic neurons by 6-hydroxydopamine (Cooper et al. 1980). It has been shown that bupropion-induced behavioral sensitization in rats is accompanied by a selective potentiation of the effects of this compound on interstitial dopamine concentrations in the nucleus accumbens (Nomikos et al. 1992). In humans, plasma concentrations of homovanillic acid, a major metabolite of dopamine, increased in patients who failed to respond to bupropion treatment, but not in clinical responders (Golden et al. 1988d).

Noradrenergic systems may also play a critical role in the mechanism of action of bupropion. In a study investigating the effects of antidepressants on noradrenergic function in hospitalized depressed patients, bupropion (along with the norepinephrine reuptake inhibitor desipramine and MAOIs) increased 24-hour excretion of 6-hydroxymelatonin, a physiological gauge of noradrenergic activity, while simultaneously reducing "whole body norepinephrine turnover" (i.e., the 24-hour excretion of norepinephrine and its metabolites) (Golden et al. 1988e). Bupropion's active metabolites, especially hydroxybupropion, inhibit the reuptake of norepinephrine into rat cortical tissue (Perumal et al. 1986).

Bupropion's metabolites may be quite important in determining clinical response. In animal models, hydroxybupropion possesses more potent antidepressant properties than the parent compound, and threo-hydrobupropion also demonstrates some antidepressant activity (Martin et al. 1990). In depressed patients, metabolite concentrations predominate over bupropion concentrations in both plasma and CSF (Golden et al. 1988c). As was mentioned previously, there is no clear relationship between plasma bupropion concentrations and clinical response; but concentrations of its metabolites, especially hydroxybupropion, are significantly greater in nonresponders than in responders. This observation may reflect untoward effects that are evoked when hydroxybupropion concentration exceeds a threshold for toxicity. On the other hand, hydroxybupropion may be responsible for bupropion's therapeutic effects, and a curvilinear plasma level response relationship (similar to that of nortriptyline) may exist. It is clear, however, that future investigations of the mechanism of action of bupropion need to consider the role played by its active metabolites.

■ Indications

Bupropion has been shown to be as effective as standard TCAs and SSRIs (and superior to placebo) in treating hospitalized or ambulatory depressed patients (Chouinard 1983; Davidson et al. 1983; Feighner et al. 1986, 1991; Mendels et al. 1983; Merideth and Feighner 1983; Pitts et al. 1983). Under double-blind conditions, bupropion was superior to placebo in treating hospitalized patients who were refractory to TCAs. In an open-label study, outpatients with either a history of nonresponse or nonresponse plus intolerance to TCAs showed marked improvement on bupropion (Stern et al. 1983).

One report suggests that bupropion may be particularly promising in treating rapid-cycling bipolar II patients (Haykal and Akiskal 1990). In that case series, all six patients showed improvement, with "dramatic" improvement in four individuals that was sustained after an average of 2 years of treatment. In addition, none of the patients developed hypomania or rapid cycling, in contrast to the experience with conventional antidepressants (Haykal and Akiskal 1990). However, there is a case report of possible bupropion precipitation of mania and a mixed affective state (Zubieta and Demitrack 1991), suggesting the need for controlled studies to assess the relative risk of inducing the "switch" process with bupropion.

In light of bupropion's enhancement of dopaminergic neurotransmission, it is not surprising that it has been prescribed for conditions where activation and other psychostimulant-like properties could be useful. Bupropion has been found to be effective in the treatment of attention-deficit hyperactivity disorder in a double-blind study in children (Casat et al. 1989) and in an open trial in adults (Wender and

Reimherr 1990). Bupropion's activating properties have led to explorations of its potential use in the treatment of chronic fatigue syndrome (Goodnick 1990; Goodnick et al. 1992).

Uncontrolled case reports have described the use of bupropion in treating social phobia (Emmanuel et al. 1991). In a double-blind placebo-controlled trial in patients with bulimia, bupropion was superior to placebo in reducing episodes of binge-eating and purging (Horne et al. 1988). However, four subjects experienced grand mal seizures during treatment; the use of bupropion to treat patients with bulimia should therefore be avoided (Horne et al. 1988).

■ Side Effects and Toxicology

Bupropion's side-effect profile is clearly different from that of conventional TCAs. It lacks anticholinergic effects, is clearly not sedating, and suppresses appetite in some patients (Rudorfer and Potter 1989). Bupropion's cardiovascular profile is especially favorable. It does not cause electrocardiogram changes and does not trigger orthostatic hypotension, even in patients with preexisting heart disease (Roose et al. 1987). Unlike several of the other second-generation antidepressants, bupropion does not cause psychosexual dysfunction (Gardner and Johnston 1985). Bupropion appears to be relatively less lethal following overdose, compared with TCAs and certain other antidepressants (Hayes and Kristoff 1986).

Many of bupropion's side effects can be predicted, based on its stimulation of dopaminergic systems. Thus, like conventional psychostimulants, bupropion can have activating effects, which are often helpful in patients with psychomotor retardation but can be experienced as agitation or insomnia in others. Appetite suppression is also seen as an advantage in some patients but a disadvantage in others. Psychotic symptoms, including hallucinations and delusions, can emerge in association with bupropion treatment (Golden et al. 1985). Since the initial description of bupropion-related psychoses, numerous case reports have described similar toxic reactions, including organic mental disorders (Ames et al. 1992), delirium (Dager and Heritch 1990), and catatonia (Jackson et al. 1992). These psychotic reactions may be a consequence of overstimulation of dopaminergic systems—one series of patients with bupropion-associated psychoses had increased plasma concentrations of homovanillic acid, a major metabolite of dopamine (Golden et al. 1985).

A rare but serious side effect of bupropion is seizure induction. A careful review by Davidson (1989) found the incidence of seizures in patients receiving bupropion at doses of 450 mg/day or less ranged from 0.33%–0.44%, depending on the method used in making the calculation. The cumulative 2-year risk in patients receiving 450 mg/day or less was 0.48%. To place these observations in the proper context, clinicians should be aware that the estimated frequency of seizures in outpatients with no predisposing factors who are receiving TCAs in modest doses (e.g., 150 mg/day or less) is 0.1% (Jick et al. 1983); at higher doses (e.g., 200 mg/day or greater), it rises to 0.6%–0.9% (Peck et al. 1983). Careful evaluation for risk factors (e.g., history of seizures, recent withdrawal from alcohol or anxiolytic drugs, concomitant therapy with other drugs that lower the seizure threshold, history of organic brain disease or abnormal electroencephalogram), conservative dose titration with a maximum dose of 450 mg/day, and use of divided (tid) dose schedules should minimize the risk for bupropion-related seizures (Davidson 1989).

■ Drug-Drug Interactions

Because bupropion undergoes extensive hepatic transformation, other drugs that induce or inhibit hepatic enzyme systems may alter its metabolism. As with most antidepressants, the combined use of bupropion with MAOIs should be approached with caution, considering the risk of a hypertensive reaction if bupropion is added to ongoing MAO inhibition. Recognizing the dopaminergic activation that bupropion provides, clinicians treating patients with both Parkinson's disease and depression can often decrease the dose of antiparkinsonian medication when bupropion is added. The combination of bupropion and antiparkinsonian medication should be administered with care. Goetz and colleagues (1984) reported the emergence of hallucinations, confusion, and dyskinesia following the addition of bupropion to previously therapeutic doses of L-dopa.

The addition of bupropion to fluoxetine treatment has coincided with the onset of delirium (Van Putten and Shaffer 1990) and a grand mal seizure (Ciraulo and Shader 1990). The combination of lithium and bupropion may affect lithium serum levels and has been linked to seizures in three patients (Goodnick 1991), although this combination has been generally safe and well tolerated in subjects in a small number of published studies (Apter and Woolfolk 1990; Goodnick, in press; Haykal and Akiskal 1990).

VENLAFAXINE

History and Discovery

Venlafaxine is a novel bicyclic compound that is chemically unrelated to the TCAs. Recognizing that TCAs displace [³H]imipramine from rat cortical binding sites with potencies paralleling their abilities to inhibit serotonin uptake, a group of pharmacologists decided to search for other MAOIs among novel compounds based on their capacity to inhibit [³H]imipramine binding in rat cortical membranes. Venlafaxine was thus identified as an interesting new compound. In preclinical studies, it demonstrated a neurochemical profile predictive of antidepressant activity, but with fewer side effects and perhaps a more rapid onset of action than the first-generation antidepressants (Muth et al. 1986). Further preclinical studies suggested that venlafaxine had in vivo antidepressant effects similar to those of the TCAs (Mitchell and Fletcher 1993). Clinical trials confirmed antidepressant efficacy and a relatively mild side-effect profile. Venlafaxine (Effexor) was released for clinical use in the United States in the spring of 1994.

Structure-Activity Relations

Venlafaxine is a bicyclic compound (Figure 10–4). It is chemically unrelated to any of the currently available antidepressants, including the heterocyclics and the SSRIs.

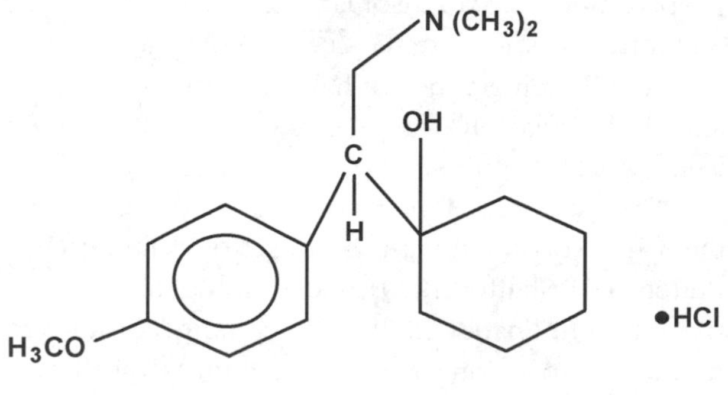

Figure 10–4. Chemical structure for venlafaxine.

Pharmacological Profile

In vitro studies have demonstrated that venlafaxine and its active metabolite O-desmethylvenlafaxine (ODV) inhibit the neuronal reuptake of serotonin, norepinephrine, and (to a lesser extent) dopamine (Bolden-Watson and Richelson 1993; Muth et al. 1986). Unlike TCAs, venlafaxine and ODV do not have substantial affinity for muscarinic, histamine-1, or α_1-adrenergic receptors. In addition, they do not inhibit MAO-A or MAO-B (Muth et al. 1986). Venlafaxine has been shown to possess antidepressant-like activity in classic animal models of antidepressant activity (Mitchell and Fletcher 1993).

Pharmacokinetics and Disposition

Venlafaxine is well absorbed from the gastrointestinal tract following oral administration and undergoes extensive first-pass metabolism in the liver to its active metabolite, ODV. Protein binding is only 27% for venlafaxine and 30% for ODV, suggesting that drug-drug interactions based on protein binding are unlikely (D. L. Albano, Wyeth Laboratories, unpublished data, April 1994). Venlafaxine and ODV display linear kinetics over the dosage range of 25–150 mg q 8 hours. Venlafaxine's elimination half-life is 4 hours and ODV's is 10 hours, shorter than those of standard TCAs (Klamerus et al. 1992). Consequently, venlafaxine should be given in divided doses to maintain acceptable plasma concentrations. There are no currently published studies examining the relationship between plasma concentrations of the parent compound and/or active metabolite and clinical response.

Mechanism of Action

The mechanism of action of venlafaxine remains unclear. The ability of venlafaxine and its active metabolite ODV to inhibit reuptake of norepinephrine and serotonin suggests that the mechanism may be similar to that of the tertiary amine TCAs. The relevance of the relatively weak inhibition of dopamine reuptake to antidepressant activity is uncertain.

Indications

Venlafaxine is approved by the U.S. Food and Drug Administration (FDA) for treatment of depression and has been shown to be effective in several acute placebo-controlled trials (D. L. Albano, Wyeth Laboratories, unpublished data, April 1994; Khan et al. 1991; Mendels et al. 1993; Schweizer et al. 1991). It has also been shown to have similar efficacy when compared with other approved antidepressants, including trazodone, fluoxetine, imipramine, and maprotiline (D. L. Albano, Wyeth Laboratories, unpublished data, April 1994; Schweizer et al. 1994).

Often, as a consequence of expanded clinical investigations, additional clinical indications for a new psychotropic medication are identified after its release. Currently there is only one published report regarding venlafaxine's use in the treatment of a condition other than depression. In that case report, a patient's OCD responded to treatment with venlafaxine. Interestingly, the depressive symptoms of this patient, who had coexistent major depression, did not improve (Zajecka et al. 1990). We anticipate additional case reports (and controlled clinical trials) examining the use of venlafaxine in the treatment of other psychiatric disorders in the near future.

■ Side Effects and Toxicology

Venlafaxine has a side-effect profile that is different from that of the TCAs and can be understood from the perspective of its neurochemical profile. Its lack of affinity for muscarinic, histamine-1, or α_1-adrenergic receptors results in a side-effect profile that is relatively mild in terms of anticholinergic side effects, sedation, and orthostatic hypotension. In controlled clinical trials, the most common side effects, which appeared in at least 5% of patients treated with venlafaxine but less than half as many placebo-treated patients, were asthenia, sweating, nausea, constipation, anorexia, vomiting, somnolence, dry mouth, dizziness, nervousness, anxiety, tremor, blurred vision, and abnormal ejaculation or orgasm and impotence in men (D. L. Albano, Wyeth Laboratories, unpublished data, April 1994). Several adverse effects of venlafaxine appear to be dose related, including nausea, diastolic hypertension, sexual dysfunction (abnormal ejaculation or orgasm), somnolence, and sweating (D. L. Albano, Wyeth Laboratories, unpublished data, April 1994; Mendels et al. 1993; Schweizer et al. 1991). Nausea and dizziness tend to diminish with continued therapy (Mendels et al. 1993).

There have been 14 reports of intentional overdose of venlafaxine taken either alone or in combination with other substances. In all cases, the amount of venlafaxine taken was only several times the standard daily dose. All 14 patients recovered without sequelae (D. L. Albano, Wyeth Laboratories, unpublished data, April 1994).

■ Drug-Drug Interactions

Venlafaxine undergoes extensive hepatic metabolism by the cytochrome $P_{450}IID6$ isoenzyme. Therefore, there is potential for an interaction between any drug that inhibits the cytochrome $P_{450}IID6$ isoenzyme and venlafaxine. Venlafaxine is not extensively protein bound, so displacement of a highly bound drug by this medication should not be a major concern.

Cimetidine can inhibit the first-pass hepatic metabolism of venlafaxine. However, cimetidine increased the overall pharmacological activity of venlafaxine and ODV only slightly, and a dosage adjustment is probably not necessary (data on file with Wyeth Laboratories).

There are limited data regarding the use of venlafaxine with other CNS active drugs, so caution should be used when combined therapies are planned. In a study of 12 healthy volunteer subjects, venlafaxine and lithium did not seem to interact with one another (D. L. Albano, Wyeth Laboratories, unpublished data, April 1994). Also, in healthy volunteers, there were no significant drug-drug interactions between venlafaxine and diazepam (D. L. Albano, Wyeth Laboratories, unpublished data, April 1994). Venlafaxine should not be used in combination with an MAOI because of the possibility of a hypertensive crisis or a "serotonin-like syndrome."

■ NEFAZODONE

■ History and Discovery

Nefazodone (Serzone) is a new antidepressant that has selective and unique effects on the 5-HT system. Its analogue trazodone was found to be an effective second-generation antidepressant but was very sedating and had a propensity to cause postural hypotension (see previous discussion). A deliberate synthetic effort to improve the pharmacological profile of trazodone using receptor-binding techniques led to the discovery of nefazodone (Taylor et al. 1986). It recently received FDA approval for the treatment of major depression, with anticipated availability for clinical use in the United States in late 1994.

■ Structure-Activity Relations

Nefazodone is a phenylpiperazine compound (Figure 10–5). It is similar in structure to trazodone (Figure 10–1).

■ Pharmacological Profile

In vitro studies have shown that nefazodone is a 5-HT$_2$ receptor antagonist but displays little affinity for α_2-, β-adrenergic, or 5-HT$_{1A}$ receptors (Eison et al. 1990). Nefazodone exhibits modest inhibition of 5-HT reuptake (with similar potency to trazodone) and norepinephrine reuptake (Taylor et al. 1986). Its affinity for the α_1-adrenergic receptor is less than that of trazodone (Eison et al. 1990). Nefazodone is inactive at most other receptor binding sites, including muscarinic, histamine-1, dopamine, benzodiazepine, γ-aminobutyric acid (GABA), μ-opiate, and calcium channel receptors (Taylor et al. 1986).

Nefazodone has two active metabolites, hydroxynefazodone and m-CPP. Hydroxynefazodone exhibits similar affinities for 5-HT$_2$ receptors and 5-HT reuptake sites compared with nefazodone, whereas m-CPP displays modest activity at 5-HT reuptake sites (Eison et al. 1990).

Nefazodone displays activity in animal models suggestive of antidepressant activity. For example, it prevents reserpine-induced ptosis in mice and reverses learned helplessness in rats (Eison et al. 1990).

■ Pharmacokinetics and Disposition

Nefazodone is rapidly and completely absorbed from the gastrointestinal tract and has an absolute bioavailability of 15%–23% because of extensive first-pass hepatic metabolism. Peak plasma levels occur between 1–3 hours, and steady state is achieved in 3–4 days with a bid dosing regimen. Nefazodone is

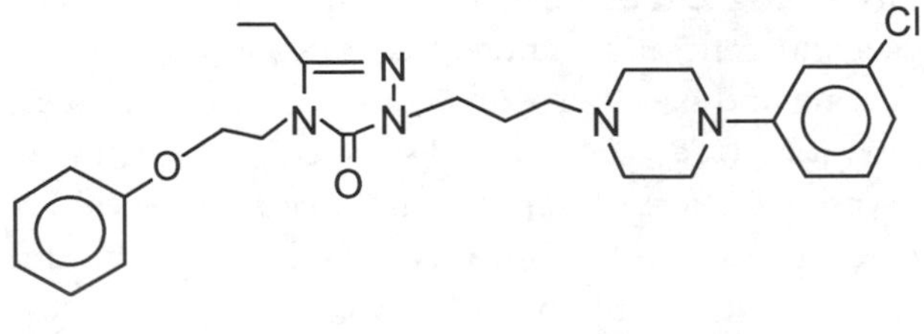

Figure 10–5. Chemical structure for nefazodone.

metabolized primarily by the liver to three metabolites: hydroxynefazodone, desmethyl-hydroxynefazodone (triazole dione), and m-CPP (only 3% of the parent compound at peak concentrations). Nefazodone exhibits nonlinear kinetics, which result in mean plasma concentrations that are greater than proportional with higher doses. Similar kinetics for nefazodone and hydroxynefazodone are seen in poor and extensive metabolizers, whereas m-CPP is eliminated more slowly by poor metabolizers. The elimination half-life is 2–4 hours for the parent compound and hydroxynefazodone, 18–33 hours for desmethyl-hydroxynefazodone, and 4–9 hours for m-CPP. Nefazodone is extensively (99%) but loosely protein bound. It does not displace chlorpromazine, desipramine, diazepam, phenytoin, lidocaine, prazosin, propranolol, verapamil, or warfarin (J. R. Ieni, Bristol-Myers Squibb Pharmaceutical Research Institute, unpublished data, June 1994).

■ Mechanism of Action

The most likely means through which nefazodone acts as an antidepressant is through its effects on serotonin neurotransmission, although these effects are complex. Nefazodone blocks serotonin reuptake, thereby increasing serotonin availability in the synapse while at the same time functioning as a 5-HT$_2$ receptor antagonist. In addition, m-CPP, nefazodone's active metabolite, functions as a serotonin agonist. In animal studies, long-term exposure to nefazodone increases the intensity of reciprocal forepaw treading induced by the 5-HT$_{1A}$ agonist 8-hydroxy-2-(di-N-propylamino)-tetralin, suggesting that nefazodone also enhances stimulation of 5-HT$_{1A}$ receptors (Eison et al. 1990). Nefazodone demonstrates effects on electrophysiological measures of serotonergic systems similar to those of many other effective antidepressants (Blier et al. 1990).

■ Indications

Nefazodone has been shown to be an effective antidepressant in eight double-blind placebo-controlled trials. There is a 72% response rate in patients meeting DSM-III-R criteria (American Psychiatric Association 1987) for major depression when treated with nefazodone at doses of 300–500 mg/day. The response rate drops to 56% with doses of 200–300 mg/day and 48% at a dose of 600 mg/day. Placebo response rates did not differ significantly from those of the low- or high-dose ranges (J. R. Ieni, Bristol-Myers Squibb Pharmaceutical Research Institute, unpublished data, June 1994). These findings suggest that nefazodone may have a therapeutic window similar to that of nortriptyline. Nefazodone has been shown to be effective in both first-episode and recurrent major depression, and several studies have shown that its efficacy is comparable to imipramine's (Feighner et al. 1989; Fontaine et al., in press).

At this point, published data regarding the use of nefazodone in the treatment of psychiatric disorders other than depression are quite limited. There is one open-label report describing nefazodone's efficacy in the treatment of late luteal phase dysphoric disorder (Freeman et al. 1994). Nefazodone has also been shown to have some analgesic properties and to potentiate morphine analgesia in animal studies, suggesting that it may have a role in pain management (Pick et al. 1992).

■ Side Effects and Toxicology

Nefazodone has been found to be safe and well tolerated in clinical trials that included approximately 2,250 patients (Fontaine 1993). It has a relatively benign side-effect profile. This is as expected given its lack of affinity for muscarinic and histaminic receptors. Its lower affinity (compared with trazodone) for α_1-adrenergic receptors suggests that it should have a lower propensity to cause orthostatic hypotension. Side effects that occur more frequently in patients who receive nefazodone compared with those receiving placebo include dizziness, asthenia, dry mouth, nausea, and constipation (Fontaine 1993). To place these observations into a clinical perspective, many of these side effects (i.e., dry mouth, constipation, sweating, and tremor) occur less often with nefazodone than with imipramine treatment. Also, there was no evidence of cardiac dysfunction or cardiotoxicity in a careful review of more than 2,000 patients. Nefazodone produced a modest reduction in resting pulse and supine blood pressure, but orthostatic hypotension was rare (Fontaine 1993).

There have been two suicide attempts by overdose with nefazodone. One person took 3,400 mg and another took 3,600 mg. Life-threatening symptoms did not occur, and both patients recovered without any sequelae (Fontaine 1993).

■ Drug-Drug Interactions

At this point, clinical experience with nefazodone has been limited; consequently, so has the opportunity for observing its interactions with other medications. In phase II and III trials, there were some changes in the kinetics of alprazolam and triazolam, but not nefazodone, when these medications were given together. There were also some small increases in the plasma concentration of digoxin with concurrent nefazodone administration. Although the observed increases in plasma digoxin concentrations were modest, the combined administration of the two drugs should be avoided in light of the narrow therapeutic index for digoxin. No significant pharmacokinetic or pharmacodynamic interactions were noted between nefazodone and cimetidine, propranolol, warfarin, or lorazepam (J. R. Ieni, Bristol-Myers Squibb Pharmaceutical Research Institute, unpublished data, June 1994).

■ OTHER AGENTS: PAST AND FUTURE

Nomifensine is a tetrahydroisoquinoline compound that inhibits the reuptake of dopamine and norepinephrine. It became available for clinical use in the United States in July 1985. It was abruptly withdrawn a few months later because of reports of relatively rare but extremely severe hemolytic anemias, which were thought to be a consequence of hypersensitivity reactions to the drug (Salama and Mueller-Eckhardt 1985).

Alprazolam is a widely prescribed anxiolytic agent that also appears to have antidepressant properties. At relatively higher doses, similar to those used in the treatment of panic disorder, alprazolam has generally been found to be as effective as TCAs and superior to placebo in several controlled studies (Warner et al. 1988). Its side-effect profile (including sedation, minimal cardiovascular effects, and lack of anticholinergic activity) is advantageous for some patients. However, the propensity for potentially severe withdrawal reactions following abrupt discontinuation needs to be considered and carefully discussed with patients (Golden et al. 1988a). With its patent due to expire in the near future, it appears unlikely that the additional studies necessary for FDA approval of alprazolam as an antidepressant will be completed. However, a related high-potency triazolobenzodiazepine, adinazolam, is currently in development as a potential antidepressant. Several double-blind studies have found its efficacy to be superior to placebo and comparable to that of conventional TCAs (Amsterdam et al. 1986; Feighner 1986; Smith and Glaudin 1986).

Gepirone is structurally related to buspirone, the nonbenzodiazepine anxiolytic. Like buspirone, gepirone is a potent 5-HT_{1A} agonist, but it has relatively less affinity for dopamine receptors (McMillen et al. 1987). Preliminary studies suggest that gepirone possesses antidepressant as well as antianxiety properties (Rausch et al. 1990).

Idazoxan is a selective α_2 receptor antagonist that should theoretically increase norepinephrine release through blockade of presynaptic negative feedback mechanisms. In a small number of severely ill, treatment-refractory patients, idazoxan produced sustained and substantial improvement while increasing plasma and CSF norepinephrine concentrations (Osman et al. 1989).

S-adenosylmethionine, an endogenous methyl donor, may enhance neurotransmitter synthesis. Several open studies have described rapid antidepressant effects following intravenous administration of S-adenosylmethionine (Carney et al. 1986; Lipinski et al. 1984). A small number of double-blind controlled studies conducted in Europe have described rapid onset of antidepressant activity with minimal side effects (Kufferle and Grunberger 1982; Muscettola et al. 1982). The development of an orally administered formulation should expedite further investigation of S-adenosylmethionine's potential as an antidepressant treatment. In an open study, the oral preparation was effective and well tolerated (Rosenbaum et al. 1990).

■ CONCLUSION

We have reviewed the pharmacological properties of several diverse antidepressants not readily cataloged within the conventional classifications of antidepressants. In addition, we have mentioned several other compounds that have been used in the past or are currently undergoing investigation as potential new antidepressants. What common themes or messages emerge from this diverse group of pharmacological agents?

One clear lesson to be learned involves our limited ability to recognize rare but potentially serious side effects in new agents before their widespread use. The most dramatic example of this in the United States is the experience with nomifensine, which was withdrawn from clinical use a few months after its introduction because of potentially fatal hematological toxicity. Similar experiences have occurred with other new agents, in which rare side effects are recognized only after the drug is widely prescribed (e.g., priapism with trazodone).

Another important theme that emerges from our review is the important advantage that an understanding of a drug's basic pharmacology provides for clinicians. Many side effects can be understood, or even predicted, based on the pharmacological profiles of the newer agents. Thus, trazodone's propensity to evoke orthostatic hypotension makes sense in light of its effects on α-adrenergic receptors, and many of the side effects associated with bupropion and amoxapine could be anticipated based on the effects that these compounds have on dopaminergic neurotransmission.

The importance of active metabolites in mediating therapeutic and/or toxic effects is underscored by each of the drugs reviewed here. Both therapeutic and toxic effects may be related as much to metabolites as to the parent compound. Careful consideration of new agents must include appropriate attention to active metabolites.

Finally, each novel antidepressant adds to our available tools for the treatment of depression. Although we do not have a "perfect" antidepressant therapy that is safe and effective for all patients, the new compounds with their varied side-effect profiles give us greater flexibility in selecting the best available approach for each patient.

■ REFERENCES

American Psychiatric Association: Diagnostic and Statistical Manual of Mental Disorders, 3rd Edition, Revised. Washington, DC, American Psychiatric Association, 1987

Ames D, Wirshing WC, Szuba MP: Organic mental disorders associated with bupropion in three patients. J Clin Psychiatry 53:53–55, 1992

Amsterdam JD, Kaplan M, Potter L, et al: Adinazolam, a new triazolobenzodiazepine, and imipramine in the treatment of major depressive disorder. Psychopharmacology 88:484–488, 1986

Anton RF, Burch EA Jr: Amoxapine versus amitriptyline combined with perphenazine in the treatment of psychotic depression. Am J Psychiatry 147:1203–1208, 1990

Apter JT, Woolfolk RL: Lithium augmentation of bupropion in refractory depression. Annals of Clinical Psychiatry 2:7–10, 1990

Arana GW, Kaplan GB: Trazodone-induced mania following desipramine-induced mania in major depressive disorders. Am J Psychiatry 142:386, 1985

Ascher J, Martin P, Colin J, et al: Bupropion's mechanism of antidepressant action: a review. J Clin Psychiatry (in press)

Ayd FJ Jr: Pharmacology update: which antidepressant to choose, II: the overdose factor. Psychiatric Annals 14:212–214, 1984

Baxter LR Jr: Two cases of obsessive-compulsive disorder with depression responsive to trazodone. J Nerv Ment Dis 173:423–433, 1985

Birkhimer LJ, Alderman AA, Schmitt CE, et al: Combined trazodone-lithium therapy for refractory depression [letter]. Am J Psychiatry 140:1382–1383, 1983

Blier P, de Montigny C, Chaput Y: A role for the serotonin system in the mechanism of action of antidepressant treatments: preclinical evidence. J Clin Psychiatry 51 (suppl 4):14–20, 1990

Bolden-Watson C, Richelson E: Blockade by newly developed antidepressants of biogenic amine uptake into rat brain synaptosomes. Life Sci 52:1023–1029, 1993

Boschmans SA, Perkin MF, Terblanche SE: Antidepressant drugs: imipramine, mianserin and trazodone. Comp Biochem Physiol [C] 86:225–232, 1987

Brogden RN, Heel RC, Speight TM, et al: Trazodone: a review of its pharmacological properties and therapeutic uses in depression and anxiety. Drugs 21:401–429, 1981

Caccia S, Ballabio M, Fanelli R, et al: Determination of plasma and brain concentrations of trazodone and its metabolite, 1-m-chlorophenylpiperazine, by gas-liquid chromatography. J Chromatogr 210:311–318, 1981

Carney MWP, Edeh J, Bottiglieri T, et al: Affective illness and S-adenosylmethionine: a preliminary report. Clin Neuropharmacol 9:379–385, 1986

Casat CD, Pleasants DZ, Schroeder DH, et al: Bupropion in children with attention deficit disorder. Psychopharmacol Bull 25:198–201, 1989

Chermat R, Simon P, Bossier JR: Amoxapine in experimental psychopharmacology: a neuroleptic or an antidepressant? Arzneimittelforschung 29:814–820, 1979

Chouinard G: Bupropion and amitriptyline in the treatment of depressed patients. J Clin Psychiatry 44:121–129, 1983

Ciraulo DA, Shader RI: Fluoxetine drug-drug interactions II. J Clin Psychopharmacol 10:213–217, 1990

Cohen ML, Fuller RW, Kurz KD: Evidence that blood pressure reduction by serotonin antagonists is related to a receptor blockade in spontaneously hypertensive rats. Hypertension 5:676–681, 1983

Cooper BR, Hester TJ, Maxwell RA: Behavioral and biochemical effects of the antidepressant bupropion (Wellbutrin): evidence for selective blockade of dopamine uptake in vivo. J Pharmacol Exp Ther 215:127–134, 1980

Dager SR, Heritch AJ: A case of bupropion-associated delirium. J Clin Psychiatry 51:307–308, 1990

Davidson J: Seizures and bupropion: a review. J Clin Psychiatry 50:256–261, 1989

Davidson J, Miller R, Fleet JVW, et al: A double-blind comparison of bupropion and amitriptyline in depressed patients. J Clin Psychiatry 44:115–117, 1983

Dorn JM: A case of phenytoin toxicity possibly precipitated by trazodone. J Clin Psychiatry 47:89–90, 1986

Eison AS, Eison MS, Torrente JR, et al: Nefazodone: preclinical pharmacology of a new antidepressant. Psychopharmacol Bull 26:311–315, 1990

Emmanuel NP, Lydiard RB, Ballenger JC: Treatment of social phobia with bupropion [letter]. J Clin Psychopharmacol 11:276–277, 1991

Feighner JP: A review of controlled studies of adinazolam mesylate in patients with major depressive disorder. Psychopharmacol Bull 22:186–191, 1986

Feighner J, Hendrickson G, Miller L, et al: Double-blind comparison of doxepin versus bupropion in outpatients with a major depressive disorder. J Clin Psychopharmacol 6:27–32, 1986

Feighner JP, Pambakian R, Fowler RC, et al: A comparison of nefazodone, imipramine, and placebo in patients with moderate to severe depression. Psychopharmacol Bull 25:219–221, 1989

Feighner JP, Gardner EA, Johnston JA, et al: Double-blind comparison of bupropion and fluoxetine in depressed outpatients. J Clin Psychiatry 52:329–335, 1991

Ferris RM, Beaman OJ: Bupropion: a new antidepressant drug, the mechanism of action of which is not associated with down-regulation of postsynaptic β-adrenergic, serotonergic (5-HT$_2$), α$_2$-adrenergic, imipramine and dopaminergic receptors in brain. Neuropharmacology 22:1257–1267, 1983

Findlay JWA, Van Wyck Fleet J, Smith PG, et al: Pharmacokinetics of bupropion, a novel antidepressant agent, following oral administration to healthy subjects. Eur J Clin Pharmacol 21:127–135, 1981

Fontaine R: Novel serotonergic mechanisms and clinical experience with nefazodone. Clin Neuropharmacol 16 (suppl 3):S45–S50, 1993

Fontaine R, Ontiveros A, Elie R, et al: A double-blind comparison of nefazodone, imipramine, and placebo in major depression. J Clin Psychiatry (in press)

Freeman EW, Rickels K, Sondheimer SJ, et al: Nefazodone in the treatment of premenstrual syndrome: a preliminary study. J Clin Psychopharmacol 14:180–186, 1994

Gamble DE, Peterson LG: Trazodone overdose: four years of experience from voluntary reports. J Clin Psychiatry 47:544–546, 1986

Garattini S: Biochemical studies with trazodone, in Trazodone: Modern Problems of Pharmacopsychiatry, Vol 9. Edited by Ban TA, Silvestrini B. Basel, Karger, 1974, pp 29–46

Gardner EA, Johnston A: Bupropion: an antidepressant without sexual pathophysiological action. J Clin Psychopharmacol 5:24–29, 1985

Gatrell N: Increased libido in women receiving trazodone. Am J Psychiatry 143:781–782, 1986

Gedye A: Serotonergic treatment for aggression in a Down's syndrome adult showing signs of Alzheimer's disease. Journal of Mental Deficiency Research 35:247–258, 1991

Gelenberg AJ, Cooper DS, Doller JC, et al: Galactorrhea and hyperprolactinemia associated with amoxapine therapy: report of a case. JAMA 242:1900–1901, 1979

Georgotas A, Forsell TL, Mann JJ, et al: Trazodone hydrochloride: a wide spectrum antidepressant with a unique pharmacological profile. Pharmacotherapy 2:255–265, 1982

Gerner RH: Geriatric depression and treatment with trazodone. Psychopathology 20:82–91, 1987

Goetz CG, Tanner CM, Klawans HL: Bupropion in Parkinson's disease. Neurology 34:1092–1094, 1984

Goldberg RJ, Huk M: Serotonin syndrome from trazodone and buspirone [letter]. Psychosomatics 33:235–236, 1992

Golden RN: Diethylpropion, bupropion, and psychoses [letter]. Br J Psychiatry 153:265–266, 1988

Golden RN: Antidepressant profile of bupropion and three metabolites: clinical and pre-clinical studies [letter]. Pharmacopsychiatry 24:68, 1991

Golden RN, James S, Sherer M, et al: Psychoses associated with bupropion treatment. Am J Psychiatry 142:1459–1462, 1985

Golden RN, Brown DO, Miller H, et al: The new antidepressants. N C Med J 49:549–554, 1988a

Golden RN, Janke I, Haggerty JJ Jr: Amoxapine treatment of psychogenic vomiting and depression. Psychosomatics 29:354, 1988b

Golden RN, DeVane L, Laizure SC, et al: Bupropion in depression: the role of metabolites in clinical outcome. Arch Gen Psychiatry 45:145–149, 1988c

Golden RN, Rudorfer MV, Sherer M, et al: Bupropion in depression: biochemical effects and clinical response. Arch Gen Psychiatry 45:139–143, 1988d

Golden RN, Markey SP, Risby ED, et al: Antidepressants reduce whole-body norepinephrine turnover while enhancing 6-hydroxymelatonin output. Arch Gen Psychiatry 45:150–154, 1988e

Goodnick PJ: Bupropion in chronic fatigue syndrome [letter]. Am J Psychiatry 147:1091, 1990

Goodnick PJ: Pharmacokinetics of second generation antidepressants: bupropion. Psychopharmacol Bull 27:513–519, 1991

Goodnick PJ: Blood levels and acute response to bupropion. Am J Psychiatry 149:399–400, 1992

Goodnick PJ: Adjunctive lithium treatment with bupropion and fluoxetine: a naturalistic report. Lithium (in press)

Goodnick PJ, Sandoval R, Brickman A, et al: Bupropion treatment of fluoxetine-resistant chronic fatigue syndrome. Biol Psychiatry 32:834–838, 1992

Greenblatt EN, Lippa AS, Osterberg AC: The neuropharmacological actions of amoxapine. Arch Int Pharmacodyn Ther 233:107–135, 1978

Greenwald BS, Marin DB, Silverman SM: Serotonergic treatment of screaming and banging in dementia. Lancet 2:1464–1465, 1986

Hayes PE, Kristoff CA: Adverse reactions to five new antidepressants. Clin Pharm 5:471–480, 1986

Haykal RF, Akiskal HS: Bupropion as a promising approach to rapid cycling bipolar II patients. J Clin Psychiatry 51:450–455, 1990

Horne RL, Ferguson JM, Pope HG Jr, et al: Treatment of bulimia with bupropion: a multicenter controlled trial. J Clin Psychiatry 49:262–266, 1988

Huang CC: Persistent tardive dyskinesia associated with amoxapine therapy. Am J Psychiatry 143:1069–1070, 1986

Hudson JI, Pope HG Jr, Keck PE Jr, et al: Treatment of bulimia nervosa with trazodone: short-term response and long-term follow-up. Clin Neuropharmacol 12 (suppl 1):38–46, 1989

Hyttel J: Citalopram-pharmacologic profile of a specific serotonin uptake inhibitor with antidepressant activity. Prog Neuropsychopharmacol Biol Psychiatry 6:277–295, 1982

Jackson CW, Head LA, Kellner CH: Catatonia associated with bupropion treatment [letter]. J Clin Psychiatry 53:210, 1992

Janowsky D, Curtis G, Zisook S, et al: Ventricular arrhythmias possibly aggravated by trazodone. Am J Psychiatry 140:796–797, 1983

Jick H, Binan B, Hunter JR, et al: Tricyclic antidepressants and convulsions. J Clin Psychopharmacol 3:128–185, 1983

Khan A, Fabre LF, Rudolphe R: Venlafaxine in depressed outpatients. Psychopharmacol Bull 27:141–144, 1991

Kim SW: Trazodone in the treatment of obsessive-compulsive disorder: a case report. J Clin Psychopharmacol 7:278–279, 1987

Klamerus KJ, Maloney K, Rudolph RL, et al: Introduction of a composite parameter to the pharmacokinetics of venlafaxine and its active O-desmethyl metabolite. J Clin Pharmacol 32:716–724, 1992

Klein HE, Muller N: Trazodone in endogenous depressed patients: a negative report and a critical evaluation of the pertaining literature. Prog Neuropsychopharmacol Biol Psychiatry 9:173–186, 1985

Knobler H: Trazodone-induced mania. Br J Psychiatry 149:787–789, 1986

Kufferle B, Grunberger J: Early clinical double-blind study with S-adenosyl-l-methionine: a new potential antidepressant, in Typical and Atypical Antidepressants: Clinical Practice. Edited by Costa E, Racagni G. New York, Raven, 1982, pp 175–177

Lader M: Recent experience with trazodone. Psycho-

pathology 20 (suppl 1):39–47, 1987

Lai AA, Schroeder DH: Clinical pharmacokinetics of bupropion: a review. J Clin Psychiatry 44:82–84, 1983

Lennhoff M: Trazodone-induced mania. J Clin Psychiatry 48:423–424, 1987

Lipinski JF, Cohen BM, Frankenburg F, et al: Open trial of S-adenosylmethionine for treatment of depression. Am J Psychiatry 141:448–450, 1984

Lippman S, Bedford P, Manshadi M, et al: Trazodone cardiotoxicity. Am J Psychiatry 140:1383, 1983

Litovitz TL, Troutman WG: Amoxapine overdose: seizures and fatalities. JAMA 250:1069–1071, 1983

Lydiard RB: Obsessive-compulsive disorder successfully treated with trazodone. Psychosomatics 27:858–859, 1986

Lydiard RB, Gelenberg AJ: Amoxapine-an antidepressant with some neuroleptic properties? Pharmacotherapy 1:163–178, 1981

Martin P, Massol J, Colin JN, et al: Antidepressant profile of bupropion and three metabolites in mice. Pharmacopsychiatry 23:187–194, 1990

Mason BJ, Kocsis JH, Frances AJ, et al: Amoxapine versus amitriptyline for continuation therapy of depression. J Clin Psychopharmacol 10:338–343, 1990

McMillen BA, Scott SM, Williams HL, et al: Effects of gepirone, an arylpiperazine anxiolytic drug, on aggressive behavior and brain monoaminergic neurotransmission. Naunyn Schmiedebergs Arch Pharmacol 335:454–464, 1987

Mehta NB: The chemistry of bupropion. J Clin Psychiatry 44:56–59, 1983

Mendels J, Amin MM, Chouinard G, et al: A comparative study of bupropion and amitriptyline in depressed outpatients. J Clin Psychiatry 44:118–120, 1983

Mendels J, Johnson R, Mattes J, et al: Efficacy and safety of b.i.d. doses of venlafaxine in a dose response study. Psychopharmacol Bull 29:169–174, 1993

Merideth CH, Feighner JP: The use of bupropion in hospitalized depressed patients. J Clin Psychiatry 44:85–87, 1983

Mitchell PJ, Fletcher A: Venlafaxine exhibits pre-clinical antidepressant activity in the resident-intruder social interaction paradigm. Neuropsychopharmacology 32:1001–1009, 1993

Monteleone P, Gnocchi G: Evidence for a linear relationship between plasma trazodone levels and clinical response in depression in the elderly. Clin Neuropharmacol 13 (suppl 1):84–89, 1990

Muscettola G, Galzenati M, Balbi A: SAMe versus placebo: a double-blind comparison in major depressive disorder, in Typical and Atypical Antidepressants: Clinical Practice. Edited by Costa E, Racagni G. New York, Raven, 1982, pp 151–156

Muth EA, Haskins JT, Moyer JA, et al: Antidepressant biochemical profile of the novel bicyclic compound WY-45,030, an ethyl cyclohexanol derivative. Biochem Pharmacol 35:4493–4497, 1986

Nambudiri DE, Mirchandani IC, Young RC: Two more cases of trazodone-related syncope in the elderly [letter]. J Geriatr Psychiatry Neurol 2:225, 1989

Nomikos GG, Damsma G, Wenkstern D, et al: Effects of chronic bupropion on interstitial concentrations of dopamine in rat nucleus accumbens and striatum. Neuropsychopharmacology 7:7–14, 1992

Osman OT, Rudorfer MV, Potter WZ: Idazoxan: a selective α_2-antagonist and effective sustained antidepressant in two bipolar depressed patients. Arch Gen Psychiatry 46:958–959, 1989

Peck AW, Stern WC, Watkinson C: Incidence of seizures during treatment with tricyclic antidepressant drugs and bupropion. J Clin Psychiatry 44:197–201, 1983

Perumal AS, Smith TM, Suckow RF, et al: Effect of plasma from patients containing bupropion and its metabolites on the uptake of norepinephrine. Neuropharmacology 25:199–202, 1986

Pick CG, Paul D, Eison, et al: Potentiation of opioid analgesia by the antidepressant nefazodone. Eur J Pharmacol 211:375–381, 1992

Pigott TA, Leheureux F, Rubenstein CS, et al: A double-blind, placebo controlled study of trazodone in patients with obsessive-compulsive disorder. J Clin Psychopharmacol 12:156–162, 1992

Pinner E, Rich CL: Effects of trazodone on aggressive behavior in seven patients with organic mental disorders. Am J Psychiatry 145:1295–1296, 1988

Pitts WM, Fann WE, Halaris AE, et al: Bupropion in depression: a tri-center placebo-controlled study. J Clin Psychiatry 44:95–100, 1983

Prasad AJ: Obsessive-compulsive disorder and trazodone. Am J Psychiatry 141:612–613, 1984

Preskorn SH: Antidepressant response and plasma concentrations of bupropion. J Clin Psychiatry 44:137–139, 1983

Preskorn SH: Should bupropion dosage be adjusted based upon therapeutic drug monitoring? Psychopharmacol Bull 27:637–643, 1991

Price WA, Giannini AJ: Withdrawal dyskinesia following amoxapine therapy [letter]. J Clin Psychiatry 47:329–330, 1986

Prusoff BA, Weissman MM, Charney D: Speed of symptom reduction in depressed outpatients treated with amoxapine and amitriptyline. Current Therapeutic Research 30:843–855, 1981

Rausch JL, Ruegg R, Moeller FG: Gepirone as a 5-HT1A agonist in the treatment of major depression. Psychopharm Bull 26:169–171, 1990

Richelson E: Biological basis of depression and therapeutic relevance. J Clin Psychiatry 52 (suppl):4–10, 1991

Roose SP, Glassman AH, Giardina EGV, et al: Cardiovascular effects of imipramine and bupropion in depressed patients with congestive heart failure. J Clin Psychopharmacol 7:247–251, 1987

Rosenbaum JF, Fava M, Falk WE, et al: The antidepressant potential of oral S-adenosyl-l-methionine. Acta Psychiatr Scand 81:432–436, 1990

Rudorfer MV, Potter WZ: Antidepressants: a comparative review of the clinical pharmacology and therapeutic use of the "newer" versus the "older" drugs. Drugs 37:713–738, 1989

Rudorfer MV, Golden RN, Potter WZ: Second generation antidepressants. Psychiatr Clin North Am 7:519–534, 1984

Salama A, Meuller-Eckhardt C: The role of metabolite-specific antibodies in nomifensine-dependent immune hemolytic anemia. N Engl J Med 313:469–474, 1985

Schatzberg AF: Trazodone: a 5-year review of antidepressant efficacy. Psychopathology 20 (suppl 1):48–56, 1987

Schuckit MA: United States experience with trazodone: a literature review. Psychopathology 20 (suppl 1):32–38, 1987

Schwartz D, Blendl M: Sedative and anxiety-reducing properties of trazodone in Trazodone: Modern Problems of Pharmacopsychiatry, Vol 9. Edited by Ban TA, Silvestrini B. Basel, Karger, 1974, pp 29–46

Schweizer E, Feighner J, Mandos LA, et al: Comparison of venlafaxine and imipramine in the acute treatment of major depression in outpatients. J Clin Psychiatry 55:104–108, 1994

Schweizer E, Weise C, Clary C, et al: Placebo-controlled trial of venlafaxine for the treatment of major depression. J Clin Psychopharmacol 11:233–

236, 1991

Shopsin B, Cassano GB, Conti L: An overview of new "second generation" antidepressant compounds: research and treatment implications, in Antidepressants: Neurochemical, Behavioral and Clinical Perspectives. Edited by Enna SJ, Molick J, Richelson E. New York, Raven, 1981, pp 219–251

Silvestrini G: Introductory remarks on trazodone and its position in treatment of psychiatric diseases, in Trazodone: A New Broad-Spectrum Antidepressant (Proceedings of the Symposium of the 11th Congress of the Collegium Internationale Neuro-Psychopharmacologicum, Vienna 1978). Edited by Gershon ES, Rickels K, Silvestrini G. Amsterdam, Excerpta Medica, 1980, pp 34–38

Silvestrini B, Lisciani R: Pharmacology of trazodone, round table discussion—trazodone: a new psychotropic agent. Current Therapeutic Research 15:749, 1973

Silvestrini B, Cioli V, Burbert S, et al: Pharmacological properties of AF 1161, a new psychotropic drug. International Journal of Neuropharmacology 7:587–599, 1968

Simpson DM, Foster DL: Improvement in organically disturbed behavior with trazodone treatment. J Clin Psychiatry 47:191–193, 1986

Smith WT, Glaudin V: Double-blind efficacy and safety study comparing adinazolam mesylate and placebo in depressed inpatients. Acta Psychiatr Scand 74:238–245, 1986

Soroko FE, Maxwell RA: The pharmacologic basis for therapeutic interest in bupropion. J Clin Psychiatry 44:67–73, 1983

Spar JE: Plasma trazodone concentrations in elderly depressed inpatients: cardiac effects and short-term efficacy. J Clin Psychopharmacol 7:406–409, 1987

Stern WC, Harto-Truax N, Bauer N: Efficacy of bupropion in tricyclic-resistant or intolerant patients. J Clin Psychiatry 44:148–152, 1983

Sternbach H: The serotonin syndrome. Am J Psychiatry 148:705–713, 1991

Sulser F: Mode of action of antidepressant drugs. J Clin Psychiatry 44:14–20, 1983

Taylor DP, Hyslop DK, Riblet A: Trazodone, a new non-tricyclic antidepressant without anticholinergic activity. Biochem Pharmacol 29:2149–2150, 1980

Taylor DP, Smith DW, Hyslop DK, et al: Receptor binding and atypical antidepressant drug discovery, in Receptor Binding in Drug Research. Edited by O'Brien RA. New York, Marcel Dekker, 1986, pp 151–165

Taylor NE, Schwartz HI: Neuroleptic malignant syndrome following amoxapine overdose. J Nerv Ment Dis 176:249–251, 1988

Thompson JW Jr, Ware MR, Blashfield RK: Psychotropic medication and priapism: a comprehensive review. J Clin Psychiatry 51:430–433, 1990

Thornton JE, Stahl SM: Case report of tardive dyskinesia and parkinsonism associated with amoxapine therapy. Am J Psychiatry 141:704–705, 1984

Van Putten T, Shaffer I: Delirium associated with bupropion. J Clin Psychopharmacol 10:234, 1990

van Zwieten PA: Inhibition of the central hypotensive effect of clonidine by trazodone, a novel antidepressant. Pharmacology 15:331–336, 1977

Warner MD, Peabody CA, Whiteford HA, et al: Alprazolam as an antidepressant. J Clin Psychiatry 49:148–150, 1988

Wender PH, Reimherr FW: Bupropion treatment of attention-deficit hyperactivity disorder in adults. Am J Psychiatry 147:1018–1020, 1990

Wheatley D: Evaluation of trazodone in the treatment of anxiety. Current Therapeutic Research 20:74–83, 1976

Yamatsu K, Kaneko T, Yamanishi Y: A possible mechanism of central action of trazodone in rats: First International Symposium on Trazodone, Montreal 1973. Mod Probl Pharmacopsychiatry 9:11–17, 1974

Zajecka JM, Fawcett J, Guy C: Coexisting major depression and obsessive-compulsive disorder treated with venlafaxine. J Clin Psychopharmacol 10:152–153, 1990

Zetin M, Aden G, Moldawsky R: Tolerance to amoxapine antidepressant effects. Clin Ther 5:638–643, 1983

Zimmer B, Daly F, Benjamin L: More on combination antidepressant therapy. Arch Gen Psychiatry 41:527–528, 1984

Zmitek A: Trazodone-induced mania. Br J Psychiatry 151:274–275, 1987

Zubieta JK, Demitrack MA: Possible bupropion precipitation of mania and a mixed affective state [letter]. J Clin Psychopharmacol 11:327–328, 1991

11

Benzodiazepines

James C. Ballenger, M.D.

■ HISTORY AND DISCOVERY

In the mid-1950s, Roche Laboratories began to investigate the development of a compound that had therapeutic properties similar to myanesin, a drug that demonstrated sedative and muscle relaxant features when tested on animals. But when myanesin was administered to humans, its effects were shown to be weak and short-acting (Randall 1982). However, this pursuit stimulated renewed interest and subsequent investigation of two compounds by Roche chemists Leo Sternbach and Earl Reeder; the compounds had initially been developed in 1955. In May 1957, when these compounds were submitted for pharmacological evaluation, laboratory tests demonstrated their superiority to meprobamate on all measures used, and to chlorpromazine on some.

The first benzodiazepine (BZ) was patented in 1959 and introduced as Librium in 1960. Known generically as methaminodiazepoxide, Librium's generic name was later changed to chlordiazepoxide (CDZ) (Sternbach 1982). Continued testing of related compounds led to the development and introduction in 1963 of diazepam (Valium), an antianxiety agent 3–10 times more potent than Librium, with a broader spectrum of activity and greater muscle relaxant properties. The study of BZ derivatives has continued, and there are now 39 BZs available on the market (Smith and Wesson 1985) derived from or related to these early compounds (Sternbach 1982). Alprazolam, a triazolobenzodiazepine, has received the most recent attention. In 1992, it was awarded the first U.S. Food and Drug Administration (FDA) approval for treatment of panic disorder (PD).

■ STRUCTURE-ACTIVITY RELATIONS

Chemically, the BZs are made up of 2-amino-benzodiazepine 4-oxides (Sternbach 1982). The first BZ developed, CDZ, was the result of a compound created by treating the quinazoline N-oxide with methylamine, a primary amine (Sternbach 1982). During early studies at Roche Laboratories, there was scientific concern regarding the chemical validity of this compound. Based on scientific knowledge of chemical interactions, the chemical process used to develop CDZ did not result in the anticipated final product. Further investigation revealed that the development of CDZ resulted from the expansion of an atypical ring in the BZ derivative—the compound contained a seven-member diazepine ring rather than a six-member pyrimidine ring (Sternbach and Reeder 1961).

Continued laboratory study and attempts to develop other related but improved compounds led to the discovery that the features shared by these compounds were the 1,4-BZ ring system, a chlorine in the 7 position, and the phenyl group in the 5 position (Sternbach 1982) (Figure 11–1). This discovery ultimately led to the development of a number of related

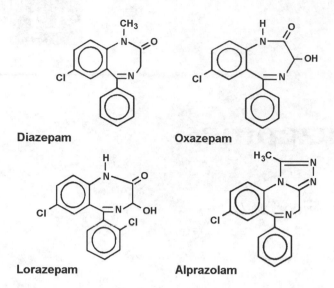

Figure 11–1. Benzodiazepine structures.
Source. Reprinted with permission of Mosby-Year Book from Bernstein 1988.

compounds, including diazepam (Valium). Most BZs have a 5-aryl and a 1,4-diazepine ring, and it is modification of the ring systems that produces BZs with somewhat different properties. The BZ currently most frequently prescribed for the treatment of anxiety, alprazolam (Xanax), is a triazolobenzodiazepine, formed by the addition of a heterocyclic ring that joins the 1 and 2 positions of the BZ ring system (Sternbach 1982).

■ PHARMACOLOGICAL PROFILE

■ Animal Studies

A number of hypotheses regarding the mechanism by which the BZs reduce anxiety have received rigorous scientific investigation using animal experimentation. Most of the animal studies conducted to predict the ability of the BZs to reduce anxiety use an anticonflict or antipunishment effect, also known as a behavioral disinhibitory or behavioral antisuppressant action (Dantzer 1977; Gray 1982; Haefely 1978; Kilts et al. 1981; Sepinwall and Cook 1978; Simon and Soubrie 1979; Thiébot and Soubrié 1983).

The Geller-Seifter test (Geller and Seifter 1960) and the Vogel punished drinking test (Vogel et al. 1971), two of the most frequently used conflict tests, predict antianxiety efficacy of BZs (or other drugs) by their ability to increase responsivity in a conflict or punishment situation. In the Geller-Seifter test, the rat

is rewarded with food for pressing a lever. However, the rat is alternately and variably given shocks when pressing the lever, thereby decreasing its willingness to depress the lever. In the Vogel punished drinking test, thirsty rats are allowed to drink water but are given shocks through either the water spout or through bars on the floor of the cage. Again, shocks alternate with no shock in a variable way in the experimental setting. In both of these tests, when rats were administered BZs, their response rate during the potential shock situation increased, but the BZ had no effect on their responsivity in a nonshock situation. The effects of the BZs were also greater after they had been administered for several days (Cook and Sepinwall 1975; File and Hyde 1978; Margules and Stein 1968).

The punished locomotion test, which was developed more recently, administers shock to the rat as it moves from one metal plate to another, alternating shock with no shock on a variable schedule. Although this test is used less frequently, the effects of BZs in the punished locomotion test is again to enhance animal movement (File 1990).

Other predictive tests have been developed that assess animal response in social situations. Rats are placed in settings that are either unfamiliar or extremely well lit, and then the setting is alternated on a variable basis. Antianxiety potency is predicted by the amount of time rats spend engaged socially. As might be anticipated, rats spend the greatest amount of time in social interaction when placed in a familiar setting without bright light. BZs have been shown to be effective in increasing the amount of time spent in social interaction in the test condition. This test has been validated behaviorally by assessing anxiety through measures associated with decreased social interaction in animals (e.g., self-grooming, defecation). Also, physiological validation was accomplished by measuring changes in adrenocorticotropic hormone (ACTH), hypothalamic noradrenaline, and corticosterone (File 1980, 1985, 1990; File and Hyde 1978, 1979).

Anxiety in the social situation has also been assessed using the elevated plus-maze, a device shaped like a plus sign and having two closed and two open arms. The BZs or other anxiolytics lead the rat to spend increased amounts of time on the open arms of the maze. This measure has also been validated physiologically and behaviorally with regard to anxiety (Pellow and File 1986; Pellow et al. 1985).

■ Pharmacological Properties

Almost all of the BZs have similar pharmacological profiles. All are sedating; in fact, it is difficult to separate the anxiety-reducing properties of the BZs from their sedating properties. They therefore have prominent hypnotic activity, and they all have anticonvulsant and muscle relaxant activity. All these actions are thought to be secondary to effects on the central nervous system (CNS).

Muscle relaxation is thought to be mediated at the spinal cord level and the antianxiety effects in cortical and perhaps in limbic areas (Lader 1987). Anticonvulsant activity appears to occur through inhibition of seizure activity by potentiation of γ-aminobutyric acid (GABA)-ergic neuronal circuits (see next section) at multiple levels of the CNS, including the brain stem.

At routine doses, BZs have little effect on the cardiovascular and respiratory systems, which probably explains their wide margin of safety. Even in overdose situations, only rarely do patients who have taken only a BZ experience respiratory depression severe enough to require attention. More commonly, serious overdoses are the result of combining a BZ with another depressant drug, usually alcohol (Finkle et al. 1979; Greenblatt et al. 1977).

The effects of BZs on sleep have been well studied and include increases in total time asleep, reduction in sleep latency, decreased awakenings, and decreases in Stages 1, 2, 3, and 4 sleep (Greenblatt and Shader 1974; Mendelson et al. 1977). BZs generally decrease time spent in rapid eye movement (REM) sleep but increase the number of REM cycles and therefore the number of dreams. When BZs are discontinued after chronic use, rebound increases in REM often occur, and patients often report increases in nightmares or bizarre dreams.

■ PHARMACOKINETICS AND DISPOSITION

Administered orally, BZs are generally well absorbed from the gastrointestinal tract and reach peak levels within 30 minutes to 6–8 hours. Only lorazepam and midazolam are predictably absorbed after intramuscular injection. The high lipid solubility of the BZs allows for easy passage into the brain (DeVane et al. 1991). This also means, however, that activity of the BZs may be prolonged in extremely overweight or elderly people, who tend to have a higher ratio of fat to lean tissue (Bernstein 1988; Harvey 1985). The BZs are predominantly bound to plasma proteins.

The BZs are metabolized primarily through the liver, with the majority being biotransformed by oxidation or Phase I metabolism. A small number of the BZs, including lorazepam, temazepam, and lormetazepam, are biotransformed by conjugation to inactive glucuronides, sulfates, and acetylated substances; this is also known as Phase II metabolism (Greenblatt et al. 1983). Some of the BZs are metabolized through both Phase I and II processes, including diazepam, chlordiazepoxide, and flurazepam (Lader 1987).

The mechanism by which these drugs are metabolized (i.e., through the liver) is of significance in prescribing the BZs for certain groups of patients. If using a BZ, those that are metabolized by Phase II alone are better tolerated in patients with impaired liver function. Patients affected include elderly people, alcoholic individuals with cirrhotic livers, and people who smoke. Metabolism of Phase I drugs slows in the aging population, and the BZs metabolized by Phase II processes only are better tolerated by elderly people (Lader 1987). However, clinicians should use caution when prescribing any of the BZs for patients who are significantly hepatically impaired, and these patients should be monitored regularly and carefully.

The BZs have widely divergent half-lives (Table 11–1). Obviously, the shorter half-life BZs require multiple daily dosing. This can be a positive clinical feature for some patients but may have negative connotations for other patients. Specifically, the recurrence of anxiety symptoms with rapid decline in blood level in those agents with short half-lives (e.g., alprazolam) can be a concern for some patients (e.g., those with PD).

The duration of action of many of the BZs is much more dependent on the half-lives of active metabolites than of the parent compounds. Perhaps the most clinically important example is flurazepam. Although its half-life is only 2–3 hours, the half-life of its primary metabolite N-desalkylflurazepam is more than 50 hours. Diazepam and its metabolite desmethyldiazepam are similar. In the case of the hypnotic flurazepam, this is often a negative feature—it can cause unwanted daytime drowsiness. When diazepam is used for anxiety relief, the long half-life of

Table 11–1.   Benzodiazepines and their metabolites (including half-life)

Drug	Half-life	Active metabolites	Half-life
Triazolam	Short (< 6 hours)	None	
Alprazolam	Intermediate (6–20 hours)	Not clinically important	
Lorazepam	Intermediate (6–20 hours)	None	
Oxazepam	Intermediate (6–20 hours)	None	
Temazepam	Intermediate (6–20 hours)	None	
Chlordiazepoxide	Intermediate (6–20 hours)	Desmethylchlordiazepoxide	Intermediate (6–20 hours)
		Demoxepam	Long (> 20 hours)
		Nordazepam	Long (> 20 hours)
Diazepam	Long (> 20 hours)	Nordazepam	Long (> 20 hours)
Clorazepate	Short (< 6 hours)	Nordazepam	Long (> 20 hours)
Halazepam	Short (< 6 hours)	Nordazepam	Long (> 20 hours)
Prazepam	Short (< 6 hours)	Nordazepam	Long (> 20 hours)
Flurazepam	Short (< 6 hours)	N-hydroxyethyl-flurazepam	Short (< 6 hours)
		N-desalkylflurazepam	Long (> 20 hours)

Source. Adapted with permission from Harvey 1985.

its principal metabolite can be a positive factor by providing smooth relief of anxiety that is not dependent on multiple daily dosing.

Other factors that affect elimination rate and half-life include the length of time that the drug is prescribed as well as the number of doses administered each day. For example, when an individual is prescribed diazepam for sleeping and takes it only qd or infrequently prn, the drug will have a much shorter half-life than that experienced by the patient who takes diazepam several times a day for an extended period (Bernstein 1988).

There are conflicting reports regarding the correlation between dose and plasma levels. Four early studies using BZs to treat patients for anxiety, sleep difficulties, or a combination of symptoms showed no correlation between plasma concentrations and patient responsivity (Bond et al. 1977; Kangas et al. 1979; Tansella et al. 1975, 1978). However, other studies in which patients were treated for anxiety have demonstrated a positive correlation between BZ plasma level and patient improvement (Bellantuono et al. 1980; Curry 1974; Dasberg et al. 1974).

Other studies have demonstrated a positive correlation between alprazolam plasma levels and treatment response in patients with PD. Lesser and colleagues (1992) studied plasma levels in 96 patients with PD who were treated with either 2 mg or 6 mg alprazolam or placebo. This study demonstrated a significant correlation between plasma level of al-

prazolam and reduction in panic and phobic symptomatology, as well as in side effects experienced. Plasma level was definitely correlated with reduction in panic attacks. However, there was wide variability among patients administered identical doses of alprazolam in terms of plasma concentration. This finding should underscore the need for individual dosing to achieve the maximum benefit with the fewest side effects.

The individual variation among patients regarding dose and plasma level in PD was replicated by Greenblatt and colleagues (1993). This study also showed a higher reduction in spontaneous panic attacks in patients with higher plasma levels of alprazolam at week 3. Reductions in situational panic attacks were also experienced by patients with higher plasma levels, but not to a significant degree. Not surprisingly, an increase in side effects was also correlated with higher plasma levels. Significantly, by week 8 of the study, plasma level was no longer correlated with symptom improvement or side effects.

■ MECHANISM OF ACTION

■ The GABA Role

The elucidation of the mechanism of action for the BZs began with the discovery that GABA serves as the major inhibitory neurotransmitter in the CNS

(Costa et al. 1975; Haefely 1985). There is now considerable evidence that the major pharmacological effects of the BZs are produced secondary to the binding of the BZs to GABA$_A$ receptors in the CNS. The pharmacological actions of BZs apparently do not involve GABA$_B$ receptors (Costa et al. 1975; Haefely 1985). Extensive research has demonstrated the critical interrelatedness of BZ actions and GABAergic mechanisms (Costa et al. 1975; Haefely et al. 1975; Polc et al. 1974). This relationship can be clearly demonstrated by the ability of the BZs to prevent or extinguish seizures caused by agents that interfere with normal GABAergic function (Haefely 1985) or by demonstration that pretreatment with antagonists of GABA (e.g., bicuculline) blocks BZ effects.

Although a definitive understanding of the way BZs produce anxiolytic effects remains to be determined, it has been shown that GABA increases the propensity of the BZs to bind to specific receptor sites on the GABA-BZ receptor complex. The converse is also true (i.e., both mutually enhance the binding of the other) (Paul and Skolnick 1982; Tallman et al. 1978, 1980). The principal action of GABA is to open the chloride ionophore on this complex. Although BZs appear to have no effect themselves on the GABA$_A$ complex or the ionophore, in the presence of GABA, BZs increase GABA's effects on the chloride ionophore—that is, they increase the number of openings of the chloride channel, which in turn causes decreased cellular excitability (Bernstein 1988; Hsiao and Potter 1990; Study and Barker 1981).

Therefore, the primary action of the BZs is thought to be to increase the frequency of the openings of the chloride channel further. Other mechanisms other than enhancement of GABA inhibition have also been suggested, including increases in calcium-dependent potassium (K$^+$) conductance (Polc 1988). Although the evidence linking the BZs and GABA is strong, other potential mechanisms may be involved. It has been hypothesized that anxiety disorders are caused by abnormalities in both GABA and brain norepinephrine, and that agents that correct these abnormalities are effective in reducing anxiety (Bernstein 1988). Oxazepam, a BZ often prescribed for anxiety, has been shown to decrease turnover of the two common transmitters serotonin and norepinephrine. It is believed that this is at least partially responsible for both its sedative and anxiolytic effects (Harvey 1985).

BZ Receptors

In the 1970s, several groups of researchers were responsible for the discovery of specific BZ binding sites in the brain (Bossman et al. 1977; Braestrup and Squires 1977; Möhler and Okada 1977a, 1977b; Squires and Braestrup 1977). The important discovery of high affinity, saturable, and stereospecific binding of BZ in the CNS provided the basis for which to explain the diverse actions of BZ. Evidence that these BZ receptors localized on neurons in the CNS mediate the pharmacological actions of the BZs is provided by the strong correlation between potencies of various BZs in displacing tritiated BZ from BZ receptors in vitro. This mediation is also demonstrated by the BZs' potencies as anticonvulsants, anxiolytics, and muscle relaxants and in various animal models of inhibited behaviors (Young and Kuhar 1980).

The GABA$_A$ receptor complex is an oligomeric glycoprotein. It was originally thought to have two subunits α and β, each with 4 segments with 20 amino acids (Barnard et al. 1988). The GABA site is apparently associated with the β subunit and the BZ receptor with the α subunit (Thomas and Tallman 1981). It also appears that there are 4 membrane spanning regions of approximately 20–30 hydrophobic amino acids in each subunit (Figure 11–2) (Zorumski and Isenberg 1991). However, cloning studies of 15 different proteins in the mammalian CNS (Seeburg et al. 1990) have demonstrated at least

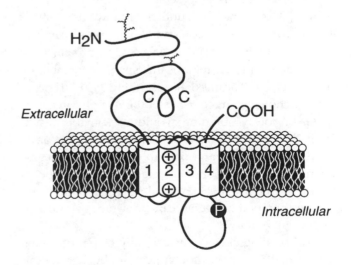

Figure 11–2. Model for GABA$_A$ receptor subunits. *Source.* Reprinted with permission from Zorumski and Isenberg 1991.

5 subunits with multiple variants within each. Although the possible number of variations in the BZ receptor probably exceeds 500, currently there are known to be 6 α, 3 β, 2 (or 3) σ, and 1 δ subunits (Lüddens and Wisden 1991). It is now known that the pharmacology of the BZ receptor varies according to the α subunit expressed. Expression of the σ2 subunit is required for the GABA$_A$ chloride channels formed to consistently and robustly respond to BZ. If the σ2 subunit is replaced by a σ1 subunit, the BZ receptors are more reminiscent of the peripheral-type BZ receptors (Ymer et al. 1990).

Although most BZs bind to GABA$_A$-BZ receptors with similar affinities throughout the brain, there are some differences for certain BZs. This has led to a characterization of BZ receptors as either Type I (with high affinity for triazolopyridazines and β-carbolines) (Nielsen and Braestrup 1980; Sieghart et al. 1985) or Type II, with lower affinities for these compounds. Type I receptors are the most common GABA$_A$ receptor class in the CNS. Type II receptors are high in the hippocampus, striatum, and spinal cord (Lo et al. 1983; Sieghart et al. 1985), whereas Type I receptors are high in cerebellum and low in hippocampus. Both subtypes are high in cortical layers (Faull and Villiger 1988; Faull et al. 1987; Olsen et al. 1990). A third class of BZ receptor is primarily located in cerebellar granule cells, involves the α6 subunit, and is relatively insensitive to BZs (Lüddens et al. 1990).

The functions of the β, σ, and δ subunits are less well known, but they do seem to be involved in agonist (GABA) binding (Lüddens and Wisden 1991). The GABA$_A$-BZ receptor complex is presumably a pentamer made up of α, β, and σ glycoprotein subunits, each with four regions that span the membrane (Figure 11–3) (Zorumski and Isenberg 1991). The actual functional characteristics of the receptor in terms of GABA or BZ binding would presumably result from whatever subunits were involved in the unit. Given the apparent and probably tremendous heterogeneity of these subunits, there appears to be a strong possibility that new and potentially more selective therapeutic agents can be synthesized using this heterogeneity.

BZ binding sites occur centrally or peripherally; however, there does not appear to be a receptor function for the peripheral type (Haefely 1985). This topic is discussed in more detail in a section later in this chapter.

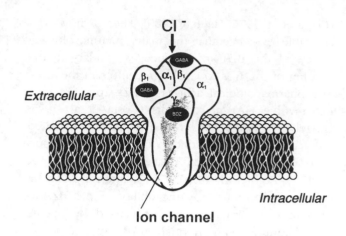

Figure 11–3. Model of the GABA-benzodiazepine receptor complex.
Source. Reprinted with permission from Zorumski and Isenberg 1991.

Ligands of the Benzodiazepine Receptor: Agonists, Antagonists, and Inverse Agonists

The BZs' action on the GABA receptor complex is mediated through the BZ receptor on this complex, but in what appears to be a unique mechanism described as positive allosteric modulation (Haefely 1990). It is worth noting that the binding site for the BZs operates differently from other neurotransmitter receptors—that is, this BZ receptor mediates the effects of different drugs that have directly opposing effects (i.e., either increasing or reducing anxiety). To further investigate the BZ GABAergic interaction, agents that have agonist, inverse agonist, and antagonist actions have been studied.

In addition to the BZs, zopiclone, triazolopyridazines, pyrazoloquinolinone derivatives, and some β-carboline derivatives have BZ agonist activity and reduce anxiety in a manner similar to the BZs. They do so by acting synergistically with GABA to increase the openings of the chloride channel (Blanchard et al. 1979; Klepner et al. 1979; Stephens et al. 1984; Yokoyama et al. 1982).

BZ antagonists block the ability of BZ agonists to amplify the effects of GABA but have no intrinsic activity themselves. The imidazobenzodiazepine derivative Ro 15-1788 is one of the most studied BZ antagonists. It has been found in both animal and human studies to have properties that enable it to totally negate all anxiety-reducing actions of BZs (Bonetti et al. 1982; Darragh et al. 1981a, 1981b,

1982a, 1982b; Haefely 1985; Hunkeler et al. 1981; Möhler et al. 1981; Polc et al. 1981). The action of Ro 15-1788 is accomplished by its ability to inhibit BZ binding to CNS neuronal binding sites (Möhler and Richards 1981; Richards et al. 1982).

The important discovery of an anxiogenic (i.e., anxiety-increasing) ligand used the social interaction test wherein it was demonstrated that ethyl-β-carboxylate (β-CCE), by acting on BZ binding sites, increased anxiety (File et al. 1982). The anxiogenic property attributed to β-CCE in animals was replicated in humans (Dorow et al. 1983) and was demonstrated in animal experimentation, as described previously (Corda et al. 1983; File and Pellow 1984; File et al. 1984; Hindley et al. 1985; Pellow and File 1986; Petersen et al. 1982, 1983; Stephens and Kehr 1985). However, it was found that although some β-carbolines are anxiogenic, others have been developed that have anxiolytic properties instead (File 1990).

Inverse agonists act directly to decrease the number of times that the chloride channel opens (Costa and Guidotti 1985; Zorumski and Isenberg 1991), giving them anxiogenic properties. These include β-carboline derivatives and the diazepam-binding inhibitor peptide (Breier and Paul 1988). This is accompanied in animals (Hommer et al. 1987) and in humans (Dorow et al. 1983) by specific physiological effects indicative of stress (e.g., elevated heart rate, blood pressure, and certain stress hormones).

Partial agonists. Partial agonists are compounds that have less functional effect after occupying the receptor than full agonists. Their ability to activate the receptor is low; therefore, a higher fraction of receptors needs to be occupied to match the action of a full agonist. A full response might not occur even with 100% receptor occupancy. Partial agonists along the entire spectrum of agonist, antagonist, and inverse agonist have now been synthesized. There is considerable excitement and clinical research now under way in this area, primarily based on the theoretical possibility that a partial agonist might have anxiolytic properties but would not be sedating or as prone to develop withdrawal symptoms. The agent under most vigorous study is abecarnil (Ballenger 1991).

Endogenous ligands. The presence of the BZ receptor argues for the existence of an endogenous ligand for this receptor (Paul et al. 1980). In theory, it could be an anxiolytic agonist or, in fact, an anxiogenic inverse agonist (see Haefely 1988 for review). However, no ligand in living humans has been found (Costa 1989). Perhaps the most likely candidate at this time is the diazepam-binding inhibitor (DBI), which is thought to have anxiogenic properties (DeRobertis et al. 1988).

It is worth noting that DeBlas and Sangameswaran (1986) isolated N-desmethyldiazepam (a metabolite of several BZs, including diazepam, chlordiazepoxide, and medazepam) from the brains of rats never exposed to BZs. Similarly, BZ metabolites were also found in human brains that were stored in the 1940s (long before development of the first BZ in the early 1960s), providing definitive evidence for the existence of endogenous BZs (File 1988). It has been hypothesized that the source of this naturally occurring BZ-like substance may come from the diet, based on evidence that BZ biosynthesis exists in fungi (Luckner 1984).

Peripheral-Type BZ Receptors

In determining exactly how the BZs affect certain behaviors and to pinpoint the specific BZ receptors in the brain, an unexpected and interesting discovery was made by Braestrup and Squires (1977). They discovered another class of BZ binding sites, the peripheral-type BZ receptors (PBRs), so named because of their discovery in peripheral tissues, which were seen first in the kidney but were subsequently identified in all tissues including the CNS (Braestrup and Squires 1977).

Although largely different from the GABA-BZ receptors, the PBRs do share some features, including their relatively high affinity for certain BZs. However, the two receptors have different binding specifications. In studies conducted on rodents, it was shown that PBRs have high affinity binding with 4'-chlorodiazepam (Krueger 1991). Conversely, GABA-BZ receptors have low affinity for this BZ derivative. Clonazepam and flumazenil have high affinity for GABA-BZ receptors, but low affinity for PBRs. Multiple studies have demonstrated that GABA-BZ receptors interact with chloride channels at synaptic terminals, whereas PBRs are localized instead in mitochondria (Anholt et al. 1986). PBRs are found in the CNS at levels as great as and in some cases even higher than the GABA-BZ receptors (Marangos et al. 1982; Villiger 1985).

PBRs make up more than 0.2% of the total mitochondrial protein (Antkiewicz-Michaluk et al. 1988). DeSouza and colleagues (1985) detected comparable receptor levels in other steroidogenic tissues. The conversion of cholesterol to pregnenolone, the initial step in the steroid synthetic pathway, takes place in the inner mitochondrial membrane. Steroid production is regulated by the transporting of cholesterol from the outer to the inner mitochondrial membranes. Hormones including adrenocorticotropin, luteinizing hormone, and follicle stimulating hormone activate cholesterol transport from the outer to the inner mitochondrial membranes (Krueger 1991). It has been confirmed that PBRs facilitate translocation of intramitochondrial cholesterol (Krueger and Papadopoulos 1990), supporting the hypothesis that PBRs are an important receptor site for certain previously unexplained physiological and behavioral actions attributed to BZs (Krueger 1991).

The work to date with PBRs indicates that BZs may bind to PBRs in the CNS, causing secondary behavioral effects (Krueger 1991). This line of reasoning and investigation is new but provides yet another hypothesis for the BZ mechanism of action. Knowing that PBRs have a primary role in steroid biosynthesis has shown at least preliminarily that agents that bind to PBRs regulate steroidogenesis, which may account for variance in pharmacological profiles and differences in tolerability among the BZs. Additional investigation is needed to determine how GABA-BZ receptors and PBRs are related in physiological regulation (Krueger 1991).

■ INDICATIONS

Because they are generally well tolerated, with minimal side effects, BZs have demonstrated efficacy for a number of conditions, most notably the treatment of anxiety and anxiety-related disorders. Indications for which BZs are used are similar to those for which barbiturates were once prescribed. However, the greater tolerability and safety profile of BZs have been responsible in large part for virtually eliminating barbiturates from being prescribed for anxiety conditions (Hollister 1982). In addition to their use as effective antianxiety agents, BZs have also been proven to be effective hypnotics, an effect that is achieved through the same pharmacological actions that block or reduce anxiety (Hollister 1982).

Flurazepam (Dalmane) has been one of the most frequently prescribed hypnotics in the United States, with demonstrated efficacy supported by rigorous scientific and clinical studies. Effective in helping patients achieve and maintain sleep, flurazepam does so with fewer of the troublesome side effects attributed to most other non-BZ hypnotics, and without the tolerance that develops to other drugs with long-term use (Kales et al. 1975). The short half-life BZ triazolam reached widespread popularity as a hypnotic largely because it was cleared from the system before morning and was therefore not associated with daytime drowsiness. However, recent concern and controversy surrounding triazolam's potential serious side effects (particularly at higher doses) has dampened enthusiasm and significantly reduced its use.

BZs are also effective when used as muscle relaxants or as anticonvulsants, during alcohol withdrawal, and as an intravenous anesthetic (Hollister 1982). Clonazepam is labeled as an anticonvulsant and is widely used for that indication, although it is also popular for treating anxiety conditions.

BZs have also become one of the most frequently used treatments for alcohol withdrawal. They are quite effective because of their cross-reactivity with alcohol, as well as their anticonvulsant properties and anxiety-reducing efficacy. Traditionally, BZs are given in a loading fashion and then rapidly tapered over the first 3–7 days of alcohol withdrawal.

The primary indications for BZs are certainly in the treatment of anxiety disorders. Eight BZs are labeled for anxiety (generalized anxiety disorder [GAD]) and alprazolam for PD, and clonazepam is also widely used for these indications. Although BZs are used as ancillary medications in the management of patients with obsessive-compulsive disorder, social phobias, and posttraumatic stress disorder (PTSD), their primary use has been in the treatment of GAD and more recently for PD.

BZs have become the primary pharmacological treatment for GAD. Although certain psychotherapeutic techniques (e.g., support, meditation, relaxation) are effective and widely used, they are often relatively unavailable or unacceptable for various reasons. Thus, BZs have become the mainstay of treatment for this condition.

GAD is characterized by excessive anxiety and worry, accompanied by motoric symptoms of anxiety (e.g., tension, autonomic hyperactivity, and vigilance). Despite the seemingly simple nature of this disorder, GAD is often chronic (Angst and Vollrath 1991) and associated with considerable impairment and distress (Croft-Jeffreys and Wilkinson 1989).

PD is characterized by recurrent severe panic attacks and persistent worry that the panic attacks will recur or that they indicate serious medical or psychiatric consequences (Ballenger and Fyer 1993). Panic is also a chronic condition in most clinical cases and is associated with even more morbidity than GAD. This includes frequent visits to the emergency room, family and occupational difficulties, financial dependency, abuse of alcohol, and even increased suicide attempts (Cowley 1992; Klerman et al. 1991; Markowitz et al. 1989; Weissman et al. 1989).

Because all BZs are apparently equally efficacious (Greenblatt and Shader 1974), the choice of a specific BZ is often influenced by physician or patient preference, side effect differences (there are actually few), and marketplace issues. Diazepam was the most popular anxiolytic through the 1970s and early 1980s, when it was supplanted by alprazolam. In part this change reflected a shift from one "type" of BZ to another. Diazepam and other BZs (e.g., chlordiazepoxide, chlorazepate) have long half-lives and therefore have considerable accumulation over time. This results in the advantages of not needing multiple daily dosing as well as having less potential for withdrawal symptomatology when abruptly discontinued. However, these same characteristics can result in excess sedation and interference with optimal functioning. Alprazolam has a shorter half-life (5–10 hours) and therefore less accumulation, a multiple daily dosing requirement, and more potential for withdrawal symptoms when abruptly discontinued. More recently, clonazepam has enjoyed increased popularity as a BZ with a longer half-life.

Early work with alprazolam in treating patients with PD suggested it might have unique efficacy. Considerable research has demonstrated its efficacy for PD patients (Ballenger et al. 1988; Cross National Collaborative Panic Study, Second Phase Investigators 1992), leading to FDA approval for this indication. However, other BZs (e.g., diazepam, lorazepam, clonazepam) are clearly also effective when taken in sufficient doses (Charney and Woods 1989; Howell et al. 1987; Noyes et al. 1984; Schweizer et al. 1988), which is again supportive of the idea that there are probably no specific indications for any one BZ.

It is probably worth emphasizing that BZ treatment of GAD or PD frequently proves to be long term, in keeping with the chronic nature of these disorders (Ballenger 1991; Romach et al. 1992; Schatzberg and Ballenger 1991). Most research experience with the BZs is short term, although longer-term treatment efficacy (i.e., up to 6 months) has been established in some trials (Cohn and Wilcox 1984; Fabre et al. 1981). In trials where the BZ is discontinued blindly, many patients experienced a return of their original anxiety symptoms (i.e., relapse), but this is not true for all patients (Rickels et al. 1980, 1983, 1990, 1991). This requires that clinicians periodically reassess the need for continued BZ therapy by tapering and discontinuing BZs.

BZs are also used to treat a number of conditions other than those previously described (Wesson 1985). The early use of BZs to treat schizophrenia-associated stress and/or anxiety proved ineffective. However, it was later postulated that the doses used were inadequate to achieve a therapeutic effect (Nestoros 1980). Because of clonazepam's rapid onset of action, it has been used as an adjunctive treatment with lithium to control the agitation seen during the acute manic phase of manic-depressive disorder (Chouinard et al. 1983). BZs have also been used to treat night terrors as well as sleep or dream disturbances in PTSD patients, because of the BZs' ability to reduce Stage 4 sleep (Friedman 1981; Kramer 1979). Clonazepam has also been used to treat nocturnal myoclonus (Boghew 1980; Matthews 1979) and tic douloureux when carbamazepine is ineffective (Court and Kase 1976).

Finally, the BZs have been used successfully in third-world countries to treat tetanus, cerebral malaria, chloroquine toxicity, and maternal eclampsia (Ward 1985).

■ SIDE EFFECTS AND TOXICOLOGY

BZs have proven efficacy for a number of conditions. Those BZs that are used for the treatment of anxiety disorders generally have a more favorable side-effect profile than the other pharmacological agents used for these indications (i.e., monoamine oxidase inhibitors and tricyclic antidepressants). Also, BZs begin to exert their therapeutic effects rapidly, with improvement generally seen in the first week of treatment.

As a class, BZs have remarkably few side effects, the principal one being sedation. Patients report feeling sedated, drowsy, and slowed down, and may fall asleep during daytime activities or have ataxia or slurred speech (Linnoila et al. 1983). In laboratory settings, slowed psychomotor performance has been observed (Hindmarch et al. 1991). Amnesia (anterograde) also occurs with intravenous administration, an effect used widely in anesthesia induction (King 1992). But it has also been reported with oral dosing, especially with the hypnotic triazolam (Greenblatt et al. 1991). Amnesia is also present in less dramatic fashion in routine use, with some patients reporting relatively minor difficulties in learning new material (Barbee 1993; Ghoneim and Mewaldt 1990; Greenblatt et al. 1991; Hindmarch et al. 1991; King 1992; Linnoila et al. 1983; Miller et al. 1988; Roth et al. 1984; Shader et al. 1986). However, these side effects are generally transient and disappear quickly (usually within days) as tolerance to these effects develops (Miller et al. 1988).

The controversy surrounding BZ administration and potential abuse or addiction in routine patient use is generally not supported by the available scientific evidence. (See Shader and Greenblatt 1993 for an excellent review of this complex area.) In a large community study of long-term alprazolam users, Romach and colleagues (1992) found that dosage did not escalate over prolonged use and that most patients used the BZs as prescribed. In fact, if deviations occurred, it was generally that a patient took less than the prescribed dosage.

Evidence regarding the use of BZs during pregnancy is inconclusive. For this reason, it is prudent to postpone pregnancy until BZ treatment has been discontinued. In addition, because BZs are excreted through breast milk and place the infant at risk for lethargy and inadequate temperature regulation, nursing mothers should also be cautioned against the use of BZs (Bernstein 1988).

■ Discontinuation

For the sake of thoroughness, a statement regarding discontinuation of the BZs is in order (see Ballenger et al. 1993; Shader and Greenblatt 1993). Numerous groups, including some medical professionals, have perpetuated the idea that if used in the long term, patients become "addicted" to the BZs, resulting in an extreme withdrawal syndrome when the medication is discontinued. Actually, what occurs with BZs is similar to the effects of other medications used for long-term treatment of a medical and/or psychiatric condition, and can be compared to what happens when a patient's cardiovascular medicine (e.g., propranolol, methyldopa) is suddenly discontinued (Garbus et al. 1979). In essence, the body goes through an adaptational process to the drug, and if medication is discontinued too abruptly, the patient can experience withdrawal symptoms. In the case of a patient treated for anxiety conditions, the patient may experience a transient recurrence of anxiety symptoms, often at levels more intense than those experienced before treatment. This is called rebound. The patient can also experience a return of symptoms that were present before treatment (relapse). However, if dosage is adjusted and gradually titrated downward, and if patients and their families are educated about what to expect during the discontinuation process, most patients can manage the transient withdrawal symptoms without much difficulty (see Ballenger et al. 1993 and Shader and Greenblatt 1993 for review).

■ DRUG-DRUG INTERACTIONS

Because BZs are frequently used for long-term treatment of conditions such as anxiety, the chances increase that at some point during treatment, the patient will receive another medication, either a prescription or over-the-counter drug. It was originally believed that BZs did not interact with other drugs; however, it is now known that this is not the case. Cimetidine and disulfiram both slow the metabolism of BZs, causing them to have enhanced and prolonged effects. This is particularly true with the longer-acting BZs, including chlordiazepoxide and diazepam (Bernstein 1988; Glassman and Salzman 1987; Ruffalo and Thompson 1980). If a patient taking diazepam is also prescribed gallamine or succinylcholine, paralysis can result (Hansten 1985). Other drugs that can exacerbate the effects of BZs include isoniazid and estrogens, an effect produced by enzyme inhibition.

Other drugs act to reduce BZ effects. These include antacids that affect BZ metabolism by reduced gastrointestinal absorption, as well as tobacco and rifampin, which interfere with enzyme induction (Bernstein 1988). When digoxin is administered to a patient taking BZs, the digoxin half-life increases; however, the mechanism by which this occurs is not known (Bernstein 1988).

At times BZs, along with other sedative and anxiety reducing medications, can cause significant sedation and CNS depression. When these drugs are taken at doses that are too high, or when they are combined with alcohol or other sedating medications, they can cause significant sedation and occasionally respiratory depression as well (Bernstein 1988).

■ REFERENCES

Angst J, Vollrath M: The natural history of anxiety disorders. Acta Psychiatr Scand 84:446–452, 1991

Anholt RRH, Pedersen PL, DeSouze EB, et al: The peripheral-type benzodiazepine receptor: localization to the mitochondrial outer membrane. J Biol Chem 261:576–583, 1986

Antkiewicz-Michaluk L, Guidotti A, Krueger KE: Molecular characterization and mitochondrial density of a recognition site for peripheral-type benzodiazepine ligands. Mol Pharmacol 34:272–278, 1988

Ballenger JC: Long-term pharmacologic treatment of panic disorder. J Clin Psychiatry 52:18–23, 1991

Ballenger JC, Fyer AJ: Examining criteria for panic disorder. Hosp Community Psychiatry 44:226–228, 1993

Ballenger JC, Burrows G, DuPont R, et al: Alprazolam in panic disorder and agoraphobia: results from a multicenter trial, I: efficacy in short-term treatment. Arch Gen Psychiatry 455:413–422, 1988

Ballenger JC, Pecknold J, Rickels K, et al: Medication discontinuation in panic disorder. J Clin Psychiatry 54 (10 suppl):15–21, 1993

Barbee JG: Memory, benzodiazepines, and anxiety: integration of theoretical and clinical perspectives. J Clin Psychiatry 54 (10 suppl):86–97, 1993

Barnard EA, Darlison MG, Fujita N, et al: Molecular biology of the $GABA_A$ receptor. Adv Exp Med Biol 236:31–45, 1988

Bellantuono C, Reggi V, Tognoni G, et al: Benzodiazepines: clinical pharmacology and therapeutic use. Drugs 19:195–219, 1980

Bernstein JG: Handbook of Drug Therapy in Psychiatry, 2nd Edition. Littleton, MA, PSG Publishing, 1988

Blanchard JC, Boireau A, Garret C, et al: In vitro and in vivo inhibition by zopiclone of benzodiazepine binding to rodent brain receptors. Life Sci 24:2417–2420, 1979

Boghew D: Successful treatment of restless legs with clonazepam [letter]. Ann Neurol 8:341, 1980

Bond AJ, Hally DM, Lader MH: Plasma concentrations of benzodiazepines. British Journal of Clinical Psychopharmacology 4:51–56, 1977

Bonetti EP, Pieri L, Cumin R, et al: Benzodiazepine antagonist Ro 15-1788: neurological and behavioral effects. Psychopharmacology (Berl) 78:8–18, 1982

Bossman HB, Case KR, DiStefano P: Diazepam receptor characterization: specific binding of a benzodiazepine to macromolecules in various areas of rat brain. FEBS Lett 82:368–372, 1977

Braestrup C, Squires RF: Specific benzodiazepine receptors in rat brain characterized by high-affinity ^3H diazepam binding. Proc Natl Acad Sci U S A 74:3805–3809, 1977

Breier A, Paul SM: Anxiety and the benzodiazepine-GABA receptor complex, in Handbook of Anxiety, Vol 1. Edited by Roth M, Noyes R, Burrows GD. Amsterdam, Elsevier, 1988, pp 193–212

Charney DS, Woods SW: Benzodiazepine treatment of panic disorder: a comparison of alprazolam and lorazepam. J Clin Psychiatry 50:418–423, 1989

Chouinard G, Young SN, Annable L: Antimanic effects of clonazepam. Biol Psychiatry 18:451–466, 1983

Cohn JB, Wilcox CS: Long-term comparison of alprazolam, lorazepam and placebo in patients with an anxiety disorder. Pharmacotherapy 4:93–98, 1984

Cook L, Sepinwall J: Behavioral analysis of the effects of and mechanisms of action of benzodiazepines, in Mechanism of Action of Benzodiazepines. Edited by Costa E, Grengard P. New York, Raven, 1975, pp 1–28

Corda MG, Blaker WD, Mendelson WB, et al: Beta-carbolines enhance shock-induced suppression of drinking rats. Proc Natl Acad Sci U S A 80:2072–2076, 1983

Costa E: Allosteric modulating centers of transmitter amino and receptors. Neuropsychopharmacology 2:167–174, 1989

Costa E, Guidotti A: Endogenous ligands for benzodiazepine recognition sites. Biochem Pharmacol 34:3399–3403, 1985

Costa E, Guidotti A, Mao CC, et al: New concepts in

the mechanism of activity of BZs. Life Sci 17:167–185, 1975

Court JE, Kase CS: Treatment of tic douloureux with a new anticonvulsant (clonazepam). J Neurol Neurosurg Psychiatry 39:297–299, 1976

Cowley DS: Alcohol abuse, substance abuse, and panic disorder. Am J Med 92 (suppl 1A):41S–48S, 1992

Croft-Jeffreys C, Wilkinson G: Estimated costs of neurotic disorder in UK general practice 1985. Psychol Med 19:549–558, 1989

Cross National Collaborative Panic Study, Second Phase Investigators: Drug treatment of panic disorder: comparative efficacy of alprazolam, imipramine, and placebo. Br J Psychiatry 160:191–202, 1992

Curry SH: Concentration-effect relationship with major and minor tranquilizers. Clin Pharmacol Ther 16:192–197, 1974

Dantzer R: Behavioral effects of benzodiazepines: a review. Biobehavioral Reviews 1:71–86, 1977

Darragh A, Lambe R, Brick I, et al: Reversal of benzodiazepine-induced sedation by intravenous Ro 15-1788. Lancet 2:1042, 1981a

Darragh A, Lambe R, Scully M, et al: Investigation in man of the efficacy of a benzodiazepine antagonist, Ro 15-1788. Lancet 2:8–10, 1981b

Darragh A, Lambe R, Brick I, et al: Antagonism of the central effects of 3-methyl-clonazepam. Br J Clin Pharmacol 14:871–872, 1982a

Darragh A, Lambe R, Kenny M, et al: Ro 15-1788 antagonizes the central effects of diazepam in man without altering diazepam bioavailability. Br J Clin Pharmacol 14:677–682, 1982b

Dasberg HH, van der Klijn E, Guelen PJR, et al: Plasma concentrations of diazepam and its metabolite N-desmethyldiazepam in relation to anxiolytic effect. Clin Pharmacol Ther 15:473–483, 1974

DeBlas A, Sangameswaran L: Demonstration and purification of an endogenous benzodiazepine from the mammalian brain with a monoclonal antibody to benzodiazepines. Life Sci 39:1927–1936, 1986

DeRobertis E, Pena C, Paladini AC, et al: New developments in the search for the endogenous ligand(s) of central benzodiazepine receptors. Neurochem Int 13:1–11, 1988

DeSouza EB, Anholt RRH, Murphy KMM, et al: Peripheral-type benzodiazepine receptors in endocrine organs: autoradiographic localization in rat pituitary, adrenal and testis. Endocrinology 116:567–573, 1985

DeVane CL, Ware MR, Lydiard RB: Pharmacokinetics, pharmacodynamics, and treatment issues of benzodiazepines: alprazolam, adinazolam, and clonazepam. Psychopharmacol Bull 27(4):463–473, 1991

Dorow R, Horowski R, Paschelke G, et al: Severe anxiety induced by FG 7142, a beta-carboline ligand for benzodiazepine receptor function. Lancet 2:98–99, 1983

Fabre LF, McLendon DM, Stephens AG: Comparison of the therapeutic effect, tolerance and safety of ketazolam and diazepam administered for six months to outpatients with chronic anxiety neurosis. J Int Med Res 9:191–198, 1981

Faull RL, Villiger JW: Benzodiazepine receptors in the human hippocampal formation: a pharmacological and quantitative autoradiographic study. Neuroscience 26:783–790, 1988

Faull RL, Villiger JW, Holford NH: Benzodiazepine receptors in the human cerebellar cortex: a quantitative autoradiographic and pharmacological study demonstrating the predominance of type I receptors. Brain Res 411:379–385, 1987

File SE: The use of social interaction as a method for detecting anxiolytic activity of chlordiazepoxide-like drugs. J Neurosci Methods 2:219–238, 1980

File SE: Animal models for predicting clinical efficacy of anxiolytic drugs: social behaviour. Neuropsychobiology 13:55–62, 1985

File SE: The benzodiazepine receptor and its role in anxiety. Br J Psychiatry 152:599–600, 1988

File SE: Preclinical studies of the mechanisms of anxiety and its treatment, in Neurobiology of Anxiety Disorders. Edited by Ballenger JC. New York, Wiley-Liss, 1990, pp 31–48

File SE, Hyde JRG: Can social interaction be used to measure anxiety? Br J Pharmacol 62:19–24, 1978

File SE, Hyde JRG: A test of anxiety that distinguishes between the actions of benzodiazepines and those of other minor tranquilizers and of stimulants. Pharmacol Biochem Behav 11:65–69, 1979

File SE, Pellow S: The anxiogenic action of PG 7142 in the social interaction test is reversed by chlordiazepoxide and Ro 15-1788 but not by CGS 8216. Arch Int Pharmacodyn Ther 271:198–205, 1984

File SE, Lister RG, Nutt DG: The anxiogenic action of benzodiazepine antagonists. Neuropharmacology 21:1033–1037, 1982

File SE, Lister RG, Maninov R, et al: Intrinsic behavioural actions of propyl beta-carboline-3-carboxylate. Neuropharmacology 23:463–466, 1984

Finkle BS, McCloskey KL, Goodman LS: Diazepam and drug associated deaths. JAMA 242:428, 1979

Friedman MJ: Post-Vietnam syndrome. Psychosomatics 22:931–941, 1981

Garbus SB, Weber MS, Priest RT, et al: The abrupt discontinuation of antihypertensive treatment. J Clin Pharmacol 19:476–486, 1979

Geller I, Seifter J: The effects of meprobamate, barbiturates, D-amphetamine, and promazine on experimentally induced conflict in the rat. Psychopharmacologia 1:482–492, 1960

Ghoneim MM, Mewaldt SP: Benzodiazepines and human memory: a review. Anesthesiology 72:926–938, 1990

Glassman R, Salzman C: Interactions between psychotropic and other drugs: an update. Hosp Community Psychiatry 38:236–242, 1987

Gray JA: The Neuropsychology of Anxiety: An Enquiry into the Functions of the Septo-Hippocampal System. Oxford, England, Clarendon, 1982

Greenblatt DJ, Shader RI: Benzodiazepines in Clinical Practice. New York, Raven, 1974

Greenblatt DJ, Allen MD, Noel BJ, et al: Acute overdose with benzodiazepine derivatives. Clin Pharmacol Ther 21:497, 1977

Greenblatt DJ, Divoll M, Abernethy DR, et al: Clinical pharmacokinetics of the newer benzodiazepines. Clin Pharmacokinet 8:233–253, 1983

Greenblatt DJ, Harmatz JS, Shapiro L, et al: Sensitivity to triazolam in the elderly. N Engl J Med 324:1691–1698, 1991

Greenblatt DJ, Harmatz JS, Shader RI: Plasma alprazolam concentrations: relation to efficacy and side effects in the treatment of panic disorder. Arch Gen Psychiatry 50:715–722, 1993

Haefely W: Behavioral and neuropharmacological aspects of drugs used in anxiety and related states, in Psychopharmacology: A Generation of Progress. Edited by Lipton MA, DiMascio A, Killam KF. New York, Raven, 1978, pp 1359–1374

Haefely W: The biological basis of benzodiazepine actions, in The Benzodiazepines: Current Standards for Medical Practice. Edited by Smith DE, Wesson DR. Hingham, MA, MTP Press, 1985, pp 7–42

Haefely W: Endogenous ligands of the benzodiazepine receptor. Pharmacopsychiatria 21:43, 1988

Haefely W: The GABA$_A$-benzodiazepine receptor: biology and pharmacology, in Handbook of Anxiety, Vol 3: The Neurobiology of Anxiety. Edited by Burrows GD, Roth M, Noyes R. Amsterdam, Elsevier Science, 1990, pp 165–188

Haefely W, Kuksar A, Möhler H, et al: Possible involvement of GABA in the central action of BZ derivatives. Adv Biochem Psychopharmacol 14:131–151, 1975

Hansten PD: Drug Interactions, 5th Edition. Philadelphia, PA, Lea & Febiger, 1985

Harvey SC: Hypnotics and sedatives, in Goodman and Gilman's The Pharmacological Basis of Therapeutics, 7th Edition. Edited by Gilman AG, Goodman LS, Rall TW. New York, Macmillan, 1985, pp 339–371

Hindley SW, Hobbs A, Paterson IA, et al: Microinjection of methyl-beta-carboline-3-carboxylate into nucleus raphe dorsalis reduces social interaction in the rat. Br J Pharmacol 86:753–761, 1985

Hindmarch I, Kerr JS, Sherwood N: The effects of alcohol and other drugs on psychomotor performance and cognitive function. Alcohol Alcohol 26:71–79, 1991

Hollister LE: Pharmacology and clinical use of benzodiazepines, in Pharmacology of Benzodiazepines. Edited by Usdin E, Skolnick P, Tallman JF Jr, et al. London, Macmillan Press, Ltd, 1982, pp 29–36

Hommer DW, Skolnick P, Paul SM: The benzodiazepine/GABA receptor complex and anxiety, in Psychopharmacology: The Third Generation of Progress. Edited by Meltzer HY. New York, Raven, 1987, pp 977–983

Howell EF, Laraia M, Ballenger JC, et al: Lorazepam treatment of panic disorder. Paper presented at the 140th annual meeting of the American Psychiatric Association, Chicago, May 1987

Hsiao JK, Potter WZ: Mechanism of action of antipanic drugs, in Clinical Aspects of Panic Disorder. Edited by Ballenger JC. New York, Wiley-Liss, 1990, pp 297–317

Hunkeler W, Möhler H, Pieri L, et al: Selective antagonists of benzodiazepines. Nature 290:514–516, 1981

Kales A, Kales JD, Bixler EO, et al: Effectiveness of hypnotic drugs with prolonged use: flurazepam and pentobarbital. Clin Pharmacol Ther 18:356–364, 1975

Kangas L, Kanto J, Lehtinen V, et al: Long-term nitrazepam treatment in psychiatric outpatients with insomnia. Psychopharmacology (Berl) 63:63–66, 1979

Kilts CD, Commissaris RL, Rech RH: Comparison of anti-conflict drug effects in three experimental animal models of anxiety. Psychopharmacology (Berl) 74:290–296, 1981

King DJ: Benzodiazepines, amnesia, and sedation: theoretical and clinical issues and controversies. Human Psychopharmacology 7:79–87, 1992

Klepner CA, Lippa AS, Benson DI, et al: Resolution of two biochemically and pharmacologically distinct benzodiazepine receptors. Pharmacol Biochem Behav 11:457–462, 1979

Klerman GL, Weissman MM, Ouellette R, et al: Panic attacks in the community: social morbidity and health care utilization. JAMA 265:742–746, 1991

Kramer M: Dream disturbances. Psychiatric Annals 9:50–68, 1979

Krueger KE: Peripheral-type benzodiazepine receptors: a second site of action for benzodiazepines. Neuropsychopharmacology 4(4):237–244, 1991

Krueger KE, Papadopoulos V: Peripheral-type benzodiazepine receptors mediate translocation of cholesterol from outer to inner mitochondrial membranes in adrenocortical cells. J Biol Chem 265:15015–15022, 1990

Lader M: Clinical pharmacology of benzodiazepines. Annu Rev Med 38:19–28, 1987

Lesser IM, Lydiard RB, Antal E, et al: Alprazolam plasma concentrations and treatment response in panic disorder and agoraphobia. Am J Psychiatry 149(11):1556–1562, 1992

Linnoila M, Erwin CW, Brendle A, et al: Psychomotor effects of diazepam in anxious patients and healthy volunteers. J Clin Psychopharmacol 3:988–996, 1983

Lo MM, Niehoff DL, Kuhar MJ, et al: Differential localization of type I and type II benzodiazepine binding sites in substantia nigra. Nature 306:57–60, 1983

Luckner M: Secondary Metabolism in Microorganisms, Plants and Animals. Berlin, Springer-Verlag, 1984, pp 272–276

Lüddens H, Wisden W: Function and pharmacology of multiple GABA$_A$ receptor subunits. Trends Pharmacol Sci 12:49–51, 1991

Lüddens H, Pritchett DB, Kohler M, et al: Cerebellar GABA$_A$ receptor selective for a behavioural alcohol antagonist. Nature 346:648–651, 1990

Marangos PJ, Patel J, Boulenger JP, et al: Character-

ization of peripheral-type benzodiazepine binding sites in brain using [^{3}H]Ro5-4864. Mol Pharmacol 22:26–32, 1982

Margules DL, Stein L: Increase of antianxiety activity and tolerance to behavioural depression during chronic administration of oxazepam. Psychopharmacology (Berl) 13:74–80, 1968

Markowitz JS, Weissman MM, Ouellette R, et al: Quality of life in panic disorder. Arch Gen Psychiatry 46:984–992, 1989

Matthews WB: Treatment of restless legs syndrome with clonazepam [letter]. British Medical Journal 1:751, 1979

Mendelson WB, Gillin JC, Wyatt RJ: Human Sleep and Its Disorders. New York, Plenum, 1977

Miller LG, Greenblatt DJ, Barnhill JG, et al: Chronic benzodiazepine administration, I: tolerance is associated with benzodiazepine receptor downregulation and decreased γ-aminobutyric acid$_A$ receptor function. J Pharmacol Exp Ther 246:170–176, 1988

Möhler H, Okada T: Properties of ^{3}H diazepam binding to benzodiazepine receptors in rat cerebral cortex. Life Sci 20:2101–2110, 1977a

Möhler H, Okada T: Benzodiazepine receptors: demonstration in the central nervous system. Science 198:849–851, 1977b

Möhler H, Richards JG: Agonist and antagonist benzodiazepine receptor interaction in vitro. Nature 294:763–764, 1981

Möhler H, Wu JY, Richards JG: Benzodiazepine receptors: autoradiographical and immunocytochemical evidence for their localization in regions of GABAergic synaptic contacts, in GABA and Benzodiazepine Receptors. Edited by Costa E, DiChaira G, Gessa GL. New York, Raven, 1981, pp 139–146

Nestoros JN: Benzodiazepines in schizophrenia: a need for reassessment. Int Pharmacopsychiatry 15:171–179, 1980

Nielsen M, Braestrup C: Ethyl β-carboline 3-carboxylate shows differential benzodiazepine receptor interaction. Nature 286:606–607, 1980

Noyes R, Anderson DJ, Clancy J, et al: Diazepam and propranolol in panic disorder and agoraphobia. Arch Gen Psychiatry 41:287–292, 1984

Olsen RW, McCabe RT, Wamsley JK: GABA$_A$ receptor subtypes: autoradiographic comparison of GABA, benzodiazepine, and convulsant binding sites in the rat central nervous system. J Chem Neuroanat

3:59–76, 1990

Paul SM, Skolnick P: Comparative neuropharmacology of antianxiety drugs. Pharmacol Biochem Behav 17 (suppl 1):37–41, 1982

Paul SM, Zatz M, Skolnick P: Demonstration of brain-specific benzodiazepine receptors in rat retina. Brain Res 187:243–246, 1980

Pellow S, File SE: Anxiolytic and anxiogenic drug effects in exploratory activity in an elevated plus-maze: a novel test of anxiety in the rat. Pharmacol Biochem Behav 24:525–529, 1986

Pellow S, Chopin P, File SE, et al: The validation of open/closed arm entries in an elevated plus-maze as a measure of anxiety in the rat. J Neurosci Methods 14:149–167, 1985

Petersen EN, Paschelke G, Kehr W, et al: Does the reversal of the anticonflict effect of phenobarbital by beta-CCE and FG 7142 indicate benzodiazepine receptor-mediated anxiogenic properties? Eur J Pharmacol 82:217–221, 1982

Petersen EN, Jensen LH, Honore T, et al: Differential pharmacological effects of benzodiazepine receptor inverse agonists, in Benzodiazepine Recognition Site Ligands: Biochemistry And Pharmacology. Edited by Biggio G, Costa E. New York, Raven, 1983, pp 57–64

Polc P: Electrophysiology of benzodiazepine receptor ligands: multiple mechanisms and sites of action. Prog Neurobiol 31(5):349–423, 1988

Polc P, Möhler H, Haefely W: The effect of diazepam on spinal cord activities: possible sites and mechanisms of action. Naunyn Schmiederbergs Arch Pharmacol 284:319–337, 1974

Polc P, Laurent JP, Scherschlicht R, et al: Electrophysiological studies on the specific benzodiazepine antagonist Ro 15-1788. Naunyn Schmiedebergs Arch Pharmacol 316:317–325, 1981

Randall LO: Discovery of benzodiazepines, in Pharmacology of Benzodiazepines. Edited by Usdin E, Skolnick P, Tallman JF Jr, et al. London, MacMillan Press, Ltd, 1982, pp 15–22

Richards JG, Möhler H, Haefely W: Benzodiazepine binding sites: receptors or acceptors? Trends Pharmacol Sci 3:233–235, 1982

Rickels K, Case WG, Diamond L: Relapse after short-term drug therapy in neurotic outpatients. International Pharmacopsychiatry 15:186–192, 1980

Rickels K, Case WG, Downing RW, et al: Long-term diazepam therapy and clinical outcome. JAMA 250:767–771, 1983

Rickels K, Schweizer E, Case WG, et al: Long-term therapeutic use of benzodiazepines, I: effects of abrupt discontinuation. Arch Gen Psychiatry 47:899–907, 1990

Rickels K, Case WG, Schweizer E, et al: Long-term benzodiazepine users 3 years after participation in a discontinuation program. Am J Psychiatry 148:757–761, 1991

Romach MK, Somer GR, Sobell LC, et al: Characteristics of long-term alprazolam users in the community. J Clin Psychopharmacol 12:316–332, 1992

Roth T, Roehrs T, Wittig R, et al: Benzodiazepines and memory. Br J Clin Pharmacol 18:45S–49S, 1984

Ruffalo RL, Thompson JF: Effect of cimetidine on the clearance of benzodiazepines. N Engl J Med 303:753–754, 1980

Schatzberg AF, Ballenger JC: Decisions for the clinician in the treatment of panic disorder: when to treat, which treatment to use, and how long to treat. J Clin Psychiatry 52:26–31, 1991

Schweizer E, Fox I, Case G, et al: Lorazepam vs alprazolam in the treatment of panic disorder. Psychopharmacol Bull 24:224–227, 1988

Seeburg PH, Wisden W, Verdoorn TA, et al: The $GABA_A$ receptor family: molecular and functional diversity. Cold Spring Harbor Symposia on Quantitative Biology 55:29–44, 1990

Sepinwall J, Cook L: Behavioral pharmacology of anti-anxiety drugs, in Handbook of Psychopharmacology, Vol 13. Edited by Iversen LL, Iversen SD, Snyder SH. New York, Plenum, 1978, pp 345–393

Shader RI, Greenblatt DJ: Use of benzodiazepines in anxiety disorders. N Engl J Med 328:1398–1405, 1993

Shader RI, Dreyfuss D, Gerrein JR, et al: Sedative effects and impaired learning and recall following single oral doses of lorazepam. Clin Pharmacol Ther 39:526–529, 1986

Sieghart W, Eichinger A, Riederer P, et al: Comparison of benzodiazepine receptor binding in membranes from human or rat brain. Neuropharmacology 24:751–759, 1985

Simon P, Soubrie P: Behavioral studies to differentiate anxiolytic and sedative activity of the tranquilizing drugs, in Modern Problems in Pharmacopsychiatry, Vol 14. Edited by Boissier JR. Basel, Karger, 1979, pp 99–142

Smith DE, Wesson DR (eds): The Benzodiazepines: Current Standards for Medical Practice. Boston,

MA, MTP Press Limited, 1985, pp 289–292

Squires RF, Braestrup CL: Benzodiazepine receptors in rat brain. Nature 266:732–734, 1977

Stephens DN, Kehr W: Beta-carbolines can enhance or antagonize the effects of punishment in mice. Psychopharmacology (Berl) 85:143–147, 1985

Stephens DN, Shearman GT, Kehr W: Discriminative stimulus properties of beta-carbolines characterized as agonists and inverse agonists at central benzodiazepine receptors. Psychopharmacology (Berl) 83:233–239, 1984

Sternbach LH: The discovery of CNS active 1,4-benzodiazepines (chemistry), in Pharmacology of Benzodiazepines. Edited by Usdin E, Skolnick, Tallman JR Jr, et al. London, Macmillan Press, Ltd., 1982, pp 7–14

Sternbach LH, Reeder E: Quinazolines and 1,4-benzodiazepines, II: the rearrangement of 6-chloro-2-chloromethyl-4-phenylquinazoline 3-oxide into 2-amino-derivatives of 7-chloro-5-phenyl-^{3}H-1,4-benzodiazepine 4-oxide. Journal of Organic Chemistry 26:1111–1118, 1961

Study RE, Barker JL: Diazepam and pentobarbital: fluctuation analysis reveals different mechanisms for potentiation of gamma-aminobutyric acid responses in cultured central neurons. Proc Natl Acad Sci U S A 78(11):7180–7184, 1981

Tallman JF, Thomas JW, Gallager DW: GABAergic modulation of benzodiazepine binding site sensitivity. Nature 274:383–385, 1978

Tallman JF, Paul SM, Skolnick P, et al: Receptors for the age of anxiety: the pharmacology of benzodiazepines. Science 207:274–281, 1980

Tansella M, Siciliani O, Burti L, et al: N-Desmethyl-diazepam and amylobarbitone sodium as hypnotics in anxious patients: plasma levels, clinical efficacy and residual effects. Psychopharmacologia 41:81–85, 1975

Tansella M, Zimmermann-Tansella CH, Ferrario L, et al: Plasma concentrations of diazepam, nordiazepam and amylobarbitone after short-term treatment of anxious patients. Pharmacopsychiatrie

Neuropsychopharmakogie 11:68–75, 1978

Thiébot MH, Soubrié P: Behavioral pharmacology of the benzodiazepines, in Benzodiazepines—Molecular Biology to Clinical Practice. Edited by Costa E. New York, Raven, 1983, pp 67–92

Thomas JW, Tallman JF: Characterization of photoaffinity labeling of benzodiazepine binding sites. J Biol Chem 156:9839–9842, 1981

Villiger JW: Characterization of peripheral-type benzodiazepine recognition sites in rat spinal cord. Neuropharmacology 24:93–98, 1985

Vogel JR, Beer B, Clody DE: A simple and reliable conflict procedure for testing antianxiety agents. Psychopharmacologia 21:1–7, 1971

Ward J: Vital uses of diazepam in third world countries, in The Benzodiazepines: Current Standards for Medical Practice. Edited by Smith DE, Wesson DR. Boston, MA, MTP Press Limited, 1985, pp 167–175

Weissman MM, Klerman GL, Markowitz JS, et al: Suicidal ideation and suicide attempts in panic disorder and attacks. N Engl J Med 321:1209–1214, 1989

Wesson DR: Additional clinical uses of benzodiazepines, in The Benzodiazepines: Current Standards for Medical Practice. Edited by Smith DE, Wesson DR. Boston, MTP Press Limited, 1985, pp 163–166

Ymer S, Draguhn A, Wisden W, et al: Structural and functional characterization of the γ_1 subunit of GABA$_A$/benzodiazepine receptors. European Molecular Biology Organization Journal 9:3261–3267, 1990

Yokoyama N, Ritter B, Neubert AD: 2-Arylpyrazolo(4,30c)quinolin-3-ones: novel agonists, partial agonists and antagonists of benzodiazepines. J Med Chem 25:337–339, 1982

Young WS, Kuhar MJ: Radiohistochemical localization of benzodiazepine receptors in rat brain. J Pharmacol Exp Ther 212:337–346, 1980

Zorumski CF, Isenberg KE: Insights into the structure and function of GABA-benzodiazepine receptors: ion channels and psychiatry. Am J Psychiatry 148:162–173, 1991

12

Nonbenzodiazepine Anxiolytics

Jonathan O. Cole, M.D., and Kimberly A. Yonkers, M.D.

Although meprobamate and buspirone are not the only nonbenzodiazepine antianxiety or hypnotic drugs used in medicine today, they represent, respectively, the first nonbarbiturate antianxiety drug to become available and the first nonsedative nonbenzodiazepine antianxiety drug to be developed and marketed. Many older barbiturates exist and are well described in earlier editions of Goodman and Gilman's *The Pharmacological Basis of Therapeutics* (e.g., Goodman and Gilman 1970), as are sedative antihistamines such as diphenhydramine and hydroxyzine. Neither class of agents has been well studied either as anxiolytics or as hypnotics. The barbiturates are presumed to be effective but are too lethal in overdose and too prone to abuse to be widely used. The antihistamines are probably less effective than appropriate benzodiazepines but have not been adequately studied. Hydroxyzine hydrochloride (Atarax) and hydroxyzine pamoate (Vistaril) are both available for prescription use. The pamoate form may cross the blood-brain barrier more efficiently. Diphenhydramine (Benadryl) is a more sedating antihistamine that is often used as a hypnotic, but its efficacy lacks validating studies.

■ MEPROBAMATE

■ History and Discovery

Meprobamate was discovered by a pharmacologist, Frank M. Berger, following an unlikely trail of findings (Berger 1970). He had been looking for an antibiotic that was effective against gram-negative or-

ganisms. One chemical compound (phenoxetol, a phenylglycol) had weak antibacterial properties that Berger's group tried to improve by lengthening its carbon chain to synthesize congeners. Berger studied drugs in this series in rodents and found the drugs to have an unusual muscle relaxant property. In mice or rats, paralysis of voluntary muscles could be produced in animals that otherwise looked calm and alert. This condition lasted variable lengths of time depending on the structure and dose used. These compounds did not show the early excitement that preceded sedation with barbiturates or anesthetics.

The only marketed drug in this group, mephenesin, was very short acting in humans, but there was some clinical evidence that it could cause tense, anxious patients to become relaxed (Dixon et al. 1950).

Berger's collaboration with B. J. Ludwig, a medicinal chemist, to create mephenesin analogues with more potency, longer duration of action, and more effect in the central nervous system (CNS) began in 1949. Meprobamate was synthesized in May 1950 and eventually received the Wallace Laboratories trade name of Miltown. Meprobamate's duration of action was eight times that of mephenesin. It had a taming effect in monkeys and some selective action on the thalamus and the limbic system as well as the muscle-relaxing and sedative effects of mephenesin. Berger made the claim that meprobamate has a sedative antianxiety effect *only* in anxious patients and does not impair performance or cause changes in subjective state in nonanxious volunteers. We believe that most current psychopharmacologists would disagree with this position, although we know of no direct tests comparing meprobamate with benzodiazepines in nonanxious control subjects (Rall 1993; Roache and Griffiths 1987).

The original approval of meprobamate (Miltown) by the U.S. Food and Drug Administration (FDA) accompanied the appearance of two positive open clinical trials in heterogeneous groups of anxious outpatients. In those days the FDA, by law, required only proof of safety, not of efficacy. Meprobamate's sales and popularity rose rapidly, and Wallace Laboratories was impelled to license Wyeth Labs to also synthesize and sell meprobamate under the trade name Equanil. Meprobamate continued in wide general use from 1955, when it was introduced, through 1972, when the benzodiazepines generally replaced it.

■ Structure-Activity Relations

Meprobamate, a bis-carbamate ester, contains two terminal amino groups and seven carbon atoms but no rings (Figure 12–1). Although it does not closely resemble any other psychoactive drug currently in general use, it does resemble carisoprodol (Soma), a drug sold as a muscle relaxant with sedative properties (Elenbaas 1980).

■ Pharmacological Profile

Meprobamate falls pharmacologically between the barbiturates and the benzodiazepines. It causes CNS

Mephenesin

Meprobamate

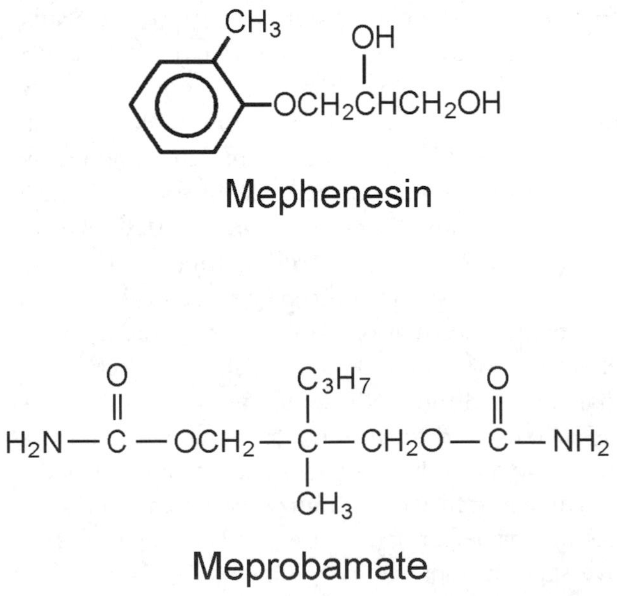

Figure 12–1. Chemical structures of mephenesin and meprobamate.

depression but does not produce anesthesia. In animals, it releases behaviors suppressed by past adverse experiences, a property it shares with all other antianxiety drugs. Meprobamate depresses polysynaptic spinal reflexes more than monosynaptic reflexes; barbiturates are less selective in this regard. This action was originally believed to be the basis of meprobamate's muscle relaxant effects. In fact, such effects are very difficult to differentiate from sedation and decreased anxiety at the human clinical level (Rall 1993).

Meprobamate has anticonvulsant properties resembling those of ethosuximide. Clinically, it suppresses absence attacks but can sometimes aggravate tonic-clonic seizures. Naloxone can block meprobamate's antianxiety effects in laboratory animals. Meprobamate may have a modest degree of analgesic action in patients with musculoskeletal pain.

■ Pharmacokinetics and Disposition

Meprobamate taken orally in humans reaches a peak blood concentration in 1–3 hours. It is not bound much to plasma proteins. Meprobamate is metabolized in the liver by hydroxylation and glucuronide formation, with a small proportion excreted unchanged. Its half-life is 6–17 hours in acute studies; with chronic administration this may increase to 24–48 hours. The exact hepatic microsomal enzymes involved and the degree to which meprobamate induces their activity are unclear.

In suicidal overdose, meprobamate tablets can form a lump (bezoar) in the patient's stomach. As the patient emerges from coma, gastric activity will break up the bezoar and reinduce the coma if gastroscopy has not been used to identify and remove the undissolved tablet mass (Rall 1993). Otherwise, suicide attempts with meprobamate are treated as one would a barbiturate overdose. The lethal dose can be as low as 30 tablets (12,000 mg), but the average lethal dose is around 28,000 mg.

■ Proposed Mechanisms

There is a presumption that meprobamate, because of its pharmacological effects, *should* work like the barbiturates, γ-aminobutyric acid (GABA), or the benzodiazepines; however, meprobamate does not bind to any of the relevant receptors (Paul et al. 1981; Rall 1993; Squires and Braestrup 1977). Three mechanisms have been proposed to explain meprobamate's action.

1. **Benzodiazepine–GABA–chloride ionophore complex.** Meprobamate is thought to exert its anxiolytic effect by interacting with the benzodiazepine–GABA–chloride ionophore complex (Paul et al. 1981). Initial studies on the benzodiazepine receptor showed that only clinically active benzodiazepines could displace ^{3}H-benzodiazepines from these receptors. Meprobamate competitively inhibits GABA-enhanced-benzodiazepine binding at the benzodiazepine receptor at concentrations fivefold lower than those required to inhibit binding to the receptor. These concentrations are also in the range of its clinical efficacy.

   Studies by Olsen (1981) and Leeb-Lundberg and Olsen (1983) suggest that the chloride ionophore may be the site of action for such inhibitory agents (Roache and Griffiths 1987). Squires and Braestrup (1977) and Polc et al. (1982) proposed that instead of acting through the benzodiazepine receptor, meprobamate may act through the barbiturate-recognition site in order to enhance benzodiazepine binding. It has also been noted that GABAergic transmission is not affected by meprobamate (Ableitner and Herz 1987). Thus, the precise site for the inhibition of the GABA-stimulated enhancement is not clear.

2. **Role of adenosine.** The central actions of meprobamate are associated with the potentiation of endogenously released adenosine (Phillis and DeLong 1984). Meprobamate has been shown to be a potent inhibitor of adenosine uptake by rat cerebral cortical synaptosomes (Phillis and DeLong 1984). This inhibitory effect results in an increase in extracellular adenosine levels (DeLong et al. 1985). In addition, meprobamate potentiates the actions of adenosine in cerebral cortical neurons, which explains its depressant effects on spinal reflexes and cortical evoked potentials and, perhaps, its antianxiety effects (Hyman and Nestler 1993). Evidence for the role of adenosine in the clinical effects of meprobamate is supported by the potent sedative actions of adenosine as well as the sedative actions of other drugs that also increase endogenous adenosine levels (DeLong et al. 1985). Adenosine antagonists (e.g., caffeine) can increase anxiety.

Further evidence for the role of adenosine in the action of meprobamate is that adenosine competitively inhibits in ^{3}H-diazepam binding to the benzodiazepine recognition site (Paul et al. 1981) through which meprobamate may act.

3. **Effect on catecholamines.** Meprobamate has been found to decrease the stress-associated increase in norepinephrine turnover in the brain (Lidbrink et al. 1972). The stress-induced decrease in turnover of dopamine in the synapses of the neostriatum is decreased further by meprobamate, but in the median eminence the dopamine turnover is increased by meprobamate. The latter finding has been difficult to interpret.

■ Abuse Liability

A relatively recent study of the human abuse liability of meprobamate compared with lorazepam and placebo was carried out on a research ward by Roache and Griffiths (1987) with drug-free persons who had formerly been addicted to sedatives. These investigators found, surprisingly, that meprobamate was preferred by subjects to lorazepam on well-tested measures of abuse liability. It resembled a barbiturate more than a benzodiazepine in that subjects on high single doses of meprobamate (or barbiturates) were aware of their deficits in psychomotor performance, whereas on lorazepam they believed they were doing well when their performance was in fact impaired.

■ Indications

The only FDA-approved indication for meprobamate is as an anxiolytic, but the drug was also widely used in the past and even studied as a hypnotic.

Meprobamate is available in 200-mg, 400-mg, and 600-mg tablets and, in combination with an anticholinergic drug, benactyzine, is also available as Deprol, which is marketed as an antidepressant.

The most recent review of efficacy studies of meprobamate, done by Greenblatt and Shader (1971), concluded that its efficacy had not been adequately proven. However, many of those studies were done in the 1950s and 1960s before the methodology for such studies was well established, and several controlled trials by Rickels's group have since demonstrated meprobamate's clear efficacy relative to placebo. It seems likely that a well-done study with an adequate sample size would show meprobamate's efficacy in generalized anxiety disorder (GAD) to be comparable to that of a standard benzodiazepine.

The appropriate initial dose of meprobamate, if used as a hypnotic, is 400 mg at bedtime, increasing to 600 mg or decreasing to 200 mg if the 400-mg dose is too weak or too sedating. In studies of meprobamate in the treatment of chronic anxiety, patients were typically started on 400 mg po tid, but starting with 200 mg po tid might be adequate. Physical dependence on meprobamate has been observed after doses as low as 3,200 mg/day. The equivalent dose in diazepam units is probably 1 mg of diazepam to 50–60 mg meprobamate.

Over the years, the senior author (J. O. C.) has encountered rare patients who became agitated (possibly akathisia) on several benzodiazepines but subsequently did well on meprobamate. In the past, a number of patients found 400 mg meprobamate at bedtime useful as a hypnotic. Studies in the 1970s reported it to be as effective as flurazepam in insomnia (Vogel et al. 1990).

Only one clinical paper on meprobamate has appeared in the past decade. A large medical screening program for people over age 65 in Dunedin, Florida (Hale et al. 1988) found a surprising amount of meprobamate use over a 2-year period ending in 1985. The proportion of these community-resident elderly people (mean age 81 years, range 72–91) taking meprobamate regularly was 1.3% as compared with 0.8% for chlordiazepoxide and 0.9% for lorazepam. Almost 90% of the patients taking meprobamate judged it "effective" or "very effective." One-half had been on meprobamate for more than 10 years. The authors of the paper were surprised that there was no evidence of dose escalation or tolerance over time and that some physicians were continuing to prescribe this inferior drug.

Conclusion

Meprobamate deserves to remain in the armamentarium of the clinical psychopharmacologist. It has no current clear advantages over newer benzodiazepines. It may be abusable, but it is not abused in the current drug culture. Occasional patients find meprobamate more effective or better tolerated than newer drugs. However, it is clearly, on the basis of present knowledge, a third- or fourth-line drug, to be tried only when more obviously effective drugs have failed.

BUSPIRONE

History and Discovery

Buspirone was developed initially by Davis Temple, Michael Eison, and others in the neuropharmacology program at Mead Johnson Pharmaceuticals after it had become part of Bristol Myers Company. Michael Eison synthesized buspirone in 1968 in a search for a better neuroleptic (A. S. Eison 1990; M. S. Eison et al. 1987). Chemically, buspirone resembles a butyrophenone antipsychotic drug more than it does any previously developed antianxiety or antidepressant drug. Buspirone blocks the conditioned avoidance response in rats, as do typical neuroleptics. It does not cause catalepsy in animals; instead, it reverses neuroleptic-induced catalepsy. It appeared, therefore, to be potentially a clozapine-like drug—an antipsychotic with few neurological side effects.

The initial phase II clinical trial in 10 newly rehospitalized schizophrenic patients (Sathananthan et al. 1975) showed little beneficial effect: two patients improved markedly, two were slightly better, and six were clearly worse. One patient showed tremor, rigidity, and akathisia. Dose was steadily raised as tolerated to an average maximum daily dose of 1,470 mg at an average duration of 24.7 days. The maximum tolerated dose was 2,400 mg/day.

Buspirone did show efficacy on some animal tests predictive of antianxiety drug actions (Riblet et al. 1982, 1984), such as inhibition of footshock-induced fighting in mice, decreased aggression in rhesus monkeys, and attenuation of conflict behavior. It was devoid of sedative/hypnotic or anticonvulsant effects.

The group at Mead Johnson decided to do clinical tests of buspirone in treatment of DSM-II (American Psychiatric Association 1968) anxiety disorders. The earliest study, by Goldberg and Finnerty (1979), was clearly positive and led to a series of double-blind placebo-controlled studies comparing buspirone with a number of benzodiazepines and placebo.

The buspirone program was tightly controlled by the company staff—the only studies permitted were those needed for a New Drug Application (NDA) for efficacy in anxiety or to show that buspirone lacked any suggestion of neuroleptic side effects or of abuse liability. On this basis, the drug received FDA approval and was marketed in 1986.

In the interim, in 1979, the same group synthesized gepirone, an analogue of buspirone that also appears to have antianxiety and antidepressant effects.

■ Structure-Activity Relations

In addition to buspirone, three other azaspirones are known to have gotten as far as clinical trials in depressed or anxious patients (M. S. Eison 1990). Gepirone, the second azaspirone developed/marketed by Bristol-Myers Squibb, was studied more as an antidepressant than as an antianxiety agent even though its pharmacology is quite similar to that of buspirone (Cott et al. 1988). Ipsapirone (Peroutka 1985) is being developed by Baye (Heller et al. 1990) and tandospirone by Pfizer (see Figure 12–2). Published controlled studies have suggested that the three newer azaspirones have efficacy similar to that of buspirone, but none of these newer agents have, to our knowledge, been marketed in any country. Gepirone was being developed by Bristol-Myers Squibb along with nefazodone, a less-sedating, less–alpha-blocking trazodone analogue. Both drugs initially looked promising, but nefazodone now has an NDA pending and gepirone's rights have been sold by the firm.

Although all three newer azaspirones share buspirone's serotonergic effects, they lack its dopaminergic effects, suggesting that the serotonergic actions are the crucial ones. Gepirone, but not buspirone, can cause a full serotonergic syndrome in mice. The newer azaspirones may have more serotonergic effects than buspirone; however, until well-designed comparative studies are completed, it will be hard to tell whether buspirone has an edge over the others.

■ Pharmacological Profile

Buspirone is believed to exert its antianxiety effect by blocking serotonin-1A ($5\text{-}HT_{1A}$) presynaptic and postsynaptic receptors. There is evidence that other specific serotonin-1 ($5\text{-}HT_1$) or -2 ($5\text{-}HT_2$) blockers (e.g., gepirone, ritanserin) have antianxiety effects and that more broadly antiserotonergic drugs (e.g., methysergide, cyproheptadine) do not. Lesions in the brain serotonergic system will block the antianxiety effects of both benzodiazepines and buspirone (A. S. Eison and M. S. Eison 1994). Buspirone is a full antagonist at presynaptic $5\text{-}HT_{1A}$ receptors but only a partial antagonist at postsynaptic $5\text{-}HT_{1A}$ receptors. It causes downregulation of $5\text{-}HT_2$ receptors.

Buspirone also prevents the increase in dopamine-2 receptors caused by standard neuroleptics (the presumed mechanism causing tardive dyskinesia [TD]) and reverses the neuroleptics' catalepsy-inducing action in rodents. In neuroradiographic studies, radioactively labeled buspirone is found on dopamine receptors throughout the brain. This is more obvious than its parallel binding to $5\text{-}HT_{1A}$ receptors. In some respects, buspirone's pharmacology early on resembled that of apomorphine—a dopamine agonist with claimed antianxiety effects—more than it did those of either the neuroleptics or the benzodiazepines (M. S. Eison et al. 1987; Ortiz et al. 1987).

Buspirone "passes" antianxiety drug tests in animals by reversing conditioned suppression of behavior, reversing "learned helplessness," and being effective in the Porsolt behavioral despair model. It reverses inhibition of conflict behavior (antianxiety) but also blocks conditioned avoidance responding (antipsychotic) (A. S. Eison et al. 1991).

Buspirone has no major effects on the benzodiazepine–GABA–chloride ionophore complex, long thought to be the major site of benzodiazepine action. Buspirone has been shown in vivo to enhance benzodiazepine binding, perhaps through a conformational change mediated by a picrotoxin-sensitive site (A. S. Eison and M. S. Eison 1984).

Buspirone lacks the benzodiazepines' sedative, muscle relaxant, or anticonvulsant actions and has no ability to affect benzodiazepine withdrawal symptoms.

Buspirone lacks abuse potential as judged by relevant animal and human studies (Cole et al. 1982; Griffith et al. 1986). In humans, it also neither impairs psychomotor performance nor potentiates the performance-impairing effects of alcohol. Benzodiazepines tend to impair performance in the above paradigms (Smiley 1987); buspirone not only does not impair performance but also improves the subject's awareness of any alcohol-induced decrements in performance (Sussman and Chou 1988).

■ Pharmacokinetics

Buspirone, taken orally at usual doses, has a short half-life ranging from 1 to 10 hours in healthy volunteers. If the drug is taken with food, first-pass metab-

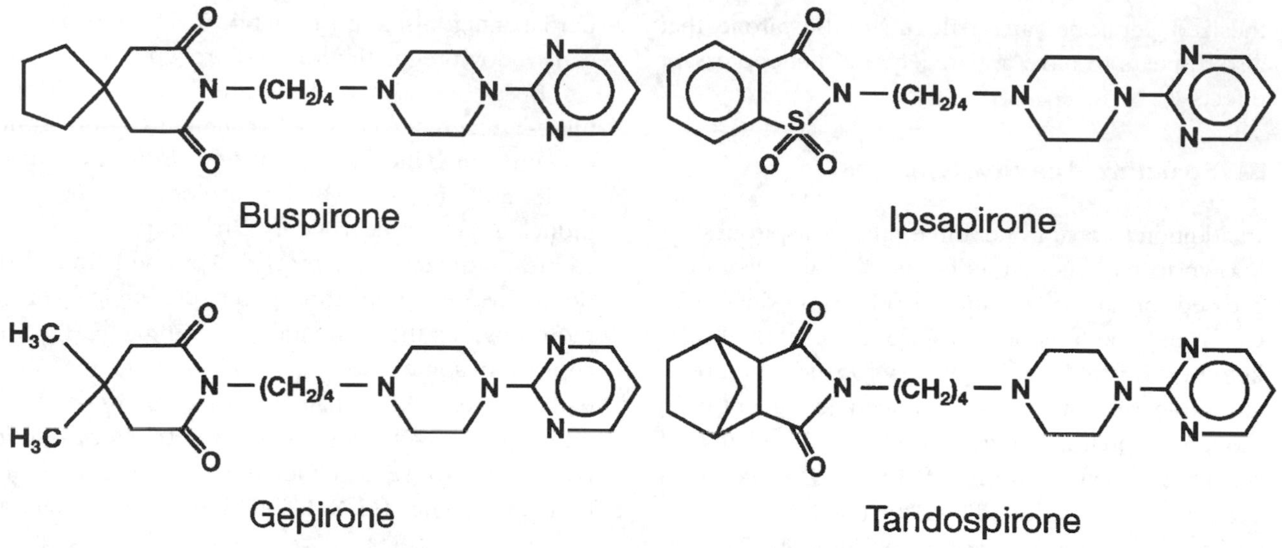

Buspirone

Ipsapirone

Gepirone

Tandospirone

Figure 12–2. Chemical structures of the azaspirones: buspirone, gepirone, ipsapirone, and tandospirone.

olism is decreased and higher "area-under-the-curve" (Jann 1988) values for buspirone blood levels are achieved.

Buspirone has multiple metabolites, mainly hydroxylated derivatives. The major metabolite is 1-pyrimidinylpiperazine (1-PP); brain levels of 1-PP can be several times higher than blood levels. 1-PP lacks buspirone's serotonergic effects but may block alpha$_2$-noradrenergic receptors and cause an increase in 3-methoxy-4-hydroxy-phenylglycol (MHPG) production. This effect is of interest because one recent study (Tollefson et al. 1991) found a strong correlation between 1-PP blood levels and buspirone's efficacy in alcoholic patients.

It is possible that the lesser efficacy of buspirone in benzodiazepine withdrawal or panic attacks may be due to the noradrenergic effects of 1-PP. If so, other azaspirones that do not form 1-PP may be better tolerated in such situations.

Buspirone's pharmacokinetics are not altered in elderly persons, in whom buspirone is probably effective both in depression and in GAD (Bohm et al. 1990; Napoliello 1986). Buspirone may have a slow onset of action (up to 7 weeks) but favorable effects in agitated patients with dementia (Gelenberg 1994).

■ Neuroendocrine Effects

Buspirone in single doses of 30–90 mg elevates plasma levels of prolactin and probably growth hormone in nonanxious subjects (Meltzer et al. 1983).

Other studies have shown less effect on prolactin levels. (For example, at 100 mg in a single dose, but not at 50 mg, levels were elevated; however, there was no effect on cortisol, aldosterone, or growth hormone levels at either dose [Cohn et al. 1986].) A study of 20 anxious patients on clinically usual buspirone dosages showed no changes in prolactin, cortisol, or growth hormone levels when the drug was given in 5- to 10-mg doses three times per day (Cohn et al. 1986).

■ Drug-Drug Interactions

Buspirone (Buspar) is surprisingly free of significant drug-drug interactions. When it was first released, it was said to have caused hypertensive states when added to monoamine oxidase inhibitors (MAOIs). These symptoms now appear to have been mild to moderate elevations in blood pressure rather than serious hypertensive or serotonergic crises of the sort elicited by selective serotonin reuptake inhibitor (SSRI)–MAOI combinations. However, it is too early to say that buspirone can be added to MAOIs with impunity. Ciraulo and Shader (1990), after reviewing all data available to Bristol-Myers on buspirone-MAOI interactions, found insufficient evidence for a total prohibition of combined buspirone-MAOI therapy; we concur.

In one study in which diazepam and buspirone were given concurrently for 2 weeks, there was a 20% elevation in desmethyldiazepam levels only

(Gammans et al. 1994). Baughman (1994), quoted in Gelenberg's (1994) summary of a recent conference on buspirone, notes that buspirone does not adversely affect parkinsonism and does not interact with the more commonly used antiparkinsonian drugs. In schizophrenic patients on neuroleptics, Baughman suggests that buspirone reduces extrapyramidal side effects (EPS) caused by neuroleptics. Buspirone has been reported to elevate haloperidol blood levels somewhat; it may also elevate cyclosporin-A levels, a clinically more important effect, because elevation of these levels may increase the risk for adverse effects on the kidneys.

Buspirone appears to improve respiratory functions and arterial pCO_2 in patients with anxiety and severe lung disease (Sussman and Chou 1988).

Gelenberg (1994) notes that buspirone may reverse sexual dysfunction caused by SSRIs. An earlier report by Othmer and Othmer (1987) found that buspirone improved sexual function in GAD patients. One drug-drug interaction that fortunately does not exist is between SSRIs and buspirone. The combination of two serotonergic drugs could cause a serotonergic syndrome but in this case does not. Several published reports (all uncontrolled studies) suggest that adding buspirone to any antidepressant, including an SSRI, will often produce a better antidepressant response (Joffe and Schuller 1993). Buspirone's bimodal action may even protect against serotonergic overamping. In other words, the presynaptic $5\text{-}HT_{1A}$ blockade increases serotonergic activity when such activity is low but reduces it by blocking postsynaptic receptors when the activity is high (M. S. Eison 1990).

■ Indications and Conundra

Use in Anxiety Disorders

Buspirone has been shown to have efficacy in GAD and has been generally available for use in that condition in the United States since 1986. The majority of the large-scale (i.e., $N > 60$) double-blind, random-assignment clinical studies have shown buspirone to be equal in efficacy to standard benzodiazepines in GAD or in less clearly specified chronic anxiety states. Buspirone often fails to show efficacy in small, short-term trials, especially those with a crossover feature (Olajide and Lader 1987), probably because patients with substantial past experience with benzodiazepines tend to respond less well to buspirone. However, the original report describing this phenom-

enon by Rickels's group (Schweizer et al. 1986) found improvement in 22 of 37 patients with previous benzodiazepine exposure; 26 of 29 patients without prior benzodiazepine exposure showed similar improvement. Thus, one cannot say that previous benzodiazepine exposure eliminates all response to buspirone. However, if a study (or an individual clinician) takes patients who have been on a short-acting benzodiazepine for months or years and transfers them "cold turkey" to buspirone, the benzodiazepine withdrawal symptoms may well be very unpleasant, even dangerous, and buspirone will have little or no effect on the patients' extended distress.

Otherwise, buspirone seems in most ways to be the ideal antianxiety drug. It lacks the benzodiazepines' sedation, ataxia, tolerance, and withdrawal symptoms; abuse liability; and propensity to interfere with complex psychomotor tasks on driving simulators and related tests. In addition, benzodiazepines are linked by association to driving accidents and to falls and injuries in the elderly (Smiley 1987; Sussman 1987; Sussman and Chou 1988). Buspirone does not impair performance; furthermore, it leaves the subject more aware of impairment resulting from alcohol ingestion than do the benzodiazepines (Sussman 1987). Buspirone lacks the ability of benzodiazepines to depress respiration, making it potentially the preferred drug in anxious pulmonary patients.

Several pilot studies have suggested that buspirone may decrease alcohol consumption in both animals and humans and may have a role in the detoxification and postdetoxification treatment of anxious alcoholic patients (Bruno 1989; Kranzler and Myers 1989; Schuckit 1993; Tollefson et al. 1991).

Buspirone has few side effects, both absolutely and versus placebo. The rates reported are 12% for dizziness, 6% for headache, 8% for nausea, 5% for nervousness, 3% for lightheadedness, and 2% for agitation (Gelenberg 1994). It is probable that tolerance develops to these side effects. They may be handled by dosage reduction. If the dose is increased slowly, side effects may be minimized.

Buspirone dosage should be started at 5 mg tid for 1 week and then increased by 5 mg every 2–4 days as tolerated until the patient is receiving 10 mg po tid. The patient should be encouraged to stay at that dose for at least 6 weeks before deciding that the drug is ineffective. It has been customary to give the drug three times per day because of its short half-life, but it is not known whether giving all or two-thirds of the dose at bedtime might work as well with better patient acceptance.

Most reviews of buspirone point out that it is not widely used by psychiatrists because it works so slowly and because it is of no value in patients who have been on benzodiazepines. It is certainly worth trying in some patients who have been on benzodiazepines. Buspirone is not effective in ameliorating benzodiazepine withdrawal symptoms if it is begun as the benzodiazepine is being stopped; however, in one study (Udelman and Udelman 1990) that started buspirone (or placebo) 2 weeks before beginning to terminate benzodiazepine use, buspirone was found to be superior to placebo in reducing symptoms. Many clinicians suggest that the best way to shift from a benzodiazepine to buspirone is to stabilize the patient on both agents for several weeks before tapering off the benzodiazepine (Sussman 1987).

It is even possible that a benzodiazepine combined with buspirone may be more effective in GAD than either alone; the two agents certainly work by different mechanisms, and many patients on long-term benzodiazepine medication have substantial degrees of residual symptomatology (Haskell et al. 1986). Udelman and Udelman (1990), in their review, identified several earlier small-sample reports suggesting improvement when buspirone is added to a benzodiazepine.

Buspirone also is likely to be more effective in relieving coexisting depressive symptoms than are the benzodiazepines, except perhaps for alprazolam. At doses in the range of 30–90 mg/day, buspirone is effective in major depressive disorder and even in such patients who qualify as melancholic. There is even one case of a patient's becoming manic on buspirone (Liegghio and Yeragani 1988), a sign that it may really be an antidepressant.

Nevertheless, buspirone has never been used clinically to the extent that its apparent safety and efficacy would support. Why? Observing the reduction in anxiety symptoms over weeks in reports of double-blind studies of buspirone versus a benzodiazepine leaves one doubting that most patients get better much faster on a benzodiazepine. Both drugs show some improvement (on the average) after 1 week, a bit more after 2 weeks, and the most by 4 weeks. Although benzodiazepine-placebo differences are often statistically significant at week 1 or 2, and benzodiazepines and buspirone both achieve significance by weeks 3 and 4, buspirone-benzodiazepine differences are not significant early in these studies.

Buspirone is presumably ineffective when given as a single dose to relieve anxiety, whereas benzodiazepines may be effective in such circumstances. The one study we have heard of—which, incidentally, was aborted (i.e., never finished or published)—compared buspirone, diazepam, and placebo in single doses in anxious patients. Neither drug was more effective than placebo over the next few hours. However, one suspects that benzodiazepines are better for insomnia early in treatment, whereas insomnia is relieved by buspirone later as part of a general improvement; benzodiazepines, as a group, are good hypnotics independent of their other effects.

Another part of the problem may be that psychiatrists, who can handle tricky drug regimens, rarely see drug-free patients with GAD or the medical patients with secondary anxiety who are the ideal candidates for buspirone, whereas primary care physicians may not have the time or motivation to explain buspirone's delayed response to their patients and then to carefully adjust the dose over several weeks until the patient is clearly better.

Buspirone's efficacy may increase over time. In one large, open study of patients with GAD, improvement rates rose from about 50% at 3 months to about 70% over 6 months (Feighner 1987). These numbers may be a little deceptive, because dropouts were reasonably numerous in this study. However, the few studies that followed patients on buspirone versus a benzodiazepine through improvement and subsequent drug withdrawal and then observed patients for several weeks after the drugs were stopped noted withdrawal agitation and relapse to benzodiazepine use in the benzodiazepine patients, whereas the buspirone patients seemed to continue to improve for several weeks after buspirone was stopped and did not require further medication (Rickels and Schweizer 1990; Rickels et al. 1988).

In other anxiety disorders, matters are less clear. Studies in panic/agoraphobia are mainly negative. Two open trials of buspirone in social phobia at dosages generally in the 30- to 60-mg/day range showed substantial improvement rates (Bruns et al. 1989; Schneier et al. 1993).

In obsessive-compulsive disorder (OCD), one incomplete crossover study comparing buspirone and clomipramine seemed to show equal efficacy in

OCD, a condition with a notoriously low rate of placebo response (Murphy et al. 1990); however, an open study of 14 OCD patients with doses of buspirone up to 60 mg/day by Jenike and Baer (1988) resulted in no improvement in any of the patients. The small studies of the effects of adding buspirone to either clomipramine or fluoxetine in OCD patients suggest that buspirone is more helpful if added to fluoxetine (Murphy et al. 1990). The role of buspirone in the treatment of OCD, alone or as an adjunct to another drug, is still far from clear.

Buspirone was found to be helpful in some anxious intravenous drug–abusing persons on methadone maintenance who had developed acquired immunodeficiency syndrome (AIDS) or AIDS-related complex (ARC) (Batki 1990). In this sample, there was no evidence of abuse of buspirone and some evidence that abuse of other drugs decreased. Buspirone was generally well tolerated and facilitated the tapering or discontinuation of benzodiazepines in most patients on benzodiazepines at the start of the study. The patients, as a group, were dubious both about trying buspirone and about decreasing benzodiazepine use, so the positive effects of buspirone occurred in spite of this resistance. Unfortunately, the positive effects of buspirone faded after a few months in one-third of the patients.

Use in Depression

The assessment of buspirone's efficacy in depression began when multisite, controlled trials comparing buspirone with a benzodiazepine showed buspirone to be superior in relieving (or preventing the emergence of) depressive symptoms in patients selected initially as having an anxiety disorder. Then Schweizer and colleagues (1986) conducted an open study of buspirone at doses between 30 and 60 mg/day in nonmelancholic depressed outpatients with favorable results. This was followed by a placebo-controlled double-blind 8-week trial (Rickels et al. 1990) in which buspirone doses were permitted to go as high as 90 mg/day. The average dose by week 8 was, in fact, 57 mg/day. The study involved 143 evaluable patients. Side effects were similar in frequency and type to those attributed to buspirone in anxiety studies. Patients completing the study showed 65% improvement on buspirone and 28% improvement on placebo.

In a larger study that probably included the Rickels et al. (1990) sample, 418 patients with major depression from five sites were randomized to buspirone or placebo and followed for 8 weeks. About one-third had major depression with melancholia, and this group showed improvement superior to that shown with placebo by the end of the first week. Patients with higher initial levels of depression or of anxiety did better versus placebo than did less-symptomatic patients. Buspirone was begun at 5 mg tid, but the dose was rapidly increased. Improvement occurred first in 21 patients (out of 101 responders) when the dose was above 60 mg/day, the current upper dose recommended for use in GAD. Those of the total sample of depressed patients who improved markedly did so at an average of 40 mg/day for initial response and of 50 mg at the end of the 8-week study. The patterns of symptom change were compatible with a full antidepressant effect, not a coincidental improvement in anxiety symptoms (Robinson et al. 1990).

Because buspirone is available in drugstores and, one assumes, most hospital pharmacies, it can be used as an antidepressant. Because no comparative studies are available contrasting buspirone with more widely used antidepressants, it is hard to guess its ultimate place in a psychopharmacologist's armamentarium compared with the now-ubiquitous SSRIs, the older tricyclic antidepressants (TCAs), or the MAOIs. Buspirone is certainly worth a trial in patients who have failed on two or three prior antidepressants, although the clinician should keep in mind the need to push the dose upward and the relative expense of the drug as well as its relatively benign side-effect profile. Again, it would be helpful if larger dosage units were available and if most or all of the dose could be given at bedtime.

One fears that, in these days of overly brief hospitalizations, buspirone will end up being one of the 12 psychoactive drugs collected by treatment-resistant depressive patients and depressive patients with personality disorders over a series of brief, inconclusive hospitalizations and fragmented outpatient trials.

Use in Neuropsychiatric Disorders

There are two negative studies (Brown et al. 1991; Goff et al. 1991) of buspirone in TD. Only a third study pushed the dose above 40 mg/day to an upper limit of 180 mg/day. Moss et al. (1993) studied buspirone treatment of eight patients who had persistent TD, with pretreatment Abnormal Involuntary

Movement Scale (AIMS) scores of 10 ± 6. These scores dropped to 6 ± 3 ($P < .02$) at 12 weeks at a mean dose of about 150 mg. The improvement in TD began at 60 mg/day and was accompanied by improvement in neuroleptic-induced parkinsonian symptoms and akathisia. Goff et al. (1991) observed a similar improvement in EPS in their sample even though buspirone raised haloperidol blood levels. Jann and colleagues (1990), in their review of movement disorders and azaspirones, noted that buspirone does not aggravate Parkinson's disease and, at higher doses, can even suppress dyskinesias caused by drugs used in the treatment of this disease.

There are a series of single case reports and several uncontrolled studies of buspirone in agitated demented, mentally retarded, or brain-damaged patients (Herrmann and Eryavec 1993). Positive effects occur in some patients—often less than half in the larger series—but the drug is sometimes quite helpful and the potential alternative drugs (e.g., neuroleptics, β-blockers, carbamazepine, lithium, clonazepam, trazodone, or SSRIs) either have not been adequately studied (Schneider and Sobin 1991) or, as with the neuroleptics, have not been very effective (Schneider et al. 1990). It is worth noting that Ratey and colleagues (1991) used buspirone in aggressive and/or anxious mentally retarded patients and found very low doses (2.5–10 mg/day) to be more effective than larger doses, suggesting a window effect.

Smiley (1987), in a review of the effects of benzodiazepines and buspirone on psychomotor performance, found either that buspirone had no deleterious effect on a wide range of tasks or, when it impaired performance, that clinically equivalent benzodiazepine doses had substantially worse effects.

■ New Antianxiety Agents

Currently, none of the "known" azaspirones—gepirone, ipsapirone, and tandospirone—appear to be anywhere near release in the United States, and publications dealing with their clinical effects are few and far between. It is even hard to tell whether they will ultimately be marketed for use in GAD, depression, or both (Borison et al. 1990; Cott et al. 1988; Harto et al. 1988; Heller et al. 1990).

Other newer drugs include those active at benzodiazepine receptors that are not chemically describable as benzodiazepines. Abecarnil is a beta-carboline-3-carboxylate that may be a partial agonist at the benzodiazepine receptor. It has side effects similar to those of the benzodiazepines but may be clinically effective at dosages free of most side effects (Ballenger 1991). Another drug, alpidem, is an imidopyridine that binds the benzodiazepine receptor; it probably has beneficial effects in GAD (Langer et al. 1988; Morselli 1990; Morton and Lader 1990) but causes benzodiazepine-like side effects.

None of these drugs seems close to release, and none shows promise of being the ideal antianxiety drug—one with rapid action, almost no side effects, and no abuse potential.

■ Conclusion

Buspirone is a novel drug with a unique probable mechanism(s) of action that, somehow, has never been as widely used as it probably deserves. It is effective in GAD and almost certainly in major depression. It seems likely that this drug may have efficacy in social phobia and in anxiety disorders accompanying various chronic medical disorders. Buspirone's side effects are mainly mildly bothersome and its drug-drug interactions are benign. It is relatively safe in overdose and free from abuse liability and performance impairment. If the drug is started cautiously with the dose raised as needed up to 60–90 mg in major disorders, it should be a major addition to our armamentarium.

It is time that some drug—perhaps a buspirone analogue with some improvements (faster onset of action, better customer acceptance but no physical or psychic dependence)—be developed or that a better understanding of how to best use buspirone be attained. It is clear that many patients who meet DSM-IV (American Psychiatric Association 1994) criteria for GAD either have relatively lifelong anxiety symptoms of GAD or have waxing and waning symptoms that could be helped by prolonged intermittent pharmacotherapy (Feighner 1987). Anxiety associated with chronic medical conditions may be similarly prolonged, recurrent, episodic, or fully chronic. Social phobia can be equally chronic, as can dysthymia, with an admixture of anxiety symptoms (Dubovsky 1990; Rickels 1987).

The benzodiazepines do work, and tolerance to their antianxiety effects does not develop over weeks or months (Rickels 1987); however, in patients with chronic anxiety it can prove difficult to test the patient's need for longer benzodiazepine therapy because withdrawal symptoms are likely to resemble or reactivate the symptoms of the patient's original condition (Lader 1987). Buspirone—or our hypothetical "super-Buspar"—could be tapered and stopped periodically without the complication of anxiety-like withdrawal symptoms.

In this chapter, various ideas were considered as to why buspirone is less widely used than it might be. More research is needed on how to optimize doctor and patient response to buspirone until an even better anxiolytic drug emerges. The relative paucity of clinical articles on newer anxiolytics makes one suspect that none of these agents are close to release in the United States or Europe.

■ REFERENCES

Ableitner A, Herz A: Influence of meprobamate and phenobarbital upon local cerebral glucose utilization: parallelism with effects of the anxiolytic diazepam. Brain Res 403:82–88, 1987

American Psychiatric Association: Diagnostic and Statistical Manual of Mental Disorders, 2nd Edition. Washington, DC, American Psychiatric Association, 1968

American Psychiatric Association: Diagnostic and Statistical Manual of Mental Disorders, 4th Edition. Washington, DC, American Psychiatric Association, 1994

Ballenger JC, McDonald S, Noyes R, et al: The first double-blind, placebo-controlled trial of a partial benzodiazepine agonist abecarnil (ZK 112–119) in generalized anxiety disorder. Psychopharmacol Bull 27:171–179, 1991

Batki SL: Buspirone in drug users with AIDS or AIDS-related complex. J Clin Psychopharmacol 10 (suppl 3):111S–115S, 1990

Baughman OL: The safety record of buspirone in generalized anxiety disorder (monograph). J Clin Psychiatry 12:37–45, 1994

Berger FM: The discovery of meprobamate, in Discoveries in Biological Psychiatry. Edited by Ayd F, Blackwell B. Philadelphia, PA, JB Lippincott, 1970, pp 115–129

Bohm C, Robinson DS, Gammans RE, et al: Buspirone therapy in anxious elderly patients: a controlled clinical trial. J Clin Psychopharmacol 10 (suppl 3):47S–51S, 1990

Borison RL, Albrecht JW, Diamond BI: Efficacy and safety of a putative anxiolytic agent: ipsapirone. Psychopharmacol Bull 26:207–210, 1990

Brown S, Fanstman W, Mone R, et al: An open-label trial of buspirone in the treatment of tardive dyskinesia (abstract). Biol Psychiatry 29:65A, 1991

Bruno F: Buspirone in the treatment of alcoholic patients. Psychopathology 22 (suppl 1):49–50, 1989

Bruns JR, Munjack DJ, Baltazar PL, et al: Buspirone for the treatment of social phobia. Family Practice Recertification (Cl. 22 Selective Therapeutic Index) 11 (no 9, suppl):46–52, 1989

Ciraulo DA, Shader RL: Question the experts: safety of buspirone with an MAOI. J Clin Psychopharmacol 10:306, 1990

Cohn JB, Wilcox CS, Meltzer HY: Neuroendocrine effects in patients with generalized anxiety disorder. Am J Med 80 (suppl 3B):36–40, 1986

Cole JO, Orzack MH, Beake B, et al: Assessment of the abuse liability of buspirone in recreational sedative users. J Clin Psychiatry 43:69–74, 1982

Cott JM, Kurtz NM, Robinson DS, et al: A 5-HT$_{1A}$ ligand with both antidepressant and anxiolytic properties. Psychopharmacol Bull 24:164–167, 1988

DeLong RE, Phillis JW, Barraco RA: A possible role of endogenous adenosine in the sedative action of meprobamate. Eur J Pharmacol 118:359–362, 1985

Dixon HH, Dickel HA, Coen R, et al: Clinical observations on tolserol in handling anxiety tension states. Am J Med Sci 220:23–29, 1950

Dubovsky SL: Generalized anxiety disorder: new concepts and psychopharmacologic therapies. J Clin Psychiatry 51 (suppl 1):3–10, 1990

Eison AS: Azapirones: history of development. J Clin Psychopharmacol 10 (suppl 3):2S–5S, 1990

Eison AS, Eison MS: Buspirone as a midbrain modulator: anxiolysis unrelated to traditional benzodiazepine mechanisms. Drug Development Research 4:109–119, 1984

Eison AS, Eison MS: Serotonergic mechanisms in anxiety. Prog Neuropsychopharmacol Biol Psychiatry 18:47–62, 1994

Eison AS, Yocca FD, Taylor DP: Mechanism of Action of Buspirone: Current Perspectives. New York, Academic Press, 1991, pp 279–326

Eison MS: Azapirones: mechanism of action in anxiety and depression. Drug Therapy Suppl, August 1990, pp 3–8

Eison MS: Serotonin: a common neurobiologic substrate in anxiety and depression. J Clin Psychopharmacol 10 (suppl 3):26S–30S, 1991

Eison MS, Taylor DP, Riblet LA: Atypical psychotropic agents—trazodone and buspirone, in Drug Discovery and Development. Edited by William M, Malick JB. Clifton, NJ, Humana Press, 1987, pp 387–407

Elenbaas JK: Centrally acting oral skeletal muscle relaxants. Am J Hosp Pharm 37:1313–1323, 1980

Feighner JP: Buspirone in the long-term treatment of generalized anxiety disorder. J Clin Psychiatry 48 (no 12, suppl):3–6, 1987

Gammans RE, Mayol RF, LaBudde JA: Metabolism and disposition of buspirone. Am J Med 80 (suppl 3B):41–51, 1986

Gelenberg AJ: Academic Highlights—Buspirone: seven year update. J Clin Psychiatry 55:222–229, 1994

Goff D, Midha K, Brotman A, et al: An open trial of buspirone added to neuroleptics in schizophrenic patients. J Clin Psychopharmacol 11:193–197, 1991

Goldberg HL, Finnerty RJ: The comparative efficacy of buspirone and diazepam in the treatment of anxiety. Am J Psychiatry 136:1184–1187, 1979

Goodman LS, Gilman A (eds): The Pharmacologic Basis of Therapeutics, 4th Edition. New York, Macmillan, 1970

Greenblatt D, Shader R: Meprobamate: a study of irrational drug use. Am J Psychiatry 127:1297–1303, 1971

Griffith JD, Jasinski DR, Casten GP, et al: Investigation of the abuse liability of buspirone in alcohol-dependent patients. Am J Med 80:30–35, 1986

Hale WE, May FE, Moore MT, et al: Meprobamate use in the elderly: a report from the Dunedin program. J Am Geriatr Soc 36:1003–1005, 1988

Harto NE, Branconnier RJ, Spera KF, et al: Clinical profile of gepirone, a nonbenzodiazepine anxiolytic. Psychopharmacol Bull 24:154–160, 1988

Haskell D, Cole JO, Schniebolk BS, et al: A survey of diazepam patients. Psychopharmacol Bull 22:434–438, 1986

Heller AH, Beneke M, Kuemmel B, et al: Ipsapirone: Evidence of efficacy in depression. Psychopharmacol Bull 26:219–222, 1990

Herrmann N, Eryavec G: Buspirone in the management of agitation and aggression associated with dementia. American Journal of Geriatric Psychiatry 1:249–253, 1993

Hyman S, Nestler E: The Molecular Foundations of Psychiatry. Washington, DC, American Psychiatric Press, 1993, pp 150–158

Jann MW: Buspirone: An update on a unique anxiolytic agent. Pharmacotherapy 8:100–116, 1988

Jann MW, Froemming JH, Borison RL: Movement disorders and new azapirone anxiolytic drugs. Journal of the American Board of Family Practitioners 3:111–119, 1990

Jenike MA, Baer L: An open trial of buspirone in obsessive-compulsive disorder. Am J Psychiatry 145:1285–1286, 1988

Joffe RT, Schuller DR: An open study of buspirone augmentation of serotonin reuptake inhibitors in refractory depression. J Clin Psychiatry 54:269–271, 1993

Kranzler HR, Myers RE: An open trial of buspirone in alcoholics. J Clin Psychopharmacol 9:379–380, 1989

Lader M: Long-term anxiolytic therapy: the issue of drug withdrawal. J Clin Psychiatry 48 (no 12, suppl):12–16, 1987

Langer SF, Feighner JP, Pambakian R, et al: Pilot study of alpidem, a novel imidazopyridine compound in anxiety. Psychopharmacol Bull 24:161–163, 1988

Leeb-Lundberg LMF, Olsen RW: Heterogeneity of benzodiazepine receptor interactions with gamma-aminobutyric acid and barbiturate receptor sites. Mol Pharmacol 23:315–325, 1983

Lidbrink P, Corrodi H, Fuxe K, et al: Barbiturates and meprobamate: decreases in catecholamine turnover of central dopamine and noradrenaline neuronal systems and the influence of immobilization stress. Brain Res 45:507–524, 1972

Liegghio NE, Yeragani VK: Buspirone-induced hypomania: a case report. J Clin Psychopharmacol 8:226–227, 1988

Meltzer HY, Flemming R, Robertson A: The effect of buspirone on prolactin and growth hormone secretion in man. Arch Gen Psychiatry 40:1099–1102, 1983

Morselli PL: On the therapeutic action of alpidem in anxiety disorders: an overview of the European data. Pharmacopsychiatry 23 (suppl):129–134, 1990

Morton S, Lader M: Studies with alpidem in normal volunteers and anxious patients. Pharmacopsychiatry 23 (suppl):120–123, 1990

Moss LE, Neppe VM, Drevets WC: Buspirone in the treatment of tardive dyskinesia. J Clin Psychopharmacol 13:204–209, 1993

Murphy DL, Pato MT, Pigott TA: Obsessive-compulsive disorder: treatment with serotonin-selective uptake inhibitors, azapirones, and other agents. J Clin Psychopharmacol 10 (suppl 3):9lS–100S, 1990

Napoliello MJ: An interim multicentre report on 677 anxious geriatric outpatients treated with buspirone. Br J Clin Pract 2:71–73, 1986

Olajide D, Lader M: A comparison of buspirone, diazepam, and placebo in patients with chronic anxiety states. J Clin Psychopharmacol 7:148–152, 1987

Olsen RW: The GABA postsynaptic membrane receptor-ionophore complex: site of action of convulsant and anticonvulsant drugs. Mol Cell Biochem 39:261–279, 1981

Ortiz A, Pohl R, Gershon S: Azaspirodecanediones in generalized anxiety disorder: buspirone. J Affect Disord 13:131–143, 1987

Othmer E, Othmer SC: Effect of buspirone on sexual dysfunction in patients with generalized anxiety disorder. J Clin Psychiatry 48:201–203, 1987

Paul S, Marangos P, Skolnick P: The benzodiazepine–GABA–chloride ionophore receptor complex: common site of minor tranquilizer action. Biol Psychiatry 16:213–229, 1981

Peroutka S: Selective interaction of novel anxiolytics with 5 HT_{1A}. Biol Psychiatry 20:971–979, 1985

Phillis JW, DeLong RE: A purinergic component in the central actions of meprobamate. Eur J Pharmacol 101:295–297, 1984

Polc P, Bonetti EP, Schaffner R, et al: A three-state model of the benzodiazepine receptor explains the interaction between the benzodiazepine antagonist to Ro 15–1788, benzodiazepine tranquilizers, β-carbolines, and phenobarbital. Naunyn Schmiedebergs Arch Pharmacol 321:256–260, 1982

Rall TW: Hypnotics and sedatives, in Goodman and Gilman's The Pharmacological Basis of Therapeutics, 8th Edition. Edited by Gilman AG, Rall TW, Nies AS, et al. New York, McGraw-Hill, 1993, pp 345–382

Ratey J, Sovner R, Park A, et al: Buspirone treatment of aggression and anxiety in mentally retarded patients: a multiple baseline placebo lead-in study. J Clin Psychiatry 52:159–162, 1991

Riblet LA, Taylor DP, Eison MS, et al: Pharmacology and neurochemistry of buspirone. J Clin Psychiatry 43:11–16, 1982

Riblet LA, Eison AS, Eison MS, et al: Neuropharma-

cology of buspirone. Psychopathology 17:69–78, 1984

Rickels K: Antianxiety therapy: potential value of long-term treatment. J Clin Psychiatry 48 (no 12, suppl):7–11, 1987

Rickels K, Schweizer E: The clinical course and long-term management of generalized anxiety disorder. J Clin Psychopharmacol 10 (suppl 3):101S–110S, 1990

Rickels K, Schweizer E, Csanalosi I, et al: Long-term treatment of anxiety and risk of withdrawal. Arch Gen Psychiatry 45:444–450, 1988

Rickels K, Amsterdam J, Clary C, et al: Buspirone in depressed outpatients: a controlled study. Psychopharmacol Bull 26:163–167, 1990

Roache J, Griffiths RR: Lorazepam and meprobamate dose effects in humans: behavioral effects and abuse liability. J Pharmacol Exp Ther 243:978–988, 1987

Robinson DS, Rickels R, Feighner J, et al: Clinical effects of the 5-HT_{1A} partial agonists in depression: a composite analysis of buspirone in the treatment of depression. J Clin Psychopharmacol 10 (suppl 3):67S–76S, 1990

Sathananthan GL, Sanghvi I, Phillips N, et al: MJ 9022: correlation between neuroleptic potential and stereotypy. Curr Ther Res 18:701–705, 1975

Schneider LS, Sobin PB: Non-neuroleptic medications in the management of agitation in Alzheimer's disease and other dementia: a selective review. International Journal of Geriatric Psychiatry 6:691–708, 1991

Schneider LS, Pollock VE, Lyness SA: A meta-analysis of controlled trials of neuroleptic treatment in dementia. J Am Geriatr Soc 38:553–563, 1990

Schneier FR, Saoud JB, Campeas R, et al: Buspirone in social phobia. J Clin Psychopharmacol 13:251–256, 1993

Schuckit MA: Buspirone: is it an effective drug for alcohol rehabilitation? Drug Abuse and Alcoholism Newsletter 22(2), April 1993

Schweizer E, Rickels K, Lucki I: Resistance to the antianxiety effect of buspirone in patients with a history of benzodiazepine use. N Engl J Med 314:719–720, 1986

Smiley A: Effects of minor tranquilizers and antidepressants on psychomotor performance. J Clin Psychiatry 48 (suppl 12):22–28, 1987

Squires R, Braestrup C: Benzodiazepine receptors in rat brain. Nature 266:732–734, 1977

Sussman N: Treatment of anxiety with buspirone. Psychiatric Annals 17:114–118, 1987

Sussman N, Chou JCY: Current issues in benzodiazepine use of anxiety disorders. Psychiatric Annals 18:139–145, 1988

Tollefson GD, Lancaster SP, Montagne-Clouse J: The association of buspirone and its metabolic 1-pyrimidinylpiperazine in the remission of comorbid anxiety with depressive features and alcohol dependency. Psychopharmacol Bull 27:163–170, 1991

Udelman HD, Udelman DL: Concurrent use of buspirone in anxious patients during withdrawal from alprazolam therapy. J Clin Psychiatry 51 (no 9, suppl):46–50, 1990

Vogel GW, Buffenstein A, Hennessey M, et al: Drug effects on REM sleep and on endogenous depression. Neurosci Biobehav Rev 14:49–63, 1990

Antipsychotics

Antipsychotic Medications

Stephen R. Marder, M.D., and Theodore Van Putten, M.D.[*]

A ntipsychotic drugs are used to treat nearly all forms of psychosis, including schizophrenia, schizoaffective disorder, affective disorders with psychosis, and psychoses associated with organic mental disorders. Although these drugs have become standard treatments in psychiatry and medicine, they have important limitations: they are not effective for all patients, they have several serious adverse effects, and even patients who respond well often continue to have serious signs and symptoms of illness.

Until recently, all effective antipsychotic drugs produced significant neurological side effects, and, for this reason, were referred to as neuroleptics. Clozapine and other new drugs are effective antipsychotics, but with fewer motor side effects than conventional antipsychotics. For this reason, the term *antipsychotic* is preferable for describing these drugs. In this chapter, we discuss the traditional antipsychotics; clozapine and the newer atypical drugs are described elsewhere.

■ HISTORY AND DISCOVERY

Henri Laborit, a French surgeon with an interest in drugs that would decrease preoperative anxiety, convinced the Rhone-Poulenc laboratories of the importance of identifying compounds that would relax patients and make surgical shock less likely. Chlorpromazine, a compound synthesized by Paul Charpentier in 1950, clearly fulfilled Laborit's goals. Patients who received doses of 50–100 mg intravenously had some drowsiness; but more importantly, they appeared relatively indifferent to the surgical procedure. Laborit realized the potential of chlorpromazine and succeeded in convincing a number of psychiatrists to administer the drug to psychotic and agitated patients. Although Delay and Deniker were not the first to observe the antipsychotic effects of chlorpromazine, their report in 1952 to the Société Medico-Psychologique is often cited as the first public report of an effective drug for the treatment of a major mental disorder.

---

[*]Deceased.

Theodore Van Putten was a clinical psychopharmacologist who made substantial contributions to our understanding of the drug treatment of schizophrenia. His lifework has reduced the suffering of innumerable patients with schizophrenia.
—S. R. M.

Within a year of chlorpromazine's introduction, the mental hospitals of Paris had changed. Restraint devices, seclusion, and the need for locked units became relatively uncommon, as they are today. The major factor that contributed to the rapid acceptance of chlorpromazine in France and subsequently in nearly every corner of the world was the absence of any other effective treatment for schizophrenia or other forms of psychosis. Chlorpromazine was relatively inexpensive to administer to large numbers of patients. Despite its side effects, it was very safe. And, because chlorpromazine was effective for a large proportion of patients to whom it was administered, its advantages became apparent to clinicians who used it in appropriate patients. Chlorpromazine also stimulated the pharmaceutical industry to develop a number of other phenothiazines during the first years after its discovery. Thioridazine and fluphenazine, as well as newer classes of drugs such as the butyrophenones (e.g., haloperidol) and the thioxanthenes (e.g., thiothixene) were developed during this time. Reserpine was also found to be an effective antipsychotic drug in the United States at about the same time that chlorpromazine was gaining acceptance. It initially became a popular alternative to chlorpromazine and other antipsychotics, but then faded from use, probably because of its side effects and the perception that it was less effective than chlorpromazine.

The side effects of chlorpromazine, particularly drug-induced parkinsonism and other extrapyramidal side effects (EPS), were reported shortly after its introduction in 1952 (Lehmann and Hanrahan 1954). The early observations of the effectiveness of chlorpromazine and other antipsychotics may have resulted in a tendency to underestimate the seriousness of their side effects. Although Delay and other early researchers of chlorpromazine found that patients usually responded to doses in the range of 200–400 mg qd, later researchers found that many individuals tolerated much higher doses. When more potent drugs such as haloperidol and fluphenazine became available, doses comparable to 2,000 mg or more of chlorpromazine (or 40 mg of haloperidol or fluphenazine) were commonly prescribed. A number of carefully designed studies have shown that these higher doses result in more side effects, but seldom in greater efficacy (Baldessarini et al. 1988). As a result, there has been a recent trend directed at treating patients with the lowest effective dose of antipsychotic.

STRUCTURE-ACTIVITY RELATIONS

Phenothiazines

The phenothiazine antipsychotics are characterized by a three-ring structure with a six-member central ring (Table 13–1). The activity of the group can be affected by substitutions at positions 2 or 10. The phenothiazines are usually categorized into three classes based on substitutions at position 10. The aliphatic class—represented by chlorpromazine—consists of drugs that have relatively low potency at D_2 receptors compared with other antipsychotics, more antimuscarinic activity, more sympathetic and parasympathetic activity, and more sedation. The piperidine class has the third carbon of the side chain and the basic nitrogen incorporated into a piperidine ring. This class—represented by thioridazine—has a similar clinical profile to the aliphatic class, with somewhat reduced potency at D_2 sites. The third class, the piperazines, have a piperazine ring substituted in the side chain. These drugs—represented by trifluoperazine and fluphenazine—have fewer antimuscarinic and autonomic effects, but greater affinity for D_2 sites, and as a result produce more EPS. For all three groups, substitutions at the 2 position can affect the drug's potency. Increasing the electron-withdrawing tendency at this position by substituting a trifluoromethyl group, for example, will increase antipsychotic potency.

Thioxanthenes

Thioxanthene antipsychotics have a three-ring structure that is similar to the phenothiazines, but with a carbon substituted for a nitrogen atom in the middle ring. Substitutions in the comparable areas of the molecule have similar effects on activity. Thioxanthenes are characterized by geometric isomerism, with the *cis* isomers having greater potency than the *trans*. Thiothixene—the most commonly prescribed thioxanthene in the United States—has a piperazine substitution at position 10, whereas chlorprothixene has an aliphatic side chain. Clopenthixol and flupentixol, which are commonly used outside of the United States, have piperazine side chains.

Table 13–1. Selected antipsychotic drugs

Drug	Routes of administration	Usual daily oral dose (mg)	Sedation	Autonomic effects	Extrapyramidal side effects	Structure
Phenothiazines						
Chlorpromazine	Oral, intramuscular, depot	200–600	+++	+++	++	
Fluphenazine	Oral, intramuscular, depot	2–20	+	+	+++	
Trifluoperazine	Oral, intramuscular	5–30	++	+	+++	
Perphenazine	Oral, intramuscular	8–64	++	+	+++	
Thioridazine	Oral	200–600	+++	+++	++	
Butyrophenones						
Haloperidol	Oral, intramuscular, depot	5–20	+	+	+++	
Thioxanthenes						
Thiothixene	Oral, intramuscular	5–30	+	+	+++	
Dihydroindolones						
Molindone	Oral	20–100	++	+	++	
Dibenzoxazepines						
Loxapine	Oral, intramuscular	20–100	++	+	++	
Benzisoxazole						
Risperidone	Oral	2–16	+	++	+	

Source. Adapted from Silver et al. 1994, pp. 901–903.

■ Butyrophenones

This class of antipsychotic drugs is characterized by a substituted phenyl ring, which is attached to a carbonyl group attached by a 3-carbon chain to a tertiary amino group. Most of the clinically useful butyrophenones have a piperidine ring attached to the tertiary amino group. Drugs in this class tend to be potent D_2 antagonists and have minimal anticholinergic and autonomic effects. Haloperidol, a substituted piperidine, is the most commonly used drug from this class.

■ Dibenzoxazepines

This class of antipsychotic drugs has a three-ring structure with a seven-member center ring. Loxapine, a dibenzoxazepine, is the only drug from this group that is available in the United States. Clozapine, a dibenzodiazepine, differs from loxapine in having a nitrogen instead of an oxygen atom in the middle ring, as well as differences in side chains. These differences have a substantial influence on clozapine's affinity for various receptors (including the D_2 receptors), which may explain its atypical antipsychotic activity.

■ Others Classes of Antipsychotics

The diphenylbutylpiperidines include pimozide, which is approved for use in the United States only for the treatment of Tourette's disorder but is used elsewhere as an antipsychotic. Fluspirilene and penfluridol are other compounds of this class that are prescribed as antipsychotics in Europe. Relatively little is understood about structure-activity relationships in the other classes of antipsychotic compounds (Baldessarini 1990).

■ PHARMACOLOGICAL PROFILE

■ Behavioral Effects

Antipsychotic drugs produce a wide spectrum of physiological actions, only some of which are essential to their antipsychotic action. Some of these effects differ among the various classes of antipsychotics. For example, aliphatic phenothiazines have potent antimuscarinic and autonomic effects, whereas others have more potent effects on dopaminergic or serotonergic systems. The effect that is common to all conventional antipsychotic agents is a high affinity for dopamine receptors. These effects are useful for defining this class of compounds.

As we mentioned in the section on history, chlorpromazine had the unusual property of inducing a state of relative indifference to stressful situations. All of the traditional antipsychotics share this property, which has been called ataraxia. The effect differs from sedation in that the individual may not be drowsy but is instead calm and relatively uninterested in the environment. Individuals who are receiving antipsychotics appear to have a decrease in their emotional responsiveness and have been described as lacking initiative. When patients are agitated or excited, these drugs may calm them without causing excessive sedation.

The calming effect of antipsychotics in humans is paralleled by their effect on the conditioned avoidance response in animals. In this research paradigm, animals are trained to make a conditioned response (e.g., moving to a safer place) following a sensory cue such as the ringing of a bell that precedes the onset of a shock. The response to the sensory cue is blocked by the antipsychotic drug, although the animal will move to a safer place when the shock is administered (Baldessarini 1990).

Traditional antipsychotics also block responses in rodents such as stereotypies and hyperactivity, which are induced by dopamine agonists such as apomorphine. This effect has been found to be a reasonably reliable predictor of antipsychotic activity in patients. Moreover, the dose-response relationships in animals provides information about the likely clinical dose range for patients. It is commonly used as a screening device to identify compounds that are likely to have clinical efficacy as antipsychotics (Gerlach 1991).

Antipsychotic drugs have other effects on animal behavior. They reduce responses to a variety of stimuli, and they reduce exploratory behavior. Antipsychotics also block self-stimulation to reward centers in the brain such as the medial forebrain bundle, and they reduce some feeding behaviors.

■ Motor Effects

When animals are administered a traditional antipsychotic in relatively high doses, they develop a syndrome with immobility, increased muscle tone, and abnormal postures called catalepsy. In addition, these agents decrease spontaneous motor activity. This motor effect is associated with a drug's tendency to cause a variety of EPS in humans. These motor effects in animals and humans are caused by dopamine receptor blockade in the striatum and inactivation of dopamine neurons in the substantia nigra (Gerlach 1991).

In humans, all of the traditional antipsychotic medications produce EPS including parkinsonism (i.e., stiffness, tremor, and shuffling gait), dystonia (i.e., abrupt onset, sometimes bizarre muscular spasms affecting mainly the musculature of the head and neck), and akathisia (with objective and subjective restlessness). These are described in greater detail in the section "Side Effects and Toxicology."

■ Endocrine Effects

Antipsychotic drugs influence the secretion of hormones in the pituitary and elsewhere mainly due to their blockade of dopamine D_2 receptors. All traditional antipsychotics increase serum prolactin concentration in the usual clinical dose range (Meltzer 1985). This occurs because prolactin secretion by the anterior pituitary is tonically inhibited by dopamine. Therefore, blockade of dopamine receptors in the tuberoinfundibular pathway results in prolactin elevation. This sometimes produces gynecomastia and galactorrhea. Antipsychotics also suppress levels of luteinizing hormone (LH) and follicle stimulating hormone (FSH) (Reichlin 1992). These changes can lead to amenorrhea and inhibition of orgasms in women. Other changes in sexual functioning are described in the section "Side Effects and Toxicology."

■ Pharmacokinetics and Disposition

All of the antipsychotics are well absorbed when they are administered orally or parenterally. Oral administration leads to less predictable absorption than parenteral administration. Liquid concentrates are absorbed slightly more rapidly than pills. In general, intramuscular preparations reach their peak concentrations sooner than oral drugs and, as a result, have an earlier onset of action. For example, intramuscular administration of most antipsychotics results in peak plasma levels in about 30 minutes, with clinical effects emerging within 15–30 minutes. Most orally administered antipsychotics result in a peak plasma

level 1–4 hours following administration. Steady state levels are reached in 3–5 days.

The bioavailability (i.e., the amount of drug reaching the site of action in the brain) is substantially greater when antipsychotics are administered parenterally. This difference may result from the incomplete absorption of the drug in the gastrointestinal tract and from extensive metabolism of oral drugs during the first pass through liver and gut. A number of factors can interfere with the gastrointestinal absorption of these drugs, including antacids, coffee, smoking, and food. The metabolism of antipsychotic drugs is largely hepatic and occurs through conjugation with glucuronic acid, hydroxylation, oxidation, demethylation, and sulfoxide formation. The metabolism of the phenothiazines and thioxanthenes is particularly complex. For example, chlorpromazine has more than 100 different potential metabolites, with some metabolites having significant amounts of pharmacological activity. Although most phenothiazine metabolites are inactive, some including 7-hydroxychlorpromazine, 7-hydroxyfluphenazine, and others may contribute to the therapeutic activity of the parent drug (Midha et al. 1993).

In the case of thioridazine, a substantial amount of the drug's activity is from metabolites that may be more active than thioridazine itself. One metabolite, mesoridazine, is also marketed as an antipsychotic. On the other hand, haloperidol has only one major metabolite, reduced haloperidol, which has substantially less antidopaminergic activity than the parent compound. However, a study demonstrated that reduced haloperidol is converted back to the parent compound and may contribute to antipsychotic activity (Chakraborty et al. 1989).

The systemic clearance of antipsychotics is high as the result of a high hepatic extraction ratio. As a result, only negligible amounts of the unchanged drug are excreted by the kidneys. Most antipsychotics have elimination half-lives of about 10–30 hours. This results, in part, from the high lipid solubility of antipsychotics, which results in large amounts of drug being stored in tissues such as fat, lung, and brain. This may explain the high concentrations of antipsychotic drugs—about twice the plasma concentration—which have been found in human and animal brain. It is also notable that the biological activity of antipsychotics may persist for periods of time that would not be predicted from their terminal half-lives. It is conceivable that the pharmacokinetics of antipsychotics in plasma may not accurately reflect the kinetics at receptor sites in the brain (Campbell and Baldessarini 1985; Hubbard et al. 1987).

Most antipsychotics are highly protein bound. For example, more than 90% of a drug such as fluphenazine or haloperidol is bound to plasma protein. The remaining unbound portion is the drug that is available for passing through the blood-brain barrier. In theory, conditions that alter the amount of plasma protein will alter the amount of bioavailable antipsychotic drug.

The pharmacokinetics of long-acting injectable antipsychotics differ markedly from those of short-acting oral and injectable drugs. Long-acting fluphenazine and haloperidol are administered as esters dissolved in sesame oil. The oil is injected into a muscle, and the drug gradually diffuses from the oily vehicle into the surrounding tissues. The rate-limiting step appears to be the rate of diffusion, because once the drug enters the tissue it is rapidly hydrolyzed and the parent compound is released. Plasma concentrations of short-acting drugs rise rather rapidly during the absorption phase and then decline during a distribution and elimination phase. Long-acting compounds, on the other hand, are absorbed continually during the interval between injections. Moreover, for patients who have received multiple injections, the drug will be absorbed from multiple injection sites simultaneously. As a result, it takes long-acting compounds much longer to reach steady state, and they are eliminated much more slowly. For example, the decanoate forms of haloperidol and fluphenazine require about 3 months to reach steady state, and substantial plasma concentrations can be detected months after therapy has been discontinued (Marder et al. 1989).

■ MECHANISM OF ACTION

Before the discovery of chlorpromazine and other antipsychotic drugs, biological research on psychosis focused on locating circulating substances that might be psychotogenic. The discovery of drugs that were effective against psychosis was a historic event; if the mechanism of action of these drugs could be understood, this could provide valuable information about the biology of psychosis.

In 1963, Carlsson and Lindquist reported that administering chlorpromazine or haloperidol to mice resulted in an accumulation of dopamine metabolites in dopamine-rich brain areas. They hypothesized that the drugs blocked receptors for dopamine and that feedback mechanisms resulted in an increase in dopamine release. Since that time, others have found that all of the effective antipsychotics bind to dopamine receptors. In 1976, Seeman and colleagues and Creese and colleagues reported that the affinity of the traditional antipsychotics for D_2 receptors is highly correlated with their effective clinical dose. In contrast, there is not a similar relationship between affinity for other receptors (e.g., muscarinic or adrenergic) and clinical effectiveness. This observation has led to the conclusion that the traditional antipsychotic drugs exert their effects against psychosis by blocking D_2 receptors.

Others have proposed that schizophrenia and other psychotic illnesses are related to an overactive dopamine system. This "dopamine hypothesis of schizophrenia" has resulted in an exhaustive search for abnormalities in the dopamine systems of schizophrenic individuals. For the most part, this search has had mixed results and remains unproven (Marder et al. 1991). The fact that antipsychotic medications relieve schizophrenic psychosis by decreasing dopamine activity does not mean that schizophrenia is caused by increased dopamine activity. It is common in medicine for illnesses to be treated through mechanisms that are unrelated to the actual cause of the illness. For example, hypertension can be treated by drugs with different biological activities that are far removed from the actual cause of hypertension. In a similar manner, schizophrenic psychosis—or any psychosis—may be attenuated by methods that are unrelated to what causes schizophrenia.

Recent information indicates that the theory that antipsychotic drugs work by blocking D_2 receptors is an oversimplification. Studies using positron-emission tomography (PET) scanning indicate that patients receiving a traditional antipsychotic improve when approximately 80% or their D_2 receptors are occupied (Farde et al. 1992). Moreover, this occurs within hours of receiving an adequate dose of drug. However, the clinical response to the medication may require days or weeks. Studies monitoring plasma homovanillic acid (HVA), a metabolite of dopamine, are consistent with the hypothesis that the delayed response may be due to a decrease in dopamine turnover. When drug-free patients receive an antipsychotic, plasma HVA increases during the first few days and then declines in some patients (Bowers 1984). Studies indicate that the decline in HVA is correlated with the amount of improvement in psychosis. Further, patients who have a high plasma HVA prior to treatment, appear to be more likely to respond to antipsychotics. These observations are supported by studies on the firing rates of midbrain dopamine neurons of rats. Treatment with haloperidol results in a short-term increase in the firing of these neurons followed by a prolonged decrease in firing that has been referred to as "depolarization inactivation" (Chiodo and Bunney 1987). It has been proposed that the antipsychotic effects of these drugs is associated with the decrease in firing. Taken together, these findings suggest that for an antipsychotic response to occur, the blockade of D_2 receptors is an initial response, that must be followed by a decrease in dopamine activity.

■ INDICATIONS

Antipsychotic medications are effective for nearly every medical and psychiatric condition that results in psychosis. In this regard, this group of drugs is antipsychotic rather than antischizophrenic. The effectiveness of these drugs is often limited by their neurological side effects. For this reason, clinicians may choose not to treat certain psychotic conditions that are either mild or transitory.

■ Acute Schizophrenia and Schizoaffective Disorders

Numerous clinical studies have demonstrated the effectiveness of antipsychotic medications for reducing psychotic symptoms in acute schizophrenia as well as schizoaffective disorders. Early studies that used doses that were too low were equivocal. Well-designed studies that used adequate doses and appropriate patient selection almost invariably found powerful drug effects.

Antipsychotic medications are effective for treating nearly all of the symptoms associated with schizophrenia, although the extent of their effectiveness is highly variable in specific patients. Symptoms such as hallucinations, delusions, and disorganized thoughts—also called positive symptoms because they were attributed to reflect abnormal function— are more likely to improve with drugs than symptoms, such as blunted affect, emotional withdrawal, and lack of social interest—also called negative symptoms because they have been attributed to the absence of normal brain function. For many patients, antipsychotics will result in substantial improvement, or even remission of positive symptoms, but negative symptoms will be minimally affected and will continue to impair the patient's social recovery. Moreover, as described under adverse effects, these drugs may result in side effects that are difficult to distinguish from negative symptoms.

All of the traditional antipsychotic medications— that is, all of the drugs except clozapine—are equally effective. Clinicians and researchers who prescribed these drugs during the years immediately following their discovery reported that certain forms or subtypes of schizophrenia improved more with particular antipsychotics. These observations have not withstood careful study. In other words, all of the traditional antipsychotic drugs are equally effective for all subtypes of schizophrenia.

There is a small population of patients with schizophrenia who should probably not be treated with antipsychotic medications. The possible justifications for withholding medications are the following: 1) their illness is unaffected or worsened by medications; 2) the patient has a history of complete recovery in a brief time without drugs; or 3) the adverse effects are too severe in proportion to the improvement that results from drug treatment. If a patient's clinical history indicates that they belong to one of these three groups, a rational decision to withhold antipsychotic medications could be made.

In certain conditions, antipsychotic drug treatment becomes problematic, and the risk-benefit shifts. Antipsychotics should be prescribed cautiously for patients with seriously impaired hepatic function since these drugs are primarily metabolized in the liver. Patients with Parkinson's disease may have difficulty tolerating traditional drugs because of EPS. Whenever possible antipsychotics should be withheld during pregnancy, particularly during the first trimester. This should be viewed as a relative contraindication since severe psychotic behavior on the part of the mother can be more serious than the effects of drugs. Moreover, alternative drug therapies such as lithium or benzodiazepines may have more serious effects on fetal development.

In the past, some senior psychotherapists reported that patients who are able to engage in intensive psychotherapy appeared to do better without antipsychotic medications. Clinicians are often impressed by an occasional patient who does extremely well without neuroleptics and sustains a complete or nearly complete recovery while receiving skilled psychotherapy. It is important not to generalize from experience with these rather rare individuals to the vastly greater number of psychotic schizophrenic patients who will be helped to a substantial degree by medication. Moreover, an extensive literature indicates that psychosocial treatments are most effective when they are administered in patients who are also receiving antipsychotics. A review by Wyatt (1991) concluded that early intervention with antipsychotics reduced long-term morbidity and decreased the number of rehospitalizations. In other words, even if a patient eventually recovers without drugs, it is possible that the amount of time spent in a psychotic state may be related to a worse long-term outcome.

It has also been claimed that patients with a very poor prognosis or those who remain psychotic on drugs should not receive them. For example, investigators have suggested that patients with "Kraepelinian schizophrenia" have poor drug responses, severe negative symptoms, a greater risk for schizophrenia in their first-degree relatives, and poor premorbid sociosexual adjustment (Keefe et al. 1990). Others have suggested that schizophrenic patients with enlarged cerebral ventricles (Weinberger et al. 1980) or other evidence of structural abnormalities of the brain (Crow 1980) are likely to respond poorly to antipsychotics. However, the fact that these patients respond to a limited extent to antipsychotics should not be seen as evidence that these patients are not helped by their medications. The evidence that structural abnormalities limit the amount of improvement is far from convincing. In my clinical experience, when severely ill, treatment-refractory patients in chronic care hospitals have their antipsychotic medications discontinued, they will deteriorate. Many of these patients may also respond to clozapine (Kane et al. 1988; Meltzer et al. 1990).

■ Maintenance Therapy in Schizophrenia

Antipsychotics have been reliably shown to decrease the frequency of relapse in schizophrenic patients who have recovered from a psychotic episode. A number of studies have randomly assigned stabilized patients to either an antipsychotic drug or a placebo.

Davis (1975) reviewed 24 double-blind studies of maintenance antipsychotic therapy and found that in all studies, many more patients relapsed on placebo than on drug. When the results were pooled, 698 out of 1,068 patients on placebo relapsed (65%), in contrast with only 639 out of 2,127 patients on drug (30%). This very large difference in survival between drug-treated and placebo-treated patients is the main reason why schizophrenic patients are commonly continued on long-term neuroleptic maintenance treatment after a schizophrenic episode. Some clinicians are often tempted to discontinue medications in patients who have been well and stable for a prolonged period. Unfortunately, these patients also have high relapse rates when their medications are discontinued (Hogarty et al. 1976).

The value of long-term antipsychotic drug treatment for well-stabilized patients has also been clarified by a series of studies by Johnson and colleagues (1983). Patients who relapsed when they were receiving antipsychotic medications had episodes that were less severe than those in patients who discontinued their drugs. Drug-maintained patients were less likely to have episodes with self-destructive behavior, violence, and antisocial acts. In addition, patients who relapsed off medications were more likely to require involuntary hospitalization. Patients who discontinued their medications actually ended up, on average, receiving more total medication, because the drug dose needed to treat relapses was much higher than the dose for relapse prevention.

In 1989, an international group of experts reached a consensus on the indications for neuroleptic relapse prevention: 1 to 2 years of maintenance antipsychotic was recommended for patients following a first episode. Although this may be somewhat longer than current practice in many settings, this was recommended because individuals at this stage of their illness often have the most to lose. Patients may be working or involved in educational programs, both of which can be jeopardized by a second psychotic episode. Moreover, the self-image of patients and their personal relationships may be permanently altered by their illness. The consensus conference also recommended that multiepisode patients receive maintenance neuroleptic treatment for at least 5 years. For patients with a history of serious suicide attempts or violent, aggressive behavior, maintenance treatment with neuroleptics may be indicated for longer than 5 years—perhaps indefinitely (Kissling 1991).

Long-Acting Depot Antipsychotics

Some antipsychotic drugs (e.g., haloperidol and fluphenazine) can be administered by injection of an esterified form given once every 2–4 weeks. The active drug is slowly released from the injection site, resulting in a fairly constant plasma level during the entire interval between injections. There are two possible advantages associated with this route of administration in comparison with oral prescribing. The first advantage is that depot drugs provide a partial solution to the problem of poor compliance in schizophrenic outpatients. Many patients who are unable to take pills reliably can be convinced to regularly receive injections. The second advantage is more theoretical. When drugs are administered through injections, a more reliable blood level is achieved than with oral drugs. This is because oral drugs may vary in the degree to which they are absorbed in the digestive system. In addition, drugs that are taken orally undergo extensive metabolism in the digestive system and liver. Both of these obstacles to drug absorption are bypassed by injectable drugs (Marder et al. 1989).

There are some indications that patients who receive depot neuroleptics have a better long-term outcome than patients who receive oral drugs. This advantage has been demonstrated in a number of uncontrolled studies but has been ambiguous in carefully designed double-blind studies. However, a close look at the later studies indicates that there may be advantages for depot antipsychotics even under these carefully controlled conditions. The best comparison was a double-blind multisite study comparing oral fluphenazine and fluphenazine decanoate over 2 years (Hogarty et al. 1979). Patients who received fluphenazine decanoate demonstrated a lower risk of relapse than those assigned to oral fluphenazine. Moreover, the best outcomes were found for patients who received fluphenazine decanoate supplemented by a form of social therapy. These results suggest that depot antipsychotics may have advantages over oral drugs for patients who are reasonably reliable as well as for patients who have a history of poor medication compliance.

Mania

All of the traditional antipsychotic drugs are effective in reducing manic excitement. In comparison with lithium and carbamazepine, antipsychotic drugs often have a more rapid onset of action. As a result, an antipsychotic may be combined with an antimanic drug during the first days of treatment of severe excited states, before the antimanic compound has its onset of action. Once lithium or the other antimanic compound has become effective, the dose of antipsychotic may be reduced and eventually discontinued. In most cases, antimanic drugs are more effective than antipsychotics for mania and are associated with fewer side effects. Some studies indicate that patients with mood disorders are more vulnerable to developing tardive dyskinesia (TD) than schizophrenic patients, suggesting the importance of using these drugs for as short a time as possible.

Depressions With Psychotic Features

Patients with major depressive episodes with psychotic features will often benefit from a combination of antipsychotic and antidepressant medications. The added benefits of antipsychotic medications are most apparent for those patients who are tormented by severe delusions. When the psychotic component of the episode has responded to treatment, the antipsychotic medications should be withdrawn.

Other Indications

Antipsychotic drugs are effective for reducing psychotic symptoms in a number of organic mental syndromes, including dementia and psychotic states due to stimulant drugs. They can be useful for controlling agitation and chorea in Huntington's disease. Both haloperidol and pimozide have been demonstrated to be helpful in treating symptoms of Tourette's disorder. Antipsychotics are occasionally useful for patients with pervasive developmental disorder and mental retardation, but there is some concern that these drugs are overprescribed for these conditions.

SIDE EFFECTS AND TOXICOLOGY

Acute Extrapyramidal Side Effects

EPS, including dystonia, tremor, akinesia, bradykinesia, rigidity, and akathisia, are the major problem in prescribing neuroleptics. The most common EPS is akathisia, which is a subjective feeling of restlessness. Patients who experience severe akathisia will often pace continuously or move their feet restlessly while they are sitting. Some complain that they are unable to feel comfortable, regardless of what they do. Severe akathisia can cause patients to feel anxious or irritable, and some reports suggest that severe akathisia can result in aggressive or suicidal acts. One study found that as many as 75% of patients treated with a conventional dose of haloperidol will experience some degree of akathisia (Van Putten et al. 1984). Other studies have found that 25% of patients experience akathisia (Braude et al. 1983). Akathisias can be difficult to assess and are frequently misdiagnosed as anxiety or agitation (Weiden et al. 1987).

Acute dystonic reactions are abrupt onset, sometimes bizarre muscular spasms affecting mainly the musculature of the head and neck. Sometimes, however, dystonias of the trunk and lower extremities lead to gait disturbances that may be confused with hysteria. Dystonia usually appears within the first few days of therapy and when patients are treated with large doses of high-potency neuroleptics such as haloperidol or fluphenazine. It almost always responds rapidly to antiparkinsonian medications and can usually be prevented by either pretreatment with these drugs or by limiting the neuroleptic dosage prescribed. Younger patients and males are more prone to develop acute dystonia (Lavin and Rifkin 1992). One study found that 21% of male subjects under 30 developed acute dystonic reactions (Swett 1975).

Parkinsonism, which has symptoms such as stiffness, tremor, and shuffling gait, affects about 30% of patients who are chronically treated with traditional antipsychotics. Patients with parkinsonism may also experience akinesia, a side effect in which affected individuals have difficulty initiating movement. In some cases, drug-induced parkinsonism can be nearly identical to Parkinson's disease (Lavin and Rifkin 1992).

For most patients, EPS can be treatable. The anticholinergic antiparkinsonian drugs such as benztropine or trihexyphenidyl are by far the most commonly used drugs for EPS. Many clinicians will prescribe these drugs routinely for patients who are receiving antipsychotics—particularly potent antipsychotics. A number of studies indicate that prescribing antiparkinsonian medications before patients demonstrate EPS can prevent dystonias (Lavin and Rifkin 1992; Winslow et al. 1986). Unfortunately, these drugs also have side effects of their own, including dry mouth, constipation, urinary retention, and blurry vision. More recent studies indicate that anticholinergic antiparkinsonian drugs can also result in some loss of memory (Gelenberg et al. 1989). This side effect is dose dependent and remits when the drug is stopped.

Other drugs for treating EPS include amantadine (a drug that is effective against parkinsonism) and propranolol (which is effective in managing akathisia). Both of these drugs can be added to anticholinergic antiparkinsonian drugs.

A number of unfortunate people are highly sensitive to EPS—particularly akathisia—at the dose that is necessary to control their psychoses. Some of these patients may agree to tolerate these side effects, at least temporarily, while their most troublesome psychotic symptoms are being treated. For others, the discomfort brought on by medication side effects may seem worse than the illness itself. These patients may be good candidates for clozapine or risperidone.

■ TARDIVE DYSKINESIA

TD is a movement disorder that may occur following chronic treatment with antipsychotic medications. Patients with TD may have any or all of a number of abnormal movements. These frequently consist of mouth and tongue movements (e.g., lip smacking, sucking, and puckering) as well as facial grimacing. Other movements may include irregular movements of the limbs, particularly choreoathetoid-like movements of the fingers and toes and slow, writhing movements of the trunk. Younger patients tend to develop slower athetoid movements of the trunk, extremities, and neck. The movements of TD tend to increase when a patient is aroused and tend to decrease when he or she is relaxed. They are typically absent during sleep. Diagnostic criteria for TD developed by Schooler and Kane (1982) require that patients have at least 3 months of antipsychotic drug exposure and that the movements persist for at least 4 weeks. Seriously disabling dyskinesia is uncommon, but a small proportion of patients may have TD that affects walking, breathing, eating, and talking.

At least 10%–20% of patients treated with neuroleptics for more than 1 year develop TD. In chronically institutionalized patients, the prevalence is

15%–20%. Recent prospective studies indicate that the cumulative incidence of TD is 5% at 1 year, 10% at 2 years, 15% at 3 years, and 19% at 4 years (Kane et al. 1986). Certain populations are at a greater risk than others for developing TD. Greater age increases risk, with elderly women being particularly vulnerable. Moreover, TD in elderly patients is less likely to remit when antipsychotics are discontinued. Patients with affective disorders may also be at a greater risk for developing TD when they are treated with antipsychotics. Other possible risk factors for TD are the dose of antipsychotic medications and the length of time on these drugs (Kane and Lieberman 1992).

Early observations of the course of TD suggested that the disorder was inevitably progressive and irreversible. In other words, once patients developed even mild dyskinesias, it was likely that they would progress toward severe TD. More recent evidence indicates otherwise. When antipsychotics are discontinued, a substantial proportion of TD patients will demonstrate a remission. This is more likely for those with a recent onset.

TD does not appear to be a progressive disorder for most patients. It seems to develop rapidly and to then stabilize and often to improve. A number of studies have followed the course of TD in patients who were continued on drugs for several years. The consensus is that most patients improve in the severity of TD, even if their antipsychotic drugs are continued. Moreover, this improvement can be clinically meaningful in some patients.

The Task Force on Tardive Dyskinesia of the American Psychiatric Association (American Psychiatric Association Task Force 1992) issued a report in which a number of recommendations for preventing and managing TD were made. These include the following:

1. Establishing objective evidence that antipsychotic medications are effective for an individual
2. Using the lowest effective dose of antipsychotic
3. Prescribing cautiously to children, elderly people, or those individuals with mood disorders
4. Examining patients on a regular basis for evidence of TD
5. When TD is diagnosed, considering alternatives to antipsychotics, obtaining informed consent, and also considering dosage reduction
6. If the TD worsens, considering a number of options, including discontinuing the antipsychotic, switching to a different drug, or considering a trial of clozapine

■ Neuroleptic Malignant Syndrome

The clinical characteristics of the neuroleptic malignant syndrome (NMS) include 1) severe muscular rigidity, 2) autonomic instability, including hyperthermia, tachycardia, increased blood pressure, tachypnea, and diaphoresis, and 3) changing levels of consciousness. A patient with NMS usually presents with muscular rigidity, and the condition progresses to elevated temperature, fluctuating consciousness, and unstable vital signs. These symptoms are often associated with elevations in creatine phosphokinase (CPK). Elevations in liver transaminases, leukocytosis, myoglobinemia, and myoglobinuria are less frequent. Acute renal failure may also occur. Mortality in well-developed cases has been reported to range from 20%–30% and may be higher when depot forms are used. More recent studies indicate that mortality from NMS has been reduced (Shalev et al. 1989).

NMS is more common when high-potency antipsychotics are prescribed in high doses and when dose is escalated rapidly. The syndrome is twice as common in males as in females and is more likely to be present in younger patients. Clinicians should be concerned about any patient who demonstrates severe muscular rigidity and a rising body temperature, because early diagnosis and treatment can be lifesaving. The most effective means for preventing NMS probably involves the early diagnosis and management of severe muscular rigidity.

When NMS is diagnosed or suspected, antipsychotics should be discontinued and supportive and symptomatic treatment begun. This may include treating EPS with antiparkinsonian medications, correcting fluid and electrolyte imbalances, treating fevers, and managing cardiovascular symptoms such as hyper- or hypotension. Gratz and colleagues (1992) suggest that when patients have fevers over 101°F, antipsychotics and anticholinergics should be discontinued. At that time, treatment with dopamine agonists such as bromocriptine should be considered, along with intensive medical monitoring if the fever exceeds 103°F. If these treatments are inadequate, dantrolene or benzodiazepines should be considered. After patients recover from NMS, they can usually be treated with a different antipsychotic drug, or even with the same drug that caused the disorder.

■ Neuroendocrine Effects

The most significant and consistent neuroendocrine effect of antipsychotic drugs is hyperprolactinemia. Some patients develop tolerance to the prolactin-elevating effects of these drugs after several weeks (Meltzer 1985). In women, elevated prolactin can lead to menstrual abnormalities, including anovulatory cycles and infertility, menses with abnormal luteal phases, or frank amenorrhea and hypoestrogenemia (Reichlin 1992). Galactorrhea is a relatively common side effect that results from the direct effect of prolactin on the breast tissue. It may be uncomfortable but is seldom of any medical significance. Female patients have also reported decreased libido and anorgasmia.

In men, elevated prolactin levels can lower testosterone levels and result in impotence. Male patients frequently report ejaculatory and erectile disturbances that are probably related to the autonomic effects of the antipsychotic. These problems tend to be most prominent with low-potency drugs and are usually dose related.

■ Cardiovascular Side Effects

Low-potency antipsychotic medications such as chlorpromazine or thioridazine can cause orthostatic hypotension through α_1-adrenergic blockade. The more potent dopamine blockers such as haloperidol or fluphenazine are less likely to cause autonomic effects. Chlorpromazine may cause prolongation of the Q-T and P-R intervals, S-T depression, and T wave blunting, and thioridazine may cause Q-T and T wave changes. Both should be used cautiously in patients with increases in their Q-T intervals.

■ Other Side Effects

Low-potency antipsychotics, particularly chlorpromazine, may cause photosensitivity reactions consisting of severe sunburn or rash. As a result, patients should be instructed to use sunscreens. These drugs can also be associated with an uncommon discoloration of the skin. Skin areas that are exposed to sunlight, particularly the face and neck, develop blue-gray metallic discoloration. This skin reaction is usually associated with long-term treatment involving high drug doses.

Patients receiving long-term treatment with chlorpromazine may develop granular deposits in the anterior lens and posterior cornea. These deposits (visualized on slit lamp examination) seldom affect the patient's vision. Changing the patient to another drug will usually result in a gradual improvement in the condition.

High doses of thioridazine (i.e., greater than 1,000 mg qd) can result in retinal pigmentation. This condition can lead to serious visual impairment or blindness. Moreover, the condition may not remit when thioridazine is discontinued. As a result, thioridazine should not be prescribed at doses over 800 mg qd.

■ Coexisting Medical Conditions

Pregnancy.   There is no clear evidence that antipsychotic drugs are associated with congenital malformations. These drugs do cross the placenta, and there are suggestions from animal studies that prenatal exposure may affect the development of the dopamine system. Clinicians should therefore attempt to discontinue these medications during the first trimester if this is feasible and should consider carefully whether the risks of prescribing these drugs during the remainder of a patient's pregnancy are justified by the likely benefits. Discontinuing antipsychotics during the weeks immediately preceding delivery should also be considered, because of the impaired drug clearance in newborns. Antipsychotics are secreted with lactation. Mothers who are being treated with these drugs should not breast feed.

Seizure disorders.   Antipsychotics lower seizure thresholds and should be prescribed with caution to patients with seizure disorders.

■ DRUG-DRUG INTERACTIONS

A number of drugs can affect the metabolism of antipsychotics including certain heterocyclic antidepressants, fluoxetine, β-blockers, and cimetidine, all of which may increase plasma levels by competing for enzyme-binding sites. Conversely, barbiturates and carbamazepine may decrease plasma levels by enhancing metabolism of the antipsychotic. A number of studies have suggested that anticholinergic antiparkinsonian medications decrease antipsychotic blood levels, but more recent and better controlled studies have concluded that antipsychotic levels are unaffected (Leipzig and Mendelowitz 1992). Levels of chlorpromazine and thioridazine increase when propranolol is also administered. Antacids can decrease the absorption of antipsychotic.

Antipsychotic drugs antagonize the effects of dopamine agonists or L-dopa when these drugs are used to treat parkinsonism. Chlorpromazine, haloperidol, and thiothixene can block the antihypertensive effects of guanethidine (Janowsky et al. 1973). Antipsychotics may also enhance the effects of CNS depressants such as analgesics, anxiolytics, and hypnotics (Leipzig and Mendelowitz 1992).

■ CONCLUSION

Antipsychotic drugs are effective agents for treating psychosis that results from schizophrenia or other illnesses. In treating schizophrenic patients, these agents are also effective in preventing relapse in stabilized individuals. However, antipsychotic medications have a number of important limitations. They have serious side effects (particularly neurological effects) that can result in severe discomfort on the one hand and prolonged abnormal movement disorders on the other. In addition, not every psychotic patient responds well to these agents. Newer antipsychotic drugs such as clozapine and risperidone appear to have milder side effects without compromising effectiveness. In the near future, these drugs may replace the conventional antipsychotic agents.

■ REFERENCES

American Psychiatric Association Task Force on Tardive Dyskinesia: Tardive Dyskinesia: A Task Force Report of the American Psychiatric Association. Washington, DC, American Psychiatric Press, 1992

Baldessarini RJ: Drugs and the treatment of psychiatric disorders, in The Pharmacological Basis of Therapeutics, 8th Edition. Edited by Gilman AG, Rall TW, Nies AS, et al. New York, Pergamon, 1990, pp 383–435

Baldessarini RJ, Cohen BM, Teicher MH: Significance of neuroleptic dose and plasma level in the pharmacological treatment of psychoses. Arch Gen Psychiatry 45:79–90, 1988

Bowers MB Jr: Homovanillic acid in caudate and prefrontal cortex following neuroleptics. Eur J Pharmacol 99:103–105, 1984

Braude WM, Barnes TRE, Gore SM, et al: Clinical characteristics of akathisia: a systematic investigation of acute psychiatric inpatient admissions. Br J Psychiatry 143:139–150, 1983

Campbell A, Baldessarini RJ: Prolonged pharmacologic activity of neuroleptics. Arch Gen Psychiatry 42:637, 1985

Carlsson A, Lindquist M: Effect of chlorpromazine or haloperidol on the formation of 3-methoxytyramine and normetanephrine in mouse brain. Acta Pharmacologica et Toxicologica 20:140–144, 1963

Chakraborty BS, Hubbard JW, Hawes EM, et al: Interconversion between haloperidol and reduced haloperidol in healthy volunteers. Eur J Clin Pharmacol 37:45–48, 1989

Chiodo LA, Bunney BS: Population response of midbrain dopaminergic neurons to neuroleptics: further studies on time course and nondopaminergic neuronal influences. J Neurosci 7:629–633, 1987

Creese I, Burt DR, Snyder SH: Dopamine receptor binding predicts clinical and pharmacologic potencies of antischizophrenic drugs. Science 192:481–483, 1976

Crow TJ: Molecular pathology of schizophrenia: more than one disease process? British Medical Journal 280:66–68, 1980

Davis J: Overview: maintenance therapy in psychiatry, I: schizophrenia. Am J Psychiatry 132:1237–1245, 1975

Farde L, Nordstrom AL, Wiesel FA, et al: Positron emission tomographic analysis of central D_1 and D_2 dopamine receptor occupancy in patients treated with classical neuroleptics and clozapine. Arch Gen Psychiatry 49:538–544, 1992

Gelenberg AJ, Van Putten T, Lavori PW, et al: Anticholinergic effects on memory: benztropine versus amantadine. J Clin Psychiatry 9:180–185, 1989

Gerlach J: New antipsychotics classification, efficacy, and adverse effects. Schizophr Bull 17(2):289–309, 1991

Gratz SS, Levinson DF, Simpson GM: Neuroleptic malignant syndrome, in Adverse Effects of Psychotropic Drugs. Edited by Kane JM, Lieberman JA. New York, Guilford, 1992, pp 266–284

Hogarty GE, Ulrich RF, Mussare F, et al: Drug discontinuation among long term, successfully maintained schizophrenic outpatients. Disorders of the Nervous System 37:494–500, 1976

Hogarty GE, Schooler N, Ulrich RF, et al: Fluphenazine and social therapy in the aftercare of schizophrenic patients: relapse analysis of two year controlled study of fluphenazine decanoate and fluphenazine hydrochloride. Arch Gen Psychiatry 36:1283–1294, 1979

Hubbard JW, Ganes DA, Midha KK: Prolonged pharmacologic activity of neuroleptic drugs. Arch Gen Psychiatry 44:99–100, 1987

Janowsky DS, El-Yousef MK, Davis JM, et al: Antagonism of guanethidine by chlorpromazine. Am J Psychiatry 130:808–812, 1973

Johnson DAW, Pasterski JM, Ludlow JM, et al: The discontinuance of maintenance neuroleptic therapy in chronic schizophrenic patients: drug and social consequences. Acta Psychiatr Scand 67:339–352, 1983

Kane JM, Lieberman J: Tardive dyskinesia, in Adverse Effects of Psychotropic Drugs. Edited by Kane JM, Lieberman JA. New York, Guilford, 1992, pp 235–245

Kane JM, Woerner M, Borenstein M: Integrating incidence and prevalence of tardive dyskinesia. Psychopharm Bull 22:254–258, 1986

Kane JM, Honigfeld G, Singer J, et al: Clozapine for the treatment-resistant schizophrenic: a double-blind comparison versus chlorpromazine/benztropine. Arch Gen Psychiatry 45:789–796, 1988

Keefe RSE, Mohs RC, Silverman JM, et al: Characteristics of Kraepelinian schizophrenia and their relation to premorbid sociosexual functioning, in The Neuroleptic Nonresponsive Patient: Characterization and Treatment. Edited by Angrist B, Schulz SC. Washington, DC, American Psychiatric Press, 1990, pp 1–21

Kissling W, Kane JM, Barnes TRE, et al: Guidelines for neuroleptic relapse prevention in schizophrenia: towards a consensus view, in Guidelines for Neuroleptic Relapse Prevention in Schizophrenia. Edited by Kissling W. Berlin, Springer-Verlag, 1991, pp 155–163

Lavin MR, Rifkin A: Neuroleptic-induced parkinsonism, in Adverse Effects of Psychotropic Drugs. Edited by Kane JM, Lieberman JA. New York, Guilford, 1992, pp 175–188

Lehmann HE, Hanrahan AE: CPZ: new inhibiting agent for psychomotor excitement and manic states. Archives of Neurology and Psychiatry 71:227–237, 1954

Leipzig RM, Mendelowitz A: Adverse psychotropic drug-drug interactions, in Adverse Effects of Psy-

chotropic Drugs. Edited by Kane JM, Lieberman JA. New York, Guilford, 1992, pp 13–76

Marder SR, Hubbard JW, Van Putten T, et al: The pharmacokinetics of long-acting injectable neuroleptic drugs: clinical implications. Psychopharmacology (Berl) 98:433–439, 1989

Marder SR, Wirshing W, Van Putten T: Drug treatment of schizophrenia: overview of recent research. Schizophr Res 4:81–90, 1991

Meltzer HY: Long-term effects of neuroleptic drugs on the neuroendocrine system. Biochemical Psychopharmacology 40:50–68, 1985

Meltzer HY, Bernett S, Bastani B, et al: Effects of six months of clozapine treatment on the quality of life of chronic schizophrenic patients. Hosp Community Psychiatry 41:892–897, 1990

Midha KK, Marder SR, Jaworski TJ, et al: Clinical perspectives of some neuroleptics through development and application of their assays. Ther Drug Monit 15:179–189, 1993

Reichlin S: Neuroendocrinology, in Williams Textbook of Endocrinology, 8th Edition. Edited by Williams RH. Orlando, FL, WB Saunders, 1992, pp 135–219

Schooler NR, Kane JM: Research diagnoses for tardive dyskinesia. Arch Gen Psychiatry 39:486–487, 1982

Seeman P, Lee T, Chau-Wong M, et al: Antipsychotic drug doses and neuroleptic/dopamine receptors. Nature 261:717–719, 1976

Shalev A, Hermesh H, Munitz H: Mortality from neuroleptic malignant syndrome. J Clin Psychiatry 51:18–25, 1989

Silver JM, Yudofsky SC, Hurowitz GI: Psychopharmacology and electroconvulsive therapy, in The American Psychiatric Press Textbook of Psychiatry, 2nd Edition. Edited by Hales RE, Yudofsky SC, Talbott JA. Washington, DC, American Psychiatric Press, 1994, pp 897–1007

Swett C: Drug-induced dystonia. Am J Psychiatry 132:532–534, 1975

Van Putten T, May PRA, Marder SR: Akathisia with haloperidol and thiothixene. Arch Gen Psychiatry 41:1036–1039, 1984

Weiden PJ, Mann JJ, Haas G, et al: Clinical nonrecognition of neuroleptic-induced movement disorders: a cautionary study. Am J Psychiatry 144:1148–1153, 1987

Weinberger DR, Bigelow LB, Kleinman JE, et al: Cerebral ventricular enlargement in chronic schizophrenia. Arch Gen Psychiatry 37:11–13, 1980

Winslow RS, Stiller V, Coons DJ, et al: Prevention of acute dystonic reactions in patients beginning high potency neuroleptics. Am J Psychiatry 143:707–710, 1986

Wyatt RJ: Neuroleptics and the natural course of schizophrenia. Schizophr Bull 17:325–351, 1991

14

Atypical Antipsychotics

Michael J. Owens, Ph.D., and S. Craig Risch, M.D.

The widely held dopamine hypothesis regarding the pathophysiology of schizophrenia is based on two main lines of evidence. First, almost all clinically useful antipsychotic drugs are dopamine receptor antagonists. Second, dopamine agonists (i.e., drugs that increase the synaptic availability of dopamine, such as dextroamphetamine) can produce positive symptoms of psychosis (i.e., hallucinations, delusions, and thought disorders) indistinguishable from paranoid schizophrenia. Indeed, the ability of neuroleptic drugs to produce an antipsychotic action, as well as extrapyramidal side effects (EPS), has been primarily attributed to their ability to block the D_2 receptor subtype in the mesolimbocortical and nigrostriatal dopamine systems, respectively. Although the inhibitory effects of these neuroleptics on classical D_2 receptors appears to correlate superbly with their clinical antipsychotic potency, this neurochemical effect alone cannot explain all the clinically relevant differences between these drugs.

Since the advent of neuroleptic use in the treatment of schizophrenia, there has been a search for superior antipsychotic drugs because the "typical," "classical," or "traditional" D_2 receptor–blocking antipsychotics often do not result in a full remission of symptoms or, in many cases, even a significant improvement. This search has focused on compounds with an improved therapeutic profile (i.e., improved efficacy on both positive and negative symptoms and decreased side effects). These compounds, of which clozapine is considered the prototypical agent, have

been termed "atypical antipsychotics." Indeed, clozapine differs from typical antipsychotics (e.g., haloperidol, chlorpromazine) in producing minimal or no EPS in humans, or catalepsy in rodents at therapeutic doses. Perhaps more importantly, clozapine (unlike typical antipsychotics) improves both positive and negative symptoms of schizophrenia. The fact that clozapine differs clinically from typical antipsychotics, together with the data showing that clozapine is a relatively weak D_2 antagonist, have been the dominant forces suggesting that the original dopamine hypothesis of schizophrenia may need revising.

Unlike other chapters in Section II of this textbook, in which many different compounds are reviewed, our discussion focuses only on clozapine, which is currently the only agent routinely used as an atypical antipsychotic (though several others may soon be available). Therefore, we begin by reviewing a number of hypotheses, based primarily on animal studies of clozapine and recent advances in molecular neuropharmacology (i.e., the cloning of a number of receptors that bind antipsychotic drugs), that have been promulgated to explain the differences between typical and atypical antipsychotics. This portion of the chapter summarizing preclinical data falls under the categories "Mechanism of Action" and "Pharmacological Profile." It is beyond the scope of our discussion in this chapter to review all the atypical antipsychotics currently under clinical investigation. We therefore focus on the clinical pharmacology and therapeutics of clozapine, the only atypical antipsychotic currently approved for use in the United States. We also make note of those atypical antipsychotics that may be approved for use in the near future.

MECHANISM(S) OF ACTION

Based on clozapine's activity, the mechanism of action of an atypical antipsychotic is thought to be through either its differential actions in various subpopulations of dopamine neurons and/or binding to different dopamine receptor subtypes or additional binding to other neurotransmitter receptors. First, we compare and contrast the neurophysiological effects of clozapine with typical antipsychotics. Some of these differences are thought to possibly confer an atypical profile on clozapine. Second, we describe the receptor-binding profile of a number of putative atypical antipsychotic agents. These differences in receptor binding are probably responsible for the neurophysiological differences between clozapine and other typical antipsychotics.

It has been suggested that clozapine, unlike other typical antipsychotics, possesses relative mesolimbic dopaminergic specificity compared with its actions on nigrostriatal dopamine neurons. This may underlie its relative lack of EPS and tardive dyskinesia (TD) liability. Much of this evidence has come from electrophysiological studies of midbrain dopamine neurons. In general, dopamine neurons originating in the ventral tegmental area (VTA; A10 cell group) project to the nucleus accumbens, amygdala, and neocortex and make up the mesolimbocortical dopamine system. These projections are thought to be responsible for the majority of symptoms associated with schizophrenia. In contrast, the dopamine cells of the substantia nigra (SN; A9 cell group) project primarily to the caudate-putamen and make up the nigrostriatal dopamine system. This pathway is thought to be involved in the motor disturbances associated with EPS and TD, although recent evidence suggests that this pathway may also be involved in the behavioral manifestations of schizophrenia.

The pioneering work of Bunney, Aghajanian, and colleagues showed that acute administration of haloperidol increases the firing rate of VTA and SN dopamine neurons (Bunney et al. 1987, 1991). This response is probably the result of a lack of negative feedback on dopamine cells following D_2 receptor

blockade. In contrast, acute clozapine administration only increases the firing rate of VTA neurons. The changes observed after chronic administration of these compounds may have more physiological significance. On a time scale similar to that in which antipsychotics exert their clinical effects, typical antipsychotics such as haloperidol significantly decrease the number of spontaneously active dopamine neurons encountered in the VTA and SN. Subsequent examination revealed that these cells enter into a state of depolarization-induced block (i.e., inactivation) and decreased dopaminergic function.

Clozapine differs from typical antipsychotics in that chronic administration does not induce depolarization block of SN dopamine neurons but does induce inactivation in dopamine neurons of the VTA (Chiodo and Bunney 1983, 1985; Hand et al. 1987). The delayed onset of depolarization block in the VTA is thought to be related to the slow onset of action of all antipsychotic drugs, including clozapine, whereas the lack of EPS with clozapine is thought to be the result of preservation of the activity of the SN neurons. Although depolarization block has been widely accepted as a primary consequence of chronic antipsychotic treatment, recent findings have raised questions about the functional importance of depolarization block in the mechanism of action of antipsychotics (clozapine included). The release of dopamine from nerve terminals may be much more independent of cell firing than was previously thought.

These electrophysiological actions are thought to result in neurochemical differences as well. Studies have shown that acute administration of typical antipsychotic drugs results in more prominent effects on dopamine metabolism in the striatum than in mesolimbocortical areas. In contrast, clozapine appears to augment dopamine turnover to a relatively greater degree in mesolimbic areas (Deutch et al. 1991). Based on the electrophysiological findings that suggest that increased firing of dopamine neurons following acute antipsychotic drug administration is secondary to a lack of negative feedback because of D_2 receptor blockade, the data suggest that clozapine preferentially alters mesolimbocortical dopamine neurons.

Using in vivo voltammetry, which can measure local catecholamine release over very short epochs, researchers have reported that clozapine preferentially blocks dopamine release in the nucleus accumbens versus the striatum. However, this was not replicated elsewhere (see Meltzer 1991). Additional studies have been reported using in vivo microdialysis, another technique that can measure local dopamine release in specific brain regions. Ichikawa and Meltzer (1991) found evidence that chronic clozapine does not interfere with either mesolimbic (i.e., nucleus accumbens) or nigrostriatal dopamine metabolism. These findings also suggest that dopamine release from nerve terminals may not be significantly affected by the presence of depolarization block. However, local tissue damage inherent in microdialysis experiments can release dopamine from neurons that are in depolarization block.

There is also evidence that clozapine may preferentially increase dopamine metabolism in the prefrontal cortex (Moghaddam and Bunney 1990). This finding, together with the relatively weaker D_2 receptor blockade produced by clozapine versus typical antipsychotics, may lead to a net increase in mesocortical dopamine activity. Indeed, the "hypofrontality" theory has been postulated, which states that the negative symptoms of schizophrenia may be the result of a cortical dopamine deficit. Thus, the ability of clozapine to benefit both negative and positive symptoms may be due to its ability to increase cortical and decrease nucleus accumbens dopamine activity, respectively. Moreover, the relative lack of effect on nigrostriatal dopamine systems may be responsible for the lack of EPS associated with clozapine.

Although it appears that there is indeed some regional specificity for clozapine versus typical antipsychotics, logic and physical chemistry dictates this must have some basis in selective binding of clozapine to certain dopamine receptor populations and/or other additional receptors. These findings are explored in the next section.

■ PHARMACOLOGICAL PROFILES

■ D_2, D_3, and D_4 Receptors

Although we stated at the outset that recent findings have suggested that the dopamine hypothesis of schizophrenia may need revision, new findings from positron-emission tomography (PET) studies have provided further proof that the D_2 receptor is involved in the pathophysiology of schizophrenia and the mechanism of action of antipsychotics. Seeman

and colleagues have found that drug-naive schizophrenic patients have increased numbers of D_2 receptors in the putamen (Seeman 1987, 1992b; Seeman et al. 1989a). Moreover, chemically distinct antipsychotics (in the case of haloperidol) occupy 65%–90% of D_2 receptors in the putamen at clinically relevant doses (Farde et al. 1986, 1988, 1993). Of special significance is the finding that, unlike typical antipsychotics, clozapine occupies only 40%–50% of D_2 receptors in the striatum, whereas 80%–90% occupancy is observed in limbic areas (Farde et al. 1989).

Although it is generally thought that it is the high affinity for D_2 receptors in the striatum that is responsible for the EPS associated with typical antipsychotics, selective D_2 antagonists may possess some atypical antipsychotic activity. Before describing some of these findings, it would be helpful to briefly characterize some properties of the D_2 receptor.

The cloning of the D_2 receptor (Bunzow et al. 1988; Grandy et al. 1989) has enabled the simultaneous visualization and distribution of D_2 receptors and messenger ribonucleic acid (mRNA) in the rat (Mansour et al. 1990; Mengod et al. 1989; Meador-Woodruff et al. 1989) and primate (Lidow et al. 1989; Meador-Woodruff et al. 1991 [Figure 14–1]). Along with the anterior pituitary, highest concentrations are observed in the nigrostriatal and mesolimbic dopamine systems, with somewhat less observed in primate cortex. D_2 receptors are located both postsynaptically and presynaptically, where they probably act as autoreceptors. Increases in D_2 receptor binding are observed following antipsychotic treatment through mechanisms that remain unclear. These mechanisms are thought to include both transcriptional (i.e., increased mRNA synthesis) and posttranscriptional (i.e., not related to changes in receptor synthesis) processes (Seeman 1992b; Srivastava et al. 1990; Van Tol et al. 1990; Xu et al. 1992).

Shortly after the initial cloning of the D_2 receptor, researchers found that different isoforms of the same receptor are synthesized through alternative RNA splicing (Chio et al. 1990; Giros et al. 1989; Monsma et al. 1989). The two different isoforms vary by 29 amino acids in the third cytoplasmic loop near the G protein recognition site. Although this difference does not appear to result in binding differences between D_2 ligands, its location near the G protein regulatory site may result in differences in intracellular transduction mechanisms.

The apparent selectivity and demonstrated efficacy of clozapine has spawned increased research efforts to develop selective mesolimbic D_2 antagonists. Such compounds may prove to have superior clinical utility by possessing good antipsychotic activity (i.e., mesolimbic D_2 blockade) and little liability for EPS (i.e., relative sparing of striatal D_2 receptors). The substituted benzamides sulpiride, raclopride, and remoxipride are the prototypical agents of this class (Ögren and Hall 1992; Wadworth and Heel 1990). These compounds show clear in vivo differences in their potency to block D_2-mediated behaviors. Thus, these compounds possess a wide separation between doses that cause catalepsy in preclinical studies and doses that block dopamine agonist–induced behaviors, indicative of antipsychotic activity. Although it has been postulated that the sub-stituted benzamides and clozapine might posses some mesolimbic specificity, there is no unequivocal description as to how this might occur. It should also be noted that the substituted benzamides can bind to other receptors as well; D_2 selectivity is a relative term. Nevertheless, some clinical trials have provided evidence of clinical efficacy with reduced propensity, but not absence, of EPS (Lewander et al. 1992).

As mentioned earlier, D_2 receptors can act presynaptically as autoreceptors located either on the somatodendritic portion of the neuron or on presynaptic terminals. Those located on presynaptic terminals inhibit the release of dopamine into the synaptic cleft when activated. Using low doses of the dopamine agonist apomorphine, Tamminga and colleagues have investigated its antipsychotic potential (Tamminga and Gerlach 1987). The main effect of apomorphine at low doses is stimulation of presynaptic dopamine autoreceptors and diminishment of dopaminergic function; at higher doses, postsynaptic agonistic actions predominate. Pursuing this line of research, chemists and pharmacologists have synthesized compounds purported to have higher affinity for autoreceptors than apomorphine, as well as reduced postsynaptic affinity. These compounds have been reported to produce less EPS in preclinical studies than typical antipsychotic agents (Carlsson 1988a, 1988b; Heffner et al. 1992; Wiedemann et al. 1992). Though these compounds are hoped to primarily decrease transmission in the mesolimbic dopamine system, it is not clear whether this can be achieved—some dopaminergic neurons do not possess autoreceptors (Bannon et al. 1981, 1982; Kilts et al. 1987).

A somewhat similar related strategy is represented by partial dopamine agonists. These compounds by definition possess a high affinity for the D_2 receptor, but limited intrinsic activity to produce a full agonist effect. Thus, in the presence of normal or increased dopaminergic stimulation (i.e., mesolimbic system, positive symptoms), such compounds would compete with endogenous dopamine and act as functional antagonists. Conversely, under conditions of low dopaminergic tone (i.e., mesocortical system, negative symptoms), partial agonists would be expected to augment dopaminergic function. For example, the S(+)-N-n-propylnoraporphines act as functional dopamine antagonists and also show an apparent limbic selectivity (Baldessarini et al. 1991;

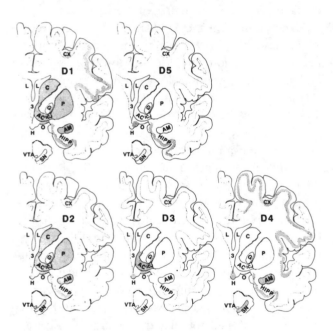

Figure 14–1. Brain region location of mRNA for dopamine receptors (grey stippled regions). The coronal view of the human brain used here is only to illustrate the various regions; in fact, most of the localization data were obtained using rat brain, with a minimum of information available on human brain. Abbreviations: Cx = cerebral cortex; L = lateral ventricle; 3 = third ventricle; C = caudate nucleus; P = putamen; G = globus pallidus; AC = nucleus accumbens; ICJ = islands of Calleja; H = hypothalamus; O = olfactory tubercle; AM = amygdala; Hipp = hippocampus; VTA = ventral tegmental area; and SN = substantia nigra.
Source. Reprinted from Seeman 1992b with permission of Elsevier Science Publishing Co., Inc. Copyright © 1992 by the American College of Neuropsychopharmacology.

Campbell et al. 1991, 1992). Partial agonists with relatively high intrinsic activity (e.g., B-HT-920) do not induce catalepsy in laboratory studies. These agonists with lower intrinsic activity (e.g., SDZ 208-912) display a clear separation of doses between those producing catalepsy and those antagonizing dopamine-mediated behaviors (Coward et al. 1990; Meltzer 1991; Naber et al. 1992). However, SDZ 208-912 was recently removed from clinical trials because it produced EPS (R. H. Baldessarini, personal communication, March 1993).

The D_3 receptor has been cloned and studied (Sokoloff et al. 1990, 1992a). This receptor displays considerable homology with the D_2 receptor but has a 10–100-fold higher affinity for dopamine than do D_2 receptors. This suggests that the effects of dopaminergic agonists and autoreceptor-selective agonists may be attributable to their actions primarily on D_3 receptors. Moreover, the D_3 receptor appears to be expressed predominantly in the mesolimbic dopaminergic system (Bouthenet et al. 1991; Buckland et al. 1992; Sokoloff et al. 1990 [Figure 14–1]).

Like the D_2 receptor, the D_3 receptor possesses a high affinity for antipsychotic drugs in vitro. Typical antipsychotics such as haloperidol are 10–20 times more potent at D_2 receptors than at D_3 receptors. However, atypical antipsychotics such as clozapine and several substituted benzamides are only 2–3 times more potent at the D_2 receptor (Schwartz et al. 1992; Sokoloff et al. 1990, 1992b). Thus, the ratio of binding in vitro toward the D_3 receptor versus the D_2 receptor is higher for several atypical antipsychotics. This (combined with the localization of D_3 receptors primarily in the mesolimbic system) might represent the ability of atypical antipsychotics such as clozapine to treat schizophrenia, while sparing the nigrostriatal dopamine system (Snyder 1990).

However, there are shortcomings to relying on drug affinities derived from in vitro binding studies. Only free drug in the extracellular water compartment is available in vivo for binding to a given receptor. This fraction of total drug is dependent on several bioavailability and pharmacokinetic considerations (e.g., the fraction protein bound, lipophilicity, metabolic half-life). Therefore, selectivity based on in vitro binding affinities may not be apparent in vivo. For example, at commonly used clinical doses, the D_2 receptors are blocked by about 80%, whereas D_3 receptors would be blocked by only 2%–40% (Seeman 1992a, 1992b). As Seeman has

pointed out, no available neuroleptics block D_3 receptors more readily than D_2 receptors. Moreover, no agonists actually discriminate between these receptors, as the affinities of agonists at the D_3 receptor are similar to that at the high-affinity state of the D_2 receptor.

Although a selective D_3 antagonist would be of considerable interest as an antipsychotic, preliminary genetic linkage studies have not found evidence for a link between D_3 receptor abnormalities and schizophrenia (Sokoloff et al. 1992c).

The D_4 receptor is the latest receptor in the D_2 receptor family to be cloned (Van Tol et al. 1991). The D_4 receptor displays similar homology with both the D_2 and D_3 receptors. In general, the D_4 receptor displays less than or equal affinities for dopamine agonists and antagonists compared with the D_2 receptor. The finding that clozapine exhibits a more than 10-fold higher affinity for the D_4 receptor than the D_2 receptor is of considerable interest. Moreover, the affinity constant of clozapine for the D_4 receptor is similar to the free concentration of clozapine observed during antipsychotic treatment (Figure 14–2 [Seeman 1992a, 1992b; Van Tol et al. 1991]). Several variants of the D_4 receptor with differing antipsychotic binding properties have been found in humans (Van Tol et al. 1992). Seeman and colleagues (1993) have reported a sixfold increase in D_4 receptors in schizophrenic striatal tissue compared with tissue from control subjects or parkinsonian subjects. D_4 receptors were determined by subtracting [^{3}H]-raclopride binding (in the presence of guanine nucleotide) from [^{3}H]-emonapride binding that label D_2 and D_3 and D_2, D_3, and D_4 receptors, respectively. This increase in D_4 receptors may actually represent the increases in D_2 receptors previously reported.

Areas of high D_4 receptor mRNA expression include the frontal cortex and other limbic regions with relatively less in the striatum (Figure 14–1). This distribution differs from the D_2 and D_3 receptors and may partly explain clozapine's lack of EPS. Additionally, the D_4 receptor may represent frontal cortical labeling observed with [^{11}C]-clozapine in a PET study (Lundberg et al. 1989).

■ D_1 and D_5 Receptors

Although researchers have known about the D_1 receptor since the late 1970s, it was not until 1990 that the receptor was cloned from rat and human tissue

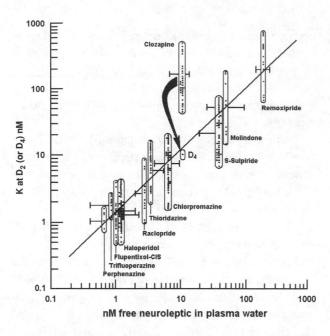

Figure 14–2. The neuroleptic dissociation constants (K) at the dopamine D_2 receptor closely match the free neuroleptic concentrations in the patients' plasma water. Each point indicates a K value. Clozapine is the only drug that does not fit the D_2 correlate, but its affinity at D_4 *(arrow)* does. The plasma molarities for *cis*-flupentixol and for *S*-sulpiride are half those published for the racemates which are used clinically.

Source. Reprinted from Seeman 1992b with permission of Elsevier Science Publishing Co., Inc. Copyright © 1992 by the American College of Neuropsychopharmacology.

(by four groups simultaneously) (Dearry et al. 1990; Monsma et al. 1990; Sunahara et al. 1990; Zhou et al. 1990). The D_1 receptor, unlike the D_2 receptor, stimulates the production of cyclic adenosine monophosphate (cAMP) and is distributed similarly to D_2 receptors (Clark and White 1987; Cortés et al. 1989; Mansour et al. 1991 [Figure 14–1]). Of particular interest is the finding that selective D_1 antagonists are effective in preclinical tests predictive of antipsychotic activity, just as with D_2 antagonists (Clark and White 1987; Waddington and Daly 1992). It has since been shown that these two receptors can interact either synergistically or antagonistically through G proteins and/or second messenger generation (Bertorello et al. 1990; Piomelli et al. 1991; Seeman et al. 1989b; Wachtel et al. 1989). Indeed, Seeman and colleagues (1989b) have found this link uncoupled in the brains of schizophrenic patients. They have suggested that a consequence of this might be excessive D_2 activity and the possible inability of antipsychotics

to bind efficiently to their receptors. Seeman and colleagues have since reported that this uncoupling is not the result of an altered amino acid sequence of the D_1 receptor as deduced from the D_1 gene (Ohara et al. 1993).

In general, most antipsychotics currently in use bind to both D_2 and D_1 receptors. No correlation has been found between the atypical nature of an antipsychotic and its D_1 affinity, although, as a group, atypical antipsychotics are less potent at the D_1 receptor (Meltzer et al. 1989). However, Farde and colleagues (1989) reported that clozapine displaces the D_1 PET ligand [^{11}C]-SCH23390 more efficiently than typical antipsychotic drugs.

In addition to preclinical antipsychotic activity, D_1 antagonists can produce catalepsy in rodents and EPS in primates. Therefore, an atypical nature attributed to these compounds is certainly not due to D_1 selectivity alone. It may be the result of the combination of low subclinical doses of a D_1 antagonist and a D_2 antagonist that may potentiate each other (see above), resulting in an antipsychotic effect without producing EPS.

A second member of the D_1 receptor subfamily, the D_5 receptor, which possesses homology similar to the D_1 receptor, has been isolated and cloned from human (Sunahara et al. 1991) and rat (Tiberi et al. 1991) tissue. Like the D_1 receptor, the D_5 receptor is linked to adenylate cyclase and cAMP production and exhibits affinities for various agonists and antagonists, much like the D_1 receptor—with the notable exception of dopamine itself, which is about 10 times more potent at the D_5 receptor. This suggests that the D_5 receptor may be important in maintaining dopaminergic tone. The D_5 receptor is expressed at much lower concentrations than the D_1 receptor, with highest concentrations found in the hippocampus and hypothalamus and lower concentrations in the striatum and cortex (Figure 14–1). Until a selective antagonist can be found, the clinical utility of D_5 ligands as antipsychotics remains unknown. Sibley and Monsma (1992) have reviewed the molecular biology of all dopamine receptors cloned to date.

■ **Serotonin Receptors**

In recent years, it has been hypothesized that clozapine's atypical actions may be due, at least in part, to its actions at other neurotransmitter receptors, such as certain serotonin (5-HT) receptor subtypes.

The involvement of 5-HT neural circuits in the mechanism of action of atypical antipsychotic drugs was postulated partly because 5-HT is known to exert a regulatory action on dopamine neurons. Relatively recent neurochemical studies suggest that 5-HT projections tonically inhibit mesolimbic and nigrostriatal dopaminergic activity. Moreover, 5-HT may directly inhibit dopamine release from striatal nerve terminals (Dray et al. 1976; Soubrie et al. 1984). These findings led to the hypothesis that 5-HT_{2A} antagonists might decrease the inhibition of dopamine activity produced by chronic neuroleptics (i.e., depolarization block, postsynaptic D_2 antagonism), functionally increasing dopaminergic activity in certain areas. This also suggests that there may be relative differences in the optimal magnitude of dopaminergic blockade needed in different brain areas. Moreover, complete dopaminergic blockade may not be beneficial for negative symptoms and may result in EPS.

Much of the data suggesting the involvement of the 5-HT_{2A} receptor have come from Meltzer and colleagues (1989), who examined the receptor-binding profile of a large series of antipsychotic drugs. They noted that typical and atypical antipsychotics can be distinguished on the basis of lower D_2 and higher 5-HT_{2A} pK_i values (a logarithmic measure of drug affinity for its receptor) of atypical compounds. Absolute potency at the 5-HT_{2A} receptor alone is not the determining factor, but atypical antipsychotics appear to have $5\text{-HT}_{2A}/D_2$ pK_i ratios of at least 1.1 (> 13-fold higher affinity). Likewise, Seeman (1992a) reported that those antipsychotics with less propensity to cause rigidity have higher $5\text{-HT}_{2A}/D_2$ ratios. However, 5-HT_{2A} blockade cannot account for the atypical actions of all purported atypical antipsychotics such as remoxipride and raclopride, because their $5\text{-HT}_{2A}/D_2$ receptor-blocking profile is similar to that of classical antipsychotics.

It has been suggested that 5-HT_{2A} antagonists be coadministered with a typical antipsychotic to determine if this would produce a clozapine-like profile. However, even low doses of typical antipsychotics produce 80%–90% D_2 receptor blockade. This makes it difficult to produce the relatively greater 5-HT_{2A} to D_2 receptor occupancy rates such as that observed with clozapine (40%–50% D_2 occupancy [Farde et al. 1989, 1993] and 80%–90% frontal cortical 5-HT_{2A} receptor occupancy [Nordstrom et al. 1993]) determined by PET studies.

In addition to the 5-HT_{2A} receptor, there is evi-

dence that other serotonin receptor subtypes may play a role in the action of atypical antipsychotics. The 5-HT_{2C} receptor (formerly the 5-HT_{1C} receptor) has been implicated in the mechanism of action of atypical antipsychotics, because clozapine has a higher affinity for 5-HT_{2C} receptors than for D_2 receptors (Canton et al. 1990). Also, in situ hybridization studies have shown that there are high densities of 5-HT_{2C} mRNA in the SN and nucleus accumbens, whereas the striatum and ventral tegmental area have lower densities (Molineaux et al. 1989). However, chlorpromazine has a higher affinity for 5-HT_{2C} receptors than D_2 receptors. Indeed, most typical and atypical antipsychotics bind weakly to 5-HT_{2C} receptors labeled with $[^3\text{H}]$-mesulergine.

5-HT_3 antagonists have also been proposed to be potential antipsychotics. Unlike other 5-HT receptors, the 5-HT_3 receptor is a component of a ligand-gated cation channel. Following binding, 5-HT rapidly increases membrane sodium and potassium conductance resulting in depolarization. 5-HT_3 receptors are found in the area postrema, where they are probably responsible for the antiemetic properties of these compounds. Receptors are also found in the nucleus of the solitary tract, entorhinal cortex, and limbic regions (Kilpatrick et al. 1987). Activation of these receptors leads to an increase in dopamine release in the mesolimbic and perhaps the nigrostriatal pathway. It is also known that clozapine binds with moderate affinity ($K_d \approx 100$ nM) to the 5-HT_3 receptor, whereas the typical antipsychotics spiperone, haloperidol, fluphenazine, and sulpiride are inactive (Bolanos et al. 1990; Watling et al. 1990). However, loxapine, which is also a typical antipsychotic, binds to 5-HT_3 receptors with the same affinity as clozapine (Hoyer et al. 1989). There is also evidence that the human nucleus accumbens and striatum may not have 5-HT_3 receptors, indicating that 5-HT_3 binding may be irrelevant to the mechanism of action of atypical antipsychotic drugs (Waeber et al. 1989). Reynolds (1992) concluded that in several clinical trials, the 5-HT_3 antagonist ondansetron was not clinically effective in the treatment of schizophrenia. However, this may have been a result of the nature of the studies' experimental design and the drug's pharmacokinetic properties more than to a lack of intrinsic efficacy.

Conflicting evidence has also been generated from electrophysiological studies examining the effect of 5-HT_3 antagonists on dopamine neuron firing rates. In a study by Sorensen and colleagues (1989), comparing MDL 73,147EF (a 5-HT$_3$ antagonist) and haloperidol, acute haloperidol administration increased dopamine firing rates in the SN and VTA, whereas acute MDL73,147EF had no effect. However, chronic treatment with both haloperidol and MDL73,147EF decreased the firing rate of neurons in both the SN and VTA, results consistent with evidence of depolarization block and likely antipsychotic efficacy. However, in vivo studies using the 5-HT$_3$ antagonist BRL 43694 showed no effect on the firing rate of dopamine neurons, acutely or chronically, in either brain region (Ashby et al. 1990). Blackburn and colleagues (1992) reported that the potent and selective 5-HT$_3$ antagonist BRL 46470A selectively reduced the number of spontaneously active dopamine neurons in the A10 area of the rat brain while having no effect on the A9 region—an action shared by clozapine. This finding suggests that BRL 46470A may possess an atypical antipsychotic profile.

Monsma and colleagues (1993) have reported the cloning of a novel 5-HT receptor linked to the stimulation of adenylate cyclase tentatively identified as the 5-HT$_6$ receptor. This receptor is localized exclusively in the central nervous system (CNS), predominantly in striatum, limbic, and cortical regions. The pharmacological profile of this receptor is of interest because clozapine displays high affinity for this site (K$_i$ 12.9 nM versus [^{125}I]-LSD), unlike dopamine or spiperone (both greater than 10 μM). However, loxapine, a typical antipsychotic, also displays relative high affinity for this site (K$_i$ 65 nM).

Sigma (σ) receptors have been implicated in schizophrenia. A stereoisomer of certain related benzopmorphans (opiates) that bind to the σ receptor possess profound psychotomimetic properties, and σ antagonists might therefore possess antipsychotic properties. Indeed, several drugs possessing preclinical antipsychotic activity, including haloperidol, bind to the σ receptor. These drugs (it is unclear whether they are agonists or antagonists), some of which bind only weakly to the D$_2$ receptor, can also alter dopaminergic firing rates (Largent et al. 1988; Snyder and Largent 1989; Steinfels et al. 1989; Taylor and Schlemmer 1992; Watchel and White 1988).

A critical review of the literature has shown that the psychotomimetic and dysphoric effects of these opiates has been attributed to the wrong stereoisomer (i.e., the psychotomimetic effects are produced by the levoenantiomer, and the dextroenantiomer is what is defined as the σ site (Itzhak and Stein 1990; Musacchio 1990; Walker et al. 1990). Additionally, classic σ ligands such as pentazocine, dextromethorphan, (+)3-PPP, and 1,3-di-o-tolyl-guanidine (DTG) do not block or cause psychotomimetic behaviors. Finally, clozapine is essentially devoid of activity at the σ receptor and σ ligands possessing preclinical antipsychotic activity may cause motor disturbances (see Walker et al. 1990).

Phencyclidine (PCP) acts as an antagonist at the N-methyl-D-aspartate (NMDA) subtype of the glutamate receptor and can cause profound schizophrenia-like symptoms. This implies that mechanisms that decrease NMDA receptor (glutaminergic) function may produce psychosis and that the glutaminergic system might be hypofunctional in schizophrenia. Based on known glutaminergic neurobiology, this is consistent with the dopamine hypothesis of schizophrenia although there is little pharmacological evidence of effective antipsychotic actions of glutamate agonists (Kalivas et al. 1989; Olney 1992; Tamminga et al. 1992).

There has been an explosion of information regarding the neurotransmitter role of neuropeptides the past decade. Indeed, opioid peptides, cholecystokinin, and neurotensin can regulate dopaminergic activity in laboratory animals. For example, haloperidol increases neurotensin and neurotensin mRNA concentrations in the mesolimbic and nigrostriatal dopamine systems, whereas the atypical antipsychotics clozapine and sertindole only increase neurotensin activity in the mesolimbic system (Kinkead et al. 1992). Unfortunately, at present few peptidergic ligands are available for detailed preclinical studies predictive of antipsychotic activity, although peptide-based drugs may hold great promise in the future.

We cite clozapine to summarize those biological characteristics that may confer an atypical nature on an antipsychotic. It appears that clozapine may be able to decrease mesolimbic dopamine activity while sparing nigrostriatal function, and possibly even increasing cortical dopamine activity. How this selectivity occurs is unknown. However, it is certain to be based on preferential binding to certain populations of dopamine receptors (i.e., mesolimbic) and/or dopamine receptor subtypes (i.e., D$_4$), along with relatively greater 5-HT$_{2A}$/D$_2$ blockade than that observed with typical antipsychotics.

HISTORY AND DISCOVERY OF CLOZAPINE

As we have discussed, over the past several decades, animal and molecular studies have begun to further elucidate the neuroanatomical and neurotransmitter circuits involved in cognition and behavior. This increased understanding of brain neurobiology had led to newer hypotheses regarding the pathophysiology of psychosis, as well as innovative approaches to psychopharmacological treatments. Specifically, putative medications exploiting differential potencies have been developed and are being studied in early clinical trails. These include those on D_1, D_2, D_3, and D_4 receptors; partial dopamine receptor agonists; σ receptor antagonists; NMDA receptor antagonists; serotonin receptor antagonists (5-HT_{2A} and 5-HT_3); muscarinic receptor antagonists; and α-adrenergic agonists.

Unfortunately, some of these agents have not proven efficacious or have had unacceptable adverse side effects, and as a result have not undergone further clinical development. However, others—including risperidone (potent 5-HT_{2A} and relatively weaker D_2 antagonistic properties) and the substituted benzamines (raclopride)—have proven efficacious and well tolerated in recent clinical studies. To date, there has not been sufficiently widespread use of these medications for a useful discussion of their clinical utility and side effects. (Excellent reviews of ongoing research studies with a wide variety of novel atypical antipsychotic medications may be found in Meltzer 1992a and Gerlach 1991.)

Currently, only clozapine among new atypical antipsychotic agents has had widespread clinical use in the United States. Clozapine received U.S. Food and Drug Administration approval for clinical use in 1990; however, it has been extensively used outside of the United States since the 1970s.

As reviewed by Hippius (1989), Austrian and German clinicians in the mid-1960s were the first to report that clozapine was an effective antipsychotic medication. It was controversial even then, because the conventional wisdom held that EPS were "necessary" for antipsychotic efficacy. Although clozapine was clearly an effective antipsychotic, it lacked EPS, causing some clinicians to question its inclusion as a "real neuroleptic." Unfortunately, in 1974, as clozapine's popularity was growing in Europe, eight patients in Finland died from a clozapine-associated agranulocytosis, and the routine use of clozapine was discontinued in many parts of the world. However, clozapine remained available in some countries, and its remarkable efficacy in otherwise refractory patients eventuated in its reemergence in the late 1980s for use in selected patients (i.e., treatment-refractory or medication-intolerant individuals) with the current laboratory monitoring system.

Structure-Activity Relations

As reviewed in detail by Baldessarini and Frankenburg (1991), clozapine is a 8-chloro-11-(4-methyl-1-piperazinyl)-5H-dibenzo[b,e]-[1,4]-diazepine originally developed in 1960 by Hünziker and colleagues (1963). No alternative has yet been developed that has the same degree of antipsychotic efficacy and lack of EPS, but with an absence of bone marrow toxicity. Clozapine is structurally similar but not identical to another antipsychotic, loxapine succinate (Loxitane), which does *not* have atypical antipsychotic properties. Clozapine's principal metabolites are believed to be N-desmethyl and N-oxide metabolites with low pharmacological activity (Baldessarini and Frankenburg 1991).

Indications and Pharmacotherapeutics

Clozapine is currently approved for use with the following patients:

1. "Treatment-refractory" schizophrenic patients (i.e., those who have failed adequate trials of several different classes of "typical" D_2 receptor blocking antipsychotic medications)
2. Patients with unmanageable EPS from "typical" D_2 receptor blocking neuroleptic medications
3. Patients with TD

However, ongoing clinical research investigations suggest the clinical utility of clozapine, alone or in combination with other psychotropics, in schizoaffective disorder and refractory bipolar (manic or depressed) patients, and during the early stages (i.e., first and second episodes) of schizophrenia. The major reason for the current restrictions on clozapine's clinical indications have been clozapine-induced agranulocytosis in approximately 1%–2% of patients, with reports of occasional fatalities. Because of this, weekly laboratory monitoring of a patient's complete and differential blood count is required for the pharmaceutical dispensing of clozapine in the United States. A number of ongoing studies are attempting to elucidate both mechanisms and predictors of clozapine-associated agranulocytosis to attempt to reduce or eliminate this potentially fatal side effect.

Clozapine has received approval for use in humans, despite its infrequent but potentially fatal adverse side effects, because 1) an increasing number of studies have suggested its antipsychotic efficacy in otherwise treatment-refractory or unresponsive schizophrenic patients, and 2) it has a markedly reduced incidence of EPS and TD when compared with "typical" antipsychotic medications.

Many open studies, and several randomized parallel design short-term (i.e., 4–6 weeks) studies (Kane et al. 1988) and crossover studies (Pickar et al. 1992b), have demonstrated a superior antipsychotic efficacy of clozapine over standard D_2 receptor blocking antipsychotic reductions (i.e., chlorpromazine, fluphenazine) in approximately one-third of treatment-refractory schizophrenic patients. The superior antipsychotic efficacy of clozapine in these studies has been demonstrated for both the "positive" symptoms of psychosis (i.e., hallucinations, delusions, thought disorder) and the "negative" symptoms of psychosis (i.e., anhedonia, asociality, blunted affect). Other preliminary studies suggest that an additional 15%–30% of patients who are unresponsive to clozapine in the first few months may show significant improvement after 6 months to 2 years of continued clozapine pharmacotherapy (Meltzer 1992b). Chronic treatment with clozapine has also been associated with improvement in "functionality," including increased vocational, social, and interpersonal adaptation in otherwise chronically impaired treatment refractory patients. This has resulted in diminished frequency and duration of hospitalizations and a greater ability among disabled patients to further their education and to reenter the workplace.

Consequently, a number of studies worldwide have indicated that clozapine therapy, despite a higher cost of medication to the individual, has resulted in significant savings to society, as evidenced by reduced hospital costs (Meltzer et al. 1993) and potentially improved economic generativity of otherwise chronically ill patients. In addition to significant clinical improvement in a large minority of otherwise treatment-refractory schizophrenic patients, an apparent complete remission of illness has been noted in a smaller subset of patients.

Unlike traditional antipsychotic medications, clozapine monotherapy is only rarely associated with EPS or TD (Lieberman et al. 1991). Furthermore, a number of investigators have observed a marked attenuation or complete elimination of EPS and TD in affected patients. Although it is not yet known whether this is simply because of withdrawal from traditional neuroleptics or a specific therapeutic effect, we have noted the disappearance of TD with clozapine treatment and its reappearance with the withdrawal of clozapine before reinstitution of other pharmacotherapy. Finally, although a few cases of neuroleptic malignant syndrome (NMS) have been reported with clozapine monotherapy, the incidence of clozapine-associated NMS would be expected to be less than that with typical antipsychotics. Of interest, clozapine has been used successfully in the antipsychotic treatment of patients who have experienced NMS associated with typical antipsychotic pharmacotherapy.

Despite its increasingly widespread clinical use, there is still a great deal of disparity among clinical practices in the administration of clozapine pharmacotherapy. When clozapine was first introduced it was recommended that candidates for clozapine pharmacotherapy have neuroleptic medication "washouts" for up to 1 week before initiation of clozapine. However, the withdrawal of typical neuroleptic medication before initiation of clozapine may sometimes be associated with significant clinical deterioration. Withdrawal should therefore be individualized.

Starting clozapine in drug-withdrawn patients is preferable; but, if necessary, low doses of a high-potency agent may be used until clozapine pharmacotherapy is established. Typically, clozapine is begun at 12.5–25 mg/day and increased in 25-mg/day increments as tolerated (see "Side Effects Management"). When patients begin to show appreciable clinical improvement, they may then be titrated off their D_2 receptor blocking "typical" neuroleptic therapy. Rarely will patients need or benefit from continued combined treatment with clozapine and a high-potency "typical" antipsychotic medication (e.g., haloperidol, fluphenazine). However, the continued use of "combination therapy" puts the patient at increased and continued risk for EPS, TD, and NMS.

As we have noted, in addition to its antipsychotic efficacy, preliminary studies suggest that clozapine also has significant antimanic and antidepressant effects in schizoaffective and bipolar patients who have failed traditional psychopharmacological regimens. Conversely, schizoaffective or bipolar patients unresponsive to clozapine monotherapy may benefit from the addition of lithium, valproic acid, or antidepressants when clozapine monotherapy does not adequately control affective symptoms. Lithium plus clozapine has been associated with a higher rate of neurological side effects, including NMS. Although any antidepressant may be used, the selective serotonin reuptake inhibitors (SSRIs) have fewer synergistic side effects (i.e., less anticholinergic, hypotensive, sedative, and decreased cardiac conduction effects). Fluoxetine administration has been reported to markedly increase clozapine plasma levels and produce toxicity through pharmacokinetic interactions (displacing serum-bound proteins and competing for hepatic microsomal enzyme metabolism). These same pharmacokinetic interactions may also occur with tricyclic antidepressant (TCA) and other antidepressant agents metabolized by the hepatic P_{450} microsomal system. The antidepressant buproprion probably should not be used in patients receiving clozapine, because both medications are associated with a significantly increased incidence of seizures. Although benzodiazepines have been used concurrently with clozapine, there have been occasional reports of severe respiratory depression or arrests. Their combined use is discouraged, especially—but not exclusively—with their concurrent initiation.

There is no universal agreement as to the "optimal" daily dosage of clozapine pharmacotherapy. Although doses in the 200–400 mg/day range have occasionally been associated with significant improvement and efficacy, greater improvement in otherwise unresponsive or partially responsive patients may occur with doses in the 500–900 mg/day range. Seizures occur with an increased incidence in clozapine-treated patients (see next section). The occurrence of seizures appears to be dose related, possibly occurring at a dosage rate of 0.7% per 100 mg. Patients experiencing seizures may be treated with concurrent anticonvulsants; carbamazepine should be avoided because of its propensity toward occasional bone marrow suppression (e.g., aplastic anemia). Although both agents (i.e., carbamazepine and clozapine) can be toxic to bone marrow, carbamazepine is thought to be directly toxic to bone marrow, and clozapine may represent an immunologic mechanism. Valproate may be the safest and best-tolerated anticonvulsant in clozapine-treated patients who experience seizures. It should be emphasized that clozapine-associated seizures do not necessarily contradict its continued use. If a patient experiences a clozapine-associated seizure, clozapine dosage may be temporarily reduced or stopped and anticonvulsants initiated. When therapeutic anticonvulsant levels are achieved, the clozapine dosage may be titrated upward to its previous therapeutic levels.

Confounding the determination of a particular patient's most effective daily dosage is the observation that some patients appear to need more time on medication rather than increased dosage for an optional therapeutic response. Thus, some patients who experience little or no improvement during the first 3 to 4 months of therapy will go on to demonstrate significant improvement after 6 months to 2 years of continued pharmacotherapy.

There is currently no consensus as to optional daily dose or adequacy of duration of trial of clozapine pharmacotherapy. Some centers recommend the titration of a patient's dosage up to approximately 450–650 mg/day during the first few months unless significant improvement occurs at lower doses. If a patient has demonstrated no appreciable improvement at 450–650 mg/day for 6 months, then titration up to a maximum of 900 mg/day with concurrent anticonvulsant administration may be considered, with a continued trial for an additional 6 months to 1 year. Other clinicians are less or more aggressive in dosage titration. However, it does appear that approximately one-third of patients will not experience significant benefit from clozapine pharmacotherapy, regardless of dosage or duration of trial.

■ Side Effects and Toxicology

In addition to an approximately 1%–2% incidence of potentially life-threatening agranulocytosis and the previously described dose-related seizures, clozapine also has a number of other undesirable but usually manageable side effects. Clozapine may frequently produce profound and often prolonged sedation, hypersalivation, enuresis (both daytime and nighttime), and anticholinergic side effects (i.e., dry mouth, blurred vision, urinary retention, and constipation). Elderly patients, and those on other medications with significant anticholinergic properties, may rarely experience anticholinergic delirium. These side effects are *usually* time limited, although they may persist for months. They are often dose related and may respond to temporary reduction in dose or to treatment with other medications with pharmacological properties opposite to the problematic side effects (i.e., caffeine for sedation, bulk increasing agents for constipation, cholinomimetic drugs for anticholinergic side effects, and anticholinergic medications for hypersalivation). Some patients may also experience urinary incontinence, either nighttime or daytime, which may also respond to anticholinergic agents. In almost all cases, these side effects eventually remit or are manageable with continued clozapine administration.

Orthostatic hypotension and tachycardia—not necessarily interrelated—occur frequently during clozapine pharmacotherapy and may respond to temporary dosage reduction or adjunctive pharmacological interventions. Both of these side effects are potentially dangerous and need careful clinical monitoring and attention to concurrently administered medication side effects that may be synergistic in toxicity.

During the first few months of clozapine pharmacotherapy, some patients will experience high "benign" fevers (100–103°F). These temperature elevations are usually not related to NMS or sepsis, nor are they anticholinergically mediated, although these etiologies must be ruled out. These temperature elevations usually remit with continued clozapine administration. When they occur, they may be managed with antipyretic agents.

As we have discussed, 1%–2% of clozapine-treated patients develop clinically significant suppression of bone marrow blood precursors, particularly the granulocyte series, but also (rarely) the erythropoid and platelet progenitors. Consequently, weekly monitoring of the complete blood count and differential is recommended throughout the duration of clozapine pharmacotherapy. Though agranulocytosis can occur at any time, its peak incidence occurs between 2–6 months of pharmacotherapy. In some cases, even more frequent monitoring may be indicated during this time if the patient is at higher risk (i.e., is older, medically ill, receiving potentially toxic concurrent medications, or experiencing large fluctuations in white blood cell [WBC] count).

It is important to note, however, that significant fluctuations in the WBC count (both increases and decreases) occur frequently early on in clozapine pharmacotherapy and do not necessarily indicate agranulocytosis or sepsis. Current laboratory monitoring recommendations include temporarily discontinuing clozapine if the WBC count drops to 3,000 or the granulocyte count falls to 1,500. Clozapine can be carefully reinstituted subsequently after complete recovery of WBC and granulocyte counts; otherwise, permanent discontinuation of clozapine is recommended if the WBC count drops to 2,000 or the granulocyte count falls to 1,000.

Patients experiencing agranulocytosis should be seen and monitored by a hematologist. Such patients usually need immediate hospital admission to a medical service for reverse isolation and aggressive monitoring and treatment. Because clozapine most frequently suppresses the granulocyte series of white blood cells, a differential cell count is recommended. Theoretically, the total WBC count could remain within normal limits despite the presence of agranulocytosis. Like any medication, clozapine may also affect other organ systems and other laboratory indices (e.g., liver function tests) should also be monitored, although less frequently if they remain normal. (More in-depth comprehensive reviews of the clinical use of clozapine are available in Kane et al. 1988, Lieberman et al. 1989, and Baldessarini and Frankenburg 1991.)

■ Mechanism of Action

Despite the abundance of side effects mentioned here, the increasingly widespread use of clozapine pharmacotherapy has generated excitement and hope in the treatment of chronically ill psychotic patients. A great deal of interest has been generated in understanding what pharmacological properties of clozapine contribute to its increased efficacy in some otherwise medication-refractory patients. As reviewed at the beginning of this chapter, a number of hypotheses have been generated to explain the increased the efficacy of certain atypical antipsychotics. Clozapine appears to have many of these properties, including an increased ratio of D_1 to D_2 blockade, greater D_3 and D_4 antagonism, 5-HT$_{2A}$ and 5-HT$_{2C}$ antagonistic properties, anticholinergic and antiadrenergic properties, and increased mesolimbic specificity with relative sparing of the nigrostriatal dopaminergic neurons. In addition to its greater effectiveness in the treatment of "positive" symptoms, clozapine has also been associated with relatively greater effectiveness in the treatment of "negative" or "deficit" symptoms of psychosis.

Many investigators have noted the association of prominent negative symptoms with relative reductions in prefrontal cortical blood flow and glucose metabolism seen during PET or single photon emission computed tomography (SPECT) scanning of schizophrenic patients (Andreasen et al. 1992; Berman et al. 1992; Buchsbaum et al. 1992; Wolkin et al. 1992). Several preliminary studies have demonstrated the ability of clozapine pharmacotherapy to improve, or at least not worsen, this relative "hypofrontality" when compared with traditional D_2 receptor blocking neuroleptics (Pickar et al. 1992a). This effect, as demonstrated in functional brain imaging, has been proffered as a possible explanation for clozapine's improvement of "negative" symptoms of psychosis. Pickar and colleagues (1992a) have preliminarily also suggested an ability of clozapine pharmacotherapy to "integrate" or increase functional interconnections of a larger number of brain "circuits" relative to that of "typical" neuroleptic agents on PET imaging.

Which, if any, of clozapine's above described pharmacological properties or combinations thereof contribute to the increased therapeutic efficacy of clozapine awaits further elucidation. However, such insights could potentially aid in the development of newer alternative atypical neuroleptic agents with fewer adverse side effects.

Current experience suggests that at least one-third of "typical" neuroleptic-refractory schizophrenic patients will *not* show appreciable benefit from clozapine pharmacotherapy. Given the considerable expense and adverse side effects associated with clozapine pharmacotherapy, it would be of considerable clinical usefulness to predict potential responders and nonresponders to clozapine a priori. In this regard, Pickar and colleagues (1992b) and Risch and Lewine (1993) have reported preliminary data suggesting that schizophrenic patients with relatively low ratios of cerebrospinal fluid (CSF) homovanillic acid (HVA) to 5-hydroxyindoleacetic acid (5-HIAA) may experience significantly greater benefit with clozapine pharmacotherapy as compared with patients who have relatively higher HVA:5-HIAA ratios.

These observations have involved only a small number of subjects and require replication in larger groups of patients. However, they add support to the theoretical hypotheses elaborated by Meltzer (1992a) and others regarding the potential importance of interactions between CNS dopaminergic and serotonergic interactions in the pathogenesis and pharmacotherapy of schizophrenia.

■ SUMMARY

Our increasingly sophisticated understanding of neurobiology has led to significant advances in the understanding of the pathophysiology of schizophrenia. These insights have led to the development of new generation "atypical" antipsychotic medications with potentially fewer adverse side effects and improved therapeutic efficacy. The prototype atypical antipsychotic agent clozapine has generated a new era of excitement and hope for the pharmacotherapy of treatment-refractory schizophrenic patients. An entire series of newer atypical antipsychotic agents that are currently undergoing clinical trials may further increase our understanding of the pathogenesis of schizophrenia and expand our treatment alternatives.

■ REFERENCES

Andreasen NC, Rezai K, Alliger R, et al: Hypofrontality in neuroleptic-naive patients and in patients with chronic schizophrenia: assessment with xenon 133 single-photon emission computed tomography and the Tower of London. Arch Gen Psychiatry 49:943–958, 1992

Ashby CR, Jiang LH, Kasser RJ, et al: Electrophysiological characterization of 5-hydroxytryptamine₃ receptors in rat medial prefrontal cortex. J Pharmacol Exp Ther 251:171–178, 1990

Baldessarini RJ, Frankenburg FR: Clozapine—a novel antipsychotic agent. N Engl J Med 324:746–754, 1991

Baldessarini RJ, Campbell A, Yeghiayan S, et al: Limbic-selective antidopaminergic effects of S(+)-aporphines compared to typical and atypical antipsychotic agents in the rat, in Biological Psychiatry, Vol 2. Edited by Racagni G, Brunello N, Fukuda T. Amsterdam, Elsevier, 1991, pp 837–840

Bannon MJ, Bunney EB, Roth RH: Mesocortical dopamine neurons: lack of autoreceptors modulating dopamine synthesis. Mol Pharmacol 19:270–275, 1981

Bannon MJ, Reinhard JF Jr, Bunney EB, et al: Unique response to antipsychotic drugs is due to absence of terminal autoreceptors in mesocortical dopamine neurons. Nature 296:444–446, 1982

Berman KF, Torrey EF, Daniel AG, et al: Regional cerebral blood flow in monozygotic twins discordant and concordant for schizophrenia. Arch Gen Psychiatry 49:927–934, 1992

Bertorello AM, Hopfield JF, Aperia A, et al: Inhibition by dopamine of $(Na^{++}K^+)$ ATPase activity in neostriatal neurons through D_1 and D_2 dopamine receptor synergism. Nature 347:386–388, 1990

Blackburn TP, Kennet G, Ashby CR, et al: BRL 46470A: a novel, potent $5\text{-}HT_3$ receptor antagonist with atypical antipsychotic properties. Proceedings of the 2nd International Symposium on Serotonin, Houston, Texas, September 1992

Bolanos FJ, Schechter LE, Miquel MC, et al: Common pharmacological and physicochemical properties of $5\text{-}HT_3$ binding sites in the rat cerebral cortex and NG 108-15 clonal cells. Biochem Pharmacol 40:1541–1550, 1990

Bouthenet ML, Souil E, Martres, MP, et al: Localization of dopamine D_3 receptor mRNA in the rat brain using in situ hybridization histochemistry: comparison with dopamine D_2 receptor mRNA. Brain Res 564:203–219, 1991

Buchsbaum MS, Haier RJ, Potkin SG, et al: Frontostriatal disorder of cerebral metabolism in never-medicated schizophrenics. Arch Gen Psychiatry 49:395–442, 1992

Buckland PR, O'Donovan MC, McGuffin P: Changes in dopamine D_1 and D_3 receptor mRNA levels in rat brain following antipsychotic treatment. Psychopharmacology (Berl) 106:479–483, 1992

Bunney BS, Sesack SR, Silva NL: Midbrain dopamine systems: neurophysiology and electrophysiological pharmacology, in Psychopharmacology: The Third Generation of Progress. Edited by Meltzer HY. New York, Raven, 1987, pp 113–126

Bunney BS, Chiodo LA, Grace AA: Midbrain dopamine system electrophysiological functioning: a review and new hypothesis. Synapse 9:79–94, 1991

Bunzow JR, Van Tol HHM, Grandy DK: Cloning and expression of a rat D_2 dopamine receptor cDNA.

Nature 336:7883–7887, 1988

Campbell A, Yeghiayan S, Baldessarini RJ, et al: Selective antidopaminergic effects of S(+)N-n-propylnoraporphine in limbic versus extrapyramidal sites in rat brain: comparisons with typical and atypical antipsychotic agents. Psychopharmacology (Berl) 103:323–329, 1991

Campbell A, Baldessarini RJ, Yeghiayan S: Antagonism of limbic and extrapyramidal actions of intracerebrally injected dopamine by ergolines with partial D_2 agonist activity in the rat. Brain Res 592:348–352, 1992

Canton H, Verriele L, Colpaert FC: Binding of typical and atypical antipsychotics to $5\text{-}HT_{1C}$ and $5\text{-}HT_2$ sites: clozapine potently interacts with $5\text{-}HT_{1C}$ sites. Eur J Pharmacol 191:93–96, 1990

Carlsson A: The current status of the dopamine hypothesis of schizophrenia. Neuropsychopharmacology 1:179–186, 1988a

Carlsson A: Dopamine autoreceptors and schizophrenia, in Receptors and Ligands in Psychiatry. Edited by Sen AK, Lee T. Cambridge, England, Cambridge University Press, 1988b, pp 1–10

Chio CL, Hess GF, Graham RS, et al: A second molecular form of D_2 dopamine receptor in rat and bovine caudate nucleus. Nature 343:266–269, 1990

Chiodo LA, Bunney BS: Typical and atypical neuroleptics: differential effects of chronic administration on the activity of A9 and A10 midbrain dopaminergic neurons. J Neurosci 3:1607–1619, 1983

Chiodo LA, Bunney BS: Possible mechanisms by which repeated clozapine administration differentially affects the activity of two subpopulations of midbrain dopamine neurons. J Neurosci 5:2539–2544, 1985

Clark D, White FJ: Review: D_1 dopamine receptor—the search for a function: a critical evaluation of the D_1/D_2 dopamine receptor classification and its functional implications. Synapse 1:247–388, 1987

Cortés R, Gueye B, Pazos A, et al: Dopamine receptors in human brain: autoradiographic distribution of D_1 sites. Neuroscience 28:263–273, 1989

Coward DM, Dixon AK, Urwyler S, et al: Partial dopamine-agonistic and atypical neuroleptic properties of the amino-erolines SDZ 208-911 and SDZ 208-912. J Pharmacol Exp Ther 252:279–285, 1990

Dearry A, Gingrich JA, Falardeau P, et al: Molecular cloning and expression of the gene for a human D_1 dopamine receptor. Nature 247:71–76, 1990

Deutch AY, Moghaddam B, Innis RB, et al: Mechanisms of action of atypical antipsychotic drugs: implications for novel therapeutic strategies for schizophrenia. Schizophr Res 4:121–156, 1991

Dray A, Gonye TJ, Oakley NR, et al: Evidence for the existence of a raphe projection to the substantia nigra in rat. Brain Res 113:45–57, 1976

Farde L, Hall H, Ehrin E, et al: Quantitative analysis of D_2 dopamine receptor binding in the living human brain by PET. Science 231:258–260, 1986

Farde L, Wiesel FA, Halldin C, et al: Central D_2-dopamine receptor occupancy in schizophrenic patients treated with antipsychotic drugs. Arch Gen Psychiatry 45:71–76, 1988

Farde L, Nordstrom AL, Weisel FA, et al: D_1 and D_2 dopamine occupancy during treatment with conventional and atypical neuroleptics. Psychopharmacology 99 (suppl):S28–S31, 1989

Farde L, Nordstrom AL, Weisel FA, et al: Positron emission tomographic analysis of central D_1 and D_2 dopamine receptor occupancy in patients treated with classical neuroleptics and clozapine. Relation to extrapyramidal side effects. Arch Gen Psychiatry 49:538–544, 1993

Gerlach J: New antipsychotics: classification, efficacy, and adverse effects. Schizophr Bull 17:289–309, 1991

Giros B, Sokoloff P, Martres MP, et al: Alternative splicing directs the expression of two D_2 dopamine receptor isoforms. Nature 342:923–926, 1989

Grandy DK, Marchionni MA, Makam H, et al: Cloning of the cDNA and gene for a human D_2 dopamine receptor. Proc Natl Acad Sci U S A 86:9762–9766, 1989

Hand TH, Hu XT, Wang RY: Differential effects of acute clozapine and haloperidol in the activity of ventral tegmental (A10) and nigrostriatal (A9) dopamine neurons. Brain Res 415:257–269, 1987

Heffner TG, Caprathe B, Davis M, et al: Effects of PD 128482, a novel dopamine autoreceptor agonist in preclinical antipsychotic tests, in Novel Antipsychotic Drugs. Edited by Meltzer HY. New York, Raven, 1992, pp 79–90

Hippius H: The history of clozapine. Psychopharmacology (Berl) 99:53–55, 1989

Hoyer D, Gozlan H, Bolanos F, et al: Interaction of psychotropic drugs with central 5-HT_3 recognition sites: fact or fiction? Eur J Pharmacol 171:137–139, 1989

Hünziker F, Künzle F, Schmutz J: Uber ein 5-Stellung basisch substituierte 5-*H*-dibenzo[b,e]-1,4-diazepine. Helv Chir Acta 46:2337–2346, 1963

Ichikawa J, Meltzer HY: Differential effects of repeated treatment with haloperidol and clozapine on dopamine release and metabolism in the striatum and the nucleus accumbens. J Pharmacol Exp Ther 256:248–357, 1991

Itzhak Y, Stein I: Sigma binding sites in the brain: an emerging concept for multiple sites and their relevance for psychiatric disorders. Life Sci 47:1073–1081, 1990

Kane J, Honigfeld G, Singer J, et al: Collaborative study group: clozapine for the treatment-resistant schizophrenic: a double-blind comparison with chlorpromazine. Arch Gen Psychiatry 45:789–796, 1988

Kalivas PW, Duffy P, Barrow J: Regulation of the mesocorticolimbic dopamine system by glutamic acid receptor subtypes. J Pharmacol Exp Ther 251:378–387, 1989

Kilpatrick GJ, Jones BJ, Tyers MB: Identification and distribution of 5-HT_3 receptors in rat brain using radioligand binding. Nature 330:746–748, 1987

Kilts CD, Anderson CM, Ely TD, et al: Absence of synthesis-modulating nerve terminal autoreceptors on mesamygdaloid and other mesolimbic dopamine neuronal populations. J Neurosci 7:3961–3975, 1987

Kinkead BL, Owens MJ, Nemeroff CB: Serotonin antagonists as antipsychotics. Proceedings of the 2nd International Symposium on Serotonin, Houston, Texas, September 1992

Largent BL, Wikström H, Snowman AM, et al: Novel antipsychotic drugs share high affinity for receptors. Eur J Pharmacol 155:345–347, 1988

Lewander T, Uppfeldt G, Köhler C, et al: Remoxipride and raclopride: pharmacological background and clinical outcome, in Novel Antipsychotic Drugs. Edited by Meltzer HY. New York, Raven, 1992, pp 67–78

Lidow MS, Goldman-Rakic PS, Rakic P, et al: Dopamine D_2 receptors in the cerebral cortex: distribution and pharmacological characterization with [^{3}H]raclopride. Proc Natl Acad Sci U S A 86:6412–6416, 1989

Lieberman JA, Kane JM, Johns CA: Clozapine: guidelines for clinical management. J Clin Psychiatry 50:329–338, 1989

Lieberman JA, Saltz BL, Johns CA, et al: The effects of clozapine on tardive dyskinesia. Br J Psychiatry

158:503–510, 1991

Lundberg T, Lindström LH, Hartvig P, et al: Striatal and frontal cortex binding of 11-C-labelled clozapine visualized by positron emission tomography (PET) in drug-free schizophrenics and healthy volunteers. Psychopharmacology (Berl) 99:8–12, 1989

Mansour A, Meador-Woodruff JH, Bunzow JR, et al: Localization of dopamine D_2 receptor mRNA and D_1 and D_2 receptor binding in the rat brain and pituitary: an in situ hybridization-receptor autoradiographic analysis. J Neurosci 10:2587–2600, 1990

Mansour A, Meador-Woodruff JH, Zhou QY, et al: A comparison of D_1 receptor binding and mRNA in rat brain using receptor autoradiographic and *in situ* hybridization techniques. Neuroscience 45:359–371, 1991

Meador-Woodruff JH, Mansour A, Bunzow JR, et al: Distribution of D_2 dopamine receptor mRNA in rat brain. Proc Natl Acad Sci U S A 86:7625–7628, 1989

Meador-Woodruff JH, Mansour A, Civelli O, et al: Distribution of D_2 dopamine receptor mRNA in the primate brain. Prog Neuropsychopharmacol Biol Psychiatry 15:885–893, 1991

Meltzer HY: The mechanism of action of novel antipsychotic drugs. Schizophr Bull 17:263–287, 1991

Meltzer HY (ed): Novel Antipsychotic Drugs. New York, Raven, 1992a

Meltzer HY: Dimensions of outcome with clozapine. Br J Psychiatry 160 (suppl 17):46–53, 1992b

Meltzer HY, Matsubara S, Lee JC: Classification of typical and atypical drugs on the basis of dopamine D_1, D_2 and serotonin$_2$ pK_i values. J Pharmacol Exp Ther 251:238–246, 1989

Meltzer HY, Cole P, Way L, et al: Cost-effectiveness of clozapine in neuroleptic resistant schizophrenia. Am J Psychiatry 150:1630–1638, 1993

Mengod G, Martinez-Mir MI, Vilaró MT, et al: Localization of the mRNA for the dopamine D_2 receptor in the rat brain by in situ hybridization histochemistry. Proc Natl Acad Sci U S A 86:8560–8564, 1989

Moghaddam B, Bunney BS: Acute effects of typical and atypical antipsychotic drugs on the release of dopamine from prefrontal cortex, nucleus accumbens, and striatum of the rat: an in vivo microdialysis study. J Neurochem 54:1755–1760, 1990

Molineaux SM, Jessell TM, Axel R, et al: 5-HT$_{1C}$ receptor is a prominent serotonin receptor subtype in the central nervous system. Proc Natl Acad Sci U S A 86:6793–6797, 1989

Monsma FJ, McVittie LD, Gerfen CR, et al: Multiple D_2 dopamine receptors produced by alternative RNA splicing. Nature 342:926–929, 1989

Monsma FJ, Mahan LC, McVittie LD, et al: Molecular cloning and expression of a D_1 dopamine receptor linked to adenylyl cyclase activation. Proc Natl Acad Sci U S A 87:6723–6727, 1990

Monsma FJ, Shen Y, Ward RP, et al: Cloning and expression of a novel serotonin receptor with high affinity for tricyclic psychotropic drugs. Mol Pharmacol 43:320–327, 1993

Musacchio JM: The psychotomimetic effects of opiates and the σ receptor. Neuropsychopharmacology 3:191–199, 1990

Naber D, Gaussares C, Moeglen JM, et al: Efficacy and tolerability of SDZ HDC 912, a partial dopamine D_2 agonist, in the treatment of schizophrenia, in Novel Antipsychotic Drugs. Edited by Meltzer HY. New York, Raven, 1992, pp 99–107

Nordstrom AL, Farde L, Halldin C: High 5-HT$_2$ receptor occupancy in clozapine treated patients demonstrated by PET. Psychopharmacology (Berl) 110:365–367, 1993

Ögren SO, Hall H: Comparison of the effects of different substituted benzamides on dopamine receptor function in the rat, in Novel Antipsychotic Drugs. Edited by Meltzer HY. New York, Raven, 1992, pp 59–66

Ohara K, Ulpian C, Seeman P, et al: Schizophrenia: dopamine D_1 receptor sequence is normal, but has DNA polymorphisms. Neuropsychopharmacology 8:131–135, 1993

Olney JW: Glutamatergic mechanisms in neuropsychiatry, in Novel Antipsychotic Drugs. Edited by Meltzer HY. New York, Raven, 1992, pp 155–169

Pickar D, Litman RE, Owen RR, et al: Predictors of treatment response to clozapine. Paper presented at the 31st annual meeting of the American College of Neuropsychopharmacology, San Juan, Puerto Rico, December 14–18, 1992a, p 48

Pickar D, Woen RR, Litman RE et al: Clinical and biologic response to clozapine in patients with schizophrenia. Arch Gen Psychiatry 49:345–353, 1992b

Piomelli D, Pilon C, Giros B, et al: Dopamine activation of the arachidonic acid cascade as a basis for D_1/D_2 receptor synergism. Nature 353:164–167, 1991

Reynolds GP: Developments in the drug treatment of schizophrenia. Trends Pharmacol Sci 13:116–121, 1992

Risch SC, Lewine RJ: Low cerebrospinal fluid homovanillic acid–5-hydroxyindoleacetic acid ratio predicts clozapine efficacy: a replication. Arch Gen Psychiatry 50:670, 1993

Schwartz JC, Sokoloff P, Giros B, et al: The dopamine D_3 receptor as a target for antipsychotics, in Novel Antipsychotic Drugs. Edited by Meltzer HY. New York, Raven, 1992, pp 135–144

Seeman P: Dopamine receptors and the dopamine hypothesis of schizophrenia. Synapse 1:133–152, 1987

Seeman P: Receptor selectivities of atypical neuroleptics, in Novel Antipsychotic Drugs. Edited by Meltzer HY. New York, Raven, 1992a, pp 145–154

Seeman P: Dopamine receptor sequences: therapeutic levels of neuroleptics occupy D_2 receptors, clozapine occupies D_4. Neuropsychopharmacology 7:261–284, 1992b

Seeman P, Guan HC, Niznik HB: Endogenous dopamine lowers the dopamine D_2 receptor density as measured by [^{3}H]raclopride: implications for positron emission tomography of the human brain. Synapse 3:96–97, 1989a

Seeman P, Niznik HB, Guan HC, et al: Link between D_1 and D_2 dopamine receptors is reduced in schizophrenia and Huntington diseased brain. Proc Natl Acad Sci U S A 86:10156–10160, 1989b

Seeman P, Hong-Chang G, Van Tol HHM: Dopamine D_4 receptors elevated in schizophrenia. Nature 365:441–445, 1993

Sibley DR, Monsma FJ: Molecular biology of dopamine receptors. Trends Pharmacol Sci 13:61–69, 1992

Snyder SH: The dopamine connection. Nature 247:121–122, 1990

Snyder SH, Largent BL: Receptor mechanisms in antipsychotic drugs action: focus on sigma receptors. J Neuropsychiatry Clin Neurosci 1:7–15, 1989

Sokoloff P, Giros B, Martres MP, et al: Molecular cloning and characterization of a novel dopamine receptor (D_3) as a target for neuroleptics. Nature 247:146–151, 1990

Sokoloff P, Martres MP, Giros B, et al: The third dopamine receptor (D_3) as a novel target for antipsychotics. Biochem Pharmacol 43:656–666, 1992a

Sokoloff P, Andrieux M, Besancon R, et al: Pharmacology of human dopamine D_3 receptor expressed in a mammalian cell line: comparison with D_2 receptor. Eur J Pharmacol 225:331–337, 1992b

Sokoloff P, Levesque D, Martres MP, et al: The dopamine D_3 receptor as a key target for antipsychotics. Clin Neuropharmacol 15 (suppl 1):456A–457A, 1992c

Sorensen SM, Humphreys TM, Palfreyman MF: Effects of acute and chronic MDL 73,147 a 5-HT$_3$ receptor antagonist, on A9 and A10 dopamine neurons. Eur J Pharmacol 163:115–120, 1989

Soubrie P, Reisine TD, Glowinski J: Functional aspects of serotonin transmission in the basal ganglia: a review and an in vivo approach using the push-pull cannula technique. Neuroscience 131:615–624, 1984

Srivastava LK, Morency MA, Bajwa SB, et al: Effect of haloperidol on expression of dopamine D_2 receptor mRNAs in rat brain. J Mol Neurosci 2:155–161, 1990

Steinfels GF, Tam SW, Cook L: Electrophysiological effects of selective σ-receptor agonists, antagonists, and the selective phencyclidine receptor agonist selective phencyclidine receptor agonist MK-801 on midbrain dopamine neurons. Neuropsychopharmacology 2:201–207, 1989

Sunahara RK, Niznik HB, Weiner DM, et al: Human dopamine D_1 receptor encoded by an intronless gene on chromosome 5. Nature 247:80–83, 1990

Sunahara RK, Guan HC, O'Dowd BF, et al: Cloning of the gene for a human dopamine D_5 receptor with higher affinity for dopamine than D_1. Nature 350:614–619, 1991

Tamminga CA, Gerlach J: New neuroleptics and experimental antipsychotics in schizophrenia, in Psychopharmacology: The Third Generation of Progress. Edited by Meltzer HY. New York, Raven, 1987, pp 1129–1140

Tamminga CA, Cascella N, Fakouhi TD, et al: Enhancement of NMDA-mediated transmission in schizophrenia: effects of milacemide, in Novel Antipsychotic Drugs. Edited by Meltzer HY. New York, Raven, 1992, pp 171–177

Taylor DP, Schlemmer RF: Sigma "antagonists": potential antipsychotics?, in Novel Antipsychotic Drugs. Edited by Meltzer HY. New York, Raven, 1992, pp 189–201

Tiberi M, Jarvie KR, Silvia C, et al: Cloning, molecular characterization, and chromosomal assignment of a gene encoding a second D_1 dopamine receptor subtype: differential expression pattern in rat brain compared with the D_{1A} receptor. Proc Natl Acad Sci U S A 88:7491–7495, 1991

Van Tol HHM, Riva M, Civelli O, et al: Lack of effect of chronic dopamine receptor blockade on D_2 dopamine receptor mRNA level. Neurosci Lett 111:303–308, 1990

Van Tol HHM, Bunzow JR, Guan H, et al: Cloning of the gene for a human dopamine D_4 receptor with high affinity for the antipsychotic clozapine. Nature 350:610–614, 1991

Van Tol HH, Wu CM, Guan HC, et al: Multiple dopamine D_4 receptor variants in the human population. Nature 358:149–152, 1992

Wachtel SR, White FJ: Electrophysiological effects of BMY 14802, a new potential antipsychotic drug, on midbrain dopamine neurons in the rat: acute and chronic studies. J Pharmacol Exp Ther 244:410–416, 1988

Wachtel SR, Hu XT, Gallaway MP, et al: D_1 dopamine receptor stimulation enables the postsynaptic, but not autoreceptor, effects of D_2 dopamine agonists in nigrostriatal and mesoaccumbens dopamine systems. Synapse 4:327–346, 1989

Waddington JL, Daly SA: The status of "second generation" selective D_1 dopamine receptor antagonists as putative atypical antipsychotic agents, in Novel Antipsychotic Drugs. Edited by Meltzer HY. New York, Raven, 1992, pp 109–115

Wadworth AN, Heel RC: Remoxipride: a review of its pharmacodynamic and pharmacokinetic properties, and therapeutic potential in schizophrenia. Drugs 40:863–879, 1990

Waeber C, Hoyer D, Palacios JM: 5-Hydroxytryptamine$_3$ receptors in the human brain: autoradiographic visualization using [^{3}H]ICS 205–930. Neuroscience 31:393–400, 1989

Walker JM, Bowen WD, Walker FD, et al: Sigma receptors: biology and function. Pharmacol Rev 42:355–402, 1990

Watling KJ, Beer MS, Stanton JA, et al: Interaction of the atypical neuroleptic clozapine with 5-HT$_3$ receptors in the cerebral cortex and superior ganglion of the rat. Eur J Pharmacol 182:465–472, 1990

Wiedemann K, Krieg JC, Loycke A: Novel dopamine autoreceptor agonists B-HT 920 and EMD 49980 in the treatment of patients with schizophrenia, in Novel Antipsychotic Drugs. Edited by Meltzer HY. New York, Raven, 1992, pp 91–98

Wolkin A, Sanfilipo M, Wolf AP, et al: Negative symptoms and hypofrontality in chronic schizophrenia. Arch Gen Psychiatry 49:959–965, 1992

Xu S, Monsma FJ, Sibley DR, et al: Regulation of D_{1A} and D_2 dopamine receptor mRNA during ontogenesis, lesion and chronin antagonist treatment. Life Sci 50:383–396, 1992

Zhou QY, Grandy DK, Thambi L, et al: Cloning and expression of human and rat D_1 dopamine receptors. Nature 347:76–80, 1990

15

Drugs to Treat
Extrapyramidal Side Effects

Joseph K. Stanilla, M.D., and George M. Simpson, M.D.

■ HISTORY OF EXTRAPYRAMIDAL SIDE EFFECTS (EPS)

The description of chlorpromazine's therapeutic properties (Delay and Deniker 1952; Laborit et al. 1952) was soon followed by the description of its tendency to produce EPS, which were generally indistinguishable from classical Parkinson's syndrome. A debate soon arose regarding the relationship between EPS and therapeutic efficacy. Flügel (1953) suggested that a therapeutic response from chlorpromazine required the development of EPS. Haase (1954) postulated that the neuroleptic dose that produced minimal, subclinical rigidity and hypokinesia—the "neuroleptic threshold"—was the minimal neuroleptic dose necessary for therapeutic antipsychotic effect and was manifested by micrographic handwriting changes. Other investigators also reported that EPS were necessary for therapeutic efficacy (Denham and Carrick 1960; Karn and Kasper 1959).

Brooks (1956), on the other hand, suggested that "signs of parkinsonism heralded the particular effect being sought" (p. 1122), but "the therapeutic effects were not dependent on extrapyramidal dysfunction. On the contrary, alleviation of such dysfunction, as

soon as it occurred, sped the progress of recovery" (p. 1122). The necessity for development of EPS for therapeutic effect was challenged by others as well. These differences in opinion about the relationship between EPS and neuroleptic efficacy can be partially attributed to differences in definitions of EPS and between methodologies of the studies (Chien and DiMascio 1967).

Haase's concept that mild, subclinical EPS manifested by handwriting changes was an indicator of a therapeutic dose was investigated further (Angus and Simpson 1970a; Simpson et al. 1970). Results from these studies indicated there was no difference in therapeutic response at doses beyond the neuroleptic threshold (i.e., patients treated with doses beyond the neuroleptic threshold received significantly larger doses of medication without further therapeutic benefit). This finding has since been discussed more fully (Baldessarini et al. 1988) and replicated (McEvoy et al. 1991).

Gross EPS can have a significant negative effect on treatment outcome by contributing to poor compliance, exacerbation of psychiatric symptoms, violence, and even to suicide (Shear et al. 1983; Van Putten et al. 1981). Akathisia, in particular, has been found to be associated with a poor clinical outcome (Levinson et al. 1990; Van Putten et al. 1984). The presence of EPS early in treatment may also be associated with an increased risk of developing tardive dyskinesia (TD) (Saltz et al. 1991).

Clearly, EPS are significant, need to be assessed, and should be minimized so that treatment may be optimized.

TYPES OF EXTRAPYRAMIDAL SIDE EFFECTS

Four types of EPS have been delineated, and the treatment of each should be individualized.

Acute dystonic reactions (ADRs) are generally the first EPS to appear—and often the most dramatic (Angus and Simpson 1970b). They are muscle spasms that occur suddenly, generally involving head and neck muscles (i.e., torticollis, facial grimacing, oculogyric crisis). The majority of ADRs occur within 1–4 days of neuroleptic initiation or dosage increase (Sramek et al. 1986).

Akathisia is the next type of EPS to appear. Akathisia, which literally means "inability to sit down," comprises both a subjective feeling of restlessness and objective, physical, restless movement. The patient with akathisia experiences the need to move. It can be difficult for a patient to explain the sensation of akathisia, and the diagnosis may thus be missed. At times, patients may display the classical movements of akathisia but not have the subjective distress. This condition has been called pseudoakathisia and may be a type of tardive syndrome (Barnes 1990).

The third type of EPS, pseudoparkinsonism, is virtually indistinguishable from classical Parkinson's syndrome. The symptoms include a generalized slowing of movement (akinesia) with masked facies, cogwheeling, rigidity, resting tremor, and hypersalivation. Parkinsonism generally occurs after a few weeks or more of neuroleptic treatment. Akinesia sometimes needs to be differentiated from primary depression and the blunted affect of schizophrenia (Rifkin et al. 1975).

Tardive syndromes, including TD and dystonia, make up the fourth group of the neuroleptic-induced extrapyramidal disorders. TD consists of irregular, stereotypical movements of the mouth, face, and tongue, and choreoathetoid movements of the fingers, arms, legs, and trunk. Respiratory dyskinesias can also occur. Unlike the other extrapyramidal syndromes, patients with TD are often unaware that they have the abnormal movements. Tardive syndromes have had generally poor response to treatment.

INCIDENCE OF EXTRAPYRAMIDAL SIDE EFFECTS

Ayd (1961) was the first to report the incidence of EPS, noting an overall incidence of 39%. Twenty-one percent of patients demonstrated akathisia, 15% had parkinsonism, and only 2% had ADRs. More recently, in a series of surveys of 721 schizophrenic patients conducted over 10 years, McCreadie (1992) found the point prevalence to be 27% for parkinsonism, 23% for akathisia or pseudoakathisia, and 29% for TD. Less than half of all patients (44%) had no movement disorder, whereas 8% had persistent TD. Varying rates of occurrence have been reported in other studies, including much higher incidences of ADRs. Higher prevalence rates have generally been associated with higher doses of neuroleptics.

ETIOLOGY OF EXTRAPYRAMIDAL SIDE EFFECTS

The mechanisms involved in the production of EPS are not completely delineated. Dopaminergic nigrostriatal tracts (in conjunction with cholinergic tracts) finely regulate the initiation and coordination of movement (Duvoisin 1967). Extrapyramidal movements traditionally have been thought to result from neuroleptic blockade of dopaminergic nigrostriatal tracts, resulting in a relative increase in cholinergic activity (Snyder et al. 1974). Drugs that decrease cholinergic activity or increase dopaminergic activity cause a reduction in EPS, presumably by restoring the two systems to their previous equilibrium. This has been demonstrated in ADRs in monkeys (Casey et al. 1980).

Increased EPS have been reported to occur in association with decreased serum calcium levels. This association may be related to the effect of calcium on the cholinergic and dopaminergic systems. Calcium is involved in the function of the cholinergic system and the metabolism of dopamine (Kuny and Binswanger 1989), and antipsychotic drugs bind to the calcium-dependent activator of several enzyme systems (calmodulin [el-Defrawi and Craig 1984]).

It has been proposed that γ-aminobutyric acid (GABA) may have an effect on EPS through feedback mechanisms of GABA on the dopamine system. In mice treated with neuroleptics, reduced GABA levels have been noted in mice that developed TD compared with those that did not, suggesting that alterations of the GABA system may contribute to TD (Gunne et al. 1984). The effect of GABA on ADR is not as clear, because ADRs in baboons were increased by drugs that increased GABA as well as drugs that decreased GABA (Casey et al. 1980).

More recent work has focused on the roles of specific neuroreceptors, particularly dopamine D_1 and D_2 receptors and serotonin (5-HT) receptors. Haloperidol, when given intravenously, has a much lower incidence of EPS, even when given at extremely high doses. Haldol is metabolized in the liver to reduced haloperidol. When administered intravenously, haloperidol would enter the central nervous system (CNS) before metabolites were produced. It has been proposed that D_2 receptor saturation by haloperidol rather than reduced haloperidol could account for the difference in EPS production (Menza et al. 1987).

Investigations of the novel antipsychotic clozapine have led to additional theories regarding mechanisms involved in development of EPS. Clozapine, unlike typical antipsychotics, has less D_2 receptor blockade, greater D_1 receptor blockade, and significant 5-HT receptor blockade, particularly of 5-HT_2. It also blocks D_3 and D_4 receptors. These differences may contribute to clozapine's favorable EPS profile.

Typical antipsychotics initially increase dopamine synthesis, turnover, and release in the striatum of baboons (Meldrum et al. 1977). This increase in dopamine production reaches a maximum 1–5 hours after a single neuroleptic injection, which corresponds, timewise, with the development of ADRs in baboons. During chronic treatment (up to 11 days), there is a marked diminution in the capacity of the antipsychotics to provoke an increased turnover of dopamine. Chronic haloperidol treatment causes decreased striatal dopaminergic neurotransmission and upregulation of postsynaptic D_2 receptors (Ichikawa and Meltzer 1991). In contrast, chronic clozapine treatment causes a slight *increase* in striatal dopaminergic neurotransmission and no changes in D_2 receptors. These differences may partly explain the occurrence of EPS and TD with typical antipsychotic

medications and the lack of such occurrence with clozapine.

D_1 receptor antagonists have a lower EPS potential than traditional D_2 neuroleptics in nonhuman primates (Coffin et al. 1989). Patients who were clinical responders to antipsychotics and who had lower D_2 receptor occupancy by positron-emission tomography (PET) analysis were found to have a lower incidence of EPS. Patients treated with clozapine had significantly lower D_2 receptor occupancy than patients treated with typical neuroleptics (Farde et al. 1992). The balanced D_1/D_2 receptor function may prevent development of EPS and TD (Gerlach and Hansen 1992).

Another putative mechanism by which clozapine produces less EPS is a high ratio of 5-HT_2 receptor to striatal D_2 receptor blockade (Meltzer et al. 1989). Evidence suggests that decreasing serotonergic neurotransmission reverses or prevents catalepsy induced by D_2 receptor blockade (Meltzer and Nash 1991).

Clozapine has a high affinity for D_3 and D_4 receptors (Sokoloff et al. 1990; Van Tol et al. 1991). The binding of clozapine to these receptors has been proposed as another possible mechanism involved in clozapine's favorable EPS profile (Meltzer 1992).

Finally, it has been proposed that α-adrenergic mechanisms may be involved in EPS—particularly with TD, akathisia, and tremor (Wilbur et al. 1988). Clozapine is a potent α_1-adrenergic receptor antagonist in the brain, causing α_1 receptor upregulation and increased noradrenalin metabolism, factors that may affect the EPS profile of clozapine (Baldessarini et al. 1992).

■ RATING EXTRAPYRAMIDAL SIDE EFFECTS

Investigations of treatment for EPS led to the need to develop instruments to evaluate and quantify them. An initial EPS scale was shown to have both clinical validity and high interrater reliability, but it did not adequately assess salivation and tremor (Simpson et al. 1964). Scores were low despite side effects such as obvious and disabling tremor or salivation, which required treatment with antiparkinsonian medication. Subsequently, the scale was expanded to include items for tremor and salivation and consists of 10 items rated on a 5-point scale (Simpson and Angus 1970). This scale has good psychometric properties and is simple to use and score. It has been modified for outpatient use by elimination of the leg rigidity item and by replacing head dropping with head rotation. Studies using this scale have shown that scores correlate with dosages and plasma levels of a neuroleptic. The scale is widely used in clinical trials and can be completed by nurses for the routine monitoring of neuroleptic treatment.

The Simpson-Angus Scale (Simpson and Angus 1970) does not include a direct rating for bradykinesia or akinesia. Mindham (1976) modified the Simpson-Angus Scale to include an item for lack of facial expression. Additional rating scales for EPS include the Chouinard Extrapyramidal Rating Scale (Chouinard et al. 1980), the Targeting of Abnormal Kinetic Effects (TAKE) Scale (Wojcik et al. 1980), and the Extrapyramidal Symptoms Scale (Adler et al. 1989).

The modified Simpson-Angus Scale mentioned here includes a single item for rating akathisia. Two more comprehensive scales were devised specifically to rate akathisia: the Barnes Akathisia Rating Scale (Barnes 1989) and the Hillside Akathisia Scale (Fleischhacker et al. 1989). Both instruments are sensitive and easy to use.

Scales have also been developed for the assessment of dyskinetic movements. These include the Abnormal Involuntary Movement Scale (AIMS) (Guy 1976) and the Simpson/Rockland Scale (Simpson et al. 1979).

■ ANTICHOLINERGIC MEDICATIONS

■ Trihexyphenidyl

History and Discovery
Antiparkinsonian medications are the agents that have primarily been used to treat EPS and include anticholinergic, antihistaminic, and dopaminergic agents (Table 15–1).

Trihexyphenidyl, a synthetic analogue of atropine, was introduced in 1949 (originally as benzhexol hydrochloride) and found to be effective in the treat-

Table 15–1. Pharmacologic agents for treatment of neuroleptic-induced parkinsonism and acute dystonic reactions

Compound	Type	Relative equivalence (mg)*	Route	Availability	Dosing	Dose range (mg)
Benztropine (Cogentin)	Anticholinergic	1	Oral Injectable	Tablets (0.5, 1, or 2 mg) Ampules (1 mg/ml [2 ml])	qd to bid q 30 minutes until symptom relief	1–12 2–8
Trihexyphenidyl (Artane)	Anticholinergic	2	Oral	Tablets (2 or 5 mg) Elixir (2 mg/ml) Sequels (5 mg [sustained release])	qd to bid	2–30
Procyclidine (Kemadrin)	Anticholinergic	2	Oral	Tablets (5 mg, scored)	bid to tid	5–20
Diphenhydramine (Benadryl)	Antihistaminic	50	Oral Injectable	Tablets (25 or 50 mg) Ampules (10 mg/ml [10 or 30 ml]), 50 mg/ml (10 ml)	bid to qid	50–200
Biperiden (Akineton)	Anticholinergic	2	Oral Injectable	Tablets (2 mg) Ampules (5 mg/ml [1 ml])	qd to tid q 30 minutes until symptom relief	2–24 2–8
Amantadine (Symmetrel)	Dopaminergic	N/A	Oral	Tablets (100 mg)	qd to bid	100–300

Source. Adapted from Klett and Caffey 1972 with permission.

ment of Parkinson's disease in a study of 411 patients (Doshay et al. 1954). Thereafter, it was also used to treat neuroleptic-induced parkinsonism (NIP) (Rashkis and Smarr 1957).

Structure-Activity Relations

Trihexyphenidyl is a tertiary amine analogue of atropine. It is a competitive antagonist of acetylcholine and other muscarinic agonists and competes for a common binding site on the muscarinic receptor. For these reasons, trihexyphenidyl is referred to as an anticholinergic, antimuscarinic, or atropine-like drug. Trihexyphenidyl exerts little blockade of acetylcholine at nicotinic receptors (Brown 1990).

Pharmacological Profile

The pharmacological properties of trihexyphenidyl are similar to those of atropine and other anticholinergic drugs, although trihexyphenidyl primarily acts centrally, with few peripheral effects and little sedative action. Anticholinergic drugs dilate the pupils through blockade of the sphincter muscle of the iris, producing mydriasis, and block accommodation of the lens, producing cycloplegia. These drugs produce mild tachycardia in the heart. In the gastrointestinal tract, they reduce gut wall motility and salivary and gastric secretions. In the respiratory system, they reduce secretions and can produce mild bronchodilation. Anticholinergic drugs inhibit the activity of sweat glands and mildly decrease contractions in the urinary and biliary tracts (Brown 1990).

Pharmacokinetics and Disposition

Peak concentration for trihexyphenidyl is reached 1–2 hours after oral administration, and its half-life is 10–12 hours (Cedarbaum and McDowell 1987). As a tertiary amine, trihexyphenidyl readily crosses the blood-brain barrier to enter the CNS.

Mechanism of Action

The presumed mechanism of action of trihexyphenidyl for treatment of EPS is the blockade of relatively high cholinergic activity in nigrostriatal tracts. This then returns the cholinergic and dopaminergic systems to a previous equilibrium.

Indications

Anticholinergic agents were reported to be effective treatment of NIP from open empiric trials (Medina et al. 1962; Rashkis and Smarr 1957). Eventually, controlled trials were conducted, but most only involved comparisons between different anticholinergics. Few trials have compared anticholinergics with placebo alone. Despite the lack of evidence of efficacy against placebo, anticholinergic agents became the mainstay of treatment for NIP and remain so today.

Daily doses of 5–30 mg have been used in studies of trihexyphenidyl in treatment of parkinsonism and NIP. The therapeutic dose must be empirically determined and can vary widely among individuals. Trihexyphenidyl has U.S. Food and Drug Administration (FDA) approval for treatment of all forms of parkinsonism, including NIP.

Side Effects and Toxicology

Peripheral side effects. Peripheral side effects of trihexyphenidyl result from parasympathetic muscarinic blockade and occur in a consistent hierarchy among different organs. They are qualitatively similar to the side effects of atropine and other available anticholinergic drugs (Brown 1990).

Anticholinergic drugs initially depress salivary and bronchial secretions and sweat production. Reduced salivation produces dry mouth and contributes to the high incidence of dental caries among chronic psychiatric patients (Winer and Bahn 1967). Treatment for this is unsatisfactory, and chewing sugar-free gum or hard candy is limited by the need for constant use. Reduced sweating can contribute to heat prostration and heat stroke, particularly in warmer ambient temperatures.

The next physiological effects occur in the eyes and heart. Pupillary dilatation and inhibition of eye accommodation lead to photophobia and blurred vision. Attacks of acute glaucoma can occur in susceptible subjects with narrow-angle glaucoma. Vagus nerve blockade leads to increased heart rate from vagal blockade and is more apparent in patients with high vagal tone (usually younger patients).

The next effects are inhibition of urinary bladder function and bowel motility, which can produce urinary retention, constipation, and obstipation. Sufficiently high doses of anticholinergics will inhibit gastric secretion and motility (Brown 1990).

Central side effects. Memory disturbance is the most common central side effect of anticholinergic medications, because memory is dependent on the cholinergic system (Drachman 1977). Patients with underlying brain pathology are more susceptible to memory disturbance (Fayen et al. 1988). Chronic psychiatric patients generally have a decreased ability to express themselves, making evaluation of verbal ability and memory more difficult. As a result, subtle memory changes can be missed or attributed to the underlying illness.

Adverse effects of anticholinergics on memory were identified in patients with Parkinson's disease (Yahr and Duvoisin 1968). Even small doses of anticholinergics can produce memory changes (Stephens 1967). Anticholinergic toxicity produces restlessness, irritability, disorientation, hallucinations, and delirium. Elderly patients are at increased risk for memory loss and toxic delirium, even at very low doses, because of the natural loss of cholinergic neurons with aging (Perry et al. 1977).

Toxic doses can produce a clinical picture similar to that of atropine poisoning, including fixed, dilated pupils; flushed face; sinus tachycardia; urinary retention; dry mouth; and fever. This condition can proceed to coma, cardiorespiratory collapse, and death.

Drug-Drug Interactions

Anticholinergic effect on neuroleptic blood levels. Some investigators have suggested anticholinergic medications can affect neuroleptic blood levels. A recent review suggested that the available data were too limited to reach a definite conclusion on this matter. The best studies indicate anticholinergic drugs do not affect neuroleptic blood levels or, at most, lowered these levels only transiently (McEvoy 1983).

Anticholinergic effect on neuroleptic activity. Haase and Janssen (1965) reported from open studies that if anticholinergic drugs were added to neuroleptic drugs given at the neuroleptic threshold, rigidity, hypokinesia, and therapeutic effects would disappear. Other studies have demonstrated no change or an improvement in scores of psychopathology with the addition of anticholinergics (Hanlon et al. 1966; Simpson et al. 1980).

Anticholinergic Abuse

Anticholinergic drugs may be abused for their euphoriant and hallucinogenic effects and may be combined with street drugs for enhanced effect.

Trihexyphenidyl reportedly is the anticholinergic most likely to be abused. Theoretically, one anticholinergic should be as effective as another, although an idiosyncratic response is possible. Abuse should be suspected if a patient becomes upset at the suggestion of substituting one anticholinergic for another (e.g., benztropine for trihexyphenidyl). The potential for abuse needs to be considered, especially in a patient with history of substance abuse.

■ Benztropine

History and Discovery

Benztropine was found to be effective in a study analyzing treatment of 302 patients with Parkinson's disease (Doshay 1956). The best results (i.e., in the control of rigidity, contracture, and tremor) were obtained in the dosage range of 1–4 mg qd for older patients and 2–8 mg qd for younger ones. Doses of 15–30 mg qd caused excessive flaccidity in some patients, to the extent that some became unable to lift their arms or raise their heads off the bed. Subsequently, benztropine was used and found to be effective for treatment of NIP (Karn and Kasper 1959).

Structure-Activity Relations

Benztropine was synthesized by uniting the tropine portion of atropine with the benzohydryl portion of diphenhydramine hydrochloride. It is a tertiary amine with activity similar to that of trihexyphenidyl.

Pharmacological Profile

Benztropine has the pharmacological properties of an anticholinergic and antihistaminic. However, it produces less sedation (in experimental animals) than diphenhydramine.

Pharmacokinetics and Disposition

Little is known about the pharmacokinetics of benztropine. A correlation between serum anticholinergic levels and the presence of EPS has been demonstrated (Tune and Coyle 1980). There is a poor correlation between total daily dose of benztropine and the serum anticholinergic level, with the range of serum activity for a given dose varying 100-fold among subjects. When treated with increased doses of anticholinergics, patients with EPS demonstrated increased serum anticholinergic activity and decreased EPS intensity. Relatively small increments in the oral dose of an anticholinergic drug resulted in significant nonlinear increases in serum anticholinergic activity levels. Benztropine has a long-acting effect and can be given once or twice a day.

Indications

Benztropine has FDA approval for treatment of all forms of parkinsonism, including NIP. Daily doses of 1–8 mg are generally used to treat NIP.

Mechanism of Action, Side Effects, and Drug Interactions

The mechanism of action and drug interactions for benztropine are similar to those of trihexyphenidyl. The side effects are also similar, but the degree of sedation produced may be different. Benztropine was reported as less stimulating or more sedating than trihexyphenidyl and other anticholinergic agents, when used to treat patients with Parkinson's disease (Doshay 1956; England and Schwab 1959). Although this has never been tested in double-blind studies, this property might account for the fact that trihexyphenidyl is the anticholinergic drug more likely to be abused.

■ Biperiden

Biperiden is an analogue of trihexyphenidyl. It has greater peripheral anticholinergic activity than trihexyphenidyl and greater activity against nicotinic receptors (Timberlake et al. 1961). Biperiden is well absorbed from the gastrointestinal tract. Its metabolism is not completely understood but involves hydroxylation in the liver. Its activity, pharmacological profile, and side effects are similar to those of other anticholinergics. It has FDA approval for use in the treatment of all forms of parkinsonism, including NIP. Daily doses of 2–24 mg have been used in studies of biperiden for treatment of parkinsonism and NIP.

■ Procyclidine

Procyclidine is an analogue of trihexyphenidyl (Schwab and Chafetz 1955). Its activity, pharmacology, and side effects are similar to those of other anticholinergics. There is little information about its pharmacokinetics. It has FDA approval for use in treating all forms of parkinsonism, including NIP. Daily doses of 5–30 mg have been used in studies of procyclidine for treatment of parkinsonism and NIP.

■ ANTIHISTAMINIC MEDICATIONS

■ Diphenhydramine

History and Discovery

Antihistaminic agents have also been used for treatment of Parkinson's disease and EPS. Although other antihistamines may have some effect in treating EPS, diphenhydramine has been the primary antihistamine studied and used in this regard.

Structure-Activity Relations

All available antihistamines are reversible, competitive inhibitors of histamine at the H_1 receptor. Only certain antihistamines inhibit the action of acetylcholine at the histamine receptor. It is believed that central anticholinergic activity is responsible for the effect of an antihistamine against EPS. Ethanolamine antihistamines (e.g., diphenhydramine, dimenhydrinate, carbinoxamine maleate) have the greatest anticholinergic activity, and ethylenediamines have the least. The newer antihistamines (i.e., terfenadine and astemizole) have no such activity. The remaining antihistamines have very mild anticholinergic activity (Garrison 1990).

Pharmacological Profile

Antihistamines inhibit the constrictor action of histamine on respiratory smooth muscle. They restrict the vasoconstrictor and vasodilatory effects of histamine on vascular smooth muscle and block histamine-induced capillary permeability. Antihistamines with CNS activity are depressants, producing diminished alertness, slowed reaction times, and somnolence. They can also block motion sickness. Antihistaminic drugs with anticholinergic activity (e.g., diphenhydramine) also possess mild pharmacological properties similar to trihexyphenidyl and other atropine-like agents (Garrison 1990).

Pharmacokinetics and Disposition

Diphenhydramine is well absorbed from the gastrointestinal tract. Peak concentrations occur 2–3 hours after oral administration. Its therapeutic effects usually last 4–6 hours, and it has a half-life of 3–9 hours. Diphenhydramine is widely distributed throughout the body, including the CNS. Age does not affect its pharmacokinetics. Diphenhydramine, a tertiary amine, undergoes demethylations in the liver and is then oxidized to carboxylic acid (Paton and Webster 1985).

Mechanism of Action

Diphenhydramine possesses some central anticholinergic activity. This is most likely the basis for its effect in the treatment of parkinsonism.

Indications

Diphenhydramine has FDA approval for all forms of parkinsonism, including NIP. Diphenhydramine is not as efficacious as the more selective anticholinergic agents for treating EPS, but it may be better tolerated in patients bothered by anticholinergic side effects, such as elderly patients. Diphenhydramine is more sedating than the anticholinergics, which can also be beneficial for some patients. Dosages generally range from 50 to 200 mg qd given in divided doses.

Side Effects and Toxicology

The primary side effect of diphenhydramine is sedation. Although other antihistamines frequently cause gastrointestinal distress, diphenhydramine has a low incidence of these effects. In general, the toxic effects are similar to those of trihexyphenidyl and other anticholinergics.

Drug-Drug Interactions

Diphenhydramine has no reported interactions with other drugs. It will have an additive depressant effect when used in combination with alcohol or other CNS depressants.

■ DOPAMINERGIC MEDICATIONS

■ Amantadine

History and Discovery

Anticholinergic side effects and inadequate treatment response eventually led to the investigation of other antiparkinsonian agents to treat EPS. Initially, both methylphenidate and intravenous caffeine were also investigated as treatments of NIP. Neither achieved general use despite apparent efficacy (Brooks 1956; Freyhan 1959).

Amantadine is an antiviral agent that is effective against A2 (Asian) influenza in animals and humans

(Wingfield et al. 1969). It was unexpectedly found to cause symptomatic improvement of patients with Parkinson's disease (Parkes et al. 1970; Schwab et al. 1969) and soon after was reported to be effective for NIP (Kelly and Abuzzahab 1971).

Structure-Activity Relations

Amantadine is a water-soluble, tricyclic amine. Its mechanism of action remains unclear.

Pharmacological Profile

Amantadine has been shown to be effective in preventing and treating illness from influenza A virus. It also reduces the symptoms of parkinsonism.

Pharmacokinetics and Disposition

In young, healthy subjects, amantadine is absorbed slowly and well from the gastrointestinal tract, with unchanged oral bioavailability over the dose range of 50–300 mg. Amantadine reaches steady state in 4–7 days. Plasma concentrations (0.12–1.12 µg/ml) may have some correlation with improvement in EPS (Greenblatt et al. 1977; Pacifici et al. 1976). It has relatively constant blood levels and long duration of action (Aoki et al. 1979) and is excreted unchanged by the kidneys. Its half-life for elimination is about 16 hours, which will be prolonged in elderly patients and those with impaired renal function (Hayden et al. 1985).

Mechanism of Action

Amantadine's mechanism of action remains unclear. Amantadine has no anticholinergic activity in tests on animals, being only 1/209,000th as potent as atropine (Grelak et al. 1970). It appears to cause the release of dopamine and other catecholamines from intraneuronal storage sites in an amphetamine-like mechanism. Amantadine has preferential selectivity for *central* catecholamine neurons (Grelak et al. 1970; Strömberg et al. 1970). Its antiviral activity appears to result from the blocking of a late stage in the assembly of the virus (Douglas 1990).

Indications

Amantadine underwent much more extensive investigation than anticholinergic agents did regarding efficacy for EPS. Various investigators have reported varying degrees of efficacy, ranging from its superiority to anticholinergics to its being no more effective than placebo (DiMascio et al. 1976; Gelenberg 1978).

The wide-ranging results can be attributed to differing methodologies and patient populations and the inherent difficulties of evaluating EPS. The conclusion that can be drawn from these studies is that amantadine is an effective agent for treating EPS, but there are no clear data to support its use prior to using anticholinergic agents. Amantadine has FDA approval for treatment of NIP and Parkinson's disease/syndrome.

Doses of 100–300 mg/day are generally used for treatment of NIP, and plasma concentrations may have some correlation with improvement. Studies of its use in patients with Parkinson's disease indicate that maximal effect is seen after 2 weeks, but it appears to lose some of its efficacy after 4 weeks (Mawdsley et al. 1972). Whether this indicates a true loss of efficacy or a progression of the condition is unknown. No such long-term studies have been conducted regarding the use of amantadine in the treatment of NIP.

Side Effects and Toxicology

At 100–300 mg qd, amantadine does not produce adverse effects as readily as anticholinergic medications do. Side effects result from CNS stimulation, with symptoms including irritability, tremor, dysarthria, ataxia, vertigo, agitation, reduced concentration, hallucinations, and delirium (Postma and Tilburg 1975). Hallucinations often are visual. Side effects are more likely to occur in elderly patients and those with reduced renal function (Borison 1979; Ing et al. 1979). Toxic effects are directly related to elevated amantadine serum levels (above 1.5 µg/ml). Resolution of toxic symptoms is dependent on renal clearance and may require dialysis in extreme cases, although less than 5% of amantadine is removed by dialysis.

Patients with congestive heart failure or peripheral edema should be monitored because of amantadine's ability to increase availability of catecholamines. Long-term use of amantadine may produce livedo reticularis in the lower extremities, from the local release of catecholamines and resulting vasoconstriction (Cedarbaum and Schleifer 1990).

Amantadine should be used with caution to treat patients with seizures because of possible increased seizure activity.

Drug-Drug Interactions

There are no reported interactions between amantadine and other drugs. There may be increased anticholinergic side effects when amantadine is used in combination with an anticholinergic agent.

■ β-Adrenergic Receptor Antagonists

History and Discovery

Propranolol is the prototype β-adrenergic receptor antagonist (β-blocker). It was reported effective for treatment of restless leg syndrome in patients with parkinsonism (Strang 1967) and later shown to be successful in treatment of neuroleptic-induced akathisia (Kulik and Wilbur 1983; Lipinski et al. 1983). Subsequently, other β-blockers have been investigated regarding their effect in treatment of EPS (Table 15–2).

Structure-Activity Relations

Competitive β-adrenergic receptor antagonism is the property common to all β-blockers. β-blockers are distinguished by additional properties such as the relative affinity for β_1 and β_2 receptors (selectivity), lipid solubility, intrinsic β-adrenergic receptor agonist ac-

Table 15–2. β-Blockers investigated in treatment of patients with akathisia

Compound	β_1 Blockade	β_2 Blockade	Lipid solubility	Effective for EPS	Dose range (mg)
Propranolol (Inderal)	++	++	++++	Yes	20–120
Nadolol (Corgard)	++	++	+	Yes	40–80
Metoprolol (Lopressor)	++	0 at low doses + at high doses	++	Yes	~300
Pindolol (Visken)	++	++	++	Yes	5
Atenolol (Tenormin)	++	0	0	No	50–100
Betaxolol (Kerlone)	++	0	+++	Yes	5–20
Sotalol	++	++	—	No	40–80

Source. Adapted from Hoffman and Lefkowitz 1990 with permission.

tivity, and blockade of α receptors (Lefkowitz et al. 1990). β-blockers with high lipid solubility readily cross the blood-brain barrier to affect the CNS. Propranolol is the most lipid-soluble β-blocker and atenolol the least.

Pharmacological Profile

β-blockers have their primary pharmacological effects on the β receptors in the cardiovascular system, pulmonary system, and organs involved in carbohydrate and lipid metabolism. Their effect on the CNS is to produce fatigue, sleep disturbance (insomnia and nightmares), and CNS depression (Drayer 1987; Gengo et al. 1987).

Pharmacokinetics and Disposition

All β-blockers, except atenolol and nadolol, are well absorbed from the gastrointestinal tract. All undergo metabolism in the liver. Propranolol and metoprolol undergo significant first-pass effect with bioavailability as low as 25%. Large interindividual variation (as much as 20-fold) leads to wide variation in clinically therapeutic doses (Hoffman and Lefkowitz 1990). Metabolites appear to have very limited β receptor antagonistic activity. Propranolol has ready access to the CNS because of its significant lipid solubility.

Mechanism of Action

The exact mechanism of action of β-blockers in the treatment of EPS is unclear. The existence of a noradrenergic pathway from the locus ceruleus to the limbic system has been proposed as a modulator involved in symptoms of TD, akathisia, and tremor (Wilbur et al. 1988). It appears that lipid solubility and the corresponding ability to enter the CNS is the most important factor determining the efficacy of a β-blocker in treating akathisia and perhaps other types of EPS (Adler et al. 1991).

Indications

There are no FDA-approved indications for the use of β-blockers in treatment of EPS. Propranolol has been approved for the treatment of familial essential tremor.

Improvement of EPS has been reported for both nonselective (β_1 and β_2 antagonism) and selective (β_1 antagonism) β-blockers (Table 15–3). The studies have usually been open trials, though with small numbers of patients and varying combinations of additional antiparkinsonian agents and benzodiaze-

Table 15–3. Risk factors leading to acute dystonic reactions

- ▼ High-potency neuroleptics
    - Haloperidol
    - Fluphenazine
    - Trifluoperazine
- ▼ High dose
- ▼ Younger age (under age 35)
    - Approaches 100% under age 20
- ▼ Intramuscular route of delivery
- ▼ Previous dystonic reaction to similar neuroleptic and dose
- ▼ Male gender

pines. The use of β-blockers for treatment of EPS has been limited primarily to treatment of akathisia. Investigations have demonstrated that propranolol is more effective than placebo and more effective than benztropine for treatment of akathisia. Propranolol was shown to be as effective as lorazepam, but with greater improvement in objective signs of akathisia. Doses up to 120 mg/day were used, and maximum effect was noted at 5 days (Adler et al. 1989; Fleischhacker et al. 1990).

All lipophilic β-blockers should be effective in treating akathisia. The choice of a particular β-blocker will be determined by the response of the patient to side effects. In patients with lung disease, betaxolol may be the β-blocker of choice because of its β_1 selectivity at lower doses (5–10 mg/day).

Side Effects and Toxicology

Side effects of β-blockers are the direct result of blockade of β receptors. Bronchospasm results from β_2 blockade of bronchial smooth muscle. Individuals with normal lung function are unlikely to develop bronchospasm. In subjects with asthma or chronic obstructive pulmonary disease and in smokers, bronchospasm is more likely to occur and can be serious. The high number of smokers encountered in the population requiring treatment for akathisia makes this an important effect.

β-blockers can produce heart failure in susceptible individuals, such as patients with compensated heart failure, acute myocardial infarction, or cardiomegaly. Abrupt cessation of β-blockers can exacerbate coronary heart disease in susceptible patients, producing angina or myocardial infarction.

Although they cause clinically insignificant bradycardia in individuals with normal heart function, β-blockers can lead to life-threatening conditions in patients with cardiac conduction defects or when combined with other drugs that impair cardiac conduction. Exercise performance can be impaired by propranolol and other β_2-blockers. Although β-blockers are hypotensive agents, they do not produce hypotension in people with normal blood pressure.

β-blockers can block the tachycardia associated with hypoglycemia, eliminating this warning sign in patients with diabetes. β_2 blockade also can inhibit glycogenolysis and glucose mobilization, interfering with recovery from hypoglycemia (Hoffman and Lefkowitz 1990).

Additional potential side effects include fatigue and major depression. Depression is probably limited only to patients with a predisposition to development of depression.

Drug-Drug Interactions

β-blockers can have significant interactions with other drugs. Additive effects on cardiac conduction and blood pressure can occur when they are used in combination with drugs of similar effect (e.g., calcium channel blockers). Phenytoin, phenobarbital, and rifampin increase the clearance of propranolol. Cimetidine increases propranolol blood levels by decreasing hepatic metabolism. Theophylline clearance is reduced by propranolol. Aluminum salts, cholestyramine, and colestipol may reduce absorption of β-blockers. Chlorpromazine in combination with propranolol may increase blood levels of both drugs (Hoffman and Lefkowitz 1990).

■ BENZODIAZEPINES

Benzodiazepines were initially shown to be effective in the treatment of restless legs syndrome (Ekbom's syndrome), which resembles the physical movements of akathisia (Ekbom 1965). Subsequently, benzodiazepines were reported to be effective for treatment of neuroleptic-induced akathisia. These reports have been small in number, primarily from open studies with few subjects and of short duration. Some studies also involved combinations of benzodiazepines and anticholinergics, which further limit definitive conclusions regarding the effectiveness of benzodiazepines for akathisia (Fleischhacker et al.

1990). There is little information regarding the long-term use of benzodiazepines for akathisia or the effect of withdrawal (Director and Muniz 1982). The benzodiazepines that have been used for EPS have been diazepam, lorazepam, and clonazepam.

Recent studies have reported clonazepam to be an effective treatment for parkinsonism, akathisia, and TD (Horiguchi and Nishimatsu 1992; Thaker et al. 1990). It is possible that larger-scale studies will eventually demonstrate benzodiazepines in general and clonazepam in particular to be a definitive treatment for EPS and TD, but there are currently no approved indications for the use of benzodiazepines to treat EPS. For a complete discussion of the use of benzodiazepines, see Chapter 11.

■ TREATMENT OF EXTRAPYRAMIDAL SIDE EFFECTS

The treatment of EPS (Table 15–4) initially involves the evaluation of dose and type of neuroleptic. Several investigators have demonstrated that an increase in dosage beyond the neuroleptic threshold brought no further improvement in therapeutic efficacy, but did lead to increased side effects (Angus and Simpson 1970a; Baldessarini et al. 1988; McEvoy et al. 1991). This suggests that EPS should be carefully monitored, with the goals of avoiding their occurrence (which is not always possible) and of eliminating them as soon as they are detected. EPS frequently can be eliminated with reduction in dose or change to a lower potency neuroleptic (Stratas et al. 1963).

Table 15–4. Treatment of extrapyramidal side effects (EPS)

Step	Action
1	Reduce dose of neuroleptic, if clinically possible.
2	Substitute a lower-potency neuroleptic.
3	Add an anticholinergic agent.
4	Titrate anticholinergic to maximum dose tolerable.
5	Add amantadine in combination with an anticholinergic or as a single agent.
6	Add a benzodiazepine or β-blocker.
7	In severe cases of EPS, stop neuroleptic temporarily and repeat process, beginning with Step 3.
8	Substitute neuroleptic with clozapine or other atypical antipsychotic.

Addition of an anticholinergic drug is the next line of treatment. Maximum therapeutic response occurs in 3–10 days, with more severe EPS taking a longer time to respond (DiMascio et al. 1976; Fann and Lake 1976). The anticholinergic dose should be increased until EPS is alleviated or an unacceptable degree of anticholinergic side effects is obtained.

EPS may remain uncontrolled despite increasing anticholinergic medications to the highest dose tolerable. At that point, amantadine can be added to the regimen, or it can be used as a single agent.

In severe cases of EPS, the neuroleptic should be temporarily stopped, because severe EPS may be a risk factor for development of neuroleptic malignant syndrome (Levinson and Simpson 1986).

For EPS that are still unresolved, β-blockers and benzodiazepines may be useful. The use of atypical antipsychotics in treatment of EPS is discussed in the next section.

Prophylaxis of EPS

Prophylactic use of antiparkinsonian agents to prevent EPS is a common (though somewhat controversial) practice. Most controlled prospective studies regarding prophylactic use of antiparkinsonian medication have shown that prophylaxis can be beneficial for certain high-risk patients but is *not* beneficial in routine use across all patient groups (Hanlon et al. 1966; Sramek et al. 1986). Studies that have demonstrated a greater general benefit across all groups have involved the use of very high doses of neuroleptics. Several retrospective studies have also demonstrated that there is a limited need for prophylaxis of EPS (Swett et al. 1977). Those retrospective studies demonstrating a greater benefit from prophylaxis also involved the use of high neuroleptic dosages (Keepers et al. 1983; Stern and Anderson 1979).

We conclude that the prophylactic use of antiparkinsonian medication is not routinely indicated for all patients but should be reserved for those patients at high risk of developing ADRs.

The risk factors for developing ADRs (Table 15–3) include younger age (under 35 years), higher doses of neuroleptic, higher potency of neuroleptic, intramuscular route of delivery, (possibly) male gender (Sramek et al. 1986), and a history of ADRs from a similar neuroleptic (Keepers and Casey 1991).

Dosages used for prophylaxis are 1–4 mg/day for benztropine, 5–15 mg/day for trihexyphenidyl, and 75–150 mg/day for diphenhydramine, although the dose required to achieve prophylaxis must be determined for each individual and is highly variable (Moleman et al. 1982; Sramek et al. 1986). Anticholinergic side effects, such as acute urinary retention or paralytic ileus, can occur even in a young patient, so high doses of anticholinergics cannot be used with impunity, even for short periods.

Prophylactic anticholinergics for ADRs need only be used for a limited time, because 85%–90% of ADRs occur within the first 4 days of treatment, and the incidence drops to nearly zero after 10 days (Keepers et al. 1983; Singh et al. 1990; Sramek et al. 1986). After this time, anticholinergics can be weaned slowly while the patient is being observed for development of parkinsonism or akathisia.

Depot Neuroleptics

In patients receiving depot neuroleptics, prophylactic anticholinergics need to be used only for a patient at high risk of developing ADRs (Idzorek 1976). The onset and characterization of EPS may be different, though, including more bizarre dystonic reactions (Simpson 1970). However, the buildup of neuroleptic levels with depot neuroleptics can lead to development of EPS at later stages of treatment, and some patients receiving fluphenazine decanoate were found to experience EPS only between days 3 and 10 following injection (McClelland et al. 1974).

Akathisia

Akathisia does not respond as well to treatment with anticholinergic medications and amantadine as do parkinsonism and ADRs (DiMascio et al. 1976; Zubenko et al. 1984). Anticholinergics are more likely to benefit akathisia if symptoms of parkinsonism are also present (Friis et al. 1983; Gagrat et al. 1978). When symptoms of parkinsonism are less prominent, studies have shown akathisia to respond less well to anticholinergic medications (Adler et al. 1987). β-blockers and (to a lesser extent) benzodiazepines have also been used with some success for treatment of akathisia (Horiguchi and Nishimatsu 1992).

Tardive Dyskinesia

Multiple different drugs have been used to treat TD, including dopaminergic agents, dopamine-depleting agents, GABAergic agents, vitamin E, calcium channel blockers, and adrenergic agents, but success has been limited (Feltner and Hertzman 1993). Clozapine has been shown to decrease symptoms of TD (Simpson et al. 1978), with the greatest improvement occurring in cases of severe TD and tardive dystonia (Lieberman et al. 1991).

Three possible mechanisms for clozapine's benefit have been proposed. Clozapine may suppress the TD movements in a fashion similar to that of typical antipsychotics. Second, TD may improve spontaneously, given that the typical neuroleptics are no longer present to cause or sustain TD. Third, clozapine may have an active therapeutic effect on TD (Lieberman et al. 1991). This issue remains to be clarified. In some patients, TD movements have recurred upon withdrawal of clozapine, but long-term follow-up studies have not been carried out. However, we would recommend clozapine for treatment of psychosis in subjects with TD.

■ Atypical Neuroleptics

In many cases, the development of EPS is the rate-limiting step in the neuroleptic treatment of psychotic patients. Clozapine, which had been shown to have potent antipsychotic effect, demonstrated that this side effect was not universal for antipsychotic activity. For patients who develop severe EPS on standard treatments, the use of clozapine would be indicated (Casey 1989). Improvement in EPS would be expected because of clozapine's low incidence of producing EPS, as well as clozapine's possibly having a direct antitremor effect on both parkinsonian (Gerlach and Simmelsgaard 1978) and essential tremors (Pakkenberg and Pakkenberg 1986). The risks involved with the use of clozapine would need to be counterbalanced against the clinical effect of EPS, whether directly through patient discomfort or indirectly with the effect of EPS on poor compliance and clinical outcome.

The recent FDA approval of risperidone will provide another method to reduce the development of EPS. Risperidone has combined 5-HT$_2$ and D$_2$ receptor antagonism, like clozapine. Risperidone would appear to produce antipsychotic effect at doses that do not produce EPS (Claus et al. 1992). Unlike clozapine, though, higher doses are associated with EPS (Chouinard et al. 1993). Risperidone does not produce agranulocytosis or require continual blood count monitoring. Whether risperidone will be as ef-

fective in preventing EPS as clozapine has been needs to be assessed in definitive studies.

Remoxipride is a third atypical antipsychotic with a favorable EPS profile. It has no effect on the serotonergic system and is a potent D$_2$ receptor antagonist. Remoxipride appears to have an antipsychotic effect equal to conventional neuroleptics, but with less propensity to produce EPS (Lewander et al. 1990). The recent reports of aplastic anemia in conjunction with the use of remoxipride may delay its entry into the market.

■ Duration of Treatment

Withdrawal Studies

The duration of treatment for EPS is an unanswered question. Studies investigating the withdrawal of antiparkinsonian agents have demonstrated that not all subjects redevelop EPS—a serendipitous finding noted when only 20% of patients withdrawn from benztropine in preparation for a trial of a new antiparkinsonian agent developed recurrent parkinsonian symptoms. This led to the suggestion that antiparkinsonian agents should be withdrawn after 2 months and their use only resumed in those patients who developed EPS again (Cahan and Parrish 1960).

Subsequently, other withdrawal studies were conducted that revealed wide-ranging rates of EPS recurrence. Differences in rates of recurrence probably are related to the varying methodologies involved in the studies, including methods of rating and the initial reason for treatment with anticholinergics—prophylaxis or active treatment (Ananth et al. 1970). The types, dosages, and combinations of neuroleptics used have also been major factors determining reoccurrence rates—the same factors that contribute to the initial development of EPS (Baker et al. 1983; McClelland et al. 1974). Additionally, there are inherent difficulties in evaluating EPS, including psychological factors and placebo effect (Ekdawi and Fowke 1966; Simpson et al. 1972; St. Jean et al. 1964).

Withdrawal Syndrome

Almost all anticholinergic withdrawal studies have involved abrupt withdrawal of the anticholinergic medications. Signs and symptoms that seemed to be related to anticholinergic withdrawal have been reported, suggesting the possibility of cholinergic sensitization and an anticholinergic withdrawal syndrome (Orlov et al. 1971). Only one study involved the gradual (rather than abrupt) withdrawal of anticholinergic agents, but the use of high neuroleptic doses and combinations of antipsychotics make it difficult to analyze the data from this study (Manos et al. 1981).

It is not known whether the use of anticholinergic agents sensitizes a patient to the subsequent development of EPS upon withdrawal of the agent. From reports of patients with no prior signs of EPS developing EPS on withdrawal of anticholinergics, there is indirect evidence that sensitization can take place (Klett and Caffey 1972). There have also been reports of an apparent generalized withdrawal syndrome (Gardos et al. 1978; Simpson et al. 1965). Sensitization, which would be expected to increase the rate and intensity of withdrawal EPS, would be significant for two reasons: 1) EPS on withdrawal might diminish over time without treatment, and 2) the possibility of development of sensitization would be another factor for limiting the routine use of prophylactic antiparkinsonian agents.

The conclusion that can be drawn from the withdrawal studies is that patients are more likely to develop EPS upon withdrawal of antiparkinsonian agents if the risk factors for developing EPS are present. If these risk factors are minimized, the rate of EPS recurrence is lowered.

In patients who develop reoccurrence, EPS generally reappears within 2 weeks, and control is easily reestablished (Klett and Caffey 1972). Patients respond rapidly and often require smaller doses of antiparkinsonian medications for control while remaining on the same dose of neuroleptic (McClelland et al. 1974).

CONCLUSION

The unique properties of chlorpromazine and other similarly active agents to ameliorate psychotic symptoms and to produce parkinsonian-like side effects were described in the early 1950s by French psychiatrists. Theories soon arose regarding the relationship between these two properties. The recognition of the benefits of reducing parkinsonian side effects led to investigations of methods to reduce EPS and instruments to measure them. The debate regarding the routine and prophylactic use of antiparkinsonian agents has continued for 30 years. It appears that pro-

phylactic antiparkinsonian agents need to be used in some situations, but probably less frequently and for briefer periods than has generally been the practice. The trend toward the use of lower dosages of neuroleptics should also lead to decreased need for use of antiparkinsonian agents. Finally, the advent of atypical antipsychotic agents has opened a new chapter in both the treatment and prevention of EPS and suggests that, in the future, EPS will be less of a problem than they have been in the past.

A summary of an American Psychiatric Association Task Force report on TD suggested that "[a] deliberate and sustained effort must be made to maintain patients on the lowest effective amount of drug and to keep the treatment regimen as simple as possible" (Baldessarini et al. 1980, p. 1168) and to discontinue anticholinergic drugs as soon as possible. Apart from a greater emphasis on avoiding the initial use of antiparkinsonian agents, this statement remains valid.

REFERENCES

Adler LA, Reiter S, Corwin J, et al: Differential effects of propranolol and benztropine in patients with neuroleptic-induced akathisia. Psychopharmacol Bull 23:519–521, 1987
Adler LA, Angrist B, Reiter S, et al: Neuroleptic-induced akathisia: a review. Psychopharmacology (Berl) 97:1–11, 1989
Adler LA, Angrist B, Weinreb H, et al: Studies on the time course and efficacy of β-blockers in neuroleptic-induced akathisia and the akathisia of idiopathic Parkinson's disease. Psychopharmacol Bull 27:107–111, 1991
Ananth JV, Horodesky S, Lehmann HE, et al: Effect of withdrawal of antiparkinsonian medication on chronically hospitalized psychiatric patients. Laval Médical 41:934–938, 1970
Angus JWS, Simpson GM: Handwriting changes and response to drugs—a controlled study. Acta Psychiatr Scand Suppl 21:28–37, 1970a
Angus JWS, Simpson GM: Hysteria and drug-induced dystonia. Acta Psychiatr Scand Suppl 21:52–58, 1970b
Aoki FY, Sitar DS, Ogilvie RI: Amantadine kinetics in healthy young subjects after long-term dosing. Clin Pharmacol Ther 26:729–736, 1979
Ayd FJ: A survey of drug-induced extrapyramidal re-

actions. JAMA 175:1054–1060, 1961

Baker LA, Cheng LY, Amara IB: The withdrawal of benztropine mesylate in chronic schizophrenic patients. Br J Psychiatry 143:584–590, 1983

Baldessarini RJ, Cole JO, Davis JM, et al: Tardive dyskinesia: summary of a task force report of the American Psychiatric Association. Am J Psychiatry 137:1163–1172, 1980

Baldessarini RJ, Cohen BM, Teicher MH: Significance of neuroleptic dose and plasma level in the pharmacological treatment of psychoses. Arch Gen Psychiatry 45:79–91, 1988

Baldessarini RJ, Huston-Lyons D, Campbell A, et al: Do central antiadrenergic actions contribute to the atypical properties of clozapine? Br J Psychiatry 160 (suppl 17):12–16, 1992

Barnes TRE: A rating scale for drug-induced akathisia. Br J Psychiatry 1564:672–676, 1989

Barnes TR: Movement disorder associated with antipsychotic drugs: the tardive syndromes. International Review of Psychiatry 2:355–366, 1990

Borison RL: Amantadine-induced psychosis in a geriatric patient with renal disease. Am J Psychiatry 136:111–112, 1979

Brooks GW: Experience with use of chlorpromazine and reserpine in psychiatry with special reference to the significance and management of extrapyramidal dysfunction. N Engl J Med 254:1119–1123, 1956

Brown JH: Atropine, scopolamine, and related antimuscarinic drugs, in Goodman and Gilman's The Pharmacological Basis of Therapeutics, 8th Edition. Edited by Gilman AG, Rall TW, Nies AS, et al. New York, Pergamon, 1990, pp 150–165

Cahan RB, Parrish DD: Reversibility of drug-induced parkinsonism. Am J Psychiatry 116:1022–1023, 1960

Casey DE: Clozapine: neuroleptic-induced EPS and tardive dyskinesia. Psychopharmacology (Berl) 99:S47–S53, 1989

Casey DE, Gerlach J, Christensson E: Dopamine, acetylcholine, and GABA effects in acute dystonia in primates. Psychopharmacologia 70:83–87, 1980

Cedarbaum JM, McDowell FH: Sixteen-year follow-up of 100 patients begun on levodopa in 1968: emerging problems, in Advances in Neurology, Vol 45: Parkinson's Disease. Edited by Yahr MD, Bergmann KJ. New York, Raven, 1987, pp 469–472

Cedarbaum JM, Schleifer LS: Drugs for Parkinson's disease, spasticity, and acute muscle spasms, in Goodman and Gilman's The Pharmacological Basis of Therapeutics, 8th Edition. Edited by Gilman AG, Rall TW, Nies AS, et al. New York, Pergamon, 1990, pp 463–484

Chien CP, DiMascio A: Drug-induced extrapyramidal symptoms and their relations to clinical efficacy. Am J Psychiatry 123:1490–1498, 1967

Chouinard G, Ross-Chouinard A, Annable L, et al: Extrapyramidal rating scale. Can J Neurol Sci 7:233, 1980

Chouinard G, Jones B, Remington G, et al: A Canadian multicenter placebo-controlled study of fixed doses of risperidone and haloperidol in the treatment of chronic schizophrenic patients [published erratum appears in J Clin Psychopharmacol 13:25–40, 1993]

Claus A, Bollen J, De Cuyper H, et al: Risperidone versus haloperidol in the treatment of chronic schizophrenic inpatients: a multicentre double-blind comparative study. Acta Psychiatr Scand 85:295–305, 1992

Coffin VL, Latranyi MB, Chipkin RE: Acute extrapyramidal syndrome in Cebus monkeys: development medicated by dopamine D_2 but not D_1 receptors. J Pharmacol Exp Ther 249:769–774, 1989

Delay J, Deniker P: Trente-huit cas de psychoses traitées par la cure prolongée et continue de 4560 RP. Léme Congrès des Alién. et Neurol. de Langue Française, Luxembourg, 21–27 juillet 1952. [Thirty-eight cases of psychoses treated with a long and continued course of 4560 RP. The Congress of the French Language for Alienists and Neurologists, Luxembourg, 21–27 July 1952.] Paris, Masson et Cie, 1952, pp 503–513

Denham J, Carrick JEL: Therapeutic importance of extra-pyramidal phenomena evoked by a new phenothiazine. Am J Psychiatry 116:927–928, 1960

DiMascio A, Bernardo DL, Greenblatt DJ, et al: A controlled trial of amantadine in drug-induced extrapyramidal disorders. Arch Gen Psychiatry 33:599–602, 1976

Director KL, Muniz CE: Diazepam in the treatment of extrapyramidal symptoms: a case report. J Clin Psychiatry 43:160–161, 1982

Doshay LJ: Five-year study of benztropine (Cogentin) methanesulfonate: outcome in three hundred two cases of paralysis agitans. JAMA 162:1031–1034, 1956

Doshay LJ, Constable K, Zier A: Five year follow-up

of treatment with trihexyphenidyl (Artane): outcome in four hundred and eleven cases of paralysis agitans. JAMA 154:1334–1336, 1954

Douglas RG Jr: Antiviral agents, in Goodman and Gilman's The Pharmacological Basis of Therapeutics, 8th Edition. Edited by Gilman AG, Rall TW, Nies AS, et al. New York, Pergamon, 1990, pp 1182–1201

Drachman DA: Memory and cognitive function in man: does the cholinergic system have a specific role? Neurology 27:783–790, 1977

Drayer DE: Lipophilicity, hydrophilicity, and the central nervous system side effects of beta blocker. Pharmacotherapy 7:87–91, 1987

Duvoisin RC: Cholinergic-anticholinergic antagonism in parkinsonism. Arch Neurol 17:124–136, 1967

Ekbom KA: Restless legs. Swedish Medical Journal 62:2376–2378, 1965

Ekdawi MY, Fowke R: A controlled trial of anti-Parkinson drugs in drug-induced parkinsonism. Br J Psychiatry 112:633–636, 1966

el-Defrawi MH, Craig TJ: Neuroleptics, extrapyramidal symptoms, and serum-calcium levels. Compr Psychiatry 25:539–545, 1984

England AC Jr, Schwab RS: Treatment in internal medicine: the management of Parkinson's disease. AMA Archives of Internal Medicine 104:439–468, 1959

Fann WE, Lake CR: Amantadine versus trihexyphenidyl in the treatment of neuroleptic-induced parkinsonism. Am J Psychiatry 133:940–943, 1976

Farde L, Nordström AL, Wiesel FA, et al: Positron emission tomographic analysis of central D_1 and D_2 dopamine receptor occupancy in patients treated with classical neuroleptics and clozapine: relation to extrapyramidal side effects. Arch Gen Psychiatry 49:538–544, 1992

Fayen M, Goldman MB, Moulthrop MA, et al: Differential memory function with dopaminergic versus anticholinergic treatment of drug-induced extrapyramidal symptoms. Am J Psychiatry 145:483–486, 1988

Feltner DE, Hertzman M: Progress in the treatment of tardive dyskinesia: theory and practice. Hosp Community Psychiatry 44:25–34, 1993

Fleischhacker W, Bergmann KJ, Perovich R, et al: the Hillside akathisia scale: a new rating instrument for neuroleptic-induced akathisia, parkinsonism and hyperkinesia. Psychopharmacol Bull 25:222–226, 1989

Fleischhacker WW, Roth SD, Kane JM: The pharmacologic treatment of neuroleptic-induced akathisia. J Clin Psychopharmacol 10:12–21, 1990

Flügel F: Neue klinische Beobachtungen zur Wirkung des Phenothiazinkorpers Megaphen auf psychische Krankheitsbidler. [Clinical observations on the effect of the phenothiazine derivative megaphen on psychic disorders in children.] Med Klin 48:1027–1029, 1953

Freyhan FA: Therapeutic implications of differential effects of new phenothiazine compounds. Am J Psychiatry 115:577–585, 1959

Friis T, Christensen TR, Gerlach J: Sodium valproate and biperiden in neuroleptic-induced akathisia, parkinsonism and hyperkinesia: a double-blind cross-over study with placebo. Acta Psychiatr Scand 67:178–187, 1983

Gagrat D, Hamilton J, Belmaker RH: Intravenous diazepam in the treatment of neuroleptic-induced acute dystonia and akathisia. Am J Psychiatry 135:1232–1233, 1978

Gardos G, Cole JO, Tarsy D: Withdrawal syndromes associated with antipsychotic drugs. Am J Psychiatry 135:1321–1324, 1978

Garrison JC: Histamine, bradykinin, 5-hydroxytryptamine, and their antagonists, in Goodman and Gilman's The Pharmacological Basis of Therapeutics, 8th Edition. Edited by Gilman AG, Rall TW, Nies AS, et al. New York, Pergamon, 1990, pp 575–599

Gelenberg AJ: Amantadine in the treatment of benztropine-refractory extrapyramidal disorders induced by antipsychotic drugs. Current Therapeutic Research, Clinical and Experimental 23:375–380, 1978

Gengo FM, Huntoon L, McHugh WB: Lipid-soluble and water-soluble beta-blockers: comparison of the central nervous system depressant effect. Arch Intern Med 147: 39–43, 1987

Gerlach J, Hansen L: Clozapine and D_1/D_2 antagonism in extrapyramidal functions. Br J Psychiatry 160 (suppl 17):34–37, 1992

Gerlach J, Simmelsgaard H: Tardive dyskinesia during and following treatment with haloperidol, haloperidol + biperiden, thioridazine and clozapine. Psychopharmacology (Berl) 59:105–112, 1978

Greenblatt DJ, DiMascio A, Harmatz JS, et al: Pharmacokinetics and clinical effects of amantadine in drug-induced extrapyramidal symptoms. J Clin Pharmacol 17:704–708, 1977

Grelak RP, Clark R, Stump JM, et al: Amantadine-dopamine interaction: possible mode of action in parkinsonism. Science 169:203–204, 1970

Gunne LM, Häggström JE, Sjöquist B: Association with persistent neuroleptic-induced dyskinesia of regional changes in brain GABA synthesis. Nature 309:347–349, 1984

Guy W: ECDEU Assessment Manual for Psychopharmacology, Revised Edition. Washington, DC, U.S. Department of Health, Education and Welfare, 1976

Haase HJ: Über Vorkommen und Deutung des psychomotorischen Parkinson-symdroms bei Megaphen-bzw, Largactil Dauer-behandlung. [The presentation and meaning of the psychomotor Parkinson syndrome during long-term treatment with megaphen, also know as Largactil.] Nervenarzt 25:486–492, 1954

Haase HJ, Janssen PAJ: The action of neuroleptic drugs. Chicago, IL, Year Book, 1965

Hanlon TE, Schoenrich C, Freinek W, et al: Perphenazine-benztropine mesylate treatment of newly admitted psychiatric patients. Psychopharmacologia 9:328–339, 1966

Hayden FG, Minocha A, Spyker DA, et al: Comparative single-dose pharmacokinetics of amantadine hydrochloride and rimantadine hydrochloride in young and elderly adults. Antimicrob Agents Chemother 28:216–221, 1985

Hoffman BB, Lefkowitz RJ: Adrenergic receptor antagonists, in Goodman and Gilman's The Pharmacological Basis of Therapeutics, 8th Edition. Edited by Gilman AG, Rall TW, Nies AS, et al. New York, Pergamon, 1990, pp 187–243

Horiguchi J, Nishimatsu O: Usefulness of antiparkinsonian drugs during neuroleptic treatment and the effect of clonazepam on akathisia and parkinsonism occurred after antiparkinsonian drug withdrawal: a double-blind study. Jpn J Psychiatry Neurol 46:733–739, 1992

Ichikawa J, Meltzer HY: Differential effects of repeated treatment with haloperidol and clozapine on dopamine release and metabolism in the striatum and the nucleus accumbens. J Pharmacol Exp Ther 256:348–357, 1991

Idzorek S: Antiparkinsonian agents and fluphenazine decanoate. Am J Psychiatry 133:80–82, 1976

Ing TS, Daugirdas JT, Soung LS, et al: Toxic effects of amantadine in patients with renal failure. Can Med Assoc J 120:695–698, 1979

Karn WN, Kasper S: Pharmacologically induced Parkinson-like signs as index of the therapeutic potential. Diseases of the Nervous System 20:119–122, 1959

Keepers GA, Casey DE: Use of neuroleptic-induced extrapyramidal symptoms to predict future vulnerability to side effects. Am J Psychiatry 148:85–89, 1991

Keepers GA, Clappison VJ, Casey DE: Initial anticholinergic prophylaxis for neuroleptic-induced extrapyramidal syndromes. Arch Gen Psychiatry 40:1113–1117, 1983

Kelly JT, Abuzzahab FS: The antiparkinson properties of amantadine in drug-induced parkinsonism. J Clin Pharmacol 11:211–214, 1971

Klett CJ, Caffey E: Evaluating the long-term need for antiparkinson drugs by chronic schizophrenics. Arch Gen Psychiatry 26:374–379, 1972

Kulik AV, Wilbur R: Case report of propranolol (Inderal) pharmacotherapy for neuroleptic-induced akathisia and tremor. Prog Neuropsychopharmacol Biol Psychiatry 7:223–225, 1983

Kuny S, Binswanger U: Neuroleptic-induced extrapyramidal symptoms and serum calcium levels. Pharmacopsychiatry 21:67–70, 1989

Laborit H, Huguenard P, Alluaume R: Un nouveau stabilisateur vegetatif (le 4560 RP). [A new vegetative stabilizer (4560 RP).] Presse Med 60:206–208, 1952

Lefkowitz RJ, Hoffman BB, Taylor P: Neurohumoral transmission: the autonomic and somatic motor nervous systems, in Goodman and Gilman's The Pharmacological Basis of Therapeutics, 8th Edition. Edited by Gilman AG, Rall TW, Nies AS, et al. New York, Pergamon, 1990, pp 84–121

Levinson DF, Simpson GM: Neuroleptic-induced extrapyramidal symptoms with fever: heterogeneity of the "Neuroleptic Malignant Syndrome." Arch Gen Psychiatry 43:839–848, 1986

Levinson DF, Simpson GM, Singh H, et al: Fluphenazine dose, clinical response, and extrapyramidal symptoms during acute treatment. Arch Gen Psychiatry 47:761–768, 1990

Lewander T, Westerbergh DE, Morrison D: Clinical profile of remoxipride—a combined analysis of a comparative double-blind multicentre trial programme. Acta Psychiatr Scand 82 (suppl 358):92–98, 1990

Lieberman JA, Saltz BL, Johns CA, et al: The effects of clozapine on tardive dyskinesia. Br J Psychiatry

158:503–510, 1991

Lipinski JF, Zubenko GS, Barreira P, et al: Propranolol in the treatment of neuroleptic-induced akathisia. Lancet 1:685–686, 1983

Manos N, Gkiouzepas J, Tzotzoras T, et al: Gradual withdrawal of antiparkinson medication in chronic schizophrenics: any better than the abrupt? J Nerv Ment Dis 169:659–661, 1981

Mawdsley C, Williams IR, Pullar IA, et al: Treatment of parkinsonism by amantadine and levodopa. Clin Pharmacol Ther 13:575–583, 1972

McClelland HA, Blessed G, Bhate S, et al: The abrupt withdrawal of antiparkinsonian drugs in schizophrenic patients. Br J Psychiatry 124:151–159, 1974

McCreadie RG: The Nithsdale schizophrenia surveys: an overview. Soc Psychiatry Psychiatr Epidemiol 27:40–45, 1992

McEvoy JP: The clinical use of anticholinergic drugs as treatment for extrapyramidal side effects of neuroleptic drugs. J Clin Psychopharmacol 3:288–302, 1983

McEvoy JP, Hogarty GE, Steingard S: Optimal dose of neuroleptic in acute schizophrenia: a controlled study of the neuroleptic threshold and higher haloperidol dose. Arch Gen Psychiatry 48:739–745, 1991

Medina C, Kramer MD, Kurland AA: Biperiden in the treatment of phenothiazine-induced extrapyramidal reactions. JAMA 182:1127–1129, 1962

Meldrum BS, Anlezark GM, Marsden CD: Acute dystonia as an idiosyncratic response to neuroleptics in baboons. Brain 100:313–326, 1977

Meltzer HY: The importance of serotonin-dopamine interactions in the action of clozapine. Br J Psychiatry 160 (suppl 17):22–29, 1992

Meltzer HY, Nash JF: Effects of antipsychotic drugs on serotonin receptors. Pharmacol Rev 43:587–604, 1991

Meltzer HY, Matsubara S, Lee JC: Classification of typical and atypical antipsychotic drugs on the basis of dopamine D-1, D-2 and serotonin$_2$ pKi values. J Pharmacol Exp Ther 251:238–246, 1989

Menza MA, Murray GB, Holmes VF, et al: Decreased extrapyramidal symptoms with intravenous haloperidol. J Clin Psychiatry 48:278–280, 1987

Mindham RHS: Assessment of drugs in schizophrenia: assessment of drug-induced extrapyramidal reactions and of drugs given for their control. Br J Clin Pharmacol 3 (suppl):395–400, 1976

Moleman P, Schmitz PJM, Ladee GA: Extrapyramidal

side effects and oral haloperidol: an analysis of explanatory patient and treatment characteristics. J Clin Psychiatry 43:492–496;1982

Orlov P, Kasparian G, DiMascio A, et al: Withdrawal of antiparkinson drugs. Arch Gen Psychiatry 25:410–412, 1971

Pacifici GM, Nardini M, Ferrari P, et al: Effect of amantadine on drug-induced parkinsonism: relationship between plasma levels and effect. Br J Clin Pharmacol 3:883–889, 1976

Pakkenberg H, Pakkenberg B: Clozapine in the treatment of tremor. Acta Neurol Scand 73:295–297, 1986

Parkes JD, Zilkha KJ, Calver DM, et al: Controlled trial of amantadine hydrochloride in Parkinson's disease. Lancet 1:259–262, 1970

Paton DM, Webster DR: Clinical pharmacokinetics of H$_1$-receptor antagonists (the antihistamines). Clin Pharmacokinet 10:477–497, 1985

Perry EK, Perry RH, Blessed G, et al: Necropsy evidence of central cholinergic deficits in senile dementia. Lancet 1:189, 1977

Postma JU, Tilburg VW: Visual hallucinations and delirium during treatment with amantadine (Symmetrel). J Am Geriatr Soc 23:212–215, 1975

Rashkis HA, Smarr ER: Protection against reserpine induced Parkinsonism. Am J Psychiatry 113:1116, 1957

Rifkin A, Quitkin F, Klein DF: Akinesia, a poorly recognized drug-induced extrapyramidal behavioral disorder. Arch Gen Psychiatry 32:672–674, 1975

Saltz BL, Woerner MG, Kane JM, et al: Prospective study of tardive dyskinesia incidence in the elderly. JAMA 266:2402–2406, 1991

Schwab RS, Chafetz ME: Kemadrin in the treatment of Parkinsonism. Neurology 5:273–277, 1955

Schwab RS, England AC, Poskanzer DC, et al: Amantadine in the treatment of Parkinson's disease. JAMA 208:1160–1170, 1969

Shear MK, Frances A, Weiden P: Suicide associated with akathisia and depot fluphenazine treatment. J Clin Psychopharmacol 3:235–236, 1983

Simpson GM: Long-acting, antipsychotic agents and extrapyramidal side effects. Diseases of the Nervous System 31 (suppl):12–14, 1970

Simpson GM, Angus JWS: A rating scale for extrapyramidal side effects. Acta Psychiatr Scand 212:11–19, 1970

Simpson GM, Amuso D, Blair JH, et al: Phenothiazine-produced extrapyramidal system disturbance. Arch Gen Psychiatry 10:199–208, 1964

Simpson GM, Amin M, Kunz E: Withdrawal effects of phenothiazines. Compr Psychiatry 6:347–351, 1965

Simpson GM, Krakov L, Mattke D, et al: A controlled comparison of the treatment of schizophrenic patients when treated according to the neuroleptic threshold or by clinical judgement. Acta Psychiatr Scand (Suppl) 212:38–43, 1970

Simpson GM, Beckles D, Isalski Z, et al: Some methodological considerations in the evaluation of drug-induced extrapyramidal disorders: a study of EX10-029, a new morphanthridine derivative. J Clin Pharmacol 12:142–152, 1972

Simpson GM, Lee JH, Shrivastava RK: Clozapine in tardive dyskinesia. Psychopharmacologia 56:75–80, 1978

Simpson GM, Lee JH, Zoubok B, et al: A rating scale for tardive dyskinesia. Psychopharmacologia 64:171–179, 1979

Simpson GM, Cooper TB, Bark N, et al: Effect of antiparkinsonian medications on plasma levels of chlorpromazine. Arch Gen Psychiatry 37:205–208, 1980

Singh H, Levinson DF, Simpson GM, et al: Acute dystonia during fixed-dose neuroleptic treatment. J Clin Psychopharmacol 10:389–396, 1990

Snyder S, Greenberg D, Yamamura HI: Anti schizophrenic drugs and brain cholinergic receptors. Arch Gen Psychiatry 31:58–61, 1974

Sokoloff P, Giros B, Martres MP, et al: Molecular cloning and characterization of a novel dopamine receptor (D_3) as a target for neuroleptics. Nature 347:146–151, 1990

Sramek JJ, Simpson GM, Morrison RL, et al: Anticholinergic agents for prophylaxis of neuroleptic-induced dystonic reactions: a prospective study. J Clin Psychiatry 47:305–309, 1986

St. Jean A, Donald MW, Ban TA: Uses and abuses of antiparkinsonian medication. Am J Psychiatry 120:801–803, 1964

Stephens DA: Psychotoxic effects of benzhexol hydrochloride (Artane). Br J Psychiatry 113:213–218, 1967

Stern TA, Anderson WH: Benztropine prophylaxis of dystonic reactions. Psychopharmacologia 61:261–262, 1979

Strang RR: The syndrome of restless legs. Med J Aust 24:1211–1213, 1967

Stratas NE, Phillips RD, Walker PA, et al: A study of

drug induced parkinsonism. Diseases of the Nervous System 24:180, 1963

Strömberg U, Svensson TH, Waldeck B: On the mode of action of amantadine. J Pharm Pharmacol 22:959–962, 1970

Swett C, Cole JO, Shapiro S, et al: Extrapyramidal side effects in chlorpromazine recipients. Arch Gen Psychiatry 34:942–943, 1977

Thaker GK, Nguyen JA, Strauss ME, et al: Clonazepam treatment of tardive dyskinesia: a practical GABAmimetic strategy. Am J Psychiatry 147:445–451, 1990

Timberlake WH, Schwab RS, England AC Jr: Biperiden (Akineton) in Parkinsonism. Arch Neurol 5:560–564, 1961

Tune L, Coyle JT: Serum levels of anticholinergic drugs in treatment of acute extrapyramidal side effects. Arch Gen Psychiatry 37:293–297, 1980

Van Putten T, May PR, Marder SR, et al: Subjective response to antipsychotic drugs. Arch Gen Psychiatry 38:187–190, 1981

Van Putten TR, May PR, Marder SR: Response to antipsychotic medication: the doctor's and the consumer's view. Am J Psychiatry 141:16–19, 1984

Van Tol H, Bunzow J, Guan H, et al: Cloning of the gene for a human dopamine D_4 receptor with high affinity for the antipsychotic clozapine. Nature 350:610–614, 1991

Wilbur R, Kulik FA, Kulik AV: Noradrenergic effects in tardive dyskinesia, akathisia and pseudoparkinsonism via the limbic system and basal ganglia. Prog Neuropsychopharmacol Biol Psychiatry 12:849–864, 1988

Winer JA, Bahn S: Loss of teeth with antidepressant drug therapy. Arch Gen Psychiatry 16:239–240, 1967

Wingfield WL, Pollack D, Grunert RR: Therapeutic efficacy of amantadine HCl and rimantadine HCl in naturally occurring influenza A2 respiratory illness in man. N Engl J Med 281:579–584, 1969

Wojcik J, Gelenberg A, La Brie RA, et al: Prevalence of tardive dyskinesia in an outpatient population. Compr Psychiatry 21:370–379, 1980

Yahr MD, Duvoisin RC: Medical therapy of parkinsonism. Modern Treatment 5:283–300, 1968

Zubenko GS, Barreira P, Lipinski JF: Development of tolerance to the therapeutic effect of amantadine on akathisia. J Clin Psychopharmacol 4:218–219, 1984

Drugs for Treatment of Bipolar Disorder

Lithium

Robert H. Lenox, M.D., and Husseini K. Manji, M.D., F.R.C.P.C.

■ HISTORY AND DISCOVERY

Lithium is an element that was discovered in 1817. For more than 150 years, lithium has been used in various formulations as a remedy for a multitude of maladies afflicting the human body (Johnson 1984). Basing his work on that of Alexander Ure in the early 1840s, 20 years later Sir Alfred Garrod was the first to introduce the oral use of lithia salts as a treatment for gout or "uric acid diathesis," which was described to encompass symptoms of "gouty mania" and "complete mental derangement" (Garrod 1859; Ure 1844/1845). During this period, Professor A. Trousseau referred to both mania and depression as being associated with uric acid diathesis (Trousseau 1868).

Although lithia salts were clearly thought to be effective as a therapy for this gouty syndrome, it was the work by the American physician John Aulde and the Danish internist Carl Lange in the late 1880s that brought attention to the prophylactic efficacy of lithium in the treatment of recurrent symptoms of depression (Aulde 1887; Lange 1886). Subsequent use of lithium salts at low concentrations in popular remedies and mineral waters around the turn of the century, and their use as a salt substitute (resulting in cases of lithium toxicity in the 1940s), led to their fall into disrepute within the medical community. It was not until lithium's serendipitous rediscovery by Cade more than 45 years ago, and seminal clinical studies by Schou in the early 1950s, that lithium was seen by modern psychiatry as an effective antimanic treatment and a prophylactic therapy for manic-depressive disorder (Cade 1949; Schou 1979a).

■ PHYSICOCHEMICAL AND PHARMACOLOGICAL PROFILE

■ Lithium—A Monovalent Cation

Lithium shares many of the physicochemical properties of the Group IA elements in the periodic table (a group that includes sodium and potassium) and is the smallest member among these alkali metals. It possesses the highest electrical field density and largest energy of hydration, giving it ready access to sodium channel transport; yet it has an ionic radius that is similar to the divalent cations magnesium and calcium (Johnson et al. 1971). The interaction and potential competition of lithium with physiological events associated with the transport and cofactor activities of these monovalent and divalent cations in cells throughout the body, especially the brain, has provided fertile ground for research over the years.

It is worth noting that there exist in nature two stable isotopes of lithium (i.e., ^{6}Li and ^{7}Li) that can readily be detected by nuclear magnetic resonance (NMR) spectroscopy (Detellier 1983). The isotope most commonly visualized using NMR spectroscopy is ^{7}Li, which constitutes almost 93% of natural lithium. Because there are reports that these two isotopes may possess small differences in biological activity, formulations of one or the other stable isotope might prove interesting in light of its relatively narrow therapeutic index as a psychotropic medication (Sherman et al. 1984). The introduction of ^{7}Li NMR techniques and magnetic resonance imaging (MRI) in vivo has permitted the determination of lithium transport and distribution in living organ or tissue, with the capability of differentiating free versus membrane-bound intracellular lithium pools in intact cell systems (i.e., erythrocytes and liposomes) as well as in brain (Detellier 1983; Renshaw and Wicklund 1988; Renshaw et al. 1986). ^{1}H NMR studies of erythrocytes in bipolar patients have demonstrated an elevation of proton spin lattice (T_1) relaxation times that normalizes relative to control subjects after a week of lithium treatment (Rosenthal et al. 1986). Similar observations have been noted in MRI studies in frontal and temporal areas of the brain in bipolar patients (Rangel-Guerra et al. 1983). These studies may be indicative of lithium effects on intracellular hydration and water transport (Ballast et al. 1986).

■ Lithium and Membrane Transport

For 40 years, it has been known that lithium undergoes active transport across cell membranes (Zerahn 1955). Numerous studies have characterized the membrane transport of lithium and its interaction with other cations in both the brain and peripheral tissues in an effort to address a potential mode of action of lithium in the treatment of manic-depressive disorder (see reviews in Bach and Gallicchio 1990; Mota de Freitas et al. 1991; Riddell 1991).

Neurons have various ion channels and pumps that serve to maintain the capacitance or resting potential across the cell membrane in preparation for rapid depolarization and subsequent neurotransmitter release (Dowling 1992; Kuffler and Nicholls 1979). Sodium-potassium-adenosine triphosphatase (Na,K-ATPase) activity requires energy and is responsible for maintaining the resting membrane potential of the neuron by preferentially extruding Na^+ ions relative to K^+ entering the cell, thus creating an electrochemical gradient with high K^+/low Na^+ intracellularly and high Na^+/low K^+ extracellularly. The voltage-gated Na^+ channel permits entry of Na^+ following an excitatory stimulus, resulting in progressive depolarization and rapid entry of Na^+, triggering an action potential. In the presence of increased intracellular Na^+ concentrations following the action potential, a Na^+-calcium ion (Ca^{2+}) exchange process permits influx of calcium and extrusion of Na^+. This leads to a cascade of events at the nerve terminal involving phosphoproteins and cytoskeletal elements, resulting in neurotransmitter release. The transient increase in calcium is buffered rapidly by calcium-binding proteins and organelles and actively pumped out of the cell by the Ca-activated, magnesium (Mg)-dependent ATPase as well as the gradient-dependent Na^+-Ca^{2+} transport system.

In excitable cells, accumulated evidence suggests that lithium influx occurs primarily through the voltage-sensitive Na^+ channel (Carmiliet 1964; El-Mallakh 1990; Keynes and Swan 1959). Upon activation of the channel, lithium entry has been shown to occur, especially during the depolarization phase wherein lithium rushes into the cells at the expense of Na^+. This property of lithium may be reflected in the increase in plasma levels of lithium occurring as a patient becomes euthymic following treatment for an acute manic episode (Degkwitz et al. 1979). Additional evidence in neuroblastoma-glioma hybrid cells indicates that lithium may also utilize the ouabain-sensitive Na,K-ATPase, but this was not observed in neurons in primary culture (Gorkin and Richelson 1981; Richelson 1977). Extrusion of lithium from the cell appears to depend on the gradient-dependent Na^+-Li^+ exchange process, wherein intracellular lithium substitutes for the intracellular Na^+ (Hitzemann et al. 1989; Sarkadi et al. 1978). However, although there is evidence that lithium enters the cell equally displacing Na^+ in excitable cells, lithium does accumulate in the cell, because removal of lithium is less efficient than Na^+ (Coppen and Shaw 1967; El-Mallakh 1990). It is thought that Na,K-ATPase may play an indirect role, because it establishes the Na^+ gradient in neurons; the greater the Na^+ gradient, the greater the rate of Na^+ efflux through the Na^+-Li^+ exchange.

The red blood cell (RBC) has served as a cell model for a series of clinical investigations over the years, as it shares lithium transport properties with neurons and is easily accessible (Bach and Gallicchio 1990; Mota de Freitas et al. 1991). At therapeutic levels, influx of lithium into the RBC occurs predominantly through passage as a cation through the "leak" or passive diffusion pathway. Additional routes of entry for lithium include a $Na^+(Li^+)$-K^+ cotransport pathway as well as the anion exchange pathway, wherein its small size and high charge density permits its anionic transport in complex with bicarbonate. Efflux of lithium occurs primarily through the Na^+-Li^+ countertransport pathway, with additional routes through the passive "leak" pathway and (to a lesser extent) the Na,K-ATPase pump. There is no evidence that lithium treatment alters the transport properties of either the "leak" or $Na^+(Li^+)$-K^+ cotransport pathways.

Over the years, clinical studies of patients with manic-depressive disorder have revealed evidence for an increase in Na^+ retention and intracellular Na^+ (Coppen and Shaw 1963; Coppen et al. 1966; Naylor et al. 1970, 1971); a decrease in Na,K-ATPase activity (Hokin-Neaverson and Jefferson 1989a, 1989b; Naylor and Smith 1981; Naylor et al. 1980; Nurnberger et al. 1982); and, most recently, evidence for an increase in intracellular calcium in peripheral blood cells in both mania and depression (Dubovsky et al. 1991a, 1992). Lithium treatment has been shown to result in a reduction of intraerythrocyte Na^+ (Hermoni et al. 1987; Hitzemann et al. 1989), and studies using Fura 2-AM fluorescence have revealed a lithium-induced reduction of Ca^{2+} in platelets of bipolar patients (Dubovsky et al. 1991b). Because free calcium ion concentration tends to parallel free sodium concentration, this may account for lithium-induced reduction in free Ca^{2+} ion concentrations noted previously (Mullins and Brinley 1977; Torok 1989).

It has been suggested that an alteration in the activity of the Na,K-ATPase pump could result in significant changes in neuronal excitability and may represent a pathogenesis for mood disorders (El-Mallakh 1983; Hokin-Neaverson et al. 1974; Naylor and Smith 1981). However, clinical studies in RBCs over the years have reported conflicting data in manic-depressive patients, with a reduction in Na,K-ATPase activity predominantly noted in the depressed phase of both unipolar and bipolar patients (Akagawa et al. 1980; Alexander et al. 1986; Choi et al. 1977; Dagher et al. 1984; El-Mallakh 1983; Glen and Reading 1973; Hokin-Neaverson and Jefferson 1989b; Hokin-Neaverson et al. 1974; Naylor et al. 1974b; Nurnberger et al. 1982; Reddy et al. 1989; Sengupta et al. 1980; Strzyzewski et al. 1984). Multiple factors such as psychotropic drugs, circulating hormones, and diet have probably contributed to much of this variability (Swann 1984, 1988; Wood et al. 1989b). Early studies in frog muscle found that lithium is a poor substrate for Na,K-ATPase (Keynes and Swan 1959). Studies in

whole brain of animals revealed an acute inhibition of lithium on Na,K-ATPase activity. There was evidence that chronic lithium treatment resulted in an inhibition of the Na,K-ATPase enzyme in synaptosomal membrane fractions from brain, which appeared to be regionally specific to the hippocampus (Guerri et al. 1981; Swann et al. 1980). Furthermore, this inhibition represented a reduction in the V_{max} of the enzyme, with no apparent change in affinity (K_m), and was selective for neurons that have the enzyme subtype with high affinity for ouabain binding. Similar observations of lithium inhibition of Na,K-ATPase have been made in peripheral neurons and have been attributed to an action of lithium competing for the intracellular Na^+ activation site of the enzyme (Ritchie and Straub 1980). On the other hand, studies of erythrocyte membranes in patients treated with lithium have revealed evidence for increased activity of Na,K-ATPase (Bunney and Garland-Bunney 1987; Dick et al. 1978; Hokin-Neaverson et al. 1976; Johnson et al. 1980; Mallinger et al. 1987; Naylor et al. 1974a, 1980; Reddy et al. 1989; Swann 1988; Wood et al. 1989a). These data may be accounted for in part by a concomitant lithium-induced inhibition, mediated through intracellular interaction with the Na^+ binding site, and activation, mediated through an extracellular K^+ site (Collard 1986; Lazarus and Muston 1978).

Although early studies suggested that the RBC/plasma lithium ratio was related to a history of bipolar disorder and that a higher ratio was associated with a clinical response to lithium treatment, it was soon evident that there was a large interindividual variation precluding adequate replication (Mendels and Frazer 1973; Ramsey et al. 1979; Richelson et al. 1986; Szentistvanyi and Janka 1979). These investigations, however, led to the hypothesis that the pathogenesis of affective disorders was related to membrane dysfunction (Ehrlich and Diamond 1980). This was followed by a series of studies using lithium transport properties in the RBC as a genetic marker, reporting a reduction in Na^+-Li^+ transport rates in a subgroup of bipolar patients and some family members (Ehrlich and Diamond 1979, 1980; Frazer et al. 1978; Ostrow et al. 1978; Pandey et al. 1977, 1978; Ramsey et al. 1979; Sarkadi et al. 1978; Shaughnessy et al. 1985; Szentistvanyi and Janka 1979). Here again, variability of data both within and between patients contributed to the failure to replicate these findings in other studies (Dagher et al. 1984; Egeland et al.

1984; Greil et al. 1977; Mallinger et al. 1983; Richelson et al. 1986). These data were also confounded by the fact that lithium treatment results in a progressive inhibition of Na^+-Li^+ countertransport (Ehrlich et al. 1981, 1983) and a history of hypertension is associated with elevated rates of Na^+-Li^+ transport (Canessa et al. 1980, 1987).

Investigators over the years have observed that chronic lithium administration will increase choline concentration in the erythrocyte by more than 10-fold (Jope et al. 1978, 1980; Lee et al. 1974; Lingsch and Martin 1976; Meltzer et al. 1982; Rybakowski et al. 1978; Stoll et al. 1991; Uney et al. 1985). This appears to be the result not only of an inhibition of choline transport but also an enhanced phospholipase D mediated degradation of choline-containing phospholipids (Chapman et al. 1982; Miller et al. 1989, 1990). The latter effect of chronic lithium use may be mediated by its action on protein kinase C (PKC), which is discussed later in this chapter. Because lithium has also been shown to inhibit choline transport in human brain (Ehrlich et al. 1980), it has been suggested that this effect of lithium may account for a lithium-induced increase in cholinergic tone in the brain, accounting for its therapeutic effects (Jope 1979; Uney and Marchbanks 1987; Uney et al. 1986). However, unlike the erythrocyte in which choline transport inhibition is irreversible, choline in the brain can be metabolized readily to acetylcholine (ACh) or incorporated into lipids. The impact of this effect of lithium is currently unknown (Diamond et al. 1982/1983; Lingsch and Martin 1976; Uney et al. 1986). Although studies have attempted to utilize intraerythrocyte choline concentration before and after lithium administration as a predictor of clinical response, the data are conflicting and need further study (Haag et al. 1984, 1987; Kuchel et al. 1984; Stoll et al. 1991).

It is of interest that lithium efflux appears to be inhibited by approximately 50% in patients after treatment with lithium for *at least* 1 week, and is associated with a threefold increase in the apparent K_m for Na^+-Li^+ pathway, with no change in the countertransport rate V_{max} (Ehrlich et al. 1981). Studies using NMR have demonstrated that uptake of lithium intracellularly is rather slow, and they confirm the increased accumulation of intraerythrocyte lithium following several days of chronic lithium exposure (Riddell 1991). Similarly, as we have noted, chronic lithium use results in a significantly elevated intracellular concentration of choline, which persists long after the levels of lithium in both plasma and RBC are no longer detectable (Lee et al. 1974; Lingsch and Martin 1976; Meltzer et al. 1982; Rybakowski et al. 1978). These effects of lithium appear to correspond to the time course of clinical efficacy of lithium treatment and have led to suggestions that chronic lithium use may induce an evolving change in membrane structure or interaction with membrane-bound enzymes (Ehrlich et al. 1983).

Although these data are of considerable interest, we must be cautious about direct extrapolation from a nonnucleated peripheral cell model to one involving excitable nucleated neuronal cells within the brain. With the evolution of molecular biological techniques and identification of critical proteins responsible for regulation of membrane transport, future studies may be able to focus more directly on molecular interactions of both acute and chronic lithium exposure at the level of these transport proteins in neuronal cells.

■ MECHANISM OF ACTION

■ Lithium and Circadian Rhythms

Although studies of circadian rhythms in patients with affective disorders have often been limited by their cross-sectional design and heterogeneous patient populations and confounded by significant variability, disturbance in biological rhythms has remained a viable hypothesis underlying the (episodic) dysregulation observed in manic-depressive illness (Goodwin and Jamison 1990). The alteration in circadian rhythms in patients appears to be manifest in an overall reduction in amplitude, possibly attributable to phase instability and a tendency to phase advance observed in rapid eye movement (REM) sleep and core temperature relative to the sleep-wake cycle. Lithium has been shown to slow circadian oscillators in a wide variety of species, ranging from plants to humans (Klemfuss and Kripke 1989). It is noteworthy that deuterium shares this property. Because both lithium and deuterium increase the density of tissue water, it has been suggested that both compounds may exert their chronotropic effects by virtue of their action on membrane processes (Hallonquist et al. 1986).

Various studies in animals have demonstrated

that lithium appears to lengthen the endogenous period of a number of circadian rhythms under free-running conditions. In the presence of environmental cues (zeitgebers) for entrainment, this lengthening of the circadian rhythm by chronic lithium administration is reflected in a delay in rhythms associated with wheel-running, sleep-wake cycle, and photoperiodic reproductive response, as well as a number of endocrine and biochemical variables. In a study of squirrel monkeys, chronic lithium administration at "therapeutic" concentrations significantly lengthened the period of free-running circadian activity rhythms (Welsh and Moore-Ede 1990). However, the effects of lithium on the regulation of hormones as well as neurotransmitter receptors in brain have not consistently demonstrated a phase delay (Kafka et al. 1983; McEachron et al. 1982; Wirz-Justice 1983; Wirz-Justice et al. 1982). Although this may reflect lithium's ability to differentially dissociate circadian rhythms similar to findings observed with antidepressants, supportive data remain weak.

Comparable studies in humans have been less convincing, undoubtedly due to the limitations associated with clinical investigations noted previously (Johnsson et al. 1983; Welsh et al. 1986; Wever 1979). Various studies have observed that lithium can phase-delay circadian rhythms in human subjects entrained to a 24-hour day schedule, consistent with its ability to lengthen the intrinsic period of a circadian oscillator (Kripke et al. 1979; Kupfer et al. 1970; Mendels and Chernik 1973). Although few studies have examined the effects of lithium on circadian rhythms in bipolar patients, one study of a bipolar patient studied in depth revealed evidence for a significant and sustained lithium-induced delay in circadian core temperature and onset of REM, with a reduction in percentage of REM during total sleep time (Campbell et al. 1989). These data were consistent with earlier electroencephalogram findings in a series of manic-depressive patients (Kupfer et al. 1970, 1974). However, it has been difficult to demonstrate a clinical correlation of change in affective state with a lithium-induced resynchronization of circadian rhythms (Campbell et al. 1989; Kripke et al. 1978; Wehr and Goodwin 1979).

It is also of interest that data from earlier studies by Lewy and colleagues (1987) have demonstrated that bipolar patients appear to be supersensitive to light-induced reduction of nocturnal plasma melatonin levels. Wever (1979) has suggested that a pacemaker that has increased sensitivity to zeitgebers might become phase advanced relative to the slower intrinsic period of the human circadian oscillator. This observation is also of interest because melatonin has been reported to promote internal and external synchronization in both animals and humans. An alteration in relative melatonin concentrations might therefore be instrumental in dissociation between different circadian rhythms (Arendt et al. 1986; Gwinner and Benzinger 1978; Rao and Mager 1987). Furthermore, studies by Seggie and colleagues (1989) examining dark adaptation threshold have documented an increased sensitivity to light in bipolar patients that appears to be reduced in male patients under chronic lithium administration. Such a lithium-induced increase in dark adaptation threshold appears to be related to effects of lithium on the adenylyl cyclase (AC) second messenger system (Carney et al. 1988; Kaschka et al. 1987).

It remains a working hypothesis that the therapeutic action of lithium can be attributed to its efficacy in correcting a putative phase advance and/or internal desynchronization of these biological rhythms in patients with manic-depressive disorder. To what extent this hypothesis is related to lithium's action in directly altering the sensitivity of the intrinsic pacemaker to environmental cues and/or the coupling process between internal oscillators, through the suprachiasmatic nucleus or melatonin secretion, has yet to be determined.

■ Lithium and Neurotransmission

Serotonin

Extensive research has been devoted to lithium's effects on brain monoaminergic systems, and a leading current theory hypothesizes that lithium's antidepressant effects are due to an augmentation of serotonin (5-HT) function in the central nervous system (CNS) (de Montigny et al. 1983, 1988; Meltzer and Lowy 1987; Price et al. 1990). Preclinical studies show that lithium's effects on 5-HT function may occur at a variety of levels, including precursor uptake, synthesis, storage, catabolism, release, receptors, and receptor-effector interaction (Bunney and Garland 1984; Bunney and Garland-Bunney 1987; Goodnick and Gershon 1985; Knapp and Mandell 1975; Price et al. 1990). Overall, there is reasonable evidence from preclinical studies that lithium enhances serotonergic neurotransmission, although its effects on 5-HT appear to vary depending on brain region, length of treatment, and 5-HT receptor subtype (Bunney and Garland 1984; Bunney and Garland-Bunney 1987; Goodnick and Gershon 1985; Price et al. 1990; Wood and Goodwin 1987). Several preclinical studies show that tryptophan uptake and/or content are increased in synaptosomes and brain tissue after short-term and long-term treatment, whereas a single dose is without effect (Berggren 1987; Goodnick and Gershon 1985; Laakso and Oja 1979; Price et al. 1990; Swann et al. 1981; Tagliamonte et al. 1971).

Studies on the effects of short-term lithium on brain concentrations of 5-HT or 5-hydroxyindole-acetic acid (5-HIAA) have yielded conflicting results, although most tend to show increases in one or both (Berggren 1987; Goodnick and Gershon 1985; Price et al. 1990; Swann et al. 1981; Tagliamonte et al. 1971). In contrast, most long-term studies tend to show that 5-HT and 5-HIAA levels decrease with lithium administration (Ahluwalia and Singhal 1980; Bunney and Garland 1984; Collard 1978; Collard and Roberts 1977; Shukla 1985; Treiser et al. 1981). Treiser and colleagues (1981) found that long-term lithium increased basal and K^+-stimulated 5-HT release in hippocampus, but not in cortex. Another study also reported that lithium increased 5-HT release in parietal cortex, hypothalamus, and hippocampus after 2–3 weeks, but not after a single injection or 1 week of treatment (Friedman and Wang 1988).

Receptor-binding studies have shown complex, regionally specific effects of acute or chronic lithium on the density of $5-HT_1$ or $5-HT_2$ receptors, although most suggest decreases in both sites, at least in the hippocampus (Godfrey et al. 1989; Goodnick and Gershon 1985; Goodwin et al. 1986b; Hotta and Yamawaki 1988; Maggi and Enna 1980; Mizuta and Segawa 1989; Newman et al. 1990; Odagaki et al. 1990; Tanimoto et al. 1983; Treiser and Kellar 1980; Treiser et al. 1981). Similarly, the reported effects of both short-term and long-term lithium treatment on $5-HT_2$–mediated head-twitch behavior and hyperactivity responses to the 5-HT precursor 5-hydroxytryptophan (5-HTP) have been inconsistent (Friedman et al. 1979a; Goodwin et al. 1986b; Grahame-Smith and Green 1974; Harrison-Read 1979). However, the PRL response to 5-HT is more consistently reported to be increased after short-term lithium administration (Koenig et al. 1984; Meltzer and Lowy 1987; Meltzer et al. 1981). Recent studies have attempted to clarify the roles of pre- versus post-

synaptic receptors in mediating the effects of lithium on 5-HT function. Investigators using a variety of methodologies have provided evidence that lithium produces a subsensitivity of presynaptic inhibitory $5-HT_{1A}$ receptors (Friedman and Wang 1988; Goodwin et al. 1986a; Hotta and Yamawaki 1988; Mork and Geisler 1989a; Newman et al. 1990; Wang and Friedman 1988), which might result in a net increase of the amount of 5-HT released per impulse.

In a series of important preclinical investigations, de Montigny used electrophysiological recordings to measure the effects of lithium on the 5-HT system. Short-term lithium did not affect the responsiveness of the postsynaptic neuron to 5-HT nor the electrical activity of the 5-HT neurons, but it enhanced the efficacy of the ascending (presynaptic) 5-HT system (Blier and de Montigny 1985; Blier et al. 1987). These observations led de Montigny and colleagues to propose that lithium might increase the efficacy of other antidepressant treatments (Blier and de Montigny 1985; Blier et al. 1987). Several open and double-blind clinical investigations have demonstrated that approximately 50% of nonresponders are converted to responders upon lithium administration within 2 weeks (de Montigny et al. 1981, 1983; Heninger et al. 1983). Although these effects have been attributed to the net effect of presynaptic facilitation of 5-HT release onto "sensitized" receptors, convincing direct evidence of enhanced 5-HT function in humans has been difficult to obtain (Cowen et al. 1989; Manji et al. 1991b).

Many early cerebrospinal fluid (CSF) studies with human subjects are difficult to interpret because of their methodology and study design, and they are most often confounded by concomitant alterations in mood state and neurovegetative symptomatology. Small increases in CSF 5-HIAA levels have been reported after subchronic lithium treatment in bipolar patients (Berrettini et al. 1985a; Bowers and Heninger 1977; Fyro et al. 1975; Goodnick 1990; Goodnick and Gershon 1985; Linnoila et al. 1984; Price et al. 1990; Swann et al. 1987), and some studies have found a significant positive correlation between pretreatment levels of CSF 5-HIAA and lithium response (Bowers and Heninger 1977; Goodnick 1990; Goodnick and Gershon 1985). Although several studies have suggested that long-term lithium treatment "normalizes" a previously low platelet 5-HT uptake in bipolar patients, which may persist for several weeks after discontinuation (Born et al. 1980; Coppen et al. 1980;

Meltzer et al. 1983; Poirier et al. 1988), the effects of lithium treatment on [^{3}H]imipramine binding in platelets remain inconclusive (Meltzer and Lowy 1987; Poirier et al. 1988; Price et al. 1990; Wood et al. 1983). Neuroendocrine studies in patients have been more consistent, showing that acute or subacute lithium treatment results in augmented prolactin and/or cortisol responses to various challenges (e.g., fenfluramine, tryptophan, 5-HTP) in affectively ill patients (Cowen et al. 1989; Glue et al. 1986; McCance et al. 1989; Meltzer et al. 1984; Muhlbauer 1984; Muhlbauer and Muller-Oerlinghausen 1985; Price et al. 1989). However, recent studies in healthy volunteer subjects after 2 weeks of "therapeutic" lithium do not reveal increased neuroendocrine responses, suggesting that lithium's effect on the serotonergic system may depend on its underlying activity (Manji et al. 1991a).

Overall, current evidence from both preclinical and clinical studies supports a role for lithium in enhancing presynaptic activity in the serotonergic system in the brain. Direct studies of lithium's effects on serotonergic neurotransmission in humans have previously been limited by a number of factors: the complexity of the widespread distribution of serotonergic fibers throughout the brain, the multiple receptor subtypes (which have only been recently recognized), the relative lack of serotonin-specific pharmacological agents and outcome variables reflecting selective serotonergic responses, and inadequate attention to effects dependent on duration of treatment and affective or physiological state of the patient. With our current understanding of the molecular neurobiology of both receptor subtypes and the transporter in the serotonergic system, we anticipate newer and more specific pharmacological probes for future preclinical and clinical investigations.

Dopamine

The effect of lithium on dopamine (DA) synthesis and transmission has been investigated extensively in preclinical studies by directly determining changes in DA or homovanillic acid (HVA) and indirectly examining lithium-induced changes in DA-linked behaviors (Bunney and Garland 1984; Bunney and Garland-Bunney 1987; Goodnick and Gershon 1985). Studies in animals suggest that lithium may differentially affect DA pathways, increasing DA turnover in hypothalamic-tuberoinfundibular dopamine (TIDA) neurons, with conflicting reports about changes in brain stem areas (Corrodi et al. 1967; Goodnick and

Gershon 1985; Murphy 1976). Lithium administration has also been found to cause a dose-dependent decrease of DA formation (Ahluwalia and Singhal 1980; Ahluwalia et al. 1981; Engel and Berggren 1980; Eroglu et al. 1981; Frances et al. 1981; Friedman and Gershon 1973; Hesketh et al. 1978), which occurs at 25% lower doses in the striatum than in the limbic forebrain (Laakso and Oja 1979; Poitou and Bohuon 1975; Segal et al. 1975).

Based on the heuristic hypothesis that supersensitive DA receptors underlie the development of manic episodes, it has been postulated that lithium would prevent DA receptor supersensitivity (Bunney and Garland 1984; Bunney and Garland-Bunney 1987; Goodnick and Gershon 1985). In a series of studies, it was found that lithium prevented haloperidol-induced DA receptor upregulation (Bunney 1981; Rosenblatt et al. 1980; Verimer et al. 1980) and supersensitivity to iontophoretically applied DA or intravenous apomorphine (Gallager et al. 1978). Lithium treatment also partially prevented the development of electrical intracranial self-stimulation usually produced by haloperidol in rats (Bunney and Garland-Bunney 1987; Goodnick and Gershon 1985; Staunton et al. 1982a, 1982b). Thus, lithium appears to be effective in blocking both the behavioral and biochemical manifestations of supersensitive DA receptors induced by receptor blockade. Interestingly, there is significantly less evidence that lithium is effective in blocking DA receptor supersensitivity induced by other methods (i.e., tyrosine hydroxylase inhibitors, reserpine, or lesions of the DA pathways) (Beckmann et al. 1975; Bloom et al. 1981; Bunney 1981; Pert et al. 1978; Rosenblatt et al. 1980; Tanimoto et al. 1983; Verimer et al. 1980).

A proposed site of action for lithium's ability to block behavioral supersensitivity is the postsynaptic receptor and the prevention of haloperidol-induced increases in DA receptors. Although this is consistent with the observation that lithium can decrease locomotor activity even in the absence of presynaptic DA terminals (Swerdlow et al. 1985), lithium treatment does not result in any consistent effects on the density of D_1 or D_2 receptors. Reports purporting to show its ability to block the increase in DA receptor density following receptor blockade are conflicting. However, a study designed to examine lithium's effects on both pre- and postsynaptic DA receptors using different doses of apomorphine suggested that the drug was equally effective at both sites (Verimer et al.

1980). Indeed, electrophysiological data examining the effects of lithium on presynaptic DA receptors in the substantia nigra are also compatible with a blockade of DA receptor supersensitivity (Gallager et al. 1978). Thus, despite significant *functional* evidence, DA receptor binding studies have remained inconclusive, suggesting a possible postreceptor site of lithium action, possibly related to receptor-effector coupling. Interestingly, a number of studies have reported a lack of effect if lithium is administered *after* the induction of DA supersensitivity (Bloom et al. 1983; Klawans et al. 1976; Staunton et al. 1982a, 1982b), suggesting that in this model lithium exerts its greatest effects prophylactically.

Among the numerous behavioral effects of lithium in animals, perhaps the best studied are those on stimulant-induced activity. Lithium's ability to antagonize increases in locomotor activity produced by amphetamine have gained much attention, perhaps because this model has been postulated to represent a better representation of lithium's effects on manic behavior (Allikmets et al. 1979; Bunney and Garland-Bunney 1987; Goodnick and Gershon 1985; Klawans et al. 1976; Pert et al. 1978; Staunton et al. 1982a). It is also of interest that lithium has been reported to attenuate the euphoriant and motor-activating effects of oral amphetamine in depressed patients, although equivocal results have been observed upon methylphenidate challenge (Huey et al. 1981; van Kammen et al. 1985). Lithium has been shown to exert an inhibitory effect on intracranial self-stimulation subacutely. However, this effect does not persist with chronic administration, suggesting a possible lack of relevance to its long-term mood-stabilizing effects (Seeger et al. 1981).

Studies of DA and its metabolites in patients' CSF before and after lithium treatment have produced conflicting results (Berrettini et al. 1985a; Bowers and Heninger 1977; Fyro et al. 1975; Goodnick and Gershon 1985; Linnoila et al. 1983; Swann et al. 1987). A longitudinal study of one unipolar and seven bipolar patients who were women found that lithium reduced the levels of 3,4-dihydrophenylacetic acid (DOPAC), DA, and HVA in all the patients (Linnoila et al. 1983). But the possible role of alterations in mood state and motor activity remains a confounding variable, as it does for all clinical investigations using this research strategy. The administration of lithium to bipolar patients or control subjects does not significantly affect serum prolactin levels (Brown et al.

1981; Lal et al. 1978; Manji et al. 1991a; Rosenblatt et al. 1979), nor does it alter prolactin response to thyrotropin-releasing hormone in control subjects. However, in manic patients, lithium does appear to enhance thyrotropin-releasing hormone–stimulated prolactin response, which is once again suggestive of a differential response in patients versus control subjects (Tanimoto et al. 1981). Although data from human investigations are sparse, lithium's postulated ability to reduce both pre- and postsynaptic aspects of DA transmission represents an attractive mechanism for its antimanic therapeutic action.

Norepinephrine

Lithium's effects on norepinephrine (NE) have been reported to be specific for both time points and brain regions (Ahluwalia and Singhal 1981; Bliss and Ailion 1970; Cameron and Smith 1980; Colburn et al. 1967; Goodnick and Gershon 1985; Katz and Kopin 1969; Katz et al. 1968; Kuriyama and Speken 1970; Poitou and Bohuon 1975; Schildkraut et al. 1969; Stern et al. 1969; Wood et al. 1985). Most early studies conducted at single time points found no alterations in the levels of NE or the rate of synthesis. Subsequent investigations revealed biphasic effects, with early increases in labeled NE uptake into rat brain synaptosomes, and increases in the rate of NE synthesis, followed by a return to baseline values following chronic treatment (Ahluwalia and Singhal 1980; Cameron and Smith 1980; Colburn et al. 1967; Kuriyama and Speken 1970; Tanimoto et al. 1981). Both acute and chronic lithium have been reported to increase (Schildkraut et al. 1966, 1969) *or not to change* the turnover of NE in some but not all regions of the brain (Ahluwalia and Singhal 1980; Ho et al. 1970). Although these results suggested that lithium may increase the activity of the enzyme monoamine oxidase (MAO) subsequent data remain conflicting (Berrettini et al. 1979; Dawood and Welch 1979; Murphy 1976; Poitou and Bohuon 1975; Segal et al. 1975).

As is the case with the other neurotransmitters, the effects of lithium on NE receptor binding studies in rodent brain have been generally inconclusive (Maggi and Enna 1980; Schultz et al. 1981; Treiser and Kellar 1979). However, significant effects have been consistently observed on β-adrenergic receptor–mediated cyclic adenosine monophosphate (cAMP) accumulation, with lithium inhibiting the response both in vivo and in vitro (discussed in detail later in this chapter). Studies have also investigated the effects of chronic lithium on drug-induced changes in β-receptor sensitivity. Lithium was unable to block antidepressant-induced downregulation (Rosenblatt et al. 1979) and in fact produced a greater subsensitivity (i.e., cAMP response) (Mork et al. 1990), but it prevented reserpine or 6-hydroxydopamine–induced β-adrenergic receptor supersensitivity (Hermoni et al. 1980; Pert et al. 1979; Treiser and Kellar 1979). Additional data from preclinical and clinical studies suggest that lithium treatment results in subsensitive α_2 receptors (Catalano et al. 1984; Goodnick and Meltzer 1984a; Goodwin et al. 1986a; Huey et al. 1981; Murphy et al. 1974). In preclinical studies, long-term lithium attenuates α_2-adrenergic mediated behavioral effects (Goodwin et al. 1986a; Smith 1988) and presynaptic α_2 inhibition of NE release (Spengler et al. 1986) while enhancing K^+-evoked NE release (Ebstein et al. 1983).

Although lithium has been reported to reduce high-affinity platelet [^{3}H]clonidine binding (Garcia-Sevilla et al. 1986; Pandey et al. 1989; Wood and Coppen 1983), compatible with a functional "uncoupling" of the receptor from the G protein (Kim and Neubig 1987; Neubig et al. 1988), interpretation of these data is confounded by the coexistence of a newly discovered imidazoline-binding site. Additional clinical investigations of lithium reported a *decrease* in growth hormone response to clonidine (an α_2 partial agonist) in control subjects (Brambilla et al. 1988; Catalano et al. 1984). Lithium also appears to reverse the blunted growth hormone response observed in depressed patients (Brambilla et al. 1988). These bidirectional effects should serve to remind us that lithium's effects may depend in part on the preexisting set point of the neural substrate—an attractive notion in view of lithium's efficacy in the treatment of manic as well as depressive episodes.

In clinical investigations, both increases and decreases in plasma and urinary NE metabolite levels have been reported after lithium treatment (Beckmann et al. 1975; Corona et al. 1982; Goodnick 1990; Greenspan et al. 1970; Grof et al. 1986; Linnoila et al. 1983; Murphy et al. 1979; Schildkraut 1973, 1974; Swann et al. 1987). Lithium has been reported to reduce excretion of NE and metabolites in manic patients while increasing excretion in depressed patients, associated with higher plasma NE concentrations in some cases (Beckmann et al. 1975; Bowers and Heninger 1977; Greenspan et al. 1970; Schildkraut 1973). However, there is also evidence that uri-

nary excretion of 3-methoxy-4-hydroxyphenylglycol (MHPG) is low during bipolar depression and elevated during mania-hypomania (Bond et al. 1972; Jones et al. 1973; Post et al. 1977; Schildkraut et al. 1973; Wehr 1977). In part, these inconsistencies may be related to the inability to adequately control for state-dependent changes in affective states, with associated changes in activity level, arousal, and sympathetic outflow. Studies have demonstrated that 2 weeks of lithium administration in control subjects resulted in increases of urinary NE, normetanephrine, fractional NE release, and a trend toward significantly increased plasma NE, suggesting an enhanced neuronal release of NE (Manji et al. 1991a). These data are compatible with similar observations of increased plasma DHPG (dihydroxyphenylglycol, a major extraneuronal NE metabolite) levels (Poirier-Littre et al. 1993). Thus, current evidence supports an action of lithium in facilitating the release of NE, possibly through effects on the presynaptic α_2 "autoreceptor," and reducing the β-adrenergic stimulated AC response, which may contribute to lithium's attenuation of the euphorigenic effects of amphetamine.

Acetylcholine

Neurochemical, behavioral, and physiological studies suggest that the cholinergic system is involved in affective illness (Dilsaver and Coffman 1989) and that lithium alters the synaptic processing of ACh in rat brain. Early studies reporting an inhibitory effect on cholinergic activity utilized toxic concentrations of lithium (Krell and Goldberg 1973; Marchbanks 1982; Miyauchi et al. 1980), which replaced sodium and interfered with high-affinity transport of choline into cholinergic terminals required for synthesis of ACh (Jope 1979; Simon and Kuhar 1976). Addition of up to 1 mM Li in vitro has no effect on ACh synthesis or release; but chronic in vivo lithium treatment appears to increase ACh synthesis, choline transport, and ACh release in rat brain (Jope 1979; Simon and Kuhar 1976). Although some investigators have reported reductions in ACh levels in rat brain following subchronic administration (Ho and Tsai 1975; Krell and Goldberg 1973; Ronai and Vizi 1975), Jope (1979) has reported increased synthesis of ACh in cortex, hippocampus, and striatum following 10 days of lithium administration.

Several laboratories have investigated lithium's effects on the density of muscarinic receptors, with conflicting results (Kafka et al. 1982; Lerer and Stanley 1985; Levy et al. 1983; Maggi and Enna 1980; Tollefson and Senogles 1982). Chronic lithium has been reported to increase (Kafka et al. 1982; Lerer and Stanley 1985; Levy et al. 1983), decrease (Tollefson and Senogles 1982), or have no effect on (Maggi and Enna 1980) the binding of [^{3}H]quinuclidinyl benzilate (QNB) in various areas of rat brain; whereas in human caudate nucleus, lithium is reported to reduce the affinity of [^{3}H]QNB binding. The effects of lithium on both up- and downregulation of muscarinic receptors in brain has also been investigated. Although there have been reports that lithium is able to abolish the increase in [^{3}H]QNB binding produced by atropine but is without effect on the downregulation induced by the cholinesterase inhibitor diisopropylfluorophosphonate (DFP), these data vary and are inconclusive (Lerer and Stanley 1985; Levy et al. 1983).

We have examined both receptor binding and muscarinic receptor–coupled phosphoinositide (PI) response in rat hippocampus during atropine-induced upregulation (Ellis and Lenox 1990) and have found that chronic treatment with atropine results in an upregulation of muscarinic receptors and a supersensitivity of the PI response in the hippocampus. Coadministration of chronic lithium prevented the development of the supersensitivity of the muscarinic receptor PI response, without significantly affecting the extent of upregulation of receptor binding sites. These findings are consistent with an effect of chronic lithium on upregulation of neuronal muscarinic receptors observed in neuroblastoma cells (Liles and Nathanson 1988). They suggest that lithium's actions are exerted at a point beyond the receptor binding site, possibly affecting the coupling of the newly upregulated receptors at the level of the signal-transducing G proteins. Thus, similar to the case for dopaminergic and β-adrenergic receptors, it has been suggested that lithium can block the development of cholinergic receptor supersensitivity.

In behavioral studies, chronic lithium is reported to enhance a number of cholinergically mediated responses, including catalepsy and hypothermia. The effect of lithium on pilocarpine-induced catalepsy and hypothermia was of the same order of magnitude as the enhancement induced by chronic scopolamine pretreatment. Combined administration of both pretreatments resulted in additive effects, suggesting that different mechanisms may be involved (Dilsaver and Hariharan 1988; Lerer and Stanley 1985; Russell et al.

1981). Of interest in this regard is a study by Dilsaver and Hariharan (1989), which reported that chronic lithium treatment results in a supersensitivity of nicotine-induced hypothermia in rats. Perhaps the most striking example of lithium's ability to potentiate muscarinic responses comes from the lithium-pilocarpine seizure model (Hirvonen et al. 1990; Honchar et al. 1983; Jope et al. 1986; Ormandy and Jope 1991; Persinger et al. 1988; Terry et al. 1990). In large doses, pilocarpine and other muscarinic agonists cause prolonged and usually lethal seizures in rats. Although lithium alone is not a convulsant, pretreatment with lithium increases the sensitivity of pilocarpine almost 20-fold (Hirvonen et al. 1990; Honchar et al. 1983; Jope et al. 1986; Ormandy and Jope 1991; Persinger et al. 1988; Terry et al. 1990). Significantly, this behavioral effect of lithium is markedly attenuated by intracerebroventricular administration of myoinositol in both rats and mice (Kofman et al. 1991; Tricklebank et al. 1991), representing perhaps the best correlation between a biochemical and behavioral effect of lithium (see section on "Phosphoinositide Turnover").

A synergism with the cholinergic system also occurs in electrophysiological studies in hippocampal slices, in which pilocarpine and lithium together (but neither alone) produce spontaneous epileptiform bursting (Jope et al. 1986; Ormandy and Jope 1991). Elegant studies of rat hippocampus have demonstrated that lithium can reverse muscarinic agonist–induced desensitization, an effect that is mediated through PI hydrolysis and can be reversed by inositol (Pontzer and Crews 1990). Studies by Evans and colleagues (1990) have suggested that lithium's role in lithium-pilocarpine seizures is to increase excitatory transmission through a presynaptic facilitatory effect. Lithium alone also augmented synaptic responses, and this effect of lithium could be blocked by a PKC inhibitor. These results suggest that lithium's effects in this model may occur through a PKC-mediated presynaptic facilitation of neurotransmitter release. Biochemical, electrophysiological, and behavioral data suggest that chronic lithium administration stimulates ACh synthesis and release in rat brain, and potentiates some cholinergic mediated physiological events. Interestingly, similar to the situation observed with the catecholaminergic system, pharmacological studies indicate that chronic lithium prevents muscarinic receptor supersensitivity, most likely through postreceptor mechanisms.

Gamma-Aminobutyric Acid (GABA) and Neuropeptides

In contrast with the abundant literature on lithium's effects on monoamine neurotransmitters, much less work has been conducted on the amino acid neurotransmitters and neuropeptides (Bernasconi 1982; Lloyd et al. 1987; Nemeroff 1991). Studies have suggested that previously low levels of plasma and CSF GABA are normalized in bipolar patients being treated with lithium (Berrettini et al. 1983, 1986), paralleling reported GABA changes observed in several regions of rat brain (Ahluwalia et al. 1981; Gottesfeld et al. 1971; Maggi and Enna 1980). It is worth noting that, following withdrawal of chronic lithium, GABA levels return to normal in striatum and midbrain but remain elevated in the pons-medulla (Ahluwalia et al. 1981), possibly due to reportedly elevated levels of the GABA-synthesizing enzyme glutamic acid decarboxylase. Lithium has also been postulated to prevent GABA uptake, and chronic lithium administration was shown to significantly decrease low affinity [³H]GABA sites in corpus striatum and hypothalamus (Maggi and Enna 1980). Because lithium has no effect on in vitro [³H]GABA binding, these receptor changes have been interpreted as downregulation secondary to activation of the GABAergic system (Maggi and Enna 1980). Although the clinical relevance of these findings remains unclear, it is significant that decreases in CSF GABA have been reported in depressed patients (Berrettini et al. 1982; Post et al. 1980b).

Among the peptides, the opioid system has been the most extensively studied. Lithium administration has been reported to produce time- and dose-dependent increases in Met-enkephalin and Leu-enkephalin levels in the basal ganglia and nucleus accumbens, and to increase dynorphin levels (as determined by immunoreactive dynorphin A [1-8] peptide) in the striatum (Sivam et al. 1986, 1988). The lithium-induced increase in dynorphin was accompanied by an increase in the abundance of prodynorphin messenger ribonucleic acid (mRNA) (Sivam et al. 1988), suggesting that the effects on the levels are at least partially mediated through increased transcription and translation (see "Discussion" section). Acute studies with lithium have demonstrated enhanced release of a number of opioid peptides from hypothalamic slices and have suggested an effect at the inhibitory presynaptic opioid autoreceptor (Burns et al. 1990). Chronic lithium ad-

ministration did not affect the basal hypothalamic release of any of the opioids, but prevented the naloxone-stimulated release of the peptides in vitro, compatible with lithium-induced autoreceptor subsensitivity (Burns et al. 1990).

Lithium is reported to decrease the affinity of opiate receptors in vitro, whereas subchronic lithium administration is reported in some but not all studies to decrease the number of opioid-binding sites in rat forebrain structures (Goodnick and Gershon 1985). Additional support for effects on the opioidergic system comes from the behavioral studies in which lithium produces aversive states in rats that can be blocked by the depletion of central pools of β-endorphin or by the blockade of μ-opioid receptors. It has also been demonstrated that chronic lithium administration abolishes both the secondary reinforcing effects of morphine and the aversive effects of the opioid antagonist naloxone (Blancquaert et al. 1987; Lieblich and Yirmiya 1987; Mucha and Herz 1985; Shippenberg and Herz 1991; Shippenberg et al. 1988).

Lithium has been shown to increase the substance P content of striatum when it is chronically administered to rats, an effect that is antagonized by the concurrent administration of haloperidol (Hong et al. 1983). More recent studies have demonstrated a lithium-induced increase in tachykinin levels that appears to be associated with an increase in transcription of the rat preprotachykinin gene (Sivam et al. 1989). Studies of the effects of subchronic lithium on regional brain concentrations of substance P, neurokinin A, calcitonin gene-related peptide (CGRP), and neuropeptide Y have demonstrated a regionally specific increase in the immunoreactivity of all the peptides except CGRP, which was significantly decreased in the pituitary gland (Mathe et al. 1990). In one of the few applicable clinical studies, CSF levels of various pro-opiomelanocortin (POMC) peptides were examined in euthymic bipolar patients before and during lithium treatment. No significant effects of lithium on the CSF levels of any of the peptides were observed (Berrettini et al. 1985b, 1987).

Similarly to carbamazepine and valproic acid, lithium may facilitate certain aspects of GABAergic neurotransmission through several mechanisms. The clinical relevance of these findings at this point remains largely unknown. However, as one of the few systems likewise affected by the other commonly used mood stabilizers, the GABAergic system is worthy of more carefully controlled investigation. With respect to the peptides, only the opioidergic system has been studied to any extent. The bulk of the evidence suggests that lithium facilitates presynaptic opioidergic function while antagonizing certain opioid-mediated effects. The preliminary reports of effects of alterations in the levels of tachykinins in the striatum may be intriguing in view of the commonly observed lithium-induced side effects of tremor.

■ Lithium and Signal Transduction

Phosphoinositide Turnover

In recent years, research on the molecular mechanisms underlying lithium's therapeutic effects has focused on intracellular second messenger generating systems, and in particular on receptor-coupled hydrolysis of phosphatidylinositol-4,5-bisphosphate (PIP_2) (Baraban et al. 1989). At therapeutically relevant concentrations in humans, lithium is a potent inhibitor of the intracellular enzyme inositol monophosphatase (K_i 0.8 mM) within the hydrolytic pathway of PIP_2, which results in an accumulation of inositol monophosphate (IP) and a reduction in the generation of free inositol (Allison and Stewart 1971; Hallcher and Sherman 1980; Sherman et al. 1986). Lithium has also been shown to have additional potential sites of action in the PI cycle, where it has been reported to inhibit the inositol polyphosphatase that dephosphorylates $I(1,3,4)P_3$ and $I(1,4)P_2$. Because the brain has limited access to inositol other than that derived from recycling of inositol phosphates, the ability of a cell to maintain sufficient supplies of myoinositol can be crucial to the resynthesis of the PIs and the maintenance and efficiency of signaling (Sherman 1991). Furthermore, because the mode of enzyme inhibition is *uncompetitive,* lithium's effects have been postulated to be most pronounced in systems undergoing the highest rate of PIP_2 hydrolysis (see reviews in Nahorski et al. 1991, 1992).

Thus, Berridge and colleagues (1982) first proposed that the physiological consequence of lithium's action is derived through the relative depletion of free inositol. Its selectivity could be attributed to its preferential action in the brain, resulting in suppression of PI hydrolysis in the most overactive receptor-mediated neuronal pathways (Berridge 1989; Berridge et al. 1989). Because several subtypes of adrenergic (e.g., α_1), cholinergic (e.g., m_1, m_3, m_5),

serotonergic (e.g., 5-HT_2, 5-HT_{1C}), and dopaminergic (e.g., D_1) receptors are coupled to PIP_2 turnover in the CNS (Fisher et al. 1992; Mahan et al. 1990; Rana and Hokin 1990; Vallar et al. 1990), this hypothesis offers a plausible explanation for lithium's therapeutic efficacy in treating both poles of manic-depressive disorder by the compensatory stabilization of an inherent biogenic amine imbalance in critical regions of the brain (Lenox 1987).

Studies have been carried out to examine the effects of lithium on receptor-mediated PI response in brain in a number of neurotransmitter systems (e.g., cholinergic, serotonergic, noradrenergic, and histaminergic). Although some investigators have found a reduction in agonist-stimulated PIP_2 hydrolysis in brain slices from rats exposed acutely and chronically to lithium, these findings have often been small, inconsistent, and subject to methodological differences (Casebolt and Jope 1989; Ellis and Lenox 1990; Godfrey et al. 1989; Kendall and Nahorski 1987; Whitworth and Kendall 1989). Muscarinic receptor–mediated PIP_2 turnover appears to be a major site of action exerted by lithium in vivo. Early studies that were later replicated have demonstrated that the increase in IP and reduction in brain myoinositol content induced by lithium is significantly enhanced by the coadministration of the cholinergic agonist pilocarpine, and blocked by pretreatment with cholinergic antagonists (i.e., atropine and scopolamine) (Allison 1978; Allison et al. 1976; Sherman et al. 1986). In addition, there are studies of rat and mouse cerebral cortical slices that have revealed potent inhibitory effects of lithium on muscarinic-stimulated IP_3 and IP_4 accumulation (Kennedy et al. 1989, 1990; Whitworth and Kendall 1988). In these cases, the effects of lithium occur after a characteristic lag of 5–10 minutes, suggesting an indirect mechanism consistent with the inositol depletion hypothesis noted previously. Furthermore, as we have also noted, studies from our laboratory have provided data in support of an indirect effect of chronic lithium in rat brain on the coupling of newly upregulated muscarinic receptor sites to the PI response (Ellis and Lenox 1990; Lenox and Ellis 1990; Lenox et al. 1991).

Several lines of evidence suggest that the action of chronic lithium may not simply be directly manifest in receptor-mediated activity coupled to this second messenger pathway. Although investigators have observed that levels of inositol in brain remain reduced in rats receiving chronic lithium (Sherman et al. 1985), it has been difficult to demonstrate that this results in a reduction in the resynthesis of PIP_2, which is the substrate for agonist-induced PI turnover. However, this may be attributable to a small, rapidly turned over signal-related pool of PIP_2, and/or recent evidence that resynthesis of inositol phospholipids may also occur through base exchange reactions from other larger pools of phospholipids such as phosphatidylcholine. An initial attempt to verify this hypothesis at this level of the PI cycle by examining the effects of lithium on muscarinic-stimulated accumulation of IP_1 in brain slices in the presence of exogenously added inositol were unsuccessful (Kendall and Nahorski 1987). More recently, studies examining the effects of chronic lithium on $I(1,4,5)P_3$ mass in cortical slices have demonstrated a time-dependent decline that is attentuated in the presence of high concentrations of inositol (Kennedy et al. 1990; Varney et al. 1992). Further evidence in support of the inositol depletion hypothesis of lithium action has been observed in studies examining the diacyl-glycerol (DAG) arm of the PIP_2 resynthesis pathway (see subsection on "Protein Kinase C").

Although pharmacological concentrations of extracellular inositol has been reported to attenuate some of lithium's biochemical, behavioral, and toxic effects, in recent animal studies, the addition of inositol appeared to *prevent* but did not *reverse* the effects of lithium on the PI system (Kennedy et al. 1990; Kofman and Belmaker 1993; Maslanski et al. 1992; Tricklebank et al. 1991). Most importantly, the therapeutic actions of lithium occur only after chronic treatment and remain in evidence long after discontinuation—actions that cannot be attributed only to inositol reductions evident in the presence of lithium. These findings suggest that although the action of lithium may initiate with alteration in receptor-coupled PI response and a relative depletion of inositol, the effects of chronic lithium administration may be mediated by resultant changes in long-term messengers on molecular targets at different levels of the signal transduction process. The possible role of G proteins and PKC as sites for the action of chronic lithium in brain is discussed later in this chapter.

Adenylyl Cyclase

The other major receptor-coupled second messenger system in which lithium has been shown to have significant effects is AC, which generates cAMP (Belmaker 1981). Cyclic AMP accumulation by vari-

ous neurotransmitters and hormones is reported to be inhibited by lithium at therapeutic concentrations both in vivo and in vitro, but the sensitivity appears to be less than that observed in the PI system (Andersen and Geisler 1984; Ebstein et al. 1980; Forn and Valdecasas 1971; Geisler and Klysner 1985; Geisler et al. 1985; Mork and Geisler 1987, 1989a, 1989b, 1989c; Newman and Belmaker 1987). NE- and adenosine-stimulated cAMP accumulation in rat cortical slices are inhibited significantly by 1–2 mM Li; in human brain tissue, the IC_{50} for lithium inhibition of NE-stimulated cAMP accumulation is approximately 5 mM (Newman et al. 1983). Studies in humans have demonstrated that lithium treatment at therapeutic levels results in an attenuation of the plasma cAMP increase in response to epinephrine (Ebstein et al. 1976; Friedman et al. 1979b), as well as evidence for an attenuation in adrenergic receptor coupling to AC in peripheral cells (Risby et al. 1991). In fact, lithium inhibition of vasopressin-sensitive or thyroid-stimulating hormone (TSH)–sensitive AC is thought to contribute to the commonly observed side effects of nephrogenic diabetes insipidus and hypothyroidism seen in patients being treated with lithium over an extended period (Dousa 1974; Wolff et al. 1970).

Lithium attenuation of β-adrenoceptor–stimulated AC activity has also been shown in membrane, slice, and synaptosomal preparations from rat brain in vitro and ex vivo (Andersen and Geisler 1984; Ebstein et al. 1980; Geisler and Klysner 1985; Geisler et al. 1985; Mork and Geisler 1987, 1989a, 1989b, 1989c; Newman and Belmaker 1987). However, Godfrey (1989) reported no change in isoproterenol-stimulated AC response in rat cortical slices after 3 days of lithium treatment. Most recently, our laboratory has demonstrated similar results using in vivo microdialysis in cortex of rats exposed to chronic lithium administration (Manji et al. 1991b; Masana et al. 1992). Postreceptor stimulation of AC (e.g., with forskolin [colforsin], fluoride, or nonhydrolyzable analogues of guanosine triphosphate [GTP]) has also been shown to be inhibited by lithium in slices and membranes from rat cerebral cortices (Andersen and Geisler 1984; Geisler et al. 1985; Mork and Geisler 1987; Newman and Belmaker 1987), and several studies have also revealed lithium-induced increases in basal cAMP.

Lithium in vitro inhibits the stimulation of AC by guanyl imidodiphosphate, or Gpp(NH)p (a poorly hydrolyzable analogue of GTP), and calcium-calmodulin, both of which can be overcome by Mg^{2+} (Andersen and Geisler 1984; Mork and Geisler 1989b; Newman and Belmaker 1987). Lithium also competes with both Mg^{2+} and Ca^{2+} for membrane-binding sites, and lithium's inhibition of solubilized catalytic unit of AC can also be overcome by Mg^{2+}. These findings suggest that lithium's inhibition of AC in vitro may be due to competition with Mg^{2+} on a site on the catalytic unit of AC (Andersen and Geisler 1984; Newman and Belmaker 1987). However, the inhibitory effects of chronic lithium treatment on rat brain AC are not reversed by Mg^{2+}, and these effects still persist after washing of the membranes but are reversed by increasing concentrations of GTP (Mork and Geisler 1989b). These results suggest that the physiologically relevant effects of lithium (i.e., those seen on chronic drug administration and not reversed immediately with drug discontinuation) may be exerted at the level of signal-transducing G proteins at a GTP-responsive step.

G Proteins

Because lithium has been shown to affect both PI turnover and AC activity, recent research has focused on mechanisms shared by these two major second messenger generating systems, namely the signal-transducing G proteins. Thus, neurotransmitter function might be modulated through alterations in intracellular signaling. Lithium might be effective because it alters the postsynaptic signal generated in response to a number of endogenous neurotransmitters (see review in Manji 1992). Multiple receptors converge onto a single G protein, but individual receptors may also "talk" to more than one G protein. Likewise, single G proteins may modulate more than one effector, and several G proteins may also converge on a single effector. Thus, the G proteins are in a position to coordinate receptor-effector activity critical to the regulation of neuronal function, thereby maintaining a functional balance between neurotransmitter systems in brain. In addition, these signaling proteins may represent attractive targets to explain lithium's efficacy in treating both poles of manic-depressive disorder.

As we have noted, experimental evidence has shown that lithium may alter receptor coupling to PI turnover in the absence of consistent changes in the density of the receptor sites themselves. Because fluoride ion will directly activate G protein–coupled sec-

ond messenger response, efforts have been made to examine the effect of lithium on sodium fluoride–stimulated PI response in brain. Although Godfrey and colleagues (1989) reported a 21% reduction of fluoride-stimulated PI response in cortical membranes of rats treated with lithium for 3 days, no change in response was observed in cortical slices from rats administered lithium for 30 days. In a more recent study of chronic lithium administration in rats, Song and Jope (1992) reported an attenuation of PI turnover in response to GTP analogues, even in the presence of labeled PI as a substrate. Avissar and colleagues (1988) reported that lithium dramatically eliminated isoproterenol- and carbachol-induced increases in $[^3H]$GTP binding in rat cerebral cortical membranes in the presence of 0.6 mM lithium chloride and in washed cortical membranes from rats treated with lithium carbonate for 2–3 weeks. In animals withdrawn from lithium for 2 days, agonist-stimulated response returned.

Follow-up studies in humans have reported a normalization of previously elevated agonist-induced $[^3H]$GTPγ S binding in leukocytes from lithium-treated euthymic bipolar patients (Schreiber et al. 1991). These studies have been of heuristic interest, and considerable data suggest an action of lithium at the level of G protein. However, such a *direct* action of lithium on G protein function has been difficult to replicate in light of several methodological problems. First, similar studies in other laboratories have been difficult in light of an inability to identify reliable agonist-induced binding of labeled GTP in the brain due to significant nonspecific binding and variable hydrolysis of the GTP. Attempts to replicate these effects of both acute and chronic lithium, not only in brain but also in other tissues, such as platelets and heart using agonist-induced release of labeled nonhydrolyzable GTP analogues were unsuccessful (Ellis and Lenox 1991). If there existed such marked sensitivity of G protein activation to the lithium ion, routine assays of coupled second messenger responses such as agonist-stimulated hydrolysis of PI in brain slices in the presence of 10 mM lithium chloride would be impossible. Furthermore, standard preparations of GTP salts are compounded with lithium and have been used for years to study G protein function.

Investigations have also addressed the role of G proteins in the action of lithium-induced attenuation of receptor-mediated AC activity in both rodents and humans. In a series of studies using in vivo microdialysis measurements of cAMP to assess lithium's effects on G proteins in the intact animal, chronic lithium treatment produced a significant increase in basal and postreceptor-stimulated (cholera toxin or forskolin [colforsin]) AC activity, while attenuating the β-adrenergic mediated effect in rat frontal cortex or hippocampus. In addition, pertussis toxin–catalyzed [^{32}P]adenosine 5′–diphosphate (ADP)-ribosylation in membranes from these brain regions of lithium-treated animals was significantly increased (Manji et al. 1991b; Masana et al. 1992). Because pertussis toxin selectively ADP-ribosylates the undissociated, inactive αβγ heterotrimeric form of G_i, these results suggest that chronic lithium administration may reduce activation of G_i through a stabilization of the inactive conformation (Manji et al. 1991b; Masana et al. 1992). If dissociation of G protein subunits were inhibited by lithium, this could decrease β-adrenergic–stimulated AC activity while simultaneously producing a relative stabilization of the receptor in a high-affinity state.

These observations in animals are supported by data from a clinical investigation of control subjects who had 2 weeks of lithium administration. Basal- and postreceptor-stimulated AC activity was increased in platelets, associated with a 40% increase in pertussis toxin catalyzed [^{32}P]ADP-ribosylation in platelet membranes (Hsiao et al. 1992). Once again, these data suggest a stabilization of the inactive undissociated αβγ heterotrimeric form of G_i. At present, the possible effects of chronic lithium administration on the absolute *levels* of $G\alpha_s$ and $G\alpha_i$ remain unclear—two independent laboratories have not observed any alterations (Li et al. 1991; Manji et al. 1991a; Masana et al. 1992), whereas another has reported small but significant decreases in the levels of the α_s, α_{i1}, and α_{i2} in rat frontal cortex (Colin et al. 1991). However, chronic lithium administration in rats has been shown to reduce the levels of mRNA for a number of G proteins in brain, including $G\alpha_{i1}$, $G\alpha_{i2}$, and $G\alpha_s$ (Colin et al. 1991; Li et al. 1991). The possibility that these intriguing effects of lithium on G protein mRNA are mediated through PKC is suggested by a study demonstrating that PKC activation produces a similar decrease in $G\alpha_s$ mRNA and $G\alpha_{i2}$ mRNA levels in cells in vitro (Thiele and Eipper 1990).

At present, the molecular mechanism(s) underlying lithium's effects on G proteins has yet to be fully established. Although there is evidence that competition with magnesium accounts for some of lithium's in vitro effects on G proteins, and speculation that an interaction with GTP binding might be relevant to the chronic effects of lithium, a *direct* effect of lithium on guanine nucleotide activation of G protein remains unsubstantiated. Long-term effects of chronic lithium on G protein may more likely be attributable to an indirect posttranslational modification of the G protein(s) and a relative change in the dynamic equilibrium of the active/inactive states of protein conformation, potentially resulting in modulation of receptor-mediated signaling in critical regions of the brain.

Protein Kinase C

The accumulating evidence discussed here suggests that at least some of lithium's critical effects are mediated through long-term processes set in motion during the brain's exposure to lithium. In this context, it is noteworthy that, as a result of inositol depletion in the presence of lithium, metabolites within the phospholipid portion of the hydrolytic pathway that include DAG, phosphatidic acid, and cytidine monophosphate-phosphatidate (CMP-PA) have been shown to be significantly elevated in a variety of cell types, including brain. This effect can be prevented in the presence of high concentrations of inositol (Brami et al. 1991a, 1991b; Downes and Stone 1986; Drummond and Raeburn 1984; Godfrey et al. 1989; Watson et al. 1990). This might be expected, because the end metabolite in this pathway (i.e., CMP-PA) requires free myoinositol to resynthesize inositol phosphates for the regeneration of PIP_2. Thus, depletion of cellular inositol interferes with the recycling of the system, resulting in the consequent accumulation of CMP-PA and its metabolite DAG. Thus, the action(s) of both acute and chronic lithium (e.g., inhibition of agonist-mediated PI turnover) may stem initially from its potent effect in inhibiting the recycling of inositol through the receptor-mediated hydrolysis of PIP_2. Ultimately, this may be explained by lithium's indirect action in accumulating DAG and subsequent changes in the activation of the family of PKC isozymes.

Evidence accumulating from various laboratories, including our own, points to a role for PKC in mediating the effects of lithium in a number of cell systems, including the brain (see review in Manji and Lenox 1994). Currently available data suggest that acute lithium exposure often mimics the action of phorbol ester and facilitates several PKC-mediated responses. Longer-term exposure results in an attenuation of phorbol ester–mediated responses, which may be accompanied by a downregulation of PKC (Anderson et al. 1988; Bitran et al. 1990; Evans et al. 1990; Lenox et al. 1992b; Lenox and Watson 1992; Manji et al. 1993; Reisine and Zatz 1987; Wang and Friedman 1989; Zatz and Reisine 1985).

Interestingly, this pattern of effects is seen both in cultured cells in vitro and in brain in vivo. Acute lithium exposure (< 2 mM) stimulates adrenocorticotropic hormone (ACTH) secretion in cultured anterior pituitary cells (AtT20), and the magnitude of the response is similar to that observed with other secretogogues, including phorbol ester. Pretreatment of the cells with lithium for 3 hours not only markedly desensitizes the ACTH response to subsequent lithium exposure, but also significantly attenuates the response to subsequent phorbol ester exposure (Reisine and Zatz 1987; Zatz and Reisine 1985). These results, accompanied by the observations that lithium pretreatment *does not* modify the ACTH response to other secretogogues (including corticotropin-releasing factor [CRF], potassium, isoproterenol, or forskolin [colforsin]), strongly suggests a role for PKC in mediating lithium's effects. Similarly, chronic (i.e., 5- to 8-day) exposure to 1 mM lithium chloride in HL60 cells markedly attenuates the Na^+/H^+ antiporter activity in response to both chemotactic receptor or phorbol ester stimulation (Bitran et al. 1990). These results are consistent with our recent observations that chronic exposure of these cells to 1 mM lithium also results in a marked and significant decrease in the immunolabeling of $PKC\alpha$ isozyme in both cytosolic and membrane fractions (Bitran et al., in press).

Biochemical studies have revealed biphasic effects of lithium on PKC-mediated events in rat hippocampus. Thus, acute (i.e., 3-day) lithium exposure augments 5-HT release, whereas chronic (i.e., 3-week) lithium exposure at "therapeutic" levels attenuates both the phorbol ester–induced cytosol to membrane PKC translocation and [^{3}H]5-HT release in hippocampus (Anderson et al. 1988; Sharp et al. 1991; Wang and Friedman 1989). In a series of studies in rat hippocampus, two major protein substrates for PKC—with apparent molecular masses of 45 kDa and 83 kDa—display reduced in vitro phosphorylation following chronic in vivo exposure to lithium (i.e.,

3–4 weeks) at therapeutic levels (Lenox et al. 1992b). Using immunoblot analysis, the 83-kDa protein has been identified as a known myristoylated alanine-rich C kinase substrate (MARCKS) implicated in presynaptic neurotransmitter release and calmodulin/calcium regulation in brain, and it has been found to be significantly reduced in hippocampus after chronic lithium exposure (Blackshear 1993; Lenox et al. 1992b). Because phorbol ester exposure has been associated with a reduction in expression of MARCKS protein in cells, these data are consistent with the mediation of the long-term action of lithium through activation of PKC (Linder et al. 1992; Wang and Friedman 1989).

Chronic administration of lithium (i.e., 5 weeks) also has been shown to result in a dramatic decrease in membrane-associated [^{3}H]PDBu (phorbol [12,13] dibutyrate) binding in both CA_1 and subicular regions of rat hippocampus, consistent with data demonstrating that chronic lithium exposure attenuates long-term potentiation in the hippocampal CA_1 region (Manji et al. 1993). Furthermore, immunoblotting revealed an isozyme-specific decrease in the amount of $PKC\alpha$, which has been particularly implicated in mediating neurohormone release that is known to be affected by chronic lithium.

Although such data provide intriguing evidence for an action of chronic lithium on long-term cellular events through changes in PKC activation, the precise mechanism remains to be demonstrated. Because PKC activation is often followed by a rapid proteolytic degradation of the enzyme, a prolonged increase in DAG levels by chronic lithium may lead to an increased membrane translocation and subsequent degradation and downregulation of PKC isozymes (Huang 1989; Kishimoto et al. 1989; Nishizuka 1992). Such a mechanism would be consistent with data indicating that lithium acutely activates PKC, whereas prolonged treatment is associated with reduced phorbol ester–mediated responses, including neurotransmitter release (Anderson et al. 1988; Bitran et al. 1990; Evans et al. 1990; Lenox et al. 1992b; Manji et al. 1993; Reisine and Zatz 1987; Sharp et al. 1991; Wang and Friedman 1989; Zatz and Reisine 1985). On the other hand, there is evidence that membrane translocation, degradation, and conversion of PKC to a constitutively active phorbol-insensitive form (PKM) may play a role in at least some of the PKC-mediated events observed following chronic lithium exposure (Manji and Lenox 1994). PKC isozymes involved in such a process may account for regulation of the expression of MARCKS observed in cells exposed to either long-term phorbol ester or chronic lithium, and they may ultimately play a role in the action of lithium at a nuclear level.

■ Lithium and Gene Expression

In recent years, it has become increasingly apparent that any relevant biochemical model of lithium's actions must account for its special clinical profile (i.e., prophylactic efficacy against the cyclic episodes of both mania and depression, which normally requires weeks to develop) (Goodwin and Jamison 1990). Biochemical changes requiring such prolonged administration of a drug suggest alterations at the genomic level. In this context, increasing evidence suggests that lithium affects gene expression, possibly through PKC-induced alterations in nuclear transcription regulatory factors responsible for modulating the expression of specific genes. Several recent studies have demonstrated that lithium alters *fos* expression in different cell systems including the brain through a PKC-mediated mechanism (reviewed in Manji and Lenox 1994). Preincubation of cultured PC12 cells (a rat pheochromocytoma cell line) with lithium for 16 hours markedly potentiates *fos* expression in response to the muscarinic agonist carbachol. Lithium pretreatment in these cells also potentiates *fos* expression in response to phorbol esters, which bypass PI turnover (Divish et al. 1991; Kalasapudi et al. 1990). Moreover, lithium's effects show a selectivity for the PKC signal transduction pathway. In this case, they do not appear to be due to a nonspecific alteration in mRNA stability, because the *fos* expression in response to AC activation is unaffected under identical conditions (Divish et al. 1991; Kalasapudi et al. 1990).

Paralleling the results observed in cell culture, a single intraperitoneal injection of lithium results in an augmentation of pilocarpine-induced *fos* gene expression in rat brain, which can be antagonized by the M_1 muscarinic antagonist pirenzepine (Weiner et al. 1991). These lithium-induced effects on the expression of *fos* mRNA, which are generally thought to represent a "master switch" that turns on a "second wave" of specific neuronal genes of functional importance, offer a mechanism for affecting long-term events in the brain.

Long-term regulation of synaptic function, as we have noted, can also result from a modification in receptors and their regulation, G proteins, effectors, proteins involved in neurotransmitter release, and enzymes involved in neurotransmitter biosynthesis. A recent study (Gao et al. 1993) has demonstrated that incubation of cerebellar granule cells with 1.5 mM lithium results in biphasic effects on the levels of both *fos* mRNA and muscarinic M_3 receptor mRNA (i.e., an early increase followed by a decline in the expression of both messages after an incubation period of several days). These data are consistent with the previously noted acute versus chronic effects of lithium on PKC-mediated responses, potentially acting through the regulation of the induction of transcriptional factors. Crucial to this discussion is evidence that *chronic,* "therapeutic," in vivo administration of lithium also significantly changes the expression of a number of genes in rat brain, several of which are known neuromodulatory peptide hormones (i.e., prodynorphin, preprotachykinin) and their receptors (i.e., glucocorticoid Type II) and peptides containing PKC-responsive elements in their gene (neuropeptide Y) (Kislauskis and Dobner 1990; Pfeiffer et al. 1991; Sivam et al. 1988, 1989; Weiner et al. 1992).

In view of lithium's proposed actions on signal-transducing systems, it is noteworthy that *chronic* lithium administration (i.e., 3–4 weeks) has been reported to alter the *expression* of various components of second messenger–generating systems, including $G\alpha_{i1}$, $G\alpha_{i2}$, and $G\alpha_s$ mRNA, and AC Type I and Type II mRNA in rat brain (Colin et al. 1991; Li et al. 1991). Long-term modulation of the genetic expression of critical proteins involved in the regulation of synaptic and transmembrane signaling in the brain offers a new strategy for unraveling the complex physiological effects of chronic lithium exposure in the prophylaxis of recurrent episodes of affective illness in patients with manic-depressive disorder.

■ INDICATIONS

■ Psychiatric Indications

Affective Disorders
As discussed elsewhere in this textbook, lithium is the most widely used treatment for bipolar disorder. Although it is far from the perfect drug, it has clearly revolutionized treatment of this disorder. Lithium has

proven useful in the treatment of acute episodes of mania and depression and, perhaps most importantly, in the long-term prophylaxis of the illness.

Treatment of Acute Mania

Lithium was approved by the U.S. Food and Drug Administration (FDA) in 1970 for the treatment of acute mania. Early uncontrolled single-blind studies, when combined, demonstrate that approximately 80% of manic patients (i.e., 334 of 413) show at least a partial response to lithium monotherapy. Subsequently, controlled double-blind studies similarly revealed a 70%–80% response rate of lithium monotherapy in the treatment of acute manic episodes (reviewed in Goodwin and Jamison 1990; Goodwin et al. 1969; Maggs 1963; Schou et al. 1954). Despite this impressive response rate and the evidence that lithium is the drug of choice for long-term prophylaxis (see below), its 5- to 10-day latency of response has limited its use as the *sole* agent in the treatment of acute manic episodes in everyday clinical practice.

A number of double-blind studies have compared lithium with neuroleptic drugs in the treatment of acute mania, suggesting that the neuroleptics are superior only in the initial management of acutely manic patients (Goodnick and Meltzer 1984b; Post et al. 1980a; Prien et al. 1972; Shopsin et al. 1971). More recent clinical studies have clearly demonstrated the efficacy of benzodiazepines such as lorazepam as an adjunct to lithium in the acute manic phase of the illness to control hyperactivity, agitation, and insomnia (Lenox et al. 1992a). This strategy affords the practical advantage of parenteral administration and limits unnecessary exposure to neuroleptics in this patient population. Thus, the majority of clinicians currently prescribe either a benzodiazepine or (when necessary) a neuroleptic in combination with lithium during the early stages of the treatment of mania, and then gradually taper the neuroleptic or benzodiazepine following stabilization of the patient's acute symptomatology. As discussed in the dosing section, clinicians frequently observe an increase in the plasma lithium levels (which often necessitates a lowering of the lithium dosage) after the manic episode has subsided. At present, it is unclear whether this is a result of increased uptake of lithium into excitable tissue during mania (as we have discussed), an increase in renal blood flow and glomerular filtration rate, or a combination thereof.

Long-Term Prophylaxis of Bipolar Disorder

Numerous placebo-controlled studies have unequivocally documented the efficacy of lithium in the long-term prophylactic treatment of bipolar disorder (reviewed in Goodwin and Jamison 1990). Lithium's beneficial effects appear to involve both a reduction in the number of episodes and in their intensity, with approximately 70%–80% of all bipolar patients showing at least a partial response to lithium. The cumulative data from 10 major double-blind studies have compared lithium prophylaxis to placebo; approximately 34% of those patients receiving lithium had relapses, compared with 81% of the patients who received placebo. Additional evidence for lithium prophylaxis is found in the studies in which successful lithium treatment was discontinued. In at least 14 studies, an average of 50% of the patients experienced relapse within 5 months of abrupt termination of treatment (Suppes et al. 1991).

Adequate lithium treatment, particularly in the context of a lithium clinic, is also reported to reduce the excessive mortality observed in the illness (Coppen and Abou-Saleh 1988; Coppen et al. 1991; Muller-Oerlinghausen et al. 1991; Vestergaard and Aagaard 1991). Debate continues as to the relative efficacy of lithium in preventing manic and depressive episodes. After careful analysis of the controlled studies, Goodwin and Jamison (1990) concluded that despite common clinical opinion, little support exists for the idea that lithium has greater prophylaxis against mania than against major depression. Nevertheless, patients *do* seem to report mild breakthrough depressive symptoms more commonly than hypomanic symptoms, although it is difficult to rule out the selective reporting of aversive symptoms by the patients. However (as is discussed in Chapter 29), data are accumulating that perhaps as many as half of all bipolar patients show an inadequate long-term response to lithium monotherapy, necessitating the addition or substitution of another agent, most commonly an anticonvulsant or an antidepressant.

Substantial research data suggest that certain features of bipolar disorder are predictive of a poor response to lithium. Patients who experience mixed states, severe stage III mania, and/or rapid cycling are all likely to show a poor response to lithium. In addition, the type and sequence of episodes may also be important—for example, patients with a manic depression/normal interval course do better with lithium than do those with a sequence of depression-mania-normalcy. The greater number of interepisode symptoms resulting from concomitant personality disorder or substance abuse, the less effective lithium response is likely to be. The potential phenomenon of "lithium discontinuation refractoriness" in certain individuals has been identified (Post et al. 1992), but more extensive study is required to assess the generalizability of the phenomenon. However, lithium is frequently discontinued for pregnant patients. Although controlled studies are lacking, refractoriness to lithium reinstitution does not appear to be a common occurrence in this population. It is more clear that abrupt lithium discontinuation after long-term maintenance treatment often results in the emergence of a manic episode, and the rate of exacerbation can be modified using a gradual discontinuation strategy (Faedda et al. 1993; Suppes et al. 1993).

It is clear that investigators studying the mechanism(s) of action of the drug and the neurobiology of bipolar affective disorder need to be cognizant of the clinical features associated with lithium response and discontinuation. These may provide clues not only about the targets of lithium's actions, but also about long-term homeostatic processes occurring during long-term lithium administration.

Acute Treatment of Depression

In addition to the well-established efficacy of lithium as a "potentiating agent" in the treatment of refractory depression (de Montigny et al. 1983; Heninger et al. 1983; Price 1989, discussed in next paragraph), there is now considerable evidence for the antidepressant efficacy of lithium monotherapy, particularly in the treatment of bipolar depressions. However, the antidepressant effects (demonstrated in placebo-controlled studies) often do not become evident until the third or fourth weeks of treatment, perhaps explaining the negative results noted in earlier studies of shorter duration (see Goodwin and Jamison 1990). Interestingly, an average of 79% of bipolar patients are reported to respond to the drug, compared with only 36% of unipolar patients. There have also been several controlled studies comparing the antidepressant efficacy of lithium to standard antidepressants. In four of five studies, lithium showed efficacy equal to that of tricyclic antidepressants (TCAs), albeit with a slower onset of action in two of the studies (Goodwin and Jamison 1990). The clinical observation of breakthrough depressions in bipolar patients despite maintenance of therapeutic lithium suggests that some patients may only experience modest antidepressant effects. Nevertheless, given the now well-documented ability of antidepressants to induce rapid cycling and precipitate manic episodes (Goodwin and Jamison 1990; Wehr and Goodwin 1987), lithium monotherapy is recommended for treatment of bipolar depressions.

Potentiation of Antidepressant Response

One of the major advances in psychopharmacology in the last decade has been the recognition of lithium augmentation as a strategy in treating depression that is refractory to monotherapy with conventional antidepressants (both TCAs and MAO inhibitors [MAOIs]). It has been established in open studies (and subsequently in controlled studies) that about half of all treatment-refractory depressed patients respond to an addition of lithium to their ongoing antidepressant regimen (with a higher response rate in bipolar subjects), usually within 1–2 weeks (de Montigny et al. 1983; Heninger et al. 1983; Price 1989). Although lithium potentiation is more efficacious in bipolar patients, it also has clear efficacy in the treatment of unipolar depressive patients. The relative safety of this strategy, and the short time needed to assess its efficacy, suggest that a trial of lithium augmentation should be considered before switching antidepressants in nonresponding depressed patients. The lithium augmentation strategy derived from de Montigny's heuristic proposal that the enhancement of ascending presynaptic serotonergic function would translate into potentiation of antidepressant efficacy (de Montigny et al. 1983). However, considerable data have shown that lithium can affect PKC, which may regulate the function of multiple neurotransmitter systems (Manji and Lenox 1994). It is tempting to speculate that it is this effect on multiple interacting neurotransmitter systems that underlies its remarkable efficacy in treating refractory depression.

Schizophrenia

Given some degree of similarity in the acute symptomatology of mania and certain forms of schizophrenia (particularly paranoid schizophrenia), it is not surprising that the efficacy of lithium has been investigated in these disorders. The results of the double-blind studies of lithium in schizophrenia have generally been disappointing, with a greater efficacy observed for neuroleptics. Lithium shows some efficacy in the treatment of the affective symptoms but is generally without benefit on the "core schizophrenic" symptoms (Atre-Vaidya and Taylor 1989; Collins et al. 1991). There is considerably more evidence for the efficacy of lithium in the treatment of schizoaffective disorder, with a meta-analysis of published findings suggesting an improvement in 77% of lithium-treated schizoaffective individuals (Delva and Letemendia 1982). Although lithium appears useful to patients with this condition, treatment with neuroleptics and other agents is usually necessary (Goodnick and Meltzer 1984b).

Aggression

The antiaggressive effect of lithium has been investigated in animal studies and in clinical studies over the past 20 years, with the preponderance of data suggesting that lithium reduces impulsive aggression (see Nilsson 1993 for an excellent review). Indeed, Schou (1987) has described lithium's antiaggressive effects as one of its best-documented effects outside of the treatment of bipolar illness. At serum levels similar to those used in the treatment of bipolar illness, lithium has generally been demonstrated to exert antiaggressive effects in psychiatric populations, in children with behavior problems, in individuals with mental retardation, and in prisoners with "uncontrolled rage outbursts" (Nilsson 1993). It should be noted that most studies have been conducted in institutions, and there is little research on the antiaggressive effects of lithium in the outpatient setting. In view of the reported association between serotonergic function and aggressive and impulsive disorders, it is not surprising that the antiaggressive properties of lithium have generally been ascribed to an enhancement of serotonergic function (Coccaro et al. 1989). Although it is not approved by the FDA for treatment of aggression, it is clear that additional studies of lithium for this purpose are warranted, not only with respect to defining the range of clinically responsive conditions but also regarding the neurobiological mechanisms underlying its efficacy.

Other Psychiatric Conditions

Although the efficacy of lithium has been investigated in the treatment of obsessive-compulsive disorder, attention-deficit hyperactivity disorder, late luteal phase dysphoric disorder, borderline personality disorder, alcoholism, Tourette's disorder, anxiety disorders, and eating disorders, there is little convincing evidence for lithium's efficacy in treating these disorders (Jefferson et al. 1983; Johnson 1987).

■ Nonpsychiatric Indications

Cluster Headache

The best established nonpsychiatric use of lithium is in the long-term prophylactic treatment of cluster headache (Bussone et al. 1990). The cyclic, recurrent nature of the illness was the original impetus for investigating lithium's efficacy. Indeed, there is general agreement that not only is lithium an effective treatment, but it should also be regarded as a first-line agent in this disorder. Interestingly, the therapeutic efficacy of lithium in cluster headache requires similar plasma levels and generally shows a 3-week latency to response (Johnson and Minnai 1993). The most interesting mechanistic studies have focused on alterations in membrane phospholipids and alterations in receptor-effector coupling by lithium (de Belleroche et al. 1984, 1986). Finally, it is noteworthy that there appear to be differences in human leukocyte antigen in patients showing responses to lithium (Giacovazzo et al. 1985, 1986). It is still unclear if the mood-stabilizing properties of lithium show a similar human leukocyte antigen association.

Effects of Lithium on Blood Cells and the Function of Granulocytes

Following therapeutic doses of lithium, fairly reproducible hematopoietic effects have been documented, especially on the granulocyte leukocytes. The observation that lithium stimulation of leukocytosis involves a true proliferative response, rather than just a shift of cell populations from the marginating to the circulatory pool of cells, led investigators to examine the bone marrow for changes in miotic cell proliferation. These studies have shown that lithium increases the number of pluripotential hematopoietic stem cells (colony-forming unit–stem cells [CFU-S]), granulocyte-macrophage progenitors (colony-forming unit–granulocyte macrophages [CFU$_{GM}$]), and megakaryocyte progenitors (colony-forming unit–megakaryocytes [CFU$_{MEG}$]) in several species, including humans. These now well-documented effects of lithium on blood cell formation have led to an investigation of this monovalent cation in the treatment of various hematopoietic disorders (particularly after anticancer or anti–acquired immunodeficiency syndrome [AIDS] chemotherapy) to ameliorate the bone marrow toxicity associated with these treatments. Although Lyman and Williams (1991) concluded after a detailed review of the literature that lithium is clearly effective in reducing both severity and duration of chemo- or radiotherapy-associated neutropenia, lithium is not routinely used as an adjunct in these conditions. Nevertheless, given the extensive clinical use of lithium worldwide and its lack of toxicity when administered at therapeutic doses, the use of lithium to ameliorate bone marrow suppression remains an area worthy of further long-term clinical investigation.

Most recently, "hematologic" studies of lithium have highlighted its potential role in modulating the hematopoietic toxicity associated with zidovudine (AZT). Despite the reported efficacy of the drug in producing immunological improvement, decreasing the incidence of opportunistic infections, and reducing AIDS mortality, its use has been associated with hematopoietic suppression manifested by anemia, neutropenia, and overall bone marrow suppression (Fischl et al. 1987). Studies have demonstrated the efficacy of clinically used doses of lithium (i.e., 1.0 mM) in attenuating the toxicity of AZT on CFU_{GM}, CFU_{MEG}, and burst-forming unit, erythroid (BFU-E) progenitor stem cells obtained from mice infected with the Rauscher leukemia virus (RLV) (Gallicchio and Hughes 1992; Gallicchio et al. 1992). The clinical studies of lithium in human immunodeficiency virus (HIV)-infected patients are much more preliminary but offer promise. In a pilot study, Roberts and associates (1988) showed that 3 of 5 AZT-treated AIDS patients receiving "therapeutic" doses of lithium (0.6–1.2 mM) showed a significant neutrophilia. Interestingly, 3 of 5 patients receiving lithium were able to tolerate higher doses of AZT. Other small studies have shown similar (albeit modest) benefit of concomitant lithium administration.

Antiviral Effects of Lithium

The use of lithium as an antiviral agent is receiving growing consideration following the demonstration about 15 years ago that lithium inhibited the replication of certain viruses under particular experimental conditions (Skinner et al. 1980). Several studies have since demonstrated that lithium inhibits the replication of several DNA viruses (see Cernescu et al. 1988). There is less agreement on RNA viruses; two RNA virus groups are not inhibited by lithium, whereas inhibition of paramyxoviruses are reported. The mechanism(s) by which lithium inhibits DNA replication through DNA polymerase in herpesvirus are presently unknown but are thought to occur through modification of intracellular second messenger systems.

In this context, it is noteworthy that the enhancement of tumor necrosis factor (TNF) cytotoxicity by lithium has been shown to be mediated by alterations in the PI second messenger system (Beyaert et al. 1993). In particular, treatment of the transformed cell line L929 with the combination of TNF and lithium induced an increase in cytidine diphosphate-DAG that preceded the onset of cell killing by approximately 1 hour, and lithium's cytotoxic effects were sensitive to the PKC inhibitor staurosporine. In vitro studies have revealed the positive effects of lithium on HIV in MT4 (a transformed lymphocyte cell line) and CEM cells (an acute lymphoblastic leukemia T cell line). Gallicchio and associates (1993) have recently investigated the effect of lithium in murine immunodeficiency virus–infected animals, demonstrating a marked reduction in the development of lymphadenopathy and splenomegaly. These investigators suggest that lithium may be effective in modulating murine immunodeficiency virus infection. They raise important questions related to the potential role lithium may play in the pathophysiological processes associated with retroviral infections.

To date, virtually all of the relevant detailed clinical studies on the potential antiviral efficacy of lithium have been directed to the treatment of herpes simplex infections. A large study of 177 subjects found that chronic lithium administration resulted in a significant reduction in the recurrence rate of these infections, with most patients reporting a reduction to less than half the pretreatment rate (Amsterdam et al. 1990a, 1990b). Other double-blind prospective studies have demonstrated a similar beneficial effect of lithium, which appears to be independent of any modulation of affective symptoms.

■ SIDE EFFECTS AND TOXICOLOGY

■ General Considerations

Lithium has a narrow therapeutic index in humans, with a currently recommended therapeutic serum concentration range of 0.8–1.2 mEq/L (Gelenberg et al. 1989; Schatzberg and Cole 1991). Side effects and toxicity become increasingly more evident at doses achieving higher serum levels (Jefferson et al. 1987). A recent review of the literature reveals that 35%–93% of patients complain about adverse side effects of lithium treatment. The most common side effects reported are noted in Table 16–1, which presents pooled data from 12 individual studies of 1,094 patients (Goodwin and Jamison 1990). It is of interest that when patients are asked about the most troublesome side effects that often lead to noncompliance with long-term lithium treatment, the most common are related to cognitive dysfunction (i.e., mental confusion, poor concentration, mental slowness, and memory problems).

The major physiological systems predisposed to lithium-induced symptomatology and toxicity include the gastrointestinal, renal, endocrine, and nervous systems as well as the teratogenicity associated with the developing fetus. Most of the side effects appear to be dose related and transient in nature (Jefferson 1990; Schou 1989; Vestergaard et al. 1988). Although sustained-release formulations of lithium may be useful in ameliorating some lithium-induced side effects, enhanced gastrointestinal symptomatology may preclude this treatment strategy. Thus, risk factors that predispose to side effects and toxicity of lithium include reduced renal clearance with age or renal disease, organic brain disorder, physical illness with vomiting and/or diarrhea, diuretic and/or other concomitant pharmacotherapy, low sodium intake and/or high sodium excretion, and pregnancy.

The vulnerability of certain organ systems to lithium-induced effects may be due not only to a preferential accumulation of lithium but also to its action as outlined above on the various ion transport, second messenger, and receptor-signaling systems shared in both the brain and periphery. The CNS, which is the apparent site of its therapeutic action, is particularly sensitive to side effects and toxicity. Studies have even reported that lithium distribution throughout brain regions can be nonuniform, resulting in relatively greater potential effects in selective regions of the brain (Sansone and Ziegler 1985). Clinical manifestations of a fine hand tremor is one of the most common reported side effects in 31%–65% of patients. This can be associated with reduced motor coordination, nystagmus, and muscular weakness most notable in the early phases of treatment (Goodwin and Jamison 1990). Evidence for cogwheel rigidity has been reported on long-term treatment with lithium alone and has been attributed to antidopaminergic effects of lithium, although this observation has been most apparent during concomitant neuroleptic exposure (Asnis et al. 1979).

■ Central Nervous System

The cognitive effects of lithium appear to be some of the most problematic for patients, yet these effects remain the least studied. Clinical reports of noncompliance with lithium over the years have attributed to lithium treatment difficulty with both creativity and productivity and a lack of drive. Yet two noted studies carried out in artists, writers, and business executives ($N = 30$) being treated with lithium revealed that more than 75% of these patients believed that lithium either enhanced or did not change their creative productivity (Marshall et al. 1970; Schou 1979b). In addition, it has been difficult to find convincing evidence for cognitive effects of lithium in animal studies. Studies of lithium-induced effects on intellectual functioning such as memory, associative processing, semantic reasoning, and rate of psychomotor and cognitive performance in bipolar patients remain contradictory (see review in Goodwin and Jamison 1990). Judd and colleagues (1987) have reported data demonstrating a "slowing of the rate of central information processing" (pp. 1467–1468) in a series of control subjects administered therapeutic doses of lithium, which supported earlier observations by

Table 16–1. Lithium side effects

Side effect	Percentage with subjective complaint[a]	Relative importance in noncompliance[b]
Excessive thirst	35.9	
Polyuria	30.4	4
Memory problems	28.2	1
Tremor	26.6	3[c]
Weight gain	18.9	2
Drowsiness/tiredness	12.4	5
Diarrhea	8.7	
Any complaint	73.8	
No complaints	26.2	

[a] Pooled percentages from 12 studies including 1,094 patients.
[b] Relative ranking of importance of side effects for lithium noncompliance in 71 patients (Goodwin and Jamison 1990).
[c] Included incoordination.

Schou (1968). However, these studies were relatively short-term, and there is evidence that accommodation to some of the cognitive effects of lithium does occur. Because lithium appears to have profound effects on PKC-mediated events in brain (as noted previously) and PKC has been implicated in long-term potentiation in hippocampus (Manji and Lenox 1994) and the subjective effects of lithium on cognition remain such an important clinical issue in compliance, further research in this area is warranted.

The neurotoxic effects of lithium that generally occur at higher serum concentrations or in patients with the risk factors we have noted are associated with increasing signs of cognitive impairment, lassitude, restlessness, and irritability (Jefferson et al. 1987). Although this symptomatology is reversible within 5–10 days, neurotoxicity can progress to frank delirium, ataxia, coarse tremors, seizures, and ultimately to coma and death. It is of interest that recent behavioral models of lithium action in brain as well as neurotoxic effect on seizure threshold have demonstrated reversibility with inositol administration, thus implicating lithium's action on PI signaling pathway in these neurobehavioral and neurotoxic events (Kofman and Belmaker 1993). Consistent with our earlier observations, these data may also implicate the PI system as a target for lithium action on a continuum from its therapeutic to its neurotoxic effects.

■ Endocrine Systems

Lithium has been demonstrated to exert effects on various endocrine systems, and interested readers are directed to excellent recent reviews of the subject (Johnson 1988; Lazarus 1986). In a study of 330 bipolar patients treated with lithium for 5 months to 3 years, Schou (1968) first reported that lithium therapy induced goiter at an overall rate of 3.6%. Lithium appears to exert antithyroid effects at different levels of thyroid function, including inhibition of hormone synthesis and release, inhibition of the action of TSH, and peripheral metabolism of thyroxine (T_4). Although reports of lithium-induced hypothyroidism range from 5%–35% due to variability in criteria for diagnosis and sensitivity of laboratory tests, it is estimated that the prevalence of clinical hypothyroidism is more likely 5% and more common in women (Jefferson 1990). It is generally accepted that approximately 30% of patients exhibit elevated levels of TSH, although most do not exhibit statistically significant

decreases in the levels of circulating thyroid hormones, suggesting that a compromised substrate may be necessary for the development of overt hypothyroidism (Amdisen and Andersen 1982; Lindstedt et al. 1977; Rogers and Whybrow 1971). Such a suggestion is supported by the studies showing that there is an increased likelihood of elevations in TSH and decreases in thyroid hormones during lithium therapy in those individuals with serum antithyroid antibodies (Calabrese et al. 1985; Myers et al. 1985).

Patients on lithium manifest a high prevalence of thyroid autoantibodies (15%–30%), suggesting a relative induction by lithium (Deniker et al. 1978; Lazarus 1986). Furthermore, low-normal T_4 levels have been associated with lethargy and cognitive impairment in patients treated with lithium for at least 6 months, and triiodothyronine (T_3) was in the low-normal range in patients who relapsed (Hatterer et al. 1989). Because lithium has been shown to suppress the cAMP formation induced by TSH stimulation, lithium-induced hypothyroidism may occur by an "uncoupling" of the TSH receptor from AC, resulting in a compensatory increased secretion of TSH (McHenry et al. 1990; Mori et al. 1989; Tseng et al. 1989). Although this is an attractive hypothesis and likely plays some role in the reduced sensitivity to the effects of TSH, it has been demonstrated that lithium also inhibits forskolin (colforsin)-stimulated iodine uptake in thyroid cells, suggesting additional effects distal to cAMP formation (e.g., protein kinase) are involved (Mori et al. 1989; Urabe et al. 1991). In this context, it is noteworthy that lithium's effects are mimicked by PKC activators and blocked by PKC inhibitors in cultured thyroid tissue, suggesting that lithium's action on both AC and PKC contributes to the observed thyroid dysfunction.

Another possible endocrine complication of lithium treatment, hyperparathyroidism, was first reported by Garfinkel and colleagues (1973) and is much less common (Nordenstrom et al. 1992; Taylor and Bell 1993). Although the clinical significance of lithium-induced primary hyperparathyroidism has remained controversial, studies have demonstrated increased parathyroid hormone (PTH) secretion in at least a subset of patients (Christiansen et al. 1978), with accompanying evidence for modest increases in serum calcium and parathyroid hyperplasia in several reports (Lazarus 1986; Mannisto 1980). Since then, hyperparathyroidism associated with lithium therapy has been reported in more than 20 cases. But the effect of lithium on PTH secretion during clinical treatment remains controversial, at least in part because of the lack of pretreatment PTH levels in most of the cases, and the inability to demonstrate an alteration in the set point for PTH secretion in healthy subjects undergoing subacute lithium administration (Spiegel et al. 1984). Nevertheless, the longitudinal studies, and the reports of parathyroid hyperplasia and elevations of serum calcium, suggest that abnormal PTH secretion may occur in at least a subset of individuals treated with lithium.

Interestingly, in vitro data in parathyroid cells exposed to lithium indicate an action on both PTH release and mitogenic properties similar to that observed with PKC activation (Saxe and Gibson 1991, 1993). Lithium at therapeutic levels appears to have diverse effects on the parathyroid gland, causing a rightward shift in the calcium-sensing set point, thereby releasing PTH abnormally. In cases of preexisting parathyroid abnormalities, lithium may serve to unmask an incipient adenoma and cause hyperplasia of the gland (Mallette et al. 1989; McHenry et al. 1991).

■ Renal Function

Lithium is excreted from the body almost entirely from the kidney, with no evidence for any significant protein binding. Lithium reversibly reduces the kidney's ability to concentrate urine primarily through effects on renal tubular function, resulting in the clinical manifestation of polyuria (> 3 L/24 hours) (Walker and Green 1982). This impairment of renal tubular concentrating ability has been associated with a reversible acute epithelial swelling and glycogen disposition in the distal nephron. It is related to both the dose and duration of lithium treatment and occurs in 20%–30% of patients treated with lithium (Goodwin and Jamison 1990; Walker 1993). Studies have indicated that once-a-day dosing of lithium may result in relatively less renal symptomatology than a multiple-dosing treatment strategy, but this still awaits further confirmation (Lauritsen et al. 1981; Schou et al. 1982). Lithium appears to inhibit the vasopressin (V2)-stimulated cAMP production, reducing water reabsorption in the distal tubules and collecting ducts, resulting in nephrogenic diabetes insipidus (Dousa and Hechter 1970a, 1970b; Jefferson 1990). There is also evidence for a dipsogenic effect of lithium through interaction with the renin-angiotensin system in the brain (Jefferson 1990). The

mechanism for the inhibition of cAMP generation probably involves an effect at the level of G proteins, and more recent studies have suggested additional mechanisms involving prostaglandin pathways and PKC (Anger et al. 1990; Yamaki et al. 1991). A more progressive development of impairment of urinary concentrating ability has been observed in patients on long-term lithium treatment, most particularly in those patients exposed to periods of lithium toxicity or concomitant exposure treatment with neuroleptics (Walker 1993). Although such patients on renal biopsy may demonstrate chronic focal interstitial nephropathy, similar lesions have been noted in psychiatric patients with no exposure to lithium. There is little evidence for a lithium-induced chronic glomerular toxicity, although there are case reports of a reversible minimal lesion nephrotic syndrome (Walker 1993). In a recent review, Gitlin (1993) cites evidence that up to 5% of lithium-treated patients may develop signs of renal insufficiency, with two reported cases demonstrating progressive renal failure. However, such data suffer from a lack of comparable statistics for rate of renal insufficiency in the general population or in untreated bipolar patients and may be related to an increased risk of renal effects of lithium observed in patients exposed to periods of acute toxicity (Schou et al. 1989; Walker 1993).

■ Less Common Side Effects

The cardiovascular effects of lithium administered orally are rather benign. Most commonly, electrocardiogram recordings demonstrate a flattening and inversion of the T wave (Tilkian et al. 1976). Lithium has been shown to prolong sinus node recovery time. Caution is recommended in patients with bradycardia or demonstrated sinus node dysfunction, as well as in those being treated concomitantly with drugs affecting sinus node conduction (Jefferson 1991; Mitchell and MacKenzie 1982; Roose et al. 1979). Because weight gain can be a significant side effect of long-term lithium treatment, the action of lithium on glucose metabolism has been examined over the years with rather conflicting results (Garland et al. 1988; Mellerup et al. 1983; Peselow et al. 1980). Consistent with lithium's ability to inhibit cAMP formation, there appears to be more consistent evidence for an insulin-like action resulting in a relative hypoglycemia (Jefferson 1991). Other lesser side effects of lithium treatment include an exacerbation of existing psoriasis, hair loss, leukocytosis, decreased libido, and altered taste sensation (Schou 1989).

■ Teratogenic Effects

Lithium treatment in humans has been associated with teratogenic properties affecting predominantly the cardiovascular development during the fetus's first trimester. Earlier studies based on the original work of Schou and colleagues (1973), which led to the development of the International Register of Lithium Babies, revealed an increased rate of Ebstein's anomaly, 400 times higher than that observed in the general population (Nora et al. 1974). More recent controlled epidemiological studies have reported an apparently reduced rate of Ebstein's anomaly in the range of 0.1%–0.7%, approximately 20–140 times greater than in the general population (Elia et al. 1987; Jacobson et al. 1992; Zalstein et al. 1990). The risk of major congenital malformations with first-trimester lithium treatment is now thought to be in the range of 4%–12%, whereas the prevalence in an untreated comparison cohort is in the range of 2%–4% (Cohen et al. 1994). Lithium is currently indicated as a category D drug in the current edition of *Drugs in Pregnancy and Lactation*, which states that "there is positive evidence of human fetal risk, but benefits from use in pregnant women may be acceptable despite the risk" (Briggs et al. 1990, pp. 357–358).

In a recent review, Cohen and colleagues (1994) recommended a reconsideration of the relative risks associated with discontinuation versus maintenance of lithium treatment during pregnancy. They outlined new guidelines for patients continuing lithium during the first trimester of pregnancy, suggesting prenatal diagnosis by fetal echocardiogram and high-resolution ultrasound examination at 16–18 weeks' gestation. Lithium passes through the placental barrier in the latter months of pregnancy and is present in breast milk, which can result in toxicity to the neonate, manifesting in lethargy, hypotonia, and cyanosis.

■ DRUG-DRUG INTERACTIONS

■ Psychotropic Drugs

Overall, lithium has surprisingly few clinically significant interactions with most routinely prescribed psy-

chotropic drugs, perhaps explaining in part why (despite its relatively low therapeutic index) a trial of adjunctive lithium therapy has been investigated in the treatment of numerous psychiatric conditions (see previous section; Table 16–2).

■ Benzodiazepines

There are few clinically relevant interactions between lithium and benzodiazepines, although certain individuals may be at greater risk for CNS depressant effects when the combination of the two drugs is used. In this context, the lithium-benzodiazepine combination has been suggested to produce an idiosyncratic reaction manifested by profound hypothermia in one individual (Naylor and McHarg 1977). Nevertheless, a combination of benzodiazepines and lithium has been used extensively in the clinical setting, with few major adverse effects noted (Jefferson et al. 1981; Lenox et al. 1992a). Indeed, in view of the potential

Table 16–2. Potentially clinically significant drug interactions with lithium

Drug	Potential manifestations
Diuretics	Affect lithium clearance
Thiazides	Alter (usually raise) plasma lithium levels
Aldosterone antagonists	
Xanthine derivatives	
Loop diuretics	Loop diuretics, potassium-sparing diuretics are less problematic than others
Potassium-sparing diuretics	
Nonsteroidal anti-inflammatory drugs	Decrease lithium clearance and raise plasma lithium levels
Diclofenac	
Indomethacin	
Ibuprofen	
Naproxen	
Phenylbutazone	
Sulindac	Sulindac *may* be less problematic than others
Neuroleptics	Worsening of EPS; Potential for neurotoxicity (high-potency agents appear to carry greater risk)
Antiarrhythmics	May potentiate cardiac conduction effects

for sleep deprivation to induce manic episodes (Wehr et al. 1987), the judicious use of a benzodiazepine is recommended in the treatment of bipolar patients experiencing sleep disruption.

■ Neuroleptics

The practice of combining neuroleptics with lithium is generally considered safe and efficacious (Goodwin and Jamison 1990), but caution is recommended, particularly with the high-potency neuroleptics. There are reports of pharmacokinetic interactions between lithium and neuroleptics, but these are generally regarded as not clinically significant (Jefferson et al. 1983). Although lithium/neuroleptic neurotoxicity is a relatively rare phenomenon, it has been most widely associated with haloperidol (Cohen and Cohen 1974), and there are more than 40 cases reported in the literature (see Ross and Coffey 1987; Werstiuk and Steiner 1987). This syndrome is characterized by altered mental status, cerebellar signs and symptoms, tremor, and extrapyramidal symptoms. Some patients also exhibit fever and elevations in serum liver enzymes, raising the possibility that these may represent atypical cases of neuroleptic malignant syndrome.

By contrast, a chart review of 425 patients treated with lithium and haloperidol revealed no greater incidence in the occurrence of side effects compared to either drug alone (Johnson 1984). Similarly, a study examining the prevalence of electroencephalogram abnormalities in patients treated with a combination of lithium and haloperidol revealed no increase compared with either drug alone (or no drug) (Abrams and Taylor 1979). Thus, overall, it appears that this *potential* interaction is relatively rare. Nevertheless, given the abundant preclinical data supporting an effect of lithium on the dopaminergic system, and the severity of the neurotoxicity, it seems prudent for clinicians to be aware of this interaction and to discontinue both drugs if toxicity develops.

■ Antidepressants

The combination of lithium and various classes of antidepressants has been used extensively in large numbers of patients. The preponderance of the data suggests that although minor side effects are common, major adverse effects are relatively uncommon (Price 1987). There are reports of increased incidence

of myoclonic jerks in patients receiving a combination of lithium and MAOIs, but this has not been extensively investigated. In view of the enhancement of serotonergic function by lithium, there is the potential for an increased risk of the so-called serotonin syndrome in individuals receiving a combination of lithium and selective serotonin reuptake inhibitors or MAOIs, but the clinical data to date are sparse.

■ Electroconvulsive Therapy

Although not a true "drug/drug" interaction, the use of lithium during a course of electroconvulsive therapy (ECT) warrants discussion. In recent years, ECT has emerged as a remarkably efficacious, potentially life-saving treatment for a number of psychiatric conditions for which lithium is also used, including severe depression and mania (Crowe 1984). There is thus a clear need to establish the safety and potential efficacy of lithium during ECT. Despite this clinical need, however, there is a dearth of adequate studies addressing this important issue (Rudorfer and Linnoila 1987).

There have been several case reports suggesting that the lithium/ECT combination may be associated with a neurotoxic syndrome characterized by confusion, disorientation, and decreased responsiveness (reviewed in Rudorfer and Linnoila 1987). However, a comprehensive retrospective review (Perry and Tsuang 1979) and a prospective, controlled double-blind study (Coppen et al. 1981) both revealed no increased morbidity for lithium/ECT. In fact, the well-known need to continue maintenance medication following ECT and lithium's latency of onset of action prompted Coppen and associates (1981) to suggest that lithium might be introduced early during the course of ECT treatment to minimize the likelihood of relapse following ECT termination. This suggestion has not been generally accepted in routine clinical practice; despite the lack of clear-cut evidence of neurotoxicity in general, it does appear that some patients are more susceptible to neurotoxic manifestations. Additionally, given the lack of obvious benefit from combining lithium and ECT in most patients, it seems prudent to discontinue lithium during the course of ECT. In cases of established lack of adequate response to either treatment alone, or in cases of known rapid relapse following ECT discontinuation, the lithium/ECT combination treatment can be conducted judiciously, by using "low therapeutic" lithium levels, avoiding other medications, and monitoring for any symptoms suggestive of neurotoxicity.

■ Nonpsychotropic Drugs

The largest single class of drugs producing a clinically significant interaction with lithium are the diuretics, several types of which can elevate lithium levels and produce toxicity. It is now well established that diuretics decrease renal lithium clearance, which frequently necessitates a reduction of the lithium dosage to avoid toxicity. Any drug capable of altering renal function should be used judiciously in patients receiving lithium, with more frequent plasma level determinations and a reduction of the dosage, if necessary. However, perhaps because of their more proximal site of action, thiazide diuretics are also sometimes used to *treat* lithium-induced nephrogenic diabetes insipidus (discussed previously). Other classes of diuretics have been less well studied. But the present data suggest that a careful monitoring of lithium levels is warranted when using osmotic diuretics, loop diuretics, aldosterone antagonists, or other potassium-sparing diuretics.

The effects of cardiac drugs that alter sinus node conduction (e.g., quinidine and digoxin) could be potentiated by lithium. It is clear that the combination of lithium with cardiac drugs requires careful monitoring, including regular electrocardiograms. Several nonsteroidal anti-inflammatory drugs (NSAIDS) can also increase plasma lithium levels, perhaps by an inhibition of renal tubular prostaglandin synthesis. Almost all of the older NSAIDS (including diclofenac, ibuprofen, indomethacin, naproxen, and phenylbutazone) have been shown to interact with lithium—often resulting in toxicity, although preliminary studies suggest that sulindac may be less frequently associated. Lithium is also known to prolong the action of neuromuscular agents, necessitating a reduction in the dose or, in the case of patients undergoing certain surgical procedures or ECT, complete cessation.

■ CONCLUSION

Lithium is a monovalent cation with complex physiological and pharmacological effects within the brain. By virtue of the ionic properties it shares with other important monovalent and divalent cations such as sodium, magnesium, and calcium, its transport into cells provides ready access to a host of intracellular enzymatic events affecting short- and long-term cell processes. It may be that, in part, the therapeutic efficacy of lithium in the treatment of both poles of manic-depressive disorder may rely on the "dirty" characteristics of its multiple sites of pharmacological interaction.

Strategic models to further delineate the mechanism(s) of action of lithium relevant to its therapeutic effects must account for a number of critical variables in experimental design. Lithium has a relatively low therapeutic index, requiring careful attention to the tissue concentrations at which effects of the drug are being observed in light of the known toxicity of lithium within the CNS. Although such a poor therapeutic index may suggest a continuum between some of the biological processes underlying therapeutic efficacy and toxicity, it may also account in part for the variability of effects of lithium observed in animal and in vitro studies. The therapeutic action of lithium is delayed, requiring more long-term administration to establish efficacy for both its treatment of acute mania and its prophylaxis of the recurrent affective episodes associated with manic-depressive disorder. Although its therapeutic effects are not reversed immediately with abrupt discontinuation, there is accumulating evidence that abrupt withdrawal of lithium may sensitize the patient's system to an episode of mania (Klein et al. 1992; Suppes et al. 1991).

The ability of lithium to stabilize an underlying dysregulation of limbic and limbic-associated function is critical to our understanding of its mechanism of action. The biological processes in the brain responsible for the episodic clinical manifestation of mania and depression may be due to an inability to mount the appropriate compensatory responses necessary to maintain homeostatic regulation, thereby resulting in sudden oscillations beyond immediate adaptive control (Depue et al. 1987; Goodwin and Jamison 1990; Mandell et al. 1984). The resultant clinical picture is reflected in disruption of behavior, circadian rhythms, neurophysiology of sleep, and neuroendocrine and biochemical regulation within the brain. Regulation of signal transduction within critical regions of the brain remains an attractive target for psychopharmacological interventions. The behavioral and physiological manifestations of the illness are complex and are mediated by a network of interconnected neurotransmitter pathways. The biogenic amines have been strongly implicated in the regulation of these physiological processes by virtue of their pharmacological actions and predominant neuroanatomical distribution within limbic-related brain regions. Thus, lithium's ability to modulate release of serotonin at presynaptic sites and affect DA-induced supersensitivity in the brain remains a relevant line of investigation into the respective action of lithium in altering the clinical manifestation of depression and mania in the bipolar patient.

However, it is at the molecular level that some of the most exciting advances in our understanding of the long-term therapeutic action of lithium will take place in the coming years. The lithium cation possesses the selective ability at clinically relevant concentrations to alter the PI second messenger system, potentially altering the activity and dynamic regulation of receptors that are coupled to this intracellular response. Subtypes of muscarinic receptors in the limbic system may represent particularly sensitive targets in this regard, especially in light of the putative role of cholinergic neurotransmission in both lithium action and affective state.

Finally, it would appear that the current studies of the long-term lithium-induced changes in PKC-mediated events (including gene expression and posttranslational modification of important phosphoproteins responsible for regulation of signal transduction in the brain) are a most promising avenue for future investigation. This is particularly significant in light of converging data from studies of chronic lithium relating its therapeutic efficacy to the regulation of membrane-related events involving cytoskeletal restructuring, such as ion transport, neurotransmitter release, and the receptor-response complex. Whether forthcoming research along these lines will lead to elucidation of a molecular basis for manic-depressive disorder remains to be determined.

■ REFERENCES

Abrams R, Taylor MA: EEG observations during combined lithium and neuroleptic treatment. Am J Psychiatry 136:336–337, 1979

Ahluwalia P, Singhal RL: Effect of low-dose lithium administration and subsequent withdrawal on biogenic amines in rat brain. Br J Pharmacol 71:601–607, 1980

Ahluwalia P, Singhal RL: Monoamine uptake into synaptosomes from various regions of rat brain following lithium administration and withdrawal. Neuropharmacology 20:483–487, 1981

Ahluwalia P, Grewaal DS, Singhal RL: Brain GABAergic and dopaminergic systems following lithium treatment and withdrawal. Progress in Neuro-Psychopharmacology 5:527–530, 1981

Akagawa K, Watanabe M, Tsukada Y: Activity of Na-K-ATPase in manic patients. J Neurochem 35:258–260, 1980

Alexander DR, Deeb M, Bitar F, et al: Sodium-potassium, magnesium, and calcium ATPase activities in erythrocyte membranes from manic-depressive patients responding to lithium. Biol Psychiatry 21:997–1007, 1986

Allikmets LH, Stanley M, Gershon S: The effect of lithium on chronic haloperidol enhanced apomorphine aggression in rats. Life Sci 25:165–170, 1979

Allison JH: Lithium and brain *myo*-inositol metabolism, in Cyclitols and Phosphoinositides. Edited by Wells WW, Eisenberg F Jr. New York, Academic Press, 1978, pp 507–519

Allison JH, Stewart MA: Reduced brain inositol in lithium treated rats. Nature: New Biology 233:267–268, 1971

Allison JH, Blisner MW, Holland WH, et al: Increased brain *myo*-inositol 1-phosphate in lithium-treated rats. Biochem Biophys Res Commun 71:664–670, 1976

Amdisen A, Andersen C: Lithium treatment of thyroid function: A survey of 237 patients in long term lithium treatment. Pharmacopsychiatria 15:149–155, 1982

Amsterdam JD, Maislin G, Rybakowski J: A possible antiviral action of lithium carbonate in herpes simplex virus infections. Biol Psychiatry 27:447–453, 1990a

Amsterdam JD, Maislin G, Potter L, et al: Reduced rate of recurrent genital herpes infections with lithium carbonate. Psychopharmacol Bull 26:343–347, 1990b

Andersen PH, Geisler A: Lithium inhibition of forskolin-stimulated adenylate cyclase. Neuropsychobiology 12:1–3, 1984

Anderson SMP, Godfrey PP, Grahame-Smith DG: The effects of phorbol esters and lithium on 5-HT release in rat hippocampal slices. Br J Pharmacol 93:96P, 1988

Anger MS, Shanley P, Mansour J, et al: Effects of lithium on cAMP generation in cultured rat inner medullary collecting tubule cells. Kidney Int 37:1211–1218, 1990

Arendt J, Aldhous M, Marks V: Alleviation of jet lag by melatonin: preliminary results of controlled double blind trial. British Medical Journal 292:1170–1174, 1986

Asnis GM, Asnis D, Dunner DL, et al: Cogwheel rigidity during chronic lithium therapy. Am J Psychiatry 136:1225–1226, 1979

Atre-Vaidya N, Taylor MA: Effectiveness of lithium in schizophrenia: do we really have an answer? J Clin Psychiatry 50:170–173, 1989

Aulde J: The use of lithium bromide in combination with solution of potassium citrate. Medical Bulletin (Philadelphia) 9:35–39, 69–72, 228–233, 1887

Avissar S, Schreiber G, Danon A, et al: Lithium inhibits adrenergic and cholinergic increases in GTP binding in rat cortex. Nature 331:440–442, 1988

Bach RO, Gallicchio VS: Lithium and Cell Physiology. New York, Springer-Verlag, 1990

Ballast CL, Sharp PR, Domino EF: Effect of lithium on RBC water permeability. Biol Psychiatry 21:426–427, 1986

Baraban JM, Worley PF, Snyder SH: Second messenger systems and psychoactive drug focus on the phosphoinositide system and lithium. Am J Psychiatry 146:1251–1260, 1989

Beckmann H, St-Laurent J, Goodwin FK: The effect of lithium on urinary MHPG in unipolar and bipolar depressed patients. Psychopharmacologia 42:277–282, 1975

Belmaker RH: Receptors, adenylate cyclase, depression, and lithium. Biol Psychiatry 16:333–350, 1981

Berggren U: Effects of short-term lithium administration on tryptophan levels and 5-hydroxytryptamine synthesis in whole brain and brain regions in rats. J Neural Transm 69:115–121, 1987

Bernasconi R: The GABA hypothesis of affective illness: influence of clinically effective antimanic drugs on GABA turnover, in Basic Mechanisms in the Action of Lithium. Edited by Emrich HM, Adenhoff JB, Lux HM. Amsterdam, Excerpta Medica, 1982, pp 183–192

Berrettini WH, Vogel WH, Ladman RK: Effects of lithium therapy on MAO in manic-depressive illness. Am J Psychiatry 136:836–838, 1979

Berrettini WH, Nurnberger JI Jr, Hare T, et al: Plasma and CSF GABA in affective illness. Br J Psychiatry 141:483–487, 1982

Berrettini WH, Nurnberger JI Jr, Hare TA, et al: Reduced plasma and CSF gamma-aminobutyric acid in affective illness. Biol Psychiatry 18:185–194, 1983

Berrettini WH, Nurnberger JI, Scheinin M, et al: Cerebrospinal fluid and plasma monoamines and their metabolites in euthymic bipolar patients. Biol Psychiatry 20:257–269, 1985a

Berrettini WH, Nurnberger JI Jr, Chan JS, et al: Proopiomelanocortin-related peptides in cerebrospinal fluid: a study of manic-depressive disorder. Psychiatry Res 16:287–302, 1985b

Berrettini WH, Nurnberger JI Jr, Hare TA, et al: CSF GABA in euthymic manic-depressive patients and controls. Biol Psychiatry 21:844–846, 1986

Berrettini WH, Nurnberger JI Jr, Zerbe RL, et al: CSF neuropeptides in euthymic bipolar patients and controls. Br J Psychiatry 150:208–212, 1987

Berridge MJ: Inositol triphosphate, calcium, lithium, and cell signaling. JAMA 262:1834–1841, 1989

Berridge MJ, Downes CP, Hanley MR: Lithium amplifies agonist-dependent phosphatidylinositol responses in brain and salivary glands. Biochem J 206:587–595, 1982

Berridge MJ, Downes CP, Hanley MR: Neural and developmental actions of lithium: a unifying hypothesis. Cell 59:411–419, 1989

Beyaert R, Heyninck K, De Valck D, et al: Enhancement of tumor necrosis factor cytotoxicity by lithium chloride is associated with increased inositol phosphate accumulation. J Immunol 151:291–300, 1993

Bitran JA, Potter WZ, Manji HK, et al: Chronic Li$^+$ attenuates agonist- and phorbol ester-mediated Na$^+$/Ha$^+$ antiporter activity in HL-60 cells. Eur J Pharmacol 188:193–202, 1990

Bitran JA, Manji HK, Potter WZ, et al: Down-regulation of PKCα by lithium in vitro. Psychopharmacol Bull (in press)

Blackshear PJ: The MARCKS family of cellular protein kinase C substrates. J Biol Chem 268:1501–1504, 1993

Blancquaert JP, Lefebvre RA, Willems JL: Antiaversive properties of opioids in the conditioned taste aversion test in the rat. Pharmacol Biochem Behav 27:437–441, 1987

Blier P, de Montigny C: Short-term lithium administration enhances serotonergic neurotransmission: electrophysiological evidence in the rat CNS. Psychopharmacology (Berl) 113:69–77, 1985

Blier P, de Montigny C, Tardif D: Short-term lithium treatment enhances responsiveness of postsynaptic 5-HT$_{1A}$ receptors without altering 5-HT autoreceptor sensitivity: an electrophysiological study in the rat brain. Synapse 1:225–232, 1987

Bliss EL, Ailion J: The effect of lithium upon brain neuroamines. Brain Res 24:305–310, 1970

Bloom FE, Rogers J, Schulman JA, et al: Receptor plasticity: inferential changes after chronic treatment with lithium desmethylimipramine or ethanol detected by electrophysiological correlates, in Neuroreceptors: Basic and Clinical Aspects. Edited by Usdin E, Bunney WE Jr, Davis JM. New York, Wiley, 1981, pp 37–53

Bloom FE, Baetge G, Deyo S, et al: Chemical and physiological aspects of the actions of lithium and antidepressant drugs. Neuropharmacology 22:359–365, 1983

Bond PA, Jenner JA, Sampson DA: Daily variation of the urine content of 3-methoxy-4-hydroxy-phenylglycol in two manic-depressive patients. Psychol Med 2:81–85, 1972

Born GVR, Grignani G, Martin K: Long-term effect of lithium on the uptake of 5-hydroxytryptamine by human platelets. Br J Clin Pharmacol 9:321–325, 1980

Bowers MB, Heninger GR: Lithium: clinical effects and cerebrospinal fluid acid monoamine metabolites. Communications in Psychopharmacology 1:135–145, 1977

Brambilla F, Catalano M, Lucca A, et al: Effect of lithium treatment on the GH-clonidine test in affective disorders. Eur J Clin Pharmacol 35:601–605, 1988

Brami BA, Leli U, Hauser G: Influence of lithium on second messenger accumulation in NG108-15 cells. Biochem Biophys Res Commun 174:606–612, 1991a

Brami BA, Leli U, Hauser G: Origin of the diacylglycerol produced in excess of inositol phosphates by lithium in NG108-15 cells. J Neurochem 57 (suppl):S9, 1991b

Briggs GG, Freeman RK, Yaffe SJ: Drugs in Pregnancy and Lactation, 3rd Edition. Baltimore, MD, Williams & Wilkins, 1990

Brown GM, Grof E, Grof P: Neuroendocrinology of depression—a discussion. Psychopharmacol Bull 17:10–12, 1981

Bunney WE Jr: Neuronal receptor function in psychiatry: strategy and theory, in Neuroreceptors: Basic and Clinical Aspects. Edited by Usdin E, Bunney WE Jr, Davis JM. New York, Wiley, 1981, pp 241–255

Bunney WE, Garland BL: Lithium and its possible modes of action, in Neurobiology of Mood Disorders. Edited by Post RM, Ballenger J. Baltimore, MD, Williams & Wilkins, 1984, pp 731–743

Bunney WE, Garland-Bunney BL: Mechanism of action of lithium in affective illness: basic and clinical implications, in Psychopharmacology: The Third Generation of Progress. Edited by Meltzer HY. New York, Raven, 1987, pp 553–565

Burns G, Herz A, Nikolarakis KE: Stimulation of hypothalamic opioid peptide release by lithium is mediated by opioid autoreceptors: evidence from a combined in vitro, ex vivo study. Neuroscience 36:691–697, 1990

Bussone G, Leone M, Peccarisi C, et al: Double blind comparison of lithium and verapamil in cluster headache prophylaxis. Headache 30:411–417, 1990

Cade JFJ: Lithium salts in the treatment of psychotic excitement. Med J Aust 36:349–352, 1949

Calabrese JR, Gulledge AD, Hahn K, et al: Autoimmune thyroiditis in manic-depressive patients treated with lithium. Am J Psychiatry 142:1318–1321, 1985

Cameron OG, Smith CB: Comparison of acute and chronic lithium treatment on ^{3}H-norepinephrine uptake by rat brain slices. Psychopharmacology (Berl) 67:81–85, 1980

Campbell SS, Gillin JC, Kripke DF, et al: Lithium delays circadian phase of temperature and REM sleep in a bipolar depressive: a case report. Psychiatry Res 27:23–29, 1989

Canessa M, Adragna N, Solomon HS, et al: Increased sodium-lithium countertransport in red cells of patients with essential hypertension. N Engl J Med 302:772–776, 1980

Canessa M, Brugnara C, Escobales N: The Li$^+$-Na$^+$ exchange and Na$^+$-K$^+$-Cl$^-$ cotransport systems in essential hypertension. Hypertension 10 (suppl I):4–10, 1987

Carmiliet EE: Influence of lithium ions on the transmembrane potential and cation content of cardiac cells. J Gen Physiol 47:501–530, 1964

Carney PA, Fitzgerald CT, Monaghan CE: Influence of climate on the prevalence of mania. Br J Psychiatry 152:820–823, 1988

Casebolt TL, Jope RS: Long-term lithium treatment selectively reduces receptor-coupled inositol phospholipid hydrolysis in rat brain. Biol Psychiatry 25:329–340, 1989

Catalano M, Bellodi L, Lucca A, et al: Lithium and alpha-2-adrenergic receptors: effects of lithium ion on clonidine-induced growth hormone release. Neuroendocrinology Letters 6:61–66, 1984

Cernescu C, Popescu L, Constantinescu S, et al: Antiviral effect of lithium chloride. Virologie 39:93–101, 1988

Chapman BE, Beilharz GR, York MJ, et al: Endogenous phospholipase and choline release in human erythrocytes: a study using ^{1}H NMR spectroscopy. Biochem Biophys Res Commun 105:1280–1287, 1982

Choi SJ, Taylor MA, Abrams R: Depression, ECT, and erythrocyte adenosinetriphosphatase activity. Biol Psychiatry 12:75–81, 1977

Christiansen C, Baastrup PC, Lindgren P, et al: Endocrine effects of lithium, II: "primary" hyperparathyroidism. Acta Endocrinol (Copen) 88:528–534, 1978

Coccaro EF, Siever LJ, Klar HM, et al: Serotonergic studies in patients with affective and personality disorders: correlates with suicidal and impulsive aggressive behavior. Arch Gen Psychiatry 46:587–599, 1989

Cohen LS, Friedman JM, Jefferson JW, et al: A reevaluation of risk of in utero exposure to lithium. JAMA 271:146–150, 1994

Cohen WJ, Cohen NJ: Lithium carbonate, haloperidol and irreversible brain damage. JAMA 230:1283–1287, 1974

Colburn RW, Goodwin FK, Bunney WE Jr, et al: Effect of lithium on the uptake of noradrenaline by synaptosomes. Nature 215:1395–1397, 1967

Colin SF, Chang HC, Mollner S, et al: Chronic lithium regulates the expression of adenylate cyclase and G_i-protein alpha subunit in rat cerebral cortex. Proc Natl Acad Sci U S A 88:10634–10637, 1991

Collard KJ: Lithium effects on brain 5-HT metabolism, in Lithium in Medical Practice. Edited by Johnson FN, Johnson S. Lancaster, United Kingdom, MTP Press, 1978, pp 123–133

Collard KJ: Effects of lithium on brain metabolism, in Endocrine and Metabolic Effects of Lithium. Edited by Lazarus JH. New York, Plenum, 1986, pp 55–98

Collard KJ, Roberts MHT: Effects of lithium on the elevation of forebrain 5-hydroxyindoles by tryptophan. Neuropharmacology 16:671–673, 1977

Collins PJ, Larkin EP, Shubsachs AP: Lithium carbonate in chronic schizophrenia: a brief trial of lithium carbonate added to neuroleptics for treatment of resistant schizophrenic patients. Acta Psychiatr Scand 84:150–154, 1991

Coppen A, Abou-Saleh MT: Lithium therapy: from clinical trials to practical management. Acta Psychiatr Scand 78:754–762, 1988

Coppen A, Shaw DM: Mineral metabolism in melancholia. British Medical Journal 2:1439–1444, 1963

Coppen A, Shaw DM: The distribution of electrolytes and water in patients after taking lithium carbonate. Lancet 2:805–806, 1967

Coppen A, Shaw DM, Malleson A, et al: Mineral metabolism in mania. British Medical Journal 1:71–75, 1966

Coppen A, Swade C, Wood K: Lithium restores abnormal platelet 5-HT transport in patients with affective disorders. Br J Psychiatry 136:235–238, 1980

Coppen A, Abou-Saleh MT, Milln P, et al: Lithium continuation therapy following electroconvulsive therapy. Br J Psychiatry 139:284–287, 1981

Coppen A, Standish-Barry H, Bailey J, et al: Does lithium reduce the mortality of recurrent mood disorders? J Affect Disord 23:1–7, 1991

Corona GL, Cucchi ML, Santagostino G, et al: Blood noradrenaline and 5-HT levels in depressed women during amitriptyline or lithium treatment. Psychopharmacology (Berl) 77:236–241, 1982

Corrodi H, Fuxe K, Hokfelt T, et al: The effect of lithium on cerebral monoamine neurons. Psychopharmacologia 11:345–353, 1967

Cowen PJ, McCance SL, Cohen PR, et al: Lithium increases 5-HT-mediated neuroendocrine responses in tricyclic resistant depression. Psychopharmacology (Berl) 99:230–232, 1989

Crowe RR: Current concepts: electroconvulsive therapy—a current perspective. N Engl J Med 311:163–167, 1984

Dagher G, Gay C, Brossard M, et al: Lithium, sodium and potassium transport in erythrocytes of manic-depressive patients. Acta Psychiatr Scand 69:24–36, 1984

Dawood I, Welch W Jr: The stimulation of rat brain monoamine oxidase by dietary lithium chloride. Experientia 35:991–992, 1979

de Belleroche J, Cook GE, Das I, et al: Erythrocyte choline concentrations and cluster headache. British Medical Journal (Clinical Research Edition) 288:268–270, 1984 de Belleroche J, Kilfeather S, Das I, et al: Abnormal membrane composition and membrane-dependent transduction mechanisms in cluster headache. Cephalalgia 6:147–153, 1986

Delva NJ, Letemendia FJ: Lithium treatment in schizophrenia and schizo-affective disorders. Br J Psychiatry 141:387–400, 1982

Degkwitz R, Koufen H, Consbruch U, et al: Untersuchungen zur lithiumbilanz wahrend der manie. [Investigation on lithium levels during mania.] International Pharmacopsychiatry 14:199–212, 1979

de Montigny C, Grunberg F, Mayer A, et al: Lithium induces rapid relief of depression in tricyclic antidepressant drug non-responders. Br J Psychiatry 138:252–256, 1981

de Montigny C, Cournoyer G, Morissette R, et al: Lithium carbonate addition in tricyclic antidepressant-resistant unipolar depression: correlations with the neurobiologic actions of tricyclic antidepressant drugs and lithium ion on the serotonin system. Arch Gen Psychiatry 40:1327–1334, 1983

de Montigny C, Chaput Y, Blier P: Lithium augmentation of antidepressant treatments: evidence for the involvement of the 5-HT system?, in New Concepts in Depression. Edited by Briley M, Fillion G. Basingstoke, United Kingdom, Macmillan, 1988, pp 144–160

Deniker P, Eygiem A, Bernheim R, et al: Thyroid antibody levels during lithium therapy. Neuropsychobiology 4:270–275, 1978

Depue RA, Karuss SP, Spoont MR: A two-dimensional threshold model of seasonal bipolar affective disorder, in Psychopathology: An Interactional Perspective. Edited by Magnusson D, Ohman A. Orlando, FL, Academic Press, 1987, pp 95–123

Detellier C: Alkali metals, in NMR of Newly Accessible Nuclei. Edited by Laszlo P. New York, Academic Press, 1983, pp 105–151

Diamond JM, Meier K, Gosenfeld LF, et al: Recovery of erythrocyte Li^+/Na^+ countertransport and choline transport from lithium therapy. J Psychiatr Res 17:385–393, 1982/1983

Dick DAT, Naylor GJ, Dick EG: Effects of lithium on sodium transport across membranes, in Lithium in Medical Practice. Edited by Johnson FN, Johnson S. Lancaster, United Kingdom, MTP Press, 1978, pp 183–192

Dilsaver SC, Coffman JA: Cholinergic hypothesis of depression: a reappraisal. J Clin Psychopharmacol

9:173–179, 1989

Dilsaver SC, Hariharan M: Amitriptyline-induced supersensitivity of a central muscarinic mechanism: lithium blocks amitriptyline-induced supersensitivity. Psychiatry Res 25:181–186, 1988

Dilsaver SC, Hariharan M: Chronic treatment with lithium produces supersensitivity to nicotine. Biol Psychiatry 25:792–795, 1989

Divish MM, Sheftel G, Boyle A, et al: Differential effect of lithium on fos protooncogene expression mediated by receptor and postreceptor activators of protein kinase C and cyclic adenosine monophosphate: model for its antimanic action. J Neurosci Res 28:40–48, 1991

Dousa TP: Interaction of lithium with vasopressin-sensitive cyclic AMP system of human renal medulla. Endocrinology 95:1359–1366, 1974

Dousa T, Hechter O: Lithium and brain adenylyl cyclase. Lancet 1:834–835, 1970a

Dousa T, Hechter O: The effect of NaCl and LiCl on vasopressin-sensitive adenyl cyclase. Life Sci 9:765–770, 1970b

Dowling JE: Neurons and Networks. Cambridge, MA, Belknap Press of Harvard University Press, 1992

Downes CP, Stone MA: Lithium-induced reduction in intracellular inositol supply in cholinergically stimulated parotid gland. Biochem J 234:199–204, 1986

Drummond AH, Raeburn CA: The interaction of lithium with thyrotropin releasing hormone-stimulated lipid metabolism in GH_3 pituitary tumor cells. Biochem J 224:129–136, 1984

Dubovsky SL, Lee C, Christiano J, et al: Elevated platelet intracellular calcium concentration in bipolar depression. Biol Psychiatry 29:441–450, 1991a

Dubovsky SL, Lee C, Christiano J, et al: Lithium lowers platelet intracellular ion concentration in bipolar patients. Lithium 2:167–174, 1991b

Dubovsky SL, Murphy J, Thomas M, et al: Abnormal intracellular calcium ion concentration in platelets and lymphocytes of bipolar patients. Am J Psychiatry 149:118–120, 1992

Ebstein R, Belmaker R, Grunhaus L, et al: Lithium inhibition of adrenaline-stimulated adenylate cyclase in humans. Nature 259:411–413, 1976

Ebstein RP, Hermoni M, Belmaker RH: The effect of lithium on noradrenaline-induced cyclic AMP accumulation in rat brain: inhibition after chronic treatment and absence of supersensitivity. J Pharmacol Exp Ther 213:161–167, 1980

Ebstein RP, Lerer B, Shlaufman M, et al: The effect of repeated electroconvulsive shock treatment and chronic lithium feeding on the release of norepinephrine from rat cortical vesicular preparations. Cell Mol Neurobiol 3:191–201, 1983

Egeland JA, Kidd JR, Frazer A, et al: Amish study V: lithium-sodium countertransport and catechol-o-methyltransferase in pedigrees of bipolar probands. Am J Psychiatry 141:1049–1054, 1984

Ehrlich BE, Diamond JM: Lithium fluxes in human erythrocytes. Am J Physiol 237:C102–C110, 1979

Ehrlich BE, Diamond JM: Lithium, membranes, and manic-depressive illness. J Membr Biol 52:187–200, 1980

Ehrlich BE, Diamond JM, Braun LD, et al: Effects of lithium on blood-brain barrier transport of the neurotransmitter precursors choline, tyrosine and tryptophan. Brain Res 193:604–607, 1980

Ehrlich BE, Diamond JM, Gosenfeld L: Lithium-induced changes in sodium-lithium countertransport. Biochem Pharmacol 30:2539–2543, 1981

Ehrlich BE, Diamond JM, Fry V, et al: Lithium's inhibition of erythrocyte cation countertransport involves a slow process in the erythrocyte. J Membr Biol 75:233–240, 1983

Elia J, Katz IR, Simpson GM: Teratogenicity of psychotherapeutic medications. Psychopharmacol Bull 23:531–586, 1987

El-Mallakh RS: The Na,K-ATPase hypothesis for manic depression. Med Hypotheses 12:253–282, 1983

El-Mallakh RS: The ionic mechanism of lithium action. Lithium 1:87–92, 1990

Ellis J, Lenox RH: Chronic lithium treatment prevents atropine-induced supersensitivity of the muscarinic phosphoinositide response in rat hippocampus. Biol Psychiatry 28:609–619, 1990

Ellis J, Lenox RH: Receptor coupling to G proteins: interactions not affected by lithium. Lithium 2:141–147, 1991

Engel J, Berggren U: Effects of lithium on behaviour and central monoamines. Acta Psychiatr Scand 61 (suppl 280):133–143, 1980

Eroglu L, Hizal A, Koyuncuoglu H: The effect of long-term concurrent administration of chlorpromazine and lithium on the striatal and frontal cortical dopamine metabolism in rats. Psychopharmacology (Berl) 73:84–86, 1981

Evans MS, Zorumski CF, Clifford DB: Lithium enhances neuronal muscarinic excitation by presynaptic facilitation. Neuroscience 38:457–468, 1990

Faedda GL, Tondo L, Baldessarini RJ: Outcome after rapid vs gradual discontinuation of lithium treatment in bipolar disorders. Arch Gen Psychiatry 50:448–455, 1993

Fischl MA, Richman DD, Grieco MH, et al: The efficacy of azidothymidine (AZT) in the treatment of patients with AIDS and AIDS-related complex: a double-blind, placebo-controlled trial. N Engl J Med 317:185–191, 1987

Fisher SK, Heacock AM, Agranoff BW: Inositol lipids and signal transduction in the nervous system: an update. J Neurochem 58:18–38, 1992

Forn J, Valdecasas FG: Effects of lithium on brain adenylyl cyclase activity. Biochem Pharmacol 20:2773–2779, 1971

Frances H, Maurin Y, Lecrubier Y, et al: Effect of chronic lithium treatment on isolation-induced behavioral and biochemical effects in mice. Eur J Pharmacol 72:337–341, 1981

Frazer A, Mendels J, Brunswick D, et al: Erythrocyte concentrations of the lithium ion: clinical correlates and mechanisms of action. Am J Psychiatry 135:1065–1069, 1978

Friedman E, Gershon S: Effect of lithium on brain dopamine. Nature 243:520–521, 1973

Friedman E, Wang HY: Effect of chronic lithium treatment on 5-hydroxytryptamine autoreceptors and release of 5-[^{3}H]hydroxytryptamine from rat brain cortical, hippocampal, and hypothalamic slices. J Neurochem 50:195–201, 1988

Friedman E, Dallob A, Levine G: The effect of long-term lithium treatment on reserpine-induced supersensitivity in dopaminergic and serotonergic transmission. Life Sci 25:1263–1266, 1979a

Friedman E, Oleshansky MA, Moy P, et al: Lithium and catecholamine-induced plasma cyclic AMP elevation, in Lithium Controversies and Unresolved Issues. Edited by Cooper TB, Gershon S, Kline NS, et al. Amsterdam, Excerpta Medica, 1979b, pp 730–736

Fyro B, Petterson U, Sedvall G: The effect of lithium treatment on manic symptoms and levels of monoamine metabolites in cerebrospinal fluid of manic depressive patients. Psychopharmacologia 44:99–103, 1975

Gallager DW, Pert A, Bunney WE Jr: Haloperidol-induced presynaptic dopamine supersensitivity is blocked by chronic lithium. Nature 273:309–312, 1978

Gallicchio VS, Hughes NK: Effective modulation of the haematopoietic toxicity associated with zidovudine exposure to murine and human haematopoietic progenitor stem cells in vitro with lithium chloride. J Intern Med 231:219–226, 1992

Gallicchio VS, Messino MJ, Hulette BC, et al: Lithium and hematopoiesis: effective experimental use of lithium as an agent to improve bone marrow transplantation. J Med 23:195–216, 1992

Gallicchio VS, Cibull ML, Hughes NK, et al: Effect of lithium in murine immunodeficiency virus infected animals. Pathobiology 61:216–221, 1993

Gao XM, Fukamauchi F, Chuang DM: Long-term biphasic effects of lithium treatment on phospholipase C-coupled M3-muscarinic acetylcholine receptors in cultured cerebellar granule cells. Neurochem Int 22:395–403, 1993

Garcia-Sevilla JA, Guimon J, Garcia-Vallejo P, et al: Biochemical and functional evidence of supersensitive platelet alpha-2-adrenoceptors in major affective disorder: effect of long-term lithium carbonate treatment. Arch Gen Psychiatry 43:51–57, 1986

Garfinkel PE, Ezrin C, Stancer HC: Hypothyroidism and hyperparathyroidism associated with lithium. Lancet 2:331–332, 1973

Garland EJ, Remick RA, Zis AP: Weight gain with antidepressants and lithium. J Clin Psychopharmacol 8:323–330, 1988

Garrod AB: The Nature and Treatment of Gout and Rheumatic Gout. London, Walton & Maberly, 1859

Geisler A, Klysner R: The effect of lithium in vitro and in vivo on dopamine-sensitive adenylate cyclase activity in dopaminergic areas of the rat brain. Acta Pharmacologica et Toxicologica (Copenhagen) 56:1–5, 1985

Geisler A, Klysner R, Andersen PH: Influence of lithium in vitro and in vivo on the catecholamine-sensitive cerebral adenylate cyclase systems. Acta Pharmacologica et Toxicologica (Copenhagen) 56:80–97, 1985

Gelenberg AJ, Kane JM, Keller MB, et al: Comparison of standard and low serum levels of lithium for maintenance treatment of bipolar disorder. N Engl J Med 321:1489–1493, 1989

Giacovazzo M, Marteletti P, Romiti, et al: Relationship between HLA antigen subtypes and lithium response in cluster headache. Headache 25:268–270, 1985

Giacovazzo M, Martelletti P, Romiti A, et al: Genetic markers of cluster headache and the links with the lithium salts therapy. Int J Clin Pharmacol Res 61:19–22, 1986

Gitlin MJ: Lithium-induced renal insufficiency. J Clin Psychopharmacol 13:276–279, 1993

Glen AIM, Reading HW: Regulatory action of lithium in manic-depressive illness. Lancet 2:1239–1241, 1973

Glue PW, Cowen PJ, Nutt DJ, et al: The effect of lithium on 5-HT mediated neuroendocrine response and platelet 5-HT receptors. Psychopharmacology (Berl) 90:398–402, 1986

Godfrey PP: Potentiation by lithium of CMP-phosphatidate formation in carbachol-stimulated rat cerebral-cortical slices and its reversal by myo-inositol. Biochem J 258:621–624, 1989

Godfrey PP, McClue SJ, White AM, et al: Subacute and chronic in vivo lithium treatment inhibits agonist- and sodium fluoride-stimulated inositol phosphate production in rat cortex. J Neurochem 52:498–506, 1989

Goodnick P: Effects of lithium on indices of 5-HT and catecholamines in the clinical content: a review. Lithium 1:65–73, 1990

Goodnick PJ, Gershon ES: Lithium, in Handbook of Neurochemistry. Edited by Lajtha A. New York, Plenum, 1985, pp 103–149

Goodnick PJ, Meltzer HY: Neurochemical changes during discontinuation of lithium prophylaxis, I: increases in clonidine-induced hypotension. Biol Psychiatry 19:883–889, 1984a

Goodnick PJ, Meltzer HY: Treatment of schizoaffective disorders. Schizophr Bull 10:30–48, 1984b

Goodwin FK, Jamison KR: Manic-Depressive Illness. New York, Oxford University Press, 1990

Goodwin FK, Murphy DL, Bunney WE: Lithium-carbonate treatment in depression and mania. Arch Gen Psychiatry 21:486–496, 1969

Goodwin GM, DeSouza RJ, Wood AJ, et al: Lithium decreases 5-HT1A and 5-HT2 receptor and alpha-2 adrenoceptor mediated function in mice. Psychopharmacology (Berl) 90:482–487, 1986a

Goodwin GM, DeSouza RJ, Wood AJ, et al: The enhancement by lithium of the 5-HT1A mediated serotonin syndrome produced by 8-OH-DPAT in the rat: evidence for a post-synaptic mechanism. Psychopharmacology (Berl) 90:488–493, 1986b

Gorkin RA, Richelson E: Lithium transport by mouse neuroblastoma cells. Neuropharmacology 20:791, 1981

Gottesfeld Z, Ebstein BS, Samuel D: Effect of lithium on concentrations of glutamate and GABA levels in amygdala and hypothalamus of rat. Nature 234:124–125, 1971

Grahame-Smith DG, Green AR: The role of brain 5-hydroxytryptamine in the hyperactivity produced in rats by lithium and monoamine oxidase inhibition. Br J Pharmacol 52:19–26, 1974

Greenspan K, Schildkraut JJ, Gordon EK, et al: Catecholamine metabolism in affective disorders, 3: MHPG and other catecholamine metabolites in patients treated with lithium carbonate. J Psychiatr Res 7:171–183, 1970

Greil W, Eisenreid F, Becker BF, et al: Interindividual differences in the Na$^+$-dependent Li$^+$ countertransport system and in the Li$^+$ distribution ratio across the red cell membrane among Li$^+$-treated patients. Psychopharmacology (Berl) 53:19–26, 1977

Grof E, Brown GM, Grof P, et al: Effects of lithium administration on plasma catecholamines. Psychiatry Res 19:87–92, 1986

Guerri C, Ribelles M, Grisolia S: Effect of lithium and lithium and alcohol administration on Na$^+$-K$^+$ ATPase. Biochem Pharmacol 30:25–30, 1981

Gwinner E, Benzinger J: Synchronization of a circadian rhythm in penealectomized European starlings by daily injections of melatonin. Journal of Comparative Physiology 127:209–213, 1978

Haag M, Haag H, Eisenried F, et al: RBC-choline: changes by lithium and relation to prophylactic response. Acta Psychiatr Scand 70:389–399, 1984

Haag M, Granzow L, Greil W, et al: RBC-choline: a biological marker of the outcome of lithium prophylaxis? Prog Neuropsychopharmacol Biol Psychiatry 11:209–212, 1987

Hallcher LM, Sherman WR: The effects of lithium ion and other agents on the activity of myoinositol-1-phosphatase from bovine brain. J Biol Chem 255:10896–10901, 1980

Hallonquist JD, Goldberg MA, Brandes JS: Affective disorders and circadian rhythms. Can J Psychiatry 31:259–272, 1986

Harrison-Read PE: Evidence from behavioural reactions to fenfluramine, 5-hydroxyptryptophan, and 5-methoxy-N,N-dimethyltryptamine for differential effects of short-term and long-term lithium on indoleaminergic mechanisms in rats. Br J Pharmacol 66:144–145, 1979

Hatterer JA, Kocsis JH, Stokes PE: Thyroid function in patients maintained on lithium. Psychiatry Res 26:249–258, 1989

Heninger GR, Charney DS, Sternberg DE: Lithium carbonate augmentation of antidepressant treatment: an effective prescription for treatment-refractory depression. Arch Gen Psychiatry 40:1335–1342, 1983

Hermoni M, Lerer B, Ebstein RP, et al: Chronic lithium prevents reserpine-induced supersensitivity of adenylate cyclase. J Pharm Pharmacol 32:510–511, 1980

Hermoni M, Barzilai A, Rahamimoff H: Modulation of the Na$^+$-Ca^{2+} antiport by its ionic environment: the effect of lithium. Isr J Med Sci 23:44–48, 1987

Hesketh JE, Nicolaou NM, Arbuthnott GW, et al: The effect of chronic lithium administration on dopamine metabolism in rat striatum. Psychopharmacology (Berl) 56:163–166, 1978

Hirvonen MR, Paljarri L, Naukkarinen A, et al: Potentiation of malaoxon-induced convulsions by lithium: early neuronal injury, phosphoinositide signaling and calcium. Toxicol Appl Pharmacol 104:276–289, 1990

Hitzemann R, Mark C, Hirschowitz J, et al: RBC lithium transport in the psychoses. Biol Psychiatry 25:296–304, 1989

Ho AKS, Tsai CS: Lithium and cthanol preference. J Pharm Pharmacol 27:58–60, 1975

Ho AKS, Loh HH, Craves F, et al: The effect of prolonged lithium treatment on the synthesis rate and turnover of monoamines in brain regions of rats. Eur J Pharmacol 10:72–78, 1970

Hokin-Neaverson M, Jefferson JW: Erythrocyte sodium pump activity in bipolar affective disorder and other psychiatric disorders. Neuropsychobiology 22:1–7, 1989a

Hokin-Neaverson M, Jefferson JW: Deficient erythrocyte Na,K-ATPase activity in different affective states in bipolar affective states in bipolar affective disorder and normalization by lithium therapy. Neuropsychobiology 22:18–25, 1989b

Hokin-Neaverson M, Spiegel DA, Lewis WC: Deficiency of erythrocyte sodium pump activity in bipolar manic-depressive psychosis. Life Sci 15:1739–1748, 1974

Hokin-Neaverson M, Burckhardt WA, Jefferson JW: Increased erythrocyte Na$^+$ pump and NaK-ATPase activity during lithium therapy. Res Commun Chem Pathol Pharmacol 14:117–126, 1976

Honchar MP, Olney JW, Sherman WR: Systemic cholinergic agents induce seizures and brain damage in lithium-treated rats. Science 220:323–325, 1983

Hong JS, Tilson HA, Yoshikawa K: Effects of lithium and haloperidol administration on the rat brain levels of Substance P. J Pharmacol Exp Ther 224:590–597, 1983

Hotta I, Yamawaki S: Possible involvement of presynaptic 5-HT autoreceptors in effect of lithium on 5-HT release in hippocampus of rat. Neuropharmacology 27:987–992, 1988

Hsiao JK, Manji HK, Chen GA, et al: Lithium administration modulates platelet G_i in humans. Life Sci 50:227–233, 1992

Huang KP: The mechanism of protein kinase C activation. Trends Neurosci 12:425–432, 1989

Huey LY, Janowsky DS, Judd LL, et al: Effects of lithium carbonate on methylphenidate-induced mood, behaviour, and cognitive processes. Psychopharmacology (Berl) 73:161–164, 1981

Jacobson SJ, Jones K, Johnson K, et al: Prospective multicentre study of pregnancy outcome after lithium exposure during first trimester. Lancet 339:530–533, 1992

Jefferson JW: Lithium: the present and the future. J Clin Psychiatry 51 (suppl 8):4–19, 1990

Jefferson JW: Update on lithium in clinical practice: an interview with James W. Jefferson, M.D. Currents in Affective Illness 10:5–14, 1991

Jefferson JW, Greist JH, Baudhiun M: Lithium: interactions with other drugs. J Clin Psychopharmacol 1:124–134, 1981

Jefferson JW, Greist JH, Ackerman DL: Lithium Encyclopedia for Clinical Practice. Washington, DC, American Psychiatric Press, 1983

Jefferson JW, Greist JH, Ackerman DL, et al: Lithium Encyclopedia for Clinical Practice, 2nd Edition. Washington, DC, American Psychiatric Press, 1987

Johnson BB, Naylor GJ, Dick EG, et al: Prediction of clinical course of bipolar manic depressive illness treated with lithium. Psychol Med 10:329–334, 1980

Johnson FN: The History of Lithium Therapy. Basingstoke, United Kingdom, Macmillan, 1984

Johnson FN: Depression and Mania: Modern Lithium Therapy. Oxford, England, IRL Press, 1987

Johnson FN: Lithium treatment of aggression, self-mutilation, and affective disorders in the context of mental handicap. Reviews in Contemporary Pharmacotherapy 1:9–18, 1988

Johnson FN, Minnai G: Potential alternative applications of oral lithium. Reviews in Contemporary Pharmacotherapy 4:237–250, 1993

Johnson G, Gershon S, Burdock EI, et al: Comparative effects of lithium and chlorpromazine in the treatment of acute manic states. Br J Psychiatry 119:267–276, 1971

Johnsson A, Engelmann W, Pflug B, et al: Period lengthening of human circadian rhythms by lithium carbonate, a prophylactic for depressive disorders. International Journal of Chronobiology (London) 8:129–147, 1983

Jones FD, Maas JW, Dekirmenjian M, et al: Urinary catecholamine metabolites during behavioural changes in a patient with manic-depressive cycles. Science 179:300–302, 1973

Jope RS: Effects of lithium treatment in vitro and in vivo on acetylcholine metabolism in rat brain. J Neurochem 33:487–495, 1979

Jope RS, Jenden DJ, Ehrlich BE, et al: Choline accumulates in erythrocytes during lithium therapy. N Engl J Med 299:833–834, 1978

Jope RS, Jenden DJ, Ehrlich BE, et al: Erythrocyte choline concentrations are elevated in manic patients. Proc Natl Acad Sci U S A 77:6144–6146, 1980

Jope RS, Morrisett RA, Snead OC: Characterization of lithium potentiation of pilocarpine induced status epilepticus in rats. Exp Neurol 91:471–480, 1986

Judd LL, Squire LR, Butters N, et al: Effects of psychotropic drugs on cognition and memory in normal humans and animals, in Psychopharmacology: The Third Generation of Progress. Edited by Meltzer HY. New York, Raven, 1987, pp 1467–1475

Kafka M, Wirz-Justice A, Naber D, et al: Effect of lithium on circadian neurotransmitter receptor rhythms. Neuropsychobiology 8:41–50, 1982

Kafka MS, Wirz-Justice A, Naber D, et al: Circadian rhythms in rat brain neurotransmitter receptors. Federation Proceedings 42:2796–2801, 1983

Kalasapudi VD, Sheftel G, Divish MM, et al: Lithium augments fos protoonocogene expression in PC12 pheochromocytoma cells: implications for therapeutic action of lithium. Brain Res 521:47–54, 1990

Kaschka WP, Mokrusch T, Korth M: Early physiological effects of lithium treatment: electro-oculographic and adaptometric findings in patients with affective and schizoaffective psychoses. Pharmacopsychiatry 20:203–207, 1987

Katz RI, Kopin KJ: Release of ^{3}H-norepinephrine and ^{3}H-serotonin evoked from brain slices by electric field stimulation: calcium dependence and the effects of lithium and tetrodotoxin. Biochem Pharmacol 18:1935–1939, 1969

Katz RI, Chase TN, Kopin IJ: Evoked release of norepinephrine and serotonin from brain slices: inhibition by lithium. Science 162:466–467, 1968

Kendall DA, Nahorski SR: Acute and chronic lithium treatments influence agonist- and depolarization-stimulated inositol phospholipid hydrolysis in rat cerebral cortex. J Pharmacol Exp Ther 241:1023–1027, 1987

Kennedy ED, Challiss RJ, Nahorski SR: Lithium reduces the accumulation of inositol polyphosphate second messengers following cholinergic stimulation of cerebral cortex slices. J Neurochem 53:1652–1655, 1989

Kennedy ED, Challiss RAJ, Ragan CI, et al: Reduced inositol polyphosphate accumulation and inositol supply induced by lithium in stimulated cerebral cortex slices. Biochem J 267:781–786, 1990

Keynes RS, Swan RC: The permeability of frog muscle fibers to lithium ions. J Physiol (Lond) 147:626–638, 1959

Kim MH, Neubig RR: Membrane reconstitution of high affinity alpha-2-adrenergic agonist binding with guanine nucleotide regulatory proteins. Biochemistry 26:3664–3672, 1987

Kishimoto A, Mikawa K, Hashimoto K, et al: Limited proteolysis of protein kinase C subspecies by calcium-dependent neutral protease (calpain). J Biol Chem 264:4088–4092, 1989

Kislauskis E, Dobner PR: Mutually dependent response elements in the cis-regulatory region of the neurotensin/neuromedin N gene integrate environmental stimuli in PC12 cells. Neuron 4:783–795, 1990

Klawans HL, Weiner WJ, Nausieda PA: The effect of lithium on an animal model of tardive dyskinesia. Progress in Neuro-Psychopharmacology 1:53–60, 1976

Klein E, Lavie P, Meiraz R, et al: Increased motor activity and recurrent manic episodes: risk factors that predict rapid relapse in remitted bipolar disorder patients after lithium discontinuation—a double blind study. Biol Psychiatry 31:279–284, 1992

Klemfuss H, Kripke DF: Effects of lithium on circadian rhythms, in Chronopharmacology, Cellular and Biochemical Interactions. Edited by Lemmer B. New York, Marcel Dekker, 1989, pp 281–297

Knapp S, Mandell AJ: Effects of lithium chloride on

parameters of biosynthetic capacity for 5-hydroxytryptamine in rat brain. J Pharmacol Exp Ther 193:812–823, 1975

Koenig JI, Meltzer HY, Gudelsky GA: Alterations of hormonal responses following lithium treatment in the rat. Proceedings of the Eighth International Congress of Endocrinology 1037, 1984

Kofman O, Belmaker RH: Biochemical, behavioral and clinical studies of the role of inositol in lithium treatment and depression. Biol Psychiatry 34:839–852, 1993

Kofman O, Belmaker RH, Grisaru N, et al: Myoinositol attenuates two specific behavioral effects of acute lithium in rats. Psychopharmacol Bull 27:185–190, 1991

Krell RD, Goldberg AM: Effect of acute and chronic administration of lithium on steady-state levels of mouse brain choline and acetylcholine. Biochem Pharmacol 22:3289–3291, 1973

Kripke DF, Mullaney DJ, Atkinson M, et al: Circadian rhythm disorders in manic-depressives. Biol Psychiatry 13:335–351, 1978

Kripke DF, Judd LL, Hubbard B, et al: The effect of lithium carbonate on the circadian rhythm of sleep in normal human subjects. Biol Psychiatry 14:545–548, 1979

Kuchel PW, Hunt GE, Johnson GFS, et al: Lithium, red blood cell choline and clinical state: a prospective study in manic-depressive patients. J Affect Disord 6:83–94, 1984

Kuffler SW, Nicholls JC: From Neuron to Brain, 2nd Edition. New York, Oxford University Press, 1979

Kupfer DJ, Wyatt RJ, Greenspan K, et al: Lithium carbonate and sleep in affective illness. Arch Gen Psychiatry 23:35–40, 1970

Kupfer DJ, Reynolds CF III, Weiss BL, et al: Lithium carbonate and sleep in affective disorders. Arch Gen Psychiatry 30:79–84, 1974

Kuriyama K, Speken R: Effect of lithium on content and uptake of norepinephrine and 5-hydroxytryptamine in mouse brain synaptosomes and mitochondria. Life Sci 9:1213–1220, 1970

Laakso ML, Oja SS: Transport of tryptophan and tyrosine in rat brain slices in the presence of lithium. Neurochem Res 4:411–423, 1979

Lal S, Nair NPV, Guyda H: Effect of lithium on hypothalamic-pituitary dopaminergic function. Acta Psychiatr Scand 57:91–96, 1978

Lange C: Om Periodiske Depressionstilstande og deres Patogenese. [About periodic depression and its pathogenesis.] Copenhagen, Jacob Lunds Forlag, 1886

Lauritsen BJ, Mellerup ET, Plenge P, et al: Serum lithium concentrations around the clock with different treatment regimens and the diurnal variation of the renal lithium clearance. Acta Psychiatr Scand 64:314–319, 1981

Lazarus JH: Endocrine and Metabolic Effects of Lithium. New York, Plenum, 1986

Lazarus JH, Muston LJ: The effect of lithium on the iodide concentrating mechanism in mouse salivary gland. Acta Pharmacologica et Toxicologica (Copenhagen) 43:55–58, 1978

Lee G, Lingsch C, Lyle PT, et al: Lithium treatment strongly inhibits choline transport in human erythrocytes. Br J Clin Pharmacol 1:365–370, 1974

Lenox RH: Role of receptor coupling to phosphoinositide metabolism in the therapeutic action of lithium, in Molecular Mechanisms of Neuronal Responsiveness. Adv Exp Biol Med. Edited by Ehrlich YH, et al. New York, Plenum, 1987, pp 515–530

Lenox RH, Ellis J: Potential targets for the action of lithium in the brain: muscarinic receptor regulation. Clin Neuropharmacol 13 (suppl):215–216, 1990

Lenox RH, Watson DG: Targets for lithium action in the brain: protein kinase C substrates and muscarinic receptor regulation. Clin Neuropharmacol 15:612A–614A, 1992

Lenox RH, Watson DG, Ellis J: Muscarinic receptor regulation and protein kinase C: sites for the action of chronic lithium in the hippocampus. Psychopharmacol Bull 27:191–199, 1991

Lenox RH, Newhouse PA, Creelman WL, et al: Adjunctive treatment of manic agitation with lorazepam versus haloperidol: a double-blind study. J Clin Psychiatry 53:47–52, 1992a

Lenox RH, Watson DG, Patel J, et al: Chronic lithium administration alters a prominent PKC substrate in rat hippocampus. Brain Res 570:333–340, 1992b

Lerer B, Stanley M: Effect of chronic lithium on cholinergically mediated responses and [^{3}H]QNB binding in rat brain. Brain Res 344:211–219, 1985

Levy A, Zohar J, Belmaker RH: The effect of chronic lithium pretreatment on rat brain muscarinic receptor regulation. Neuropharmacology 21:1199–1201, 1983

Lewy AJ, Sack RL, Miller LS, et al: Antidepressant and circadian phase-shifting effects of light. Science 235:352–354, 1987

Li PP, Tam YK, Young LT, et al: Lithium decreases Gs, Gi-$_1$ and Gi-$_2$ alpha-subunit mRNA levels in rat cortex. Eur J Pharmacol 206:165–166, 1991

Lieblich I, Yirmiya R: Naltrexone reverses a long term depressive effect of a toxic lithium injection on saccharin preference. Physiol Behav 39:547–550, 1987

Liles WC, Nathanson NM: Alteration in the regulation of neuronal muscarinic acetylcholine receptor number induces by chronic lithium in neuroblastoma cells. Brain Res 439:88–94, 1988

Linder D, Gschwendt M, Marks F: Phorbol ester-induced down-regulation of the 80-kDa myristoylated alanine-rich C-kinase substrate-related protein in Swiss 3T3 fibroblasts. J Biol Chem 267:24–26, 1992

Lindstedt G, Nilsson L, Walinder J, et al: On the prevalence, diagnosis and management of lithium-induced hypothyroidism in psychiatric patients. Br J Psychiatry 130:452–458, 1977

Lingsch C, Martin K: An irreversible effect of lithium administration to patients. Br J Pharmacol 57:323–327, 1976

Linnoila M, Karoum F, Rosenthal N, et al: Electroconvulsive treatment and lithium carbonate. Arch Gen Psychiatry 40:677–680, 1983

Linnoila M, Miller TL, Barko J, et al: Five antidepressant treatments in depressed patients. Arch Gen Psychiatry 41:688–692, 1984

Lloyd KG, Morselli PL, Bartholini G: GABA and affective disorders. Medical Biology (Helsinki) 65:159–165, 1987

Lyman GH, Williams CC: Lithium attenuation of leukopenia associated with cancer chemotherapy, in Lithium and the Blood. Edited by Gallicchio VS. Basel, Switzerland, Karger, 1991, pp 30–45

Maggi A, Enna SJ: Regional alterations in rat brain neurotransmitter systems following chronic lithium treatment. J Neurochem 34:888–892, 1980

Maggs R: Treatment of manic illness with lithium carbonate. Br J Psychiatry 109:56–65, 1963

Mahan LC, Burch RM, Monsma FJ Jr, et al: Expression of striatal D$_1$ dopamine receptors coupled to inositol phosphate production and Ca^{2+} mobilization in Xenopus oocytes. Proc Natl Acad Sci U S A 87:2196–2200, 1990

Mallette LE, Khouri K, Zengotita H, et al: Lithium treatment increases intact and midregion parathyroid hormone and parathyroid volume. J Clin Endocrinol Metab 68:654–660, 1989

Mallinger AG, Mallinger J, Himmelhoch JM, et al: Essential hypertension and membrane lithium transport in depressed patients. Psychiatry Res 10:11–16, 1983

Mallinger AG, Hanin I, Himmelhoch JM, et al: Stimulation of cell membrane sodium transport activity by lithium: possible relationship to therapeutic action. Psychiatry Res 22:49–59, 1987

Mandell AJ, Knapp S, Ehlers C, et al: The stability of constrained randomness: lithium prophylaxis at several neurobiological levels, in Neurobiology of Mood Disorders. Edited by Post RM, Ballenger JC. Baltimore, MD, Williams & Wilkins, 1984, pp 744–776

Manji HK: G proteins: implications for psychiatry. Am J Psychiatry 149:746–760, 1992

Manji HK, Lenox RH: Long-term action of lithium: a role for transcriptional and posttranscriptional factors regulated by protein kinase C. Synapse 16:11–28, 1994

Manji HK, Bitran JA, Masana MI, et al: Signal transduction modulation by lithium: cell culture, cerebral microdialysis and human studies. Psychopharmacol Bull 27:199–208, 1991a

Manji HK, Hsiao JK, Risby ED, et al: The mechanisms of action of lithium. Arch Gen Psychiatry 48:505–512, 1991b

Manji HK, Etcheberrigaray R, Chen G, et al: Lithium dramatically decreases membrane-associated PKC in the hippocampus: selectivity for the alpha isozyme. J Neurochem 61:2303–2310, 1993

Mannisto PT: Endocrine side-effects of lithium, in Handbook of Lithium Therapy. Edited by Johnson FN. Baltimore, MD, University Park Press, 1980, pp 310–322

Marchbanks RM: The activation of presynaptic choline uptake by acetylcholine release. J Physiol (Paris) 78:373–378, 1982

Marshall MH, Neumann CP, Robinson M: Lithium, creativity, and manic-depressive illness: review and prospectus. Psychosomatics 11:406–488, 1970

Masana MI, Bitran JA, Hsiao JK, et al: In vivo evidence that lithium inactivates G_i modulation of adenylate cyclase in brain. J Neurochem 59:200–205, 1992

Maslanski JA, Leshko L, Busa WB: Lithium-sensitive production of inositol phosphates during amphibian embryonic mesoderm induction. Science 256:243–245, 1992

Mathe AA, Jousisto-Hanson J, Stenfors C, et al: Effect of lithium on tachykinins, calcitonin gene-related peptide, and neuropeptide Y in rat brain. J Neurosci Res 26:233–237, 1990

McCance SL, Cohen PR, Cowen PJ: Lithium increases 5-HT-mediated prolactin release. Psychopharmacology (Berl) 99:276–281, 1989

McEachron DL, Kripke DF, Hawkins R, et al: Lithium delays biochemical circadian rhythms in rats. Neuropsychobiology 8:12–29, 1982

McHenry CR, Rosen IB, Rotstein LE, et al: Lithiumogenic disorders of the thyroid and parathyroid glands as surgical disease. Surgery 108:1001–1005, 1990

McHenry CR, Racke F, Meister M, et al: Lithium effects on dispersed bovine parathyroid cells grown in tissue culture. Surgery 110:1061–1066, 1991

Mellerup ET, Dam H, Wildschiotz G, et al: Diurnal variation of blood glucose during lithium treatment. J Affect Disord 5:341–347, 1983

Meltzer HY, Lowy MT: The serotonin hypothesis of depression, in Psychopharmacology: The Third Generation of Progress. Edited by Meltzer HY. New York, Raven, 1987, pp 513–526

Meltzer HY, Simonovic M, Sturgeon RD, et al: Effect of antidepressants, lithium and electroconvulsive treatment on rat serum prolactin levels. Acta Psychiatr Scand 63 (suppl 290):100–121, 1981

Meltzer HL, Kassir S, Dunner DL, et al: Repression of a lithium pump as a consequence of lithium ingestion by manic-depressive subjects. Psychopharmacology (Berl) 54:113–118, 1982

Meltzer HY, Arora RC, Goodnick P: Effect of lithium carbonate on serotonin uptake in blood platelets of patients with affective disorders. J Affect Disord 5:215–221, 1983

Meltzer HY, Lowy M, Robertson A, et al: Effect of 5-hydroxytryptophan on serum cortisol levels in major affective disorders, III: Effect of antidepressants and lithium carbonate. Arch Gen Psychiatry 41:391–397, 1984

Mendels J, Chernik DA: The effect of lithium carbonate on the sleep of depressed patients. International Pharmacopsychiatry 8:184–192, 1973

Mendels J, Frazer A: Intracellular lithium concentration and clinical response: towards a membrane theory of depression. J Psychiatr Res 10:9–18, 1973

Miller BL, Jenden DJ, Tang C, et al: Factors influencing erythrocyte choline concentrations. Life Sci 44:477–482, 1989

Miller BL, Lin KM, Djenderedjian A, et al: Changes in red blood cell choline and choline-bound lipids with oral lithium. Experientia 46:454–456, 1990

Mitchell JE, MacKenzie TB: Cardiac effects of lithium therapy in man: a review. J Clin Psychiatry 43:47–51, 1982

Miyauchi T, Okiawa S, Kitada Y: Effects of lithium chloride on the cholinergic system in different brain regions in mice. Biochem Pharmacol 29:654–657, 1980

Mizuta T, Segawa T: Chronic effects of imipramine and lithium on 5-HT receptor subtypes in rat frontal cortex, hippocampus and choroid plexus: quantitative receptor autoradiographic analysis. Jpn J Pharmacol 50:315–326, 1989

Mori M, Tajima K, Oda Y, et al: Inhibitory effect of lithium on the release of thyroid hormones from thyrotropin-stimulated mouse thyroids in a perifusion system. Endocrinology 124:1365–1369, 1989

Mork A, Geisler A: Mode of action of lithium on the catalytic unit of adenylate cyclase from rat brain. Pharmacol Toxicol 60:241–248, 1987

Mork A, Geisler A: Effects of GTP on hormone-stimulated adenylate cyclase activity in cerebral cortex, striatum, and hippocampus from rats treated chronically with lithium. Biol Psychiatry 26:279–288, 1989a

Mork A, Geisler A: The effects of lithium in vitro and ex vivo on adenylate cyclase in brain are exerted by distinct mechanisms. Neuropharmacology 28:307–311, 1989b

Mork A, Geisler A: Effects of lithium ex vivo on the GTP-mediated inhibition of calcium-stimulated adenylate cyclase activity in rat brain. Eur J Pharmacol 168:347–354, 1989c

Mork A, Klysner R, Geisler A: Effects of treatment with a lithium-imipramine combination on components of adenylate cyclase in the cerebral cortex of the rat. Neuropharmacology 29:261–267, 1990

Mota de Freitas DE, Espanol MT, Dorus E: Lithium transport in red blood cells of bipolar patients, in Lithium and the Blood. Edited by Gallicchio VS. Farmington, CT, Karger, 1991, pp 96–120

Mucha RF, Herz A: Motivational properties of kappa and mu opioid receptor agonists studied with place and taste preference conditioning. Psychopharmacology (Berl) 86:274–280, 1985

Muhlbauer HD: The influence of fenfluramine stimulation on prolactin plasma levels in lithium long-term-treated manic-depressive patients and healthy subjects. Pharmacopsychiatry 17:191–193, 1984

Muhlbauer HD, Muller-Oerlinghausen B: Fenfluramine stimulation of serum cortisol in patients with major affective disorders and healthy controls: further evidence for a central serotonergic action of lithium in man. J Neural Transm 61:81–94, 1985

Muller-Oerlinghausen B, Ahrens B, Volk J, et al: Reduced mortality of manic-depressive patients in long-term lithium treatment: an international collaborative study by IGSLI. Psychiatry Res 36:329–331, 1991

Mullins LJ, Brinley FJ: Calcium binding and regulation in nerve fibers, in Calcium Binding Protein and Calcium Function. Edited by Wasserman RH, Corradino RA, Carafoli E. New York, North-Holland, 1977, pp 87–95

Murphy DL: Effects of lithium on catecholamines and other brain neurotransmitters. Neuroscience Research Progress Bulletin 14:165–169, 1976

Murphy DL, Donnelly C, Moskowitz J: Inhibition by lithium of prostaglandin E1 and norepinephrine effects on cyclic adenosine monophosphate production in human platelets. Clin Pharmacol Ther 14:810–814, 1974

Murphy DL, Lake CR, Slater S, et al: Psychoactive drug effects on plasma norepinephrine and plasma dopamine beta-hydroxylase in man, in Catecholamines: Basic and Clinical Frontiers. Edited by Usdin E, Kopin IJ, Barchas J. New York, Pergamon, 1979, pp 918–920

Myers DH, Carter RA, Burns BH, et al: A prospective study of the effects of lithium on thyroid function and on the prevalence of antithyroid antibodies. Psychol Med 15:55–61, 1985

Nahorski SR, Ragan CI, Challiss RAJ: Lithium and the phosphoinositide cycle: an example of uncompetitive inhibition and its pharmacological consequences. Trends Pharmacol Sci 12:297–303, 1991

Nahorski SR, Jenkinson S, Challiss RA: Disruption of phosphoinositide signalling by lithium. Biochem Soc Trans 20:430–434, 1992

Naylor GJ, McHarg A: Profound hypothermia on combined lithium carbonate and diazepam treatment. British Medical Journal 2:22, 1977

Naylor GJ, Smith AHW: Defective genetic control of sodium-pump density in manic depressive psychosis. Psychol Med 11:257–263, 1981

Naylor GJ, McNamee HB, Moody JP: Erythrocyte sodium and potassium in depressive illness. J Psychosom Res 14:173–177, 1970

Naylor GJ, McNamee HB, Moody JP: Changes in

erythrocyte sodium and potassium on recovery from depressive illness. Br J Psychiatry 118:219–223, 1971

Naylor GJ, Dick DAT, Dick EG, et al: Lithium therapy and erythrocyte membrane cation carrier. Psychopharmacologia 37:81–86, 1974a

Naylor GJ, Dick DAT, Dick EG, et al: Erythrocyte membrane cation carrier in mania. Psychol Med 6:659–663, 1974b

Naylor GJ, Smith AHW, Dick EG, et al: Erythrocyte membrane cation carrier in manic-depressive psychosis. Psychol Med 10:521–525, 1980

Nemeroff CB: Neuropeptides and Psychiatric Disorders. Washington, DC, American Psychiatric Press, 1991

Neubig RR, Gantzos RD, Thomsen WJ: Mechanism of agonist and antagonist binding to alpha-2-adrenergic receptors: evidence for a precoupled receptor-guanine nucleotide protein complex. Biochemistry 27:2374–2384, 1988

Newman ME, Belmaker RH: Effects of lithium in vitro and ex vivo on components of the adenylate cyclase system in membranes from the cerebral cortex of the rat. Neuropharmacology 26:211–217, 1987

Newman M, Klein E, Birmaher B, et al: Lithium at therapeutic concentrations inhibits human brain noradrenaline sensitive cyclic AMP accumulation. Brain Res 278:380–381, 1983

Newman ME, Drummer D, Lerer B: Single and combined effects of desipramine and lithium on serotonergic receptor number and second messenger function in rat brain. J Pharmacol Exp Ther 252:826–831, 1990

Nilsson A: The anti-aggressive actions of lithium. Reviews in Contemporary Pharmacotherapy 4:269–285, 1993

Nishizuka Y: Intracellular signaling by hydrolysis of phospholipids and activation of protein kinase C. Science 258:607–614, 1992

Nora JJ, Nora AH, Toews WH: Lithium, Ebstein's anomaly and other congenital heart defects. Lancet 1:594–595, 1974

Nordenstrom J, Strigard K, Perbeck L, et al: Hyperparathyroidism associated with treatment of manic-depressive disorders by lithium. Eur J Surg 158:207–211, 1992

Nurnberger J Jr, Jimerson DC, Allen JR, et al: Red cell ouabain-sensitive Na^+-K^+-adenosine triphosphatase: a state marker in affective disorder inversely related to plasma cortisol. Biol Psychiatry 17:981–992, 1982

Odagaki Y, Koyama T, Matsubara S, et al: Effects of chronic lithium treatment on serotonin binding sites in rat brain. J Psychiatr Res 24:271–277, 1990

Ormandy G, Jope RS: Analysis of the convulsant-potentiating effects of lithium in rats. Exp Neurol 111:356–361, 1991

Ostrow DG, Pandey GN, Davis JM, et al: A heritable disorder of lithium transport in erythrocytes of a subpopulation of manic-depressive patients. Am J Psychiatry 135:1070–1078, 1978

Pandey GN, Ostrow DG, Haas M, et al: Abnormal lithium and sodium transport in erythrocytes of a manic patient and some members of his family. Proc Natl Acad Sci U S A 74:3607–3611, 1977

Pandey GN, Sarkadi M, Haas M, et al: Lithium transport pathways in human red blood cells. J Gen Physiol 72:233–247, 1978

Pandey GN, Janicak PG, Javaid JI, et al: Increased ^{3}H-clonidine binding in the platelets of patients with depressive and schizophrenic disorders. Psychiatry Res 28:73–88, 1989

Perry P, Tsuang MT: Treatment of unipolar depression following electroconvulsive therapy: relapse rate comparisons between lithium and tricyclics therapies following ECT. J Affect Disord 1:123–129, 1979

Persinger MA, Makarec K, Bradley JC: Characteristics of limbic seizures evoked by peripheral injections of lithium and pilocarpine. Physiol Behav 44:27–37, 1988

Pert A, Rosenblatt JE, Sivit C, et al: Long-term treatment with lithium prevents the development of dopamine receptor supersensitivity. Science 201:171–173, 1978

Pert CB, Pert A, Rosenblatt JE, et al: Catecholamine receptor stabilization: a possible mode of lithium's antimanic action, in Catecholamines: Basic and Clinical Frontiers. Edited by Usdin E, Kopin IJ, Barchas JD. New York, Pergamon, 1979, pp 583–585

Peselow ED, Dunner DL, Fieve RR, et al: Lithium carbonate and weight gain. J Affect Disord 2:303–310, 1980

Pfeiffer A, Veilleux S, Barden N: Antidepressant and other centrally acting drugs regulate glucocorticoid receptor messenger RNA levels in rat brain. Psychoneuroendocrinology 16:505–515, 1991

Poirier MF, Galzin AM, Pimoule C, et al: Short-term

lithium administration to healthy volunteers produces long-lasting pronounced changes in platelet serotonin uptake but not imipramine binding. Psychopharmacology (Berl) 94:521–526, 1988

Poirier-Littre MF, Loo H, Dennis T, et al: Lithium treatment increases norepinephrine turnover in the plasma of healthy subjects [letter]. Arch Gen Psychiatry 50:72–73, 1993

Poitou P, Bohuon C: Catecholamine metabolism in the rat brain after short and long term lithium administration. J Neurochem 25:535–537, 1975

Pontzer NJ, Crews FT: Desensitization of muscarinic stimulated hippocampal cell firing is related to phosphoinositide hydrolysis and inhibited by lithium. J Pharmacol Exp Ther 253:921–929, 1990

Post RM, Stoddard FJ, Gillin JC, et al: Alterations in motor activity, sleep, and biochemistry in a cycling manic-depressive patient. Arch Gen Psychiatry 34:470–477, 1977

Post RM, Jimerson DC, Bunney WE Jr, et al: Dopamine and mania: behavioral and biochemical effects of the dopamine receptor blocker pimozide. Psychopharmacology (Berl) 67:297–305, 1980a

Post RM, Ballenger JC, Hare TA, et al: Cerebrospinal fluid GABA in normals and patients with affective disorders. Brain Res Bull 5 (suppl 2):755–759, 1980b

Post RM, Leverich GS, Altshuler L, et al: Lithium-discontinuation-induced refractoriness: preliminary observations. Am J Psychiatry 149:1727–1729, 1992

Price LH: Antidepressants, in Depression and Mania: Modern Lithium Therapy. Edited by Johnson FN. Oxford, England, IRL Press, 1987, pp 161–166

Price LH: Lithium augmentation in tricyclic-resistant depression, in Treatment of Tricyclic-Resistant Depression. Edited by Extein IL. Washington, DC, American Psychiatric Press, 1989, pp 49–79

Price LH, Charney DS, Delgado PL, et al: Lithium treatment and serotoninergic function. Arch Gen Psychiatry 46:13–19, 1989

Price LH, Charney DS, Delgado PL, et al: Lithium and serotonin function: implications for the serotonin hypothesis of depression. Psychopharmacology (Berl) 100:3–12, 1990

Prien RF, Caffey EM Jr, Klett CJ: Comparison of lithium carbonate and chlorpromazine in the treatment of mania: report of the Veterans Administration and National Institute of Mental Health Collaborative Study Group. Arch Gen Psychiatry 26:146–153, 1972

Ramsey TA, Frazer A, Mendels J, et al: The erythrocyte lithium-plasma lithium ratio in patients with primary affective disorder. Arch Gen Psychiatry 36:457–461, 1979

Rana RS, Hokin LE: Role of phosphoinositides in transmembrane signaling. Physiol Rev 70:115–164, 1990

Rangel-Guerra RA, Perez-Payan H, Minkoff L, et al: Nuclear magnetic resonance in bipolar disorders. AJNR Am J Neuroradiol 4:229–231, 1983

Rao ML, Mager T: Influence of the pineal gland on the pituitary function in humans. Psychoendocrinology 12:141–147, 1987

Reddy PL, Khanna S, Subhash MN, et al: Erythrocyte membrane Na-K ATPase activity in affective disorder. Biol Psychiatry 26:533–537, 1989

Reisine T, Zatz M: Interactions between lithium, calcium, diacylglycerides and phorbol esters in the regulation of ACTH release from AtT-20 cells. J Neurochem 49:884–889, 1987

Renshaw PF, Wicklund S: In vivo measurement of lithium in humans by nuclear magnetic resonance spectroscopy. Biol Psychiatry 23:465–475, 1988

Renshaw PF, Haselgrove JC, Bolinger L, et al: Relaxation and imaging of lithium in vivo. Magn Reson Imaging 4:193–198, 1986

Richelson E: Lithium ion entry through the sodium channel of cultured mouse neuroblastoma cells: a biochemical study. Science 196:1001–1002, 1977

Richelson E, Snyder K, Carlson J, et al: Lithium ion transport in erythrocytes of randomly selected blood donors and manic-depressive patients: lack of association with affective illness. Am J Psychiatry 143:457–462, 1986

Riddell FG: Studies on Li$^+$ transport using ^{7}Li and ^{6}Li nuclear magnetic resonance, in Lithium and the Cell. Edited by Birch NJ. San Diego, CA, Academic Press, 1991, pp 85–98

Risby ED, Hsiao JK, Manji HK, et al: The mechanisms of action of lithium. Arch Gen Psychiatry 48:513–524, 1991

Ritchie JM, Straub RW: Observations on the mechanism for the active extrusion of lithium in mammalian non-myelinated nerve fibres. J Physiol 304:123–124, 1980

Roberts DE, Berman SM, Nakasato S, et al: Effect of lithium carbonate on zidovudine-associated neutropenia in the acquired immunodeficiency syndrome. Am J Med 85:428–431, 1988

Rogers M, Whybrow P: Clinical hypothyroidism occurring during lithium treatment: two case histories and a review of thyroid function in 19 patients. Am J Psychiatry 128:150–155, 1971

Ronai AZ, Vizi SE: The effect of lithium treatment on the acetylcholine content of rat brain. Biochem Pharmacol 24:1819–1820, 1975

Roose SP, Bone S, Haidorfer C, et al: Lithium treatment in older patients. Am J Psychiatry 136:843–844, 1979

Rosenblatt JE, Pert CB, Tallman JF, et al: The effect of imipramine and lithium on alpha- and beta-receptor binding in rat brain. Brain Res 160:186–191, 1979

Rosenblatt JE, Pert A, Layton B, et al: Chronic lithium reduced ^{3}H-spiroperidol binding in rat striatum. Eur J Pharmacol 67:321–322, 1980

Rosenthal J, Strauss A, Minkoff L, et al: Identifying lithium-responsive bipolar depressed patients using nuclear magnetic resonance. Am J Psychiatry 143:779–780, 1986

Ross DR, Coffey CE: Neuroleptics and anxiolytics, in Depression and Mania: Modern Lithium Therapy. Edited by Johnson FN. Oxford, England, IRL Press, 1987, pp 167–171

Rudorfer MV, Linnoila M: Electroconvulsive therapy, in Lithium Combination Treatment. Edited by Johnson FN. Basel, Switzerland, Karger, 1987, pp 164–178

Russell RW, Pechnick R, Jope RS: Effects of lithium on behavioral reactivity: relation to increases in brain cholinergic activity. Psychopharmacology (Berl) 73:120–125, 1981

Rybakowski J, Frazer A, Mendels J: Lithium efflux from erythrocytes incubated in vitro during lithium carbonate administration. Communications in Psychopharmacology 2:105–112, 1978

Sansone MEG, Ziegler DK: Lithium toxicity: a review of neurologic complications. Clin Neuropharmacol 8:242–248, 1985

Sarkadi B, Alifimoff JK, Gunn RB, et al: Kinetics and stoichiometry of Na-dependent Li transport in human red blood cells. J Gen Physiol 72:249–265, 1978

Saxe AW, Gibson G: Lithium increases tritiated thymidine uptake by abnormal human parathyroid tissue. Surgery 110:1067–1076, 1991

Saxe A, Gibson G: Effect of lithium on incorporation of bromodeoxyuridine and tritiated thymidine into human parathyroid cells. Arch Surg 128:865–869, 1993

Schatzberg AF, Cole JO: Manual of Clinical Psychopharmacology, 2nd Edition. Washington, DC, American Psychiatric Press, 1991

Schildkraut JJ: The effects of lithium on norepinephrine turnover and metabolism: basic and clinical studies, in Lithium: Its Role in Psychiatric Research and Treatment. Edited by Gershon S, Shopsin B. New York, Plenum, 1973, pp 51–73

Schildkraut JJ: The effects of lithium on norepinephrine turnover and metabolism: basic and clinical studies. J Nerv Ment Dis 158:348–360, 1974

Schildkraut JJ, Schanberg SM, Kopin IJ: The effects of lithium ion on ^{3}H-norepinephrine metabolism in brain. Life Sci 16:1479–1483, 1966

Schildkraut JJ, Logue MA, Dodge GA: The effect of lithium salts on the turnover and metabolism of norepinephrine in rat brain. Psychopharmacologia 14:135–141, 1969

Schildkraut JJ, Keeler BA, Grob EL, et al: MHPG excretion and clinical classification in depressive disorders. Lancet 1:1251–1252, 1973

Schou M: Lithium in psychiatric therapy and prophylaxis. J Psychiatr Res 6:67–95, 1968

Schou M: Lithium research at the Psychopharmacology Research Unit, Risskov, Denmark: a historical account, in Origin, Prevention and Treatment of Affective Disorders. Edited by Schou M, Stromgren E. London, Academic Press, 1979a, pp 1–8

Schou M: Artistic productivity and lithium prophylaxis in manic-depressive illness. Br J Psychiatry 135:97–103, 1979b

Schou M: Use in other psychiatric conditions, in Depression and Mania: Modern Lithium Therapy. Edited by Johnson FN. Oxford, England, IRL Press, 1987, pp 44–50

Schou M: Lithium Treatment of Manic-Depressive Illness, 4th Edition, Revised. Basel, Switzerland, Karger, 1989

Schou M, Juel-Neilsen N, Stromberg E, et al: The treatment of manic psychoses by the administration of lithium salts. J Neurol Neurosurg Psychiatry 17:250–260, 1954

Schou M, Goldfield MD, Weinstein MR, et al: Lithium and pregnancy, I: report from the Register of Lithium Babies. British Medical Journal 2:135–136, 1973

Schou M, Amdisen A, Thomsen K, et al: Lithium treatment regimen and renal water handling: the significance of dosage pattern and tablet type examined through comparison of results from two clinics with different treatment regimens. Psychopharmacology (Berl) 77:387–390, 1982

Schou M, Hansen HE, Thomsen K, et al: Lithium treatment in Aarhus, 2: risk of renal failure and of intoxication. Pharmacopsychiatry 22:101–103, 1989

Schreiber G, Avissar S, Danon A, et al: Hyperfunctional G proteins in mononuclear leukocytes of patients with mania. Biol Psychiatry 29:273–280, 1991

Schultz JE, Siggins GR, Schocker FW, et al: Effects of prolonged treatment with lithium and tricyclic antidepressants on discharge frequency, norepinephrine responses and beta receptor binding in rat cerebellum: electrophysiological and biochemical comparison. J Pharmacol Exp Ther 216:28–38, 1981

Seeger TF, Gardner EL, Bridger WF: Increase in mesolimbic electrical self-stimulation after chronic haloperidol: reversal by L-dopa or lithium. Brain Res 215:404–409, 1981

Segal DS, Callaghan M, Mandell AJ: Alterations in behaviour and catecholamine biosynthesis induced by lithium. Nature 254:58–59, 1975

Seggie J, Carney PA, Parker J, et al: Effect of chronic lithium on sensitivity to light in male and female bipolar patients. Prog Neuropsychopharmacol Biol Psychiatry 13:543–549, 1989

Sengupta N, Datta SC, Sengupta D, et al: Platelet and erythrocyte membrane ATPase activity in depression and mania. Psychiatry Res 3:337–344, 1980

Sharp T, Bramwell SR, Lambert P, et al: Effect of short- and long-term administration of lithium on the release of endogenous 5-HT in the hippocampus of the rat in vivo and in vitro. Neuropharmacology 30:977–984, 1991

Shaughnessy R, Greene SC, Pandey GN, et al: Red-cell lithium transport and affective disorders in a multigeneration pedigree: evidence for genetic transmission of affective disorders. Biol Psychiatry 20:451–460, 1985

Sherman WR: Lithium and the phosphoinositide signalling system, in Lithium and the Cell. Edited by Birch NJ. London, Academic Press, 1991, pp 121–157

Sherman WR, Munsell LY, Wong YHH: Differential uptake of lithium isotopes by rat cerebral cortex and its effect on inositol phosphate metabolism. J Neurochem 42:880–882, 1984

Sherman WR, Munsell LY, Gish BG, et al: Effects of systemically administered lithium on phosphoinositide metabolism in rat brain, kidney, and testis. J Neurochem 44:798–807, 1985

Sherman WR, Gish BG, Honchar MP, et al: Effects of lithium on phosphoinositide metabolism in vivo. Federation Proceedings 45:2639–2646, 1986

Shippenberg TS, Herz A: Influence of chronic lithium treatment upon the motivational effects of opioids: alteration in the effects of mu- but not kappa-opioid receptor ligands. J Pharmacol Exp Ther 256:1101–1106, 1991

Shippenberg TS, Millan MJ, Mucha RF, et al: Involvement of beta-endorphin and mu-opioid receptors in mediating the aversive effect of lithium in the rat. Eur J Pharmacol 154:135–144, 1988

Shopsin B, Kim SS, Gershon S: A controlled study of lithium vs. chlorpromazine in acute schizophrenics. Br J Psychiatry 119:435–440, 1971

Shukla GS: Combined lithium and valproate treatment and subsequent withdrawal: serotonergic mechanism of their interaction in discrete brain regions. Prog Neuropsychopharmacol Biol Psychiatry 9:153–156, 1985

Simon JR, Kuhar MJ: High affinity choline uptake: ionic and energy requirement. J Neurochem 27:93–99, 1976

Sivam SP, Strunk C, Smith DR, et al: Proenkephalin-A gene regulation in the rat striatum: influence of lithium and haloperidol. Mol Pharmacol 30:186–191, 1986

Sivam SP, Takeuchi K, Li S, et al: Lithium increases dynorphin A(1-8) and prodynorphin mRNA levels in the basal ganglia of rats. Brain Res 427:155–163, 1988

Sivam SP, Krause JE, Takeuchi K, et al: Lithium increases rat striatal beta- and gamma-preprotachykinin messenger FNAs. J Pharmacol Exp Ther 248:1297–1301, 1989

Skinner GR, Hartley C, Buchan A, et al: The effect of lithium chloride on the replication of herpes simplex virus. Med Microbiol Immunol (Berl) 168:139–148, 1980

Smith DF: Lithium attenuates clonidine-induced hypoactivity: further studies in inbred mouse strains. Psychopharmacology (Berl) 94:428–430, 1988

Song L, Jope R: Chronic lithium treatment impairs phosphatidylinositol hydrolysis in membranes from rat brain regions. J Neurochem 58:2200–2206, 1992

Spengler RN, Hollingsworth PJ, Smith CB: Effects of long-term lithium and desipramine treatment upon clonidine-induced inhibition of ^{3}H-norepinephrine release from rat hippocampal slices. Federation Proceedings 45:681, 1986

Spiegel AM, Rudorfer MV, Marx SJ, et al: The effect of short term lithium administration on suppressibility of parathyroid hormone secretion by calcium in vivo. J Clin Endocrinol Metab 59:354–357, 1984

Staunton DA, Magistretti PJ, Shoemaker WJ, et al: Effects of chronic lithium treatment on dopamine receptors in the rat corpus striatum, I: locomotor activity and behavioral supersensitivity. Brain Res 232:391–400, 1982a

Staunton DA, Magistretti PJ, Shoemaker WJ, et al: Effects of chronic lithium treatment on dopamine receptors in the rat corpus striatum, II: no effect on denervation or neuroleptic-induced supersensitivity. Brain Res 232:401–412, 1982b

Stern DN, Fieve RR, Neff NH, et al: The effect of lithium chloride administration on brain and heart norepinephrine turnover rates. Psychopharmacologia 14:315–322, 1969

Stoll AL, Cohen BM, Snyder MB, et al: Erythrocyte choline concentration in bipolar disorder: a predictor of clinical course and medication response. Biol Psychiatry 29:1171–1180, 1991

Strzyzewski W, Rybakowski J, Potok E, et al: Erythrocyte cation transport in endogenous depression: clinical and psychophysiological correlates. Acta Psychiatr Scand 70:248–253, 1984

Suppes T, Baldessarini RJ, Faedda GL, et al: Risk of recurrence following discontinuation of lithium treatment in bipolar disorder. Arch Gen Psychiatry 48:1082–1088, 1991

Suppes T, Baldessarini RJ, Faedda GL, et al: Discontinuation of maintenance treatment in bipolar disorder: risks and implications. Harvard Reviews in Psychiatry 1:131–144, 1993

Swann AC: Caloric intake and (Na$^+$,K$^+$)-ATPase: differential regulation by alpha-1 and beta noradrenergic receptors. Am J Physiol 247:R449–R455, 1984

Swann AC: Norepinephrine and (Na$^+$,K$^+$)-ATPase: evidence for stabilization by lithium or imipramine. Neuropharmacology 27:261–267, 1988

Swann AC, Marini JL, Sheard MH, et al: Effects of chronic dietary lithium on activity and regulation of [Na$^+$,K$^+$]-adenosine triphosphatase in rat brain. Biochem Pharmacol 29:2819–2823, 1980

Swann AC, Heninger GR, Roth RH, et al: Differential effects of short and long term lithium on tryptophan uptake and serotonergic function in cat brain. Life Sci 28:347–354, 1981

Swann AC, Koslow SH, Katz MM, et al: Lithium carbonate treatment of mania. Arch Gen Psychiatry 44:345–354, 1987

Swerdlow NR, Lee D, Koob GF, et al: Effects of chronic dietary lithium on behavioral indices of dopamine denervation supersensitivity in the rat. J Pharmacol Exp Ther 235:324–329, 1985

Szentistvanyi I, Janka Z: Correlation between lithium ratio and Na-dependent Li transport in red blood cells during lithium prophylaxis. Biol Psychiatry 14:973–977, 1979

Tagliamonte A, Tagliamonte P, Perez-Cruet J, et al: Effect of psychotropic drugs on tryptophan concentration in the rat brain. J Pharmacol Exp Ther 177:475–480, 1971

Tanimoto K, Maeda K, Yamaguchi N, et al: Effect of lithium on prolactin responses to thyrotropin releasing hormone in patients with manic state. Psychopharmacology (Berl) 72:129–133, 1981

Tanimoto K, Maeda K, Terada T: Inhibitory effect of lithium on neuroleptic and serotonin receptors in rat brain. Brain Res 265:148–151, 1983

Taylor JW, Bell AJ: Lithium-induced parathyroid dysfunction: a case report and review of the literature. Ann Pharmacother 27:1040–1043, 1993

Terry JB, Padzernik TL, Nelson SR: Effect of LiCl pretreatment on cholinomimetic-induced seizures and seizure-induced brain edema in rats. Neurosci Lett 114:123–127, 1990

Thiele EA, Eipper BA: Effect of secretogogues on components of the secretory system in AtT-20 cells. Endocrinology 126:809–817, 1990

Tilkian AG, Schroder JS, Kao J, et al: Effect of lithium on cardiovascular performance: report on extended ambulatory monitoring and exercise testing before and during lithium therapy. Am J Cardiol 38:701–708, 1976

Tollefson GD, Senogles S: A cholinergic role in the mechanism of lithium in mania. Biol Psychiatry 18:467–479, 1982

Torok TL: Neurochemical transmission and the sodium pump. Prog Neurobiol 32:11–76, 1989

Treiser S, Kellar KJ: Lithium effects on adrenergic receptor supersensitivity in rat brain. Eur J Pharmacol 58:85–86, 1979

Treiser S, Kellar KJ: Lithium: effects on serotonin receptors in rat brain. Eur J Pharmacol 64:183–185, 1980

Treiser SL, Cascio CS, O'Donohue TL, et al: Lithium increases serotonin release and decreases serotonin receptors in the hippocampus. Science 213:1529–1531, 1981

Tricklebank MD, Singh L, Jackson A, et al: Evidence that a proconvulsant action of lithium is mediated by inhibition of myo-inositol phosphatase in mouse brain. Brain Res 558:145–148, 1991

Trousseau A: Clinique Medicale de l'Hôtel-Dieu de Paris, 3rd Edition. Paris, JB Balliere et Fils, 1868

Tseng FY, Pasquali D, Field JB: Effects of lithium on stimulated metabolic parameters in dog thyroid slices. Acta Endocrinol (Copenh) 121:615–620, 1989

Uney JB, Marchbanks RM: Inhibition of choline transport in human brain by lithium treatment, in Cellular and Molecular Basis of Cholinergic Function. Edited by Dowdall MJ, Hawthorne JN. New York, VCH Publishers, 1987, pp 774–780

Uney JB, Marchbanks RM, Marsh A: The effect of lithium on choline transport in human erythrocytes. J Neurol Neurosurg Psychiatry 48:229–233, 1985

Uney JB, Marchbanks RM, Reynolds GP, et al: Lithium prophylaxis inhibits choline transport in postmortem brain. Lancet 2:458, 1986

Urabe M, Hershman JM, Pang XP, et al: Effect of lithium on function and growth of thyroid cells in vitro. Endocrinology 129:807–814, 1991

Ure A: Researches on gout. Medical Times 11:145, 1844/1845

Vallar L, Muca C, Magni M, et al: Differential coupling of dopaminergic receptors expressed in different cell types: stimulation of phosphatidylinositol 4,5-bisphosphate hydrolysis in LtK- fibroblasts, hyperpolarization, and cytosolic-free Ca^{2+} concentration decrease in GH_4Cl cells. J Biol Chem 265:10320–10326, 1990

van Kammen DP, Docherty JP, Marder SR, et al: Lithium attenuates the activation-euphoria but not the psychosis induced by d-amphetamine in schizophrenia. Psychopharmacology (Berl) 87:111–115, 1985

Varney MA, Godfrey PP, Drummond AH, et al: Chronic lithium treatment inhibits basal and agonist-stimulated responses in rat cerebral cortex and GH_3 pituitary cells. Mol Pharmacol 4:671–678, 1992

Verimer T, Goodale DB, Long JP, et al: Lithium effects

on haloperidol-induced pre- and postsynaptic dopamine receptor supersensitivity. J Pharm Pharmacol 32:665–666, 1980

Vestergaard P, Aagaard J: Five-year mortality in lithium-treated manic-depressive patients. J Affect Disord 21:33–38, 1991

Vestergaard P, Poulstrup I, Schou M: Prospective studies on a lithium cohort, 3: tremor, weight gain, diarrhea, psychological complaints. Acta Psychiatr Scand 78:434–441, 1988

Walker E, Green M: Soft signs of neurological dysfunction in schizophrenia: an investigation of lateral performance. Biol Psychiatry 17:381–386, 1982

Walker RG: Lithium nephrotoxicity. Kidney Int 44 (suppl 42):S93–S98, 1993

Wang HY, Friedman E: Chronic lithium: desensitization of autoreceptors mediating serotonin release. Psychopharmacology (Berl) 94:312–314, 1988

Wang HY, Friedman E: Lithium inhibition of protein kinase C activation-induced serotonin release. Psychopharmacology (Berl) 99:213–218, 1989

Watson SP, Shipman L, Godfrey PP: Lithium potentiates agonist formation of [^{3}H]CDP-diacylglycerol in human platelets. Eur J Pharmacol 188:273–276, 1990

Wehr TA: Phase and biorhythm studies in affective illness. Ann Intern Med 87:319–335, 1977

Wehr TA, Goodwin FK: Rapid cycling in manic-depressives induced by tricyclic antidepressants. Arch Gen Psychiatry 36:555–559, 1979

Wehr TA, Goodwin FK: Can antidepressants cause mania and worsen the course of affective illness? Am J Psychiatry 144:1403–1411, 1987

Wehr TA, Sack DA, Rosenthal NE: Sleep reduction as a final common pathway in the genesis of mania. Am J Psychiatry 144:201–204, 1987

Weiner ED, Kalaaspudi VD, Papolos DF, et al: Lithium augments pilocarpine-induced fos gene expression in brain. Brain Res 553:117–122, 1991

Weiner ED, Mallat AM, Papolos DF, et al: Acute lithium treatment enhances neuropeptide Y gene expression in rat hippocampus. Brain Res Mol Brain Res 12:209–214, 1992

Welsh DK, Moore-Ede MC: Lithium lengthens circadian period in a diurnal primate, *Saimiri sciureus*. Biol Psychiatry 28:117–126, 1990

Welsh DK, Nino-Murcia G, Gander PH, et al: Regular 48-hour cycling of sleep duration and mood in a 35-year-old woman: use of lithium in time isolation. Biol Psychiatry 21:527–537, 1986

Werstiuk ES, Steiner M: Anti-psychotics, II: butyrophenones, in Lithium Combination Treatment. Edited by Johnson FN. Basel, Switzerland, Karger, 1987, pp 84–104

Wever RA: The Circadian System of Man. New York, Springer-Verlag, 1979

Whitworth P, Kendall DA: Lithium selectively inhibits muscarinic receptor-stimulated inositol tetrakisphosphate accumulation in mouse cerebral cortex slices. J Neurochem 51:258–265, 1988

Whitworth P, Kendall DA: Effects of lithium on inositol phospholipid hydrolysis and inhibition of dopamine D_1 receptor-mediated cyclic AMP formation by carbachol in rat brain slices. J Neurochem 53:536–541, 1989

Wirz-Justice A: Antidepressant drugs: effects on the circadian system, in Circadian Rhythms in Psychiatry. Edited by Wehr TA, Goodwin FK. Pacific Grove, CA, Boxwood, 1983, pp 235–264

Wirz-Justice A, Groos GA, Wehr TA: The neuropharmacology of circadian timekeeping in mammals, in Vertebrate Circadian Systems: Structure and Physiology. Edited by Aschoff J, Daan S, Groos GA. New York, Springer-Verlag, 1982, pp 1–26

Wolff J, Berens SC, Jones AB: Inhibition of thyrotropin-stimulated adenylyl cyclase activity of beef thyroid membranes by low concentration of lithium ion. Biochem Biophys Res Commun 39:77–82, 1970

Wood AJ, Goodwin GM: A review of the biochemical and neuropharmacological actions of lithium. Psychol Med 17:579–600, 1987

Wood AJ, Elphick M, Aronson JK, et al: The effect of lithium on cation transport measured in vivo in patients suffering from bipolar affective illness. Br J Psychiatry 155:504–510, 1989a

Wood AJ, Elphick M, Grahame-Smith DG: Effect of lithium and of other drugs used in the treatment of manic illness on the cation-transporting properties of Na^+,K^+-ATPase in mouse brain synaptosomes. J Neurochem 52:1042–1049, 1989b

Wood K, Coppen A: Prophylactic lithium treatment of patients with affective disorder is associated with decreased platelet ^{3}H-dihydroergocryptine binding. J Affect Disord 5:253–258, 1983

Wood K, Swade C, Abou-Saleh M, et al: Drug plasma levels and platelet 5-HT uptake inhibition during long-term treatment with fluvoxamine or lithium in patients with affective disorder. Br J Clin Pharmacol 15:365S–368S, 1983

Wood K, Swade C, Abou-Salch MT, et al: Apparent supersensitivity of platelet 5-HT receptors in lithium-treated patients. J Affect Disord 8:69–72, 1985

Yamaki M, Kusano E, Tetsuka T, et al: Cellular mechanism of lithium-induced nephrogenic diabetes insipidus in rats. Am J Physiol 261:F505–F511, 1991

Zalstein E, Koren G, Einarson T, et al: A case-control study on the association between first trimester exposure to lithium and Ebstein's anomaly. Am J Cardiol 65:817–818, 1990

Zatz M, Reisine TD: Lithium induces corticotropin secretion and desensitization in cultured anterior pituitary cells. Proc Natl Acad Sci U S A 82:1286–1290, 1985

Zerahn K: Studies on the active transport of lithium in the isolated frog skin. Acta Physiol Scand 33:347–358, 1955

17

Antiepileptic Drugs

Susan L. McElroy, M.D., and Paul E. Keck, Jr., M.D.

An increasing number of studies performed over the past several decades have shown that many drugs with antiepileptic properties are effective in the acute and prophylactic treatment of some patients with bipolar disorder, including those inadequately responsive to or intolerant of treatment with lithium. These agents include a number of standard antiepileptics (e.g., carbamazepine, valproate, and phenytoin), the investigational antiepileptic oxcarbazepine, and the benzodiazepines clonazepam and lorazepam (Keck et al. 1992a; McElroy and Pope 1988; McElroy et al. 1992b; Post 1988, 1990; Post et al. 1991; Prien and Gelenberg 1989). The expanding body of research showing that carbamazepine and valproate have both acute antimanic and long-term mood-stabilizing effects has led some authorities to recommend that they be considered second-line agents to lithium in the treatment of bipolar disorder when lithium is either ineffective or not tolerated, and as first-line agents in specific patients (e.g., those with psoriasis, renal impairment, dysphoric mania, or rapid cycling) (Gerner and Stanton 1992; McElroy and Keck 1993).

Although it has not been definitively proven that benzodiazepines possess specific antimanic or mood-stabilizing effects separate from their nonspecific sedative effects, clinical experience indicates that these agents are effective in the treatment of acute manic agitation in place of, or in conjunction with, antipsychotic drugs, prior to the onset of action of primary mood stabilizers (Lenox et al. 1992).

Benzodiazepines are also useful for the treatment of catatonia (which, in many cases, is a manifestation of the manic phase of bipolar disorder) (Bodken 1990; Rosebush et al. 1990).

In this chapter, we review the pharmacology of carbamazepine and valproate, as well as the research supporting their efficacy in the treatment of bipolar disorder. Research examining the efficacy of benzodiazepines and other antiepileptic agents in bipolar disorder is also summarized. Moreover, issues such as predictors of response, use of these agents in combination with other psychotropics, and antiepileptic resistance are addressed.

■ CARBAMAZEPINE

■ History and Discovery

Carbamazepine was developed in the late 1950s in the laboratories of J.R. Geigy AG in Basel, Switzerland. Its synthesis was described by Schindler in 1961, its antiepileptic properties were first reported by Theobald and Kunz in 1963, and its efficacy in patients with epilepsy and paroxysmal pain syndromes was first demonstrated in Europe in the early 1960s (Kutt 1989; Levy et al. 1989; Loiseau and Duche 1989; Rall and Schleifer 1985). Reports of carbamazepine having beneficial psychotropic effects in patients with epilepsy appeared in the early 1960s (Dalby 1971). The first report of its therapeutic effects in bipolar disorder appeared in Japan in 1971 (Takezaki and Hanaoka 1971). The association of carbamazepine with blood dyscrasias delayed its use in North America. However, once the rarity of this serious adverse effect became apparent, the U.S. Food and Drug Administration (FDA) approved carbamazepine in 1974 as an antiepileptic for adults, in 1978 as an antiepileptic for children older than age 6, and in 1987 as an antiepileptic without age limitations. Carbamazepine is currently considered a major antiepileptic, and it continues to be increasingly prescribed because it possesses less psychological and neurological toxicity than either phenytoin or phenobarbital (Loiseau and Duche 1989).

■ Structure-Activity Relations

Carbamazepine (5-carbamyl-5H-dibenzo[b,f]azepine or 5H-dibenzo[b,f]azepine-5-carboxamide) is an iminostilbene derivative with a tricyclic structure similar to that of the tricyclic antidepressant (TCA) imipramine (Kutt 1989; Levy et al. 1989; Rall and Schleifer 1985 [see Figure 17–1]). Iminodibenzyl (a precursor of carbamazepine) and a number of iminodibenzyl derivatives possess local anesthetic as well as antihistaminic properties but only modest antiepileptic activity. When a carbamyl (carboxamide) group is added at the 5 position of iminodibenzyl, considerable antiepileptic activity is conferred. However, the strongest antiepileptic effects occur when the carbamyl side chain is combined with iminostilbene to make carbamazepine, the structure of which is similar to iminodibenzyl except for a double bond between the 10 and 11 positions (see Figure 17–1).

■ Pharmacological Profile

Carbamazepine has an antiepileptic profile similar to that of phenytoin, and is effective against maximal electroshock seizures at nontoxic doses but ineffective against pentylenetetrazole-induced seizures (Macdonald 1989). However, carbamazepine is more effective than phenytoin in reducing stimulus-induced discharges in the amygdala of kindled rats (Albright and Burnham 1980). Also, carbamazepine has antidiuretic effects that may be associated with reduced serum antidiuretic hormone (ADH) concentrations, and (with chronic administration) is associated with decreases in peripheral thyroid function indices, increased urinary free cortisol secretion, and

a high incidence of escape from dexamethasone suppression (Post et al. 1991).

In humans, carbamazepine has been shown to be effective in the treatment of simple partial, complex partial, and generalized tonic-clonic seizures. Carbamazepine is ineffective against and may even exacerbate absence seizures. It is also effective in the treatment of paroxysmal pain syndromes such as trigeminal neuralgia (Blom 1963).

■ Pharmacokinetics and Disposition

After oral ingestion, the absorption of carbamazepine is slow, erratic, and unpredictable, although absorption in patients with epilepsy may be more rapid than in healthy volunteer subjects and there is minimal first-pass metabolism (Morselli 1989). Peak plasma concentrations are generally attained 4–8 hours after ingestion, but peaks as late as 26 hours have been reported (see Table 17–1). The time of administration may have a significant effect on the absorption rate, with absorption being slower with evening rather than morning doses. Carbamazepine's irregular absorption has been attributed to a very slow dissolution rate in gastrointestinal fluid and to the anticholinergic properties of the drug modifying gastrointestinal transit time. Precise data on the absolute bioavailability of carbamazepine do not exist (because of the lack of an injectable formulation), but ranges of 75% to 85% have been estimated from studies using the ^{14}C-labeled molecule. Solutions, suspensions, syrups, and the newly developed chewable and slow-release formulations of carbamazepine seem to have similar bioavailability. The slow-release

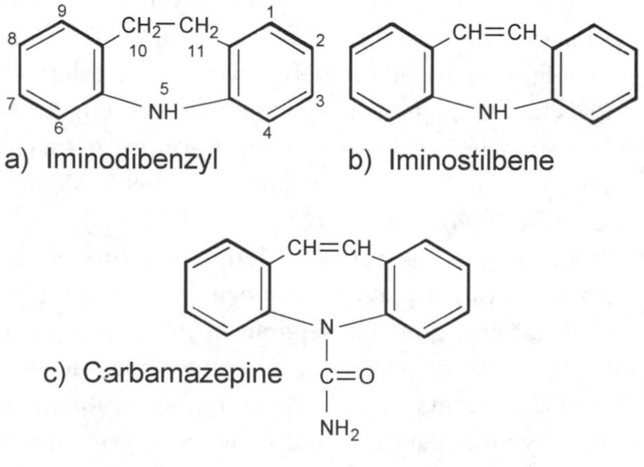

Figure 17–1. Carbamazepine and its precursors.
Source. Reproduced from Kutt 1989 with permission.

formulations, however, give rise to more stable plasma concentrations. It is worth noting that, in cases of massive overdose, peak plasma carbamazepine concentrations have been reached during the second or third day after ingestion.

Carbamazepine distributes rapidly into all tissues, with 75%–78% bound to plasma proteins, including proteins other than albumin. Concentrations of carbamazepine in cerebrospinal fluid (CSF) correspond with concentrations of free drug in plasma, and range from 17%–31% of those in plasma.

Carbamazepine undergoes almost complete biotransformation in humans and is metabolized in the liver by the cytochrome P_{450} system to a wide number of metabolites, many of which have antiepileptic activity (see Figure 17–2). The predominant pathway of metabolism in humans involves conversion to the 10,11-epoxide (see Figure 17–3). This metabolite is as active as carbamazepine and has neurotoxic side effects. Its concentrations in plasma and brain may reach 50% of those of carbamazepine. The 10,11-epoxide is metabolized further to inactive compounds that are excreted in the urine principally as glucuronides. Carbamazepine is also inactivated by conjugation and hydroxylation. Less than 3% of the drug is excreted in the urine as the parent compound or the epoxide.

Carbamazepine's elimination half-life ranges from 18 to 55 hours. During long-term treatment, carbamazepine may induce its own metabolism (a phenomenon called autoinduction), and its half-life may be decreased to 5–26 hours (see Figure 17–4). The half-life of the 10,11-epoxide is much shorter than that of the parent compound (6–7 hours).

Treatment with carbamazepine for epilepsy, trigeminal neuralgia, and mania is usually started at a dosage of 100–200 mg taken either qd or bid. The dosage is increased (usually by 100 mg or 200 mg every few days) according to the patient's response and side effects, usually to serum concentrations

ranging from 4–15 µg/ml. Although there is no clear relationship between carbamazepine serum concentration and response, therapeutic concentrations for epilepsy, paroxysmal pain syndromes, and mania are

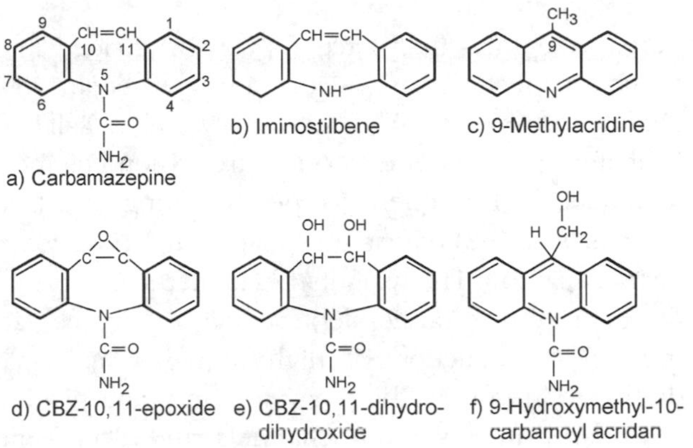

Figure 17–2. Carbamazepine (CBZ) and its metabolites and breakdown products.
Source. Reproduced from Kutt 1989 with permission.

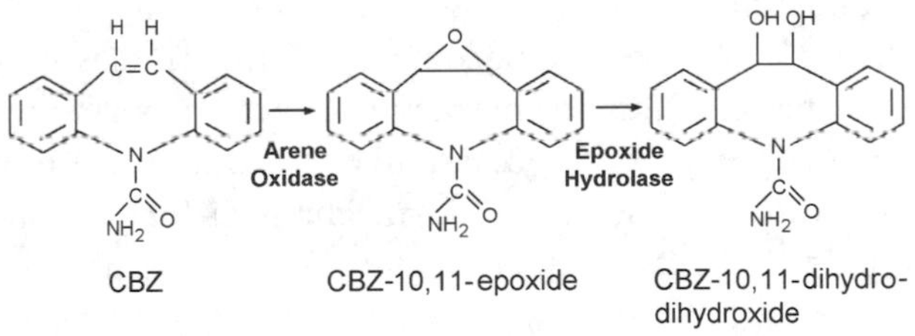

Figure 17–3. Major pathway of carbamazepine (CBZ) metabolism. This pathway of CBZ metabolism produces a CBZ-10,11-epoxide, a compound that possesses both anticonvulsant and toxic properties. The CBZ-10,11-epoxide is further metabolized by epoxide hydrolase. The action of epoxide hydrolase is blocked by valproate (VPA); therefore, when VPA is dosed concurrently with CBZ, the CBZ-10,11-epoxide metabolite accumulates.
Source. Reproduced from Wilder 1992 with permission.

Table 17–1. Population data for valproate (VPA) and carbamazepine (CBZ)

	Peak absorption (hours)	Elimination half-life (hours)	Time to steady state (days)	Protein binding (%)	Therapeutic range (µg/ml)
CBZ	2–8	2–17	2–4	73–88	3–14
VPA	1–4	5–20	2–4	70–95	50–150

Source. Reproduced with permission from Wilder 1992.

reported to be 4–15 µg/ml. Significantly, neurological side effects become more frequent at serum concentrations above 9 µg/ml.

■ Mechanism of Action

Carbamazepine's many actions can be divided into two basic mechanisms (reviewed in Levy et al. 1989; Mcdonald 1989; Post et al. 1984a, 1991, 1992; Rall and Schleifer 1985): 1) effects on neuronal ion channels to reduce high-frequency repetitive firing of action potentials, and 2) effects on synaptic and postsynaptic transmission. The weight of evidence suggests that carbamazepine's antiepileptic action can be attributed to reduction of high-frequency neuronal discharge through binding to and inactivating voltage-sensitive sodium channels and decreasing sodium influx in a voltage-, frequency-, and use-dependent fashion (Mcdonald 1989; Post et al. 1992). Because carbamazepine's effects on sodium channels are acute, and because its antiepileptic and antinociceptive effects are more rapid in onset than its antimanic or antidepressant effects, Post and colleagues (1992) have speculated that the drug's sodium channel effects do not account for its mood-stabilizing properties. Recent noteworthy studies suggest that carbamazepine may also act on potassium channels to increase potassium conductance, thereby providing another possible mechanism for its antiepileptic effects (Post et al. 1992; Zona et al. 1990).

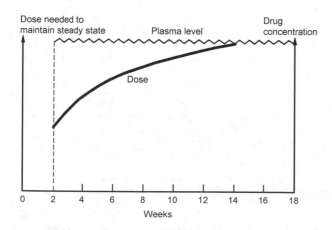

Figure 17–4. Carbamazepine (CBZ) dosage adjustments versus time to compensate for autoinduction. The clearance of CBZ approximately doubles in the first 2–3 months of therapy. To maintain therapeutic plasma levels, the daily dose must be increased, often by 100%. *Source.* Reproduced from Wilder 1992 with permission.

Regarding synaptic and postsynaptic actions, carbamazepine has been reported to alter neurotransmitter concentrations, metabolism, receptors, and second messenger systems. Indeed, the drug affects a multiplicity of neurotransmitter systems implicated in the pathophysiology of mood disorders. The primary neurotransmitters thus far shown to be altered by carbamazepine include adenosine, norepinephrine, dopamine, serotonin, acetylcholine, γ-aminobutyric acid (GABA), glutamate, substance P, and aspartate (Macdonald 1989; Post et al. 1991, 1992). Carbamazepine binds to adenosine receptors and acts as an adenosine receptor antagonist. However, studies suggest that this property of carbamazepine is not responsible for its antiepileptic effects. Carbamazepine acutely increases locus ceruleus firing and decreases glutamate release; subchronic treatment decreases norepinephrine, dopamine, and GABA turnover, and blocks adenylate cyclase activity stimulated by norepinephrine, dopamine, and adenosine. Chronic carbamazepine administration is associated with increases in adenosine receptors, substance P sensitivity and levels, and plasma free tryptophan; decreases in CSF somatostatin; and greater decreases in GABA turnover (Post et al. 1991, 1992).

It is unclear whether the drug's activities on these systems play a role in its antiepileptic properties. However, carbamazepine's ability to decrease release of the excitatory amino acid aspartate and its effects on α$_2$-adrenergic receptors have been implicated in its antiepileptic activity (Post et al. 1992). Also, although carbamazepine is not active at the central-type benzodiazepine receptor (which is linked to chloride channels and related to the antiepileptic effects of diazepam, clonazepam, and lorazepam), it may exert some of its antiepileptic effects by acutely binding to and acting as an antagonist at the "peripheral-type" benzodiazepine receptor, which appears linked to calcium channels (Post et al. 1992). Carbamazepine does not modify GABA-A receptors, but it may have effects at the GABA-B receptor. Although these effects probably do not contribute to the drug's antiepileptic properties, they may contribute to its antinociceptive effects. Finally, some of carbamazepine's effects on second messenger systems include decreased activity of adenylate and guanylate cyclase and reductions of some aspects of phosphoinositide turnover (Post et al. 1992).

Thus far, none of these mechanisms has been

linked with the psychotropic effects of carbamazepine, and it remains unknown whether the actions underlying the drug's antiepileptic effects are also responsible for its mood-stabilizing properties. Indeed, Post and colleagues (1992) have speculated that different biochemical effects of carbamazepine may underlie its efficacy in different seizure types. It is noteworthy that carbamazepine does not block either stimulant-induced hyperactivity in animals or dopamine receptors in vitro. Thus, it exerts its antimanic effects through a mechanism other than dopamine receptor antagonism (Post et al. 1991).

■ Indications

Carbamazepine is currently approved in the United States for the treatment of complex partial seizures, generalized tonic-clonic seizures, and other minor or partial seizure disorders (reviewed in Levy et al. 1989; Loiseau and Duche 1989; Mattson et al. 1992). Controlled studies have shown that carbamazepine has the following characteristics:

1. It is as effective as phenytoin and valproate in the treatment of primary tonic-clonic and secondarily generalized tonic-clonic seizures.
2. It is comparable to or better than phenobarbital and primidone in suppressing primary tonic-clonic and secondarily generalized tonic-clonic seizures.
3. It is comparable to or better than all of these drugs in controlling the entire range of partial seizures (i.e., simple and complex seizures, with or without secondary generalization). Indeed, it is a drug of first choice in symptomatic location-related (partial) epilepsy with partial or secondary generalized tonic-clonic seizures. However, carbamazepine is ineffective in, and may even exacerbate, absence seizures.

Carbamazepine is also approved for use in a variety of paroxysmal pain syndromes, including trigeminal neuralgia. Although not formally approved for use in bipolar disorder, carbamazepine is frequently used as an alternative or adjunct to lithium in lithium-resistant or -intolerant patients. Research supporting its efficacy in bipolar disorder is summarized later in this chapter.

Carbamazepine in Acute Mania

To date, at least 11 double-blind studies have shown that carbamazepine is superior to placebo and comparable to lithium and antipsychotics in the short-term treatment of acute mania, with approximately two-thirds of patients showing significant improvement (Ballenger and Post 1978; Brown et al. 1987; Desai et al. 1987; Grossi et al. 1984; Keck et al. 1992a; Lenzi et al. 1986; Lerer et al. 1987; Lusznat et al. 1988; Möller et al. 1989; Müller and Stoll 1984; Okuma et al. 1979, 1990; Post 1990; Post et al. 1984a; Small 1990; Small et al. 1991 [see Table 17–2]). However, only six studies (Ballenger and Post 1978; Okuma et al. 1979; Grossi et al. 1984; Lerer et al. 1987; Post et al. 1984a; Small et al. 1991) are unconfounded by concurrent lithium and neuroleptic administration, and thus allow for more meaningful interpretation.

Pooled data from these latter studies reveal an overall response rate for carbamazepine in acute mania of 50%, compared with 56% for lithium monotherapy and 61% for neuroleptic monotherapy (differences not significant) (Keck et al. 1992a). These studies further indicate that carbamazepine has an onset of acute antimanic action comparable to that of neuroleptics and perhaps slightly more rapid than that of lithium (with significant antimanic effects usually evident within 1–2 weeks of treatment) and that it is generally better tolerated than neuroleptics and lithium (with fewer extrapyramidal side effects [EPS]). Moreover, its antimanic effects may be augmented by or synergistic with concurrent administration of other mood-stabilizing agents (including lithium and valproate) and neuroleptics (Keck et al. 1992b; Ketter et al. 1992). In responders, therapeutic serum concentrations are similar to those for epilepsy, generally 4–15 µg/ml, with carbamazepine doses of 200–2,000 mg/day.

Carbamazepine in Acute Major Depression

Only three controlled studies have examined the efficacy of carbamazepine in the treatment of patients with unipolar or bipolar major depression (see Table 17–3). In the first study (Neumann et al. 1984), 10 patients (bipolar and unipolar) were randomly assigned to treatment with carbamazepine ($n = 5$) or trimipramine ($n = 5$). Both treatments were associated with significant antidepressant effects, and no significant differences were found between the two groups. In the second study (Post et al. 1985), 12 (34%) of 35 bi-

Table 17–2. Controlled studies of carbamazepine in treatment of acute mania

Study	N	Design	Concomitant medications	Duration (days)	Outcome
Placebo-Controlled					
Ballenger and Post 1978; Post et al. 1984a	19	B-A-B-A; CBZ v. P	None	11–56	63% response on CBZ; significant relapse on placebo
Placebo + Neuroleptic					
Klein et al. 1984	14	CBZ + HAL v. P + HAL; CBZ + HAL	HAL 15–45 mg/day HAL	35	71% response CBZ + HAL; 54% response P + HAL; both groups improved, but CBZ + HAL group's improvement was greater
Müller and Stoll 1984	6	P + HAL		21	
Möller et al. 1989	11 CBZ; 9 P	CBZ + HAL v. P + HAL	HAL 24 mg/day; levomepromazine prn	21	No significant difference
Placebo + Lithium					
Desai et al. 1987	5	CBZ + L v. P + L	L; ND	28	CBZ + L response > P + L response by 14
Lithium-Controlled					
Lerer et al. 1987	14 CBZ; 14 L	CBZ v. L	None	28	79% response L > 29% response CBZ
Small et al. 1991	24 CBZ; 24 L	CBZ v. L	None	56	33% response rate for both groups
Neuroleptic-Controlled					
Grossi et al. 1984	18 CBZ; 19 CPZ	CBZ v. CPZ	ND	21	67% response on CPZ; 59% response on CBZ
Okuma et al. 1979	32 CBZ; 28 CPZ	CBZ v. CPZ	None	21–35	66% response on CBZ; 54% response on CPZ
Neuroleptic + Neuroleptic					
Brown et al. 1987	8 CBZ; 9 HAL	CBZ + CPZ HAL + CPZ	CPZ	28	HAL group had higher dropout rate because of EPS
Lithium + Neuroleptic					
Lusznat et al. 1988	22	CBZ + CPZ; HAL v. L + CPZ, HAL	HAL, CPZ	42	No significant difference
Lenzi et al. 1986	22	CBZ + CPZ v. L + CPZ	CPZ	19	73% response for both groups
Okuma et al. 1990	101	CBZ + neuroleptics (80%); neuroleptics	Neuroleptics	28	62% response on CBZ; 59% response on mean level 0.46 mEq/L

Note. CBZ = carbamazepine; P = placebo; HAL = haloperidol; L = lithium; ND = not documented; EPS = extrapyramidal side effects; CPZ = chlorpromazine.
Source. Adapted from Keck et al. 1992a with permission.

polar and unipolar patients with treatment-resistant depression displayed a marked antidepressant response to treatment with carbamazepine alone. Fifty-four percent of patients ($n = 19$) showed at least a mild degree of improvement. Substitution of carbamazepine with placebo was associated with loss of response in some carbamazepine responders. Also, the time course of antidepressant response to carbamazepine in responders was longer than that in pa-

tients with mania, and comparable to that of standard antidepressants: patients began to exhibit antidepressant effects after 2–3 weeks of treatment and exhibited maximal antidepressant effects after 4–6 weeks.

In the third study (Small 1990), patients with treatment-resistant unipolar or bipolar depression were randomized to a 4-week trial of lithium, carbamazepine, or a combination of both drugs. Patients randomized to carbamazepine or the combination

Table 17–3. Controlled studies of carbamazepine in acute depression

Study	N	Design	Concomitant medications	Duration (days)	Outcome
Neumann et al. 1984	10 (bipolar & unipolar)	CBZ v.TRI	None	28	CBZ and TRI equally effective
Post et al. 1985	24 bipolar 11 unipolar	B-A-B-A	None	Median 45	34% marked response CBZ; 54% response overall
Small 1990	4 bipolar 24 unipolar	L v. CBZ v. L + CBZ	None	28, then L + CBZ for 28	32% response CBZ, CBZ + L; 13% response L

Note. CBZ = carbamazepine; L = lithium; TRI = trimipramine.
Source. Adapted from Keck et al. 1992a with permission.

displayed 32% moderate or marked improvement compared with the lithium-treated patients, who displayed 13% improvement. Significantly, one small controlled study suggests that carbamazepine's acute antidepressant effects may be augmented by lithium. Of 15 patients with major depression refractory to carbamazepine alone, 8 (53%) displayed a rapid onset of antidepressant response (within a mean of 4 days) following the blind addition of lithium (Kramlinger and Post 1989). Finally, open studies indicate that carbamazepine may sometimes be effective in treatment-resistant depression. For instance, in a retrospective review of 16 patients with treatment-resistant melancholic depression who were treated with carbamazepine either alone or in conjunction with other psychotropics, 7 (44%) displayed moderate or marked improvement (Cullen et al. 1991).

Carbamazepine in the Prophylactic Treatment of Bipolar Disorder

Five controlled studies have examined the efficacy of carbamazepine in the long-term treatment of patients with bipolar disorder, with approximately two-thirds of patients displaying a significant prophylactic response over 1–2 years (Bellaire et al. 1988; Lusznat et al. 1988; Okuma et al. 1981; Placidi et al. 1986; Watkins et al. 1987). In the only placebo-controlled study (Okuma et al. 1981), 60% of patients had not relapsed with carbamazepine treatment at 1-year follow-up, as compared with 22% of patients receiving placebo. In the other four controlled studies, carbamazepine appeared comparable to lithium in reducing affective episodes and prolonging euthymic intervals. Also, carbamazepine's mood-stabilizing effects have been reported to be augmented by the concurrent administration of lithium, valproate, thyroid hormone, antipsychotics, and antidepressants.

The drug's prophylactic effects, however, may be better for mania than for depression, are often incomplete even in responders, and may display tachyphylaxis in some patients (Frankenburg et al. 1988; Post et al. 1990). For example, of 24 lithium-refractory affectively ill patients displaying a marked acute response to carbamazepine who were subsequently followed up for a mean of 4 years, 50% displayed significant breakthrough episodes during the second or third year of treatment despite adequate serum concentrations (Post et al. 1990). This apparent loss of efficacy has been hypothesized to be due to the development of contingent tolerance or to the progression of the underlying illness. On the other hand, Murphy and colleagues (1989) have suggested that the methodological limitations of the controlled trials cast doubt on the prophylactic efficacy of carbamazepine.

Predictors of Response

Early studies suggested that certain factors associated with poor response to lithium might be associated with favorable antimanic response to carbamazepine. These factors included more severe mania, rapid cycling (the occurrence of four or more mood episodes within 1 year), greater dysphoria or depression during mania (so-called mixed or dysphoric mania), and a lower incidence of familial bipolar disorder (Goodwin 1990; Kishimoto et al. 1983; McElroy et al. 1992a; Post et al. 1987, 1991). However, recent studies indicate that decreasing or stable episode frequencies (Post et al. 1990) and decreasing mania severity

(Small et al. 1991) correlate with favorable carbamazepine response. Factors not associated with antimanic response to carbamazepine include the presence of psychosensory symptoms and response to other antiepileptics (Post et al. 1991). For instance, manic patients failing to respond to valproate and phenytoin have been reported to respond to carbamazepine (Post et al. 1984b).

Factors possibly associated with favorable antidepressant response to carbamazepine in one study included more severe depression at the time of treatment, a history of more discrete episodes of depression, and a history of less chronicity (Post et al. 1985, 1991). In this study, the patients displaying the greatest degree of thyroid hormone decrement (either thyroxine [T_4] or free T_4) while receiving carbamazepine exhibited the best antidepressant response. A trend toward greater improvement was observed in bipolar rather than unipolar patients. Factors such as family history, mild electroencephalogram (EEG) abnormalities, and psychosensory symptoms, however, did not predict antidepressant response.

■ Side Effects and Toxicology

Carbamazepine possesses a favorable side effect profile compared with lithium, antipsychotics, and other antiepileptics (Andrews et al. 1990; Gram and Jensen 1989; Levy et al. 1989; Mattson et al. 1992; Pellock 1987; Pellock and Willmore 1991; Post et al. 1991; Rall and Schleifer 1985; Smith and Bleck 1991). Notably, the drug rarely causes EPS or renal side effects. It is associated with less cognitive and neurological toxicity than are phenytoin and phenobarbital; was associated with less weight gain, hair changes, and tremor than was valproate in one study of a large group of patients with epilepsy (Mattson et al. 1992); and, in another study, was associated with less memory impairment than was lithium in a group of patients with mood disorders (Andrews et al. 1990). However, 33%–50% of patients receiving carbamazepine experience side effects. These most commonly include neurological symptoms such as diplopia, blurred vision, fatigue, nausea, vertigo, nystagmus, and ataxia. These neurological side effects are dose-related, usually transient, and reversible with dose reduction. Elderly patients, however, may be more sensitive to them.

Less frequent side effects of carbamazepine include transient leukopenia occurring in approximately 10%–12% of patients; transient thrombocytopenia; rash occurring in up to 10%–12% of patients; hyponatremia and, less commonly, hypoosmolality; liver enzyme elevations in 5%–15% of patients; and other central nervous system (CNS) toxicities such as mild peripheral polyneuropathies and involuntary movement disorders. The leukopenia primarily involves granulocytes but does not predispose patients to infection, is not related to the serious idiopathic dyscrasias agranulocytosis and aplastic anemia, and usually resolves spontaneously despite continuation of medication. In the event of asymptomatic leukopenia, thrombocytopenia, or elevated liver enzymes, the carbamazepine dosage can be reduced or (in cases with severe changes) the drug discontinued. Once the abnormalities normalize, carbamazepine may be increased or restarted at a lower dose. If rash develops, carbamazepine may be continued as long as there is no associated fever, bleeding, exfoliative skin lesions, or other signs or symptoms of hypersensitivity. Also, carbamazepine-induced rash can be successfully treated with steroids.

Hyponatremia is most likely the result of water retention resulting from carbamazepine's antidiuretic effect. It occurs in 6%–31% of patients, is rare in children but probably more common in elderly people, occasionally occurs many months after the initiation of carbamazepine treatment, and often necessitates withdrawal from the drug. Carbamazepine may also decrease total and free thyroxine levels and increase free cortisol levels, but these effects are rarely clinically relevant.

Rare, nondose-related, idiosyncratic, and unpredictable but serious and potentially fatal carbamazepine side effects include blood dyscrasias (agranulocytosis and aplastic anemia), hepatic failure, exfoliative dermatitis (e.g., Stevens-Johnson syndrome), and pancreatitis. Other rare side effects include systemic hypersensitivity reactions, conduction disturbances (sometimes resulting in bradycardia or Stokes-Adams syndrome), psychological disturbances (e.g., sporadic cases of psychosis and mania), and (very rarely) renal effects (e.g., renal failure, oliguria, hematuria, and proteinuria). The development of a severe blood dyscrasia due to carbamazepine occurs in 2 in 575,000 treated patients per year, with a mortality rate of approximately 1 in 575,000 (Seetharam and Pellock 1991). Although most cases occur within the first 3–6 months of treatment, some have occurred after more extended periods of exposure. It is worth noting that transient leukopenia, thrombocytopenia, or hepatic enzyme elevations are not related to these life-threatening reactions. Routine blood monitoring does not permit anticipation of blood dyscrasias, hepatic failure, or exfoliative dermatitis (Pellock and Willmore 1991). Thus, educating the patient about the signs and symptoms of hepatic, hematologic, or dermatologic reactions and instructing him or her to report these signs and symptoms if they occur, along with careful monitoring of the patient's clinical status, is probably better than routine laboratory screening for detecting these serious side effects.

Carbamazepine has teratogenic effects (Jones et al. 1989; Levy et al. 1989; Rosa 1991). First-trimester exposure is associated with an increased risk of neural tube defects, craniofacial defects, fingernail hypoplasia, and developmental delay. Fortunately, the frequency of neural tube defects in general, as well as those associated with in utero antiepileptic exposure, may be reduced by prophylactic treatment with high doses of folate—ideally begun well before conception occurs (Centers for Disease Control 1991; Delcado-Escveta and Janz 1992).

Early signs of carbamazepine toxicity typically develop several hours after a given dose and include dizziness, ataxia, sedation, and diplopia. Higher concentrations are associated with nystagmus and obtundation. Acute intoxication can result in hyperirritability, stupor, or coma. Carbamazepine can be fatal in overdose: of 311 reported overdoses, 9 resulted in death, with the lethal doses of carbamazepine being 4–60 grams (Gram and Jensen 1989). The most common symptoms of carbamazepine overdose are nystagmus, ophthalmoplegia, cerebellar signs and EPS, impairment of consciousness, convulsions, and respiratory dysfunction. Cardiac symptoms include tachycardia, arrhythmia, conduction disturbances, and hypotension. Gastrointestinal and anticholinergic symptoms may also occur. Coma may develop with serum carbamazepine concentrations as low as 80 μmol/L.

In carbamazepine intoxication, the concentration of the 10,11-epoxide may exceed that of the parent compound. Indeed, it has been suggested that the course of intoxication correlates more closely with the course of the 10,11-epoxide serum concentrations than with the concentrations of carbamazepine itself. Treatment of carbamazepine intoxication includes symptomatic treatment, gastric lavage (which should be undertaken up to 12 hours after ingestion), and hemoperfusion, which may accelerate carbamazepine's elimination. Forced diuresis, peritoneal dialysis, and hemodialysis, however, are not recommended (Gram and Jensen 1989).

■ Drug-Drug Interactions

Carbamazepine has important interactions with a variety of other drugs (Ketter et al. 1991a, 1991b; Levy et al. 1989). First, because carbamazepine is a potent inducer of catabolic enzymes, it stimulates the metabolism and decreases the plasma levels of many other metabolized medications, including haloperidol and other antipsychotics, methadone, antiasthmatics (e.g., prednisone, methylprednisolone, and theophylline), warfarin, valproate, TCAs, benzodiazepines, and hormonal contraceptives. Indeed, although failure of oral contraceptives is more common in women using phenytoin and/or phenobarbital, instances in patients receiving carbamazepine have been reported (Mattson et al. 1986).

Second, because the metabolism of carbamazepine is exclusively hepatic, certain enzyme inhibitors can inhibit carbamazepine metabolism, increase serum carbamazepine concentrations, and precipitate carbamazepine toxicity. These medications include acetazolamide, the calcium channel blockers diltiazem and verapamil (but not nifedipine), danazol, dextropropoxyphene, propoxyphene, erythromycin, isoniazid, and valproate.

Third, combinations of carbamazepine with other enzyme-inducing agents, including antiepileptics, can increase carbamazepine-10,11-epoxide concentrations and result in signs of toxicity at normally tolerable serum concentrations. Indeed, some studies indicate a connection between plasma 10,11-epoxide concentrations and side effects; neurological side effects are also more frequent in patients receiving carbamazepine with other antiepileptics (Gram and Jensen 1989).

Finally, the potential exists for pharmacodynamic interactions with other neurotoxic drugs. Thus, although most patients tolerate carbamazepine when it is given in conjunction with lithium or antipsychotics, cases of enhanced neurotoxicity have been reported with both combinations (Fogel 1988). In one study, the combination of carbamazepine and lithium caused greater memory impairment than either drug alone (Andrews et al. 1990).

VALPROATE

History and Discovery

Valproic acid was first synthesized by Burton in the United States in 1882 and subsequently used as an organic solvent. The drug's antiepileptic properties were discovered serendipitously by Meunier in 1963 in France. Employing it as a vehicle for other compounds that were being screened for anticpileptic activity, Meunier found that compounds that did not demonstrate antiepileptic properties when administered alone inhibited seizure activity when dissolved in valproic acid, and concluded that the antiepileptic activity was due to the solvent, valproic acid, rather than to the test drugs (Fariello and Smith 1989; Levy et al. 1989; Penry and Dean 1989).

Initial clinical trials confirming valproate's efficacy in epilepsy were conducted in Europe in the mid-1960s with the sodium salt of the drug. Valproate was first introduced as an antiepileptic in France in 1967. It has been used in Holland and Germany since 1968, in the United Kingdom since 1973, and became available in the United States in 1978. An enteric-coated formulation, divalproex sodium, was introduced to the United States market in 1983, and a formulation consisting of a capsule containing coated particles of divalproex sodium was introduced in 1989. Interestingly, the first report of valproate having therapeutic effects in bipolar disorder appeared in France in 1966 (Lambert et al. 1966).

Structure-Activity Relations

Valproic acid (dipropylacetic acid) is a simple branched-chain carboxylic acid structurally distinct from other existing antiepileptic and psychotropic compounds (see Figure 17–5 [Levy et al. 1989; Rimmer and Richens 1985]). Although straight chain acids have little or no antiepileptic activity, other branched-chain carboxylic acids have potencies similar to that of valproate in antagonizing pentylenetetrazole-induced seizures. However, increasing the number of carbon atoms to nine introduces marked sedative properties. The primary amide of valproic acid (valpromide, which is available in Europe but not the United States) has been reported to be about twice as potent as the parent compound.

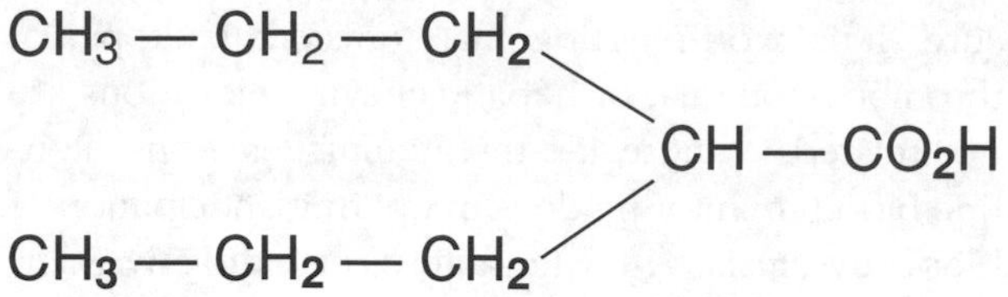

$$CH_3 - CH_2 - CH_2 \diagdown$$
$$CH - CO_2H$$
$$CH_3 - CH_2 - CH_2 \diagup$$

Figure 17–5. Structure of valproic acid (2-propyl-pentanoic acid).
Source. Reproduced from Kupferberg 1989 with permission.

Pharmacologic Profile

Valproate blocks pentylenetetrazole-induced and maximal electroshock seizures in a variety of animals (with somewhat better efficacy in the former than in the latter), and suppresses secondarily generalized seizures without affecting focal activity in cortical cobalt and alumina lesioned animals (Fariello and Smith 1989). Valproate also has antikindling properties—preventing the spread of epileptiform activity in cats without affecting focal seizures (Leveil and Nanquet 1977). In humans, valproate has activity against a wide variety of epilepsy types while causing only minimal sedation and other CNS side effects.

Pharmacokinetics and Disposition

Valproate is presently commercially available in the United States in four oral preparations: divalproex sodium, an enteric-coated stable coordination compound containing equal proportions of valproic acid and sodium valproate in a 1:1 molar ratio; valproic acid; sodium valproate; and divalproex sodium sprinkle capsules containing coated particles of divalproex sodium that can be ingested intact or pulled apart and sprinkled on food. Valproate is also available in suppository form for rectal administration, and an intravenous preparation is currently under development. As mentioned, valpromide, the amide of valproic acid, is available in Europe. There are only minor differences in the pharmacokinetics of these preparations, and valproic acid is the common compound in plasma (see Table 17–1).

The bioavailability of valproate approaches 100% with all preparations (Levy et al. 1989; Penry and Dean 1989; Wilder 1992). All preparations taken po, except divalproex sodium, are rapidly absorbed after oral ingestion, attaining peak serum concentrations within two hours (see Table 17–1). Divalproex sodium reaches peak serum concentrations within 3–8 hours. The divalproex sodium sprinkle formulation has an earlier onset of absorption but a slower rate of absorption than divalproex sodium tablets (see Figure 17–6). Absorption can also be delayed if the drug is taken with food.

Valproate is highly protein bound, predominantly to serum albumin and proportional to the albumin concentration. Although patients with low levels of albumin will have a higher fraction of unbound drug, the steady state level of total drug is not altered. Only the unbound drug crosses the blood brain barrier and is bioactive. Thus, when valproate is displaced from protein binding sites through drug interactions, the total drug concentration may not change; however, the pharmacologically active unbound drug does increase and may produce signs and symptoms of toxicity. Moreover, when the plasma concentration of valproate increases in response to increased dosing, the amount of unbound (active) valproate increases disproportionately and is metabolized with an apparent increase in clearance of total drug, yielding lower than expected total plasma concentrations (Levy et al. 1989; Wilder 1992 [see Figures 17–7 and 17–8]). In addition, valproate protein binding is increased by low fat diets and decreased by high fat diets.

The correlation between valproate serum concentration and both its antiepileptic and antimanic effects is poor, but the concentration range generally required for good clinical effect is approximately 50 to 125 or 150 µg/ml. There appears to be a response threshold at 50 µg/ml—the approximate valproate serum concentration at which plasma albumin sites begin to become saturated—as valproate concentrations equal to or greater than 50 µg/ml are more often associated with response than are lower concentrations (Rimmer and Richens 1985). However, some patients with epilepsy or mania display clinical response only with serum concentrations well above 100 µg/ml, and in some cases, with serum concentrations approaching 200 µg/ml (McElroy et al. 1992b). Conversely, patients with cyclothymia may respond to serum valproate concentrations below 50 µg/ml (Jacobsen 1993).

Valproate is metabolized primarily in the liver by two metabolic pathways to a large number of metabolites, some of which have antiepileptic and/or toxic effects (Levy et al. 1989; Penry and Dean 1989;

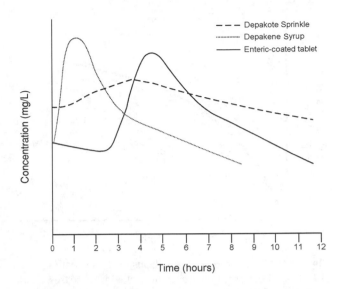

Figure 17–6. Absorption of three valproate (VPA) formulations after oral dosing in patients taking chronic VPA therapy: valproic acid (Depakene Syrup) versus enteric-coated divalproex sodium tablets versus divalproex sodium sprinkle capsules.
Source. Reproduced from Wilder 1992 with permission.

Rimmer and Richens 1985; Wilder 1992 [see Figure 17–9]). These two metabolic pathways are 1) mitochondrial β-oxidation to 3-OH-valproate, 3-oxo-valproate, and 2-en-valproate; and 2) P_{450} microsomal metabolism to the toxic 4-en- and 2,4-en metabolites, and to a number of inactive metabolites that are conjugated with glucuronide. Of note, the 2-en-valproate metabolite is considered an active antiepileptic with a long half-life (Wilder 1992). Less than 3% of valproate is excreted unchanged in the urine and feces. Valproate's elimination half-life is typically 5–20 hours and can be altered by agents that affect the mitochondrial and/or microsomal enzymes systems responsible for its metabolism. Mitochondrial β-oxidation (the pathway used extensively for processing fatty acids) is the more important pathway for valproate's metabolism, especially when valproate is administered alone. However, P_{450} microsomal metabolism is increased (along with the toxic metabolites it generates) when valproate is administered with other drugs that induce the P_{450} system, thereby increasing chances of adverse effects, including (extremely rarely and primarily in children) liver necrosis.

Treatment with valproate for epilepsy or bipolar disorder is usually begun at a dosage of 15 mg/kg/day (usually 500–1,000/day in 2–4 divided

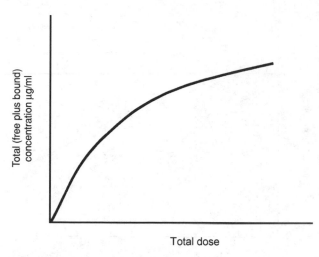

Figure 17–7. Accelerated metabolism of valproate (VPA). As the plasma concentration of VPA increases, clearance of VPA also increases. This increased clearance is secondary to the disproportionate concentration of unbound VPA produced at high levels that becomes available for metabolism (see Figure 17–8).
Source. Reproduced from Wilder 1992 with permission.

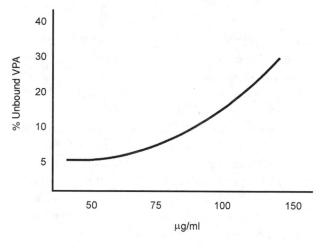

Figure 17–8. Total valproate (VPA) concentrations. As the total concentration of VPA increases, protein-binding sites become saturated, and the percentage of unbound to bound VPA increases.
Source. Reproduced from Wilder 1992 with permission.

doses). The drug can be "orally loaded" at 20 mg/kg/day in status epilepticus and acute mania to induce more rapid response. As with carbamazepine, valproate dosage is increased according to the patient's response and side effects, usually by 250–500 mg/day every 1–3 days and to serum concentrations of 50–150 μg/ml. Of note, neurological side effects become more frequent at serum concentrations above 100 μg/ml. Once the patient is stabi-

Valproate metabolism

$$VPA \xrightarrow{\substack{\text{mitochondrial} \\ \beta\text{-oxidation}}} \begin{array}{l} \text{3-OH-VPA} \\ \text{3-OXO-VPA} \\ \Delta^2 \text{ VPA*} \end{array}$$

*Active anticonvulsant—Long $T_{1/2}$

$$VPA \xrightarrow{\substack{\text{microsomal} \\ P_{450} \text{ pathway}}} \begin{array}{l} \Delta^4 \text{ VPA and other} \\ \text{inactive metabolites} \\ \Delta^{2,4} \text{ VPA} \end{array}$$

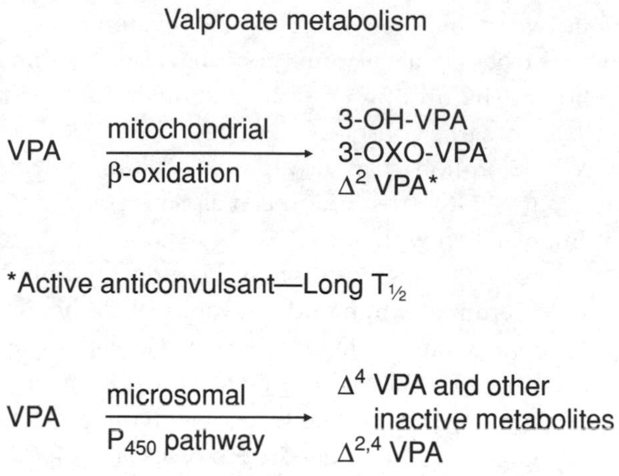

Figure 17–9. Two pathways for metabolism of valproate (VPA). VPA is metabolized within the mitochondria by the β-oxidative pathway, which metabolizes medium- and long-chain fatty acids. This is the major metabolic pathway used by patients taking VPA as monotherapy. VPA is also metabolized by the microsomal P_{450} pathway, which occurs outside the mitochondria and is increased when VPA is dosed in combination with enzyme-inducing drugs (i.e., carbamazepine).
Source. Reproduced from Wilder 1992 with permission.

lized, the entire valproate dosage may be taken as one daily dose before sleep to enhance convenience and compliance.

■ Mechanism of Action

Like carbamazepine, valproate has many effects, and the mechanisms underlying its antiepileptic and mood-stabilizing actions are unknown. One theory is that valproate induces its antiepileptic and possibly its mood-stabilizing effects by changes in the metabolism of GABA, the major inhibitory neurotransmitter in mammalian CNS (Emrich et al. 1981; Fariello and Smith 1989; Post et al. 1992; Rimmer and Richens 1985). Valproate inhibits the catabolism of GABA, increases its release, decreases GABA turnover, increases GABA-B receptor density, and may also enhance neuronal responsiveness to GABA. Studies have suggested that valproate-induced increased brain levels of GABA and improved neuronal responsiveness to GABA are associated with seizure control. Other research, however, suggests that valproate exerts its antiepileptic effects by direct neuronal effects (i.e., reducing sodium influx and increasing potassium efflux). Yet other effects of valproate include decreased dopamine turnover, decreased N-methyl-

D-aspartate (NMDA)-mediated currents, decreased release of aspartate, and decreased CSF somatostatin concentrations. It is noteworthy that, unlike carbamazepine, valproate does not bind to the peripheral-type benzodiazepine receptor (except at high concentrations) (Post et al. 1992).

■ Indications

Indications for valproate currently recognized by the FDA are for sole and adjunctive therapy in the treatment of simple and complex absence seizures, and adjunctive therapy in multiple seizures types that include absence seizures. Controlled studies have also shown that valproate is highly effective in other primarily generalized epilepsies, including generalized tonic-clonic and myoclonic seizures, as well as in secondarily generalized tonic-clonic seizures, infantile spasms, photosensitive epilepsy, and febrile seizures (Anonymous 1988; Bourgeois 1989; Rimmer and Richens 1985).

Valproate also has some efficacy in partial seizures (including complex partial seizures), but a controlled trial suggests that it may not be as effective as carbamazepine (Mattson et al. 1992). Valproate is not currently approved by the FDA for use in treatment of any psychiatric disorder. However, the drug is becoming widely used in the acute and prophylactic treatment of patients with recurrent manic and depressive episodes who are unable to tolerate or who are resistant to lithium and/or carbamazepine. Also, Abbott Laboratories, the manufacturer of divalproex sodium, has filed for an indication for the drug with the FDA for the manic phase of bipolar disorder.

Valproate in Acute Mania

Numerous open studies and six controlled trials (four placebo-controlled, one lithium-controlled, and one placebo- and lithium-controlled) indicate that valproate is effective in the treatment of acute mania (Bowden et al. 1994; McElroy et al. 1992b). In the controlled trials (Bowden et al. 1994; Brennan et al. 1984; Emrich et al. 1985; Freeman et al. 1992; Pope et al. 1991; Post et al. 1984b), valproate was superior to placebo and comparable to lithium in the short-term treatment of acute mania, with 61 of 113 patients (54%) receiving valproate displaying a moderate or marked reduction in acute manic symptoms (see Table 17–4). In these studies, the antimanic response to valproate occurred within several days to 2 weeks of achieving a serum valproate concentration equal to or greater than 50 µg/ml. Indeed, in an open-label rater-blind study of valproate administration via an oral loading dosage of 20 mg/kg/day to 19 patients with acute mania, 10 (53%) patients displayed a significant response within 5 days of treatment with minimal side effects (Keck et al. 1993). In contrast, preliminary open data indicate that the hypomanic episodes of cyclothymia and possibly bipolar II disorder may respond to lower valproate doses and serum concentrations (i.e., doses of 125–500 mg/day and serum concentrations of 20–45 µg/ml) (Jacobsen 1993). Open reports also suggest that the acute antimanic effects of valproate may be augmented by lith-

Table 17–4. Controlled studies of valproate in acute mania

Study	N	Design	Concomitant medications	Duration (days)	Outcome
Emrich et al. 1985	5	A-B-A	None	Variable	4/5 marked response; 1/5 no response
Brennan et al. 1984	8	A-B-A	None	14	6/8 marked response; 2/8 no response
Post et al. 1984b	1	Crossover to P, CPZ, VPA; Phenytoin	None	Variable	Marked response to CBZ only
Pope et al. 1991	36	VPA v. P	Lorazepam	21	VPA > P on all scales
Freeman et al. 1992	27	VPA v. L	None	21	92% response to L; 63% response to VPA
Bowden et al. 1994	179	VPA v. L v. P	Lorazepam, chloral hydrate	21	VPA > P, L > P, VPA = L

Note. VPA = valproate; P = placebo; CBZ = carbamazepine; L = lithium.
Source. Adapted from Keck et al. 1992a with permission.

ium, carbamazepine, and antipsychotics, including clozapine (Keck et al. 1992b; Ketter et al. 1992; McElroy et al. 1988a; Suppes et al. 1992).

Valproate in Acute Major Depression

There are no controlled studies of valproate in the treatment of acute unipolar or bipolar major depression. Open studies suggest that valproate is less effective in the treatment of acute depression than in the treatment of acute mania. Of 195 acutely depressed patients receiving valproate in 4 open trials, 58 (30%) displayed a significant acute antidepressant response (McElroy et al. 1992b). However, open data also suggest that valproate may be more effective in ameliorating depression when administered over longer periods of time (Hayes 1989); that its prophylactic antidepressant effects may be superior to its acute antidepressant effects (Calabrese and Delucchi 1990; Calabrese et al. 1992); and/or that it may be more likely to exert antidepressant effects in certain subtypes of bipolar patients—including, for example, those with bipolar II disorder (Puzynski and Klosiewicz 1984).

Valproate in the Prophylactic Treatment of Bipolar Disorder

No controlled studies have tested the efficacy of valproate in the long-term treatment of bipolar disorder. However, open studies suggest that the drug reduces the frequency and intensity of manic and depressive episodes over extended periods in some patients, including those with rapid cycling, mixed bipolar disorder, bipolar II disorder, and schizoaffective disorder (Calabrese and Delucchi 1990; Calabrese et al. 1992; Emrich and Wolf 1992; Hayes 1989; McElroy et al. 1992b; Puzynski and Klosiewicz 1984; Suppes et al. 1992). These studies also indicate that valproate may be more effective in the prevention of manic and mixed episodes than depressive episodes. The drug's mood-stabilizing effects may also be augmented by concurrent treatment with lithium, carbamazepine, standard antipsychotics, antidepressants, thyroid hormone, and clozapine.

Predictors of Response to Valproate

Although inconsistencies exist, a variety of factors are emerging as possibly being associated with a favorable antimanic or mood-stabilizing response to valproate. These factors include rapid cycling, dysphoric or mixed mania, a later age at onset and/or shorter duration of illness, and possibly mania due to or associated with medical or neurological illness (McElroy et al. 1988a, 1988b, 1992a, 1992b). For instance, in an open-label prospective study of valproate in 101 rapid-cycling bipolar I and II patients followed for a mean of 17.2 months, 52 of 58 (90%) patients displayed a marked or moderate antimanic response, 88 of 94 (94%) a prophylactic antimanic response, 13 of 15 (87%) an acute anti–mixed state response, and 17 of 18 (94%) a prophylactic anti–mixed state response (Calabrese et al. 1993). Moreover, among these patients, antimanic response was associated with decreasing or stable episode frequencies and nonpsychotic mania; antidepressant response was associated with worsening nonpsychotic mania and the absence of borderline personality disorder.

In a controlled comparison of valproate and lithium in 27 bipolar patients with acute mania, high depression scores during acute mania were associated with a favorable antimanic response to valproate (Clothier et al. 1992; Freeman et al. 1992). However, in a double-blind placebo-controlled trial performed by Pope and colleagues (1991) of valproate in acutely manic bipolar patients, the 12 patients who responded to valproate did not differ with respect to frequency of rapid cycling from the 5 valproate-treated patients who displayed no response (McElroy et al. 1991). Also, antimanic response to valproate was not correlated with the degree of depression during mania. Similarly, in the double-blind placebo-controlled trial conducted by Bowden and colleagues (1994), valproate was as effective in rapid-cycling manic patients (defined in this study as patients with four manic episodes within the past year) as in non-rapid-cycling manic patients. It therefore is currently unclear whether valproate is more effective in mixed mania and rapid cycling than it is in pure mania or nonrapid cycling, or whether it is more effective than lithium in these variants.

Evidence suggesting that secondary or complicated mania responds well to valproate is similarly mixed. In an open study of 56 valproate-treated patients with mania, response was associated with the presence of nonparoxysmal EEG abnormalities, but not with neurological soft signs or brain computerized axial tomography scan abnormalities (McElroy et al. 1988b). Nevertheless, there was a trend for responders to have histories of closed head trauma antedating the onset of their affective symptoms (Pope et al. 1988). Furthermore, case reports describe successful valproate treatment of patients with organic brain syndromes with affective features (Kahn et al. 1988) and mentally retarded patients with bipolar disorder or symptoms (Kastner et al. 1993; Sovner 1989).

In primarily open and retrospective studies, factors such as sex, presence of psychotic symptoms, family history of mood or neurological disorder, and response to lithium and to other antiepileptics showed no significant association with antimanic response to valproate. However, the diagnosis of schizoaffective disorder, bipolar type has been associated with a less favorable valproate response compared with the diagnosis of bipolar disorder (McElroy et al. 1992b).

■ Side Effects and Toxicology

Valproate is generally well-tolerated, with a low incidence of adverse effects and a favorable side effect profile compared with other antiepileptics, lithium, and antipsychotics (Anonymous 1988; Beghi et al. 1986; Dreifuss 1989; Smith and Bleck 1991). For instance, valproate is less likely to cause cognitive impairment compared with other antiepileptics (Beghi et al. 1986; Vining 1987) and has been associated with a lower incidence of side effects than lithium in bipolar patients (Vencovsky et al. 1983). For example, in the double-blind placebo-controlled trial of valproate versus lithium conducted by Bowden and colleagues (1994), the rate of premature termination for intolerance in the lithium group was 11% compared with 6% for valproate and 3% for placebo. Like carbamazepine, valproate rarely causes renal side effects or EPS. Unlike carbamazepine, it rarely causes thyroid, cardiac, dermatologic, or allergic effects. However, the drug is associated with both benign and potentially fatal side effects (for thorough reviews, see Beghi et al. 1986; Pellock and Willmore 1991; Rimmer and Richens 1985; Smith and Bleck 1991). Common dose-related side effects are gastrointestinal distress (e.g., anorexia, nausea, dyspepsia, indigestion, vomiting, and diarrhea), benign hepatic transaminase elevations, and neurological symptoms (most commonly, tremor and sedation). Gastrointestinal complaints, benign hepatic transaminase elevations, and sedation are more likely to occur at the initiation of treatment and usually subside with dosage reduction and/or over time.

Significantly, gastrointestinal complaints are more frequent with valproic acid and sodium valproate than with the enteric-coated divalproex sodium formulation (Wilder et al. 1983). However, gastrointestinal complaints that persist despite dosage reduction may be relieved by using divalproex sprinkle capsules or by the addition of a histamine-2 receptor antagonist (e.g., famotidine or cimetidine) (Stoll et al. 1991). Tremor can be managed with dosage reduction or treatment with β-blockers. Coagulopathies, impaired platelet function, and transient thrombocytopenia (which are reversible with drug discontinuation) occur less frequently. Fairly frequent side effects that are often bothersome to patients include hair loss (which is usually transient), increased appetite, and weight gain. Hair loss may be minimized by cotreatment with a multivitamin containing zinc and selenium (Hurd et al. 1984).

Rare, idiosyncratic adverse effects that are not dose-related but could potentially be fatal include irreversible hepatic failure, acute hemorrhagic pancreatitis, and (extremely rarely) agranulocytosis. Clear-cut risk factors for development of valproate-associated irreversible hepatic failure have been identified in patients with epilepsy and include 1) young age (especially 2 years or younger), 2) administration of valproate in conjunction with other antiepileptics, and 3) the presence of other medical or neurological abnormalities in addition to epilepsy. Since these factors were identified, the rate of valproate-associated fatal hepatic toxicity has decreased despite increased use of the drug. Thus, the overall rate of fatal hepatic toxicity decreased from 1 in 10,000 between 1978 and 1984 to 1 in 49,000 in 1985 and 1986. Furthermore, no hepatic fatalities have been reported to date in patients over age 10 receiving valproate as antiepileptic monotherapy (Dreifuss et al. 1989).

Other serious side effects of valproate include teratogenicity (particularly neural tube defects with first-trimester exposure) and coma and death when taken in overdose. Offspring of mothers receiving valproate have been reported to have an incidence of neural tube defects of 1%–1.5%. Minor dysmorphic syndromes have also been reported. Although the mechanism of valproate's teratogenicity is unknown, free radical formation during the microsomal metabolism of valproate has been implicated. Valproate depletes selenium, a necessary component for the synthesis of glutathione peroxidase, which is an important free radical scavenger and antioxidant (Wilder 1992). Thus, multivitamins with trace metals (as well as folinic acid) have been recommended for women of childbearing potential who are taking valproate (and other antiepileptics) (Wilder 1992).

Regarding overdose, recovery from coma has occurred with serum valproate concentrations above 2,000 μg/ml. Also, serum valproate concentrations have been reduced by hemodialysis and hemoprofusion, and valproate-induced coma has been reversed with naloxone (Rimmer and Richens 1985). Because transient hepatic enzyme elevations, leukopenia, and thrombocytopenia are not predictive of life-threatening reactions (and thus, routine blood monitoring does not permit anticipation of hepatic failure or blood dyscrasias), routine blood monitoring of hematologic and hepatic function in epileptic patients receiving chronic antiepileptic medication is generally not necessary (Pellock and Willmore 1991). Educating patients about the signs and symptoms of hepatic or hematologic dysfunction and instructing them to report these symptoms if they occur, in conjunction with careful monitoring of the patient's clinical status, is superior to routine laboratory screening. Nevertheless, because clinical experience with valproate in the treatment of psychiatric patients is not as extensive as it is for epileptic patients, many authorities recommend that hepatic and hematologic parameters be monitored periodically when using valproate to treat psychiatric illness. In general, our group monitors these tests several times during initiation of treatment, and once the patient is stable, every 6 to 24 months thereafter as long as the patient remains on the drug.

■ Drug-Drug Interactions

Because valproate is highly protein bound and extensively metabolized by the liver, a number of potential drug-drug interactions may occur with other protein-bound or metabolized drugs (Fogel 1988; Levy et al. 1989; Rall and Schleifer 1985; Rimmer and Richens 1985). Thus, serum valproate free fraction concentrations can be increased and valproate toxicity precipitated by coadministration of other highly protein-bound drugs (e.g., aspirin) that can displace valproate from its protein-binding sites. Because valproate tends to inhibit drug oxidation—it is the only major antiepileptic that does not induce hepatic microsomal enzymes—serum concentrations of a number of metabolized drugs can be increased by the coadministration of valproate. Thus, valproate has

been reported to increase serum concentrations of phenobarbital, phenytoin, and TCAs. Conversely, valproate's metabolism can be increased, and valproate serum concentrations subsequently decreased, by coadministration of microsomal enzyme-inducing drugs such as carbamazepine; drugs that inhibit metabolism may increase serum valproate concentrations. Fluoxetine, for instance, has been reported to boost valproate concentrations (Sovner and Davis 1991).

Finally, neurological reactions may occur when valproate is administered with other neurotoxic drugs. For example, increased sedation and (extremely rarely) delirium have been reported when valproate is administered with antipsychotics. However, an initial report of the combination of valproate and clonazepam inducing absence status in 3 patients with absence epilepsy has not been replicated. Indeed, in our experience, patients in general tolerate the combination of valproate with antipsychotics and benzodiazepines, including clonazepam, very well.

■ BENZODIAZEPINES

The benzodiazepines as a class are discussed in detail in Chapter 11. Because these drugs have antiepileptic properties (i.e., diazepam in status epilepticus and clonazepam in absence epilepsy), their use in the treatment of bipolar disorder is briefly reviewed here.

In general, studies examining the efficacy of benzodiazepines in bipolar disorder are inconsistent. Of four controlled studies evaluating clonazepam in the treatment of acute mania (summarized in Table 17–5), clonazepam was found to be superior to placebo in one, superior to lithium in another, and comparable to haloperidol in a third (Chouinard 1987; Chouinard et al. 1983; Edwards et al. 1991). In the fourth study (Bradwejn et al. 1990), lorazepam was superior to clonazepam, which had no significant antimanic effects. All of these studies were confounded by small sample sizes, short durations of treatment, and difficulties in distinguishing putative specific antimanic effects from nonspecific sedative effects. Moreover, the first two studies were further confounded by the coadministration of neuroleptics.

However, in a controlled study comparing lorazepam with haloperidol as adjuncts to lithium in the treatment of acute manic agitation, the two treat-

Table 17–5. Controlled studies of clonazepam and lorazepam in acute mania

Study	N	Design	Concomitant medications	Duration (days)	Outcome
Chouinard et al. 1983	12	Crossover with L	HAL	10	CPM > L
Edwards et al. 1991	40	CPM v. P	CPZ	5	CPM > P
Chouinard 1987	12	CPM v. HAL	None	7	CPM, HAL comparable
Bradwejn et al. 1990	24	CPM v. LPM	None	14	61% response to LPM; 18% response to CPM

Note. CPM = clonazepam; LPM = lorazepam; HAL = haloperidol; L = lithium.
Source. Adapted from Keck et al. 1992a with permission.

ments appeared comparable (Lenox et al. 1992). This suggests that lorazepam (and perhaps other benzodiazepines) may be safe, effective alternatives to neuroleptics in the initial or early management of manic agitation while awaiting the effects of the primary mood-stabilizing agent to become apparent. Also, open studies suggest that lorazepam may have beneficial effects in the short-term treatment of catatonia, which is often a manifestation of the manic phase of bipolar disorder (Bodken 1990; Rosebush et al. 1990).

Although there are no controlled studies of benzodiazepines in the treatment of bipolar depression, one open study reported the successful treatment of 21 of 25 depressed patients (84%) with open-label clonazepam (maximum daily doses of 1.5–6.0 mg/day) (Kishimoto et al. 1983). Of this group, 18 had major depression and 9 had bipolar depression, including 8 who had failed to respond to previous treatment with two or more antidepressants. However, treatment of panic disorder with various benzodiazepines has been associated with treatment-emergent depression (Tesar 1990).

Two studies have examined the prophylactic efficacy of benzodiazepines in bipolar disorder. In the first, bipolar patients requiring combined maintenance treatment with lithium and haloperidol did equally well when their regimens were changed to lithium and clonazepam (Sachs et al. 1990). However, the second study (the only study to date attempting to assess the efficacy of clonazepam alone as a maintenance treatment) had to be prematurely terminated after the first five patients enrolled relapsed within the first 2–15 weeks of treatment (Aronson et al. 1989). Of note, the poor results observed in this study may have been due in part to inclusion of lithium-refractory patients and to rapid taper of antipsychotics before initiation of clonazepam (Chouinard 1989).

In summary, available studies have not yet definitively proven that benzodiazepines possess specific antimanic, antidepressant, or long-term mood-stabilizing properties apart from their nonspecific sedative effects. However, benzodiazepines may be extremely useful in the treatment of acute manic agitation either in place of or in conjunction with antipsychotics 1) while awaiting the effects of other primary mood-stabilizing agents to become apparent; 2) in the short-term treatment of insomnia, anxiety, or catatonia associated with either mania or depression; and perhaps 3) as adjunctive maintenance agents in combination with lithium, carbamazepine, or valproate.

OTHER ANTIEPILEPTICS

Oxcarbazepine

Available in Europe but not yet available in the United States, oxcarbazepine (10,11-dihydro-10-oxo-carbamazepine), the 10-keto analogue of carbamazepine, has a chemical structure and antiepileptic profile similar to that of carbamazepine (Anonymous 1989; Dam and Jensen 1989). Oxcarbazepine has been shown to be as effective as carbamazepine in suppressing generalized tonic-clonic seizures and partial seizures, with and without secondary generalization. Preliminary reports also suggest that it may have antineuralgic effects. However, oxcarbazepine and carbamazepine have significantly different pharmacokinetic profiles. Unlike carbamazepine, oxcarbazepine does not appear to induce the hepatic microsomal P_{450} enzyme system, and it is not metabolized to an epoxide with neurotoxic effects. Rather, oxcarbazepine is rapidly and extensively converted to the 10-hydroxy metabolite, an active metabolite responsible for most of the drug's antiepileptic effects. These differences suggest that oxcarbazepine may be an easier drug to administer, with fewer drug-drug interactions, and easier to tolerate with less neurotoxicity. Nevertheless, oxcarbazepine's most common side effects are tiredness, headache, dizziness, and ataxia. Also, it has been reported to cause allergic reactions and hyponatremia, although less frequently than does carbamazepine.

Four controlled studies assessing the efficacy of oxcarbazepine in the treatment of acute mania have shown that oxcarbazepine is superior to placebo and comparable to haloperidol and lithium after 14 days of treatment (Emrich 1990; Emrich et al. 1985; Müller and Stoll 1984 [see Table 17–6]). In these studies, oxcarbazepine was better tolerated than haloperidol and of comparable tolerability to lithium. These results are limited, however, by the concomitant use of haloperidol (and in some cases lithium) in both treatment groups in the two largest studies (Emrich 1990). Also, although the average oxcarbazepine dosage used in these studies was 1,400–2,400 mg/day, the optimal dosage range for the antimanic effects of oxcarbazepine has not yet been established.

Oxcarbazepine has not been tested in the treatment of acute major depression. However, two controlled studies have compared the prophylactic efficacy of oxcarbazepine with that of lithium in patients with bipolar disorder (see Table 17–7). The first study, using an oxcarbazepine dosage of only 900 mg/day, found significant decreases in the rates of recurrent manic and depressive episodes in both the oxcarbazepine- and lithium-treated groups (Cabrera et al. 1986). The second study found a higher rate of relapse in patients maintained on ox-

carbazepine as compared to patients receiving lithium (Wildgrube 1990). However, the subjects in the oxcarbazepine-treated group were significantly older and more severely ill at the initiation of treatment than those in the group randomized to lithium. The small sample size in each study makes further interpretation of their data difficult, and larger studies are needed to establish the optimal dosage and therapeutic efficacy of oxcarbazepine as a maintenance agent for bipolar disorder.

■ Phenytoin

Although there are no controlled studies of phenytoin in the treatment of bipolar disorder, open studies performed in the late 1940s and early 1950s indicate that phenytoin may sometimes be helpful in psychiatric patients with acute mania or manic-like presentations (e.g., "excited psychoses") (Gutierrez-Esteinou and Cole 1988). For instance, in an open-label study of phenytoin in 60 state hospital psychiatric patients, the best results were observed in the "excited" group, with 73% of patients with "excited schizophrenia" ($n = 22$) and 89% of those with mania ($n = 9$) showing improvement (Kalinowsky and Putnam 1943). In a similar open-label trial of phenytoin in 73 psychotic patients, 11 of whom had manic-depressive illness, 5 of 9 patients in the manic phase and 1 of 2 in the depressive phase showed improvement (Kubanek and Rowell 1946). The authors concluded that phenytoin was useful in the treatment of "excited chronic psychoses." In yet another one-label study involving 45 chronic patients with a wide range of diagnoses, 1 patient with mania and some patients with schizophrenia (only those

Table 17–6.   Controlled studies of oxcarbazepine in acute mania

Study	N	Design	Concomitant medications	Duration (days)	Outcome
Emrich et al. 1985	6	A-B-A	None	Variable	4/6 (67% had > 50% decrease in IMPS scores)
Müller & Stoll 1984	10 OX; 10 HAL	OX v. HAL	None	14	Mean decrease of 55% in BRMAS scores in both groups
Emrich 1990	19 OX; 19 HAL	OX v. HAL	HAL, L	14	Mean decrease of 64% in BRMAS scores in both groups
Emrich 1990	28 OX; 24 L	OX v. L	HAL	14	Mean decrease of 63% in BRMAS scores in both groups

Note. OX = oxcarbazepine; IMPS = Inpatient Multidimensional Psychiatric Scale (Lorr et al. 1962); BRMAS = Bech-Raefelson Mania Scale (Bech et al. 1986); HAL = haloperidol; L = lithium.
Source. Adapted from Keck et al. 1992a with permission.

with catatonia) showed improvement (Freyhan 1945). In short, although these studies are methodologically flawed and there are as yet no controlled data indicating that phenytoin is effective in the treatment of mania, it may be considered as a treatment alternative for some patients resistant to lithium, carbamazepine, and valproate.

■ Progabide

Open studies and one controlled comparison with imipramine suggest that progabide and its congeners (effective antiepileptics that act as indirect potentiators of GABA) may have acute antidepressant effects (Post et al. 1991). Although not yet studied in the treatment of mania, studies of these drugs in patients with bipolar disorder would appear warranted in light of GABA's potential role in the pathogenesis of mood disorder.

■ Barbiturate Antiepileptics

Barbiturate antiepileptics have not been well studied in the treatment of bipolar disorder. However, in an open study of primidone and/or mephobarbital in 27 patients with mood disorders refractory to lithium, carbamazepine, valproate, and phenytoin, 9 patients

displayed sustained positive effects with primidone and 3 displayed positive effects with mephobarbital after failing with primidone (Hayes 1993).

■ Acetazolamide

Inoue and colleagues in Japan (1984) reported that acetazolamide (a diuretic with antiepileptic properties) was effective in patients with atypical psychoses characterized by dreamy or confusional states and often associated with the premenstrual or puerperal period. Testing of this drug in bipolar patients— especially those with associated confusion or perimenstrual or puerperal exacerbation of their symptoms—would therefore appear warranted.

■ CONCLUSION

Growing evidence indicates that a variety of antiepileptic drugs have beneficial effects in bipolar disorder. To date, the antiepileptics best studied in the treatment of bipolar disorder are carbamazepine and valproate. These drugs have acute antimanic and long-term mood-stabilizing effects (and possibly acute antidepressant effects) in some bipolar pa-

Table 17–7. Controlled studies of carbamazepine and oxcarbazepine as preventive therapy in patients with bipolar disorder

Study	N	Design	Concomitant medications	Duration (years)	Outcome
Okuma et al. 1981	12 CBZ; 10 P	CBZ v. P	Not specified, but permitted for breakthrough episodes	1	40% relapse on CBZ; 78% relapse on P
Placidi et al. 1986	20 CBZ; 16 L	CBZ v. L	TCAs, CPZ for breakthrough episodes	to 3	67% response rate for both groups
Watkins et al. 1987	19 CBZ; 18 L	CBZ v. L	Neuroleptics, antidepressants for breakthrough episodes	1.5	Mean time in remission: CBZ 16 months, L 9.4 months
Lusznat et al. 1988	20 CBZ; 21 L	CBZ v. L	Neuroleptics, antidepressants for breakthrough episodes	to 1	45% CBZ patients at 12 months, 25% L patients at 12 months; 25% CBZ rehospitalized, 50% L rehospitalized
Bellaire et al. 1988	46 CBZ; 52 L	CBZ v. L	ND	1	Mean reduction in number of episodes comparable: 1.8/year to 0.67/year CBZ, 1.7/year to 0.7/year L
Cabrera et al. 1986	4 OX; 6 L	OX v. L	Neuroleptics (1 OX, 2 L)	Up to 22	3/4 OX, 6/6 L had significant decrease in affective episodes
Wildgrube 1990	8 OX; 7 L	OX v. L	ND	Up to 33	6/9 OX, 3/9 L treatment failures

Note. CBZ = carbamazepine; OX = oxcarbazepine; ND = not described; TCAs = tricyclic antidepressants; CPZ = chlorpromazine; L = lithium.
Source. Reproduced from Keck et al. 1992a with permission.

tients, including those patients inadequately responsive to or intolerant of lithium. Despite lacking formal FDA indications for bipolar disorder, carbamazepine and valproate are considered by many authorities to be second-line agents to lithium for lithium-refractory or lithium-intolerant patients. Moveover, in light of preliminary data indicating that carbamazepine and valproate may be effective in rapid cycling and dysphoric mania (bipolar variants known to be poorly responsive to lithium), some clinicians use these antiepileptics as first-line treatments for such patients. Indeed, our group considers carbamazepine and valproate along with lithium as first-line treatments for bipolar disorder. Other less well-studied antiepileptic compounds, including oxcarbazepine and phenytoin, may also have mood-stabilizing effects. Although it is unclear whether benzodiazepines have specific mood-stabilizing effects, they are useful adjuncts to primary mood stabilizers in the treatment of acute manic agitation and catatonia.

It is important to remember that the antiepileptics may be synergistic with other mood-stabilizing agents—including each other—in the treatment of bipolar patients inadequately responsive to monotherapy. Indeed, although viewed together as a class of drugs, the antiepileptics are in fact very different agents—possessing different chemical structures, pharmacological properties, pharmacokinetics, side effects, and efficacies in epilepsy. Thus, even though carbamazepine and valproate may share similar predictors of response for bipolar disorder (e.g., dysphoric mania), different bipolar patients may respond to one agent but not to the other or tolerate one agent better than the other, as is the case for patients with epilepsy. Clinicians therefore have a wide range of medications and combinations of medications to choose from when treating the bipolar patient. Furthermore, although the actions underlying the antiepileptic properties of these drugs may or may not be responsible for their mood-stabilizing effects, any future drugs with antiepileptic activity should be screened as putative antimanic, mood-stabilizing, or antidepressant agents.

■ REFERENCES

Albright PS, Burnham WM: Development of a new pharmacological seizure model: effects of anticonvulsants on cortical and amygdala-kindled seizures in the rat. Epilepsia 21:681–689, 1980

Andrews DG, Schweitzer I, Marshall N: The comparative side effects of lithium, carbamazepine and combined lithium-carbamazepine in patients treated for affective disorders. Human Psychopharmacology 5:41–45, 1990

Anonymous: Sodium valproate. Lancet 2:1229–1231, 1988

Anonymous: Oxcarbazepine. Lancet 2:196–198, 1989

Aronson TA, Skukla S, Hirschowitz J: Clonazepam treatment of five lithium-refractory patients with bipolar disorder. Am J Psychiatry 146:77–80, 1989

Ballenger JC, Post RM: Therapeutic effects of carbamazepine in affective illness: a preliminary report. Communications in Psychopharmacology 2:159–175, 1978

Bech P, Kastrup M, Rafaelsen OJ: Mini-compendium of rating scales for anxiety, depression, mania, schizophrenia, with corresponding DSM-III syndromes. Acta Psychiatr Scand 73 (S236):29–31, 1986

Beghi E, DiMascio R, Sasanelli F, et al: Adverse reactions to antiepileptic drugs: a multicenter survey of clinical practice. Epilepsia 27:323–330, 1986

Bellaire W, Demish K, Stoll KD: Carbamazepine versus lithium in prophylaxis of recurrent affective disorders. Psychopharmacology (Berl) 96:2875, 1988

Blom S: Tic douloureux treated with a new anticonvulsant: experiences with G 32883. Arch Neurol 2:357–366, 1963

Bodken JA: Emerging uses for high-potency benzodiazepines in psychotic disorders. J Clin Psychiatry 51:41S–46S, 1990

Bourgeois BFD: Valproate: clinical use, in Antiepileptic Drugs, 3rd Edition. Edited by Levy RH, Dreifuss FE, Mattson RH, et al. New York, Raven, 1989, pp 633–642

Bowden CL, Brugger AM, Swann AC, et al: Efficacy of divalproex vs lithium and placebo in the treatment of mania. JAMA 271:918–924, 1994

Bradwejn J, Shriqui C, Koszycki D, et al: Double-blind comparison of the effects of clonazepam and lorazepam in mania. J Clin Psychopharmacol 10:403–408, 1990

Brennan MJW, Sandyk R, Borsook D: Use of sodium valproate in the management of affective disorders: basic and clinical aspects, in Anticonvulsants in Affective Disorders. Edited by Emrich HM, Okuma T, Müller AA. Amsterdam, Excerpta Medica, 1984, pp 56–65

Brown D, Silverstone T, Cookson J: Carbamazepine compared to haloperidol in acute mania. International Journal of Clinical Psychopharmacology 48:89–93, 1987

Cabrera JF, Muhlbauer HD, Schley J, et al: Long-term randomized clinical trial of oxcarbazepine vs. lithium in bipolar and schizoaffective disorders: preliminary results. Pharmacopsychiatry 19:282–283, 1986

Calabrese JR, Delucchi GA: Spectrum of efficacy of valproate in 55 rapid-cycling manic depressives. Am J Psychiatry 147:431–434, 1990

Calabrese JR, Markovitz PJ, Kimmel SE, et al: Spectrum of efficacy of valproate in 78 rapid-cycling bipolar patients. J Clin Psychopharmacol 12:53S–56S, 1992

Calabrese JR, Woyshville MJ, Kimmel SE, et al: Predictors of valproate response in bipolar rapid cycling. J Clin Psychopharmacol 13:280–283, 1993

Centers for Disease Control: Use of folic acid for prevention of spina bifida and other neural tube defects. JAMA 266:1190–1191, 1991

Chouinard G: Clonazepam in acute and maintenance treatment of bipolar affective disorder. J Clin Psychiatry 48:29S–36S, 1987

Chouinard G: Clonazepam in treatment of bipolar psychotic patients after discontinuation of neuroleptics [letter]. Am J Psychiatry 146:1642, 1989

Chouinard G, Young SN, Annable L: Antimanic effect of clonazepam. Biol Psychiatry 18:451–486, 1983

Clothier J, Swann AC, Freeman T: Dysphoric mania. J Clin Psychopharmacol 12:13S–16S, 1992

Cullen M, Mitchell P, Brodaty H, et al: Carbamazepine for treatment-resistant melancholia. J Clin Psychiatry 52:472–476, 1991

Dalby MA: Antiepileptic and psychotropic effect of carbamazepine (Tegretol) in the treatment of psychomotor epilepsy. Epilepsia 12:325–334, 1971

Dam M, Jensen PK: Potential antiepileptic drugs: oxcarbazepine, in Antiepileptic Drugs, 3rd Edition. Edited by Levy RH, Dreifuss FE, Mattson RH, et al. New York, Raven, 1989, pp 913–924

Delcado-Escveta AV, Janz D: Consensus guidelines: preconception counseling management, and care of the pregnant woman with epilepsy. Neurology 42:149–160, 1992

Desai NG, Gangadhar BN, Channabasavanna SM, et al: Carbamazepine hastens therapeutic action of lithium in mania, in Proceedings of the International Conference of New Directions in Affective Disorders, Jerusalem, Israel, 1987

Dreifuss FE: Valproate toxicity, in Antiepileptic Drugs, 3rd Edition. Edited by Levy RH, Dreifuss FE, Mattson RH, et al. New York, Raven, 1989, pp 643–651

Dreifuss FE, Langer DH, Moline KA, et al: Valproic acid hepatic fatalities, II: US experience since 1984. Neurology 39:201–207, 1989

Edwards R, Stephenson U, Flewett T: Clonazepam in acute mania: a double-blind trial. Aust N Z J Psychiatry 25:238–242, 1991

Emrich HM: Studies with oxcarbazepine (Trileptal) in acute mania. Int Clin Psychopharmacol 5:83S–88S, 1990

Emrich HM, Wolf R: Valproate treatment of mania. Prog Neuropsychopharmacol Biol Psychiatry 16:691–701, 1992

Emrich HM, von Zerssen D, Kissling W, et al: On a possible role of GABA in mania: therapeutic efficacy of sodium valproate, in GABA and Benzodiazepine Receptors. Edited by Costa E, Dicharia G, Gessa GL. New York, Raven, 1981, pp 287–296

Emrich HM, Dose M, von Zerssen D: The use of sodium valproate, carbamazepine, and oxcarbazepine in patients with affective disorders. J Affect Disord 8:243–250, 1985

Fariello R, Smith MC: Valproate: mechanisms of action, in Antiepileptic Drugs, 3rd Edition. Edited by Levy RH, Dreifuss FE, Mattson RH, et al. New York, Raven, 1989, pp 567–575

Fogel BS: Combining anticonvulsants with conventional psychopharmacologic agents, in Use of Anticonvulsants in Psychiatry: Recent Advances. Edited by McElroy SL, Pope HG Jr. Clifton, NJ, Oxford Health Care, 1988, pp 77–94

Frankenburg FR, Tohen M, Cohen BM, et al: Long-term response to carbamazepine: a retrospective study. J Clin Psychopharmacol 8:130–132, 1988

Freeman TW, Clothier JL, Pazzaglia P, et al: A double-blind comparison of valproate and lithium in the treatment of acute mania. Am J Psychiatry 149:108–111, 1992

Freyhan FA: Effectiveness of diphenylhydantoin in management of nonepileptic psychomotor excitement states. Arch Neurol Psychiatry 53:370–374, 1945

Gerner RH, Stanton A: Algorithm for patient management of acute manic states: lithium, valproate, or carbamazepine? J Clin Psychopharmacol 12:57S–

63S, 1992

Goodwin FK: Medical treatment of manic episodes, in Manic-Depressive Illness. Edited by Goodwin FK, Jamison KR. New York, Oxford University Press, 1990, pp 603–629

Gram L, Jensen PK: Carbamazepine toxicity, in Antiepileptic Drugs, 3rd Edition. Edited by Levy RH, Dreifuss FE, Mattson RH, et al. New York, Raven, 1989, pp 555–565

Grossi E, Sacchetti E, Vita A, et al: Carbamazepine vs. chlorpromazine in mania: a double-blind trial, in Anticonvulsants in Affective Disorders. Edited by Emrich HM, Okuma T, Müller AA. Amsterdam, Excerpta Medica, 1984, pp 177–187

Gutierrez-Esteinou R, Cole JO: Psychiatric effects of phenytoin and ethosuximide, in Use of Anticonvulsants in Psychiatry: Recent Advances. Edited by McElroy SL, Pope HG Jr. Clifton, NJ, Oxford Health Care, 1988, pp 59–76

Hayes SG: Long-term use of valproate in primary psychiatric disorders. J Clin Psychiatry 50:35S–39S, 1989

Hayes SG: Barbiturate anticonvulsants in refractory affective disorders. Annals of Clinical Psychiatry 5:35–44, 1993

Hurd RW, Van Rinsvelt HA, Wilder BJ, et al: Selenium, zinc, and copper changes with valproic acid: possible relation to drug side effects. Neurology 34:1394–1395, 1984

Inoue H, Hazama H, Hamazoe K, et al: Antipsychotic and prophylactic effects of acetazolamide (Diamox) on atypical psychosis. Folia Psychiatrica et Neurologica Japonica 38:425–436, 1984

Jacobsen FM: Low-dose valproate: a new treatment for cyclothymia, mild rapid-cycling disorders, and premenstrual syndrome. J Clin Psychiatry 54:229–234, 1993

Jones KL, Lacro RV, Johnson KA, et al: Pattern of malformations in the children of women treated with carbamazepine during pregnancy. N Engl J Med 320:186–188, 1989

Kahn D, Stevenson E, Douglas CJ: Effect of sodium valproate in three patients with organic brain syndromes. Am J Psychiatry 145:1010–1011, 1988

Kalinowsky LB, Putnam TJ: Attempts at treatment of schizophrenia and other non-epileptic psychoses with Dilantin. Archives of Neurology and Psychiatry 49:414–420, 1943

Kastner T, Finesmith R, Walsh K: Brief report: long-term administration of valproic acid in the treatment of affective symptoms in people with mental retardation. J Clin Psychopharmacol 13:448–451, 1993

Keck PE Jr, McElroy SL, Nemeroff CB: Anticonvulsants in the treatment of bipolar disorder. J Neuropsychiatry Clin Neurosci 4:395–405, 1992a

Keck PE Jr, McElroy SL, Vuckovic A, et al: Combined valproate and carbamazepine treatment of bipolar disorder. J Neuropsychiatry Clin Neurosci 4:319–322, 1992b

Keck PE Jr, McElroy SL, Tugrul KC, et al: Valproate oral loading in the treatment of acute mania. J Clin Psychiatry 54:305–308, 1993

Ketter JA, Pazzaglia PJ, Post RM: Synergy of carbamazepine and valproate in affective illness: case report and review of the literature. J Clin Psychopharmacol 12:276–281, 1992

Ketter TA, Post RM, Worthington K: Principles of clinically important drug interactions with carbamazepine, part I. J Clin Psychopharmacol 11:198–203, 1991a

Ketter TA, Post RM, Worthington K: Principles of clinically important drug interactions with carbamazepine, part II. J Clin Psychopharmacol 11:306–313, 1991b

Kishimoto A, Ogura C, Hazama H, et al: Long-term prophylactic effects of carbamazepine in affective disorder. Br J Psychiatry 143:327–331, 1983

Klein E, Bental E, Lerer B, et al: Carbamazepine and haloperidol in excited psychoses. Arch Gen Psychiatry 41:165–170, 1984

Kramlinger KG, Post RM: The addition of lithium to carbamazepine. Antidepressant efficacy in treatment-resistant depression. Arch Gen Psychiatry 46:794–800, 1989

Kubanek JL, Rowell RC: The use of Dilantin in the treatment of psychotic patients unresponsive to other treatments. Diseases of the Nervous System 7:47–50, 1946

Kupferberg AJ: Valproate: chemistry and methods of determination, in Antiepileptic Drugs, 3rd Edition. Edited by Levy RH, Dreifuss FE, Mattson RH, et al. New York, Raven, 1989, pp 577–582

Kutt H: Carbamazepine: chemistry and methods of determination, in Antiepileptic Drugs, 3rd Edition. Edited by Levy RH, Dreifuss FE, Mattson RH, et al. New York, Raven, 1989, pp 457–471

Lambert PA, Cavaz G, Borselli S, et al: Action neuropsychotrope d'un nouvel anti-épileptique: le Dépamide. Ann Med Psychol (Paris) 1:707–710,

1966

Lenox RH, Newhouse PA, Creelman WL, et al: Adjunctive treatment of manic agitation with lorazepam vs haloperidol: a double blind study. J Clin Psychiatry 53:47–52, 1992

Lenzi A, Lazzerini F, Grossi E, et al: Use of carbamazepine in acute psychosis: a controlled study. J Int Med Res 14:78–84, 1986

Lerer B, Moore N, Meyendorff E, et al: Carbamazepine versus lithium in mania: a double-blind study. J Clin Psychiatry 48:89–93, 1987

Leveil V, Nanquet R: A study of the action of calproic acid on the kindling effect. Epilepsia 18:229–234, 1977

Levy RH, Dreifuss FE, Mattson RH, et al (eds): Antiepileptic Drugs, 3rd Edition. New York, Raven, 1989

Loiseau P, Duche B: Carbamazepine: clinical use, in Antiepileptic Drugs, 3rd Edition. Edited by Levy RH, Dreifuss FE, Mattson RH, et al. New York, Raven, 1989, pp 533–554

Lorr M, Klett CJ, McNair DM, et al: Inpatient Multidimensional Psychiatric Scale. Palo Alto, CA, Consulting Psychologists Press, 1962

Lusznat RM, Murphy DP, Nunn CMH: Carbamazepine vs. lithium in the treatment of prophylaxis of mania. Br J Psychiatry 153:198–204, 1988

Macdonald RL: Carbamazepine: mechanisms of action, in Antiepileptic Drugs, 3rd Edition. Edited by Levy RH, Dreifuss FII, Mattson RH, et al. New York, Raven, 1989, pp 447–455

Mattson RH, Cramer JA, Darney PD, et al: Use of oral contraceptives by women with epilepsy. JAMA 2556:238–240, 1986

Mattson RH, Cramer JA, Collins JF, et al: A comparison of valproate with carbamazepine for the treatment of complex partial seizures and secondarily generalized tonic-clonic seizures in adult. N Engl J Med 327:765–771, 1992

McElroy SL, Keck PE Jr: Valproate treatment of bipolar and schizoaffective disorder. Can J Psychiatry 38:62S–66S, 1993

McElroy SL, Pope HG Jr (eds): Use of Anticonvulsants in Psychiatry: Recent Advances. Clifton, NJ, Oxford Health Care, 1988

McElroy SL, Keck PE Jr, Pope HG Jr, et al: Valproate in the treatment of rapid-cycling bipolar disorder. J Clin Psychopharmacol 8:275–279, 1988a

McElroy SL, Pope HG Jr, Keck PE Jr, et al: Treatment of psychiatric disorders with valproate: a series of 73 cases. Psychiatrie Psychobiologie 3:81–85, 1988b

McElroy SL, Keck PE Jr, Pope HG Jr, et al: Correlates of antimanic response to valproate. Psychopharmacol Bull 27:127–133, 1991

McElroy SL, Keck PE Jr, Pope HG Jr, et al: Clinical and research implications of the diagnosis of dysphoric or mixed mania or hypomania. Am J Psychiatry 149:1633–1644, 1992a

McElroy SL, Keck PE Jr, Pope HG Jr, et al: Valproate in bipolar disorder: literature review and treatment guidelines. J Clin Psychopharmacol 12:42S–52S, 1992b

Möller MJ, Kissling W, Riehl T, et al: Double-blind evaluation of the antimanic properties of carbamazepine as a comedication to haloperidol. Prog Neuropsychopharmacol Biol Psychiatry 13:127–136, 1989

Morselli PL: Carbamazepine: absorption, distribution, and excretion, in Antiepileptic Drugs, 3rd Edition. Edited by Levy RH, Dreifuss FE, Mattson RH, et al. New York, Raven, 1989, pp 473–490

Müller AA, Stoll KD: Carbamazepine and oxcarbazepine in the treatment of manic syndromes: studies in Germany, in Anticonvulsants in Affective Disorders. Edited by Emrich HM, Okuma T, Müller AA. Amsterdam, Excerpta Medica, 1984, pp 134–147

Murphy DJ, Gannon MA, McGennis A: Carbamazepine in bipolar affective disorder. Lancet 2:1151–1152, 1989

Neumann J, Seidel K, Wunderlich HP: Comparative studies of the effect of carbamazepine and trimipramine in depression, in Anticonvulsants in Affective Disorders. Edited by Emrich HM, Okuma T, Müller AA. Amsterdam, Excerpta Medica, 1984, pp 160–166

Okuma T, Inanaga K, Otsuki S, et al: Comparison of the antimanic efficacy of carbamazepine and chlorpromazine. Psychopharmacology (Berl) 66:211–217, 1979

Okuma T, Inanaga K, Otsuki S, et al: A preliminary double-blind study on the efficacy in prophylaxis of manic depressive illness. Psychopharmacology (Berl) 73:95–96, 1981

Okuma T, Yamashita I, Takahasi R, et al: Comparison of the antimanic efficacy of carbamazepine and lithium carbonate by double-blind controlled study. Pharmacopsychiatry 23:143–150, 1990

Pellock JM: Carbamazepine side effects in children and adults. Epilepsia 28:564S–570S, 1987

Pellock JM, Willmore LJ: A rational guide to routine blood monitoring in patients receiving antiepileptic drugs. Neurology 41:961–964, 1991

Penry JK, Dean JC: The scope and use of valproate in epilepsy. J Clin Psychiatry 40:17S–22S, 1989

Placidi GF, Lenzi A, Lazzerini F, et al: The comparative efficacy and safety of carbamazepine versus lithium: a randomized, double-blind 3 year trial in 83 patients. J Clin Psychiatry 47:490–494, 1986

Pope HG Jr, McElroy SL, Satlin A, et al: Head injury, bipolar disorder, and response to valproate. Compr Psychiatry 29:34–38, 1988

Pope HG Jr, McElroy SL, Keck PE Jr, et al: Valproate in the treatment of acute mania: a placebo-controlled study. Arch Gen Psychiatry 48:62–68, 1991

Post RM: Approaches to treatment-resistant bipolar affectively ill patients. Clin Neuropharmacol 11:93–104, 1988

Post RM: Non-lithium treatment for bipolar disorder. J Clin Psychiatry 51:9S–16S, 1990

Post RM, Ballenger JC, Uhde TW, et al: Efficacy of carbamazepine in manic-depressive illness: implications for underlying mechanisms, in Neurobiology of Mood Disorders. Edited by Post RM, Ballenger JC. Baltimore, MD, Williams & Wilkins, 1984a, pp 77–816

Post RM, Berettini W, Uhde TW, et al: Selective response to the anticonvulsant carbamazepine in manic depressive illness: a case study. J Clin Psychopharmacol 4:178–185, 1984b

Post RM, Uhde TW, Roy-Byrne PP, et al: Antidepressant effects of carbamazepine. Am J Psychiatry 143:29–34, 1985

Post RM, Uhde TW, Roy-Byrne PP, et al: Correlates of antimanic response to carbamazepine. Psychiatry Res 21:71–83, 1987

Post RM, Leverich GS, Rosoff AS, et al: Carbamazepine prophylaxis in refractory affective disorders: a focus on long-term follow-up. J Clin Psychopharmacol 10:318–327, 1990

Post RM, Altshuler LL, Ketter TA, et al: Antiepileptic drugs in affective illness: clinical and theoretical implications, in Advances in Neurology, Vol 55. Edited by Smith D, Treiman D, Trimble M. New York, Raven, 1991, pp 239–277

Post RM, Weiss SRB, Chuang DM: Mechanisms of action of anticonvulsants in affective disorders: comparison with lithium. J Clin Psychopharmacol 12:23S–35S, 1992

Prien RF, Gelenberg AJ: Alternatives to lithium for preventive treatment of bipolar disorder. Am J Psychiatry 146:840–848, 1989

Puzynski S, Klosiewicz L: Valproic Acid amid as a prophylactic agent in affective and schizoaffective disorders. Psychopharmacol Bull 20:151–159, 1984

Rall TW, Schleifer LS: Drugs effective in the therapy of the epilepsies, in The Pharmacological Basis of Therapeutics. Edited by Gilman AG, Goodman LS, Rall TW, et al. New York, Macmillan, 1985, pp 446–472

Rimmer E, Richens A: An update on sodium valproate. Pharmacotherapy 5:171–184, 1985

Rosa FWL: Spina bifida in infants of women treated with carbamazepine during pregnancy. N Engl J Med 324:674–677, 1991

Rosebush PI, Hildeband AM, Furlong BG, et al: Catatonic syndrome in a general psychiatric inpatient population: frequency, clinical presentation, and response to lorazepam. J Clin Psychiatry 51:357–362, 1990

Sachs GS, Weilburg JB, Rosebaum JF: Clonazepam vs. neuroleptics as adjuncts to lithium maintenance. Psychopharmacol Bull 26:137–143, 1990

Seetharam MN, Pellock JM: Risk-benefit assessment of carbamazepine in children. Drug Saf 6:148–158, 1991

Small JG: Anticonvulsants in affective disorders. Psychopharmacol Bull 26:25–36, 1990

Small JG, Klapper MH, Milstein V, et al: Carbamazepine compared with lithium in the treatment of mania. Arch Gen Psychiatry 48:915–921, 1991

Smith MC, Bleck TP: Convulsive disorders: toxicity of anticonvulsants. Clin Neuropharmacol 14:97–115, 1991

Sovner R: The use of valproate in the treatment of mentally retarded persons with typical and atypical bipolar disorders. J Clin Psychiatry 50:40S–43S, 1989

Sovner R, Davis JM: A potential drug interaction between fluoxetine and valproic acid. J Clin Psychopharmacol 11:389, 1991

Stoll AL, Vuckovic A, McElroy SL: Histamine 2-receptor antagonists for the treatment of valproate-induced gastrointestinal distress. Annals of Clinical Psychiatry 3:301–304, 1991

Suppes T, McElroy SL, Gilbert J, et al: Clozapine in the treatment of dysphoric mania. Biol Psychiatry 32:270–280, 1992

Takezaki H, Hanaoka M: The use of carbamazepine

(Tegretol) in the control of manic-depressive psychosis and other manic, depressive states. Clinical Psychiatry 13:173–182, 1971

Tesar GE: High potency benzodiazepines for short-term management of panic disorder: the U.S. experience. J Clin Psychiatry 51:4S–10S, 1990

Vencovsky E, Soucek K, Žatecká I: Comparison of side effects of lithium and dipropylacetamide (Depamide). Ceskoslovenská Psychiatrie 79:223–227, 1983

Vining EPG: Cognitive dysfunction associated with antiepileptic drug therapy. Epilepsia 28:18S–22S, 1987

Watkins SE, Callender K, Thomas DR, et al: The effect of carbamazepine and lithium on remission from affective illness. Br J Psychiatry 150:180–182, 1987

Wilder BJ: Pharmacokinetics of valproate and carbamazepine. J Clin Psychopharmacol 12:64S–68S, 1992

Wilder BJ, Karas BJ, Penry JK, et al: Gastrointestinal tolerance of divalproex sodium. Neurology 33:808–811, 1983

Wildgrube C: Case studies on prophylactic long-term effects of oxcarbazepine in recurrent affective disorders. Int Clin Psychopharmacol 5:89S–94S, 1990

Zona C, Tancredi V, Palma E, et al: Potassium currents in rat cortical neurons in culture are enhanced by the antiepileptic drug carbamazepine. Can J Physiol Pharmacol 68:545–547, 1990

18

Calcium Channel Antagonists as Novel Agents for Manic-Depressive Disorder

Steven L. Dubovsky, M.D.

The introduction of the anticonvulsants carbamazepine and divalproex sodium has greatly expanded psychiatric treatment options for bipolar illness (see Chapter 17). However, the anticonvulsants are not always effective for the 25%–33% of bipolar patients who are at least partially unresponsive to lithium (Aronson et al. 1989; Post 1988; Prien and Gelenberg 1989). Many patients cannot tolerate lithium side effects or the regular monitoring that taking the drug requires, leading up to 50% of them to discontinue or reduce the dose of the drug even if it is effective (Prien and Gelenberg 1989). The anticonvulsants are also not without significant side effects, as well as requirements for routine blood tests that can reduce compliance. In addition, lithium, carbamazepine, and valproate are all problematic medications for pregnant patients.

The calcium channel antagonists or calcium channel blockers (CCBs), a novel class of medications currently being investigated as possible antimanic agents, have a favorable side-effect profile, do not require routine blood level monitoring, and may be safer during pregnancy. In addition, some of these medications could prove to be effective in bipolar subtypes that do not respond completely to standard treatments. Studying the spectrum of response to some of these medications could reveal phenotypic (e.g., rapid cycling) or biological markers (e.g., alterations of intracellular calcium ion concentration) of preferential response to these medications. Conversely, commonalities of action of CCBs, lithium, and anticonvulsants could provide new insights into the pathophysiology of bipolar illness.

Many clinicians are less familiar with the CCBs than with the anticonvulsants as alternatives or supplements to lithium. One reason for this discrepancy may be that new treatments such as the CCBs are usually first tried with patients who are unresponsive to lithium; however, such patients may be no more likely to respond to the CCBs. Another issue is that the combination of growing pressure on clinical services to confine all reimbursed care to treatments that will result in rapid discharge, as well as constraints on independent funding for trials of innovative therapies, have forced investigators to rely increasingly on pharmaceutical manufacturers for research support. Whereas industry support has been an important factor in the investigation and popularization of the antimanic potential of the anticonvulsants, manufacturers of the CCBs have largely been uninterested in this application (Dubovsky 1994).

Despite slower research into uses of CCBs as potential antimanic drugs, there is mounting evidence that they may have important psychiatric applications. In this chapter, I review the pharmacology of the CCBs and the evidence supporting their efficacy in the treatment of bipolar illness. Clinical guidelines for the use of CCBs are also offered.

■ HISTORY AND DISCOVERY

Verapamil, the first calcium channel antagonist to be introduced, was synthesized in 1962 (Morris et al. 1992). A derivative of papaverine (Bigger and Hoffman 1991), verapamil was found to have negative inotropic effects that in 1967 were postulated to be due to reduction of excitation-contraction coupling caused by inhibition of calcium influx into cardiac cells (Fleckenstein et al. 1967). In addition to blocking calcium influx, the intracellular action of the calcium ion (Ca^{2+}) may be inhibited by substances that enhance efflux, intracellular storage, or binding of Ca^{2+} to inactivating proteins, or that activate second messengers with contradictory actions. However, the CCBs are the only drugs in widespread clinical use for their calcium antagonist activities.

As noted in Table 18–1, three additional classes of CCBs have been developed since the introduction of the phenylalkylamine verapamil (Cohan 1990; Freedman and Waters 1987; Morris et al. 1992; Murad 1991). These medications are heterogeneous in their structure and actions and are not interchangeable (Triggle 1992). However, they all have the capacity to reduce excessive excitability of diverse cellular systems. As a result, many of the CCBs have been used to treat various forms of angina, hypertension, migraine headaches, Raynaud's phenomenon, esophageal spasm, premature labor, and epilepsy (Bigger and Hoffman 1991; Kim 1991; Murad 1991). Verapamil and diltiazem, but not the 1,4-dihydropyridines

Table 18–1. Calcium channel blocker classes

Class	Examples
Phenylalkylamine	Verapamil, norverapamil, D600
1,4-Dihydropyridine	Nifedipine, nicardipine, nimodipine, amlodipine, nisoldipine, felodipine, nitrendipine
Benzothiazepine	Diltiazem
Diphenylpiperazine	Flunarizine, cinnarizine

(DHPs), have Class IV antiarrhythmic activity and are used to treat supraventricular arrhythmias (Triggle 1992). Several CCBs have been found to retard the development of atherosclerosis in animals (Freedman and Waters 1987). The DHP nimodipine, which is used to block cerebral arteriospasm following subarachnoid hemorrhage, may be useful in the treatment of Alzheimer's disease (Bigger and Hoffman 1991; Ikeda et al. 1992). The role of elevated free intracellular calcium ion concentration ($[Ca^{2+}]_i$) in neuronal death may also make the CCBs useful in reducing brain damage after anoxia (Cohan 1990). The use of nifedipine (chewed up and placed under the tongue) to treat hypertensive crises associated with monoamine oxidase inhibitors (Clary and Schweizer 1987; Kim 1991) has been criticized on the grounds that absorption of nifedipine is inadequate from the buccal mucosa (Gerber and Nies 1991).

The first type of calcium antagonist used in psychiatry was calcitonin, which lowers $[Ca^{2+}]_i$ by driving Ca^{2+} into intracellular storage sites. Carman and Wyatt (1979) found that three manic patients had a temporary reduction of agitation after injections of subcutaneous salmon calcitonin, but not of placebo. After receiving an unstated dose of salmon calcitonin for 20 days, a group of 9 patients with chronic "psychopathological suffering" (Mussini et al. 1984), a state accompanied by depression or anxiety but no formal diagnoses, felt tranquilized and demonstrated a reduction of Brief Psychiatric Rating Scale (Overall and Gorham 1962) scores.

The first report of the use of a CCB in the treatment of mania was a double-blind placebo-controlled trial of verapamil in a single manic patient (Dubovsky et al. 1982). The decision to investigate this use of a CCB was based on observations that the intracellular calcium ion is involved in the regulation of many processes implicated in bipolar affective disorders and that lithium might interfere with the intracellular action of Ca^{2+} (Dubovsky and Franks 1983). Verapamil was chosen because its cardiovascular effects were being studied by a colleague, and the manufacturer was willing to make it available to the investigators at a time at which none of the CCBs had yet been approved for use in the United States.

Subsequently, case reports of 27 patients and open and double-blind studies involving approximately 180 patients with bipolar disorder (reviewed in Dubovsky 1993) have indicated the antimanic efficacy of verapamil compared with placebo or with no treatment, and two studies have reported equivalent antimanic efficacy with lithium (Garza-Trevino et al. 1992; Hoschl and Kozemy 1989). However, with the exception of a few studies (Dubovsky et al. 1986; Garza-Trevino et al. 1992; Hoschl and Kozemy 1989; Hoschl et al. 1986), patients in most studies have only been moderately ill, trials have been brief, and additional medications (especially neuroleptics) have been employed as needed. A 2-week open trial of diltiazem in 7 manic patients (Caillard 1985), a 3-year follow-up of a bipolar patient for whom flunarizine was successfully substituted for lithium (Lindelius and Nilsson 1992), a 1-week trial of nimodipine (Brunet et al. 1990), and a prolonged double-blind follow-up of 3 bipolar patients receiving high doses of nimodipine (Post et al. 1993) suggest possible antimanic applications of these medications.

As is true of lithium, the usefulness of CCBs in the treatment of depression is not as clear as its applications in mania. Nifedipine reduces immobility in the behavioral despair test, which is thought to be an animal model of antidepressant activity (Mogilnicka et al. 1987). Flunarizine was thought to reduce depressive recurrences in one patient (Lindelius and Nilsson 1992), and one patient with recurrent brief depression responded to blind trials of both nimodipine and verapamil (Post et al. 1993). Verapamil may have acute antidepressant properties in some bipolar patients (J. Berlant, unpublished data, April 1994; Deicken 1990; Dubovsky et al. 1992a) and psychotically depressed patients (Jacques and Cox 1991). Hoschl and Kozemy (1989) found that, overall, verapamil was no more effective than placebo and was inferior to amitriptyline in the treatment of depression. However, a few patients did seem to have a genuine antidepressant response to verapamil in this study and in a previous report by the same authors (Hoschl et al. 1986). Because the investigators did not differentiate between bipolar and unipolar depression, it is possible that—as would be expected with lithium—those subjects with bipolar depression were more likely to respond to verapamil. Verapamil appeared to augment the antidepressant action of imipramine in a patient with unipolar depression who had previously responded to lithium augmentation. When imipramine was discontinued 6 months later, the patient remained euthymic on verapamil alone (Pollack and Rosenbaum 1987). Conversely, Eccleston and Cole (1990) thought that nifedipine either

gave rise to depression itself or to resistance to antidepressants in 5 unipolar depressed patients.

■ STRUCTURE-ACTIVITY RELATIONSHIPS

Different classes of calcium channel antagonists have significantly different structures (Figure 18–1) leading to differential activity in various tissues. This differential activity depends on interactions with ion-specific channels in the cell membrane. A consideration of the structure of calcium channels is therefore central to an understanding of the structural specificity of the medications that act on them.

Extracellular calcium ions enter the cytosol through channels gated by receptors for hormones and transmitters such as the excitatory amino acids and through potential dependent channels gated by membrane potential. Additional pathways for calcium entry include a "leak" through an ungated chan-

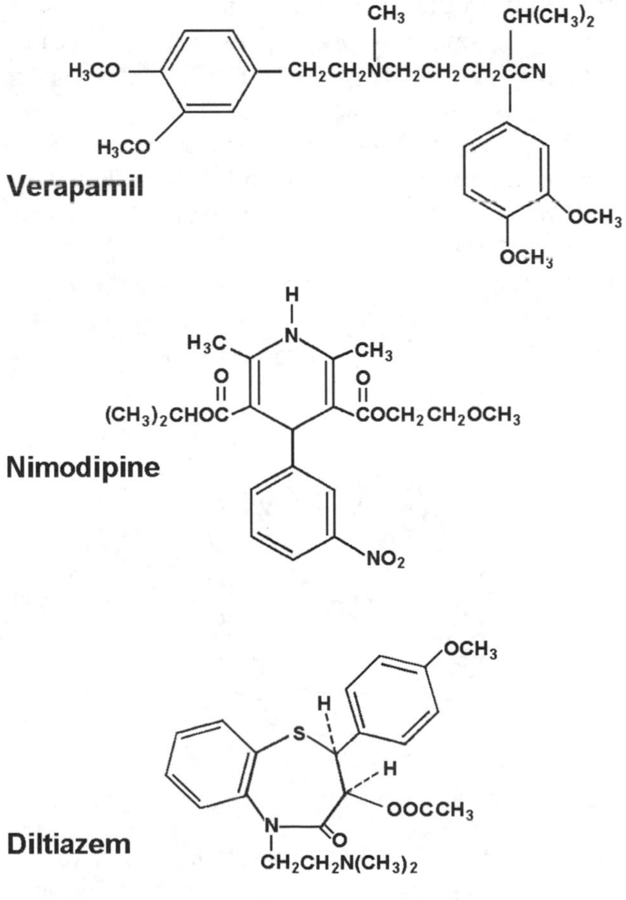

Figure 18–1. Structures of some calcium channel blockers.

nel and exchange of extracellular calcium ions for intracellular sodium ions (Na^+) (Cohan 1990; Rosenberg 1991; Triggle 1992). Under physiological conditions, potential dependent channels can be regulated by receptor-mediated events such as the production of inositol triphosphate (Bergamaschi et al. 1990; Janis and Triggle 1991), and receptor operated channels can be gated by voltage-dependent events (Bergamaschi et al. 1990). In addition, extracellular Ca^{2+} entering the cell may release calcium ions from intracellular stores, and "triggered" amounts of calcium ions released from intracellular stores may facilitate calcium channel opening (Dubovsky and Franks 1983; Murad 1991). Even subtle alterations of the function of one kind of calcium channel may therefore have significant effects on the overall balance of calcium-dependent cellular activity.

CCBs interact with the potential dependent channel (PDC). This type of channel consists of five allosterically linked subunits, α_1, α_2, β, γ, and δ; the α_1 channel has a hydrophobic region that spans the cell membrane and outlines the actual calcium pore (Figure 18–2). In the brain, PDCs for calcium are localized in regions rich in synapses, perhaps because high $[Ca^{2+}]_i$ must be produced rapidly to regulate neurotransmitter release (Fox et al. 1991). Endogenous regulators unrelated to neurotransmitters appear to modulate PDC gating and CCB binding (Janis and Triggle 1991) and may be altered in disease states (Triggle 1992).

Four subtypes of PDCs have been identified (Fox et al. 1991; Janis and Triggle 1991; Kenny et al. 1991; Murad 1991; Siesjo 1990; Triggle 1992):

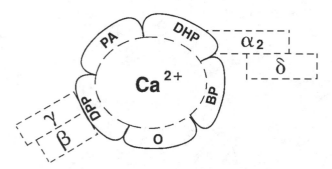

Figure 18–2. Structure of the calcium channel blocker (CCB) binding site.
PA = phenylalkylamine binding site; DHP = 1,4-dihydropyridine binding site; BP = benzothiazepine binding site; DPP = diphenylpiperazine binding site; O = other binding sites.

1. The L (or long-lasting) channel, the only PDC shown definitely to bind CCBs, requires significant depolarization for Ca^{2+} entry and inactivates slowly.
2. The T (or transient) channel is activated by small depolarizations and inactivates rapidly.
3. The N (neither L nor T) channel, which is primarily found on central nervous system neurons, is unresponsive to CCBs.
4. A rapidly inactivating P (Purkinje cell) channel identified in cerebellar Purkinje cells is insensitive to the DHP CCBs.

N and P channels may participate in release of neurotransmitters in response to the action potential, whereas the role of L channels is less certain. Studies of actions of specific CCBs on L channels may be complicated by differential binding of CCBs by the same channels in different tissues, alteration of findings by slight changes in experimental conditions, and confusion of N and L channels (Janis and Triggle 1991; Kenny et al. 1991).

CCBs bind primarily to L channels (Bigger and Hoffman 1991). Nimodipine, nicardipine, methoxyverapamil, flunarizine, and cinnarazine may also antagonize T channels (Cohan 1990; Janis and Triggle 1991), and a phenylalkylamine binding site exists on the inner mitochondrial membrane (Zernig 1992).

As noted in Figure 18–2, at least four and possibly seven or more distinct binding sites for different classes of CCBs exist on the L channel α_1 subunit (Kenny et al. 1991; Murad 1991), allosterically linked to each other and to the Ca^{2+} gating site and capable of regulation by circulating factors (Janis and Triggle 1991). The other subunits may allosterically modify the CCB affinity of the α_1 subunit (Kenny et al. 1991). Activity of guanine nucleotide-binding proteins (G proteins), phosphorylation dependent on cyclic adenosine monophosphate (cAMP), calcium-calmodulin and calcium–protein kinase C, and binding of Ca^{2+} to the α_1 subunit can all alter the conformation of the subunit, changing the affinity of the L channel for a given CCB (Bergamaschi et al. 1990).

Thus far, four separate genes coding for the α_1 subunit have been identified, producing different versions of CCB-binding sites (Triggle 1992). Depending on the distribution of binding sites for a given chemical class of CCBs, that class may be more or less active in a particular tissue or region. Variations in CCB structure produce variations in potency at different L channels in various tissues (Janis and Triggle 1991). For example, DHPs are more selective for vascular tissue, whereas verapamil and diltiazem have more prominent antiarrhythmic properties (Triggle 1992).

Several additional features of the calcium channel contribute to activity profiles of CCBs of different structure (Janis and Triggle 1991; Triggle 1992). Along with allosteric regulation and the influence of circulating modulators, membrane potential determines the conformation (and thus the affinity) of CCB-binding sites. DHP binding is enhanced by membrane depolarization, the CCB stabilizing the channel in an inactivated state. Most DHPs are uncharged at physiological pH and easily gain access to the receptor through the cell membrane if it is sufficiently depolarized. Charged DHPs such as amlodipine have slower onsets of action because of interactions with negatively charged phosphate headgroups in the cell membrane. Verapamil and diltiazem, which are also charged at physiological pH, gain access to the receptor through open channels and are therefore more active when channel openings are more frequent. The activity dependence of both charged and uncharged CCBs make these drugs much more potent in hyperactive than in normal tissue. Actions measured in normal cell preparations may not reflect activity in pathological states.

Figure 18–3 describes further structure-activity relationships that have been defined for the DHP CCBs (Janis and Triggle 1991). The activity of the (–) enantiomer of verapamil is greater than the activity of the (+) enantiomer. Micromolar concentrations of Ca^{2+} are required for binding of the DHPs, whereas the same Ca^{2+} concentrations inhibit receptor binding of phenylalkylamines and diltiazem (Janis and Triggle 1991). The structure-activity relationships that have been defined for the CCBs apply to activity at L channels in various tissues and have not been specifically correlated with clinical effects.

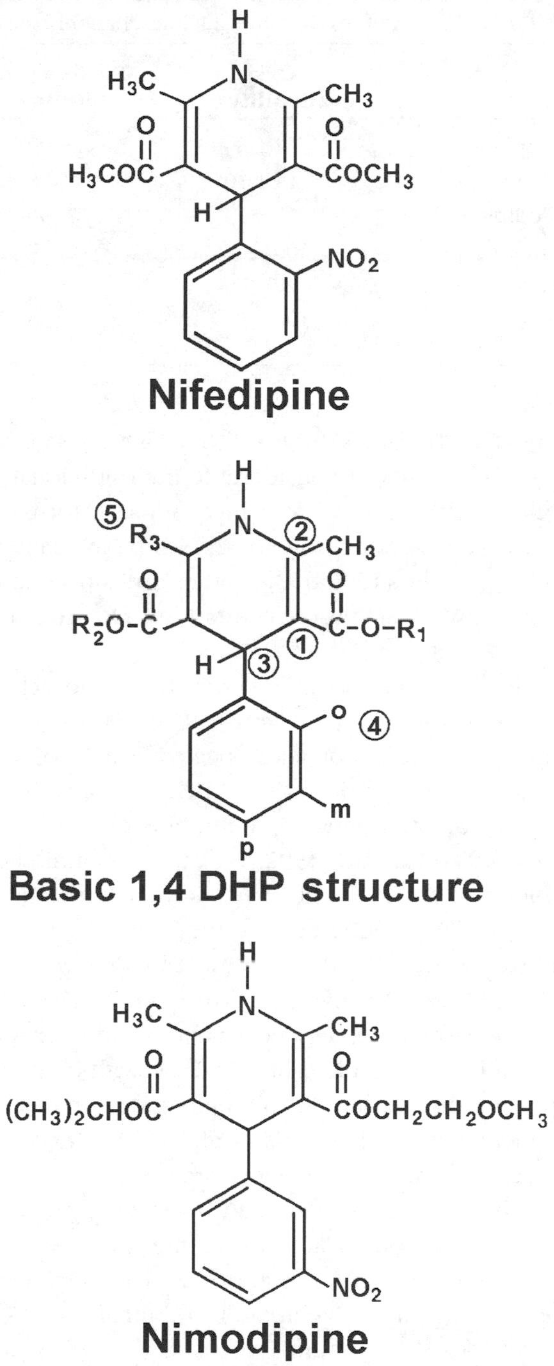

■ PHARMACOLOGICAL PROFILE

Absorption, fate, and excretion of some CCBs compared with lithium, carbamazepine, and valproate are summarized in Table 18–2 (Benet and Williams 1991; Kim 1991; Morris et al. 1992). The CCBs are nearly completely absorbed after oral administration, but bioavailability is decreased by extensive first-pass he-

Figure 18–3. Structure-activity relationships for 1,4-dihydropyridines (DHPs).
1. $CO_2R > COCH_3 > CN > H$.
2. Basic substituent in this position (e.g., amlodipine) results in slow onset, long duration of action, and high stereoselectivity.
3. Torsion angle of aryl ring influences activity.
4. $o \geq m > p$.
5. Greater activity with R = small alkyl, amine, or aminoalkyl.
Source. Adapted from Janis and Triggle 1991; Triggle 1992.

Table 18–2. Profiles of some calcium channel blockers and antimanic drugs

Drug	Oral availability (%)	Plasma protein binding (%)	Volume of distribution (L/kg)	Half-life (hours)	Effective concentration
Verapamil	22 ± 8	90	5 ± 2.1	4 ± 1.5	40–120 ng/ml
Diltiazem	44 ± 10	78	3.1 ± 1.2	3.7 ± 1.2	Unknown
Nifedipine	50 ± 13	96	0.78 ± 0.22	2.5 ± 1.3	27–67 ng/ml
Lithium	100	0	0.79 ± 0.34	22 ± 8	0.5–1.5 mEq/L
Carbamazepine	70	74	1.4 ± 0.4	15 ± 5	4–10 µg/ml
Valproate	100	93	0.22 ± 0.07	14 ± 3	50–125 µg/ml

patic metabolism (Murad 1991). First-pass metabolism also results in considerable interindividual variability in blood level at a given dose (Morris et al. 1992). As noted in Table 18–2, oral bioavailability of the CCBs is less than that of other drugs used to treat mania, but effective concentrations are an order of magnitude lower.

Peak plasma levels of most CCBs are achieved within 30 minutes to 3 hours after oral dosing, but amlodipine does not reach peak plasma concentrations for 6 hours (Morris et al. 1992). Most CCBs have elimination half-lives in the range of 1.3–6 hours (Kim 1991; Murad 1991) except for amlodipine, which has a half-life of 35–50 hours (Benet and Williams 1991). Although amlodipine can be given once daily, the short half-lives of most CCBs require multiple dosing. However, because repeated administration saturates hepatic metabolizing enzymes, bioavailability and half-life increase with chronic administration and the dosing interval can be increased (Benet et al. 1991; Morris et al. 1992). All CCBs are extensively bound to plasma proteins.

Verapamil is metabolized by *D*-dealkylation and *O*-demethylation to at least 12 metabolites. One of these, norverapamil, has about 20% as much cardiovascular activity as verapamil in animal models and a half-life of 10 hours (Morris et al. 1992; Murad 1991). After oral administration, verapamil and norverapamil can be recovered from human cerebrospinal fluid (Doran et al. 1985), although penetration of the more lipophilic nimodipine across the blood-brain barrier is better (Freedman and Waters 1987). One piece of experimental evidence that the concentration of phenylalkylamines in the brain is sufficient for a therapeutic effect is the protective effect of this class after cerebral ischemia in rats (Rosenberg 1991).

Diltiazem, which is metabolized by *O*-deacetylation or *N*-demethylation, has active metabolites that do not appear to be clinically important (Morris et al. 1992). Nifedipine, nicardipine, and most of the other DHPs have inactive metabolites. Most people are rapid metabolizers of nifedipine and possibly other DHPs; about 17% are slow metabolizers.

■ MECHANISMS OF ACTION

Free intracellular Ca^{2+} concentration is normally regulated very tightly at around 100 nM, or 1/10,000th the Ca^{2+} concentration in the extracellular fluid (Fox et al. 1991). The regulation of $[Ca^{2+}]_i$ is complex, depending on calcium influx pathways (described previously) as well as extrusion of Ca^{2+} from the cell by a calcium-ATPase membrane pump, uptake of Ca^{2+} into intracellular stores, and complexing with intracellular proteins. Calcium influx in the brain is determined by the membrane potential, receptor activity, availability of excitatory amino acids, and the intracellular Na^+ concentration (Rosenberg 1991; Triggle 1992). Elevations of $[Ca^{2+}]_i$ produced by increased Ca^{2+} influx from the extracellular space and/or release of Ca^{2+} from intracellular stores provide a bidirectional intracellular signal that may stimulate cellular processes at moderate elevations and inhibit the same processes at further elevations or at different phases of the cell cycle (Dubovsky et al. 1992a).

Significant elevations of $[Ca^{2+}]_i$ have been found in blood platelets (Dubovsky et al. 1989, 1991a, 1991b, 1992b; Tan et al. 1990) and lymphocytes (Dubovsky et al. 1992b) of manic and bipolar depressed patients who are affectively ill, but not in platelets of unipolar depressed patients, control subjects, or bipolar patients who are euthymic after treatment with various medications or electroconvulsive therapy (ECT). Elevated $[Ca^{2+}]_i$ could reflect a primary alteration in intracellular Ca^{2+} homeostasis, or it could be a downstream result of elevated activity of G proteins gated to influx or release mechanisms. Consistent with the latter possibility are observations of hyperactive receptor-linked G proteins in mononuclear leukocyte membrane preparations of untreated manic patients (but not in lithium-treated euthymic bipolar patients) (van Calker et al. 1993) and heightened activation of the platelet phosphatidylinositol system that is linked to G proteins and that mobilizes influx and release of Ca^{2+} (Brown et al. 1993). Whether produced by excessive receptor activation of G proteins or some other mechanism, excess elevations of $[Ca^{2+}]_i$ could be the effector arm that produces the mixtures and alternations of elevated and inhibited cellular activity that are characteristic of bipolar illness (Dubovsky et al. 1992a).

Lithium treatment normalizes platelet $[Ca^{2+}]_i$ (Dubovsky et al. 1989, 1991a), leukocyte G protein response to agonists (van Calker et al. 1993), and agonist-induced accumulation of inositol phosphates (Greil et al. 1991). In addition, in vitro incubation with lithium was found to inhibit coupling of muscarinic cholinergic and β-adrenergic receptors to their G proteins (Avissar and Schreiber 1992) and to lower platelet $[Ca^{2+}]_i$ significantly in ill bipolar patients but in not control subjects (Dubovsky et al. 1991b). Lithium had no effect on platelet $[Ca^{2+}]_i$ in another study (Tan et al. 1990), but patients were euthymic and the action of lithium on intracellular Ca^{2+} dynamics may differ between the ill and well states (Dubovsky et al. 1992a). Carbamazepine inhibits Ca^{2+} currents in a variety of models, and the time course of suppression of calcium-dependent potentials is comparable to that produced by verapamil (Messing et al. 1985; Schirrmacher et al. 1993; Walden et al. 1992). This anticonvulsant may alter influx through N-methyl-D-aspartate receptor-gated channels (Post et al. 1993). Lithium, carbamazepine, and CCBs could all correct elevated Ca^{2+} influx. Reduction of Ca^{2+} influx produced by CCBs could also alter intracellular Ca^{2+} homeostasis sufficiently to compensate for dysregulated intracellular signaling associated with other mechanisms.

Several objections can be raised to the hypothesis that attenuation of excessive rises in $[Ca^{2+}]_i$ produced by stimulation of neurons with hypersensitivity of this or a related messenger system is a mechanism of action of CCBs in bipolar illness. First, L channels do not appear to be involved in the action potential–dependent release of neurotransmitters (Janis and Triggle 1991). However, neurotransmitters activate L channels, making them an important component of neuronal signaling (Fox et al. 1991). Another problem is that low concentrations of CCBs do not affect neurotransmitter release or neuronal Ca^{2+} currents; depolarization in these cells is normally too brief to permit sufficient binding of the CCBs (Triggle 1992). In response to these objections, higher concentrations of CCBs may alter neuronal activity, and some negative reports may be the result of confusing L channels with other channels that do not respond to CCBs. CCBs do have significant effects on neurons with prolonged or marked depolarization (Janis and Triggle 1991). This may be why the effects of antimanic drugs such as lithium on $[Ca^{2+}]_i$ are evident in hyperactive peripheral cells from bipolar patients but not in normally active cells from control subjects (Dubovsky et al. 1992a).

It could also be argued that it is the anticonvulsant property of CCBs (Janis and Triggle 1991) and not their effect on Ca^{2+} currents that accounts for the CCBs' antimanic activity (Post et al. 1993). Although reduction of neuronal excitability does convey anticonvulsant effects to the CCBs, these effects do not appear to be in proportion to their antimanic potential. In addition, the anticonvulsant potency of many of the CCBs is manifest mainly in animal models and is not as apparent in humans with epilepsy or electrically induced seizures.

INDICATIONS

Available data suggest that CCBs are most useful for manic patients who are responsive to lithium but cannot tolerate it, whereas acutely manic patients who do not respond to lithium seem less likely to respond to verapamil (Barton and Gitlin 1987; Kennedy et al. 1986). In the few reported cases in which verapamil (Dubovsky et al. 1982, 1986) or diltiazem (Caillard 1985) was administered to manic patients with brain damage, the CCBs were well tolerated. CCBs might be considered in the treatment of patients with physical conditions for which other medications would be more dangerous (e.g., pregnancy) or for which a CCB might be helpful (e.g., hypertension, migraine headaches, tardive dyskinesia [TD], Tourette's syndrome, or supraventricular arrhythmias) (Amery et al. 1981; Leys et al. 1988; Litzinger et al. 1985; Reiter et al. 1989; Walsh et al. 1986; Yamawaki and Yanagawa 1986).

Most manic patients enrolled in studies of verapamil either have responded to lithium or, not having received lithium, cannot be said to have been unresponsive to it. A few rapid-cycling patients have benefited from verapamil, and addition of verapamil to lithium has been helpful to some patients who did not respond to lithium alone (Brotman et al. 1986). However, most patients with complex or treatment-refractory bipolar illness should probably be treated first with anticonvulsants with or without lithium, as there has been more published positive experience with these drug combinations in such situations.

Verapamil has been noted to prevent antidepressant-induced hypomania (Barton and Gitlin 1987; Dubovsky et al. 1986; Gitlin and Weiss 1984; Solomon and Williamson 1986). Extended follow-up of several patients demonstrated the usefulness of nimodipine in maintenance therapy for bipolar illness (Manna 1991; Post et al. 1993), and verapamil also has been found effective in the clinical setting in preventing affective recurrence. As noted previously, CCBs do not have impressive antidepressant properties; but they may be helpful in some cases of bipolar or highly recurrent depression (Hoschl et al. 1986; Jacques and Cox 1991; Lindelius and Nilsson 1992; Post et al. 1993).

The heterogeneity of CCB-binding sites provides for different spectra of action of various CCBs, and it is possible that patients who do not respond to one class of drug may have a good response to another (Post et al. 1993). Combinations of CCBs with one other and with other antimanic drugs could also produce additive effects on Ca^{2+}-dependent mechanisms that could make such combinations useful in treatment-refractory states. However, such possibilities have not been investigated formally.

The CCBs do not appear helpful for treatment of chronic, treatment-refractory schizophrenia (Grebb et al. 1986; Pickar et al. 1987; Uhr et al. 1988), although they may reduce signs of TD (Leys et al. 1988; Reiter et al. 1989). Verapamil in doses of 240–480 mg qd produced modest improvement in panic disorder in 11 patients and marked improvement in 4 (Klein and Uhde 1988). Although further studies for this indication have not been reported, clinicians sometimes find that adding verapamil to antidepressants and/or benzodiazepines enhances the antipanic efficacy of these drugs.

Available preparations and recommended maximum doses of some CCBs are summarized in Table 18–3 (Murad 1991). The usual daily doses of verapamil in the treatment of mania have been 240–480 mg qd, although some patients may need higher doses. The sustained release preparation often is not as effective as standard preparations, possibly because blood levels are inadequate. The reported daily dose of nimodipine in the treatment of bipolar illness has ranged from 360 mg (Brunet et al. 1990) to considerably higher doses (Post et al. 1993) that were substantially above the maximum dose approved by the U.S. Food and Drug Administration (Table 18–3).

■ SIDE EFFECTS AND TOXICOLOGY

Verapamil is safe for long-term administration (Mauritson et al. 1982). Possibly because of compensatory changes in calcium channels or CCB receptors, tachyphylaxis and withdrawal do not occur (Murad 1991). CCBs do not alter exercise tolerance (Gerber and Nies 1991).

The most common CCB side effects involve consequences of excessive vasodilatation (e.g., dizziness, headache, skin flushing, tachycardia, nausea, and digital dysesthesia); aggravation of myocardial ischemia may rarely occur (Bigger and Hoffman 1991; Gerber and Nies 1991; Murad 1991). Precapillary dilatation with reflex postcapillary constriction can increase capillary hydrostatic pressure and cause peripheral edema (Gerber and Nies 1991). The highest incidence of vascular side effects occurs with the DHPs (Gerber and Nies 1991). Verapamil and diltiazem are more likely than other preparations to produce sinus bradycardia and atrioventricular block

Table 18–3. Some calcium channel blocker preparations and doses

Drug	Trade name	Size supplied (mg)	Usual daily dose, mg (maximum)
Verapamil	Calan, Isoptin	40, 80, 120, 240 SR	120–480 (480)
Nimodipine	Nimotop	30	60–120 (180)
Nifedipine	Procardia, Adalat	10, 20	30–120 (180)
Nicardipine	Cardene	20, 30	60–120 (120)
Diltiazem	Cardizem	30	30–120 (360)

Note. SR = sustained release.

and may aggravate heart failure. Coughing, wheezing, rashes, somnolence, constipation, and (very rarely) psychosis may be caused by the CCBs (Bigger and Hoffman 1991; Freedman and Waters 1987; Gerber and Nies 1991; Kim 1991; Murad 1991). Akathisia (Jacobs 1983), parkinsonism (Chouza et al. 1986), and delirium (Jacobsen et al. 1987) have occasionally been associated with use of calcium channel antagonists. Toxic serum concentrations of CCBs have not been defined as they have for lithium and anticonvulsants (Benet and Williams 1991).

■ DRUG-DRUG INTERACTIONS

Adding CCBs to β-adrenergic blocking agents can depress ventricular function and produce cardiac slowing and atrioventricular block (Murad 1991), whereas additive effects with α-adrenergic blocking agents may produce hypotension (Morris et al. 1992). Verapamil and nitrendipine increase plasma concentrations of digoxin and produce bradycardia, hypotension, or atrioventricular block (Bigger and Hoffman 1991; Gerber and Nies 1991). Pharmacokinetic and pharmacodynamic interactions with other drugs used to treat mania are noted in Table 18–4 (Brodie and MacPhee 1986; Chouza et al. 1986; Dubovsky et al. 1987; Jacobs 1983; Kumana and Mahon 1981; Kupersmith and Slater 1985; MacPhee et al. 1986; Morris et al. 1992; Valdiserri 1985; Weinrauch et al. 1984).

■ CONCLUSION

Possibly because of the differential interest of pharmaceutical companies in supporting research and educational programs (Dubovsky 1994), the efficacy of the CCBs as alternatives to lithium in the treatment of bipolar affective disorder has not been as widely appreciated as has that of the anticonvulsants. The CCBs may be particularly useful for patients who cannot tolerate the other antimanic drugs, patients with brain damage, and pregnant patients. The use of these medications in maintenance therapy and in complicated illnesses such as rapid cycling has not been the subject of extended prospective double-blind studies, but the same is true of the anticonvulsants. As with the latter medications, clinical experience suggests that combining a CCB with another antimanic drug may be helpful for some treatment-refractory patients, but this application also has not been studied formally. In view of differences in CCB-binding sites as well as in the pharmacology of the CCBs, it seems likely that different preparations will have different spectra of action, at least in some cases. However, until more research is available, the CCBs should be considered second- or third-line treatments for bipolar illness.

The CCBs were initially studied as antimanic drugs, because it was thought that intracellular Ca^{2+} signaling might be unstable in patients with bipolar disorder. Patients who have peripheral evidence of increased $[Ca^{2+}]_i$ may be more likely to respond to this class of medication (Dubovsky et al. 1991b), whereas those who do not may have abnormalities of different or additional signaling mechanisms. Regardless of the specific clinical uses of the CCBs that will eventually be demonstrated, studying them may be one of a number of new approaches to understanding intracellular mechanisms in mood disorders. As these mechanisms are better understood, treatments that act more specifically on one or another intracellular effector may accompany biological and clinical measurements that predict their efficacy in a given bipolar subtype.

Table 18–4. Some calcium channel blocker interactions

Drug	Interaction effects
Lithium	Neurotoxicity
	Choreoathetosis
	Parkinsonism
	Cardiac slowing
	Decreased lithium levels (?)
Carbamazepine	Increased carbamazepine levels
	Neurotoxicity
Neuroleptics	Increased parkinsonism

■ REFERENCES

Amery WK, Wauquier A, Van Neuten JM, et al: The anti-migrainous pharmacology of flunarizine (R14 950), a calcium antagonist. Drugs Exp Clin Res 7:1–10, 1981

Aronson TA, Shukla S, Hirschowitz J: Clonazepam treatment of five lithium-refractory patients with bipolar disorder. Am J Psychiatry 146:77–80, 1989

Avissar S, Schreiber G: The involvement of guanine

nucleotide binding proteins in the pathogenesis and treatment of affective disorders. Biol Psychiatry 31:435–459, 1992

Barton BM, Gitlin MJ: Verapamil in treatment-resistant mania: an open trial. J Clin Psychopharmacol 7:101–103, 1987

Benet LZ, Williams RL: Design and optimization of dosage regimens: pharmacokinetic data, in Goodman and Gilman's The Pharmacological Basis of Therapeutics, 8th Edition. Edited by Gilman AG, Rall TW, Nies AS, et al. New York, Pergamon, 1991, pp 1650–1735

Benet LZ, Mitchell JR, Sheiner LB: Pharmacokinetics: the dynamics of drug absorption, distribution, and elimination, in Goodman and Gilman's The Pharmacological Basis of Therapeutics, 8th Edition. Edited by Gilman AG, Rall TW, Nies AS, et al. New York, Pergamon, 1991, pp 3–32

Bergamaschi S, Trabucchi M, Battaini F, et al: Modulation of dihydropyridine-sensitive calcium channels: a role for G proteins. Eur Neurol 30 (suppl 2):16–20, 1990

Bigger JT, Hoffman BF: Antiarrhythmic drugs, in Goodman and Gilman's The Pharmacological Basis of Therapeutics, 8th Edition. Edited by Gilman AG, Rall TW, Nies AS, et al. New York, Pergamon, 1991, pp 840–873

Brodie MJ, MacPhee GJA: Carbamazepine neurotoxicity precipitated by diltiazem. British Medical Journal 292:1170–1171, 1986

Brotman AW, Farhadi AM, Gelenberg AJ: Verapamil treatment of acute mania. J Clin Psychiatry 47:136–138, 1986

Brown AS, Mallinger AG, Renbaum LC: Elevated platelet membrane phosphatidylinositol-4,5-biphosphate in bipolar mania. Am J Psychiatry 150:1252–1254, 1993

Brunet G, Cerlich B, Robert P, et al: Open trial of a calcium antagonist, nimodipine, in acute mania. Clin Neuropharmacol 13:224–228, 1990

Caillard V: Treatment of mania using a calcium antagonist—preliminary trial. Neuropsychobiology 14:23–26, 1985

Carman JS, Wyatt RJ: Calcium: pacesetting the periodic psychoses. Am J Psychiatry 136:1035–1039, 1979

Chouza C, Scaramelli A, Carmano JL, et al: Parkinsonism, tardive dyskinesia, akathisia and depression induced by flunarizine. Lancet 1:1303–1304, 1986

Clary C, Schweizer E: Treatment of MAOI hypertensive crisis with sublingual nifedipine. J Clin Psychiatry 48:249–250, 1987

Cohan SL: Pharmacology of calcium antagonists: clinical relevance in neurology. Eur Neurol 30 (suppl 2):28–30, 1990

Deicken RF: Verapamil treatment of bipolar depression [letter]. J Clin Psychopharmacol 10:148–149, 1990

Doran AR, Narang PK, Meigs CY, et al: Verapamil concentrations in cerebrospinal fluid after oral administration [letter]. N Engl J Med 312:1261–1262, 1985

Dubovsky SL: Calcium antagonists in manic-depressive illness. Neuropsychobiology 27:184–192, 1993

Dubovsky SL: Why don't we hear more about the calcium antagonists? Biol Psychiatry 35:149–150, 1994

Dubovsky SL, Franks RD: Intracellular calcium ions in affective disorders: a review and an hypothesis. Biol Psychiatry 18:781–797, 1983

Dubovsky SL, Franks RD, Lifschitz M, et al: Effectiveness of verapamil in the treatment of a manic patient. Am J Psychiatry 139:502–504, 1982

Dubovsky SL, Franks RD, Allen S, et al: Calcium antagonists in mania: a double-blind study of verapamil. Psychiatry Res 18:309–320, 1986

Dubovsky SL, Franks RD, Allen S: Verapamil: a new antimanic drug with potential interactions with lithium. J Clin Psychiatry 48:371–372, 1987

Dubovsky SL, Christiano J, Daniell LC, et al: Increased platelet intracellular calcium concentration in patients with bipolar affective disorders. Arch Gen Psychiatry 46:632–638, 1989

Dubovsky SL, Lee C, Christiano J, et al: Elevated intracellular calcium ion concentration in bipolar depression. Biol Psychiatry 29:441–450, 1991a

Dubovsky SL, Lee C, Christiano J, et al: Lithium decreases platelet intracellular calcium ion concentrations in bipolar patients. Lithium 2:167–174, 1991b

Dubovsky SL, Murphy J, Christiano J, et al: The calcium second messenger system in bipolar disorders: data supporting new research directions. J Neuropsychiatry Clin Neurosci 4:3–14, 1992a

Dubovsky SL, Murphy J, Thomas M, et al: Abnormal intracellular calcium ion concentration in platelets and lymphocytes in bipolar patients. Am J Psychiatry 149:118–120, 1992b

Eccleston D, Cole AJ: Calcium-channel blockade and depressive illness. Br J Psychiatry 156:889–891,

1990

Fleckenstein JA, Kammermeier H, Doring H, et al: Zum Wirkungs-Mechanismus neurartiger Koronardilalatoren mit gleichzeitig Sauerstoffeinsparenden, myokard-Effekten, Prenylamin und Iproveratril. Zeitschrift für Kreislaufforschung 56:716–744, 1967

Fox AP, Hirning LD, Mogul DJ, et al: Modulation of calcium channels by neurotransmitters, hormones and second messengers, in Calcium Channels: Their Properties, Functions, Regulation, and Clinical Relevance. Edited by Hurwitz L, Partridge LD, Leach JK. Boca Raton, FL, CRC Press, 1991, pp 251–263

Freedman DD, Waters DD: "Second generation" dihydropyridine calcium antagonists: greater vascular selectivity and some unique applications. Drugs 34:578–598, 1987

Garza-Trevino ES, Overall JE, Hollister LE: Verapamil versus lithium in acute mania. Am J Psychiatry 149:121–122, 1992

Gerber JS, Nies AS: Antihypertensive agents and the drug therapy of hypertension, in Goodman and Gilman's The Pharmacological Basis of Therapeutics, 8th Edition. Edited by Gilman AG, Rall TW, Nies AS, et al. New York, Pergamon, 1991, pp 784–813

Gitlin MJ, Weiss J: Verapamil as maintenance treatment in bipolar illness: a case report. J Clin Psychopharmacol 4:341–343, 1984

Grebb JA, Shelton RC, Taylor EH, et al: A negative, double-blind placebo-controlled clinical trial of verapamil in chronic schizophrenia. Biol Psychiatry 21:691–694, 1986

Greil W, Steber R, van Calker D: The agonist-stimulated accumulation of inositol phosphates is attenuated in neutrophils from male patients under chronic lithium therapy. Biol Psychiatry 30:443–451, 1991

Hoschl C, Kozemy J: Verapamil in affective disorders: a controlled, double-blind study. Biol Psychiatry 25:128–140, 1989

Hoschl C, Blahos J, Kabes J: The use of calcium channel blockers in psychiatry, in Biological Psychiatry 1985. Edited by Shagass CE, Josiassen RC, Bridger WH, et al. New York, Elsevier, 1986, pp 330–332

Ikeda M, Dewar D, McCulloch J: A correlative study of calcium channel antagonist binding and local neuropathological features in the hippocampus in Alzheimer's disease. Brain Res 589:313–319, 1992

Jacobs MB: Diltiazem and akathisia. Ann Intern Med 99:794–795, 1983

Jacobsen FM, Sack DA, James SP: Delirium induced by verapamil [letter]. Am J Psychiatry 144:248, 1987

Jacques RM, Cox SJ: Verapamil in major (psychotic) depression. Br J Psychiatry 158:124–125, 1991

Janis RA, Triggle DJ: Drugs acting on calcium channels, in Calcium Channels: Their Properties, Functions, Regulation, and Clinical Relevance. Edited by Hurwitz L, Partridge LD, Leach JK. Boca Raton, FL, CRC Press, 1991, pp 195–249

Kennedy S, Ozersky S, Robillard M: Refractory bipolar illness may not respond to verapamil [letter]. J Clin Psychopharmacol 6:316–317, 1986

Kenny BA, Kilpatrick AT, Spedding M: Quantification of the affinity of drugs acting at the calcium channel, in Cellular Calcium: A Practical Approach. Edited by McCormack JG, Cobbold PH. Oxford, England, IRL Press, 1991, pp 267–282

Kim KE: Comparative clinical pharmacology of calcium channel blockers. Am Fam Physician 43:583–588, 1991

Klein E, Uhde TW: Controlled study of verapamil for treatment of panic disorder. Am J Psychiatry 145:431–434, 1988

Kumana CR, Mahon WA: Bizarre perceptual disorder of extremities in patients taking verapamil [letter]. Lancet 1:1324–1325, 1981

Kupersmith J, Slater W: Calcium channel blockers: pharmacologic basis for therapeutic properties. Hospital Formulary 20:184–195, 1985

Leys D, Vermersch P, Daniel T, et al: Diltiazem for tardive dyskinesia. Lancet 1:250–251, 1988

Lindelius R, Nilsson CG: Flunarizine as maintenance treatment of a patient with bipolar disorder [letter]. Am J Psychiatry 149:139, 1992

Litzinger M, Nelson PG, Pun RYK: Does nitrendipine block calcium channels in mammalian neurons? implications for treatment of ischemic cell death. Neurology 35 (suppl 1):141, 1985

MacPhee G, McInnes GT, Thompson G, et al: Verapamil potentiates carbamazepine neurotoxicity: a clinically important inhibitory interaction. Lancet 1:700–703, 1986

Mauritson DR, Winniford MD, Walker WS, et al: Oral verapamil for paroxysmal supraventricular tachycardia: a long-term double blind randomized trial. Ann Intern Med 96:409–412, 1982

Manna V: Disturbi affettivi bipolari e ruolo del calcio intraneuronale: effetti terapeutici del trattamento con sali di litio e/o calcio antagonista in pazienti con rapida inversione di polarita. Minerva Med 82:757–763, 1991

Messing RO, Carpenter CL, Greenberg DA: Mechanism of calcium channel inhibition by phenytoin: comparison with classical calcium channel antagonists. J Pharmacol Exp Ther 235:407–411, 1985

Mogilnicka E, Czyzak A, Maj J: Dihydropyridine calcium channel antagonists reduce immobility in the mouse behavioral despair test; antidepressants facilitate nifedipine action. Eur J Pharmacol 138:413–416, 1987

Morris AD, Meredith PA, Reid JL: Pharmacokinetics of calcium antagonists: implications for therapy, in Calcium Antagonists in Clinical Medicine. Edited by Epstein M. Philadelphia, PA, Hanley & Belfus, 1992, pp 49–67

Murad F: Drugs used for the treatment of angina: organic nitrates, calcium-channel blockers, and β-adrenergic agents, in Goodman and Gilman's The Pharmacological Basis of Therapeutics, 8th Edition. Edited by Gilman AG, Rall TW, Nies AS, et al. New York, Pergamon, 1991, pp 764–783

Mussini M, Agricola R, Moia GC, et al: A preliminary study on the use of calcitonin in clinical psychopathology. J Int Med Res 12:23–29, 1984

Overall JE, Gorham DR: The Brief Psychiatric Rating Scale. Psychol Rep 10:799–812, 1962

Pickar D, Wolkowitz O, Doran A: Clinical and biochemical effects of verapamil administration to schizophrenic patients. Arch Gen Psychiatry 44:113–119, 1987

Pollack MH, Rosenbaum JF: Verapamil in the treatment of recurrent unipolar depression. Biol Psychiatry 22:779–782, 1987

Post RM: Approaches to treatment-resistant bipolar affectively ill patients. Clin Neuropharmacol 11:93–104, 1988

Post RM, Ketter TA, Pazzaglia PJ, et al: New developments in the use of anticonvulsants as mood stabilizers. Neuropsychobiology 27:132–137, 1993

Prien RF, Gelenberg AJ: Alternatives to lithium for preventive treatment of bipolar disorder. Am J Psychiatry 146:840–848, 1989

Reiter S, Adler R, Angrist B: Effect of verapamil on tardive dyskinesia and psychosis in schizophrenic patients. J Clin Psychiatry 50:26–27, 1989

Rosenberg GA: Calcium channel blockers in neurological disorders, in Calcium Channels: Their Properties, Functions, Regulation, and Clinical Relevance. Edited by Hurwitz L, Partridge LD, Leach JK. Boca Raton, FL, CRC Press, 1991, pp 377–384

Schirrmacher K, Mayer A, Walden J, et al: Effects of carbamazepine on action potentials and calcium currents in rat spinal ganglion cells in vitro. Neuropsychobiology 27:176–179, 1993

Siesjo BK: Calcium in the brain under physiological and pathological conditions. Eur Neurol 30 (suppl 2):3–9, 1990

Solomon L, Williamson P: Verapamil in bipolar illness. Can J Psychiatry 31:442–444, 1986

Tan CH, Javors MA, Seleshi E, et al: Effects of lithium on platelet ionic intracellular calcium concentration in patients with bipolar (manic-depressive) disorder and healthy controls. Life Sci 46:1175–1180, 1990

Triggle DJ: Biochemical and pharmacologic differences among calcium channel antagonists: clinical implications, in Calcium Antagonists in Clinical Medicine. Edited by Epstein M. Philadelphia, PA, Hanley & Belfus, 1992, pp 1–27

Uhr SB, Jackson K, Berger PA: Effects of verapamil administration on negative symptoms of chronic schizophrenia. Psychiatry Res 23:351–352, 1988

Valdiserri EV: A possible interaction between lithium and diltiazem: case report. J Clin Psychiatry 46:540–541, 1985

van Calker D, Forstner U, Bohus M, et al: Increased sensitivity to agonist stimulation of the Ca^{2+} response in neutrophils of manic-depressive patients: effect of lithium therapy. Neuropsychobiology 27:180–183, 1993

Walden J, Grunze H, Bingmann D, et al: Calcium antagonistic effects of carbamazepine as a mechanism of action in neuropsychiatric disorders: studies in calcium dependent model epilepsies. Eur Neuropsychopharmacol 2:455–462, 1992

Walsh TL, Lavenstein B, Licamele WL, et al: Calcium antagonists in the treatment of Tourette's disorder. Am J Psychiatry 143:1467–1468, 1986

Weinrauch LA, Belok S, D'Elia JA: Decreased serum lithium during verapamil therapy. Am Heart J 108:1378–1380, 1984

Yamawaki S, Yanagawa K: Possible central effect of dantrolene sodium in neuroleptic malignant syndrome. J Clin Psychopharmacol 6:378–379, 1986

Zernig G: Photoaffinity labeling of the partially purified mitochondrial phenylalkylamine calcium antagonist receptor. Mol Pharmacol 42:1010–1013, 1992

Other Agents

19

Cognitive Enhancers

Deborah B. Marin, M.D., Kenneth L. Davis, M.D., and
Albert J. Speranza, Jr., M.D.

Identification of neurotransmitter deficits in the brains of patients with Alzheimer's disease (AD) has fostered the development of pharmacological strategies to alleviate these deficits (Davies and Maloney 1976). Consistent demonstration of central cholinergic depletion in AD, in conjunction with the cholinergic system's involvement in learning, generated many studies that focused on cholinergic enhancement. Although the cholinergic approach has yielded some promising findings, the results to date have not yet revealed a consistently robust treatment for the cognitive disturbances in AD (Chatellier and Lacomblez 1990; Davis et al. 1992; Farlow et al. 1992; Tariot et al. 1987a). It can be hypothesized that the variable results with the cholinergic replacement strategy in AD may be due in part to the deficiencies in other neurotransmitters. If so, correction of deficits in multiple neurotransmitters would be expected to be more efficacious than a purely cholinergic approach.

An alternative to the palliative treatment of AD with neurotransmitter replacement strategies is the development of treatments that could slow the neurodegenerative process of AD and consequent cognitive decline. In this chapter, we review the cholinergic and combined neurotransmitter approaches and discuss strategies designed to modify the course of AD through their presumed alteration of the fundamental pathophysiological processes in the disease.

■ CHOLINERGIC AGENTS

Multiple lines of evidence support a critical role for cholinergic mechanisms in AD, including the following findings:

1. Centrally active anticholinergic agents produce cognitive deficits in humans (Drachman and Leavitt 1974; Dundee and Pandit 1972).
2. Cholinergic neurotransmission modulates memory and learning (Deutsch 1971).
3. Lesions of the central cholinergic system create learning and memory impairments that can, in turn, be reversed with cholinomimetic administration (Bartus et al. 1987; Collerton 1986; Olton and Wenk 1987).
4. Postmortem studies of patients with AD document cholinergic cell loss in the septum and nucleus basalis of Meynert, decreased concentrations of choline acetyltransferase and acetylcholinesterase, and a correlation between these changes and degree of cognitive impairment (Davies and Maloney 1976; Perry et al. 1977, 1978).

Improvement of the overall functioning of the central cholinergic system could theoretically result from prevention of neuronal degeneration, increasing acetylcholine availability, and activation of postsynaptic cholinergic receptors. Of the several possible methods that could achieve these goals, three strategies have been clinically used: acetylcholine precursors, cholinesterase inhibitors, and postsynaptic agonists.

It has been reasoned that enhancing the availability of acetylcholine precursors could increase acetylcholine synthesis, thereby providing an increased pool of neurotransmitter for cholinergic transmission. Acetylcholine precursor treatments with choline or lecithin represented early attempts to enhance cholinergic transmission in AD. Because the choline uptake system is saturated under normal conditions, increases in extracellular choline will not enhance acetylcholine synthesis or release. Nonetheless, increased extracellular choline availability may be beneficial during intense cholinergic activity and greater demand for precursor. Acetylcholine precursor therapy could therefore enhance cognitive performance in patients with AD if there exist insufficient amounts of acetylcholine precursor. However, there is little evidence to support the efficacy of the precursor loading approach (for review, see Bartus et al. 1985).

■ Cholinesterase Inhibitors

Physostigmine

History and discovery. The use of physostigmine and other cholinesterase inhibitors is based on the goal of enhancing cholinergic neurotransmission through inhibiting the breakdown of acetylcholine.

Structure. Physostigmine is a natural alkaloid that contains a tertiary amine.

Pharmacological profile. Physostigmine is a reversible anticholinesterase that effectively increases the concentration of acetylcholine at the sites of cholinergic transmission.

Pharmacokinetics and disposition. Physostigmine is absorbed in the gastrointestinal tract, subcutaneous tissue, and mucous membranes. It is hydrolyzed and inactivated within 2 hours, thus requiring multiple dosings each day. Physostigmine readily crosses the blood-brain barrier.

Mechanism of action. Physostigmine enhances cholinergic transmission through its increasing acetylcholine availability in the central nervous system (CNS).

Indications. Most studies using parenteral administration of physostigmine have demonstrated transient cognitive improvement in at least a subgroup of patients with AD (Mohs and Davis 1987). Oral administration of the compound has also been shown to have some efficacy. Some have speculated that long-term treatment with physostigmine may delay deterioration in AD. Four out of five patients who received the medication over a 3-year period did not significantly deteriorate in their performances on the Buschke selective reminding task (Beller et al. 1988). Two out of six patients treated with oral physostigmine for 29 months also did not show deterioration, whereas all six control subjects did (Jenike et al. 1990).

Physostigmine's limited efficacy may reflect the biological heterogeneity of patients and the pharmacological properties of the medication. There is significant interindividual variability in gastrointestinal absorption, hepatic catabolism, hydrolysis, and CNS penetration with this compound (Whelpton and Hurst 1985). The unpredictable blood (and therefore CNS) concentrations achieved with a given dose necessitate individual titration of medication dosing. The peripheral to brain partitioning of physostigmine also hampers its clinical utility. Blood levels required to achieve CNS concentrations necessary for cognitive enhancement may be associated with significant adverse effects, including gastrointestinal distress, hypotension, and bradycardia. It is therefore possible that ineffective CNS penetration has led to the lack of response in some patients tested with this drug. Novel drug delivery systems that overcome the blood-brain barrier problem have yet to be systematically tested. The medication's short half-life is also problematic, because this characteristic causes continuous fluctuations in blood levels. Because of the inverted U-shape dose-response curve observed with physostigmine, nonoptimal blood levels could also limit the beneficial effects observed with this agent.

Side effects. The side effects observed with physostigmine include depressed mood, anxiety, salivation, bradycardia, and gastrointestinal distress.

Drug-drug interactions. Physostigmine has been used primarily as a single agent for treating AD. As we describe later in this chapter, physostigmine has been shown to be safely administered in conjunction with L-deprenyl.

Tetrahydroaminoacridine

History and discovery. Two pilot studies in patients with a diagnosis of AD suggested that 9-amino-1,2,3,4,-tetrahydroacridine (THA) administration alone or in combination with lecithin was associated with improvement in performances on psychometric tests and global assessments (Kaye et al. 1982; Summers et al. 1981). Summers and colleagues (1986) documented significant improvement in global status and psychometric performance in 16 subjects treated with THA. These earlier studies led to several multicenter trials to evaluate the efficacy of THA in AD.

Structure. THA is an aminoacridine compound that is a reversible synthetic acetylcholinesterase inhibitor. It has an empirical formula of $C_{13}H_{14}N_2 \cdot HCl \cdot H_2O$.

Pharmacological profile. In vitro studies demonstrate that THA inhibits plasma cholinesterase and tissue acetylcholinesterase (Adem 1992). Unlike physostigmine that interacts with the catalytic site of acetylcholinesterase, THA produces allosteric inhibition by binding to a hydrophobic region on the active surface of the enzyme (Adem 1992). THA has also been shown to interact with muscarinic and nicotinic receptors (Adem 1992). THA increases presynaptic acetylcholine release through blocking slow potassium channels and increases postsynaptic monoaminergic stimulation by interfering with noradrenaline and serotonin uptake (Drukarch et al. 1987, 1988). These latter characteristics of THA occur at concentrations higher than those required for acetylcholinesterase inhibition and therefore probably do not contribute to the drug's clinical effects.

Pharmacokinetics and disposition. THA is rapidly absorbed after oral administration. Maximal plasma concentration occurs within 1–2 hours. THA is about 55% bound by plasma proteins and is metabolized by the cytochrome p_{450} system to multiple metabolites. Following aromatic ring hydroxylation, THA's metabolites undergo glucuronidation. The elimination half-life is 2–4 hours. THA is concentrated 10-fold in the brain, in part because of its high lipid solubility (Nielsen et al. 1989).

Mechanism of action. THA enhances cholinergic transmission through its increasing acetylcholine availability in the CNS.

Indications. Four double-blind placebo-controlled studies have assessed the therapeutic efficacy of THA in larger patient samples. THA and lecithin administration produced minimal cognitive improvement in a study of 67 subjects (Chatellier and Lacomblez 1990), and statistically significant improvement in the Mini-Mental State Examination score (Folstein et al. 1975) in another investigation of 39 patients (Gauthier et al. 1990). A 6-week crossover trial that used an enriched-population design with 215 patients (Davis et al. 1992) demonstrated that the THA-treated group showed significantly less decline in cognitive function than the placebo-treated group, as assessed by the cognitive subscale of the Alzheimer's Disease Assessment Scale (Rosen et al. 1984). A 12-week parallel group design that included 273 patients demonstrated a significant dose-related improvement in cognition with THA treatment (Farlow et al. 1992).

In reviewing THA's efficacy, we must consider the outcome measures used to assess medication response. For example, use of the Clinical Global Assessment Scale (Guy 1976) does not necessarily identify whether improvement with THA was the result of cognitive enhancement (Davis et al. 1992; Farlow et al. 1992). Different methods of administration of the Clinical Global Assessment Scale could also lead to discrepant results (Davis et al. 1992; Farlow et al. 1992).

Side effects and toxicity. Side effects most often associated with THA include nausea, abdominal distress, tachycardia, and liver toxicity. Despite earlier reports of significant hepatic toxicity, THA is relatively safe (Summers et al. 1989). Hepatic toxicity is dose dependent and reversible.

Drug-drug interactions. Because THA undergoes extensive hepatic metabolism by the P_{450} system, drug-drug interactions may occur when this agent is given concurrently with others that undergo extensive metabolism through cytochrome P_{450}. Coadministration of THA and theophylline has been shown to double theophylline's elimination half-life and plasma concentration.

HP 029

History and discovery. HP 029 has been investigated as another potential treatment of AD. Animal studies demonstrate that HP 029 significantly enhances long-term potentiation (considered an electrophysiological model for memory formation within the hippocampus) (Tanaka et al. 1989). The drug also reverses scopolamine or lesion-induced memory impairment in rodents (Fielding et al. 1989).

Structure. HP 029 (velnacrine maleate) is the maleate salt of an alcohol derivative of THA (Puri et al. 1989).

Pharmacological profile. HP 029 inhibits both true cholinesterase and pseudocholinesterase and does not cause release of acetylcholine or act as a muscarinic agonist.

Pharmacokinetics and disposition. HP 029 is well absorbed after oral administration. Mean peak plasma levels are attained 0.75–1.2 hours after dosing. The mean half-life range is 1.6–2.0 hours. Most of the HP 029 is conjugated before excretion.

Indications. AD patients show marked intersubject variability in drug tolerance within the therapeutic dose range (Cutler et al. 1990). A double-blind placebo-controlled enriched population design consisting of a 7-week dose-ranging phase followed by a 6-week dose-replication phase demonstrated modest clinical improvement in a subset of the 195 patients with AD (Murphy et al. 1991).

Side effects and toxicity. Side effects of HP 029 include dizziness, diarrhea, and headache. Reversible liver toxicity is observed in a dose-dependent manner with this compound (Murphy et al. 1991).

Drug-drug interactions. No specific drug-drug interactions have been observed with HP 029 that are still undergoing clinical evaluation.

Galanthamine

History and discovery. Galanthamine has been used clinically since the early 1960s in the treatment of paresis, paralysis, and myasthenia gravis (Mihailova et al. 1989). It has also been shown to reverse spatial memory deficits in hypocholinergic mice (Sweeney et al. 1988).

Structure. Galanthamine is a tertiary amine of the phenthrene group.

Pharmacological profile. Galanthamine is a potent inhibitor of acetylcholinesterase. In vivo, maximal inhibition of acetylcholinesterase is approached 30 minutes after oral administration (Thomsen et al. 1990).

Pharmacokinetics and disposition. Galanthamine is rapidly absorbed after oral administration. Cerebral concentrations that are three times higher than its plasma level are observed after its administration. Galanthamine's half-life of 7 hours is longer than that of THA or physostigmine (Thomsen et al. 1990). Metabolites include epigalanthamine and galanthaminone (Mihailova et al. 1989).

Indications. Eighteen patients with possible AD who received galanthamine for up to 6 months showed no statistically significant improvement on neuropsychological measures (Dal-Bianco et al. 1991).

Side effects and toxicity. Administration of galanthamine has been associated with agitation, sleeplessness, and irritability (Thomsen et al. 1990).

■ Summary

Several methodological issues must be considered in interpreting the studies using cholinesterase inhibitors. Intersubject variability in bioavailability and inadequate dosing could attenuate response patterns. For example, a given dosing regimen may be less than optimal for one patient, yet therapeutic for another. Crossover designs may include carryover effects that detract from the drug's effect in comparison to placebo. Repeated assessments lead to learning effects that can erroneously inflate a patient's response to medication and can produce carryover effects with discontinuation of the drug. A perfect test would be free of such effects and would involve multiple ways of asking the relevant questions. The majority of outcome measures used in therapeutic trials assess memory, yet AD is also a disease of learning. Finally, another problem is the shifting baseline resulting from the progression of the severity of AD. The longer the study, the more this becomes a factor that needs to be addressed.

Overall, the THA studies suggest some therapeutic efficacy with this agent. The percentage of patients who improve with THA is dependent on dosing, with

50% of patients showing improvement at a dose of 80 mg/day (Farlow et al. 1992). These findings suggest that anticholinesterase therapy is likely to benefit a subgroup of AD patients.

■ Cholinergic Agonists

The use of muscarinic agonists for cognitive enhancement is supported by their beneficial effects on memory and learning in hypocholinergic animals (Haroutunian et al. 1985). The use of postsynaptic agonists is of interest because of the observed depletion of presynaptic (M2) receptors in conjunction with the relative preservation of postsynaptic (M1) sites in AD (Whitehouse and Kellar 1987).

Significant advances have been made in identifying muscarinic receptor subtypes. Research using molecular biology techniques have demonstrated the presence of five muscarinic receptor subtypes, m1 through m5 (Ashkenazi et al. 1989; Birdsall et al. 1989; Bonner 1989; Bonner et al. 1987; Fukada et al. 1989). Studies with pharmacological antagonists have identified three classes of muscarinic receptors, M1, M2, and M3. The m1–m5 and M1–M3 systems do overlap. Activation of the m1, m3, and m5 receptors causes cellular excitation, whereas activation of the m2 and m4 subtypes produces inhibitory effects (Ashkenazi et al. 1989; Bonner 1989). Although the exact locations of the m1–m5 receptors are not known, the distribution of messenger ribonucleic acid (mRNA) for these sites has been determined (Buckley et al. 1988). For example, most mRNA located in the cerebral cortex and hippocampus is for m1 and m3 receptors, making these sites potentially most important for pharmacological enhancement of cognition.

Although muscarinic receptors play a significant role in memory, there is evidence to suggest involvement of the nicotinic system in AD. The nicotinic receptors can be divided into the super-high–, high-, and low-affinity subtypes (Nordberg et al. 1992). Brains of patients with AD demonstrate decrements in the high-affinity nicotinic sites (Nordberg et al. 1992). In animal studies, the nicotinic antagonist mecamylamine produces a dose-dependent impairment of memory comparable to what is observed with scopolamine (Elrod and Buccafusco 1991).

The nicotinic and muscarinic systems appear to jointly modulate performance in learning and memory (Riekkinen et al. 1990). Animal data suggest that presynaptic nicotinic receptors mediate a positive feedback mechanism that modulates cholinergic activity (Elrod and Buccafusco 1991). Incomplete information exists regarding the contributions of different nicotinic and muscarinic subtypes in cognition and the pathophysiology of AD. To date, the development and implementation of pharmacological treatments for AD patients have not approached the basic science findings.

RS-86. RS-86 (2-ethyl-8-methyl-2,8-diazospiro-4,5-decan-1,3-dionhydrobromide) is a muscarinic receptor agonist that has a relatively higher affinity for M1 than for M2 sites.

The postsynaptic effects of RS-86 are hypothesized to enhance cholinergic neurotransmission. Oral administration of RS-86 produced minimal effects in AD patients (Wettstein and Spiegal 1984) or none at all (Bruno et al. 1985; Mouradian et al. 1988). A 2-week double-blind placebo-controlled trial including a best-dose finding phase also demonstrated no therapeutic drug effects in AD (Hollander et al. 1987).

Bethanechol. Bethanechol is a synthetic β-methyl analogue of acetylcholine. Bethanechol's agonist effects on M1 and M2 cholinergic receptors are believed to enhance cholinergic neurotransmission. Studies conducted on AD patients have reported modest improvement with this agent (Harbaugh et al. 1989; Penn et al. 1988; Read et al. 1990). Variable dose responses may contribute to the heterogeneous response patterns (Read et al. 1990). Bethanechol must be administered by an intracerebroventricular (ICV) route, because it does not cross the blood-brain barrier. ICV administration carries substantial risks, including perioperative complications, pneumocephalus, seizures, and chronic subdural hematoma (Gauthier et al. 1986; Penn et al. 1988). Thus, ICV bethanechol treatment is not a viable option for cholinergic enhancement in AD patients.

Arecoline. Arecoline is a natural alkaloid that has both muscarinic and nicotinic agonist properties. Its cholinergic agonist properties are thought to be responsible for its enhancing cholinergic transmission. Arecoline has been shown to improve learning in healthy volunteer subjects (Sitaram et al. 1978). Modest improvement in picture recognition, verbal memory, and visuospatial construction after arecoline infusion have been observed in patients with AD (Christie et al. 1981; Raffaele et al. 1991; Tariot et al. 1988a).

Oxotremorine. Oxotremorine is a synthetic cholinergic agonist with a half-life of several hours. Oxotremorine administered to AD patients produced no cognitive enhancing effects and significant side effects, including panic and depression (Davis et al. 1987).

AF102B. AF102B [(±) cis-2-methyl-spiro(1,3-oxathiolane-5,3′)quinuclidine] is a structurally rigid analogue of acetylcholine. Unlike most of the cholinergic agents described previously, AF102B is a selective M1 agonist (Potter 1987). This characteristic is desirable, because activation of the M2 autoreceptors can result in decreased acetylcholine release. In addition, M1 receptors are present in the hippocampus and cerebral cortex and may play a significant role in cognitive processes (Potter 1987). Like other cholinergic agonists, AF102B effectively reverses the cognitive impairments observed in hypocholinergic animals (Nakahara et al. 1988).

Azaspirodecanes. Azaspirodecanes (2-methyl-1,3-dioxaazaspiro[4,5]decanes) are a group of muscarinic compounds that are analogues of the tertiary amine AF-30. Some of these analogues are potent muscarinic agonists that have yet to be clinically tested (Saunders et al. 1988).

Nicotine. The reduction in nicotinic receptors in brains of AD subjects suggests the potential usefulness of strategies to provide additional stimulation of the remaining nicotinic receptors to enhance cognition in AD patients (Sugaya et al. 1990). Nicotine administration has been shown to improve both the attentional component and facilitate retention of the memory process (Warburton and Wesnes 1984). Intramuscular nicotine administration to primates improved performance on a delayed matching-to-sample task (Buccafusco and Jackson 1991).

Intravenous nicotine administration to six patients with AD has been shown to improve performance in recall (Newhouse et al. 1988). Unfortunately, the anxiety and depressive symptoms associated with nicotine administration represent toxic effects that lessen the clinical utility of this compound.

■ Summary

None of the cholinergic agonist approaches tested to date has yielded the clinical benefit initially anticipated. Yet it may very well be that the potential benefits of postsynaptic enhancement have not been adequately tested. The diverse physiological effects of muscarinic and nicotinic activation limit the clinical usefulness of the agents currently employed. Arecoline, RS-86, and bethanechol probably do not have much effect on the m1 and m3 receptor sites in the cortex (Potter et al. 1991). The importance of targeting the appropriate site is exemplified by the compound oxotremorine, which actually decreases acetylcholine release through its action on the presynaptic m2 receptor. Development of therapies that are directed specifically at the receptors involved in cognition will enhance therapeutic efficacy and avoid undesirable side effects. Future directions in cholinergic enhancement may include manipulation of specific subtypes of both the muscarinic and nicotinic receptors. Postsynaptic therapy is also limited by the fact that agonist administration provides a nonphysiological tonic stimulation, whereas the physiological state is characterized by phasic mechanisms.

■ OTHER NEUROTRANSMITTER SYSTEMS

The heterogenous nature of the neurochemical deficits in AD may significantly contribute to variable response patterns observed with anticholinesterases. Animal studies also demonstrate the involvement of multiple neurotransmitter systems in learning and memory. For example, noradrenergic brain lesions negate cholinomimetic enhancement of memory. Clonidine administration restores the efficacy of cholinomimetic treatment in animals with combined noradrenergic and cholinergic lesions (Haroutunian et al. 1990). Postmortem studies demonstrate major neurotransmitter losses of the noradrenergic and somatostatinergic systems in AD patients. These findings suggest that anticholinesterase administration (in conjunction with an agent that augments another neurotransmitter system found to be deficient in AD) may be a more appropriate strategy for some patients.

L-*Deprenyl*

History and discovery. L-Deprenyl has been used for the treatment of depression and Parkinson's disease. Use of L-deprenyl for cognitive enhancement in AD is based on the following:

1. The monoaminergic system is involved in cognitive behaviors and AD.
2. L-Deprenyl's antioxidant effect, through its inhibition of monoamine oxidase B (MAO-B), may prevent cell death.
3. L-Deprenyl interferes with the increased activity of MAO-B that is observed in AD patients (Oreland and Gottfries 1986).

Structure. L-Deprenyl [(R)-(–)-N,2-dimethyl-N-2-propynylphenethylamine hydrochloride] is a levorotatory acetylenic derivative of phenethylamine.

Pharmacological profile. L-Deprenyl is an irreversible monoamine oxidase inhibitor (MAOI) that selectively inhibits MAO-B at low doses.

Pharmacokinetics and elimination. L-Deprenyl is absorbed readily after oral administration. Three metabolites—N-desmethyl-deprenyl (mean half-life 2 hours), amphetamine (mean half-life 18 hours), and methamphetamine (mean half-life 21 hours)—are found in the serum and urine.

Indications. Four double-blind placebo-controlled trials with small patient samples suggest that subchronic treatment with L-deprenyl at 10 mg/day improves performance on attention, memory, and learning tasks (Agnoli et al. 1990; Mangoni et al. 1991; Piccinin et al. 1990; Tariot et al. 1987a, 1987b). Higher doses of L-deprenyl were not as efficacious and were associated with more side effects (Tariot et al. 1987b). The beneficial effects of L-deprenyl do not appear to result from its antidepressant action, because the MAO-A inhibitor tranylcypromine does not improve cognitive performance (Tariot et al. 1988b). The L-deprenyl results need to be replicated with larger patient samples and longer treatment trials to determine if this agent will have clinically significant effects on cognition in AD patients.

Side effects and toxicity. At low doses (10 mg/day), L-deprenyl administration is not associated with tyramine sensitivity. L-Deprenyl is well tolerated at low doses. Side effects include nausea, dizziness, abdominal discomfort, and dry mouth.

Drug-drug interactions. L-Deprenyl administration to patients on levodopa may lead to an exacerbation of levodopa-associated side effects. These effects may be reduced by lowering the dosage of levodopa.

Combined Treatment Approaches

Animal and postmortem human studies suggest that the combined treatment approach employing cholinergic-noradrenergic combinations may be more efficacious than cholinomimetic or monoaminergic agents alone. A pilot study with clonidine and physostigmine treatment in nine patients demonstrated the safety of combining these agents in AD (Davidson et al. 1989). One study noted that the combination of L-deprenyl and a cholinesterase inhibitor was superior to administration of a cholinesterase alone, whereas another investigation did not demonstrate significant cognitive improvement with the combination of physostigmine and deprenyl (Schneider et al. 1993; Sunderland et al. 1992). Inadequate physostigmine levels achieved in the latter trial may have lead to spuriously poor results. Future studies are needed to determine the potential efficacy of combination treatments.

■ NEW APPROACHES

The approaches described here generally offer palliative treatment to augment the functioning of deficient neurotransmitter systems in AD. Advances in the understanding of the biology of AD permit development of strategies that may alter its underlying pathophysiology.

Glutamatergic Agents

Glutamatergic agents have not been systematically used for the treatment of AD. However, in this section we review the rationale for and provide examples of potential glutamatergic agents for the treatment of AD.

History and background. Glutamate is the major excitatory neurotransmitter of pyramidal neurons (Fonnum 1984). The postsynaptic effects of glutamate are mediated via several different receptor subtypes. These receptors can be classified according to their prototypic agonists (i.e., N-methyl-D-aspartate [NMDA], quisqualate [QUIS], and kainate [KAIN]) (Foster and Fagg 1987).

The different receptor subtypes of the glutamatergic system have been implicated in memory processing. NMDA receptor blockade with aminophosphonopentanoic acid (AP-5) in the CA_1 region of the hippocampus prevents long-term potentiation (Collingridge and Bliss 1987). AP-5 binding to NMDA receptors disrupts spatial learning in a manner similar to what is observed with hippocampal lesioning (Morris et al. 1986). Antagonist binding to QUIS and KAIN receptors interferes with passive avoidance training in rodents (Danysz et al. 1988). Extensive loss of NMDA sites has been demonstrated in brains of AD patients (Greenamyre et al. 1985). Increased KAIN receptor binding has been observed in postmortem studies (Geddes et al. 1985). Glutamate can induce neurotoxicity (Rothman and Olney 1987). The excitatory and neurotoxic effects of glutamate can occur through both NMDA and non-NMDA receptors (Greenamyre and Young 1989). NMDA and non-NMDA antagonists protect against injury caused by ischemia (Greenamyre and Young 1989; Rothman and Olney 1987). Thus, glutamate's wide CNS distribution and its neurotoxic properties implicate it as a potential contributor to the pathogenesis of several CNS neurodegenerative disorders.

Given that glutamate can enhance learning as well as produce neurotoxicity, determination of the optimal glutamatergic strategy must consider the complex functions of glutamate and the various glutamatergic receptors. Both NMDA sites and non-NMDA sites could be potential targets for therapeutic approaches. A strategy that enhances glutamatergic transmission is supported by the presynaptic glutamatergic losses observed in AD and glutamate's role in cognition. However, excessive augmentation of glutamatergic functioning could be neurotoxic. Glutamatergic blockade could protect against neurotoxic effects yet may potentially interfere with memory processing.

Glycine Site Inhibitors

Antagonism of the glycine modulatory site of the NMDA receptor could decrease neurotoxicity mediated by glutamate. 1-Hydroxy-3-amino-2-pyrrolidone (HA-966) and L-aminocyclobutane (ACB) appear to inhibit NMDA-specific binding and block NMDA responses (Hood et al. 1989; Watson et al. 1989). The glycine antagonists kynurenic acid (KYNA) and 7-chloro-kynurenic acid (7-Cl-KYNA) do not interfere with passive avoidance in mice. These findings indicate that antagonism at the glycine site may interfere with glutamate's neurotoxicity without causing cognitive impairment (Chiamulera et al. 1991), a finding whose relevance to altering the course of AD is dependent upon glutamate's involvement in cell death in AD.

Non-NMDA Antagonists

Non-NMDA antagonism may provide a potential therapeutic strategy to decrease glutamatergic functioning and neurotoxicity. Antagonists of the non-NMDA receptors include 2,3-dihydroxy-6-nitro-7-sulfamoyl-benzo(F)quinoxaline (NBQX), 6,7-dinitroquinoxaline-2,3-dione (DNQX), and 6-cyano-7-nitroquioxaline-2,3-dione (CNQX) (Honore et al. 1988; Sheardon et al. 1990). These agents have been shown to protect against the effects of ischemia by blocking non-NMDA sites (Sheardon et al. 1990). Clinical trials are necessary to determine whether these agents can interfere with cell death and alter the course of AD.

Partial Agonists

Given the complex sequelae of glutamatergic activation, a partial agonist approach is optimal. The glycine agonist milacemide enhances learning in normal and amnestic rodents (Handelmann et al. 1989). One clinical trial of this drug, however, did not enhance cognition and was accompanied by significant liver toxicity (Pomara et al. 1991). The partial glycine agonist D-cycloserine has also been shown to reverse memory impairments caused by scopolamine in healthy subjects (Jones et al. 1992). As with other glutamatergic modulating agents, further clinical studies are necessary to test their potential efficacy.

■ Summary

Modulation of the glutamatergic system may provide several therapeutic strategies to enhance cognition and diminish neuronal toxicity observed in AD. No large-scale clinical trials have yet been conducted with glutamatergic modulators that have found these agents to prevent neuronal damage, enhance memory, and have acceptable side-effect profiles.

Antiinflammatory Agents

History and discovery. As with glutamatergic strategies, antiinflammatory agents have not been widely tested in the treatment of AD. However, basic science and epidemiological findings suggest the utility of these agents for AD treatment.

Several lines of evidence demonstrate the involvement of the immune system and inflammation in AD. Involvement of the immune system in AD and other CNS disorders refutes the long-held belief that the brain is immunologically privileged. Histochemical studies demonstrate the presence of several markers of inflammation in brains of AD subjects (Bauer et al. 1991; McGeer et al. 1989b; Styren et al. 1990). Furthermore, the immune response in the CNS has been shown to colocalize with senile plaques, suggesting a role for the immune response in the pathophysiology of AD (McGeer et al. 1989a).

Increased numbers of reactive glia and microglia (believed to be related to macrophages) have been observed in several postmortem studies of brains of AD subjects (Styren et al. 1990). Activated T lymphocytes, a hallmark of the cell-mediated response observed in chronic inflammatory states, have also been observed in postmortem studies of AD cases (McGeer et al. 1989b; Rogers et al. 1988). Complement proteins (including the membrane attack components) associated with the classical pathway have also been identified in senile plaques and tangles (McGeer et al. 1989a). The implications of the presence of complement proteins is that host cells can be inadvertently attacked and destroyed by these molecules.

Elevated concentrations of interleukins, agents that signal cell proliferation and the production of mediators of the inflammatory response, have also been noted in AD patients. Specifically, elevated concentrations of tumor necrosis factor (TNF), interleukin 1 (IL-1), and interleukin 6 (IL-6) have been demonstrated in AD patients (Altstiel and Sperber 1991; Bauer et al. 1991; Fillit et al. 1991). The role of cytokines in amyloidogenesis is supported by their ability to stimulate amyloid precursor protein (APP) synthesis (Goldgaber et al. 1989).

Acute phase proteins—inflammatory response molecules that are induced by interleukins—have also been shown to be elevated in AD (Heinrich et al. 1990). C-reactive protein, α_2-macroglobulin, and α_1 antichymotripsin (ACT) concentrations are in-creased in AD patients compared to age-matched control subjects (Abraham et al. 1988; Bauer et al. 1991; Matsubara et al. 1990; Rozmuller et al. 1990). Increased ACT concentrations are particularly intriguing, because the ACT molecule is a component of senile plaques (Bauer et al. 1991). ACT may contribute to abnormal processing of APP, leading to β-amyloid deposition (Bauer et al. 1991).

It has been suggested that the immune system response in AD originates in the CNS. Evidence to support this hypothesis includes the following:

1. Astrocyte expression of IL-1 and IL-6 receptors have been demonstrated (Frei et al. 1989; Guilian et al. 1986).
2. IL-6 induces neurite formation in pheochromocytoma cell lines (Satoh et al. 1988), suggesting the presence of IL-6 receptors on neurons.
3. Microglia and astrocytes can secrete IL-1 and IL-6, respectively (Frei et al. 1989).

The question that needs to be answered is what CNS events cause cytokine production. It is not known whether local brain injury, an immunological process, or an autoimmune phenomenon induces the acute phase response. Nonetheless, there definitely is an immune response in AD that could lead to cell death and enhance β-amyloid deposition. These data suggest that anti-inflammatory therapy may slow progression of the illness.

Evidence suggests that chronic exposure to antiinflammatory agents is protective against the development of AD. The prevalence of AD among patients at rheumatoid arthritis clinics—a population likely to have received chronic antiinflammatory therapy—was shown to be significantly less than that observed in the general population over age 64 (McGeer et al. 1992a). Elderly leprosy patients who had been treated with the antiinflammatory agent dapsone had significantly lower rates of dementia than that observed in drug-free patients (McGeer et al. 1992b). A 6-month double-blind trial with the nonsteroidal antiinflammatory agent indomethacin documented that the conditions of AD patients who received active drug declined significantly less than those of patients who received placebo (Rogers et al. 1988). Future studies with antiinflammatory agents in AD patients are necessary to determine the usefulness of antiinflammatory strategies.

■ CONCLUSION

Several strategies for cognitive enhancement have been attempted with AD patients. An adequate acetylcholinesterase inhibitor has not yet been tested with all the necessary parameters. Combined neuro-transmitter therapies have also not been adequately tested to determine the level of efficacy that could be achieved with this approach. Strategies to delay progression of AD are now being explored and may provide the most effective means to treat the cognitive deterioration observed in patients with AD.

■ REFERENCES

Abraham CR, Selkoe DJ, Potter H: Immuno-histochemical identification of the serine protease inhibitor alpha-1 antichymotrypsin in the brain amyloid deposits of Alzheimer's disease. Cell 52:487–501, 1988

Adem A: Putative mechanisms of action of tacrine in Alzheimer's disease. Acta Neurol Scand 139:69–74, 1992

Agnoli A, Martucci N, Fabbrini G, et al: Monoamine oxidase and dementia: treatment with an inhibitor of MAO-B activity. Dementia 1:109–114, 1990

Altstiel LD, Sperber K: Cytokines in Alzheimer's disease. Prog Neuropsychopharmacol Biol Psychiatry 15:481–495, 1991

Ashkenazi A, Peralta EG, Winslow JW, et al: Functional diversity of muscarinic receptor subtypes in cellular signal transduction and growth. Trends Pharmacol Sci Suppl 10:16–22, 1989

Bartus RT, Dean RL, Pontecorvo MJ, et al: The cholinergic hypothesis: a historical overview, current perspective and future directions. Ann N Y Acad Sci 444:332–358, 1985

Bartus RT, Dean RL, Flicker C: Cholinergic psychopharmacology: an integration of human and animal research on memory, in Psychopharmacology: The Third Generation of Progress. Edited by Meltzer HY. New York, Raven, 1987, pp 219–232

Bauer J, Strauss S, Schreiter-Gasser U, et al: Interleukin-6 and alpha-2-macroglobulin indicate an acute phase response in the Alzheimer's disease cortices. FEBS Lett 285:111–114, 1991

Beller SA, Overall JE, Rhoades HM, et al: Long term outpatient treatment of senile dementia with oral physostigmine. J Clin Psychiatry 49:400–404, 1988

Birdsall N, Buckley N, Doods H: Nomenclature for muscarinic receptor subtypes recommended by symposium. Trends Pharmacol Sci Suppl 10:7, 1989

Bonner TI: New subtypes of muscarinic acetylcholine receptors. Trends Pharmacol Sci Suppl 10:11–15, 1989

Bonner TI, Buckley A, Young AC, et al: Identification of a family of muscarinic acetylcholine receptor genes. Science 237:527–532, 1987

Bruno G, Mohr E, Gillepsie M, et al: RS-86 therapy of Alzheimer's disease. Arch Neurol 43:659–661, 1985

Buccafusco JJ, Jackson W: Beneficial effects of nicotine administered prior to a delayed matching-to-sample task in young and aged monkeys. Neurobiol Aging 12:233–238, 1991

Buckley NJ, Bonner TI, Brann MR: Localization of a family of muscarinic receptor mRNAs in rat brain. J Neurosci 4646–4652, 1988

Chatellier G, Lacomblez L: Tacrine (tetrahydro-aminoacridine; THA) and lecithin in senile dementia of the Alzheimer's type: a multi-center trial. BMJ 300:495–499, 1990

Chiamulera C, Costa S, Reggiani A: Effect of NMDA and strychnine-insensitive glycine site antagonist on NMDA-mediated convulsions and learning. Psychopharmacology 102:551–552, 1991

Christie JE, Shering A, Ferguson J, et al: Physostigmine and arecoline: effects of intravenous infusions in Alzheimer's presenile dementia. Br J Psychiatry 138:46–50, 1981

Collerton D: Cholinergic function and intellectual decline in Alzheimer's disease. Neuroscience 19:1–28, 1986

Collingridge GL, Bliss TVP: NMDA receptors—their role in long-term potentiation. Trends Neurosci 10:288–293, 1987

Cutler NR, Murphy MF, Nash RJ, et al: Clinical safety, tolerance and plasma levels of the oral anticholinesterase 1,2,3,4-tetrahydro-9-aminoacradin-l-olmaleate (HP 029) in Alzheimer's disease: preliminary findings. J Clin Pharmacol 39:556–561, 1990

Dal-Bianco P, Maly J, Wober C, et al: Galanthamine treatment in Alzheimer's disease. J Neural Transm Suppl 33:59–63, 1991

Danysz W, Wroblewski JT, Costa E: Learning impairment in rats by N-methyl-D-aspartate receptor antagonist. Neuropharmacology 27:653–656, 1988

Davidson M, Bierer LM, Kaminsky R, et al: Combined

administration of physostigmine and clonidine to patients with dementia of the Alzheimer type: a pilot safety study. Alzheimer Dis Assoc Disord 1:1–4, 1989

Davies P, Maloney AJ: Selective loss of central cholinergic neurons in Alzheimer's disease. Lancet 2:1403–1405, 1976

Davis KL, Hollander E, Davidson M, et al: Induction of depression with oxotremorine in Alzheimer's disease patients. Am J Psychiatry 144:468–471, 1987

Davis KL, Thal LJ, Gamzu ER, et al: A double blind, placebo-controlled multicenter study of tacrine in Alzheimer's disease. N Engl J Med 327:1253–1259, 1992

Deutsch JA: The cholinergic synapse and the site of memory. Science 174:788–794, 1971

Drachman DA, Leavitt J: Human memory and the cholinergic system. Arch Neurol 30:113–121, 1974

Drukarch B, Kits S, Van der Meer EG, et al: 9-amino-1,2,3,4-tetrahydroacridine (THA), an alleged drug for the treatment of Alzheimer's disease, inhibits acetylcholinesterase activity and slows outward K^+ current. Eur J Pharmacol 141:153–157, 1987

Drukarch B, Leysen JE, Stoof JC: Further analysis of the neuropharmacological profile of 9-amino-1,2,3,4-tetrahydroacridine (THA), an alleged drug for the treatment of Alzheimer's disease. Life Sci 42:1011–1017, 1988

Dundee JW, Pandit SK: Anterograde amnesic effects of pethidine, hyoscine, and diazepam in adults. Br J Pharmacol 44:140–144, 1972

Elrod K, Buccafusco JJ: Correlation of the amnestic effects of nicotinic antagonists with inhibition of regional brain acetylcholine synthesis in rats. J Pharmacol Exp Ther 258:403–409, 1991

Farlow M, Gracon SI, Hershey LA, et al: A controlled trial of tacrine in Alzheimer's disease. JAMA 268:2523–2529, 1992

Fielding S, Cornfeldt ML, Szewczak MR, et al: HP-029, a new drug for the treatment of Alzheimer's disease: its pharmacological profile. Paper presented at the 4th World Conference on Clinical Pharmacology and Therapeutics, West Berlin, July 28–30, 1989

Fillit H, Ding W, Buee L, et al: Elevated circulating tumor necrosis factor levels in Alzheimer's disease. Neurosci Lett 129:318–320, 1991

Folstein MF, Folstein SE, McHugh PR: Mini-Mental State: a practical method for grading the cognitive state of patients for the clinician. J Psychiatr Res 12:189–198, 1975

Fonnum F: Glutamate: a neurotransmitter in mammalian brain. J Neurochem 42:1–11, 1984

Foster AC, Fagg GE: Taking apart the NMDA receptor. Nature 329:395–396, 1987

Frei K, Malipiero UV, Leist TP, et al: On the cellular source and function of interleukin 6 produced in the central nervous system in viral diseases. Eur J Immunol 19:689–694, 1989

Fukada K, Kubo T, Maeda A, et al: Selective effector coupling of muscarinic acetylcholine receptor subtypes. Trends Pharmacol Sci Suppl 10:4–10, 1989

Gauthier S, Leblanc R, Quirion R, et al: Transmitter-replacement therapy in Alzheimer's disease using intracerebroventricular infusions of receptor agonists. Can J Neurol Sci 13:394–402, 1986

Gauthier S, Bouchard R, Lamontagne A, et al: Tetrahydroaminoacridine-lecithin combination treatment in patients with intermediate-stage Alzheimer's disease. N Engl J Med 1272–1276, 1990

Geddes JW, Monaghan DT, Cotman CW, et al: Plasticity of hippocampal circuitry in Alzheimer's disease. Science 230:1179–1181, 1985

Goldgaber D, Harris H, Hal T, et al: Interleukin-1 regulates synthesis of amyloid beta protein precursor mRNA in human endothelial cells. Proc Natl Acad Sci U S A 86:7606–7610, 1989

Greenamyre JT, Young AB: Excitatory amino acids and Alzheimer's disease. Neurobiol Aging 10:593–602, 1989

Greenamyre JT, Penney JB, Young AB: Alterations in L-glutamate binding in Alzheimer's and Huntington's diseases. Science 227:1496–1498, 1985

Guilian D, Baker TJ, Shin LN, et al: Interleukin-1 of the central nervous system is produced by ameboid microglia. J Exp Med 164:594–604, 1986

Guy W (ed): Clinical Global Assessment Scale (CGI), in ECDEU Assessment Manual for Psychopharmacology (DHEW Publ No ADM-76-338). Washington, DC, U.S. Government Printing Office, 1976, pp 218–222

Handelmann GE, Nevins ME, Mueller LL, et al: Milacemide, a glycine prodrug, enhances performance of learning tasks in normal and amnestic rodents. Pharmacol Biochem Behav 34:823–838, 1989

Haroutunian V, Kanof PD, Davis KL: Pharmacological alleviation of cholinergic lesion induced memory deficits in rats. Life Sci 37:945–952, 1985

Haroutunian V, Kanof PD, Tsuboyama G, et al: Restoration of cholinomimetic activity by clonidine in cholinergic plus adrenergic lesioned rats. Brain Res 507:261–266, 1990

Harbaugh RE, Reeder TM, Senter HJ, et al: Intracerebroventricular bethanechol chloride administration in Alzheimer's disease: results of a collaborative double blind study. J Neurosurg 71:481–486, 1989

Heinrich PC, Castell JV, Andus T: Interleukin-6 and the acute phase response. Biochem J 265:621–636, 1990

Hollander E, Davidson M, Mohs RC, et al: RS 86 in the treatment of Alzheimer's disease: cognitive and biological effects. Biol Psychiatry 22:1067–1078, 1987

Honore T, Davies SN, Drejer J, et al: Quinoxalinediones: potent competitive non-NMDA glutamate receptor antagonist. Science 241:701–703, 1988

Hood WF, Sun ET, Compton RP, et al: 1-Aminocyclobutane 1-carboxylate (ACBC): a specific antagonist of the N-methyl-D-aspartate receptor coupled glycine receptor. Eur J Pharmacol 161:281–282, 1989

Jenike MA, Albert MS, Baer L: Oral physostigmine as treatment for Alzheimer's disease: a long term outpatient trial. Alzheimer Dis Assoc Disord 4:226–231, 1990

Jones RW, Wesnes KA, Kirby J: Effects of NMDA modulation in scopolamine dementia. Ann N Y Acad Sci 64:241–244, 1992

Kaye WH, Sitaram H, Weingartner H, et al: Modest facilitation of memory in dementia with combined lecithin and anticholinesterase treatment. Biol Psychiatry 17:275–280, 1982

Mangoni A, Grassi MP, Frattola L, et al: Effects of a MAO-B inhibitor in the treatment of Alzheimer disease. Eur Neurol 31:100–107, 1991

Matsubara E, Hirai S, Amari M, et al: Alpha-1 antichymotrypsin as a possible biochemical marker for Alzheimer-type dementia. Ann Neurol 28:561–567, 1990

McGeer PL, Akiyama H, Itagaki S, et al: Activation of the classical complement pathway in brain tissue of Alzheimer patients. Neurosci Lett 107:341–346, 1989a

McGeer PL, Akiyama H, Itagaki S, et al: Immune system response in Alzheimer's disease. Can J Neurol Sci 16:516–527, 1989b

McGeer PL, McGeer EG, Rogers J, et al: Does anti-inflammatory treatment protect against Alzheimer's disease? in Alzheimer's Disease: New Treatment Strategies. Edited by Khachaturian ZS, Blass JP. New York, Marcel Dekker, 1992a, pp 165–171

McGeer PL, Harada N, Kimura H, et al: Prevalence of dementia amongst elderly Japanese with leprosy: apparent effect of chronic drug therapy. Dementia 3:146–149, 1992b

Mihailova D, Yamboliev I, Zhivkova Z, et al: Pharmacokinetics of galanthamine hydrobromide after single subcutaneous and oral dosage in humans. Pharmacology 39:50–58, 1989

Mohs RC, Davis KL: The experimental pharmacology of Alzheimer's disease and related dementias, in Psychopharmacology: The Third Generation of Progress. Edited by Meltzer HY. New York, Raven, 1987, pp 921–928

Morris RGM, Anderson E, Lynch GS, et al: Selective impairment of learning and blockade of long-term potentiation by an N-methyl-D-aspartate receptor antagonist, AP5. Nature 319:774–776, 1986

Mouradian MM, Mohr E, Williams AJ, et al: No response to high dose muscarinic agonist therapy in Alzheimer's disease. Neurology 38:606–608, 1988

Murphy MF, Hardiman ST, Nash RJ, et al: Evaluation of HP 029 (Velnacrine Maleate) in Alzheimer's disease. Ann N Y Acad Sci 640:253–262, 1991

Nakahara N, Iga Y, Mizobe F, et al: Amelioration of experimental amnesia (passive avoidance failure) in rodents by selective M[1] agonist AF102B. Jpn J Pharmacol 48:502–505, 1988

Newhouse PA, Sunderland T, Tariot PN, et al: Intravenous nicotine in Alzheimer's disease: a pilot study. Psychopharmacology (Berl) 95:171–175, 1988

Nielsen JA, Mena JEE, Williams IH, et al: correlation of brain levels of 9-amino-1,2,3,4-tetrahydroaminoacridine (THA) with neurochemical and behavioral changes. Eur J Pharmacol 173:53–64, 1989

Nordberg A, Alafuzoff I, Winblad B: Nicotinic and muscarinic subtypes in the human brain: changes with aging and dementia. J Neurosci Res 31:103–111, 1992

Olton DS, Wenk GL: Dementia: animal models of the cognitive impairments produced by degeneration of the basal forebrain cholinergic system, in Psychopharmacology: The Third Generation of Progress. Edited by Meltzer HY. New York, Raven, 1987, pp 941–953

Oreland L, Gottfries CG: Brain and monoamine oxidase in aging and in dementia of Alzheimer's type. Prog Neuropsychopharmacol Biol Psychiatry 10:533–540, 1986

Penn RD, Martin EM, Wilson RS, et al: Intraventricular bethanechol infusion in Alzheimer's disease: results of double blind and escalating dose trials. Neurology 38:219–222, 1988

Perry EK, Perry RH, Blessed G, et al: Necropsy evidence of central cholinergic deficits in senile dementia. Lancet 1:189, 1977

Perry EK, Tomlinson BE, Blessed G, et al: Correlation of cholinergic abnormalities with senile plaques and mental test scores in senile dementia. British Medical Journal 2:1457–1459, 1978

Piccinin FL, Finali G, Piccirilli M: Neuropsychological effects of L-deprenyl in Alzheimer's type dementia. Clin Neuropharmacol 13:147–163, 1990

Pomara N, Mendels J, Lewitt PA, et al: Multicenter trial of milacemide in the treatment of Alzheimer's disease. Biol Psychiatry 29 (suppl):718, 1991

Potter LT: Muscarinic receptors in the cortex and hippocampus in relation to the treatment of Alzheimer's disease, in International Symposium on Muscarinic Cholinergic Mechanisms. Edited by Cohen S, Sokolovsky M. London, Freud Publishing Ltd, 1987, pp 294–301

Potter LT, Ballesteros LA, Bichajian LH, et al: Evidence of paired M2 muscarinic receptors. Mol Pharmacol 39:211–212, 1991

Puri SK, Hsu R, Ho I: Single dose safety, tolerance and pharmacokinetics of HP 029 in healthy young men: a potential Alzheimer's agent. J Clin Pharmacol 29:278–284, 1989

Raffaele KC, Berardi A, Morris P, et al: Effects of acute infusion of the muscarinic cholinergic agonist arecoline on verbal and visuo-spatial function in dementia of the Alzheimer type. Prog Neuropsychopharmacol Biol Psychiatry 15:643–648, 1991

Read SL, Frazee J, Shapira J, et al: Intracerebroventricular bethanechol for Alzheimer's disease: variable dose-related responses. Arch Neurol 47:1025–1030, 1990

Riekkinen P Jr, Sirvio J, Aaltonen M, et al: Effects of concurrent manipulations of nicotinic and muscarinic receptors on spatial and passive avoidance learning. Pharmacol Biochem Behav 54:405–410, 1990

Rogers J, Luber-Narod J, Styren SD, et al: Expression of immune-system-associated antigens by cells of the human central nervous system:relationship to the pathology of Alzheimer's disease. Neurobiol Aging 9:339–349, 1988

Rosen WG, Mohs RC, Davis K: A new rating scale for Alzheimer's disease. Am J Psychiatry 141:1356–1364, 1984

Rothman SM, Olney JW: Excitoxicity and the NMDA receptor. Trends Neurosci 7:299–302, 1987

Rozmuller JM, Stam FC, Eikelenboom P: Acute phase proteins are present in amorphous plaques in the cerebral but not in the cerebellar cortex of patients with Alzheimer's disease. Neurosci Lett 109:75–78, 1990

Satoh T, Makamura S, Taga T, et al: Induction of neuronal differentiation in PC12 cells by B-cell stimulatory factor 2/interleukin 6. Mol Cell Biol 8:3546–3549, 1988

Saunders J, Showell GA, Snow J, et al: 2-methyl-1, 3-dioxaazaspiro[4, 5]decanes as novel muscarinic cholinergic agonists. J Med Chem 31:487–491, 1988

Schneider LS, Olin JT, Pawluczyk S: A double blind crossover pilot study of L-deprenyl (Selegiline) combined with cholinesterase inhibitors in Alzheimer's disease. Am J Psychiatry 150:321–323, 1993

Sheardon MJ, Nielsoen EO, Hansen AJ, et al: 2,3-Dihydroxy-6-nitro-7-sulfamoyl-benzo(F)quinoxaline: a neuroprotectant for cerebral ischemia. Science 247:571–574, 1990

Sitaram N, Weingartner H, Gillin JC: Human serial learning: enhancement with arecoline and impairment with scopolamine correlated with performance on placebo. Science 201:274–276, 1978

Styren SD, Civin WH, Rogers J: Molecular cellular and pathologic characterization of HLA-DR immunoreactivity in normal elderly and Alzheimer's disease brain. Exp Neurol 110:93–104, 1990

Sugaya K, Giacobini E, Chiappinelli VA: Nicotinic acetylcholine receptor subtypes in human frontal cortex:changes in Alzheimer's disease. J Neurosci Res 27:349–359, 1990

Summers WK, Viesselman JO, Marsh GM, et al: Use of THA in treatment of Alzheimer-like dementia: pilot study in twelve patients. Biol Psychiatry 16:145–153, 1981

Summers WK, Majovski LV, Marsh GM, et al: Oral tetrahydroaminoacridine in long term treatment of senile dementia of the Alzheimer type. N Engl J Med 315:1241–1245, 1986

Summers WK, Koehler AL, Marsh GM, et al: Long-term hepatoxicity of tacrine. Lancet 1:729, 1989

Sunderland T, Molchan S, Lawlor B, et al: A strategy of "combination chemotherapy" in Alzheimer's disease: rationale and preliminary results with physostigmine plus deprenyl. Int Psychogeriatr 4 (suppl 2):291–309, 1992

Sweeney JE, Hohmann CF, Moran TM, et al: A long-acting cholinesterase inhibitor reverses spatial memory deficits in mice. Pharmacol Biochem Behav 31:141–147, 1988

Tanaka Y, Sakurai M, Hayashi S: Effect of scopolamine and HP 029, a cholinesterase inhibitor, on long term potentiation in hippocampal slices of the guinea pig. Neurosci Lett 98:179–183, 1989

Tariot PN, Cohen RM, Sunderland T, et al: L-Deprenyl in Alzheimer's disease. Arch Gen Psychiatry 44:427–433, 1987a

Tariot PN, Sunderland T, Weingartner H, et al: Cognitive effects of L-deprenyl in Alzheimer's disease. Psychopharmacology (Berl) 91:489–495, 1987b

Tariot PN, Cohen RM, Welkowitz JA, et al: Multiple-dose arecoline infusions in Alzheimer's disease. Arch Gen Psychiatry 45:901–905, 1988a

Tariot PN, Sunderland T, Cohen RM, et al: Tranylcypromine compared with L-deprenyl in Alzheimer's

disease. J Clin Psychopharmacol 8:23–27, 1988b

Thomsen T, Bickel U, Fischer JP, et al: Stereoselectivity of cholinesterase inhibition by galanthamine and tolerance in humans. Eur J Clin Pharmacol 39:603–605, 1990

Warburton DM, Wesnes K: Drugs as research tools in psychology: Cholinergic drugs and information processing. Neuropsychobiology 11:121–132, 1984

Watson GB, Bolanowski MA, Baganoff MP, et al: Glycine antagonist action of 1-aminocyclobutane-1-carboxylate (ACBC) in *Xenopus* oocytes injected with rat brain mRNA. Eur J Pharmacol 167:291–294, 1989

Wettstein A, Spiegal R: Clinical studies with the cholinergic drug RS-86 in Alzheimer's disease (AD) and senile dementia of the Alzheimer type (SDAT). Psychopharmacology (Berl) 84:572–573, 1984

Whelpton R, Hurst P: Bioavailability of oral physostigmine [letter]. N Engl J Med 313:1293–1294, 1985

Whitehouse PJ, Kellar KJ: Nicotinic and muscarinic cholinergic receptors in Alzheimer's disease and related disorders. J Neural Transm Suppl 24:175–182, 1987

Sedative-Hypnotics

Seiji Nishino, M.D., Ph.D., Emmanuel Mignot, M.D., Ph.D., and William C. Dement, M.D., Ph.D.

I n this chapter, we examine some of the pharmacological properties of barbiturates, benzodiazepines, and other sedative-hypnotic compounds. Sedative drugs moderate excitement, decrease activity, and induce calmness, whereas hypnotic drugs produce drowsiness and facilitate the onset and maintenance of a state resembling natural sleep in its electroencephalographic characteristics. Although these agents have the effects of central nervous system (CNS) depressants, they usually produce therapeutic effects at far lower doses than those causing substantial generalized depression of CNS, such as induction of coma.

Some sedative-hypnotic drugs retain other therapeutic uses, such as muscle relaxants (especially benzodiazepines), antiepileptics, and preanesthetic medication. Although the benzodiazepines are used widely as antianxiety drugs, it is still not certain whether their effect on anxiety is truly distinct from their effect on sleepiness.

The sedative-hypnotics are of significant interest to neuroscientists. These substances seem to be able to selectively modulate basic behaviors such as arousal and stress response. An understanding of these actions will help elucidate neurochemical and neurophysiological control of these behaviors.

■ BARBITURATES

■ History

Before 1900, a few agents such as bromide, chloral hydrate, paraldehyde, urethan, and sulfonal were used as sedatives and hypnotics. Barbital, one of the derivatives of barbituric acid, was introduced in 1903 and soon became extremely popular in clinical medicine because of its sleep-inducing and anxiolytic effects (Maynert 1965). In 1912, phenobarbital was introduced. In addition to its use as a sedative-hypnotic, phenobarbital has become one of the most important pharmacological treatments for epilepsy. Since then, more than 2,500 barbiturate analogues have been synthesized, about 50 of which have been made commercially available and only 20 of which are still on the market.

The success of the partial separation of anticonvulsant from sedative-hypnotic properties led to the development of nonsedative anticonvulsants such as phenytoin in the late 1930s and trimethadione in the early 1940s. The success of barbiturates as sedative-hypnotics was largely overshadowed by the discovery of benzodiazepines in the late 1960s. With pharmacological properties very similar to those of

405

barbiturates, these compounds have a much safer pharmacological profile. Benzodiazepines have therefore replaced barbiturates in many of these areas, especially in psychiatric cases in which there is a possibility of suicide.

■ Structure-Activity Relations

Barbituric acid (2,4,6-trioxohexahydropyrimidine) is the parent compound of the barbiturates. This structure lacks central depressant activity, but if alkyl or aryl groups are present at position 5, sedative-hypnotic properties are conferred (Figure 20–1).

Compounds with side chains exceeding 6–7 carbon atoms lose their hypnotic activity and have a convulsant effect. In contrast, introduction of aryl or reactive alkyl side chains impairs anticonvulsant activity (Rall 1990).

The barbituric acid derivatives do not dissolve readily in water but are quite soluble in nonpolar solvents, a feature they share with most other organic compounds that depress the CNS. In general, structural changes that increase liposolubility also decrease duration of action, decrease latency to onset of activity, accelerate metabolic degradation, and often increase hypnotic potency.

Derivatives with large aliphatic groups at position 5 have greater activity than those with methyl groups, but shorter duration of action. However, groups larger than seven carbons tend to confer convulsant activity. Methylation of the 1-N atom increases liposolubility and shortens duration of action, and desmethylation may increase the duration of action (Rall 1990).

■ Pharmacokinetics and Disposition

For hypnotic use, barbiturates are usually administered orally. Barbiturates are rapidly absorbed in the stomach, and their absorption decreases when the stomach is full. The sodium salts are more rapidly absorbed than the free acids because of rapid dissolution.

The main metabolic pathway of barbiturates is in the liver. Oxidation of the larger of the two side chains at position 5 is the major pathway and generally produces inactive polar metabolites that are rapidly excreted in the urine (Rall 1990). Thus, changes in liver function can markedly alter the rate at which these compounds are inactivated. On the contrary, even quite low or infrequent doses of barbiturates can stimulate the activity of liver degradation enzymes, leading to tolerance (see the section "Drug-Drug Interactions").

The rate of penetration of barbiturates into the CNS varies according to their lipophilicity. In general, liposolubility decreases latency to onset of action and makes compounds shorter-lasting ones. Thiopentone, for example, enters the CNS rapidly and is used to rapidly induce anesthesia, whereas barbitone crosses into the brain so slowly that it is inappropriate as a hypnotic.

■ Pharmacology

The main effects of barbiturates are sedation, sleep induction, and anesthesia. Some of the barbiturates such as phenobarbital also have selective anticonvulsant properties. The mechanisms of action of barbiturates are complex and still not fully understood. Nonanesthetic doses of barbiturates preferentially suppress polysynaptic responses. Pertinent to their sedative-hypnotic effects is the fact that the mesencephalic reticular activating system is extremely sensi-

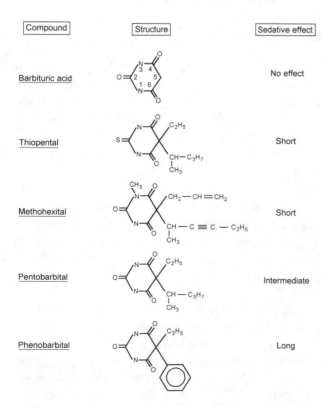

Figure 20–1. Structure-activity relationships among barbiturates.

tive to these drugs (Killam 1962). The synaptic site of inhibition is either postsynaptic (e.g., at cortical and cerebellar pyramidal cells and in the cuneate nucleus, substantia nigra, and thalamus relay neurons) or presynaptic (e.g., in the spinal cord). This inhibition occurs only at synapses where physiological inhibition is γ-aminobutyric acid (GABA)ergic and not glycinergic or monoaminergic. Thus barbiturates, like benzodiazepines, potentiate GABA-mediated inhibitory processes in the brain. However, it is still unclear whether all of the effects of barbiturates are entirely mediated by GABAergic mechanisms.

Barbiturates do not displace benzodiazepines from their binding sites; instead, they enhance benzodiazepine binding by increasing the affinity of the receptor for benzodiazepines (Leeb-Lumberg et al. 1980). They also enhance the binding of GABA and its agonists to specific binding sites (Asano and Ogasawara 1981). These effects are almost completely dependent on the presence of chloride or other anions known to permeate through chloride channels associated with the GABA receptor complex, and they are competitively antagonized by picrotoxin, a convulsant (Olsen et al. 1978). Taken together, these observations suggest that the macromolecular complex composed of $GABA_A$-ergic receptors, chloride ionophores, and binding sites for benzodiazepines (ω-site) is an important site of action for depressant barbiturates.

Although both barbiturates and benzodiazepines are capable of potentiating the GABA-induced increase in chloride conductance, barbiturates appear to increase the duration of the open state of chloride channels regulated by $GABA_A$-ergic receptors. In contrast, benzodiazepines increase the frequency of channel openings with little effect on duration. It has been suggested that barbiturates may prolong the activation of the channel by acting directly on the ion channel (Enna and Möhler 1987; Richter and Holman 1982).

Effects on stages of sleep. Barbiturates decrease sleep latency; however, they slightly increase fast electroencephalographic activity and decrease body movement during sleep. Stage 2 sleep is increased, while Stages 3 and 4 (slow wave sleep [SWS]) are generally shortened, except in some patients with anxiety and in patients who are addicted to barbiturates. Rapid eye movement (REM) sleep latency is prolonged, and the total time spent in REM sleep and the number of REM cycles (i.e., REM density) are both diminished. With repeated nightly administration, drug tolerance to the effects on sleep occurs in a few days. Discontinuation of barbiturates may lead to insomnia (mainly a decrease in Stage 2 sleep), with increases of REM sleep (Kay et al. 1976).

■ Indications

Although clinical trials have shown that the barbiturates have sedative and hypnotic properties, they generally compare poorly with benzodiazepines. The patient feels "drugged" the next day, and there is always the risk of fatal overdose because of the depressant effect on respiration. As a result, many clinicians have stopped using barbiturates as hypnotics and sedatives (except to treat severe psychomotor excitation) and prescribe them only as anticonvulsants.

Barbiturates suppress respiration, and their therapeutic dose may cause fatal respiratory depression in sleep apnea patients. Patients with sleep apnea should therefore avoid taking barbiturates.

Barbiturates have also been used intravenously to facilitate interviewing patients (i.e., amobarbital interview). This technique is also helpful in 1) mobilizing catatonic patients who are in a stupor, 2) aiding the diagnosis of intellectual impairment, and 3) lessening disturbance associated with previous negative experiences (i.e., abreactions).

These drugs are contraindicated in patients with porphyria because barbiturates enhance porphyrin synthesis. Liver function should be checked before and during drug administration. Liver dysfunction can significantly prolong the sedative effects of these drugs and may lead to overdose.

■ Side Effects and Toxicology

In treating many patients who are prescribed barbiturates, it is difficult to control symptoms without oversedation. Patients typically oscillate between anxiety and torpor. Mental performance is usually impaired, and patients should not drive or operate dangerous machinery.

Patients who have been stabilized for years on barbiturates must be considered dependent. Withdrawal leads to anxiety, agitation, trembling, and even convulsions. Substitution of a benzodiazepine that can be withdrawn more easily later is often successful.

In some patients, barbiturates repeatedly produce excitement rather than depression (i.e., paradoxical excitement), and the patients may appear to be intoxicated.

Hypersensitive reactions (especially of the skin) sometimes occur, and instances of megaloblastic anemia has been reported.

Overdosage. An overdose of barbiturates leads to fatal respiratory and cardiovascular depression. Suicide attempts frequently involve overdoses of barbiturates, either taken alone or in combination with alcohol or other psychotropic drugs, particularly tricyclic antidepressants. These suicide attempts are often successful.

Depending on factors such as proximity to a hospital and expertise of staff in intensive emergency care, death occurs in 0.5%–10% of overdose cases. Severe poisoning is likely at 10 times the hypnotic dose, and twice that amount may be fatal.

■ Tolerance and Dependence

Tolerance to barbiturates occurs rapidly and is due both to pharmacokinetic factors (e.g., liver-enzyme induction) and to pharmacodynamic factors (e.g., neuronal adaptation to chronic drug administration). Cross-tolerance develops with alcohol, gas anesthetics, and other sedatives, including benzodiazepines.

Psychological dependence (i.e., drug-seeking behavior) is common. Patients will visit several physicians to obtain more barbiturates. Physical dependence may be induced by doses of 500 mg/day. Intoxication may occur, as evidenced by impaired mental functioning, emotional instability, and neurological signs. Abrupt discontinuation after high dosage is likely to induce convulsions and delirium. After normal dosage, withdrawal phenomena include anxiety, insomnia, restlessness, agitation, tremor, muscle twitching, nausea and vomiting, orthostatic hypotension, and weight loss.

■ Drug-Drug Interactions

Barbiturates used with other CNS depressants can cause severe depression. Ethanol is the drug most frequently used, and interactions with antihistaminic compounds are also common. Monoamine oxidase inhibitors and methylphenidate also increase the CNS-depressant effect of barbiturates.

Barbiturates may increase the activity of hepatic microsomal enzymes two- or threefold. Clinically, this change is particularly important for patients who are also receiving metabolic competitors such as warfarin or digitoxin, for which careful control of plasma concentrations is vital (Rall 1990).

■ BENZODIAZEPINES

■ History

Benzodiazepines were first synthesized in the 1930s but were not systematically evaluated until 20 years later. The introduction of chlorpromazine and meprobamate in the early 1950s, which had sedative effects in animals, led to increasingly sophisticated methods being used to evaluate the behavioral effects of benzodiazepines in animals. Since the introduction of chlordiazepoxide (which was synthesized by Sternbach in 1957) into clinical medicine, more than 3,000 benzodiazepines have been synthesized. About 40 are in clinical use.

Recently, several drugs chemically unrelated to the benzodiazepines have been shown to have sedative-hypnotic effects with a benzodiazepine-like profile, and it has been demonstrated that these drugs act through the benzodiazepine receptor.

Most of the benzodiazepines on the market were selected for their high anxiolytic potential relative to CNS depression. Nevertheless, the benzodiazepines all possess sedative-hypnotic properties to various degrees, and the compounds that facilitate sleep have been used as hypnotics.

Mainly because of their remarkably low capacity to produce fatal CNS depression, benzodiazepines have displaced barbiturates as sedative-hypnotic agents.

■ Structure-Activity Relations

The term *benzodiazepine* refers to the portion of the structure composed of a benzene ring (A) fused to a seven-member diazepine ring (B) (Figure 20–2). However, most of the older benzodiazepines contain a 5-aryl substituent (ring C) and a 1,4-diazepine ring, and the term has come to mean 1,4-benzodiazepines.

A substituent (most often chloride) at position 7 is essential for biological activity. A carbonyl at position 2 enhances activity and is generally present.

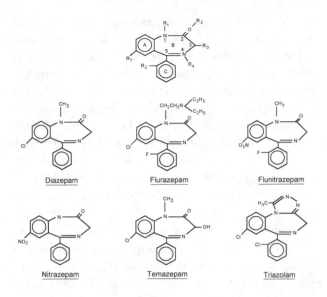

Figure 20–2. Chemical structure of some commonly used benzodiazepines.

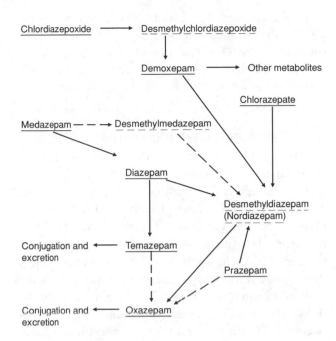

Figure 20–3. Metabolic pathways of some 1,4-benzodiazepines (solid and broken arrows denote major and minor pathways, respectively; commercially available drugs are underscored). Flunazepam, flunitrazepam, nitrazepam, and triazolam have separate metabolic pathways.

Most of the newest products also substitute the 2′ position, as with flurazepam. These general features are important for the metabolic fate of the compounds. Because the 7 and 2′ positions of the molecule are resistant to the major degradative pathways, many of the metabolites retain substantial pharmacological activity.

■ **Pharmacokinetics and Disposition**

Benzodiazepines are generally absorbed rapidly and completely. Plasma binding is high (i.e., about 98% for diazepam). Benzodiazepines are very lipophilic (except for oxazepam), and penetration into the brain is rapid.

The major metabolic pathways for the 1,4-benzodiazepines are shown in Figure 20–3. Medazepam is metabolized to diazepam, which in turn is N-demethylated to desmethyldiazepam. Chlordiazepoxide is also partly converted to desmethyldiazepam. Clorazepate is transformed to desmethyldiazepam.

Desmethyldiazepam is an important metabolite for biological activity because of its long half-life of more than 72 hours. Because diazepam's half-life is about 36 hours, the concentration of its desmethyl derivative soon exceeds that of diazepam during chronic administration. Desmethyldiazepam undergoes oxidation to oxazepam, which (like its 3-hydroxy analogue temazepam) is rapidly conjugated with glucuronic acid and excreted.

Among various benzodiazepines, triazolam has a particularly short half-life of less than 4 hours, and flurazepam and nitrazepam both have a long half-life—particularly a major active metabolite of flurazepam, N-desalkylflurazepam, which has a half-life of about 100 hours.

Because benzodiazepines are often prescribed for long periods, their long-term pharmacokinetics are important. Diazepam and desmethyldiazepam reach plateau levels after a few weeks. Diazepam concentrations may then fall somewhat without much change in the concentration of the desmethyl metabolite.

Although benzodiazepines can induce liver enzymes in animals, induction is of little clinical significance in humans.

■ **Pharmacology**

The benzodiazepines share with the barbiturates anticonvulsant as well as sedative-hypnotic effects. In addition, they possess the remarkable ability to reduce anxiety and aggression (Cook and Sepinwall 1975). Several lines of evidence suggest that benzodiazepines are powerful potentiators of GABA. Although this hypothesis is elegant and generally accepted, other neurotransmitters may also be involved in these actions.

Schmidt and colleagues in 1967 were the first to show that diazepam could potentiate the inhibitory effects of GABA on spinal cords in cats. Later, it was shown that the effect of diazepam could be abolished if the endogenous content of GABA was depleted. This established that diazepam (and related benzodiazepines) did not act directly through GABA receptors but modulated inhibitory transmission through GABA in some way. It was subsequently demonstrated that benzodiazepines bind specifically to neural elements in mammalian brain with high affinity. There is, in fact, an excellent correlation between their affinity for these specific binding sites and their in vivo pharmacological potencies (Möhler and Okada 1977; Squires and Braestrup 1977). The binding of a benzodiazepine to this receptor site is enhanced by the presence of GABA or a GABA agonist, thereby suggesting that a functional (but independent) relationship exists between the GABA receptor and the benzodiazepine receptor (Tallman et al. 1987).

Barbiturates (and to some extent alcohol) also seem to produce their anxiolytic and sedative effects at least by partly facilitating GABAergic transmission (see the section "Barbiturates"). This common action of chemically unrelated compounds can be explained by their ability to stimulate specific sites in the $GABA_A$ receptor complex.

Benzodiazepines bind with high affinity to the ω-site so that the action of GABA on its receptor is allosterically enhanced. This enables GABA to produce stronger inhibition of the postsynaptic neuron than would occur without a benzodiazepine.

The inhibitory effect of GABA is mediated by chloride ion channels. When the $GABA_A$ receptor is occupied by GABA or GABA agonists such as muscimol, the chloride channels open and chloride ions diffuse into the cell. One of the binding sites on the chloride ion channel is activated by barbiturates. As was described previously, barbiturates appear to increase the duration of the open state of the chloride channels, whereas benzodiazepines increase the frequency of channel openings with little effect on the duration of the open site.

It may thus be concluded that ω (benzodiazepine) agonists act as sedative-hypnotics by activating a specific benzodiazepine receptor that facilitates inhibitory GABAergic transmission. Other sedative-hypnotics, such as barbiturates and alcohol, also facilitate GABAergic transmission by acting on sites associated more directly with the chloride channel (Figure 20–4). It is therefore also assumed that ω (benzodiazepine) agonists potentiate only the ongoing, physiologically initiated action of GABA (at $GABA_A$ receptors), whereas barbiturates can cause inhibition at all GABAergic synapses, whether or not these synapses are physiologically active. This fundamental difference between the allosteric effects of benzodiazepines within the $GABA_A$ receptor complex, and the conducive effects of barbiturates on the chloride ion channel, may explain why low doses of barbiturates display a pharmacological profile similar to benzodiazepines, whereas high doses of these drugs cause a profound and sometimes fatal suppression of CNS function.

Recent cloning of the $GABA_A$ receptor has suggested that there are many distinct structural classes (α_{1-6}, β_{1-3}, γ_{1-3}, δ), implying that the brain may contain a truly astonishing variety of $GABA_A$ receptor subtypes (Lüddens and Wisden 1991). The functional significance of these subunits is not well established and needs to be studied further to better understand the site of drug action and possibly the pathology of some psychiatric and sleep disorders.

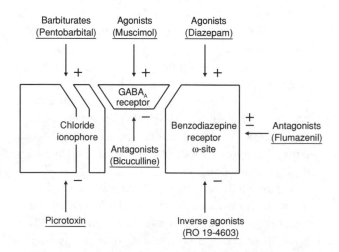

Figure 20–4. Diagrammatic representation of the complex macromolecular components of the GABAergic receptor, chloride ionophores, and benzodiazepine binding sites.

Nonbenzodiazepine hypnotics (acting on the benzodiazepine receptor). Until about 1980, it was widely accepted that the benzodiazepine structure was a prerequisite for the anxiolytic profile and for recognition of and binding to the benzodiazepine receptor. However, more recently two chemically unrelated drugs, the imidazopyridine zolpidem and the cyclopyrrolone zopiclone, have been shown to be useful sedative-hypnotics with benzodiazepine-like profiles. Other chemical classes of drugs that are structurally dissimilar to the benzodiazepines (e.g., triazolopyridazines) that have also been developed and have been shown to have anxiolytic activity in humans act through the benzodiazepine receptor (Figure 20–5).

Zolpidem and zopiclone have short half-lives—about 3 hours and 6 hours, respectively. It was originally claimed that these drugs do not appreciably affect the REM sleep pattern, whereas the quality of SWS may be slightly increased (Jovanovic and Dreyfus 1983; Shlarf 1992). Rebound effects (e.g., insomnia, anxiety), which are commonly seen following withdrawal of short-acting benzodiazepines, are minimal. These compounds also induce little respiratory depression and have little abuse potential. However, much longer clinical trials are needed to show whether the imidazopyridines or cyclopyrrolones have any significant advantage over the short to medium half-life benzodiazepines in the treatment of insomnia.

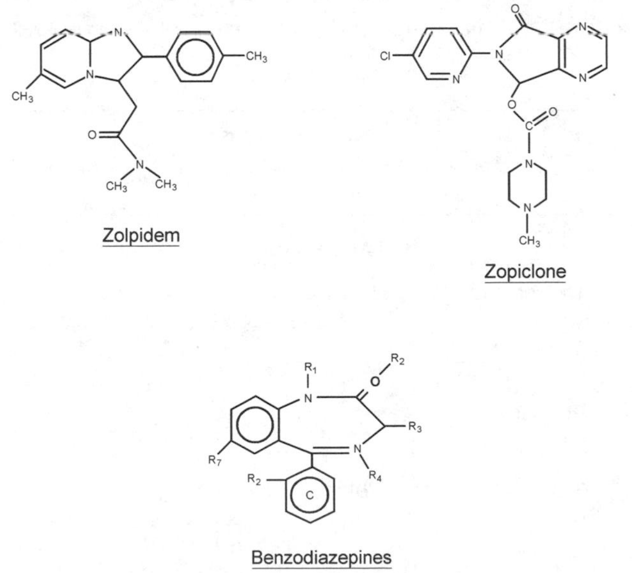

Benzodiazepine antagonists, partial agonists, and inverse agonists. Increased knowledge about the relationship between the structure of benzodiazepine receptor ligands and their pharmacological properties has given rise to the development of potent receptor agonists that stimulate the receptor and produce pharmacological effects qualitatively similar to classic benzodiazepines. Antagonists, which block the effects of the agonists without having any effects themselves, and a group of drugs that have a mixture of agonistic and antagonistic properties (i.e., partial agonists), have also been introduced (Haefley 1988). Partial agonists may be particularly important as sedative-hypnotics that lack common side effects such as ataxia or amnesia.

At the molecular level, the benzodiazepine agonists are drugs that induce a conformational change of the receptor molecule that produces functional consequences in terms of cellular changes, whereas antagonists only occupy binding sites. Braestrup and Nielsen (1986) found that a group of nonbenzodiazepine compounds, the β-carbolines, not only antagonized the action of the full agonists but also had intrinsic activity themselves. These compounds are called benzodiazepine inverse agonists because they have biological effects exactly opposite to those of the pure agonists while also having intrinsic activity like agonists. Their effects are blocked by antagonists; thus, the benzodiazepine receptor is particularly unique in that it has a bidirectional function (Figure 20–6).

Figure 20–5. Nonbenzodiazepine hypnotics. Two nonbenzodiazepine compounds—zolpidem (an imidazopyridine) and zopiclone (a cyclopyrrolone)—have recently been shown to be useful sedative-hypnotics with benzodiazepine-like profiles.

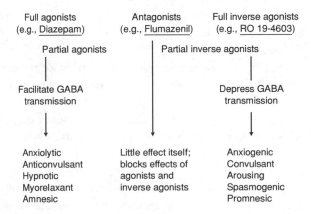

Figure 20–6. Properties of benzodiazepine agonists, antagonists, and inverse agonists.

Natural ligands for benzodiazepine receptors in the brain. The presence of benzodiazepine receptors in the brain suggests that there are natural ligands present that modulate these receptors. A specific compound has not yet been identified, but a number of endogenous ligands for the benzodiazepine binding site of GABA$_A$ receptor have been reported and termed *endozepines* (Rothstein et al. 1992a). Their intrinsic action, like that of diazepam, is to potentiate GABA$_A$ receptor function by acting as positive allosteric modulators of this receptor. They are present in the CNS in pharmacologically relevant concentrations. Several lines of experimental evidence suggest that these substances play a part in normal CNS processes (e.g., memory and learning) and in pathological processes (e.g., panic disorders) (Nutt et al. 1990) or hepatic encephalopathy (Mullen et al. 1990). Furthermore, Rothstein and colleagues (1992b) demonstrated that one of the endozepines is involved in a newly reported central nervous syndrome, idiopathic recurring stupor, characterized by recurrent episodes of stupor or coma in the absence of known toxic, metabolic, or structural brain damage. Thus, further knowledge of the roles of endozepine in physiological and pathological processes should be forthcoming.

■ Effects on Stages of Sleep

The hypnotic effects of benzodiazepines might be attributed to the modulatory effects on the GABAergic system of the raphe projections and locus ceruleus, although the precise mechanism whereby these drugs induce sleep is not known. However, recent studies of the effects of benzodiazepines on suprachiasmatic nucleus (SCN)-lesioned animals have shed new light on the mechanisms of hypnotic action, especially in relation to the homeostatic control of sleep (Edgar et al. 1993). SCN-lesioned animals show no consolidated activity or sleep-wake patterns under free-running conditions. The squirrel monkeys studied exhibited substantially increased total sleep time after lesioning. The benzodiazepine treatment, which is very effective in control animals, did not increase sleep in SCN-lesioned animals. When SCN-lesioned animals were once sleep deprived, the hypnotic effect of benzodiazepine reappeared in these animals. Thus, benzodiazepines may facilitate the release of the sleep debt accumulated during the previous wake period (Mignot et al. 1992).

There are many studies on the effects of benzodiazepines on sleep architecture in humans. Most benzodiazepines decrease sleep latency, especially when first used, and diminish the number of awakenings (Table 20–1). All benzodiazepines increase time spent in Stage 2 sleep. Benzodiazepines also affect the quality of the SWS pattern. Thus Stage 3 and Stage 4 sleep are suppressed and remain so during the period of drug administration. The decrease in Stage 4 sleep is accompanied by a reduction in nightmares.

Most benzodiazepines increase REM latency. The time spent in REM sleep is usually shortened; however, the reduction of percentage REM sleep is minimal, because the number of cycles of REM sleep usually increases late in sleep time. Despite the shortening of SWS and REM sleep, the net effect of administration of benzodiazepines is usually an increase in total sleep time, so that the individual feels that the quality of sleep under the hypnotics has improved. Furthermore, the hypnotic effect is greatest in subjects with the shortest baseline total sleep time.

If the benzodiazepine is discontinued after 3–4 weeks of nightly use, there may be a considerable rebound in the amount and density of REM sleep and SWS. However, this is not a consistent finding.

Because the long-acting benzodiazepine hypnotics induce impairment of daytime performance and increase the risk of falls in geriatric patients, several shorter-acting compounds have been introduced and

Table 20–1. Comparative properties of benzodiazepines and barbiturates on sleep parameters

	Benzodiazepines	**Barbiturates**
Total sleep time	↑ tolerance with short-acting agents	↑ rapid tolerance
Stage 2 %	↑	↑
SWS (Stages 3 and 4) %	↓	↓ (slight)
REM latency	↑	↑
REM %	↓ (slight)	↓
Withdrawal	Rebound insomnia with short-acting agents	Rebound decrease in stage 2
	Carryover effectiveness with long-acting agents	Total sleep time
	REM rebound (slight)	REM rebound

are the preferred choice for treatment of elderly patients. However, it has since been found that short-acting benzodiazepines induce rebound insomnia (a worsening of sleep difficulty beyond baseline levels on discontinuation of a hypnotic) (Kales et al. 1979), rebound anxiety, anterograde amnesia, and even paradoxical rage (Figure 20–7). Many other factors, such as the diagnosis of subjects, the dosage and duration of treatment, and the duration of action of the compounds, may also influence occurrence of these rebound phenomena. Nevertheless, enthusiasm for the shorter-acting compounds has been tempered.

■ Indications

Benzodiazepines are the treatment of choice in the management of anxiety, insomnia, and stress-related conditions. Although none of the currently available compounds has any significant advantage over the others, some choices can be made to fit the patient's symptom patterns to the pharmacokinetics of the various drugs. If a patient has a persistent high level of anxiety, one of the precursors of desmethyldiazepam such as diazepam or clorazepate is most appropriate. A patient with fluctuating anxiety may prefer to take a shorter-acting compound, such as oxazepam or lorazepam, when stressful circumstances occur or are expected.

Hypnotics should induce sleep rapidly, and their effects should preferably not be present upon waking. Both flurazepam and nitrazepam are inappropriately long acting unless a persistent anxiolytic effect is desired the next day. Even in such situations, diazepam given in one dose at night may be preferable. Oxazepam penetrates too slowly for a dependable hypnotic effect. Both lorazepam and temazepam are appropriate for patients with insomnia. Triazolam is the shortest-acting hypnotic available. When administered to patients with insomnia, very small doses of benzodiazepines (which were assumed to have no significant hypnotic action) were found to greatly improve their feelings of sleep quality.

Benzodiazepines can increase the frequency of apnea and severity of oxygen desaturation in control subjects and in subjects with chronic bronchitis (Geddes et al. 1976). Although there are many reports concerning the effects and safety of benzodiazepines on patients with sleep apnea syndrome, the results are still unclear. It therefore seems wise for sleep apnea patients to avoid using benzodiazepines.

Lorazepam and diazepam can also be used for relaxation procedures, preoperative medication, and sedation during minor operations and investigations, but often cause retrograde amnesia.

The benzodiazepines have been used for managing alcohol withdrawal because cross-tolerance usu-

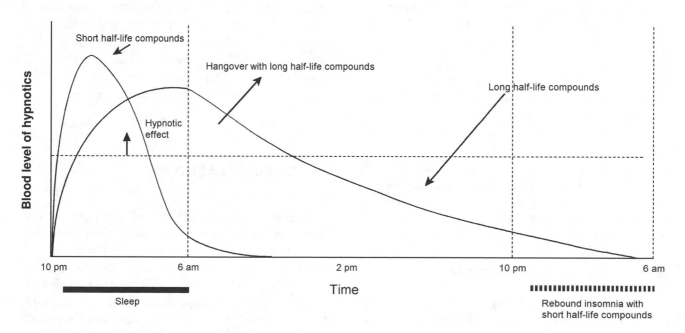

Figure 20–7. Duration of hypnotics and hangover and rebound insomnia. Hypnotics with a long half-life may induce impairment of daytime performance on the second day of administration, whereas short half-life compounds may induce rebound insomnia on discontinuation.

ally exists, but large doses are often needed to suppress the withdrawal syndrome.

The use of diazepam in status epilepticus is well established.

■ Side Effects and Toxicology

When a benzodiazepine is taken at high doses, tiredness, drowsiness, and profound feelings of detachment are common but can be minimized by careful adjustment of dosage. Headache, dizziness, ataxia, confusion, and disorientation are less common, but may affect the elderly. Marked potentiation of the depressant effect of alcohol occurs. Other less common side effects include weight gain, skin rash, menstrual irregularities, impairment of sexual function, and, rarely, agranulocytosis.

Although normal subjects clearly show mental impairment with the benzodiazepines, the situation with anxious patients is more complex. Because anxiety itself interferes with mental performance, alleviation of the anxiety may result in improved functioning that more than compensates for the direct drug-related decrement. The effects in some patients may be complicated and unpredictable, even at low dosages.

Because the safety of benzodiazepines in early pregnancy is not established, they should be avoided unless absolutely necessary. Diazepam is known to be secreted in breast milk and may make the baby sleepy, unresponsive, and slow to feed.

Overdosage. The benzodiazepines are extremely widely prescribed, so it is not surprising that they are used in many suicide attempts. For adults, overdoses of benzodiazepines reportedly are not fatal unless other psychotropic drugs or alcohol are taken at the same time. Typically, the patient falls asleep but is arousable and wakes after 24–48 hours. Treatment is supportive. A stomach pump is usually more punitive than therapeutic, and dialysis is usually useless because of high plasma binding.

■ Tolerance and Dependence

Dependence, both psychological and physical, occurs with benzodiazepines as with other drugs in the sedative-hypnotics class. Abrupt discontinuation results in withdrawal phenomena such as anxiety, agitation, restlessness, and tension, which are usually delayed for several days because of the long half-life of the major metabolite, desmethyldiazepam. Even with the normal dosage, some patients show withdrawal effects. The fact that some patients gradually increase the dose suggests tolerance, with increases in dose sometimes being related to particularly stressful crises.

Psychological dependence is also common, judging by the high incidence of repeat prescriptions. But it is mild, and drug-seeking behavior is much less insistent than with barbiturates.

■ ALCOHOL-TYPE HYPNOTICS

The alcohol type of hypnotics include the chloral derivatives; chloral hydrate, chlomethiazole, and ethchlorvynol are still occasionally used to treat elderly patients. Chloral hydrate is metabolized to another active sedative-hypnotic, trichloroethanol. These are drugs with a short half-life (about 4–6 hours) that decrease sleep latency and number of awakenings; SWS is slightly depressed, whereas overall REM sleep time is largely unaffected. Chloral hydrate and its metabolite have an unpleasant taste and cause epigastric distress and nausea. Undesirable side effects include lightheadedness, ataxia, and nightmares. Chronic use of these drugs can lead to tolerance and occasionally to physical dependence. As with barbiturates, overdosage can lead to respiratory and cardiovascular depression, and therapeutic use of these drugs has largely been superseded by benzodiazepines.

■ ANTIHISTAMINES

Antihistamines such as diphenhydramine or doxylamine are sometimes prescribed as sleep inducers. They decrease sleep latency but do not increase total sleep time (Reite et al. 1990). These compounds are especially useful for patients who cannot sleep well because of acute allergic reactions or itching. Sedative antihistamines may also be prescribed for people who have demonstrated tendencies to abuse psychoactive drugs, because these agents have not been shown to have abuse potential.

■ CONCLUSION

The recent progress toward an understanding of the biochemical actions of barbiturates and benzodiazepines, especially in relation to GABAergic systems, confirms a continuing need for basic research. Most of the important findings about the mechanism of action have become available only in the last several years. This progress is mainly due to new technologies in neuroscience research and our expanding knowledge of the GABAergic system. However, many questions remain unanswered. Considering the tremendous importance of benzodiazepines in psychiatry and general medicine, these questions, when resolved, should result in development of better treatments.

■ REFERENCES

Asano T, Ogasawara N: Chloride-dependent stimulation of GABA and benzodiazepine receptor binding by pentobarbital. Brain Res 225:212–216, 1981

Braestrup C, Nielsen M: Benzodiazepine binding in vivo and efficacy, in Benzodiazepine/GABA Receptors and Chloride Channels: Structural and Functional Properties. New York, Alan R Liss, 1986, pp 167–184

Cook L, Sepinwall J: Behavioral analysis of the effects and mechanisms of action of benzodiazepines. Adv Biochem Psycopharmacol 14:1–28, 1975

Edgar DM, Dement WC, Fuller CA: Effect of SCN lesions on sleep in squirrel monkeys: evidence for opponent processes in sleep-wake regulation. J Neurosci 13:1065–1079, 1993

Enna SJ, Möhler H: γ-Aminobutyric acid (GABA) receptors and their association with benzodiazepine recognition sites, in Psychopharmacology: The Third Generation of Progress. Edited by Meltzer HY. New York, Raven, 1987, pp 265–272

Geddes DM, Rudof M, Saunders KB: Effect of nitrazepam and flurazepam on the ventilatory response to carbon dioxide. Thorax 31:548–551, 1976

Haefley W: Partial agonists of the benzodiazepine receptor: from animal data to results in patients, in Chloride Channels and Their Modulation by Neurotransmission and Drugs. Edited by Biggio G, Costa E. New York, Raven, 1988, pp 275–292

Jovanovic UJ, Dreyfus JF: Polygraphical sleep recording in insomniac patients under zopiclone or nitrazepam. Pharmacology 27 (suppl 2):136–145, 1983

Kales A, Shlarf MB, Kales JD, et al: Rebound insomnia: a potential hazard following withdrawal of certain benzodiazepines. JAMA 241:1691–1695, 1979

Kay DC, Blackburn AB, Buckingham JA, et al: Human pharmacology of sleep, in Pharmacology of Sleep. Edited by Williams RL, Karakan I. New York, Wiley, 1976, pp 83–210

Killam K: Drug action on the brainstem reticular formation. Pharmacol Rev 14:175–224, 1962

Leeb-Lumberg F, Snowman A, Olsen RW: Barbiturate receptor sites are coupled to benzodiazepine receptors. Proc Natl Acad Sci U S A 77:7468–7472, 1980

Lüddens H, Wisden W: Function and pharmacology of multiple GABA$_A$ receptor subunit. Trends Pharmacol Sci 12:49–51, 1991

Maynert EW: Sedative and hypnotics, II: barbiturates, in Drill's Pharmacology in Medicine. Edited by DiPalma JR. New York, McGraw-Hill, 1965, pp 188–209

Mignot E, Edgar DM, Miller JD, et al: Strategies for the development of new treatments in sleep disorders medicine, in Target Receptors for Anxiolytics and Hypnotics: From Molecular Pharmacology to Therapeutics. Edited by Mendelewicz J, Racagni G. Basel, Karger, 1992, pp 129–150

Möhler H, Okada T: Benzodiazepine receptors: demonstration in the central nervous system. Science 198:849–851, 1977

Mullen KD, Szauter KM, Kaminsky-Russ K: "Endogenous" benzodiazepine activity in physiological fluids of patients with hepatic encephalopathy. Lancet 336:81–83, 1990

Nutt DJ, Glue P, Lawson C, et al: Flumazenil provocation of panic attacks. Arch Gen Psychiatry 47:917–925, 1990

Olsen RW, Ticku MK, Miller T: Dihydropicrotoxinin binding to crayfish muscle sites possibly related to γ-aminobutyric acid receptor-ionophores. Mol Pharmacol 14:381–390, 1978

Rall TR: Hypnotics and sedatives: ethanol, in The Pharmacological Basis of Therapeutics, 8th Edition. Edited by Gilman AG, Rall TW, Niles AS, et al. New York, Pergamon, 1990, pp 345–382

Reite ML, Nagel KE, Ruddy JR: The Evaluation and Management of Sleep Disorders. Washington, DC,

American Psychiatric Press, 1990

Richter JA, Holman JR Jr: Barbiturates: their in vivo effects and potential biochemical mechanisms. Prog Neurobiol 18:275–319, 1982

Rothstein JD, Garland W, Puia G, et al: Purification and characterization of naturally occurring benzodiazepine receptor ligands. J Neurochem 58:2102–2115, 1992a

Rothstein JD, Guidotti A, Tinuper P, et al: Endogenous benzodiazepine receptor ligands in idiopathic recurring stupor. Lancet 340:1002–1004, 1992b

Schmidt RF, Vogel ME, Zimmerman M: Die wirkung von diazepam auf de prasynaptishe hemmung und andere ruckensnarksreflexe. [Effect of diazepam on presynaptic inhibition and other spinal reflexes.] Naunyn Schmiedebergs Arch Exp Pathol Pharmacol 258:69–82, 1967

Shlarf MB: Pharmacology of classic and novel hypnotic drugs, in Target Receptors for Anxiolytics and Hypnotics: From Molecular Pharmacology to Therapeutics. Edited by Mendelwicz J, Racagni G. Basel, Karger, 1992, pp 109–116

Squires RF, Braestrup C: Benzodiazepine receptors in rat brains. Nature 266:732–734, 1977

Tallman JF, Thomas JW, Gallagher DW: GABAergic modulation of benzodiazepine binding site sensitivity. Nature 274:383–385, 1987

Stimulants in Psychiatry

Jan Fawcett, M.D., and Katie A. Busch, M.D.

The colorful history of stimulants began with the discovery of the psychoactive effects of cocaine, which has pharmacological properties remarkably similar to those of amphetamine despite their dissimilar chemical structures. Amphetamine, like cocaine, was introduced in medicine because of its effect of temporarily alleviating fatigue and its enhancement of mental and physical performance. The marked and varied effects of amphetamine, despite its relatively simple structure and its potential for abuse and dependence, have made it a topic of interest and controversy since it was first synthesized in 1887.

Today, the major areas of medical use of stimulants are the treatment of narcolepsy, for which amphetamine or methylphenidate (MPH) is used to relieve the symptoms of sleepiness and involuntary sleeping without affecting the etiology of the illness, and in the treatment of attention-deficit hyperactivity disorder (ADHD) in children, which continues to generate scientific, medical, and public controversy. They are also of possible value in treating adult attention deficit disorder or residual ADHD, and they are still used in the treatment of obesity, despite significant medical and scientific doubts as to their long-term benefits in maintaining weight loss and concerns over liability to abuse and dependence. Other proposed uses of stimulants include the treatment of affective disorders. This is discussed later in this chapter and is somewhat controversial, on the grounds of the stimulants' efficacy when used alone, as well as risks of abuse and dependency. Studies

that stated that stimulants had no place in general psychiatry were based on work done in the 1960s that is considered flawed by some (Chiarello and Cole 1987) and valid by others (Satel and Nelson 1989). On the other hand, open case reports of the effectiveness of stimulants in medically ill patients, poststroke patients, and acquired immunodeficiency syndrome (AIDS) patients with depression, as well as recent reports of the use of the stimulants to potentiate antidepressant medications in treatment-resistant patients (i.e., partial responders) or treatment-refractory (i.e., total nonresponding) patients, and evidence that certain patients may require more dopaminergic effects for effective antidepressant treatment, leave open the question of the usefulness of stimulants in these and other areas of psychiatry.

Dextroamphetamine (DAMPH) and MPH are the two most commonly used stimulants in psychiatry and medicine and demonstrate both similarities and differences in effect. In this chapter, we focus on these two compounds as primary examples of stimulant medications and consider their mechanisms of action and the current evidence concerning their therapeutic effects, their adverse effects, and hazards associated with their use.

■ HISTORY

The first known stimulant, cocaine, was isolated in the mid-eighteenth century. In 1884, cocaine was given to Bavarian soldiers who reported that it decreased fatigue (Patrick 1977). Amphetamine was first synthesized in 1887 and has certain similarities to cocaine in its potent psychomotor stimulant activity. Amphetamine was studied by Alles (1933), who wanted to find a synthetic substitute for ephedrine after Chen and Schmidt rediscovered ephedrine, which had been isolated from the *Ephedra vulgaris* plant in 1925. Alles and Leake developed techniques for evaluating toxicity and activity of phenylalkylamines. The most active compound was *d,l-*phenylisopropylamine or amphetamine, of which the dextro isomer was found to increase alertness and wakefulness and to promote improved physical and mental performance in people who are fatigued or bored, as well as to suppress appetite (Patrick 1977). Amphetamines were used by both sides in World War II. It is contended that Japan had large supplies of amphetamines that were placed on the open market after the war, leading to an epidemic of amphetamine abuse and cases of amphetamine psychosis, first in Japan in the 1950s and then in the United States in the 1960s (Fischman 1987). Patrick (1977) mentioned that it is "one of the ironies in history of psychopharmacology that the Haight-Ashbury amphetamine epidemic took place less than a mile from the University of California San Francisco Medical Center, where Alles and Leake had synthesized amphetamines more than 40 years earlier" (p. 335). In 1958, the piperazine derivative of amphetamine, MPH, was first introduced to treat hyperactivity in children (Anders and Ciaranello 1977).

In an excellent historical review published in 1968, Connell observed that there were more than 50 preparations of "amphetamine substances" either alone as derivatives or in combination with other drugs (notably barbiturates) on the market. At that time, Connell reviewed the status of the clinical uses of amphetamines in a wide range of conditions. Narcolepsy was probably the first condition for which amphetamine was used clinically (Prinzmetal and Bloomberg 1935). It revolutionized therapy for this condition and, although it was not curative, it was noted that "the drug may enable the patient to become symptom free" (Connell 1968, p. 235). The effective dose ranged as large as 30–50 mg, taken in divided doses bid or tid.

The use of amphetamine in treating parkinsonism dates back to 1937, when it was used for muscular rigidity and postencephalitic parkinsonism. By 1968, its use in the treatment of this condition had been largely superseded by more effective agents (Connell 1968). Connell observed that amphetamine was first used in treating epilepsy because of its action in antagonizing the sedative effect of narcotics. It was later found that amphetamine itself may have beneficial effects, particularly in the milder epileptic states, and has been used as the sole method of medication with varying results. Connell pointed out that in 1968, it was more common for amphetamine to be used in combination with other anticonvulsant drugs than by itself. This is in accordance with the observations of Hoffman and Lefkowitz (1993) that amphetamine "can obtund the maximal electroshock seizure discharge" (p. 211).

Connell (1968) noted that the role of amphetamine in the treatment of barbiturate poisoning had changed over the previous 25 years, observing that Riishede (1950) found a lower mortality in patients treated with amphetamine than those treated with nikethamide. Methylamphetamine, because of its greater vasoconstricting action, together with a more marked stimulating effect on respiration and muscle tone, was often preferred. Connell (1968) observed that the use of amphetamines in barbiturate poisoning had "been superseded by other drugs and other methods of treatment" (p. 235). Amphetamines were widely used in the treatment of drug addiction and alcoholism to offset sleepiness and lethargy. This continued until a realization of the dangers of amphetamine dependence and abuse of amphetamines, "together with the vicious cycle of amphetamine to counteract effect of sedatives followed by sedatives to counteract the use of amphetamines (e.g., insomnia)" (Connell 1968, p. 235), led to a discontinuation of amphetamine use in the treatment of these conditions.

Amphetamines were used to treat "psychopathic states" based on their effects on electroencephalogram tracings and the clinical state of adults with aggressive psychopathology (Hill 1947; Hill and Watterson 1942). Researchers described these states as including very deep sleep, excessive sexual appetite, a history of long-continuing nocturnal enuresis, epilepsy, and occasional convulsive seizures in the patient. Connell (1968) noted that the "paradoxical" effect of "quieting the emotional behavior, in which the patient tolerated high doses without disturbance of sleep" (p. 235) was of great interest. He concluded that using amphetamines to treat psychopathic states and delinquency showed results that were "variable and somewhat unpredictable" (p. 235). Connell mentioned that Bradley and Bowen (1941) had reported the use of amphetamines to modify antisocial behavior in children. He summarized clinical observations of the effects of amphetamine as showing that "when children are withdrawn or lethargic, the amphetamines tended to make them more alert, more accessible to persons and the environment" (Connell 1968, p. 236).

Conversely, the "paradoxical" effect noted in psychopathic adults was also seen in aggressive, noisy children, with those children who were hyperactive tending to move more quietly, to be calmer, and to quarrel less. These observations appear to precede the observations of the effect of amphetamine and MPH in the hyperkinetic child diagnosed with what is now called ADHD. Amphetamines were used to treat enuresis, based on observations that there was a group of enuretic patients who slept very deeply (Connell 1968). A regimen was worked out by Hodge and Hutchings (1952) that used a starting dose of 2.5 mg at bedtime for 1 week, increasing to 5 mg per week and subsequently raising the dose every week until the patient is sleeping more lightly. Connell (1968) commented that this method of treatment may result in failure as commonly as in success.

The next historical use of amphetamines, and perhaps one of its commonest uses, was in the treatment of obesity. Connell (1968) commented that there was "an increasing body of opinion suggesting that the contribution of amphetamines to the long-term treatment of obesity is small or nonexistent and does not justify their use now that the dangers of dependency and abuse are so much better known" (p. 236). He mentioned the possibility that diethylpropion and fenfluramine have fewer reports of abuse potential and of side effects such as stimulation of the nervous system.

Connell (1968) noted that

the value of amphetamines in the treatment of depressive disorder has been the subject of considerable controversy, but it would seem that there is an increasing number of psychiatrists who maintain that it has no use at all in the treatment of depression and that the dangers of dependence and abuse prohibit its use not only in depression but in psychiatric practice. (p. 237)

This is very similar to the position taken by Wheatley (1969) based on the use of amphetamines prescribed by general practitioners to treat depression. Shaw (1964) stated that the "amphetamine drugs hold a very doubtful place in the treatment of depression" (p. 28). Connell (1968) also observed that methamphetamine (MAMP) was being used less and less in psychiatric practice as an abreactive agent to treat neurotic conditions and as an aid in the diagnosis of psychiatric disorders. The amphetamine abuse epidemic peaked in the United States in the 1960s and 1970s and was in decline by 1978, when the cocaine epidemic was well under way (Foltin and Fischman 1991). In 1970, amphetamine and its derivatives were scheduled under the Controlled Substances Act.

From the perspective of the history of stimulants, the indications for their use has considerably narrowed over the years. Some reasons for this would probably include the realization of the risks of abuse and dependence on these agents, that newer and more effective agents have been shown to work in treating some of these conditions, or that the stimulants have simply been shown to be ineffective and fallen into disuse. At the same time, an interest in the clinical use of stimulants in psychiatry still exists, as evidenced by case reports of positive treatment responses in patients with particular types of affective disorders and some other psychiatric conditions. These areas of possible effectiveness for the stimulants are reviewed in the "Indications" section.

■ STRUCTURE-ACTIVITY RELATIONSHIPS

Phenylisopropylamine (amphetamine) is a relatively simple structure and forms the template for a wide variety of pharmacologically active substances. Although amphetamine is a central stimulant, minor modifications result in agents that can produce a broad spectrum of effects, including decongestant, anorexiant, antidepressant (the monoamine oxidase inhibitor [MAOI] tranylcypromine, and bupropion), and hallucinogenic agents (Glennon 1987). As Glennon noted, although it may be assumed by health professionals and the lay public that all amphetamine derivatives could possess amphetamine-like character, this is not necessarily the case. Though amphetamine itself has (most notably) central stimulant, anorexiant, and vasoconstrictor properties, a review of its structure-activity relationships shows that amphetamine's major properties (plus psychomimetic, MAO inhibition, and neurotransmitter uptake effects) can be enhanced by structural modification at the expense of other effects.

With respect to the behavioral properties of the simple phenylisopropylamines, two general groups can be considered: the central stimulant and hallucinogenic properties. The phenylisopropylamine molecule can be arbitrarily divided into three structural components: 1) the aromatic nucleus, 2) the terminal amine, and 3) the isopropyl side chain. In general, substitution on the aromatic nucleus of amphetamine results in agents that are less potent or inactive as central nervous system (CNS) stimulants (Glennon 1987). The substitution of two or more methoxy groups plus ethyl, methyl, or bromine groups on the aromatic nucleus creates hallucinogens of various potencies. Several popular hallucinogens of abuse result from the substitution of methylenedioxy substitutions on two carbons of the aromatic ring. This results in 2,3-methylenedioxyamphetamine (MDA) or 3,4-MDA, known as MDA or the "love drug," which has behavioral properties distinct from those of either amphetamine or other typical hallucinogens. The end monomethyl analogue of 3,4-MDA, MDMA or "XTC" (Ecstasy), is perhaps one of the best known contemporary stimulant hallucinogens of abuse (Glennon 1987). These compounds have often been called designer drugs, because structure-activity relationships have been applied to design new derivatives of a known agent, with the resulting drugs not yet covered under the Controlled Substances Act of 1970.

Substitution on the terminal amine group of amphetamine tends to reduce the hallucinogenic potency of phenylisoproplyamines. It is believed that MAMP may have stronger central stimulant properties than amphetamine. The d-isomer of amphetamine has been generally found to be far more potent in its central stimulant effects than the l-isomer. In contrast to this, the l-isomers of hallucinogenic phenylisopropylamines are more potent with respect to hallucinogenic effects (Glennon 1987). Removal of an α-methyl group of amphetamine leads to the formation of phenylethylamine that has little central stimulating effects because of its rapid breakdown by MAO-B. The removal of an α-methyl group of a hallucinogenic phenylisopropylamine usually results in

retention of activity but a decrease in potency. In contrast, 3,4-MDA is unique, because it seems to possess both stimulant and hallucinogenic effects and may produce effects that are distinct from these properties. However, it is also unique in that it possesses a methylene dioxy group on the aromatic ring in the 3,4 position. The addition of a methyl group to the terminal chain to produce MDMA appears to increase central stimulant potency while decreasing its hallucinogenic activity somewhat (Glennon 1987).

There have been contradictory reports in the literature concerning the relative effects of d- and l-isomers of amphetamine on mood activation, neurohormone responses, and effects presumed to be increasing norepinephrine (NE) and dopamine (DA) system effects. Smith and Davis (1977) showed in control subjects that DAMPH was more efficacious than MPH, which was more efficacious than l-amphetamine in increasing euphoric and activating moods, presumably reflecting the potency of DA actions. This was in contrast to the finding of Janowsky and Davis (1976) that MPH had 1.5 times the ability of DAMPH to increase activation of psychosis in schizophrenic patients. In both studies, DAMPH was about twice as effective as l-amphetamine. The drugs were given orally in the former study and intravenously in the latter, which could explain the difference. In terms of d- and l-isomer effects on growth hormone, adrenocorticotropic hormone (ACTH), cortisol, and prolactin secretion, findings have varied in both animals and humans and are therefore inconclusive.

MPH piperazine–substituted phenylisopropylamine containing a methyl ester possesses "two chiral centers that give rise to four optical isomers: d-threo, l-threo, d-erythro, and l-erythro" (Patrick et al. 1987, p. 1387). The present pharmaceutical product of MPH contains only the threo racemate in the d-l form. The d-threo enantiomer of MPH is believed to be responsible for the therapeutic activity. Patrick and colleagues (1981) synthesized pure d-l threo-p-hydroxy MPH and found that the locomotor-inducing activity in the rat after intracerebral ventricular administration was nearly twice that of the parent compound. In a review of the pharmacokinetics of MPH, the researchers suggest that "it is possible that the individual therapeutic response to racemic MPH may in part depend on the enantiomeric disposition of circulating MPH (i.e., responders may metabolize MPH with enantioselectivity differing from nonresponders, thereby producing a different profile of effects)" (Patrick et al. 1987, p. 1394). An example provided by MPH suggests how enantioselective metabolism may alter enantiomorphic structure-activity relationships and produce different response patterns in individual patients.

■ PHARMACOLOGICAL PROFILE

Amphetamine produces stimulating effects on the CNS such as arousal, wakefulness, euphoria, lessening of fatigue, and increased energy and self-confidence. Another central action is the inhibition of appetite. In humans, both cocaine and amphetamine produce behaviors characterized by repetitious arrangement of objects. Such behaviors may be analogous to stereotyped behaviors induced by amphetamines in animals (Patrick et al. 1981). Amphetamine is a weak base; one theory for its mechanism of action is its dissipation of the pH gradient intracellularly (see next section on "Mechanism of Action").

The metabolism of amphetamine can occur by either aromatic or aliphatic hydroxylation, yielding parahydroxyamphetamine or norephedrine, respectively, both of which are biologically active (Williams et al. 1973). Amphetamine is excreted unchanged in the urine (34% in human control subjects). It is also metabolized to benzoic acid (23%), which is subsequently converted to hippuric acid or to parahydroxyamphetamine (2%). This is in turn converted to parahydroxynorefedron (0.4%) (see Figure 21–1). Because of the basic nature of amphetamine and its excretion pattern, both hydration and the use of ammonium chloride 500 mg q 3–4 hours to acidify the urine will accelerate its excretion and possibly shorten the duration of the amphetamine reaction. Urine pH should be kept below 5 (Tinklenburg and Berger 1977). Metabolism of MPH is shown in Figure 21–2. The major metabolite of MPH is ritalinic acid, which is inactive. A thin-layer chromatographic analysis of human plasma collected 2 hours after administration of labeled MPH indicates that more than 75% of the total radioactivity is ritalinic acid, whereas compounds appearing to be parahydroxyritalinic acid and 6-oxoritalinic acid make up approximately 1%–2% of the activity, respectively (Patrick et al. 1987).

"Since MPH is a basic drug, plasma protein binding would be expected to be associated with α-acid glycoprotein and lypoprotein fractions, not primarily with albumin, which generally binds acidic drugs" (Patrick et al. 1987, p. 1388). Binding of MPH in an albumin solution of pH 7.4 is 12%, comparable to binding in whole plasma of 15%. The clinical blood concentrations of MPH are 2–20 ng/ml, which is below that of most psychotherapeutic agents. Such a minute amount requires sensitive analytical meth-

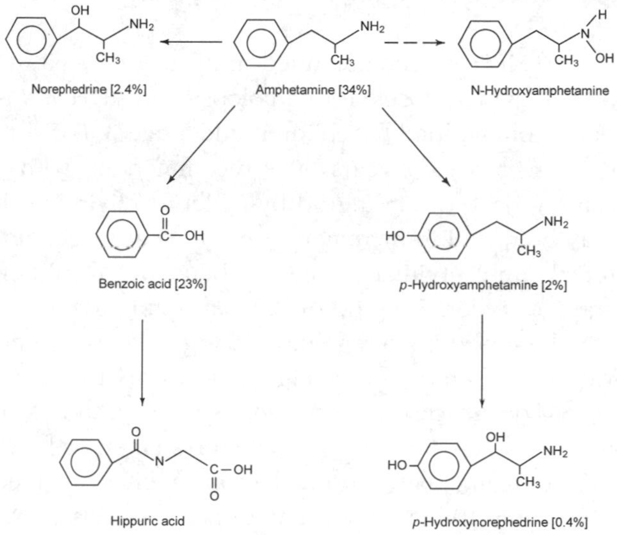

Figure 21–1. Metabolic pathway for amphetamine in humans.
Source. Reprinted from Patrick 1977 with permission.

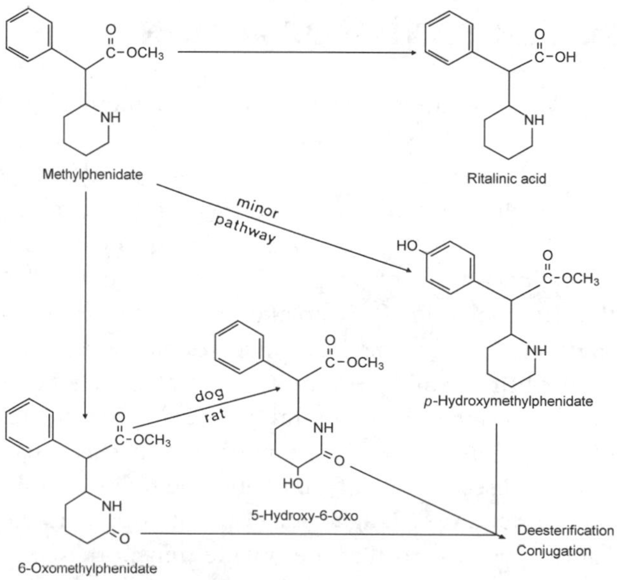

Figure 21–2. Metabolic pathway for methylphenidate.
Source. Reprinted from Patrick et al. 1987 with permission.

odology for therapeutic drug monitoring, often requiring gas chromatography/mass spectrometry methods. Like amphetamine, MPH accumulates in highly perfused tissues, and accumulates rapidly in the brain within 1–5 minutes after intravenous administration. Although typical doses of amphetamine result in significantly higher plasma concentrations than do typical doses of MPH, it appears that the pharmacological actions of MPH in humans can be attributed solely to the parent compound (Patrick et al. 1987).

DAMPH is recommended in doses of 50–60 mg qd (in divided doses) for narcolepsy and ADHD. It is not recommended for children under age 3. For children ages 3 to 5 years, it is recommended with a starting dose of 2.5 mg qd by tablet or elixir, which may be raised in increments of 2.5 mg at weekly intervals until optimal dosage is obtained. In children age 6 or older, 5 mg qd or bid is a starting dose that may be raised in increments of 5 mg at weekly intervals. Only in rare cases will it be necessary to exceed 40 mg qd. In cases of exogenous obesity, the usual dosage is 10–15 mg in spansule form taken daily, or up to 30 mg daily in tablet form taken in divided doses of 5–10 mg 30–60 minutes before meals. However, it is not recommended for this use in children under age 12 years (Physicians' Desk Reference 1994).

■ MECHANISM OF ACTION

The two prototypic stimulants amphetamine and MPH, though they have some similar net effects, also show differences in structure-activity relationships and mechanisms of action. As noted by Seiden and colleagues (1993), "Both the releasing and uptake-inhibiting actions of [amphetamine] are mediated by the catecholamine [CA] uptake transporter" (p. 640). In 1959, Axelrod and colleagues demonstrated that epinephrine could be rapidly and selectively taken up by the heart, spleen, and glandular organs, each of which has sympathetic innervation. It was subsequently discovered that NE-containing neurons could bind or take up NE against a concentration gradient; later, it was found that the uptake transporter could release CAs as well as reclaim them back into the nerve terminals. Further investigation revealed that amphetamine apparently inhibits the uptake and release of DA, NE, or both. The CA transporter nor-

mally moves DA from outside to inside of the cell. However, in the presence of some drugs such as amphetamine, the direction of transport appears to be reversed. DA is moved from inside the cell to outside of it through a mechanism called exchange diffusion, which occurs at low doses (1–5 mg/kg) of amphetamine. Moderate to high doses of amphetamine (> 5 mg/kg) cause the release of DA through exchange diffusion across the cell membrane, passive diffusion of amphetamine into the cell, and an interaction between amphetamine and the vesicle membrane transporter. A passive diffusion of amphetamine into the storage vesicle, causing alkylization of the vesicle, results in the release of DA from the vesicles as well, which is then subject to release by the cell membrane. These mechanisms, as well as a blocking of reuptake of DA by amphetamine, all lead to an increase of synaptic NE and DA. Other antidepressant medications acting on CAs, including both DA and NE, tend to exert their action by simply blocking the reuptake mechanism.

MPH appears to release DA stored in the vesicles alone, whereas amphetamine releases DA from newly synthesized pools and increases DA diffusion from the vesicles into the cell. This mechanism appears to distinguish amphetamine from antidepressant medication in terms of its rapidity of onset of effect and from MPH in terms of its potency. Further support for these differentiations include the findings that blocking CA synthesis by α-methyl-p-tyrosine (AMPT) will interfere with DA release by both amphetamine and MPH, whereas reserpine, which releases DA from storage sites in vesicles, only interferes significantly with MPH effect but does not totally inhibit amphetamine effects. This again differentiates between the two DA storage pools—vesicular storage, which is dependent on an inward proton pump and the maintenance of low intravesicular pH; and cytoplasmic storage, which has neither of these requirements (Seiden et al. 1993).

The structure of amphetamine is similar to that of both NE and DA. Part of the mechanism related to the vesicular action of amphetamine is that it is a weak base and causes alkylinization of the storage vesicles. Amphetamine also induces the release of [³H]serotonin (5-HT) from chromaffin granules from the adrenal medulla (Sulzer and Rayport 1990). Although amphetamine competitively inhibits MAO in vitro, it appears to be a weak MAOI in moderate doses in vivo. In high doses, there is evidence that amphetamine may act as a competitive inhibitor for MAO-A (Mantle et al. 1976; Miller et al. 1980). This effect seems to be less significant physiologically than the CA-releasing effects of the drugs.

Brown and colleagues (1978) have shown that, although amphetamine given in doses of 20 mg to control subjects causes stimulation of both growth hormone and cortisol, MPH in the same dose causes only growth hormone stimulation. The elation caused by MPH was found to be correlated with growth hormone elevation. This led Brown and colleagues to suggest that the elation response may be related to the DA effects of both stimulants, whereas the cortisol response may be related to the NE effects of amphetamine alone. The NE effects of amphetamine may explain its higher incidence of increased pulse and hypertension.

In studies with human subjects, Nurnberger and colleagues (1984) showed that DAMPH-induced excitation is due to central DA stimulation, whereas cardiovascular effects, increased blood pressure, and increased serum NE result from noradrenergic effects that can be blocked by propranolol. Sloviter and colleagues (1978) first noticed the similarity between the effects of high-dose DAMPH in rats and the behavioral syndrome caused by intense 5-HT receptor activation. The researchers pursued studies showing that responsiveness of the amphetamine syndrome could be blocked by either 5-HT synthesis inhibition or receptor blockade. This suggests that amphetamine acts indirectly through the 5-HT system by activating 5-HT receptors, possibly through the displacement of endogenous 5-HT.

■ INDICATIONS

The *Physicians' Desk Reference* (1994) lists two indications approved by the U.S. Food and Drug Administration for Dexedrine: 1) narcolepsy and 2) ADHD. The indications listed in the *Physicians' Desk Reference* for MPH are 1) attention-deficit disorders in children and 2) narcolepsy. Other therapeutic uses of stimulant medications are controversial, principally because they have become drugs of abuse when sold illicitly or prescribed irresponsibly. As a result, amphetamine is therefore a schedule II and MPH a schedule III substance under the Controlled Substances Act of 1970. Moreover, certain states (e.g., Wisconsin) have passed even more restrictive legis-

lation limiting the use of stimulants to specific indications. Stimulants are prohibited in some European countries. Are stimulants ineffective in comparison to their risks and thus without a place in psychiatric practice? Or has concern over the abuse potential of these drugs in certain vulnerable populations led to a suppression of their use in cases in which they could be medically useful (and even possibly life-saving), as in severe treatment-refractory depression?

Since 1987, there have been three published reviews of the use of psychostimulants and several reviews preliminary to case reports. Of the major reviews, Chiarello and Cole (1987) dealt with the use of stimulants in general psychiatry, Satel and Nelson (1989) focused on the use of psychostimulants in the treatment of affective disorders, and Ayd and Zohar (1987) emphasized the role of stimulants in treatment-resistant affective disorders. Based on these reviews, it can be seen that the efficacy of DAMPH alone in treating patients with affective disorders is controversial. This is based on the fact that there have been no double-blind studies since 1962. Many of the studies that were reported had high placebo response rates not exceeded by the DAMPH effects, and the studies were done on a short-term basis. Chiarello and Cole (1987) have pointed out that the studies were not done adequately enough to conclude whether DAMPH did in fact have therapeutic effects for some patients, and data may have been analyzed in such a way as to miss positive effects by their authors. However, Satel and Nelson (1989) observed that studies of imipramine (IMI) versus placebo carried out at approximately the same time, presumably with similar methodology and interpretation, showed IMI to be superior to placebo in 15 out of 24 studies—a more robust outcome than could be drawn from the 3 or 4 double-blind placebo-controlled studies conducted using DAMPH with doses ranging from 10–30 mg qd. There is presently no evidence to justify the use of DAMPH, or any other stimulant as a first-line or routine treatment in patients with depressive illness.

MPH was studied in four reported double-blind studies in the late 1960s and early 1970s, in doses up to 30–40 mg qd, showing modest responses in comparison to placebo. There was evidence of clinical effects in some patients. Pemoline has also been given in double-blind placebo-controlled studies in the mid- to late 1970s, with modest effects when given as a sole treatment. The studies of these three major stimulants and critical reviews of these studies seem to echo the conclusion that although some effects might be noted in some patients, the evidence as to whether these responses will persist over time is mixed. There is not good evidence that would establish stimulants as a responsible first-line treatment when their benefits in placebo-controlled studies are compared with those of other available antidepressant medications.

Open studies have a significant disadvantage compared with placebo-controlled studies in that they do not account for placebo response. (These studies also tend to be published more often if they are positive than if they turn out to have negative results.) On the other hand, open studies tend to have more flexible dose ranges and may provide useful information about the type of clinical responses seen and in what type of patients, because they may not treat groups of more highly selected patients. There have been five open studies of either amphetamine, benzedrine, or MAMP involving 185 subjects, ranging from hospitalized patients with retardation or agitation to patients diagnosed with neurotic depressions. Judged by various criteria, improvement was seen in 30%–76% of the subjects. In two open studies of MPH in treating subjects with various types of depressive disorders at doses of 30–60 mg qd, 76%–82% improvement was reported.

A number of uncontrolled studies and case reports have been cited using MPH for treatment of depression in various types of medically ill patients. Between 1956 and 1991, studies of medically ill patients involving 159 patients were reported showing positive responses in 68%–98% of patients (Kraus and Burch 1992). A study in adult patients with cancer showed a 77% response in 30 patients, whereas 17 patients presented with an average response of 85% (Fernandez et al. 1987). From 1988 to 1992, four studies presented 38 case reports of patients with human immunodeficiency virus (HIV)-related neuropsychiatric symptoms, including depression, with 86% of subjects showing some improvement and 65% showing moderate to marked improvement (Angrist et al. 1992; Fernandez et al. 1988a, 1988b; Holmes et al. 1989). There are two studies with case reports of response to MPH in poststroke depression patients, one showing 70% of subjects improving and the other showing 80% improving, on doses ranging from 5 mg bid to total doses of 40 mg qd (Johnson et al. 1992;

Lazarus et al. 1992). Reviewing open series or case reports of medically ill patients with varying diagnoses showed two important advantages for the stimulants. One was the rapidity of response, with most authors agreeing that response was evident within 2–3 days—much earlier than seen on average for other antidepressants. The second advantage frequently cited was the dearth of side effects compared with other antidepressant medications, especially in medically ill patients. (The question of side effects and hazards is reviewed in the section on "Side Effects and Toxicology.")

■ Stimulants as Potentiation for Antidepressant Medications

In 1971, Wharton and colleagues published a paper that had been read at the annual meeting of the American Psychiatric Association in 1969. The researchers reported on seven patients with recurrent refractory psychotic depressive illness, five of whom had had repeated courses of electroconvulsive therapy (ECT). Five of these patients recovered within 2 weeks of receiving IMI at 150 mg qd and Ritalin 10 mg bid (Wharton et al. 1971). The other two patients recovered more gradually without requiring ECT. Wharton and colleagues documented a rise in serum IMI levels following the addition of Ritalin, and they hypothesized that this rapid increase in blood levels might possibly be related to the enhanced response. Five of the patients who could be followed up maintained their response for 2–3 years. Subsequently, in a letter to the *American Journal of Psychiatry,* Flemenbaum (1971) reported "six to ten" patients (p. 239) treated with MPH-IMI combinations, noting a rapid onset of effect and correction of hypotension associated with the tricyclic antidepressant (TCA) medication. However, Flemenbaum did note three cases of young patients with labile hypertension who had hypertensive episodes associated with the MPH-IMI combination.

Cooper and Simpson (1973) reported another case of a 61-year-old patient with a 19-year history of depressive disorder. The patient had not benefited from various treatment modalities and sustained a partial response on 300 mg qd of IMI but still required hospitalization; however, there was marked improvement with the addition of 40 mg maximum of MPH. Cooper and Simpson reported an almost 20-fold increase in IMI levels and a 50% increase in desipramine (DMI). In this case, within 2 weeks after MPH was withdrawn, plasma IMI and DMI levels had returned to baseline values, and the patient apparently relapsed. The authors presented this as a confirmation of the observation by Perel and associates (1969) that IMI metabolism was inhibited by MPH.

Drimmer and colleagues (1983) presented the case of a patient with a diagnosis of bipolar depression with hypomania who had had a depressive episode and was not helped by up to 350 mg qd of amoxapine. The patient was then treated with DMI 200 mg qd and sustained marked improvement in mood and agitation within 3 days of the addition of MPH 10 mg bid (Drimmer et al. 1983). The patient experienced a relapse after MPH was withdrawn gradually, and again responded to its reinstatement at up to 40 mg qd. No significant increases in DMI levels were noted in this patient. The authors believed that the rapidity of response when MPH was added to DMI, as well as the lack of DMI increase, argued against a mechanism of enhancement of TCA levels for the potentiating effect of MPH. Rather, Drimmer and colleagues argued that the dopaminergic effects of MPH were more likely to be the basis for its potentiating effects on IMI and DMI treatment.

Myers and Stewart (1989) further commented on the rapidity of onset of a DMI-MPH combination in the case of a 69-year-old male patient admitted for the treatment of transitional cell carcinoma of the bladder. The patient had developed suicidal ideation and was threatening to jump out of his fourth floor hospital window. However, within 2 days of administration of this combination, he was no longer suicidal and was able to enjoy watching television. He relapsed within 4 days of discontinuation of MPH but then responded to 400 mg qd of DMI (Myers and Stewart 1989). Although the mechanism of action of the IMI-DMI plus MPH combination is unclear, the case reports available suggest that it may be an effective combination for patients with treatment-resistant depression. This combination has the advantage of rapid response and relatively few hazards, except for the possibility of elevated blood pressure in patients with histories of labile hypertension.

In 1989, Linet reported on a 36-year-old male patient who did not improve on 300 mg qd of IMI despite potentiation with triiodothyronine, tryptophan 8,000 mg qd, and L-thyroxine 0.15 mg qd as well as

DAMPH augmentation up to a dose of 45 mg tid (Linet 1989). The patient's IMI dosage was discontinued, and he subsequently had no particular response to 60 mg qd of fluoxetine until the addition of 45 mg tid of DAMPH, which resulted in "significant and sustained clinical improvement" (p. 804) after 2½ years of depression. His response was maintained for 5 months, and he relapsed on four subsequent occasions when attempts were made to taper DAMPH and increase the dose of fluoxetine.

Metz and Shader (1991) reported four cases of patients refractory to TCA, three of whom obtained either partial responses to fluoxetine or who relapsed on fluoxetine under stress but improved when 9.375–18.75 mg qd of pemoline was added. These responses were monitored and observed to have lasted for 9–23 months. The addition of either DAMPH or pemoline to fluoxetine is suggested by these case reports as a way of treating partial responses in patients on fluoxetine or patients who have relapsed in treatment. Although the use of stimulants with other antidepressants has not been documented in a double-blind study (which is not surprising, considering the expense of double-blind placebo-controlled studies, the lack of commercial interest in these older stimulants, and the relatively small percentage of patients treated with antidepressants who require stimulant potentiation), published case reports suggest the efficacy and probable safety of this combination in patients with depression that has been resistant to successful treatment with existing antidepressant agents.

MAOIs are currently used mainly to treat patients with depression that has proven refractory to other antidepressant medications, some patients with "atypical depression," and patients with severe panic or anxiety disorders unresponsive to other pharmacological therapies. Because of their potential for interactions with dietary substances and other medications as well as their frequent side effects, MAOIs are usually not used until after other medications have failed. However, the clinicians who see patients with depressive illnesses that are resistant to conventional pharmacological treatment still see patients who not only require MAOIs but who may have also failed to respond to these agents as well as to ECT. In patients with highly resistant depression, the stakes become higher in many cases, because hopelessness induced by the depressive illness is augmented by the reality of a lack of response with a further increased risk of suicide.

In 1985, Feighner and colleagues reported on the use of a combination of MAOI, TCA, and stimulant therapy for treatment-resistant depression. The researchers cited 16 subjects, 13 of whom improved when various MAOIs were potentiated by either DAMPH or MPH. Fawcett and colleagues (1991) presented 32 cases of patients who were refractory to long series of trials with TCAs, selective serotonin reuptake inhibitors (SSRIs) (in some cases), and (in 14 cases) ECT without a response to treatment. Seventy-eight percent of these patients responded with the addition of either pemoline or DAMPH to one to four different MAOIs in their maximal tolerated doses. DAMPH was given in doses of 10–40 mg qd and pemoline in doses of 18.75–37.50 mg tid to patients receiving maximal tolerated doses of 40–120 mg of MAOIs. The patients ranged in age from 20 to the early 80s (Fawcett et al. 1991). Neither of these two reports of stimulant potentiation of MAOIs reported any serious side effects except for the possible switching of several patients into hypomania or mania in the series conducted by Fawcett and colleagues. Both studies reviewed older literature in which three cases of death had ensued after the administration of MAOIs potentiated with DAMPH (Dally 1962; Krisko et al. 1969; Lloyd and Walker 1965; Mason 1962; Smilkstein et al. 1987; Stockley 1973; Zeck 1961). Two of these three cases involved elevation of blood pressure, hyperpyrexia, seizures, and death; one case did not show elevation of blood pressure but did show hyperpyrexia, seizures, and death. These cases were reported in the literature in the early to late 1960s.

Although it was noted that the use of stimulants is contraindicated in *Physicians' Desk Reference* recommendations, in addition to the observations of Feighner and colleagues (1985), it is noted that in some patients with high-risk depression for whom all other treatments have failed, the use of stimulants to potentiate MAOIs has proved helpful and even lifesaving.

As in the case with other uses of stimulants in treating depression (such as their use in treating medically ill stroke patients, elderly patients, or treatment-resistant patients), with the potentiating effects presented with the TCAs, fluoxetine, and potentially other antidepressant medications, and even the use of stimulants to potentiate MAOIs in patients with highly treatment-resistant depressive illness, the decision to prescribe stimulants should be based on clinical history of treatment resistance or treatment-refractory illness. Noncompliance should be ruled out as a factor, as well as the patient's medical status and his or her capacity for careful compliance with the regimen prescribed. In making these clinical decisions, careful clinical judgment in evaluating the risk-benefit analysis of what is best for an individual patient is important.

Although the use of stimulants may not be necessary in the average patient, it is our opinion that though the continual addition of new antidepressant medications may increase patients' chances of being treatment responsive, there are still a significant percentage of patients who do not respond at all to these medications (finding themselves stuck in severe states of impairment or even at risk for death by suicide) or who cannot tolerate various effects of some of the drugs available, because of idiosyncratic differences or medical conditions. These patients may benefit from the use of stimulants alone or in combination, to potentiate other available antidepressant medications. It is important that the clinical literature concerning the possible usefulness of stimulants is available to psychiatrists as well as to those who legislate the use of these substances. The latter group may be motivated more by their concern for potential danger and may not be fully aware of the potential benefits of psychostimulants to patients who may not otherwise recover and regain control of their lives.

In 1971, Fawcett and Siomopoulos reported the use of DAMPH (Dexedrine) to predict antidepressant response, showing data suggesting that patients who were responsive to 10 mg bid of Dexedrine were more likely to respond to DMI. This predictive effect of Dexedrine was confirmed by van Kammen and Murphy (1978). In 1983, Sabelli and colleagues reported the use of MPH to predict DMI response as opposed to nortriptyline response in patients with major depression. In a paper entitled "Challenging the Amphetamine Challenge Test," Kravitz and colleagues (1990) reviewed this issue based on new data. These data suggested that although Dexedrine challenge did tend to predict DMI response about 70% of the time, the degree of correct prediction might not be powerful enough in the individual patient to justify the use of the stimulant challenge test as a routine procedure.

■ Summary of the Use of Stimulants in Depression

Although double-blind studies done in the 1960s did not produce data strongly supporting the efficacy of stimulants in treating a broad range of depressed patients, it is important to recognize that the design of these studies was highly flawed. Placebo response rates were extremely high, making it difficult for stimulants to show a higher rate of effectiveness. Though these studies do not offer support for the efficacy of stimulants used alone in the treatment of depression, they certainly do not convincingly rule out the possibility that stimulants may be effective for some patients. Open studies point in a slightly different direction, emphasizing the value of stimulants in treating patients with severe medical illnesses, poststroke patients, elderly patients, patients with severe heart disease, and AIDS patients, all of whom had concurrent depression and increased risks associated with side effects to antidepressant medications.

In general, these case reports were positive, showing a high rate of improvement in patients with a relatively low rate of side effects and a rapid response time of 2–3 days. It has been noted that case reports are generally published when they are positive; thus, the efficacy of stimulants in these patients may be overestimated. The use of stimulants to potentiate other antidepressant medications in patients with either treatment-resistant depression or partial response has been raised in several studies—including their use with MAOIs, despite *Physicians' Desk Reference* warnings against this practice. The use of stimulants to predict TCA response showed some theoretical interest, but the movement to more widespread use of SSRIs diminishes the significance and value of this early research.

Some studies have reviewed the hypothesis that DA hypofunction may play a significant role in depressive illness. D'haenen and Bossuyt (1994) reported an increased D_2 receptor density in depressed patients. These studies, when viewed in the context of antidepressant effects reported with the use of DA agonists bromocriptine, piribedil, and pergolide, further strengthen the hypothesis that the DA system is an important mechanism in at least some depressed patients (Bouckoms and Mangini 1993; Post et al. 1978; Theohar et al. 1981). The therapeutic use of stimulants in some of these selected patients appears to have a growing theoretical and empirical basis, particularly in view of the limited dopaminergic effects of most standard antidepressant medications.

■ Other Uses of Stimulants in Psychiatry and Medicine

The use of psychostimulants—particularly MPH, DAMPH, MAMP, and pemoline—in the treatment of children with ADHD has been a continually accepted indication for the use of these substances. This use has not been without some social controversy involving the use of drugs in children and the possibilities of adverse side effects. Possible effects include growth retardation, which has not been substantiated, and the possible negative cognitive effects that seem to result from overdosage in some children, as well as overuse or inappropriate use as the result of poor clinical diagnosis. In 1977, Barkley reviewed 15 studies of the use of amphetamines in children with ADHD, involving 915 patients. The studies had varying designs, including using hospital staff, teachers, clinicians, and parents as judges of response. They showed an average response of 74% of subjects improving and 26% unchanged or worsening. Fourteen studies of MPH, involving 866 patients and using clinicians, parents, and teachers as judges of outcome, were studied. These studies showed an average of 77% improvement among subjects, with 23% unchanged or worsened. Pemoline was used in two studies with 105 subjects. These studies used clinicians and teachers as judges of outcome, with 73% of subjects improving and 27% unchanged or worsening. In another 8 studies, 417 children were shown to have a mean improvement rate of 39% versus a 61% mean percentage unchanged or worsened. It was concluded in this review that most children are judged as improved on the psychostimulant medications, whereas a small percentage are not. At that time Barkley (1977) concluded that follow-up studies find the long-term psychosocial adjustment of these children to be essentially unaffected by stimulant treatment. Barkley then noted that the search needed to consider specific variables for measures of improvement rather than just general improvement, as many studies up until that time had tended to do.

More recently, Schachar and Tannock (1993) looked for evidence of sustained effect of stimulant treatment in children with ADHD. Eighteen studies were identified with a duration of at least 3 months. Seventeen were studies of MPH and 1 was a study of

DAMPH; none involved pemoline or slow-release stimulants. Eleven of these studies were randomized controlled trials, whereas 7 employed quasi-experimental designs without randomization. The results of randomized controlled trials showed that psychostimulants provide a greater benefit than did nonrandomized trials. This suggested to the researchers that "efficacy of extended treatment may have been underestimated because more seriously disturbed children were assigned to medication treatment than to control treatments in nonrandomized trials" (p. 81). Reviewing 11 randomized controlled studies that collectively involve 271 children medicated for an average of 6 months, the authors found that "results of 8 out of the 11 randomized controlled trials indicate clear beneficial effects of prolonged treatment with MPH on the core behavioral features of ADHD, that is, poor sustained attention, impulsiveness, and excessive motor activity" (p. 89).

Of the three studies that failed to find efficacy of extended stimulant treatment, one study was discounted because of an attrition rate of more than 50%. The results of a second study indicated prolonged MPH treatment did reduce the severity of poor symptoms, but the improvements were comparable in magnitude to those obtained with IMI. Another study found that behavioral improvements obtained with MPH were no longer discernible when medication was discontinued. Schachar and Tannock (1993) concluded that there is no evidence that

> longer term benefits of MPH are greater than those of treatment with the TCA IMI, nor are they potentiated by adjunctive pharmacological treatment with thioridazine or nonpharmacological therapy such as cognitive training, educational tutoring or the combination of parent training and self-control training. (p. 90)

It was also shown that the beneficial effects of treatment dissipate rapidly when treatment is terminated. Stimulant treatment did not appear to reduce symptoms to those considered to be in the range of normal behavior. It was concluded that few children made sufficient progress to become symptom free at the end of the trial. In addition, although short-term treatment produced a significant impact on social and academic symptoms, extended treatment produced a far less clear result. Schachar and Tannock (1993) further concluded that future extended treatment studies must address questions about the development of drug tolerance, as well as concerns about long-term adverse effects, such as abnormal movement and dysphoria.

The modest effectiveness of MPH indicated by these studies suggests a need to combine medication with educational interventions and psychological therapies. Although indirect evidence for the superior effectiveness of combining intensive multimodal therapy and MPH over the use of medication alone has been shown by Satterfield and colleagues (1987), no direct evidence exists in longer-term studies to support this contention (Satterfield et al. 1981, 1987; Schachar and Tannock 1993). Psychostimulants have been shown to be helpful in treating the core symptoms of ADHD in children, both acutely and over at least a 6-month period. It is also clear that the effect of psychostimulants is toward improvement and not total suppression of symptoms—the symptoms return when medications are discontinued. There is still concern about long-term effects of these medications and the long-term effects of ADHD itself in terms of delinquency and other conduct disturbances.

Wender and colleagues (1985) described the use of stimulants in adults with similar problems of attention, concentration, and focus, terming this syndrome "adult attention deficit disorder." These investigators have found that although pemoline was not more effective than placebo, MPH produced improvement in core symptoms. In patients meeting the Utah criteria for ADHD (Wender et al. 1985), this improvement occurred (and sometimes in a dramatic nature) in 57% of subjects, compared with improvements in 11% in response to placebo. The Utah criteria for residual ADHD included a history of core symptoms of childhood ADHD being reported by a parent using the Conners Teacher Rating Scale (Sprague et al. 1974).

Stimulants have long been accepted as valuable in treating narcolepsy, which is often treated by psychiatrists as well as by neurologists and general physicians. The chronic use of stimulants will frequently reduce episodes of daytime sleepiness. This use can cause impairment and danger, especially if the sleepiness occurs while the patient is driving. Stimulants do not reverse the cataplexy that some narcoleptic patients experience, but either TCAs or SSRIs in combination with stimulants may be helpful for this.

Although there have been several studies suggesting that stimulants may improve negative symptoms in schizophrenic patients, there have also been studies showing that stimulants may worsen positive symptoms of schizophrenia, such as delusions and hallucinations (Lieberman et al. 1990). There is also evidence that schizophrenic patients have high rates of comorbid substance abuse, perhaps as a consequence of the blunted affectivity associated with negative symptoms of the disease.

In one report, Insel and colleagues (1983) reported positive effects from Dexedrine given to patients with obsessive-compulsive disorder in terms of their disorder's severity. The experience of Insel and colleagues suggests that these patients also had lower levels of anxiety when Dexedrine was used.

In 1984, Khantzian and colleagues presented three cases of cocaine abuse treated with MPH, all three of whom demonstrated improvement. This led to an hypothesis of the presence of dysthymic disorder or chronic depression without the full neurovegetative symptomatology of major depression, in association with cocaine abuse. It was further hypothesized that the "normalizing effect of MPH with the pilot cases makes a compelling argument for more extensive clinical study to test the possibility that a minimal brain dysfunction syndrome or attention deficit disorder or a variant contributes to cocaine dependence" (pp. 110–111). This hypothesis was also based on the fact that the patients did not develop tolerance to MPH. It was also mentioned that the authors had treated four other subjects who had abused cocaine and who did not have attention deficit disorder symptoms. Khantzian and colleagues (1984) observed dosage escalations without prolonged facilitation of cocaine abstinence. Hence, initial observations indicated that only a subpopulation of abusers respond favorably to MPH treatment of cocaine abuse. This has led to a proposal for further study of the use of MPH in cocaine abusers with ADHD symptoms (H. D. Kleber, personal communication, May 1993).

■ SIDE EFFECTS AND TOXICITY

The effects of amphetamine include alpha and beta actions common to sympathomimetic drugs that act indirectly. Amphetamine given orally raises both systolic and diastolic blood pressure. Heart rate is often reflexly slowed and, with large doses, cardiac arrhythmias may occur. Cardiac output is not enhanced by therapeutic doses, and cerebral blood flow is little changed (Hoffman and Lefkowitz 1993). Smooth muscles respond to amphetamine in general as they do to other sympathomimetic drugs. There is a contractile effect on the urinary bladder sphincter, an effect that has been used in treating enuresis and incontinence. Pain and difficulty in micturition can therefore occur. Amphetamine may cause relaxation of the intestine and delay the movement of intestinal contents, but the opposite effect may also be seen. The response of the human uterus varies, but usually an increase in tone occurs.

Side effects noted when therapeutic doses of amphetamine are taken also include mild gastrointestinal disturbance, anorexia, dryness of mouth, tachycardia, cardiac arrhythmias, insomnia, and restlessness (Meyler 1966). Headache, palpitations, dizziness, vasomotor disturbances, agitation, confusion, dysphoria, apprehension, and delirium are also mentioned. Other side effects that have been documented include flushing, pallor, a sensation of swaying, excessive sweating, and muscular pains. Tiredness and sleepiness as well as lethargy and listlessness may occur when the effect wears off, together with a mild depression of mood.

The unsupervised use of amphetamine or the abuse of this substance results in the taking of doses in excess of therapeutic doses, based on the patient's wish to experience the psychological effects of the drug, such as euphoria. This also leads to a tendency to loquaciousness and diminution of inhibitions. Tolerance is progressive in some individuals, and drug dependence may occur.

The effects of large dosages of amphetamine include marked euphoria and overcheerfulness, restlessness, and rapid and slurred speech, as well as tension, anxiety, and irritability. Excessively dry mouth with a tendency to rub the tongue along the inside of the lower lip as well as tachycardia and cardiac arrhythmias, brisk reflexes, dilation of pupils, and, occasionally, a sluggish response to light as well as a fine tremor of the limbs and evidence of weight loss may occur. Amphetamine psychosis has been described in detail (Connell 1968). The psychosis presents as a paranoid psychosis in a setting of clear consciousness. A rare confusional state may occur for a short time, but this is usually short lived. After withdrawal in a patient who has taken large quantities of amphetamine, excessive tiredness and sleepiness may be noted. More importantly, however, the patient may experience severe depression with suicidal ideation and the danger of suicidal attempts.

Although most studies of stimulants in general psychiatry have emphasized the lack of side effects or adverse events associated with their use, some reports have suggested caution and careful monitoring in prescribing stimulant medications for psychiatric patients. Several reports have suggested the possibility of hypertension as a side effect, particularly in patients with hypertension illness or labile hypertension. There have been an increasing number of reports of cerebral hemorrhage and cerebral angiitis using intravenous stimulants or after ingesting large amounts. However, it appears that in these cases, self-administered overdoses were either being taken by individuals who were abusing drugs, or the medications were not being given under medical supervision (Bergstrom and Keller 1992; Brust 1992; Carson et al. 1987; Citron et al. 1970; Harrington et al. 1983; Imanse and Vanneste 1990; Kalant and Kalant 1975; Lazarus et al. 1992; Ragland et al. 1993; Rumbaugh et al. 1971a, 1971b; Trugman 1988). Also, increasing reports of cardiomyopathy and myocardial infarction have been noted regarding patients who had abused stimulants intravenously and, less commonly, with high oral doses (Call et al. 1982; O'Neill et al. 1983; Packe et al. 1990). The amphetamine epidemic of the 1960s and subsequent abuse of stimulants both orally and intravenously, as well as the rise of designer drugs with both stimulant and hallucinogenic potency, have underscored the risks of abuse and dependence that have focused attention on the availability and possibly misuse of psychostimulant drugs.

Findings of high rates of comorbidity of alcohol, cocaine, opiate, and (in some cases) stimulant abuse in patients with Axis I disorders were reported in the Epidemiologic Catchment Area (ECA) study sampled in 1980–1984 by Regier and colleagues (1990). The ECA survey found the 6-month prevalence of amphetamine abuse or dependence to be 0.2%, whereas the lifetime prevalence was 1.7%. Sixth-three percent of patients who exhibited amphetamine abuse or dependence had a comorbid mental disorder, with 33% having a comorbid affective disorder and 33% a comorbid anxiety disorder. A 1971 study by Blumberg and colleagues reported the findings of chromatographic examination of urine samples in 332 young psychiatric patients and demonstrated that 24.1% of patients had positive tests for amphetamines at least

once. Robinson and Wolkind (1970) reported that 16 out of 54 patients (29.6%) in a psychiatric hospital were shown to have nonprescribed amphetamines in their urine. These studies (albeit from a period when stimulant abuse was close to its peak in the late 1960s) demonstrate the high rate of abuse of stimulant medications among psychiatric patients.

On the other hand, we are aware of few, if any, reports of stimulant abuse among patients without prior histories of drug or alcohol abuse who are being medically supervised in psychostimulant use for treatment of psychiatric disorders such as major depression.

■ Risk of Abuse or Addiction

The basis for the classification of stimulants as Class II or III narcotic substances requiring regulation (and in some cases triplicate prescription) are based on the recognition of the addictive potential of these stimulants. The concern about addictiveness is also reflected in some state laws contraindicating stimulant use in any treatment indication such as depression or other psychiatric indications other than those that are specifically spelled out in the individual state's laws. On the other hand, clinical reports of the use of stimulants in practice have provided very few reports of diagnosed patients increasing the dose, becoming dependent, or abusing stimulant medications. Metz and Shader (1991) mentioned one case of a patient who abused MPH who had a history of stimulant abuse. Several authors and reviewers of the literature on stimulants have stated that there simply are no studies showing that patients being treated for depression or other specific psychiatric syndromes are prone to abuse or to become addicted to stimulants.

Although it is recognized more and more that comorbidity certainly exists between affective disorders, personality disorders, and even addictive disorders such as alcoholism (and though clinical discretion is certainly always indicated), it has yet to be demonstrated that patients with depression or other specific medical or psychiatric indications for the use of stimulants are at any higher risk of abuse or addiction to these agents. It would therefore seem that concerns about abuse or addictiveness of these drugs need not automatically be interpreted as constituting a risk for patients who might benefit from stimulants used under the care of a skilled psychiatrist. This question needs to be examined in terms of the risks and benefits related to the clinical state of the particular patient. It should be recognized that there is still a significant percentage of patients with severe debilitating and even life-threatening depressive illnesses who do not respond to available antidepressant medications. We will consider some theoretical reasons why stimulants may add an ingredient of response in these patients when other medications fail.

A report from the Drug Abuse Warning Network (DAWN) (Carabillo 1978) presented a collection of episodic reports obtained from hospital emergency rooms, medical examiners, and crisis intervention centers in the continental United States. These reports documented incidents conforming to the definition of the term "drug abuse," or the nonmedical use of a substance for psychic effects, dependence, or self-destruction. Drug abuse was further defined as the use of prescription drugs in a manner inconsistent with accepted medical practice. This survey of incidents from July 1, 1973, through September 30, 1976, showed a marked difference in reporting of abuse of various stimulants in the anorexiant class. Amphetamine, MAMP, and phenmetrazine were ranked highest, whereas mazindol and phenteramine were in the middle ranges and mazindol and chlorphentermine were ranked at the bottom of the list.

When the relation of cumulative DAWN incidents of anorexiant drugs to dosage units prescribed for these drugs was tabulated for the time period July 1, 1973, to December 30, 1975, amphetamine and MAMP were still the highest ranked, by rate as well as by mention, whereas phenteramine and chlorphentermine were in the middle range and diethylproprion, fenfluramine, mazindol, and benzphetamine were at the low end. A comparison of DAWN-reported incidents and total prescriptions for various anorexiants from July 1973 to December 1975 again showed amphetamine preparations five times that of phenmetrazine, which was five times that of diethylproprion, phenteramine, benzphetamine, and mazindol. Some of the anorexiants such as diethylproprion may be less abused because of patterns of metabolic conversion of limited capacity to form the primary metabolites seen with modest dosage. It is considered unlikely, in view of this, that the rapid incremental effects seen with increasing doses of DAMPH would be obtainable with diethylproprion, according to this report.

When tested for self-administration and "liking,"

amphetamine and cocaine score at the top of all such measures. Phenmetrazine and diethylproprion are also chosen above placebo 60%–80% of the time, with 40%–60% of subjects exclusively choosing active drug. Phenylpropanolamine and mazindol were chosen at placebo levels despite their identification as stimulants by subjects discriminating between them and placebo. Caffeine, despite its widespread consumption in caffeinated beverages, resulted in experimentally low doses being chosen above placebo levels by about half of the subjects tested. High doses (i.e., the equivalent of more than 3 cups) were avoided by most of the subjects tested (Foltin and Fischman 1991).

It can therefore be readily seen that stimulant drugs do present hazards of abuse and dependence. However, patients with specific psychiatric disorders such as major depression and adult attention hyperactivity disorder may have a decreased risk of abuse, particularly in medically supervised environments.

■ DRUG-DRUG INTERACTIONS

Burrell and colleagues (1969) reported on the possibility of interference with the metabolism of drugs such as IMI in the presence of MPH. This was supported by Cooper and Simpson (1973) as well as in the original report by Wharton and colleagues (1971). This might suggest that the mechanism for this effect with DMI may be through inhibition of cytochrome P_{450} enzyme systems, suggesting a possible increase of other drugs metabolized by various subfamilies of this system. A second possible drug interaction is the use of stimulants with other potential stimulant drugs taken for other purposes, such as phenylpropanolamine used as a decongestant and other over-the-counter medicines that might produce significant hypertension. Cerebral hemorrhage has been reported in a few cases of patients taking phenylpropanolamine alone, and the combination with psychostimulants might prove hazardous for some patients through this mechanism.

Although we have reported the use of stimulants with MAOIs and found no apparent interactions, any such use should be carefully monitored for the possibility of hypertensive reactions or hyperpyrexia. There have been three or four reported cases of severe interactions producing hypertension, hyperpyrexia, convulsions, and death. The use of psychostimulants in significant doses may overwhelm the effect of antihypertensive medications and produce clinically significant hypertension in some individuals. Psychostimulants are potent substances and should be used only after careful clinical diagnosis (both psychiatric and medical) is considered. This use should be followed with great clinical care in selected patients. The informed and careful use of these substances may produce benefits for individuals with significant psychiatric disorders who are not responsive to currently available treatment. Stimulants should be prescribed by skilled clinicians who are familiar with potential clinical and medical side effects and potential side effects, toxic effects, and drug-drug interactions.

■ REFERENCES

Alles GA: The comparative physiological actions of *dl*-beta-phenylisopropylamines. J Pharmacol Exp Ther 47:339–354, 1933

Anders TF, Ciaranello RD: Pharmacologic treatment of minimal brain dysfunction syndrome, in Psychopharmacology: From Theory to Practice. Edited by Barchas JD, Berger PA, Ciaranello RD, et al. New York, Oxford University Press, 1977, pp 425–435

Angrist B, D'Hollosy M, Sanfilipo M, et al: Central nervous system stimulants as symptomatic treatments for AIDS-related neuropsychiatric impairment. J Clin Psychopharmacol 12:268–272, 1992

Axelrod J, Weil-Malherbe H, Tomchick R: The physiological disposition of ^{3}H-epinephrine and its metabolite metanephrine. J Pharmacol Exp Ther 127:251–256, 1959

Ayd FJ, Zohar J: Psychostimulant (amphetamine or methylphenidate) therapy for chronic and treatment-resistant depression, in Treating Resistant Depression. Edited by Zohar J, Belmaker RH. New York, PMA Publishing Corp, 1987, pp 343–355

Barkley RA: A review of stimulant drug research with hyperactive children. J Child Psychol Psychiatry 18:137–165, 1977

Bergstrom DL, Keller C: Drug-induced myocardial ischemia and acute myocardial infarction. Critical Care Nursing Clinics of North America 4(2):273–278, 1992

Blumberg AG, Cohen M, Heaton AM, et al: Covert drug abuse among voluntary hospitalized psychiatric patients. JAMA 217:1659–1661, 1971

Bouckoms A, Mangini L: Pergolide: an antidepressant adjuvant for mood disorders? Psychopharmacol Bull 29:207–211, 1993

Bradley C, Bowen M: Amphetamine (benzedrine) therapy of children's behavior disorders. Am J Orthopsychiatry 11:92–103, 1941

Brown WA, Corriveau DP, Ebert MH: Acute psychologic and neuroendocrine effects of dextro-amphetamine and methylphenidate. Psychopharmacology (Berl) 58:189–195, 1978

Brust JCM: Stroke and substance abuse, in Stroke: Pathophysiology, Diagnosis, and Management, 2nd Edition. Edited by Barnett HJM, Mohr JP, Stein BM, et al. New York, Churchill Livingstone, 1992, pp 875–893

Burrell JM, Black M, Wharton RN, et al: Inhibition of imipramine metabolism by methylphenidate. Federation Proceedings 28:418, 1969

Call TD, Hartneck J, Dickinson WA, et al: Acute cardiomyopathy secondary to intravenous amphetamine abuse. Ann Intern Med 97:559–560, 1982

Carabillo EA: U.S.A. Drug Abuse Warning Network, in Central Mechanisms of Anorectic Drugs. Edited by Garattini S, Samanin R. New York, Raven, 1978, pp 461–471

Carson P, Oldroyd K, Phadke K: Myocardial infarction due to amphetamine. British Medical Journal 294:1525–1526, 1987

Chiarello RJ, Cole JO: The use of psychostimulants in general psychiatry. Arch Gen Psychiatry 44:286–295, 1987

Citron BP, Halpert M, McCarron M, et al: Necrotizing angiitis associated with drug abuse. N Engl J Med 283:1003–1011, 1970

Connell PH: The use and abuse of amphetamines. Practitioner 200:234–243, 1968

Cooper TB, Simpson GM: Concomitant imipramine and methylphenidate administration: a case report. Am J Psychiatry 130:6, 1973

Dally PJ: Fatal reaction associated with tranylcypromine and methylamphetamine. Lancet 1:1235–1236, 1962

D'haenen HA, Bossuyt A: Dopamine D_2 receptor density in depression measured with single photon emission computed tomography. Biol Psychiatry 35:128–132, 1994

Drimmer EJ, Gitlin MJ, Gwirtsman HE: Desipramine and methylphenidate combination treatment for depression: case report. Am J Psychiatry 140:241–

242, 1983

Fawcett J, Siomopoulos V: Dextroamphetamine response as a possible predictor of improvement with tricyclic therapy in depression. Arch Gen Psychiatry 25:247–255, 1971

Fawcett J, Kravitz HM, Zajecka JM, et al: CNS stimulant potentiation of monoamine oxidase inhibitors in treatment-refractory depression. J Clin Psychopharmacol 11:127–132, 1991

Feighner JP, Herbstein J, Damlouji N: Combined MAOI, TCA and direct stimulant therapy of treatment resistant depression. J Clin Psychiatry 46:206–209, 1985

Fernandez F, Adams F, Holmes VF, et al: Methylphenidate for depressive disorders in cancer patients. Psychosomatics 28:455–459, 1987

Fernandez F, Adams F, Levy JK, et al: Cognitive impairment due to AIDS-related complex and its response to psychostimulants. Psychosomatics 29(1):38–46, 1988a

Fernandez F, Levy JK, Galizzi H: Response of HIV-related depression to psychostimulants: case reports. Hosp Community Psychiatry 39:628–631, 1988b

Fischman MW: Cocaine and the amphetamines, in Psychopharmacology: The Third Generation of Progress. Edited by Meltzer HY. New York, Raven, 1987, pp 1543–1553

Flemenbaum A: Methylphenidate: a catalyst for the tricyclic antidepressants? Am J Psychiatry 128:239, 1971

Foltin RW, Fischman MW: Assessment of abuse liability of stimulant drugs in humans: a methodological survey. Drug Alcohol Depend 28:3–48, 1991

Glennon RA: Psychoactive phenylisopropylamines, in Psychopharmacology: The Third Generation of Progress. Edited by Meltzer HY. New York, Raven, 1987, p 1627

Harrington H, Heller HA, Dawson D, et al: Intracerebral hemorrhage and oral amphetamine. Arch Neurol 40:503–507, 1983

Hill D: Amphetamine in psychopathic states. British Journal of Addiction 44:50–54, 1947

Hill D, Watterson D: Electro-encephalographic studies of psychopathic personalities. Journal of Neurology and Psychiatry 5:47–65, 1942

Hodge RS, Hutchings HM: Enuresis: a brief review, a tentative theory and a suggested treatment. Arch Dis Child 27:498–504, 1952

Hoffman BB, Lefkowitz RJ: Catecholamines and sympathomimetic drugs, in The Pharmacological Basis of Therapeutics, 8th Edition. Edited by Gilman AG, Goodman LS, Rall TW, et al. New York, Macmillan, 1993, pp 187–220

Holmes VF, Fernandez F, Levy JK: Psychostimulant response in AIDS-related complex patients. J Clin Psychiatry 50(1):5–8, 1989

Imanse J, Vanneste J: Intraventricular hemorrhage following amphetamine abuse. Neurology 40:1318, 1990

Insel TR, Hamilton JA, Guttmacher LB, et al: d-Amphetamine in obsessive-compulsive disorder. Psychopharmacology (Berl) 80:231–235, 1983

Janowsky D, Davis JM: Methylphenidate, dextroamphetamine, and levoamphetamine. Arch Gen Psychiatry 33:304–308, 1976

Johnson ML, Roberts MD, Rossa R, et al: Methylphenidate in stroke patients with depression. Am J Phys Med Rehabil 71:239–241, 1992

Kalant H, Kalant OJ: Death in amphetamine users: causes and rates. Can Med Assoc J 112:299–304, 1975

Khantzian EJ, Gawin F, Kleber HD, et al: Methylphenidate (Ritalin®) treatment of cocaine dependence—a preliminary report. J Subst Abuse Treat 1:107–112, 1984

Kraus MF, Burch EA: Methylphenidate hydrochloride as an antidepressant: controversy, case studies and review. South Med J 85:985–991, 1992

Kravitz HM, Edwards JH, Fawcett J, et al: Challenging the amphetamine challenge test: report of an antidepressant study. J Affect Disord 20:121–128, 1990

Krisko I, Lewis E, Johnston JE: Severe hyperpyrexia due to tranylcypromine-amphetamine toxicity. Ann Intern Med 70:559–564, 1969

Lazarus LW, Winemiller DR, Lingam VR, et al: Efficacy and side effects of methylphenidate for post-stroke depression. J Clin Psychiatry 53:447–449, 1992

Lieberman JA, Kinon BJ, Loebel AD: Dopaminergic mechanisms in idiopathic and drug-induced psychoses. Schizophr Bull 16:97–110, 1990

Linet LS: Treatment of a refractory depression with a combination of fluoxetine and d-amphetamine. Am J Psychiatry 146(6):803–804, 1989

Lloyd JTA, Walker DRH: Death after combine dexamphetamine and phenelzine. British Medical Journal 2:168–169, 1965

Mantle TJ, Tipton KF, Garrett NJ: Inhibition of monoamine oxidase by amphetamine and related compounds. Biochem Pharmacol 25:2073–2077, 1976

Mason A: Fatal reaction associated with tranylcypromine and methylamphetamine. Lancet 1:1073, 1962

Metz A, Shader RI: Combination of fluoxetine with pemoline in the treatment of major depressive disorder. Int Clin Psychopharmacol 6:93–96, 1991

Meyler L: The Side Effects of Drugs. Amsterdam, Excerpta Medica Foundation, 1966

Miller HH, Shore PA, Clarke DE: In vivo monoamine oxidase inhibition by d-amphetamine. Biochem Pharmacol 29:1347–1354, 1980

Myers WC, Stewart JT: Use of methylphenidate. Hosp Community Psychiatry 40:754, 1989

Nurnberger JI, Simmons-Alling S, Kessler L, et al: Separate mechanisms for behavioral, cardiovascular, and hormonal responses to dextroamphetamine in man. Psychopharmacology (Berl) 84:200–204, 1984

O'Neill ME, Arnolda LF, Coles DM, et al: Acute amphetamine cardiomyopathy in a drug addict. Clin Cardiol 6:189–191, 1983

Packe GE, Garton MJ, Jennings K: Acute myocardial infarction caused by intravenous amphetamine abuse. Br Heart J 64(1):23–24, 1990

Patrick KS, Kilts CD, Breese GR: Synthesis and pharmacology of hydroxylated metabolites of methylphenidate. J Med Chem 24:1237–1240, 1981

Patrick KS, Mueller RA, Gualtieri CT, et al: Pharmacokinetics and actions of methyl-phenidate, in Psychopharmacology: The Third Generation of Progress. Edited by Meltzer H. New York, Raven, 1987, pp 1387–1395

Patrick RL: Amphetamine and cocaine: biological mechanisms, in Psychopharmacology: From Theory to Practice. Edited by Barchas JD, Berger PA, Ciaranello RD, et al. New York, Oxford University Press, 1977, pp 331–340

Perel JM, Black N, Wharton RN, et al: Inhibition of imipramine metabolism by methylphenidate. Federation Proceedings 28:418, 1969

Physicians' Desk Reference, 48th Edition. Montvale, NJ, Medical Economics Data Production Company, 1994

Post RM, Gerner RH, Carman JS: Effects of a dopamine agonist piribedil in depressed patients. Arch Gen Psychiatry 35:609–615, 1978

Prinzmetal M, Bloomberg W: The use of benzedrine for the treatment of narcolepsy. JAMA 105:2051–2054, 1935

Ragland AS, Ismail Y, Arsura EL: Myocardial infarction after amphetamine use. Am Heart J 125:247–249, 1993

Regier DA, Farmer ME, Rae DS, et al: Comorbidity of mental disorders with alcohol and other drug abuse: results from the Epidemiologic Catchment Area (ECA) study. JAMA 264:2511–2518, 1990

Riishede J: Treatment of acute barbiturate poisoning; a comparison of nikethamide and amphetamine. Lancet 2:789–792, 1950

Robinson AE, Wolkind SN: Amphetamine abuse amongst psychiatric inpatients: the use of gas chromatography. Br J Psychiatry 116:643–644, 1970

Rumbaugh CL, Bergeron RT, Fang HCH, et al: Cerebral angiographic changes in the drug abuse patient. Radiology 101:335–344, 1971a

Rumbaugh DL, Bergeron RT, Scanlan RL, et al: Cerebral vascular changes secondary to amphetamine abuse in the experimental animal. Radiology 101:345–351, 1971b

Sabelli HC, Fawcett J, Javaid JI, et al: The methylphenidate test for differentiating desipramine-responsive from nortriptyline-responsive depression. Am J Psychiatry 140:212–214, 1983

Satel SL, Nelson JC: Stimulants in the treatment of depression: a critical overview. J Clin Psychiatry 59:241–249, 1989

Satterfield JH, Satterfield BT, Cantwell DP: Three multi-modal treatment of 100 hyperactive boys. Behavioral Pediatrics 98:650–655, 1981

Satterfield JH, Satterfield BT, Shell AM: Therapeutic interventions to prevent delinquency in hyperactive boys. J Am Acad Child Adolesc Psychiatry 26:56–64, 1987

Schachar R, Tannock R: Childhood hyperactivity and psychostimulants: a review of extended treatment studies. Journal of Child and Adolescent Psychopharmacology 3:81–97, 1993

Seiden LS, Sabol KE, Ricaurte GA: Amphetamine: Effects on catecholamine systems and behavior. Annu Rev Pharmacol Toxicol 32:639–677, 1993

Shaw DM: Antidepressant drugs. Practitioner 192:28–32, 1964

Sloviter E, Drust EG, Connor JD: Evidence that serotonin mediates some behavioral effects of amphetamine. J Pharmacol Exp Ther 206:348–352, 1978

Smilkstein MJ, Smolinske SC, Rumack BH: A case of MAO inhibitor/MDMA interaction: agony after ecstasy. Clinical Toxicology 25:149–152, 1987

Smith RC, Davis JM: Comparative effects of d-amphetamine/amphetamine and methylphenidate on mood in man. Psychopharmacology (Berl) 53:1–12, 1977

Sprague RL, Cohen M, Werry JS: Normative data on the Conners Teacher's Rating Scale and Abbreviated Scale (technical report). Urbana-Champaign, University of Illinois Children's Research Center, 1974

Stockley IH: Drug interactions 10: monoamine oxidase inhibitors; part 1: interactions with sympathomimetic amines. The Pharmaceutical Journal 210:590–594, 1973

Sulzer D, Rayport S: Amphetamine and other psychostimulants reduce pH gradients in midbrain dopaminergic neurons and chromaffin granules: a mechanism of action. Neuron 5:797–808, 1990

Theohar C, Fischer-Cornelssen K, Akesson H, et al: Bromocriptine as antidepressant: double-blind comparative study with imipramine in psychogenic and endogenous depression. Current Therapeutic Research 30(6):830–842, 1981

Tinklenburg JR, Berger PA: Treatment of abusers of non-addictive drugs, in Psychopharmacology: From Theory to Practice. Edited by Barchas JD, Berger PA, Ciaranello RD, et al. New York, Oxford University Press, 1977, pp 386–403

Trugman JM: Cerebral arteritis and oral methylphenidate. Lancet 1:584–585, 1988

van Kammen DP, Murphy DL: Prediction of antidepressant response by a one day d-amphetamine trial. Am J Psychiatry 135:1179–1184, 1978

Wender PH, Reimherr FW, Wood D, et al: A controlled study of methylphenidate in the treatment of attention deficit disorder, residual type, in adults. Am J Psychiatry 142:547–552, 1985

Wharton RN, Perel JM, Dayton PG, et al: A potential clinical use for methylphenidate with tricyclic antidepressants. Am J Psychiatry 127:1619–1625, 1971

Wheatley D: Amphetamines in general practice: their use in depression and anxiety. Seminars in Psychiatry 1:163–173, 1969

Williams RT, Caldwell RJ, Dreng LG: Comparative metabolism of some amphetamine in various species, in Frontiers of Catecholamine Research. Edited by Schneider SH, Esdin E. Oxford, England, Pergamon, 1973, pp 927–932

Zeck P: The dangers of some antidepressant drugs. Med J Aust 2:607–608, 1961

Clinical Psychobiology and Psychiatric Syndromes

David J. Kupfer, M.D., Section Editor

22

Biology of Mood Disorders

Kalpana I. Nathan, M.D., Dominique L. Musselman, M.D.,
Alan F. Schatzberg, M.D., and Charles B. Nemeroff, M.D., Ph.D.

■ HISTORICAL CONSIDERATIONS

The fundamental concept of psychobiology in psychiatry was posited by Adolf Meyer (1866–1950) in the early twentieth century. In an era of exceptional contributions from Kraepelin, who empirically outlined the classification of mood and schizophrenic disorders, and from Freud, whose work delineated important psychodynamic processes and their role in symptom generation, Meyer undertook the difficult task of integrating the psychological and biological approaches to understanding disorders of the mind. However, in the post–World War II era, biological psychiatry retreated with the preeminence of psychoanalytic theory and practice. The reemergence of interest in the biological perspective began in the 1950s after the introduction of chlorpromazine as an effective antipsychotic agent. Interest in the biology of depression was fostered by the introduction of effective antidepressants.

The earliest hypothesis of mood disorders focused on biogenic amine metabolism playing a key role in the pathogenesis of depression. Pioneering work in this area was done in the United States by Bunney and Davis (1965), Prange (1964), and Schildkraut (1965), who focused on catecholamine physiology. Schildkraut (1965) originated the catecholamine hypothesis, which has inspired much of the biological research that continues to this day. However, substantial data have implicated alterations in several other neuromodulary systems in mood disorders.

European researchers began their investigation of the serotonergic system in the 1960s with a hypothesis that serotonergic deficiency produced depressive symptoms (Coppen 1968; Lapin and Oxenkrug 1969). This area of research was bolstered by the observations of Asberg and colleagues (1976a), who noted that depressed patients with low cerebrospinal fluid (CSF) concentrations of 5-hydroxyindoleacetic acid (5-HIAA) were at greater risk for attempting or committing suicide, particularly by violent means. The association between indices of low serotonin (5-HT) turnover and impulsive violent behavior has been consistently replicated in several studies (Roy et al. 1989; Traskman et al. 1981; Van Praag 1982), although it does not appear to be specific to depression (Linnoila and Virkkunen 1992; Virkkunen et al. 1994). Interest in 5-HT systems in depression has been supported by the introduction of selective serotonin reuptake inhibitors (SSRIs) (e.g., fluoxetine, sertraline).

Janowsky and colleagues (1972) hypothesized that adrenergic-cholinergic imbalances were responsible for pronounced variations in mood. A relative increase in acetylcholine (ACh) activity in comparison to norepinephrine (NE) activity was associated with depression and a relative increase in NE activity in comparison to ACh activity was associated with mania.

Several of these hypotheses originally arose in part from important pharmacological observations. Reserpine, a rauwolfia alkaloid antihypertensive agent, was found to produce depressive symptoms in patients—symptoms resulting from depletion of available biogenic amines. Reserpine also produced symptoms suggestive of increased ACh activity. The antidepressant action of monoamine oxidase inhibitors (MAOIs) was discovered by the chance observation of the effects of iproniazid, a drug that was developed for the treatment of tuberculosis. Monoamine oxidase (MAO) was known to degrade intraneuronal NE and 5-HT, and MAOIs alleviated depressive symptoms. Imipramine, a tricyclic compound, was originally developed for the treatment of schizophrenia, but it was found to elevate mood rather than relieve psychosis. Tricyclic antidepressants (TCAs) blocked the reuptake of NE into presynaptic neurons. Additionally, they had anticholinergic properties. 5-HT was also shown to play a potential role in the therapeutic action of antidepressant drugs. For example, Shopsin and colleagues (1975, 1976) found that administration of p-chlorophenylalanine, an inhibitor of 5-HT synthesis, reversed the antidepressant action of imipramine (a TCA) as well as tranylcypromine (an MAOI).

Clinical endocrinopathies have been long associated with disturbances in mood, especially those affecting the adrenocortical and thyroid functions. Patients with Cushing's disease often have symptoms of depression, mania, and impaired cognitive function. Administration of corticosteroids is also known to precipitate psychiatric syndromes. In the late 1950s, hypercortisolemia was noted as a feature of depression; this led to considerable research in the past 20 years on the relationship between hypothalamic-pituitary-adrenal (HPA) axis activity and depression. Multiple studies have shown that 40%–50% of patients with endogenous depression demonstrate resistance to dexamethasone-induced HPA axis suppression, in the so-called dexamethasone suppression test (DST) (Brown et al. 1979; Carroll and Davies 1970). Although research on the DST often emphasizes its use as a biological test, more recently our respective research groups have been interested in the role of increased HPA axis activity in the pathogenesis of specific symptoms.

Recent data also suggest subtle thyroid dysfunction may play important roles in the etiology of depression. The thyrotropin-releasing hormone (TRH) stimulation test, which measures the release of pituitary thyroid-stimulating hormone (TSH) following TRH administration, has been studied extensively in affective disorders. A blunted TSH response to TRH in 25%–30% of depressed patients was originally reported in the 1970s by several research groups (Kastin et al. 1972; Prange et al. 1972; Takahashi et al. 1973). In this chapter, we review recent advances in neurotransmitter physiology, psychoneuroendocrinology, psychoneuroimmunology, genetics, and imaging.

■ NOSOLOGY

Standardized diagnostic criteria of mood disorders not only assist in the detection and recognition of disorders such as major depression and bipolar disorder but also provide estimation of their prevalence. Moreover, reliable diagnostic criteria can be used to systematically evaluate treatment modalities, identify risk factors leading to development of a mood disorder, and herald preventive measures. The *Diagnostic and Statistical Manual of Mental Disorders, Fourth Edition* (American Psychiatric Association 1994) has updated the classification of mood disorders. We briefly review the DSM-IV section on mood disorders and focus on changes in the spectrum of depressive and manic syndromes that were previously defined in accordance with DSM-III-R (American Psychiatric Association 1987) criteria.

The DSM-IV section on mood disorders is divided into three parts, with the first part describing mood episodes, including major depressive, manic, mixed, and hypomanic episodes. The second part sets criteria for mood disorders, including depressive and bipolar disorders, mood disorder due to a general medical condition, and substance-induced mood disorder. The third part includes the specifiers that describe either the most recent mood episode or the course of recurrent episodes.

The major depressive disorders have severity, psychotic, and remission specifiers; additional categories include catatonic, melancholic, and atypical features, as well as postpartum onset. The recurrent major depressive disorders have longitudinal course specifiers (with and without interepisode recovery), as well as specifications for seasonal pattern and rapid cycling.

The depressive disorder not otherwise specified has been expanded to include premenstrual dysphoric disorder, minor depressive disorder (depressive symptoms subthreshold in severity to major depression), recurrent brief depressive disorder (episodes that occur at least once a month for 12 months, lasting from 2 days to 2 weeks), postpsychotic depressive disorder of schizophrenia, and major depressive disorder superimposed on psychotic disorders. The inclusion of these disorders makes it possible to validate depressive syndromes that fall short of DSM-III-R thresholds for depressive disorders. Because these patients exhibit clinically significant impairment (as measured by health care utilization and functional disability), these syndromes of depression have been included in DSM-IV. In fact, recurrent brief depressive disorder is currently included in the International Statistical Classification of Diseases and Related Health Problems, Tenth Revision (ICD-10 [World Health Organization 1992]; APA Task Force on DSM-IV 1991).

Criteria for bipolar mood disorder spectrum has undergone substantial revision. There is now a clear specification of the period of abnormally elevated, expansive, or irritable mood, which should last at least 1 week, or of any duration if hospitalization is necessary. There are six separate criteria sets for bipolar disorder, which include single manic episode, most recent episode hypomanic, most recent episode manic, most recent episode mixed, most recent episode depressed, and most recent episode unspecified. Bipolar II disorder has been included, which specifies recurrent depressive episodes with hypomanic episodes.

The DSM-III-R criteria for mixed subtype of bipolar disorder describe two very different types of presentations: depressive and manic symptoms that are "intermixed" and those "rapidly alternating every few days." DSM-IV has differentiated between and described these two different patient populations. There is a rapid-cycling course specifier to describe those patients with rapidly alternating symptoms, whereas "intermixed" presentations are now reclassified as mixed episode.

The unipolar and bipolar mood syndromes have each subsumed the overinclusive and ambiguous diagnosis of organic mood disorder. This diagnosis was listed in two different sections of DSM-III-R (organic mental disorders associated with Axis III physical disorders or conditions, and psychoactive substance–induced organic mental disorders). As multiple factors (biological, psychological, and social) contribute to the presentation of most mental disorders, the dichotomy between "organic" and "nonorganic" has become obsolete. The term *organic* has been re-

placed by the term *mood disorder due to . . .,* and the related nonpsychiatric medical condition is included as part of the name of the disorder and included on Axis I (e.g., "mood disorder due to autoimmune thyroiditis, with hypomanic episode"). This subtyping scheme allows the clinician to indicate whether the individual has met specific diagnostic criteria for major depression or manic episode or whether he or she has a subthreshold or mixed presentation (American Psychiatric Association Task Force on DSM-IV 1991; American Psychiatric Association 1994).

Organic mood disorder had been listed within yet another section of DSM-III-R, psychoactive substance–induced organic mental disorders. In DSM-IV, substance-induced mood disorder has been placed within the mood disorders section. The specific substance used, the context in which the substance-induced mood disorder has developed (i.e., during intoxication or withdrawal), and the specific mood disorder are described (e.g., "cocaine withdrawal mood disorder, with major depressive episode"). The categorization of substance-induced mood disorder and mood disorder due to a nonpsychiatric medical condition under the rubric of mood disorders facilitates differential diagnosis while eliminating the anachronistic "organic" classification.

The "course specifiers" offered by DSM-IV (e.g., "with seasonal pattern," "postpartum mood disturbance," "with/without full interepisode recovery") for both the unipolar and bipolar mood syndromes provide further diagnostic refinements. With each successive edition of DSM, identification of phenomenologically defined subsets of patients progresses, in the hope of improving identification, treatment, and even prevention of chronic and disabling mood disorders.

◼ EPIDEMIOLOGY AND GENETICS

◼ Epidemiology

Over the past 30 years, epidemiological studies of the major mood disorders have reported considerable variation in the prevalence of depression and bipolar mood disorder. This variability may be explained by the differing methodology of these surveys: sampling of the populations at risk, the particular diagnostic system used, the method for obtaining information about symptoms, and the time when information is obtained (Weissman et al. 1992).

The most extensive survey completed after publication of DSM-III (American Psychiatric Association 1980) is the Epidemiologic Catchment Area (ECA) study sponsored by the National Institute of Mental Health (NIMH). Between 1980 and 1984, 20,291 adults ages 18 and older were interviewed using the Diagnostic Interview Schedule (DIS) (Robins et al. 1981) in a variety of settings: community households, long-term treatment mental hospitals, nursing homes, and correctional institutions. The ECA study indicated the following 1-month prevalence rates (a guide in determining the number in the population with a disorder at a given point in time) per 100 persons: major depression (1.8), dysthymia (3.3), bipolar I (0.4), and bipolar II disorder (0.2). Lifetime prevalence rates (or risk of acquiring the disorder over a lifetime) per 100 persons were major depression (4.9), dysthymia (3.3), bipolar I (0.8), and bipolar II disorder (0.5) (Regier et al. 1988).

■ Genetics of Affective Disorder

The probability that a person will have an affective disorder is probably influenced by a number of factors, including premature parental loss, inadequate rearing by parents, a history of traumatic events, certain personality traits, previous history of affective episodes, the extent of social support, and recent stressful life events (Kendler et al. 1993b). The scrutiny of major depression and bipolar disorder in family, twin, and adoption studies demonstrates that genetic influences undoubtedly play a substantial role in the etiology of affective disorder. Understanding this genetic contribution may help provide genetic counseling, early identification of those at risk, and clues about the specific genetic defect(s) associated with or responsible for vulnerability to these disorders (Michels and Marzuk 1993). We present a brief review of the steps necessary to clarify the role of genetic factors in a particular psychiatric disorder, and the multiple methods of evaluating the data.

Family studies can provide initial evidence of genetic contributions. Morbid risk (i.e., adjusted prevalence) of the disorder is determined within the affected families, and the rate for patients' relatives is compared with that for relatives of control groups or for the general population. First-degree relatives (i.e., parents, siblings, and offspring) of patients with bipolar affective disorder are reported to be at least 24

times more likely to develop bipolar affective disorder than relatives of control subjects (Weissman et al. 1984). However, family studies cannot establish that an disorder is hereditary. Familial aggregation may reflect a shared environment—for example, common exposure to a particular culture or to a virus (Pardes et al. 1989).

Twin studies compare the concordance rate for illness in pairs of monozygotic (identical) twins versus the rate in dizygotic (nonidentical) twins. The rationale is that monozygotic twins share identical genes, whereas dizygotic twins share only half of their genes. It is also assumed that both types of twins are exposed to the same prenatal and postnatal environment. Thus, if monozygotic twins show a greater concordance rate for a particular psychiatric disorder than dizygotic twins, this is believed to be firm evidence for a strong genetic contribution to development of the disorder. However, the extent to which environmental factors can be considered equal for monozygotic and dizygotic twins is arguable. In utero, monozygotic twins share the identical placental circulation; dizygotic twins do not. Moreover, monozygotic twins may also elicit similar treatment from the environment by virtue of their similar appearance. Therefore, monozygotic twins have different life experiences than do dizygotic twins. However, the marked difference in concordance rates between monozygotic and dizygotic twins strongly supports the hypothesis of a major genetic component in unipolar depression (Kendler et al. 1992, 1993a; McGuffin et al. 1991; Tsuang and Faraone 1990) and in bipolar disorder (Bertelson et al. 1977; Mendlewicz 1988).

Adoption studies attempt to elucidate the contribution of environment ("nurture") and genetic contribution ("nature") by studying children raised away from their biological parents. Cases of adopted children developing the affective disorder of their biological parent and, conversely, of adoptive children *not* developing the mood disorder of the parents with the disorder support the hypothesis of heritable diathesis. However, one of the limitations of adoption studies is the environmental factors (including the in utero environment) that have already affected the adopted child. Nevertheless, adoption studies show a greater prevalence rate of bipolar disorder among biological relatives versus adopted relatives of bipolar patients (Mendlewicz and Rainier 1977; Wender et al. 1986). Despite their respective limitations, family, twin, and adoption studies all demonstrate a significant contribution of hereditary factors in the pathogenesis of affective disorder.

There are three major models regarding the mode of inheritance (i.e., *how* an illness is genetically transmitted and *what* constitutes the factor that is inherited). About one-quarter of the more than 4,000 illnesses transmitted through *monogenic inheritance* (i.e., caused by defects in a single major gene and transmitted according to a Mendelian pattern: dominant, recessive, or sex-linked) affect mental functioning. However, the prevalence rates of any of these diseases (e.g., Lesch-Nyhan syndrome and phenylketonuria) is uncommon (McKusick 1992). In contrast, other illnesses (e.g., atherosclerosis and diabetes) are believed to be caused by combined defects of several genes, or *polygenic inheritance.* The other mode of inheritance is *multifactorial inheritance,* based on major and minor gene effects in combination *and* also on the interaction between the environment and heredity.

Statistical analysis, including segregation and linkage analysis, are used to search for both the mode of inheritance and for the chromosomal location of the genes predisposing to the particular disorder under study. Segregation analysis compares the observed frequency of an illness in a pedigree (ancestral relationships of individuals of a family over two or more generations) with the pattern that would occur if a hypothesized mode of inheritance (i.e., monogenic versus polygenic transmission) were true (McKusick 1992).

Another mode of analysis is linkage analysis (Gershon and Goldin 1987), which tests whether the observed co-occurrence of a disease and a marker for a genetic locus within a given pedigree are compatible with that locus contributing to disease susceptibility (Kauffman and Malaspina 1993). Linkage analysis may proceed along one of three possible lines—identification of an abnormal protein, or a particular nucleic acid sequence, or "biological marker" gene that is consistently transmitted or "linked" with the gene(s) responsible for the affective illness. The "protein-gene" approach posits that when an abnormal protein is found to accompany a particular illness, this abnormal protein can be used to track the accompanying abnormal gene. (Unfortunately, specific neurochemical disturbances associated with many psychiatric illnesses are unknown.) Second, linkage analysis can proceed by the "gene-protein"

approach. If a specific DNA sequence of the genome (the DNA content of a cell) is consistently transmitted or "linked" with the disease, the approximate chromosomal location of the abnormal gene is revealed (this is discussed in more detail later in this chapter).

Finally, the third approach is to study "candidate" genes, which are already implicated in the pathogenesis or pathophysiology of a particular disease. If a disease has a particular "biological marker" or an associated biological abnormality, it may derive from either an abnormal gene and/or from a gene "linked" (in close proximity) to it (Pardes et al. 1989). If the genomic region that codes for the biological marker is known, it permits a more direct search for the gene causing the disease (Botstein et al. 1980). Clearly, researchers would more usefully study a trait marker than a state marker for the illness of interest. Unfortunately, most biological markers of affective disorder identified thus far are state markers.

Linkage analysis uses a variety of genetic markers. The recent advances in molecular genetics include the remarkable paper by Botstein and colleagues (1980), who proposed treating differences in DNA sequence like allelic variants of a gene and to use these variations in DNA as markers for mapping of the genome. These variations in the sequence of nucleotide base pairs between individuals are called polymorphisms. These polymorphisms between individuals or interindividual differences in DNA can be detected by using restriction enzymes, which are bacterial molecules that recognize and cut at specific nucleic acid sequences within a strand of DNA, thereby producing DNA "restriction fragments" of characteristic lengths.

Polymorphisms—the variations in nucleotide base pair sequences—cause restriction fragments to vary in length. Radiolabeled single strands of DNA ("probes") are then used to bind to homologous sequences of restriction fragment DNA. The radiolabeled probe–restriction fragment combination is known as a restriction fragment length polymorphism (RFLP). The size differences of the RFLPs lead to a differential migration in electrophoresis (Southern 1975) and are visible as different banding patterns on X-ray film. When an RFLP cosegregates with an illness in members of a family, it could represent a gene mutation or a marker linked to the gene causing the disorder. In this way, the general chromosomal location of a disease-associated gene is established, and more specific localization can begin. If the messenger RNA derived from the gene has a disease-appropriate neuroanatomical distribution, this increases the likelihood that the gene is a contributor to the psychiatric illness. Putative RFLPs have been identified in bipolar disorder, and it is hoped that the gene defects will be elucidated in the near future.

RFLPs are based on single nucleotide changes. Another polymorphism is known as the variable number of tandem repeats (VNTRs) (also known as "minisatellites") of a relatively short oligonucleotide sequence (Nakamura et al. 1987). In these polymorphisms, the variation in length of the DNA restriction fragments stems from differences in the number of short oligonucleotide sequences found between two adjacent restriction fragment sites. For example, a sequence with 100 base pairs can be repeated multiple times between two adjacent restriction fragment sites. The number of tandem repeats is inherited in Mendelian fashion and typically has numerous alleles (each one defined by a unique number of the repeated sequence). A VNTR locus is genotyped using the identical techniques as for an RFLP locus. Because VNTRs cluster at the ends of chromosomes and are not evenly spaced throughout the human genome (Royle et al. 1988), researchers have used another polymorphism, simple sequence repeat (SSR) markers.

SSR markers (also known as "microsatellites") are similar to VNTRs, because they are based on a variable number of a sequence of nucleotides repeated in tandem. Unlike VNTRs, microsatellites are abundant and evenly distributed across the human genome (Weber and May 1989). The repeated sequence usually consists of 2–5 nucleotides (often —$(CA)_n$—, —$(AG)_n$—, or —$(AAAT)_n$—). If this sequence repeated in tandem consists of at least 20 uninterrupted units, then the locus is likely to show 60%–70% heterozygosity, based on inherited differences in the number of units repeated in tandem. These short stretches of DNA can be synthesized using the polymerase chain reaction (PCR) technique. The "amplified" amount of microsatellite is then detected by autoradiography, with allele sizes varying according to the number (n) of the repeated nucleotide sequence (Berrettini 1992).

Segregation and linkage analysis studies have not yet produced definitive results in the study of the major psychiatric disorders. Two teams of investigators have reported two different genes responsible for producing manic-depressive disorder. In a Pennsylvania Amish community, the gene reported to produce manic-depressive disorder was found to be positioned on chromosome 11 and inherited by autosomal dominant transmission (Egeland et al. 1987). Unfortunately, subsequent analysis has not confirmed this finding in an expanded data set of the same population (Kelsoe et al. 1989). Moreover, other groups reported that the chromosome 11 marker was not linked with bipolar disorder (Detera-Wadleigh et al. 1987; Hodgkinson et al. 1987). In an Israeli population, Baron and colleagues (1987) localized another gene responsible for bipolar disorder on the long arm of the X chromosome. Taken together, these reports suggest that bipolar illness exhibits *nonallelic genetic heterogeneity*—different genes are affected in different individuals yet produce a similar clinical disorder (Baron et al. 1987, 1993; Detera-Wadleigh et al. 1987; Egeland et al. 1987; Hodgkinson et al. 1987).

Further puzzles arise when *non*genetic cases of an illness occur in the disease spectrum of depression or bipolar disorder; these nongenetic cases are known as phenocopies. Phenocopies present a clinical picture similar to that of a hereditary form; they have been reported in cases of major depression and manic-depressive disorder (Price et al. 1987) and with other psychiatric disorders. If nongenetic forms of an illness can be detected and excluded, linkage studies can determine the linked markers that cosegregate with a disease in the remaining pedigrees.

Another obstacle in determining the genetic contribution to an affective illness is the degree of *penetrance* (i.e., the likelihood that the genetic disturbance will be expressed). In monozygotic twins discordant for bipolar disorder, it is likely that both twins are at genetic risk, even if bipolar disorder remains unexpressed in the unaffected twin (Pardes et al. 1989).

Yet another conundrum is variable expressivity. The gene conferring susceptibility to a major mood disorder may be capable of producing a spectrum of clinical manifestations. One research group has reported that major affective disorder and anorexia nervosa cosegregate in families (Gershon et al. 1983). In relatives of patients with anorexia nervosa, there is a significantly higher rate of major affective illness than in the relatives of control subjects; thus, a genetic variant of affective illness may be anorexia nervosa. The statistical techniques of segregation and linkage analyses are limited by several factors. Nevertheless, diagnostic refinement of the subtypes of depression and bipolar mood disorder offers the hope that new biological markers associated with these syndromes may be identified. Phenomenologically defined subsets of patients (with clear-cut presentations such as characteristic age at onset, symptoms, and response to medication) will undoubtedly provide genetic researchers with more uniform populations with which to modify existing models or produce new, more accurate paradigms regarding the contribution of genetic factors to the development of mood disorders.

NEUROENDOCRINE AND NEUROPEPTIDE HYPOTHESES

Several psychiatric disorders, including the major mood disorders, are associated with specific, highly reproducible neuroendocrine alterations. Conversely, certain endocrine disorders (e.g., hypothyroidism and Cushing's disease) are associated with higher than expected rates of psychiatric morbidity. Neuroendocrine abnormalities have long been thought to provide a unique "window to the brain," revealing clues about the pathophysiology of central nervous system (CNS) dysfunction in the particular psychiatric disorder under study. This so-called "neuroendocrine window strategy" is based on extensive literature that indicates that the secretion of the peripheral endocrine organs is largely controlled by their respective pituitary trophic hormone. This, in turn, is controlled primarily by the secretion of the hypothalamic release and release-inhibiting hormones. Unipolar depression (and to a lesser extent bipolar disorder) are associated with multiple alterations, specifically of the HPA, hypothalamic-pituitary-thyroid (HPT), and growth hormone (GH) axes.

There is now considerable evidence that the secretion of these hypothalamic hypophysiotropic hormones is controlled by many of the classical neurotransmitters such as 5-HT, ACh, and NE—all previously posited to be involved in the pathophysiology of mood as well as anxiety disorders. Also, there is mounting evidence that components of neuroendocrine axes (e.g., corticotropin-releasing factor [CRF]) may themselves contribute to depressive symptomatology.

Hypothalamic-Pituitary-Adrenal Axis

The HPA axis is the most intensely studied neuroendocrine axis in depression. CRF, which is made up of 41 amino acids, is the primary physiological mediator of adrenocorticotropic hormone (ACTH) and β-endorphin secretion from the anterior pituitary (Vale et al. 1981). Within the hypothalamus, CRF-containing neurons project from the paraventricular nucleus to the median eminence (Swanson et al. 1983).

Activation of this CRF-containing neural circuit occurs in response to stress, resulting in an increase in synthesis and release of ACTH, β-endorphin, and other pro-opiomelanocortin (POMC) products. There are numerous reports documenting HPA axis hyperactivity in drug-free depressed and bipolar depressed patients, including CNS (i.e., CRF), pituitary (i.e., ACTH), and adrenal (i.e., glucocorticoid) involvement (Tables 22–1 and 22–2). There is considerable

---

Table 22–1. Alterations in the activity of the hypothalamic-pituitary-adrenal (HPA) axis in depression

↑ Corticotropin-releasing factor (CRF) in cerebrospinal fluid[a,b]

Blunted adrenocorticotropic hormone (ACTH), β-endorphin to CRF stimulation[a]

↓ Density of CRF receptors in frontal cortex of patients who commit suicide

Pituitary gland enlargement in depressed patients[b]

Adrenal gland enlargement in depressed patients and patients who commit suicide[b]

↑ Cortisol production during depression[a]

Plasma glucocorticoid, ACTH, and β-endorphin nonsuppression after dexamethasone administration[a]

↑ Urinary free cortisol concentrations

[a] State-dependent.
[b] Significantly correlated to postdexamethasone cortisol concentrations.

Table 22–2. Alterations in the activity of the hypothalamic-pituitary-adrenal (HPA) axis in bipolar disorder

↑ Plasma cortisol concentrations

Blunted diurnal variation of plasma cortisol

↑ Cerebrospinal cortisol

Nonsuppression of plasma glucocorticoid after dexamethasone

evidence that CRF-containing circuits throughout the nervous system coordinate the endocrine, behavioral, autonomic, and immune responses to stress in mammals (Table 22–1).

Involvement of the CNS in the pathophysiology of depression is suggested by elevated CRF concentrations in CSF, which have been documented in multiple studies of drug-free patients with major depression (Arato et al. 1986; Banki et al. 1987, 1992; France et al. 1988; Nemeroff et al. 1984; Risch et al. 1992) as well as in depressed people who committed suicide (Arato et al. 1989), although not all studies agree (Roy et al. 1987). These elevations of CRF concentrations in CSF are believed to be due to central CRF hypersecretion (Post et al. 1982). Reduction of CRF concentrations in CSF has been reported in healthy volunteer subjects following administration of desipramine (Veith et al. 1992).

One method to assess the activity of the HPA axis is by the use of the CRF stimulation test. CRF is administered intravenously (usually in a 1 mg/kg dose), and the ensuing ACTH (or β-endorphin) and cortisol response is measured over a 2- to 3-hour period (Hermus et al. 1984; Watson et al. 1986). In drug-free depressed patients, the ACTH and β-endorphin response to exogenously administered ovine CRF (oCRF) is blunted compared with that of nondepressed subjects (Amsterdam et al. 1987; Gold et al. 1984, 1986; Holsboer et al. 1984a; Kathol et al. 1989; Young et al. 1990). This phenomenon has been shown to occur in depressed DST nonsuppressors but not in DST suppressors (Krishnan et al. 1993). The attenuated ACTH response to CRH is likely to be due (at least in part) to chronic hypersecretion of CRF from the nerve terminals in the median eminence. This results in downregulation of anterior pituitary CRF receptor density with resultant decreased pituitary responsivity to CRF, as has previously been demonstrated in laboratory animals (Aguilera et al. 1986; Holmes et al. 1987; Wynn et al. 1983, 1984, 1988). Furthermore, decreased density of CRF receptors in the frontal cortex has been reported in postmortem studies of people who committed suicide (Nemeroff et al. 1988).

Not only do neurochemical alterations of the HPA axis occur in depression, but structural changes have been reported as well. Perhaps at least partly in response to the hypersecretion of CRF, depressed patients demonstrate pituitary gland enlargement (Krishnan et al. 1991), which significantly correlates to postdexamethasone cortisol concentrations, another measure of HPA axis hyperactivity (Axelson et al. 1992). Another morphological change, enlargement of the adrenal gland, has been reported postmortem in people who committed suicide (Zis and Zis 1987) and in depressed patients (Amsterdam et al. 1987; Nemeroff et al. 1992). This is most likely due to chronic ACTH hypersecretion.

This adrenal hypertrophy probably explains the fact that, unlike the blunted ACTH and β-endorphin response to CRF, the plasma cortisol response in depressed patients and nondepressed control subjects does not differ (Amsterdam et al. 1987; Gold et al. 1984, 1986; Holsboer et al. 1984b; Kathol et al. 1989; Young et al. 1990). Thus, for each pulse of ACTH, depressed patients with an enlarged adrenal cortex would be expected to secrete greater quantities of cortisol than would nondepressed control subjects. Adrenocortical hypertrophy could also explain the heightened cortisol response to pharmacological doses of ACTH (Amsterdam et al. 1983; Jaeckle et al. 1987; Kalin et al. 1982; Krishnan et al. 1990b; Linkowski et al. 1985).

Another indication of HPA axis hyperactivity in depression is cortisol hypersecretion, which is reflected in elevated plasma corticosteroid concentrations (Carpenter and Bunney 1971; Gibbons and McHugh 1962), increased levels of cortisol metabolites (Sachar et al. 1970), elevated 24-hour urinary free cortisol (UFC) concentrations and nonsuppression of plasma hydroxycorticosteroid levels after the administration of dexamethasone (the DST). Since Carroll's initial report (1968) and subsequent claims for diagnostic utility (Carroll 1982), the DST has generated considerable controversy (Arana and Mossman 1988). The rate of cortisol nonsuppression after dexamethasone administration has been generally found to be correlated with the severity of the subtype of depression (i.e., nearly all patients with major depression with psychotic features exhibit DST nonsuppression) (Arana et al. 1985; Evans and Nemeroff 1983a; Krishnan et al. 1985; Schatzberg et al. 1984). Moreover, DST nonsuppressors have been found to have elevated CRF concentrations in CSF (Pitts et al. 1990; Roy et al. 1987).

One factor that may contribute to DST nonsuppression is the more rapid metabolism of dexamethasone that occurs in depressed patients (Ritchie et al. 1990). Therefore, the many reports of HPA hyperactivity in depressed patients could be explained by hypersecretion of CRF during and/or immediately preceding a depressive episode, with secondary pituitary and adrenal gland hypertrophy. The DST usually normalizes after recovery from depression (Carroll 1968; Nemeroff and Evans 1984) and may help predict early relapse or poor prognosis (Arana et al. 1985). DST nonsuppression, like hypercortisolemia (Sachar et al. 1970), hypersecretion of CRF (Nemeroff et al. 1991a), blunting of the ACTH response to CRF (Amsterdam et al. 1988), and adrenal gland hypertrophy (Rubin et al. 1992b), all appear to be state dependent.

Alterations of the HPA axis have also been documented in patients with bipolar affective disorder (Kiriike et al. 1988; Stokes and Sikes 1987). This increased HPA activity has been associated with mixed states (Evans and Nemeroff 1983b; Krishnan et al. 1983; Swann et al. 1992), mania (Godwin et al. 1984), and depression in rapid-cycling patients (Kennedy et al. 1989) (Table 22–2). (For a discussion of the interaction of the amines and the HPA axis, see the following sections on NE, ACh, and 5-HT.)

■ Hypothalamic-Pituitary-Thyroid Axis

The HPT axis has also been closely scrutinized in patients with mood disorders. Hypothyroidism has long been known to be frequently associated with markedly depressed mood. Moreover, many patients with rapid-cycling bipolar disorder have evidence of hypothyroidism, with some responding to thyroid hormone treatment (Bauer and Whybrow 1990a, 1990b; Cowdry et al. 1983). Use of thyroid hormone supplementation (usually triiodothyronine [T_3]) has been reported to increase the rapidity of action of TCA agents (Prange et al. 1969, 1980) and is as effective as lithium in converting depressed TCA nonresponders into responders (Joffe et al. 1993).

Discovered in 1970, TRH is a tripeptide (pGlu-His-Pro-NH$_2$) found in the hypothalamus, where it acts as a hypothalamic hypophysiotropic hormone. Released from the median eminence, TRH is transported in the vessels of the hypothalamo-hypophyseal portal system to the anterior pituitary. At the adenohypophysis, TRH binds to the TRH receptors on the pituitary thyrotrophs, increasing the synthesis and release of TSH by activation of the phosphatidylinositol (PIP) hydrolysis second messenger system. Released into the general circulation, TSH binds to TSH receptors in the thyroid gland and causes the release of the thyroid hormones T_3 and thyroxine (T_4). In turn, thyroid hormones act at the anterior pituitary to inhibit TSH release and at the hypothalamus to inhibit the synthesis and secretion of TRH. TRH is widely distributed in extrahypothalamic brain areas, where it functions as a CNS neuroregulator. Thyroid hormone receptors are also widely distributed throughout the mammalian brain.

The initial report of elevated CSF concentrations of TRH in depressed patients was published more than 15 years ago (Kirkegaard et al. 1979) and subsequently confirmed by Banki and colleagues (1988). Elevated CSF concentrations of TRH are believed to be a reflection of increased intracellular fluid concentrations of the tripeptide, probably the result of central TRH hypersecretion (Post et al. 1982). The increase in pituitary gland size reported in depressed patients (Krishnan et al. 1991) may be due in part to TRH hypersecretion. Hatterer and colleagues (1993) have reported low levels of transthyretin, the thyroid transport globulin in the CSF of refractory depressive patients, suggesting this could be a factor in low central thyroid hormone and high central TRH level.

Considered one of the most sensitive measures of HPT function, the TSH response to TRH (200–500 µg intravenously) is greater than normal in hypothyroidism and more attenuated than normal in hyperthyroidism. More than 20 years ago, it was established that about 25% of depressed patients with major depression exhibit a blunted TSH response to TRH (Kastin et al. 1972; Prange et al. 1972). In fact, depressed patients have been shown to exhibit considerably reduced CSF concentrations of somatostatin-release inhibiting factor (SRIF) compared with nondepressed control subjects (Bissette et al. 1986; Rubinow et al. 1983). The blunted TSH response to exogenously administered TRH is probably due to chronic hypersecretion of TRH from median eminence (i.e., elevated TRH release from the hypothalamus, causing downregulation of anterior pituitary TRH receptors), with resultant diminished anterior pituitary responsiveness to TRH. Following chronic administration of TRH, blunting of the TSH response to TRH stimulation has been observed in rats (Nemeroff et al. 1980). Adinoff and colleagues (1991) found an inverse relationship between the blunted TSH response to TRH and CSF TRH concentrations in 13 drug-free male alcoholic subjects. Moreover, Maeda and colleagues (1993) demonstrated that repeated TRH administration in humans produces the blunted

TSH response to TRH observed in depressed patients. Further studies documenting TRH hypersecretion and TRH receptor downregulation are needed.

Two HPT markers have demonstrated potentially improved sensitivity in depression when compared with the standard TRH stimulation test (Table 22–3). Duval and colleagues (1990) performed a standard TRH (200 μg) stimulation test on subjects at 8 A.M. and 11 P.M. The difference between the 11 P.M. ΔTSH and the 8 A.M. ΔTSH, designated the ΔΔTSH, is markedly lower in depressed patients when compared with control subjects, with a diagnostic specificity of 95% and a diagnostic sensitivity of 89%. Another purportedly more sensitive indicator of depression than the TRH stimulation test is diminished nocturnal plasma TSH concentrations (Bartalena et al. 1990; Goldstein et al. 1980; Weeke and Weeke 1980).

In contradistinction to the blunted TSH response to TRH, 15% of depressed patients exhibit an exaggerated TSH response to TRH (Extein et al. 1981). Patients with normal levels of T_3, T_4, and TSH who exhibit an exaggerated TSH response to TRH are defined as having Grade III hypothyroidism (Table 22–4). (In Grade I hypothyroidism, plasma concentrations of T_3 and T_4 are decreased, plasma TSH concentrations are elevated because of the loss of the negative feedback on the pituitary, and the TSH response to TRH is markedly exaggerated. In Grade II hypothyroidism, plasma concentrations of thyroid hormones are normal, but basal plasma TSH concentration is elevated, and the TSH response to TRH is exaggerated.)

Depressed patients have also been reported to have a higher than expected occurrence of symptomless autoimmune thyroiditis (SAT), as defined by the abnormal presence of circulating antimicrosomal thyroid and/or antithyroglobulin antibodies (Gold et al. 1982; Nemeroff et al. 1985; Reus et al. 1986). Moreover, there is a higher incidence of SAT (i.e., 50%) in depressed patients who are DST nonsuppressors (Haggerty et al. 1987; Reus et al. 1986). These patients may be designated as having Grade IV hypothyroidism (Table 22–4)—that is, they have positive antithyroid antibodies, but normal T_3, T_4, TSH, and TRH-induced TSH response (Haggerty et al. 1990).

Abnormalities of the HPT axis (e.g., hypothyroidism) have also been reported in patients with bipolar disorder, as demonstrated by an exaggerated TSH response to TRH and elevated basal plasma concentrations of TSH (Haggerty et al. 1987; Loosen and

Table 22–3. Alterations in the activity of the hypothalamic-pituitary-thyroid (HPT) axis in depression

↑ Cerebrospinal thyrotropin-releasing hormone (TRH) in depressed patients

↓ Nocturnal plasma thyroid-stimulating hormone (TSH)

Blunted TSH in response to TRH stimulation[a]

Exaggerated TSH response to TRH stimulation

↓ ΔΔTSH (difference between 11 P.M. ΔTSH and 8 A.M. ΔTSH after TRH administration)

Presence of antimicrosomal thyroid and/or antithyroglobulin antibodies[b]

[a] State-dependent.
[b] Correlated to postdexamethasone cortisol concentrations.

Table 22–4. Grades of hypothyroidism

Grade	T_3, T_4	Basal TSH	TSH to TRH	Antithyroid antibodies
I	↓	↑	↑	Often present
II	Normal	↑	↑	Often present
III	Normal	Normal	↑	Often present
IV	Normal	Normal	Normal	Present

T_3 = triiodothyronine; T_4 = thyroxine; TRH = thyrotropin-releasing hormone; TSH = thyroid-stimulating hormone.

Prange 1982). In fact, two groups have reported a higher prevalence rate of hypothyroidism (Grades I, II, and III) in bipolar patients who experience rapid cycling of their mood than in bipolar patients who do not have frequent mood cycling (Bauer et al. 1990a; Cowdry et al. 1983). Other abnormalities of the thyroid axis have been documented in bipolar patients, including a blunted TSH response to TRH, a blunted or absent nocturnal surge in concentrations of plasma TSH (Sack et al. 1988; Souetre et al. 1988), and the presence of antithyroid microsomal and/or antithyroglobulin antibodies (Lazarus et al. 1986; Myers et al. 1985) (Table 22–5). The presence of antithyroid antibodies is apparently not a result of lithium treatment, although lithium can exacerbate the process (Calabrese et al. 1985).

■ Hypothalamic–Growth Hormone Axis

Mood disorders are also associated with alterations in the activity of the GH axis. GH is synthesized and secreted from the somatotroph cells of the anterior pituitary. Its secretion is modulated by two hypothalamic hypophysiotropic hormones, growth-hormone–releasing factor (GRF) and SRIF, as well as by the classical neurotransmitters (e.g., dopamine [DA], NE, and serotonin) that innervate the GRF-containing neurons. Located primarily in the arcuate nucleus of the hypothalamus, GRF stimulates the synthesis and release of GH. Inhibition of the GH release is mediated primarily by SRIF, which is found predominantly in the periventricular nucleus of the hypothalamus. Unlike GRF, SRIF is widely distributed in extrahypothalamic brain regions, including the cerebral cortex, hippocampus, and amygdala. Both GRF and SRIF are released from nerve terminals in the median eminence and transported via the hypothalamic-pituitary portal system to act on the GH-producing somatotrophs of the anterior pituitary.

Release of GH is stimulated by L-dopa (Boyd et al. 1970), a DA precursor, and by apomorphine, a centrally active DA agonist (Lal et al. 1975). GH release also occurs following the administration of the 5-HT precursors L-tryptophan and 5-hydroxytryptophan (5-HTP) (Imura et al. 1973; Muller et al. 1974). The 5-HT receptor antagonists methysergide and cyproheptadine interfere with the GH response to hypoglycemia (Toivola et al. 1972). NE and clonidine, a central α-adrenergic agonist, inhibit GH secretion (Toivola et al. 1972), which varies in a daily circadian pattern that decreases in magnitude as a person ages. Under normal basal conditions, GH is secreted in pulses that are highest during the initial hours of the night (Finkelstein et al. 1972). In depressed patients, multiple findings indicate dysregulation of the secretion of GH (Table 22–6); nocturnal GH secretion is diminished in these individuals (Schilkrut et al. 1975),

whereas in unipolar and bipolar depressed patients, daylight GH secretion is exaggerated (Mendlewicz et al. 1985). Furthermore, multiple studies have reported a marked attenuation of the GH response to clonidine (and, to a lesser extent, apomorphine) in depressed patients (Charney et al. 1982; Checkley et al. 1981; Matussek et al. 1980; Siever et al. 1982). (For further discussion, see the section on adrenergic receptors.)

GH response to stimulation by GRF has been studied in depressed patients, and the results are discordant. Two research groups have reported a diminished GH response to GRF in depressed patients (Lesch et al. 1987a, 1987b; Risch et al. 1991). However, Krishnan and colleagues (1988) found minimal differences between depressed patients and nondepressed control subjects in the plasma concentrations of GH following GRF stimulation. These discordant findings could be explained by various other factors that can influence GH response to GRF, including sex, age, menstrual cycle, plasma somatomedin concentrations, and body weight (Krishnan et al. 1988). Further studies using GRF will assist in the development of a standard GRF stimulation test and further clarify the response of GH to GRF in depressed patients. SRIF, the tetrapeptide hypothalamic GH release-inhibiting hormone, inhibits secretion of both CRF and ACTH (Brown et al. 1984; Heisler et al. 1982; Richardson and Schonbrunn 1981). Remarkably, in several studies CSF concentrations of SRIF have been reported to be relatively low in depressed patients (Agren and Lundqvist 1984; Bissette et al. 1986; Gerner and Yamada 1982; Rubinow et al. 1983, 1984). These decreased CSF concentrations of SRIF correlate inversely with postdexamethasone plasma cortisol concentrations (Rubinow 1986); in fact, exogenous glucocorticoids reduce SRIF concentrations in CSF (Wolkowitz et al. 1987). In patients with bipolar disorder, blunting of noradrenergic-stimulated GH has been observed during mania (Dinan et al. 1991). Table 22–6 presents a summary of the alterations of the hypothalamic-GH axis in depression.

■ Hypothalamic-Pituitary-Gonadal Axis

Despite the higher incidence of depression in women and the purportedly increased occurrence of depression during and after menopause, the data on the hypothalamic-pituitary-gonadal (HPG) axis in patients with mood disorders are limited. As with the

---

Table 22–5. Alterations in the activity of the hypothalamic-pituitary-thyroid (HPT) axis in bipolar disorder

Blunting of the plasma thyroid-stimulating hormone (TSH) response to thyrotropin-releasing hormone (TRH) stimulation

Exaggeration of the plasma TSH response to TRH stimulation

Blunted or absent nocturnal surge in plasma TSH concentration

Presence of antimicrosomal thyroid and/or antithyroglobulin antibodies

HPA and HPT axes, the HPG axis is organized in a "hierarchical" fashion. Driven by a "pulse generator" in the arcuate nucleus of the hypothalamus, gonado-tropin-releasing hormone (GnRH) secretion occurs in a pulsatile fashion (Knobil 1990). GnRH causes secretion of luteinizing hormone (LH) and follicle stimulating hormone (FSH) from gonadotrophs in the anterior pituitary (Midgely and Jaffe 1971). The ebb and flow of LH concentration in the peripheral circulation is used as an indication of pulses of GnRH secretion (Clarke and Cummins 1982). In the follicular phase of the menstrual cycle, LH pulses of nearly constant amplitude occur with regular frequency (i.e., every 1–2 hours) (Reame et al. 1984). In the luteal phase, LH pulse amplitude (reflecting GnRH secretion) is more variable, with pulse frequency declining to one pulse every 2–6 hours (Jaffe et al. 1990). Through negative feedback, gonadal steroids inhibit the secretion of GnRH from the hypothalamus as well as the secretion of LH and FSH from the pituitary. GnRH secretion is also inhibited by CRF (Jaffe et al. 1990) and β-endorphin (Ferin and Van de Wiele 1984).

In early studies, no significant differences were reported in plasma concentrations of LH and FSH in depressed postmenopausal women compared with nondepressed matched control subjects (Sachar et al. 1972). But in another study, decreased plasma LH concentrations were observed in depressed post-menopausal women who were compared with matched control subjects (Brambilla et al. 1990). Rather than measure baseline plasma levels of the pituitary gonadotrophins in depressed patients, other investigators have studied the response of the pituitary to exogenous administration of GnRH. Normal LH and FSH responses to a high dose of GnRH (i.e., 250 μg) have been reported in male depressed and female depressed (pre- and postmenopausal) patients (Winokur et al. 1982), whereas decreased LH response to a lower dose of GnRH (150 μg) has been reported in premenopausal and postmenopausal depressed patients (Brambilla et al. 1990). In a depressed cohort including both sexes (analyses of men and premenopausal versus postmenopausal depressed women were not separately performed), Unden and colleagues (1988) observed no change in baseline or TRH/LH-releasing hormone (LHRH)-stimulated LH or FSH concentrations (200 μg TRH and 100 μg LHRH combined, intravenously). Notably, plasma LH concentrations are increased in those individuals who have recovered from a manic state—possibly a trait phenomenon (Whalley et al. 1987). Additional research on the HPG axis in depression is clearly warranted.

Investigation of other CNS peptides has proceeded as well, including the neurohypophyseal hormone vasopressin. Arginine vasopressin, a nonpeptide that stimulates ACTH secretion (Landon et al. 1965), also potentiates release of ACTH stimulated by CRF (Von Bardeleben et al. 1985). Unlike the ACTH response to CRF, the ACTH response to arginine vasopressin is unchanged in depression (Carroll et al. 1993).

■ ROLE OF NEUROTRANSMITTERS AND RECEPTORS

The basic neurology of neurotransmitter function is discussed in detail in Chapters 1 and 3 of this textbook. Various approaches have been taken to the study of neurotransmitters in humans. These include measurement of levels of neurotransmitters and metabolites in peripheral blood and CSF, as well as in postmortem brain tissue; direct study of neurotransmitter receptors in platelets, leukocytes, and cell cultures of fibroblasts, as well as in postmortem brain; and neuroendocrine responses to receptor agonists and antagonists.

■ Norepinephrine

NE, epinephrine, and DA are all catecholamines, because they derive from catechol or 1,2-dihydroxy-benzene. The catecholamine hypothesis of affective disorders proposed that some forms of depression are associated with a deficiency of catecholamine ac-

---

Table 22–6. Alterations in the activity of the GH axis in depression

↓ Nocturnal growth hormone (GH) in depression

↑ GH during the day (unipolar and bipolar)

↓ Response of GH to clonidine and apomorphine in depression

↓ Somatostatin in cerebrospinal fluid[a]

?↓ GH response to growth-hormone–releasing factor (GRF)

[a] Significantly correlated to postdexamethasone cortisol concentrations.

tivity (particularly NE) at functionally important adrenergic receptor sites in the brain, whereas mania was associated with a relative excess of catecholamines (Schildkraut 1965). In initial reports, urinary levels of 3-methoxy-4-hydroxyphenylglycol (MHPG), the major metabolite of CNS NE, were found to be significantly lower in depressed patients compared with those found in control subjects (Maas et al. 1972). MHPG also appeared to be elevated in bipolar patients when they were manic compared with the levels when these patients were depressed (Halaris 1978). Table 22–7 presents a summary of the known alterations of the NE system in depression.

Much research in the area of NE activity has emphasized the use of catecholamine measures to discriminate among subtypes of depressed patients. Early reports indicated that, as a group, bipolar depressed patients demonstrated significantly lower urinary MHPG levels than did unipolar patients or healthy control subjects (Schildkraut et al. 1978a). More recent studies indicate that low urinary MHPG levels are characteristic of bipolar I depressive patients, but not of bipolar II depressive patients who have MHPG levels similar to those of unipolar patients (Muscettola et al. 1984; Schatzberg et al. 1989). Although as a group unipolar depressive patients have higher urinary MHPG levels than do bipolar I patients, some unipolar patients do demonstrate low MHPG levels. Preliminary data suggest that these patients may be more likely to develop hypomania or mania than unipolar patients with high MHPG levels (Schatzberg et al. 1989).

Overall, with regard to catecholamine excretion, unipolar depressed patients are more heterogeneous than are bipolar I patients, with unipolar patients demonstrating MHPG levels over a wide range of values. MHPG levels may help to biochemically classify unipolar depressed patients (Schatzberg et al. 1982; Schildkraut et al. 1981). The subtype with low MHPG

Table 22–7. Alterations in the norepinephrine system in depression

↑ or ↓ 3-methoxy-4-hydroxyphenylglycol (MHPG)

↑ α_2-adrenergic binding in platelets

Blunted growth hormone response to clonidine

↑ β-adrenergic receptors in postmortem brain of patients who committed suicide

? Downregulation of β-adrenergic receptors after treatment

levels may have low NE output or relea[...] tients appear to respond well to noradre[...] tive antidepressants such as imipramin[...] 1972), although this finding has not always been replicated (Janicak et al. 1986). More recent data suggest low-MHPG patients also respond to treatment with fluoxetine (Rosenbaum et al. 1992). De Ballis and colleagues (1993) reported that MHPG levels in CSF for 9 depressed patients, which were no different from those of control subjects, decreased significantly after treatment with the serotonergic antidepressant fluoxetine, which suggests this drug may effect NE turnover. The subtype with intermediate MHPG levels may have another neurochemical abnormality other than one involving NE activity.

Patients with high MHPG levels have high NE output, which may reflect receptor dysfunction or may be secondary to cholinergic hyperactivity (Schildkraut et al. 1984). Such patients demonstrate elevated cortisol levels and respond poorly to both noradrenergic TCAs and fluoxetine.

Mooney and colleagues (1988) reported that depressed patients with high catecholamine output respond to treatment with alprazolam, a triazolobenzodiazepine. High catecholamine output was associated with heterologous desensitization of the platelet receptor–G protein–adenylate cyclase (AC) complex. Alprazolam appeared to decrease catecholamine output and to correct the desensitization of the receptor complex.

Schildkraut and colleagues (1978b) reported that discriminant function analysis of urinary catecholamines and metabolites yielded a depression-type (D-type) score that more clearly separated unipolar nonendogenous depressions from bipolar depressions than did urinary MHPG levels alone. In a subsequent report (Schatzberg et al. 1989), D-type scores provided greater sensitivity and specificity in differentiating among depressed patients with bipolar or schizoaffective disorder and those individuals with unipolar depression and all other depressions than were seen using individual catecholamine and metabolite measures, or the sum of the catecholamines and their metabolites. Specifically, bipolar I depressed patients demonstrated significantly lower D-type scores than did subjects with all other depressive subtypes, including those with bipolar type II depression. Patients with bipolar II disorders demonstrated D-type scores similar to those individuals with unipolar depression. D-type scores also have been reported to provide more precise discrimination between responders and nonresponders to imipramine or alprazolam than do urinary MHPG levels alone (Mooney et al. 1991).

NE may also play an important role in the control of cortisol secretion. Several studies have reported on the relationship between measurements of the HPA axis and catecholamine systems. Early hypotheses suggested that NE may have an inhibitory effect on HPA activity. However, investigators have reported significant positive correlations between cortisol and MHPG levels in depressed patients (Rosenbaum et al. 1983; Stokes et al. 1981). Similar findings have been reported for cortisol and epinephrine levels (Stokes et al. 1981). These data suggest that simultaneous elevation of HPA axis and NE activity is a feature of some depressed patients. This simultaneous increase in activity could be explained by increased ACh or CRF activity.

More recently, catecholamine levels have been examined in patients who are in manic phases of bipolar disorder. Bipolar patients during manic episodes demonstrated significantly higher plasma NE and epinephrine levels than when they were depressed or euthymic (Maj et al. 1984). Swann and colleagues (1987) reported that MHPG and urinary NE levels in CSF were significantly higher in manic patients than in either depressed patients or control subjects. Other researchers have reported that plasma MHPG was higher during the manic rather than the depressive phase in bipolar patients (Halaris 1978). In a later report, Swann and colleagues (1990) noted that environmental sensitivity had a significant effect on urinary NE excretion. Manic patients whose episodes were "environmentally sensitive" demonstrated elevated NE excretion, compared with patients with manic episodes that were unrelated to external stressors. Future research that simultaneously explores the relationship of stress to neurotransmitter measures in mood disorders would be relevant to treatment interventions.

■ Adrenergic Receptors

The α_1 receptor is not coupled to the AC system but is linked to processes that regulate cellular calcium ion fluxes. α_2 receptors exist in both pre- and postsynaptic subtypes that are inhibitory to the AC system. The presynaptic α_2 receptor has been shown to have an inhibitory effect on the release of NE in the brain. Increased binding occurs at α_2 receptor sites in the platelet membrane in depressed patients (Halaris and Piletz 1990). There is also increased α_2 receptor density in the brains of people who committed suicide (Meana et al. 1992). These studies support the theory of supersensitivity of α_2 receptors in depression, although these findings have not been consistently replicated. Also partially supporting this hypothesis is the observation that treatment with antidepressants has been associated with decreases in the density and sensitivity of these receptors.

Activation of the α_2 receptor inhibits AC and produces a decrease in cyclic adenosine monophosphate (cAMP), which mediates several physiological responses, one of which is platelet aggregation. Garcia-Sevilla and colleagues (1990) assessed the functional status of α_2 receptors in depressed patients by measuring both inhibition of AC activity and induction of platelet aggregation. They reported that these two responses represent different phenomena of α_2 receptor activation and argued that platelet aggregation may be a better marker to assess receptor changes in depression. Mooney and colleagues (1988) reported that some depressed patients frequently demonstrate decreased responsivity of α_2 receptors to inhibition by epinephrine.

An indirect method for studying α_2 receptors is to challenge subjects with the α_2 receptor agonist clonidine. Administration of clonidine induces GH secretion, primarily through postsynaptic receptors. Several abnormalities in GH release in depression have been reported, as we have discussed previously. GH response to clonidine is blunted in unipolar depressed patients (Matussek et al. 1980; Siever et al. 1984), supporting the concept of decreased responsiveness of postsynaptic α_2-adrenergic receptors in depressed patients. Siever and colleagues (1992) reported that GH response to clonidine was significantly blunted in both acute and remitted patients compared with control subjects, suggesting that blunted GH response to clonidine may be a trait marker in some forms of depression. The significance of this finding vis-à-vis α_2 receptor activity is not entirely clear. Clonidine can bind to nonadrenergic sites on platelets, and GH responses to clonidine may involve other systems (e.g., somatostatin).

The β_1- and β_2-adrenergic receptor subtypes are postsynaptic and stimulate the AC system. Measurement of these receptors in depressed patients has yielded mixed results. Mann and colleagues (1986) reported increased β-adrenergic receptor density in the postmortem brains of people who committed suicide. However, Crow and colleagues (1984) demonstrated decreased density of hippocampal β receptors in the postmortem brains of depressed patients who had been hospitalized. It is possible that previous antidepressant treatment may have induced receptor downregulation in these patients.

The receptor downregulation hypothesis posits that the mode of action of clinically effective antidepressants is to decrease the number of or downregulate the β-adrenergic receptor sites. However, this is based on animal studies that have shown that antidepressants produce desensitization of the adrenergic receptor. Sharma and colleagues (1990) investigated three biochemical indices, urinary MHPG levels, platelet MAO activity, and leukocyte β-adrenergic receptor functions in 36 depressed patients treated with phenelzine. They did not find any change in the β-adrenergic receptor. There were significant reductions in MAO activity and MHPG levels in all patients treated with phenelzine, of whom 15 responded and 16 did not (only 32 patients completed the study and 1 patient was excluded). Pretreatment MHPG levels did not predict clinical response to phenelzine. Because the leukocyte β-adrenergic receptor does not have a presynaptic component, it may not reflect central activity, particularly changes in brain postsynaptic receptors that may be secondary to changes in presynaptic NE release or reuptake. This might explain the differences between this study and the downregulation of postsynaptic receptors found in rat brain after chronic antidepressant treatment.

■ Serotonin

It was hypothesized more than 20 years ago that indoleamines play a role in the pathogenesis of affective illness (Coppen et al. 1972). There has been a steadily increasing research effort in this area, in part because of the introduction of SSRIs that are effective antidepressants. The permissive hypothesis of serotonin function postulated that the deficit in the central serotonergic transmission permits the expression of bipolar affective disorder but is not sufficient enough to cause it (Prange et al. 1974). According to this theory, both the manic and depressive phases are characterized by low central 5-HT function but differ in high versus low NE activity.

Several studies have demonstrated that there is

reduction in CSF concentrations of 5-HIAA, principal metabolite of 5-HT, in some depressed patients (Asberg et al. 1976a, 1976b; Gibbons and Roy et al. 1989). The most attention has been paid to the relationship between low concentrations of CSF 5-HIAA and suicidal behavior in depressed patients. Asberg and colleagues (1976a) suggested that low concentrations of 5-HIAA may be a marker for suicidal behavior and for suicide risk in depressed patients. Several subsequent studies have replicated these observations and have suggested that decreased CSF 5-HIAA may predict suicidal behavior (Banki et al. 1984; Brown et al. 1982; Traskman et al. 1981). Low CSF 5-HIAA levels appear to be associated with more impulsive or aggressive methods of suicide (Traskman-Bendz et al. 1992), suggesting an association between decreased levels of 5-HIAA and suicide, aggression, or poor impulse control. Indeed, such low levels of 5-HIAA have also been associated with aggression or poor impulse control in impulsive violent criminal offenders (Linnoila et al. 1983) and arsonists (Virkkunen et al. 1987). Linnoila and Virkkunen (1992) describe a low–5-HT syndrome model, with associations between low 5-HIAA, hypoglycemia, early-onset alcoholism (Type II) and impulsive violent behavior, suggesting low 5-HIAA levels may describe a behavioral dimension that goes beyond depression. Recent data strengthen the association between central serotonergic deficit, impulsivity, alcoholism, and hypoglycemia (Virkkunen et al. 1994).

Drugs that target the 5-HT transporter site, thereby selectively inhibiting reuptake of 5-HT (e.g., fluoxetine, sertraline, paroxetine, and fluvoxamine) have been shown to be effective antidepressants in research and clinical settings. In addition to SSRIs, there is growing interest in agents that influence the many 5-HT receptor subtypes that mediate the various regulatory functions of 5-HT (Figure 22–1).

Several different 5-HT receptor subtypes have been identified in recent years, reflecting an increased sophistication of biochemical techniques. Subtyping is based in part on the characteristics of binding to 5-HT or other antagonists. There are three main classes: 5-HT_1, 5-HT_2, and 5-HT_3 receptors, which are further subdivided into 5-HT_{1A}, 5-HT_{1B}, 5-HT_{1D}, 5-HT_{1E}, and 5-HT_{1F} subtypes. The 5-HT_2 receptor appears to be virtually identical to the 5-HT_{1C} receptors, and this class may be divided into 5-HT_{2A} and 5-HT_{2B} subtypes. The 5-HT_{1A} receptor in particular has been implicated in the pathophysiology of depression and anxiety. This receptor has a high affinity for 5-HT, and chronic treatment with antidepressants in rats results in reduction of $5-HT_{1A}$ receptor sensitivity. Similar results have been reported for low-affinity $5-HT_2$ receptors, which have also been implicated in depression and anxiety, though their role is not entirely clear.

Antidepressants decrease the number of $5-HT_2$ receptors, yet electroconvulsive therapy (ECT) increases them (Gonzalez-Heydrich and Peroutka 1990). Mann and colleagues (1986) reported an increased number of postsynaptic $5-HT_2$ receptors in the brains of depressed patients. This suggests that a functional deficiency of presynaptic serotonergic neurotransmitter activity in depression may lead to an increased number or upregulation of postsynaptic

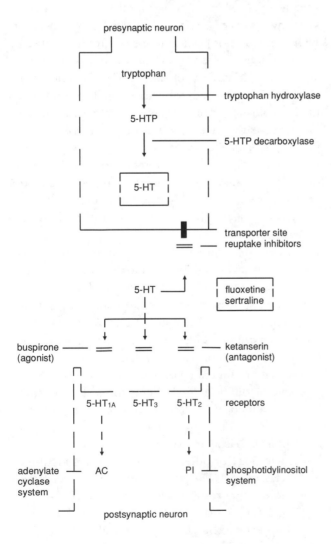

Figure 22–1. Schematic diagram of serotonergic action at the synapse.

$5-HT_2$ serotonergic receptors (Risch et al. 1992).

Binding to platelet membranes and 5-HT–induced shape change and aggregation have been commonly used to study $5-HT_2$ receptors. Beigon and colleagues (1990) suggested that serotonin $5-HT_2$ receptor binding on platelets may be viewed as a state-dependent marker in major depression. In their study of 15 depressed patients, receptor binding was measured at baseline, and again after 1 and 3 weeks of treatment with maprotiline. A significant decrease in $5-HT_2$ receptor binding was seen in responders; in contrast, there was increase or no change in receptor binding in the nonresponders.

The human platelet concentrates 5-HT from plasma via the 5-HT transporter in a fashion similar to that seen in the brain, and it may therefore serve as a model for the central 5-HT neurons. [3H]imipramine binds to the 5-HT transporter on the presynaptic nerve terminal and in the platelet. A reduction in the number of platelet [3H]imipramine binding sites in depressed patients has been reported by several groups (Briley et al. 1980; Langer and Raisman 1983; Lewis and McChesney 1985). Also, Perry and colleagues (1983) reported decreased density of [3H]imipramine binding sites in the hippocampus and occipital cortex of depressed patients.

In contrast, the report of the World Health Organization Collaborative Study (1990) argued that [3H]imipramine binding is not a valid biological marker of endogenous depression. This multicenter study investigated data from 154 depressed patients and 130 control subjects. It found no significant difference in [3H]imipramine binding capacity between depressed patients and control subjects. There were marked discrepancies in findings among different centers, perhaps reflecting different biochemical techniques used for platelet isolation and membrane preparation. A meta-analysis of all the platelet [3H]imipramine binding data has revealed a reduction in the density of 5-HT transporter in depressed patients when compared with that of control subjects (Ellis and Salmond, in press).

In recent years, [3H]imipramine has been found to have less specificity than [3H]paroxetine (Nemeroff et al. 1991b). Nemeroff and colleagues (in press) reported that [3H]paroxetine binding sites are reduced in the platelets of depressed patients. This may ultimately prove a more useful tool than [3H]imipramine.

Serotonergic systems are involved in the regulation of a variety of neuroendocrine hormones including cortisol, prolactin, and GH. Administration of the 5-HT releasing agent fenfluramine results in an increase in plasma concentrations of ACTH, cortisol, and prolactin, as well as an increase in body temperature. Stahl and colleagues (1992) reported that fenfluramine-induced hyperthermic responses were blunted in unmedicated patients with major depression. Pindolol, a 5-HT$_1$ and β-adrenergic antagonist, failed to block fenfluramine's temperature or neuroendocrine responses. This suggests that fenfluramine mediates its actions via receptors other than the 5-HT$_1$ subtype. 5-HT$_2$ and 5-HT$_{1C}$ receptors have been implicated, because ritanserin, a 5-HT$_2$ or 5-HT$_{1C}$ antagonist, can block d-fenfluramine's neuroendocrine effects. Clinical response of depressed patients treated with nortriptyline, but not with adinazolam (a triazolobenzodiazepine), is associated with downregulation of 5-IIT$_2$ or 5-IIT$_{1C}$ receptors.

5-HT agonists are effective stimulants of prolactin release. In nondepressed subjects, administration of L-tryptophan, a 5-HT precursor, produces a robust increase in plasma prolactin concentrations. Prolactin response to L-tryptophan and to the 5-HT releasing agent fenfluramine is blunted in depression (Cowen and Charig 1987; Siever et al. 1984). This response may be due to abnormal 5-HT receptors (particularly 5-IIT$_{1C}$ and 5-IIT$_2$) or to the effect of high cortisol on 5-HT$_1$ receptor function (Deakin et al. 1990). Because other types of patients also demonstrate blunted prolactin response to fenfluramine, the specificity and sensitivity of the blunted prolactin response in depression needs to be studied further before it can be of clinical use.

The 5-HTP–induced cortisol response has been found to be enhanced in unmedicated depressed patients and to decrease following treatment with antidepressants (Koyama and Meltzer 1986). Noting a significant negative correlation between baseline plasma cortisol levels and the cortisol response to 5-HTP in nondepressed control subjects, Koyama and Meltzer (1986) postulated that 5-HT may play an important role in the stimulation of basal plasma cortisol secretion. In this study, the dose of 5-HTP administered (i.e., 2–4 mg/kg) did not significantly affect plasma levels of homovanillic acid (HVA), the major DA metabolite, in either depressed patients or control subjects. However, it has been suggested that high doses of 5-HTP may displace NE and DA from catecholaminergic neurons.

As a potent stimulator of the HPA axis, increased 5-HT activity could play a role in the increased HPA axis activity and pathogenesis of psychotic depression. Indeed, in a review of the literature, Schatzberg and Rothschild (1992) noted that increased 5-HT uptake into platelets and increased CSF levels of 5-HIAA have both been reported in patients with psychotic major depression. These findings point to the need for further studies on increased serotonergic activity in psychotic depression. Table 22–8 summarizes the alterations in the 5-HT system in depression.

■ Dopamine and Dopamine β-Hydroxylase: Monoamine Oxidase

Enhanced dopaminergic activity may also play a role in the pathogenesis of psychotic depression. Compared with nonpsychotic depressed patients, psychotically depressed patients have been reported to have lower levels of serum DA β-hydroxylase (DBH) activity and higher levels of plasma DA and HVA (Devanand et al. 1985; Schatzberg et al. 1985a; Sweeney et al. 1978).

Several recent studies suggest that increased DA activity may occur as a result of increased corticosteroid activity. Glucocorticoids may induce tyrosine hydroxylase activity, the rate-limiting step in the biosynthesis of DA and NE. The administration of dexamethasone can significantly increase plasma free DA and HVA in healthy control subjects (Rothchild et al. 1984; Wolkowitz et al. 1985), and the administration of corticosterone or dexamethasone to rats significantly increases central DA activity (Rothchild et al. 1985; Wolkowitz et al. 1986). Schatzberg and colleagues (1985a) hypothesized that the glucocorticoids' enhancement of dopaminergic activity may explain the development of psychosis or delusional thinking in depressed patients.

Platelet MAO activity has been studied as a possible biological marker in mood disorders. Bipolar probands and their relatives have demonstrated

Table 22–8. Alterations in the serotonin (5-HT) system in depression

↓ Cerebrospinal 5-hydroxyindoleacetic acid (5-HIAA)
↑ 5-HIAA in psychotic depression
↑ Postsynaptic 5-HT$_2$ receptors
?↓ [^{3}H]imipramine binding
↓ [^{3}H]paroxetine binding
Blunted prolactin response to fenfluramine

lower MAO activity than unipolar patients or control subjects (Gershon et al. 1980; Leckman et al. 1977; Samson et al. 1985). Low MAO levels are found primarily in bipolar I and not in bipolar II subjects (Samson et al. 1985). Although studies have suggested that MAO activity is under strong genetic control and is linked to affective pathology, these results have not been replicated elsewhere (Maubach et al. 1981). Schatzberg and colleagues (1987) reported that MAO activity was significantly higher in patients with psychotic depression than in those with nonpsychotic depression or in healthy control subjects.

High platelet MAO activity has been found to correlate with elevated UFC levels and nonsuppression on the DST (Agren and Oreland 1982; Schatzberg et al. 1985b). The association between high platelet MAO activity and DST nonsuppression has been replicated by several groups (Meltzer et al. 1988; Pandey et al. 1992). MAO activity correlated with nonsuppression on the DST. Mean 4 P.M. postdexamethasone cortisol levels are significantly higher in patients with high MAO activity. Several hypotheses have been put forth for this finding. MAO could be a genetic marker for a risk for nonsuppression in the face of developing depression. If elevated MAO activity were correlated with a corresponding increase in hypothalamic MAO, a decrease in central noradrenergic tonic inhibition of HPA axis activity could then result in nonsuppression to dexamethasone challenge. Also, increased central MAO activity could be associated with serotonergic supersensitivity and elevated HPA axis activity. Conversely, it is possible that increased glucocorticoid activity is associated with elevated levels of catecholamines, which then results in an increase in platelet MAO activity. Further studies are needed to ferret out the biological underpinnings of this relationship.

DBH catalyzes the hydroxylation of DA to NE. Several studies have looked at DBH activity in major psychiatric disorders, such as schizophrenia and affective disorders. However, results have been generally consistent only for unipolar psychotic depressive patients, who have been reported to demonstrate low levels. For example, Sapru and colleagues (1989) investigated DBH activity in 280 adult male psychiatric patients with no previous exposure to psychoactive drugs. The researchers reported significantly lower serum DBH activity in patients with psychotic major depression compared with control subjects, but there were no differences between values for control sub-

jects and those for patients with schizophrenia, bipolar manic disorder, or nonpsychotic major depression. Low DBH activity has been hypothesized to be a risk factor for developing psychotic depression.

■ Gamma-Aminobutyric Acid (GABA)

GABA exerts inhibitory, hyperpolarizing synaptic effects in almost all areas of the CNS. GABA is a major regulator of many CNS functions such as seizure threshold, and it also has inhibitory input into other neurotransmitter systems such as NE and DA. Clinical and pharmacological data suggest that GABA metabolism may be altered in affective disorders.

Two types of GABA receptors, GABA-A and GABA-B, have been identified. GABA-A receptors are coupled to chloride ion channels and are associated with benzodiazepine-binding sites, whereas GABA-B receptors are associated with calcium ion transport. GABA-B agonists such as baclofen enhance cAMP production during exposure to other neurotransmitters such as NE, although they themselves have little effect on the second messenger response. It is possible that a decrease in the activity of GABAergic systems can play a role in depression by regulating receptor responses to catecholamines. For example, with the addition of baclofen to imipramine, downregulation of β-adrenergic receptor number and activity occurs more rapidly (Enna et al. 1986).

The role of the GABA system in convulsive disorders has been extensively studied, and the antiepileptic drugs appear to have direct or indirect action on GABA. The antiepileptic agents valproic acid and carbamazepine were serendipitously noted to have a mood-stabilizing effect, decreasing the intensity and frequency of both manic and depressive phases of bipolar disorder. In addition to valproic acid, other antimanic agents (e.g., lithium and carbamazepine) appear to stabilize mood by increasing GABAergic transmission, leading to the hypothesis that GABA deficiency can play a role in mania (Bernasconi 1982). In addition to its potential antimanic effects, GABA has been shown to have antidepressant effects as well, thus playing a significant role in mood regulation and stabilization.

Gold and colleagues (1980) showed that CSF GABA in depressed patients is significantly lower than in nondepressed control subjects, and several studies have replicated these findings in plasma concentrations of GABA as well (Petty and Schlesser

1981; Petty and Sherman 1984). Honig and colleagues (1989) directly measured GABA in brain tissue from patients undergoing cingulotomy for intractable depression, and found that GABA was inversely correlated with severity of depression, with the lowest levels of cortical GABA concentrations occurring in those with the most severe depression. However, GABA is altered by extraneous coincidental factors such as exercise, menstrual cycle, season of the year, or time of day, and may not be clinically applicable as a potential marker for mood disorders. Low levels of GABA are not specific to cases of depression or mania but are also seen in alcoholism (Petty 1994). The potential use of GABA measures as biological markers requires further study.

■ Acetylcholine

Janowsky and colleagues (1972) postulated that an increased ratio of cholinergic to adrenergic activity may underlie depression, and the reverse may be true in mania. Pharmacologically induced changes in ACh activity have resulted in alterations in mood. Increases in cholinergic activity (induced by cholinergic agonists such as arecoline, and cholinesterase inhibitors such as physostigmine) may reduce certain manic symptoms in bipolar patients, or intensify specific depressive symptoms in depressed patients.

Based on more recent research, Schatzberg and Mooney (1991) have offered a slightly different perspective on ACh and catecholamine interactions in depression. Increased ACh activity may result in increased catecholamine output as well as the commonly co-occurring elevation in cortisol activity in a subgroup of depressed patients. Thus, ACh activity may not be reciprocal to catecholamine activity.

Sitaram and colleagues (1984) proposed that primary affective illness (specifically bipolar disorder) may be characterized by a state-independent cholinergic hypersensitivity in conjunction with a state-dependent noradrenergic supersensitivity (during late depression and early mania), which return to normal during remission. The researchers intravenously administered arecoline during the second nonrapid eye movement (NREM) sleep period of the night, which resulted in significantly more rapid onset of rapid eye movement (REM) sleep in currently depressed as well as in remitted depressive patients than was seen in control subjects. This research group has replicated this finding of supersen-

sitive cholinergic response in patients with major depressive disorder (Dube et al. 1985; Jones et al. 1985). These findings also suggest that cholinergic sensitivity may play a key role in the pathogenesis of depression.

■ Pineal Function and Circadian Rhythm

The pineal gland, which is regulated by adrenergic input, produces the hormone melatonin, a marker for human circadian rhythm. The light/dark cycle synchronizes circadian melatonin secretion, with light acting as a suppressant. Seasonal changes of light and dark durations throughout the year produce corresponding changes in melatonin regulation. Alteration in the circadian rhythms of sleep and body temperature as well as plasma melatonin, prolactin, and cortisol concentrations have been reported in depressed patients. These may occur because of desynchronization of rhythms or phase advancement of certain rhythms in affective disorders.

The nocturnal secretion of melatonin is primarily induced by increased noradrenergic neurotransmission, resulting in increased activity of N-acetyltransferase, the rate-limiting step in conversion of 5-HT to melatonin. Several studies have shown low nocturnal output of melatonin in depressed patients (Boyce 1985; Nair and Hariharasubramanian 1984). Beck-Friis and colleagues (1985) reported that depressed patients with abnormal DSTs demonstrate lower melatonin levels than those with normal DSTs. This suggests that low melatonin states in depression occur in conjunction with abnormal DST results and 24-hour cortisol rhythm, but these data have not been replicated by other studies. Indeed, in a study of 38 depressed patients, Rubin and colleagues (1992a) reported a trend toward elevated average nocturnal melatonin secretion, primarily accounted for in the study by 14 premenopausal subjects. Melatonin measures were not consistently related to HPA axis measures.

■ Second Messenger Systems

The cAMP system and the phosphoinositide system are major second messenger systems. They are stimulated via guanine nucleotide-binding proteins (G proteins) and phosphorylating enzymes (Figure 22–2).

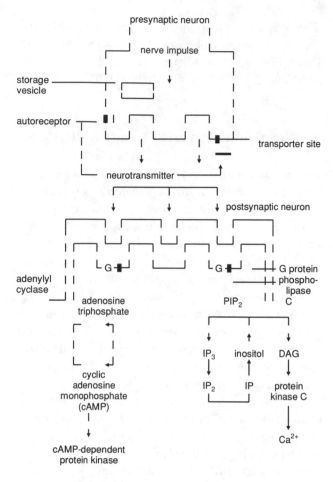

Figure 22–2. First and second messenger systems. Phosphotidylinositol-bisphosphate (PIP$_2$) generates inositol triphosphate (IP$_3$) and diacylglycerol (DAG), after hydrolysis by phospholipase C. IP$_3$ in turn produces inositol biphosphate (IP$_2$) and then inositol phosphate (IP), which generates inositol. Free inositol forms phosphotidylinositol, which is phosphorylated to PIP$_2$.

Guanine nucleotide-binding proteins. Distinct G proteins mediate effects on AC: G$_s$ for stimulation and G$_i$ for inhibition. These differential effects are mediated through the subunits of G protein, namely α, β, and γ. AC is directly activated by the α subunit of G$_s$. When the α subunit is bound to β and γ subunits, the G protein is inactive. When the transmitter-receptor complex binds to the G protein, guanosine triphosphate (GTP) interacts with the G protein, triggering dissociation of β and γ units from the G$_s$ protein. The resultant α subunit activates AC, and through its intrinsic GTPase activity cleaves GTP to GDP. The β and γ subunits then reassociate with the α unit, terminating activation of AC. In addition to regulating AC activity, G proteins can influence so-

dium and potassium ion channels (Baraban et al. 1989).

Avissar and colleagues (1992) proposed that hyperactivity of G proteins, either as a trait marker or as a state function, leads to an unstable dynamic system in bipolar disorder. Lithium treatment is hypothesized to attenuate G protein function, dampen the oscillatory system, and stabilize both manic and depressed mood states.

Adenylate cyclase system. There are two types of desensitization of the AC system: heterologous and homologous. Homologous desensitization is agonist-specific and occurs within seconds to minutes after exposure to the agonist. Heterologous desensitization, on the other hand, requires a longer duration of exposure to an agonist-type hormone or neurotransmitter, but it is by definition not specific to the agonist.

Mooney and colleagues (1988) proposed that prostaglandins, in conjunction with catecholamines, may produce heterologous desensitization of the platelet receptor—G protein—AC complex. In a study of 17 depressed patients and 10 control subjects, the researchers found significant inverse correlations between 24-hour urinary catecholamine levels and various measures of receptor-mediated (prostaglandin D$_2$ and epinephrine) and postreceptor (sodium fluoride)-mediated platelet AC activity. They postulated that increased catecholamine output may be partly due to increased output of several prostaglandins of the E, I, and D series, any one of which can also produce heterologous desensitization of the receptor complex in platelets. As we have indicated, depressed patients who had favorable antidepressant responses to alprazolam had significantly higher pretreatment urinary catecholamine output and lower receptor- and nonreceptor-mediated platelet AC enzyme activities compared with control subjects (Mooney et al. 1988). These findings normalized early in treatment of patients who were responders to treatment.

Phosphoinositide system and calcium. Receptor stimulation of the phosphinositide second messenger system activates a phospholipase C (PLC) enzyme that triggers the formation of inositol triphosphate (IP$_3$), as well as diacylglycerol (DAG). IP$_3$ binds to a unique receptor on the endoplasmic reticulum within the cell to trigger the release of calcium, which in turn regulates cell function. Lithium has been found to alter the phosphoinositide turnover and metabolism (Baraban et al. 1989). The phosphoinositide turnover system has been shown to be inversely linked to the AC cAMP second messenger system.

Pandey and colleagues (1991) examined whether the mode of action of antidepressants is related to their interaction with the phosphoinositide system by studying the effect of TCAs (i.e., desipramine, imipramine, and amitriptyline) and iprindole, an atypical antidepressant, on thrombin-stimulated formation of inositol phosphate in human platelets. These antidepressants decreased thrombin-stimulated inositol phosphate formation and increased the level of [^{3}H]inositol-labeled phospholipids, most likely mediated through the inhibition of PLC. Their findings suggest that antidepressants may cause changes in the phosphoinositide signaling system and that changes in receptors caused by antidepressants may be related to their effects on membrane phospholipids.

Calcium plays an important role in regulation of neuronal processes, including synthesis and release of neurotransmitters and modulation of ion channels that determine action potentials. Several studies have implicated hyperactivity of calcium in bipolar disorder. For example, intracellular calcium is significantly higher in untreated depressed bipolar patients than in untreated unipolar depressed patients (Dubovsky et al. 1991). Because calcium levels did not differ when euthymic-treated bipolar patients and control subjects were compared, this suggested that calcium activity may be a state-dependent marker in bipolar patients.

■ BRAIN IMAGING STUDIES

Investigation of the etiology of the major mood disorders has used a variety of approaches, including genetic and family studies, measurement of neurochemical and neuroendocrine parameters, electrophysiological studies, study of the actions of antidepressant drugs, and (most recently) brain imaging methods. As early as 1937, Papez proposed the limbic system as the location of the "seat of human emotions" (p. 725). Early study of CNS morphology and its relationship to affective disorder was limited to animal models and postmortem studies of humans. With the advent of computed tomography (CT) im-

aging and then magnetic resonance imaging (MRI), invaluable tools emerged for investigating the neural substrate(s) thought to be involved in the regulation of affect and/or the pathophysiology of affective disorder.

The fundamental assumptions underpinning the use of brain imaging in the investigation of mental illness include the following:

1. *Dysfunction* of the CNS contributes to the pathogenesis and pathophysiology of the major mood disorders.
2. This dysfunction is associated with specific *structural* brain abnormalities.
3. Those particular structural brain abnormalities *reflect* functional CNS alterations.

In recent years, imaging of in vivo brain function (or dysfunction) became possible with single photon emission computed tomography (SPECT), positron-emission tomography (PET), and magnetic resonance spectroscopy (MRS). These methods assume that brain function is reflected in neuronal activity and that such activity can be characterized by measurement of cerebral blood flow (CBF), oxygen uptake, or utilization of glucose. Through the use of radiopharmaceuticals such as [^{123}I]iofetamine (Spectamine) and [^{99m}Tc]HMPAO (Ceretec), SPECT provides measurement of CBF and is quantified in relative (rather than absolute) terms. Image resolution is as precise as 12 mm. SPECT is available in almost all clinical nuclear medicine facilities. In contrast, PET has better image resolution (down to 5 mm) and measures not only CBF but also glucose utilization. This can be quantified in absolute measurements reflecting neurochemical activity; rate of CBF; and location, density, and activity levels of receptors. A nearby cyclotron must produce the short-lived isotopes such as radioactively labeled oxygen and glucose analogues that PET requires. Because of the cost of the isotopes, equipment, and trained technicians, PET is quite expensive and usually found only in research centers. Both PET and SPECT also have the capability to measure neurotransmitter receptor occupancy in the CNS.

In this section, we review the controlled structural (CT and MRI) and functional (PET and SPECT) imaging studies of patients with affective disorder. Even though there are many reports of ventriculomegaly in patients with schizophrenia, the literature is replete with CT and MRI studies reporting increased ventricle size in patients with unipolar and bipolar mood disorders. However, these studies are confounded by numerous methodological problems. As extensively reviewed by Figiel and colleagues (in press), most of these studies *estimate* lateral ventricle size by using a ventricular brain ratio (VBR). Unfortunately, few conclusions can be drawn from the CT literature on ventricular enlargement in affective disorder. More consistent, however, are the CT and MRI studies of increased ventricular size in depression in geriatric patients (those individuals over age 65) (Tables 22–9 and 22–10).

Hyperintensities of gray and white matter (Table 22–10) have been reported in multiple MRI studies of geriatric patients with affective disorder, particularly those with "late-onset depression" (i.e., elderly depressed patients experiencing their first depression after age 60). Subcortical hyperintensities in the elderly are age dependent and may reflect pathological changes stemming from genetic, perinatal, posttraumatic, demyelinating, and infectious factors (Valk and van der Knaap 1989), or from infarctions stemming from arteriosclerotic involvement of the small lacunar arterioles that supply the basal ganglia and subcortical white matter (Roman 1987). Study of nondepressed control subjects has revealed that increasing age is also associated with reduction of the size of the putamen (Husain et al. 1991b) and caudate nuclei (Krishnan et al. 1990a), as well as of the size of the midbrain (Shah et al. 1992) and pituitary gland (Krishnan et al. 1991; Lurie et al. 1990).

To assess if abnormal brain structure is associated with abnormal brain *function,* investigators

have used CT and MRI studies of the CNS in association with neuroendocrine stimulation tests and neuropsychological testing, monitoring their patients' clinical course, response to treatment, and so on. For example, postdexamethasone cortisol levels are significantly correlated with VBR (Rao et al. 1989) and pituitary volume (Axelson et al. 1992). Furthermore, in depressed elderly patients, caudate hyperintensities are associated with an increased risk for the development of TCA- and ECT-induced delirium (Figiel et al. 1989, 1990, 1991a) as well as neuroleptic-induced parkinsonism (Figiel et al. 1991b).

As was previously mentioned, in vivo brain func-

Table 22–9. Alterations on brain computed tomography

Major depression

↑ Lateral ventricular size (geriatric depression[a]) (Abas et al. 1990; Jacoby and Levy 1980; Pearlson et al. 1989)

↑ Third ventricular width (Iacono et al. 1988; Schlegel et al. 1989)

↔ Cortical atrophy

Bipolar disorder

↔ Cortical atrophy

No cerebral asymmetry

Cerebellar atrophy (also in schizophrenic patients) (Lippman et al. 1982)

---

[a] Geriatric depression = depression in patients over age 65 years.

Table 22–10. Alterations on brain magnetic resonance imaging

Major depression

↑ Ventricular size (geriatric depression[a]) (Abas et al. 1990; Jacoby and Levy 1980; Pearlson et al. 1989; Rabins et al. 1991)

↑ Prevalence of subcortical (grey and white matter) hyperintensities (geriatric depression[a]) (Coffey et al. 1990) (late-onset depression[b]) (Figiel et al. 1991c)

↑ Prevalence of periventricular hyperintensities (geriatric depression[a]) (Coffey et al. 1990)

↑ Prevalence of hyperintensities of the basal ganglia (late-onset depression[b]) (Figiel and Nemeroff 1993; Figiel et al. 1991c)

↓ Cerebellar volume and smaller cerebellar vermis (Shah et al. 1992)

Smaller brain stem and medulla (Shah et al. 1992)

Smaller temporal lobe (Hauser et al. 1989a)

No significant structural changes in corpus callosum (Husain et al. 1991a)

↓ Caudate volume (Figiel and Nemeroff 1993; Krishnan et al. 1992)

↑ Prevalence of hyperintensities of the caudate (geriatric depression[a]) (Coffey et al. 1990; Rabins et al. 1991)

Smaller putamen volume (Husain et al. 1991b)

Larger pituitary gland volume (Krishnan et al. 1991)

Bipolar disorder

Smaller temporal lobe volume bilaterally (Altshuler et al. 1991)

No significant structural changes in corpus callosum (Hauser et al. 1989b)

↑ Incidence of subcortical hyperintensities (Dupont et al. 1990; Figiel et al. 1991; Swayze et al. 1990)

---

[a] Geriatric depression = depression in patients over age 65 years.
[b] Late-onset depression = depression that first appears in a patient after age 60.

tion can now be assessed by PET, MRS, and SPECT. Indeed, alterations of neuronal activity are associated with major depression and bipolar disorder. The controlled PET studies are summarized in Table 22–11.

Of particular interest is the decreased neuronal activity of the caudate and putamen associated with unipolar and bipolar depression. This is consistent with the MRI-documented morphological abnormalities of the basal ganglia (i.e., reduced size and increased prevalence of hyperintensities within these structures). The subcortical structures that constitute the basal ganglia are the caudate, putamen, and globus pallidus; most investigators also include the amygdala. The basal ganglia can be visualized as the motor behavioral effector mechanism that underlies the cognitive expression of emotion. Vulnerability to affective dysfunction might derive from disruption of connections between the basal ganglia or from interruption of pathways connecting the basal ganglia to other parts of the brain, specifically the limbic system and prefrontal cortex (Alexander et al. 1986; Krishnan 1991). This speculation would be consistent with the findings of subcortical hyperintensities (deep white matter and periventricular) found on MRI and the abnormal cortical neuronal activity reported in patients with depression and mania.

Undoubtedly, structures within the basal ganglia circuit requiring further scrutiny include the globus pallidus and amygdala, as well as brain structures with neuronal pathways leading to or from the basal ganglia: the thalamus, subthalamic nucleus, hippocampus, and relevant cortical areas. Further research is required to determine the diagnostic specificity of morphological and functional abnormalities associated with the major mood disorders. Furthermore, the stability or state dependency of these alterations is not known (e.g., the ventriculomegaly associated

Table 22–11.   Alterations on brain positron-emission tomography

Major depression

↓ Cerebral glucose metabolic rates in the basal ganglia (Baxter et al. 1985; Buchsbaum et al. 1986)

Bipolar disorder

↓ Global cerebral activity during depression (Baxter et al. 1989)

↑ Global cerebral activity during depression (Kishimoto et al. 1987)

with major depression). One prospective study by Vita and colleagues (1988) reports VBRs increased in size over a 3-year period in depressed patients. Yet one retrospective study found no significant increase in VBR in bipolar patients (Woods et al. 1990). Prospective longitudinal studies might help determine whether patients afflicted with a major mood disorder exhibit structural and functional brain alterations before, during, or as a result of affective episodes and, furthermore, whether these findings "normalize" with clinical improvement. Undoubtedly, brain imaging will continue to make an invaluable contribution to further understanding of the pathophysiology and treatment of unipolar and bipolar mood disorder.

■ PSYCHONEUROIMMUNOLOGY

It has long been speculated that "stress" can modulate immune responses. This is supported by a growing body of evidence that supportive and behavioral treatment strategies may enhance immune function. The field of psychoimmunology was in a sense first defined and explored by Solomon and Moos (1964). In recent years, psychoneuroimmunology has emerged as a major research area involving the study of interactions among behavioral, neural, endocrine, and immune processes of adaptation, each serving homeostatic and regulatory functions. Immune functions are primarily mediated by lymphocytes, which interact with the nervous system through direct neuronal connections and neuroendocrine pathways.

T lymphocytes, which mature in the thymus, may be classified as T-helper (CD^{4+}), T-suppressor (CD^{8+}), and T-cytotoxic (CD^{8+}) cells. B lymphocytes, which mature in the bone marrow, mediate immune processes through the production of immunoglobulins. The helper T lymphocytes regulate the differentiation of B cells into antibody-secreting cells, whereas the cytotoxic cells lyse those cells that they recognize as having pathogens. Suppressor T cells suppress immune responses by regulating B cells and T-helper and T-cytotoxic cells. Natural killer (NK) cells are a heterogeneous subset of lymphocytes involved in the recognition and destruction of malignant and virus-infected cells. T lymphocytes are predominantly regulatory cells. They exert their effect on target cells such as B cells by releasing soluble molecules called lymphokines that include the interleukins (IL) -2, -3,

-4, -5, -6, and -7, as well as γ-interferon (IFN). When activated by an antigen, the B lymphocytes proliferate, differentiate, and express the immunoglobulin (Ig) specific for that antigen. Macrophages, which originate from monocytes, present the antigen to T and B lymphocytes and secrete prostaglandins, thromboxane, and monokines, including IL-1, tumor necrosis factor-α (TNF), and α- and β-IFN. The lymphokines and the monokines have been studied extensively and were originally thought to function exclusively within the framework of immunological response. Evidence now indicates that these substances seem to function more like hormones, acting on target sites outside the immune system, especially the endocrine system.

The monokine IL-1 and the lymphokine IL-2 mediate the complex interactions between the endocrine and immune systems. IL-1, which is one of the chief mediators of inflammation, activates arachidonic acid release and prostaglandin production. On the other hand, small doses of IL-1, when injected into the lateral ventricle of rat brain, has been shown to produce immunosuppression. IL-1 stimulates the HPA axis, but this immunosuppresive effect seems to be in part independent of a glucocorticoid effect. For example, Weiss and colleagues (1989) reported that IL-1 infused into adrenalectomized animals still suppressed NK cell activity, T-cell mitogenesis, and IL-2 production. IL-2 (initially called T-cell growth factor) causes the proliferation of activated T cells and also augments induction of NK cell activity. It is possible that stress-induced suppression of T-cell mitogenesis and NK cells may be mediated by IL-2. However, Weiss and colleagues (1989) reported that the addition of IL-2 to adrenalectomized rats who were given IL-1 intraventricularly was not able to restore the suppressed mitogenic response to normal.

Gorman (1991) has taken a Darwinian approach in linking the CNS and the immune system, speculating that in distant phylogeny the immune system was part of the brain. The interaction between the two systems is evident in several ways:

1. The sympathetic fibers from the CNS directly innervate peripheral immune system organs, such as spleen, thymus, lymph nodes, and bone marrow.
2. The immune system cells produce chemical messengers—cytokines—which are polypeptides that are released by activated lymphocytes (such as IL-2, IL-6, and IFN) and activated macrophages (such as IL-1 and TNF).
3. The cells of the immune system bear specific surface receptors for a wide array of neurotransmitters, neurohormones, and neuropeptides. By virtue of sharing common receptors, the nervous, endocrine, and immune systems can potentially interact in several ways.

A neuroimmunological perspective has been used to study several psychiatric disorders, including schizophrenia and depression. Early studies reported increased prevalence and titers of herpes simplex virus (HSV) in psychotic depression (Halonen et al. 1974; Rimon and Halonen 1969). However, when the effect of age was controlled for, significant differences were not found, because HSV titers correlate with age (King et al. 1985). The association between Epstein-Barr virus (EBV) infection and mood disorders has received considerable attention. But there are no significant differences between titers of EBV antibodies in depressed patients compared with those in nondepressed control subjects (Amsterdam et al. 1986; King and Cooper 1989). More recently, the association between human immunodeficiency virus type 1 (HIV-1) infection and mood alterations have also been studied. Depression is thought to potentially result from one of various processes: a psychological response to knowledge of the infection, a direct neurotropic effect of the virus, and/or an indirect CNS effect secondary to viral activation of the immune system (Stein et al. 1991). However, the prevalence of major depression or mania is not particularly elevated in HIV-positive subjects; rather, there may be an increase in subsyndromal depressive symptoms.

■ Immune Function and Depression

Although depression has long been thought to have an immunosuppresive effect, recently there have been reports of enhanced immune response in depressed patients. Researchers investigating the immune alterations in depressive disorder have used enumerative techniques (e.g., numbers of lymphocytes and their T-cell and B-cell subsets), or more functional studies that have focused on the lymphocyte proliferative response to mitogens and the NK cell assay. Stein and colleagues (1991) have reviewed several of these studies and noted some methodological and conceptual concerns. Many of the studies failed to distinguish between subtypes of depression (e.g., melancholic or psychotic), and few studies distinguished between bipolar and unipolar depressed patients. Sample size has been small in the majority of the studies, and most did not include age- and sex-matched control subjects. Of eight studies that examined the total number of lymphocytes, only one found any difference between depressed patients and control subjects (Schleifer et al. 1984). The researchers reported lymphopenia (a decrease in the total number of lymphocytes) in depressed patients compared with nondepressed control subjects. However, other studies have not replicated these findings (Albrecht et al. 1985; Schleifer et al. 1985). Studies on T-cell and B-cell subsets in depression have also not produced consistent results.

Lymphocyte proliferative response to mitogens has been to access immune activity in depressed disorders. Stein and colleagues (1991) listed 12 studies that examined the lymphocyte response to one or more of the mitogens phytohemagglutinin antigen (PHA), concanavalin A (Con A), and pokeweed mitogen (PWM). Some studies found the mitogen-stimulated responses to be decreased in depressed patients (Kronfol et al. 1983; Schleifer et al. 1984), whereas others found no differences between depressive subjects and control subjects (Darko et al. 1989; Schleifer et al. 1985). Mitogen assays are technically complicated to perform and the interassay variability in functional assays tends to be high, raising possible methodological explanations for the lack of consistent findings.

Suppression of immune responses is described as the typical effect observed in humans and animals when exposed to stressful situations. However, more recent research has revealed that stressful conditions might not always be immunosuppressive; rather, they may produce an enhancement of cellular immune responses. Maes and colleagues (1992c) reported leukocytosis in major depression, characterized by neutrophilia and monocytosis (phagocytic cells), supporting the hypothesis that there is an ongoing inflammatory process in depression. Maes and colleagues (1993) have also reported significantly increased expression of T cell activation receptors (CD^{7+} and CD^{25+}) and the appearance of previously unexpressed T-cell surface markers (CD^{2+} $HLADR^+$) in depressed patients, with a sensitivity of 64% and a specificity of 91%. This theory of an inflammatory

response in depression with T-cell activation, polyclonal B-cell proliferation (Maes et al. 1992b), and monocytosis is not supported by other studies that have in fact reported immunosuppression.

IL-2 activates T lymphocytes through the IL-2 receptor. During T-cell activation, there is both an increase in membrane-bound receptor and in release of plasma soluble IL-1 (S-IL-2). Elevated levels of S-IL-2 have been reported in autoimmune disorders such as systemic lupus erythematosus and rheumatoid arthritis. Increased concentrations of plasma soluble IL-2 receptor (S-IL-2R) in plasma samples from medication-free individuals who attempted suicide have been reported (Nassberger and Traskman-Bendz 1993). In that study, significant associations between postdexamethasone plasma cortisol, 24-hour urinary cortisol, and plasma S-IL-2R were not observed.

Maes and colleagues (1992a) studied the leukocyte T helper (CD^{4+}) and T suppressor-cytotoxic (CD^{8+}) cell profile in 91 depressed patients and 21 control subjects. Depressed subjects had a significantly higher CD^{4+}/CD^{8+} ratio compared with nondepressed subjects. This T-cell activation corresponds with previous data from the Maes group that severe depression is characterized by a systemic immune activation. Darko and colleagues (1988) had previously reported a similar increase in CD^{4+}/CD^{8+} ratio in major depression.

There have been several reports of mitogen-induced lymphoproliferative responses in depressed patients (Kronfol et al. 1983; Maes et al. 1989; Schleifer et al. 1984). Lymphocyte stimulation responses to the mitogens PHA, Con A, and PWM have been reported to be lowered in depression, as well as in bereaved individuals. However, other studies have not reported such differences. For example, Darko and colleagues (1989) reported that there were no significant differences in the dose-response curves for Con A and PHA stimulation between 20 depressed patients and matched control subjects.

NK activity has been reported to be impaired in depression, with especially low NK activity observed in the morning. Pettito and colleagues (1992) tested the hypothesis that depressed patients have abnormal diurnal variation of NK cell activity by examining circulating Leu-11 NK cell phenotypes and NK activity in depressed patients and control subjects. Significantly less diurnal variation in NK activity was observed in the depressed patients. Irwin and colleagues (1992) assessed NK activity in depressed patients at intake and at follow-up 6 months after discharge from the hospital. At intake, NK cytotoxicity was significantly decreased in these patients compared with control subjects. At the 6-month follow-up, the NK activity had increased significantly, whereas the depression scores had decreased with treatment. Darko and colleagues (1992) found that both plasma β-endorphin and NK cell activity were reduced in depressed patients compared with age-matched control subjects; this suggests that β-endorphin may play a role in the enhancement of NK cell activity.

■ Glucocorticoids and the Immune System

The relationship between HPA axis activity and the immune system has been studied extensively, especially in mood disorders. Cytokines stimulate various regions of the brain, including the hypothalamus, causing release of CRF. Corticosteroids suppress inflammation and immune response, increasing the number of neutrophils while decreasing lymphocytes and monocytes. They also suppress mitogen and antigen responsivity, T-cell cytotoxicity, NK cell activity, and allogenic and autologous mixed leukocyte reactivity.

However, the HPA system alone is not fully responsible for the regulation of the immune system in response to stress. Keller and colleagues (1983) studied the effect of stress on immune function in intact and adrenalectomized rats. Although there was stress-induced lymphopenia in association with stress-induced secretion of corticosteroids in intact rats, lymphocyte response to mitogen PHA stimulation in adrenelectomized animals was suppressed. This effect on lymphocyte stimulation occurs independent of the HPA system and is possibly due to effects of another neuroendocrine or neurotransmitter system.

In conclusion, the immune system and the CNS interact in a complex manner to bring about immune responses. There are diverse reports from studies that have examined effects of acute stress, bereavement, and depression on the immune system. As research strives to elucidate the physiological mechanisms underlying these complex responses, it may shed more light on the relevance of immune system activity to the pathogenesis of mood disorders.

■ CONCLUSION

We have attempted to review several biological hypotheses of mood disorders and recent findings from relevant research studies. It is not unlikely that mood disorders are heterogenous, with pathophysiological changes occurring at neurochemical, neuroendocrinological, and neuroimmunological levels, manifesting in multiple systems and at different levels in each system. Interpretation of the individual biological studies is difficult, but over time, integrating them will help in the overall understanding of these complex disorders. Future research in delineating specific and sensitive biological mechanisms in mood disorders would contribute greatly to our understanding of pathophysiology and could also lead to breakthroughs in strategies for better treatment and, ultimately, prevention.

■ REFERENCES

Abas MA, Sahakian BJ, Levy et al: Neuropsychological deficits and CT scan changes in elderly depressives. Psychol Med 20:507–520, 1990

Adinoff B, Nemeroff CB, Bissette G, et al: Inverse relationship between CSF TRH concentrations and the TSH response to TRH in abstinent alcohol-dependent patients. Am J Psychiatry 148:1586–1588, 1991

Agren H, Lundqvist G: Low levels of somatostatin in human CSF mark depressive episodes. Psychoneuroendocrinology 9:233–248, 1984

Agren H, Oreland L: Early morning awakening in unipolar depressives with higher levels of platelet MAO activity. Psychiatry Res 7:245–254, 1982

Aguilera G, Wynn PC, Harwood JP, et al: Receptor-mediated actions of corticotropin-releasing factor in pituitary gland and nervous system. Neuroendocrinology 43:79–88, 1986

Albrecht J, Helderman J, Schlesser M, et al: A controlled study of cellular immune function in affective disorders before and during somatic therapy. Psychiatry Res 15:185–193, 1985

Alexander GE, Delong MR, Strick PL: Parallel organization of functionally segregated circuits linking basal ganglia and cortex. Annu Rev Neurosci 9:357–381, 1986

Altshuler LL, Conrad A, Hauser P, et al: Reduction of temporal lobe volume in bipolar disorder: a preliminary report of magnetic resonance imaging. Arch Gen Psychiatry 48:482–483, 1991

American Psychiatric Association: Diagnostic and Statistical Manual of Mental Disorders, 3rd Edition. Washington, DC, American Psychiatric Association, 1980

American Psychiatric Association: Diagnostic and Statistical Manual of Mental Disorders, 3rd Edition, Revised. Washington, DC, American Psychiatric Association, 1987

American Psychiatric Association: Task Force on DSM-IV Options Book: Work in Progress 9/1/91. Washington, DC, American Psychiatric Press, 1991

American Psychiatric Association: Diagnostic and Statistical Manual of Mental Disorders, 4th Edition. Washington, DC, American Psychiatric Association, 1994

Amsterdam JD, Winokur A, Abelman E, et al: Cosyntropin (ACTH) stimulation test in depressed patients and healthy subjects. Am J Psychiatry 140:907, 1983

Amsterdam JD, Henle W, Winokur A, et al: Serum antibodies to Epstein-Barr virus in patients with major depressive disorder. Am J Psychiatry 143:1593–1596, 1986

Amsterdam JD, Marinelli DL, Arger P, et al: Assessment of adrenal gland volume by computed tomography in depressed patients and healthy volunteers: a pilot study. Psychiatry Res 21:189–197, 1987

Amsterdam JD, Maislin G, Winokur A, et al: The oCRF test before and after clinical recovery from depression. J Affect Disord 14:213–222, 1988

Arana GW, Mossman D: The DST and depression: approaches to the use of a laboratory test in psychiatry. Neurol Clin 6:21–39, 1988

Arana GW, Baldessarini RJ, Ornsteen M: The dexamethasone suppression test for diagnosis and prognosis in psychiatry. Arch Gen Psychiatry 42:1193–1204, 1985

Arato M, Banki CM, Nemeroff CB, et al: Hypothalamic-pituitary-adrenal axis and suicide. Ann N Y Acad Sci 487:263–270, 1986

Arato M, Banki CM, Bissette G, et al: Elevated CSF CRF in suicide victims. Biol Psychiatry 25:355–359, 1989

Asberg M, Traskman L, Thoren P: 5-HIAA in the cerebrospinal fluid: a biochemical suicide predictor? Arch Gen Psychiatry 33:1193–1197, 1976a

Asberg M, Thoren P, Traskman L, et al: "Serotonin depression"—a biochemical subgroup within the affective disorders? Science 191:478–483, 1976b

Avissar S, Schreiber G: The involvement of guanine nucleotide binding proteins in the pathogenesis and treatment of affective disorders. Biol Psychiatry 31:435–459, 1992

Axelson DA, Doraiswamy PM, Boyko OB, et al: In vivo assessment of pituitary volume using MRI and systemic stereology: relationship to dexamethasone suppression test results in patients with affective disorder. Psychiatry Res 46:63–70, 1992

Banki CM, Arato M, Papp Z, et al: Biochemical markers in suicidal patients: investigations with cerebrospinal fluid amine metabolites and neuroendocrine tests. J Affect Disord 6:341–350, 1984

Banki CM, Bissette G, Arato M, et al: Cerebrospinal fluid corticotropin-releasing factor-like immunoreactivity in depression and schizophrenia. Am J Psychiatry 144:873–877, 1987

Banki CM, Bissette G, Arato M, et al: Elevation of immunoreactive CSF TRH in depressed patients. Am J Psychiatry 145:1526–1531, 1988

Banki CB, Karmacsi L, Bissette G, et al: CSF corticotropin-releasing hormone and somatostatin in major depression: response to antidepressant treatment and relapse. Eur Neuropsychopharmacol 2:107–113, 1992

Baraban JM, Worley PF, Snyder SH: Second messenger systems and psychoactive drug action: focus on the phosphoinositide system and lithium. Am J Psychiatry 146:1251–1260, 1989

Baron M, Risch N, Hamburger R, et al: Genetic linkage between X-chromosome markers and bipolar affective illness. Nature 326:289–292, 1987

Baron M, Freimer NF, Risch N: Diminished support for linkage between manic depressive illness and X-chromosome markers in three Israeli pedigrees. Nature Genetics 3:49–55, 1993

Bartalena L, Placidi GF, Martino E, et al: Nocturnal serum thyrotropin (TSH) surge and the TSH response to TSH-releasing hormone: dissociated behavior in untreated depressives. J Clin Endocrinol Metab 71:650–655, 1990

Bauer MS, Whybrow PC: Rapid cycling bipolar affective disorder, I: association with grade I hypothyroidism. Arch Gen Psychiatry 47:427–432, 1990a

Bauer MS, Whybrow PC: Rapid cycling bipolar affective disorder, II: treatment of refractory rapid cycling with high-dose levothyroxine: a preliminary study. Arch Gen Psychiatry 47:435–447, 1990b

Baxter LR, Phelps MC, Mazziotta JC, et al: Cerebral metabolic rates for glucose in mood disorders studied with positron emission tomography (PET) and (F-18)-fluro-2-deoxyglucose (FDG). Arch Gen Psychiatry 42:441–447, 1985

Baxter LR, Schwartz JM, Phelps ME, et al: Reduction of prefrontal cortex glucose metabolism common to three types of depression. Arch Gen Psychiatry 46:243–250, 1989

Beck-Friis J, Kjellman BF, Ljunggren JG, et al: The pineal gland and melatonin in affective disorder, in The Pineal Gland: Endocrine Aspects (Advances in Bioscience, Vol 53). Edited by Brown GM, Wainwright SD. Oxford, England, Pergamon, 1985, pp 313–325

Beigon A, Essar N, Israeli M, et al: Serotonin 5-HT2 receptor binding on blood platelets as a state dependent marker in major affective disorder. Psychopharmacology (Berl) 102:73–75, 1990

Bernasconi R: The GABA hypothesis of affective illness: influence of clinically effective antimanic drugs on GABA turnover, in Basic Mechanisms in the Action of Lithium. Edited by Emrich HM, Aldenhoff JB, Lux HD. Amsterdam, Elsevier, 1982, pp 183–192

Berrettini WH: Genetics in psychiatry. Paper presented at the annual meeting of the American Psychiatric Association, Washington, DC, May 1992

Bertelson A, Harvald B, Hauge M: A Danish twin study of manic depressive disorders. Br J Psychiatry 130:330–351, 1977

Bissette G, Widerlov E, Walleus H, et al: Alterations in cerebrospinal fluid concentrations of somatostatin-like immunoreactivity in neuropsychiatric disorders. Arch Gen Psychiatry 43:1148–1151, 1986

Botstein D, White RL, Skolnick M, et al: Construction of a genetic linkage map in man using restriction fragment length polymorphisms. Am J Hum Genet 32:314–331, 1980

Boyce PM: 6-Sulphatoxy melatonin in melancholia. Am J Psychiatry 142:125–127, 1985

Boyd AE, Levovitz HE, Pfeiffer JB: Stimulation of growth hormone secretion by L-dopa. N Engl J Med 283:1425–1429, 1970

Brambilla F, Maggioni M, Ferrari E, et al: Tonic and dynamic gonadotropin secretion in depressive and normothymic phases of affective disorders. Psychiatry Res 32:229–239, 1990

Briley M, Langer SZ, Raiseman R, et al: Tritiated im-

ipramine binding sites are decreased in platelets of untreated depressed patients. Science 209:303–305, 1980

Brown GL, Ebert MH, Goyer PF et al: Aggression, suicide, and serotonin: relationships to CSF amine metabolites. Am J Psychiatry 139:741–746, 1982

Brown MR, Rivier C, Vale W, et al: Central nervous system regulation of adrenocorticotropin secretion: role of somatostatins. Endocrinology 114:1546–1549, 1984

Brown WA, Johnson R, Mayfield D: 24 hour dexamethasone suppression test in a clinical setting: relationship to diagnosis, symptoms and responses to treatment. Am J Psychiatry 136:543–547, 1979

Buchsbaum MS, Wu J, DeLisi LE, et al: Frontal cortex and basal ganglia metabolic rates assessed by positron emission tomography with F2-deoxyglucose in affective illness. J Affect Disord 10:137–152, 1986

Bunney WE Jr, Davis M: Norepinephrine in depressive reactions. Arch Gen Psychiatry 13:483–494, 1965

Calabrese JR, Gulledge AD, Hahn K, et al: Autoimmune thyroiditis in manic-depressive patients treated with lithium. Am J Psychiatry 142:1318–1321, 1985

Carpenter W, Bunney W: Adrenal cortical activity in depressive illness. Am J Psychiatry 128:31–40, 1971

Carroll BJ: Pituitary-adrenal function in depression. Lancet 1:1373–1374, 1968

Carroll BJ: Use of the dexamethasone test in depression. J Clin Psychiatry 43:44–50, 1982

Carroll BJ, Davies B: Clinical associations of 11-hydroxy-corticosteroid suppression and nonsuppression in severe depressive illness. British Medical Journal 3:285–287, 1970

Carroll BT, Meller WH, Kathol RG, et al: Pituitary-adrenal axis response to arginine vasopressin in patients with major depression. Psychiatry Res 46:119–126, 1993

Charney DS, Henninger GR, Steinberg DE, et al: Adrenergic receptor sensitivity in depression: effects of clonidine in depressed patients and healthy controls. Arch Gen Psychiatry 39:290–294, 1982

Checkley SA, Slade AP, Shur P: Growth hormone and other responses to clonidine in patients with endogenous depression. Br J Psychiatry 138:51–55, 1981

Clarke IJ, Cummins JT: The temporal relationship between gonadotropin releasing hormone (GnRH) and luteinizing hormone (LH) secretion in ovariectomized ewes. Endocrinology 111:1737–1739, 1982

Coffey CE, Figiel GS, Djang WT, et al: Subcortical hyperintensity on magnetic resonance imaging: a comparison of normal and depressed elderly subjects. Am J Psychiatry 147:187–189, 1990

Coppen A: Depressive states and indolealkylamines, in Advances in Pharmacology, Vol 6. Edited by Garattini S, Shore PA. New York, Academic Press, 1968, pp 283–291

Coppen A, Prange AJ Jr, Whybrow PC, et al: Abnormalities of indoleamines in affective disorders. Arch Gen Psychiatry 26:474–478, 1972

Cowdry RW, Wehr TA, Zis AP, et al: Thyroid abnormalities associated with rapid-cycling bipolar illness. Arch Gen Psychiatry 40:414–420, 1983

Cowen PJ, Charig EM: Neuroendocrine responses to tryptophan in major depression. Arch Gen Psychiatry 44:958–966, 1987

Crow TJ, Cross AJ, Cooper SJ, et al: Neurotransmitter receptors and monoamine metabolites in the brains of patients with Alzheimer-type dementia and depression, and suicides. Neuropharmacology 23:1561–1569, 1984

Darko DF, Lucas AII, Gillin JC, et al: Cellular immunity and the hypothalamic-pituitary-adrenal axis in major affective disorder: a preliminary study. Psychiatry Res 25:1–10, 1988

Darko DF, Gillin JC, Risch SC, et al: Mitogen-stimulated lymphocyte proliferation and pituitary hormones in major depression. Biol Psychiatry 26:145–155, 1989

Darko DF, Irwin MR, Risch SC, et al: Plasma beta-endorphin and natural killer cell activity in major depression: a preliminary study. Psychiatry Res 43(2):111–119, 1992

Deakin JFW, Pennell I, Upadhyaya AJ, et al: A neuroendocrine study of 5-HT function in depression: evidence for biological mechanisms of endogenous and psychosocial causation. Psychopharmacology (Berl) 101:85–92, 1990

De Ballis MD, Geracioti TD Jr, Altemus M, et al: Cerebrospinal fluid monoamine metabolites in fluoxetine-treated patients with major depression and in healthy volunteers. Biol Psychiatry 33:636–641, 1993

Detera-Wadleigh SD, Berrettini WH, Goldin LR, et al: Close linkage of c-Harvey-ras-1 and the insulin gene to affective disorder is ruled out in three North American pedigrees. Nature 325:806–808, 1987

Devanand DP, Bowers MB, Hoffman FJ, et al: Elevated plasma homovanillic acid in depressed females with melancholia and psychosis. Psychiatry Res 15:1–4, 1985

Dinan TG, Yatham LN, O'Keane VO, et al: Blunting of noradrenergic-stimulated growth hormone release in mania. Am J Psychiatry 148:936–938, 1991

Dube S, Kumar N, Ettedgui E, et al: Cholinergic REM induction response: separation of anxiety and depression. Biol Psychiatry 20:408–418, 1985

Dubovsky SL, Lee C, Christiano J, et al: Elevated platelet intracellular calcium concentration in bipolar depression. Biol Psychiatry 29:441–450, 1991

Dupont RM, Jernigan TL, Butters N, et al: Subcortical abnormalities detected in bipolar affective disorder using magnetic resonance imaging: clinical and neuropsychological difference. Arch Gen Psychiatry 1:55–60, 1990

Duval F, Macher JP, Mokrani MC: Difference between evening and morning thyrotropin responses to protirelin in major depressive episode. Arch Gen Psychiatry 47:443–448, 1990

Egeland JA, Gerhard DS, Pauls DL, et al: Bipolar affective disorders linked to DNA markers on chromosome 11. Nature 325:783–787, 1987

Ellis PM, Salmond C: Is platelet imipramine binding reduced in depression? a meta-analysis. Biol Psychiatry (in press)

Enna SJ, Karbon EW, Duman RS: GABA-B agonist and imipramine-induced modifications in rat brain beta-adrenergic receptor binding and function, in GABA and Mood Disorders: Experimental and Clinical Research. Edited by Bartholini G, Lloyd KG, Morselli PL. New York, Raven, 1986, pp 23–49

Evans DL, Nemeroff CB: Use of dexamethasone suppression test using DSM III criteria on an inpatient psychiatric unit. Biol Psychiatry 18:505–511, 1983a

Evans DL, Nemeroff CB: The dexamethasone suppression test in mixed bipolar disorder. Am J Psychiatry 140:615–617, 1983b

Extein I, Pottash ALC, Gold MS: The thyrotropin-releasing hormone test in the diagnosis of unipolar depression. Psychiatry Res 5:311–316, 1981

Ferin M, Van de Wiele R: Endogenous opioid peptides and the control of the menstrual cycle. Eur J Obstet Gynecol Reprod Biol 18:365–373, 1984

Figiel GS, Nemeroff CB: The mesolimbic motor circuit

and its role in neuropsychiatric disorders, in Vol 4: Advances in Physiology. Edited by Kalivas PW, Barnes CD. Boca Raton, FL, CRC Press, 1993, pp 351–357

Figiel GS, Krishnan KRR, Brenner JC, et al: Radiologic correlates of antidepressant-induced delirium: the possible significance of basal ganglia lesions. J Neuropsychiatry Clin Neurosci 1:188–190, 1989

Figiel GS, Coffey CE, Djang WT, et al: Brain magnetic resonance imaging findings in ECT-induced delirium. J Neuropsychiatry Clin Neurosci 2:53–58, 1990

Figiel GS, Krishnan KRR, Doraiswamy PM: Subcortical structural changes in ECT-induced delirium. J Geriatr Psychiatry Neurol 3:172–176, 1991a

Figiel GS, Krishnan KRR, Doraiswamy PM, et al: Caudate hypertensities in elderly depressed patients with neuroleptic-induced parkinsonism. J Geriatr Psychiatry Neurol 4:86–89, 1991b

Figiel GS, Krishnan KRR, Doraiswamy PM, et al: Subcortical hyperintensities on brain magnetic resonance imaging: a comparison between late age onset and early onset elderly depressed subjects. Neurobiol Aging 12:245–247, 1991c

Figiel GS, Botteron KN, Doraiswamy PM, et al: Structural brain changes in affective disorder: a review. J Neuropsychiatry Clin Neurosci (in press)

Finkelstein JW, Roffwarg HP, Boyar RM, et al: Age-related changes in the twenty-four-hour spontaneous secretion of growth hormone. J Clin Endocrinol Metab 35:665–670, 1972

France RD, Urban B, Krishnan KRR, et al: CSF corticotropin-releasing factor-like immunoreactivity in chronic pain patients with and without major depression. Biol Psychiatry 23:86–88, 1988

Garcia-Sevilla JA, Padro D, Giralt T, et al: Alpha-2 adrenoceptor-mediated inhibition of platelet adenyl cyclase and induction of aggregation in major depression. Arch Gen Psychiatry 47:125–132, 1990

Gerner RH, Yamada T: Altered neuropeptide concentrations in cerebrospinal fluid of psychiatric patients. Brain Res 238:298–302, 1982

Gershon ES, Goldin LR: The outlook for linkage research in psychiatric disorders. J Psychiatr Res 21:541–550, 1987

Gershon ES, Goldin LR, Lake CR, et al: Genetics of plasma dopamine-β-hydroxylase, erythrocyte catechol-O-methyltransferase and platelet monoamine oxidase in pedigrees of patients with affective disorders, in Enzymes and Neurotransmitters in Mental Disease. Edited by Usdin E, Sourkes L, Young MBH. New York, Wiley, 1980, pp 281–299

Gershon ES, Hamovit JR, Schreiber JL: Anorexia nervosa and major affective disorders associated in families: a preliminary report, in Childhood Psychopathology and Development. Edited by Guze SB, Earls FJ, Barrett JE. New York, Raven, 1983

Gibbons JL, McHugh PR: Plasma cortisol in depressive illness. J Psychiatr Res 1:162–171, 1962

Gibbons RD, Davis JM: Consistent evidence for a biological subtype of depression characterized by low CSF monoamine levels. Acta Psychiatr Scand 74:8–12, 1986

Godwin CD, Greenberg LB, Shukla S: Predictive value of the dexamethasone suppression test in mania. Am J Psychiatry 141:1610–1612, 1984

Gold BI, Bowers MB, Roth RH, et al: GABA levels in CSF of patients with psychiatric disorders. Am J Psychiatry 137:362–364, 1980

Gold MS, Pottash AC, Extein I: Symptomless autoimmune thyroiditis in depression. Psychiatry Res 6:261–269, 1982

Gold PW, Chrousos GP, Kellner C, et al: Psychiatric implications of basic and clinical studies with corticotropin-releasing factor. Am J Psychiatry 141:619–627, 1984

Gold PW, Loriaux DL, Roy A, et al: Responses to corticotropin releasing hormone in the hypercortisolism of depression and Cushing's disease: pathophysiologic and diagnosis implications. N Engl J Med 314:1329–1335, 1986

Goldstein J, Van Cauter E, Linkowski P, et al: Thyrotropin nyctohemeral pattern in primary depression: difference between unipolar and bipolar women. Life Sci 27:1695–1703, 1980

Gonzalez-Heydrich J, Peroutka SJ: Serotonin receptors and reuptake sites: pharmacologic significance. J Clin Psychiatry 51 (suppl):5–12, 1990

Gorman JM: Psychoimmunology: a Darwinian approach, in Psychoimmunology Update. Edited by Gorman JM, Kertzner RM. Washington, DC, American Psychiatric Press, 1991, pp 1–8

Haggerty JJ, Evans DL, Golden RN, et al: The presence of anti-thyroid antibodies in patients with affective and non-affective psychiatric disorders. Biol Psychiatry 27:51–60, 1990

Haggerty JJ, Simon JS, Evans DL, et al: Relationship of serum TSH concentration and antithyroid antibodies to diagnosis and DST response in psychiatric inpatients. Am J Psychiatry 144:1491–1493, 1987

Halaris A, Piletz J: Platelet adrenoceptor binding as a marker in neuropsychiatric disorders. Abstracts of 17th CINP Congress, 1990, p 28

Halaris AE: Plasma 3-methoxy-4-hydroxyphenylglycol in manic psychosis. Am J Psychiatry 135:493–494, 1978

Halonen PE, Rimon R, Arohonka K: Antibody levels to herpes simplex type 1, measles and rubella viruses in psychiatric patients. Br J Psychiatry 125:461–465, 1974

Hatterer JA, Herbert J, Hidaka C, et al: CSF transthyretin in patients with depression. Am J Psychiatry 150:813–815, 1993

Hauser PH, Altshuler LL, Berrettini W, et al: Temporal lobe measurement in primary affective disorder by magnetic resonance imaging. J Neuropsychiatry Clin Neurosci 1:128–134, 1989a

Hauser PH, Dauphinais D, Berrettini W, et al: Corpus callosum dimensions measured by magnetic resonance imaging in bipolar affective disorder and schizophrenia. Biol Psychiatry 26:659–668, 1989b

Heisler S, Reisine T, Hook V, et al: Somatostatin inhibits multireceptor stimulation of cyclic AMP formation and adrenocorticotropin secretion in mouse pituitary tumor cells. Proc Natl Acad Sci U S A 79:6502–6507, 1982

Hermus AR, Pieters GF, Smals AG, et al: Plasma adrenocorticoptropin, cortisol, and aldosterone responses to corticotropin-releasing factor: modulatory effect of basal cortisol levels. J Clin Endocrinol Metab 58:187–191, 1984

Hodgkinson S, Sherrington R, Gurlin H, et al: Molecular genetic evidence for heterogeneity in manic depression. Nature 325:805–806, 1987

Holmes MC, Catt KJ, Aguilera G: Involvement of vasopressin in the down-regulation of pituitary corticotropin-releasing factor receptors after adrenalectomy. Endocrinology 121:2093–2098, 1987

Holsboer F, Haack D, Gerken A, et al: Plasma dexamethasone concentrations and different suppression response of cortisol and corticosterone in depressives and controls. Biol Psychiatry 19:281–291, 1984a

Holsboer F, Von Bardeleben U, Gerken A, et al: Blunted corticotropin and normal cortisol response to human corticotropin-releasing factor in depression [letter]. N Engl J Med 311:1127, 1984b

Honig A, Bartlett JR, Bouras N, et al: Amino acid levels in depression: a preliminary investigation. J Psychiatr Res 22:159–164, 1989

Husain MM, Figiel GS, Lurie SN, et al: MRI of corpus callosum and septum pellucidum in depression. Biol Psychiatry 29:300–301, 1991a

Husain MM, McDonald WM, Doraiswamy PM, et al: A magnetic resonance imaging study of putamen nuclei in major depression. Psychiatry Res 40:95–99, 1991b

Iacono WG, Smith GN, Moreau M, et al: Ventricular and sulcal size at the onset of psychosis. Am J Psychiatry 145:820–824, 1988

Imura H, Nakai Y, Hoshimi T: Effect of 5-hydroxytryptophan (5-HTP) on growth hormone and ACTH release in man. J Clin Endocrinol Metab 36:204–206, 1973

Irwin M, Lacher U, Caldwell C: Depression and reduced natural killer cytotoxicity: a longitudinal study of depressed patients and control subjects. Psychol Med 22:1045–1050, 1992

Jacoby RJ, Levy R: Computed tomography in the elderly: affective disorder. Br J Psychiatry 136:270–275, 1980

Jaeckle RS, Kathol RG, Lopez JF, et al: Enhanced adrenal sensitivity to exogenous ACTH stimulation in major depression. Arch Gen Psychiatry 44:233–240, 1987

Jaffe RB, Plosker S, Marshall L, et al: Neuromodulatory regulation of gonadotropin-releasing hormone pulsatile discharge in women. Am J Obstet Gynecol 163:1727–1731, 1990

Janicak PG, Davis JM, Chan C, et al: Failure of urinary MHPG levels to predict treatment response in patients with unipolar depression. Am J Psychiatry 143:1398–1402, 1986

Janowsky DS, El-Yousef MK, Davis JM, et al: A cholinergic-adrenergic hypothesis of mania and depression. Lancet 2:573–577, 1972

Joffe RT, Singer W, Levitt AJ, et al: A placebo-controlled comparison of lithium and triiodothyronine augmentation of tricyclic antidepressants in unipolar refractory depression. Arch Gen Psychiatry 50:387–394, 1993

Jones D, Kelwala S, Bell J, et al: Cholinergic REM sleep induction response correlation with endogenous major depressive type. Psychiatry Res 14:99–110, 1985

Kalin NH, Risch SC, Janowsky DS, et al: Plasma ACTH and cortisol concentrations before and after dexamethasone. Psychiatry Res 7:87–92, 1982

Kastin AJ, Ehrensing RH, Schalch DS, et al: Improvement in mental depression with decreased thyrotropin response after administration of thyrotropin-releasing hormone. Lancet 2:740–742, 1972

Kathol RG, Jaeckle RS, Lopez JR, et al: Consistent reduction of ACTH responses to stimulation with CRH, vasopressin and hypoglycaemia in patients with depression. Br J Psychiatry 155:468–478, 1989

Kauffman CA, Malaspina D: Molecular genetics of schizophrenia. Psychiatric Annals 23:111–122, 1993

Keller SE, Weiss JM, Schleifer SJ, et al: Stress-induced suppression of immunity in adrenalectomized rats. Science 221:1301–1304, 1983

Kelsoe JR, Ginns EI, Egeland JA, et al: Re-evaluation of the linkage relationship between chromosome 11p loci and the gene for bipolar affective disorder in the Old Order Amish. Nature 342:238–243, 1989

Kendler KS, Neale MC, Kessler RC, et al: A population-based twin study of major depression in women: the impact of varying definitions of illness. Arch Gen Psychiatry 49:257–266, 1992

Kendler KS, Pedersen N, Johnson L, et al: A pilot Swedish twin study of affective illness, including hospital- and population-ascertained subsamples. Arch Gen Psychiatry 50:699–706, 1993a

Kendler KS, Kessler RC, Neale MC, et al: The prediction of major depression in women: toward an integrated etiologic model. Am J Psychiatry 150:1139–1148, 1993b

Kennedy SH, Tighe S, McVey G, et al: Melatonin and cortisol "switches" during mania, depression, and euthymia in a drug-free bipolar patient. J Nerv Ment Dis 177:300–303, 1989

King DJ, Cooper SJ: Viruses, immunity and mental disorder. Br J Psychiatry 154:1–7, 1989

King DJ, Cooper SJ, Earle JAP: A survey of serum antibodies to eight common viruses in psychiatric patients. Br J Psychiatry 147:137–144, 1985

Kiriike N, Izumiya Y, Nishiwaki S, et al: TRH test and DST in schizoaffective mania, mania, and schizophrenia. Biol Psychiatry 24:415–422, 1988

Kirkegaard CJ, Faber J, Hummer L, et al: Increased levels of TRH in cerebrospinal fluid from patients with endogenous depression. Psychoneuroendocrinology 4:227–235, 1979

Kishimoto H, Takazu O, Ohno S, et al: 11C-glucose metabolism in manic and depressed patients. Psychiatry Res 22:81–88, 1987

Knobil E: The GnRH pulse generator. Am J Obstet Gynecol 163:1721–1727, 1990

Koyama T, Meltzer HY: A biochemical and neuroendocrine study of the serotonergic system in depression, in New Results in Depression Research. Edited by Hippius H, Klerman GL, Matussek N. New York, Springer-Verlag New York, 1986, pp 169–188

Krishnan KRR: Organic bases of depression in the elderly. Annu Rev Med 42:261–266, 1991

Krishnan KRR, Maltbie AA, Davidson JRT: Abnormal cortisol suppression in bipolar patients with simultaneous manic and depressive symptoms. Am J Psychiatry 140:203–205, 1983

Krishnan KRR, France RD, Pelton S, et al: What does the dexamethasone suppression test identify? Biol Psychiatry 20:957–964, 1985

Krishnan KR, Manepalli AN, Ritchie JC, et al: Growth hormone-releasing factor stimulation test in depression. Am J Psychiatry 145:190–2, 1988

Krishnan KRR, Husain MM, McDonald WM, et al: In vivo assessment of caudate volume in man: effect of normal aging. Life Sci 47:1325–1329, 1990a

Krishnan KRR, Ritchie JC, Saunders WB, et al: Adrenocortical sensitivity to low dose ACTH administration in depressed patients. Biol Psychiatry 27:930–933, 1990b

Krishnan KRR, Doraiswamy PM, Lurie SN, et al: Pituitary size in depression. J Clin Endocrinol Metab 72:256–259, 1991

Krishnan KRR, McDonald WM, Escalona PR, et al: Magnetic resonance imaging of the caudate nuclei in depression. Arch Gen Psychiatry 49:553–557, 1992

Krishnan KRR, Rayasam K, Reed D, et al: The CRF corticotropin-releasing factor stimulation test in patients with major depression: relationship to dexamethasone suppression test results. Depression 1:133–136, 1993

Kronfol Z, Silva J, Greden J, et al: Impaired lymphocyte function in depressive illness. Life Sci 33:241–247, 1983

Langer SZ, Raisman R: Binding of [³H]imipramine and [³H]desipramine as biochemical tools for studies in depression. Neuropharmacology 22:407–413, 1983

Lal S, Martin JB, de la Vega C, et al: Comparison of the effect of apomorphine and L-dopa on serum growth hormone levels in man. Clin Endocrinol (Oxf) 4:277–285, 1975

Landon J, James VHT, Stoker DJ: Plasma cortisol response to lysine-vasopressin in comparison with other tests of human pituitary-adrenocortical function. Lancet 2:1156–1159, 1965

Langer SZ, Raisman R: Binding of [3H]imipramine and [^{3}H]desipramine as biochemical tools for studies in depression. Neuropharmacology 22:407–413, 1983

Lapin I, Oxenkrug G: Intensification of the central serotonergic process as a possible determinant of thymoleptic effect. Lancet 1:132–136, 1969

Lazarus JH, McGregor AM, Ludgate M, et al: Effect of lithium carbonate therapy on thyroid immune status in manic depressive patients: a prospective study. J Affect Disord 11:155–160, 1986

Leckman JF, Gershon ES, Nichols AS, et al: Reduced MAO activity in first-degree relatives of individuals with bipolar affective disorders: a preliminary report. Arch Gen Psychiatry 34:601–606,1977

Lesch KP, Laux G, Erb A, et al: Attenuated growth hormone response to growth hormone RH in major depressive disorder. Biol Psychiatry 22:1495–1499, 1987a

Lesch KP, Laux G, Pfuller H, et al: Growth hormone response to GH-releasing hormone in depression. J Clin Endocrinol Metab 65:1278–1281, 1987b

Lewis DA, McChesney C: Tritiated imipramine binding distinguishes among subtypes of depression. Arch Gen Psychiatry 42:485–488, 1985

Linkowski P, Mendlewicz J, LeClercq R, et al: The 24 hour profile of ACTH and cortisol in major depressive illness. J Clin Endocrinol Metab 61:429–438, 1985

Linnoila VM, Virkkunen M: Aggression, suicidality and serotonin. J Clin Psychiatry 53 (suppl):46–51, 1992

Linnoila VM, Virkkunen M, Scheinin M, et al: Low cerebrospinal fluid 5-hydroxyindoleacetic acid concentration differentiates impulsive from non-impulsive violent behavior. Life Sci 33:2609–2614, 1983

Lippman S, Manshadi M, Baldwin H, et al: Cerebellar vermis dimensions on computerized tomographic scans of schizophrenia and bipolar patients. Am J Psychiatry 139:667–668, 1982

Loosen PT, Prange Jr AJ: Serum thyrotropin response to thyrotropin-releasing hormone in psychiatric patients: a review. Am J Psychiatry 139:405–416, 1982

Lurie SN, Doraiswamy PM, Figiel GS, et al: In vivo assessment of pituitary gland volume with MRI: effect of age. J Clin Endocrinol Metab 71:505–508, 1990

Maas JW, Fawcett JA, Dekirmenjian H: Catecholamine metabolism, depressive illness and drug response. Arch Gen Psychiatry 26:252–262, 1972

Maeda K, Yoshimoto Y, Yamadori A: Blunted TSH and unaltered PRL responses to TRH following repeated administration of TRH in neurologic patients: a replication of neuroendocrine features of major depression. Biol Psychiatry 33:277–283, 1993

Maes M, Bosmans E, Suy E, et al: The impaired mitogen lymphocyte stimulation in severely depressed patients: a complex interface between HPA-axis hyperfunction, noradrenergic activity, and aging process. Br J Psychiatry 155:793–798, 1989

Maes M, Stevens W, DeClerck L, et al: Immune disorders in depression: higher T helper/T suppressor-cytotoxic cell ratio. Acta Psychiatrica Scand 86:423–431, 1992a

Maes M, Stevens WJ, DeClerck LS, et al: A significantly increased number and percentage of B cells in depressed subjects: results of flow cytometric measurements. J Affect Disord 24:127–134, 1992b

Maes M, Van Der Planken M, Stevens WJ, et al: Leucocytosis, monocytosis and neutrophilia: hallmarks of severe depression. J Psychiatr Res 26:125–134, 1992c

Maes M, Stevens W, DeClerck L, et al: Significantly increased expression of T-cell activation markers (interleukin-2 and HLA-DR) in depression: further evidence for an inflammatory process during that illness. Prog Neuropsychopharmacol Biol Psychiatry 17:241–255, 1993

Maj M, Ariano MG, Arena F, et al: Plasma cortisol, catecholamine and cyclic AMP levels, response to dexamethasone suppression test and platelet MAO activity in manic-depressive patients: a longitudinal study. Neuropsychobiology 11:168–173, 1984

Mann JJ, Stanley M, McBride PA, et al: Increased serotonin 2 and β-adrenergic receptor binding in the frontal cortices of suicide victims. Arch Gen Psychiatry 43:954–959, 1986

Matussek N, Ackenheil M, Hippius H, et al: Effects of clonidine on growth hormone release in psychiatric patients and controls. Psychiatry Res 2:25–36, 1980

Maubach M, Dieblod K, Fried W, et al: Platelet MAO activity in patients with affective psychosis and their first-degree relatives. Pharmacopsychiatry 14:87–93, 1981

McGuffin P, Katz R, Rutherford J: Nature, nurture and depression: a twin study. Psychol Med 21:329–335, 1991

McKusick V: Mendelian Inheritance in Man, 10th Edition. Baltimore, MD, Johns Hopkins University Press, 1992

Meana JJ, Barturen F, Garcia-Sevilla JA: Alpha$_2$-adrenoceptors in the brain of suicide victims: increased receptor density associated with major depression. Biol Psychiatry 31:471–490, 1992

Meltzer HY, Lowy MT, Locascio JJ: Platelet MAO activity and the cortisol response to dexamethasone in major depression. Biol Psychiatry 24:129–142, 1988

Mendlewicz J: Genetics of depression and mania, in Depression and Mania. Edited by Georgotas A, Cancro R. New York, Elsevier, 1988, pp 197–212

Mendlewicz J, Rainier J: Adoption study supporting genetic transmission in manic-depressive illness. Nature 268:326–329, 1977

Mendlewicz J, Linkowski P, Kerkhofs M, et al: Diurnal hypersecretion of growth hormone in depression. J Clin Endocrinol Metab 60:505–512, 1985

Michels R, Marzuk P: Progress in psychiatry, I. N Engl J Med 329:552–560, 1993

Midgely AR, Jaffe RB: Regulation of human gonadotropins: episodic fluctuation of LH during the menstrual cycle. J Clin Endocrinol Metab 33:962–969, 1971

Mooney JJ, Schatzberg AF, Cole JO, et al: Rapid antidepressant response to alprazolam in depressed patients with high catecholamine output and heterologous desensitization of platelet adenyl cyclase. Biol Psychiatry 23:543–559, 1988

Mooney JJ, Schatzberg AF, Cole JO, et al: Urinary 3-methoxy-4-hydroxyphenylglycol and the depression-type score as predictors of differential responses to antidepressants. J Clin Psychopharmacol 11:339–343, 1991

Muller EE, Brambilla F, Cavagnini F, et al: Slight effect of L-tryptophan on growth hormone release in normal human subjects. J Clin Endocrinol Metab 39:1–5, 1974

Muscettola G, Potter WZ, Pickar D, et al: Urinary 3-methoxy-4-hydroxyphenylglycol and major affective disorders: a replication and new findings. Arch Gen Psychiatry 41:337–342, 1984

Myers DH, Carter RA, Burns BH, et al: A prospective study of the effects of lithium on thyroid function and on the prevalence of antithyroid antibodies. Psychol Med 15:55–61, 1985

Nair PNV, Hariharasubramanian N: Pilapil circadian rhythm of melatonin in endogenous depression. Prog Neuropsychopharmacol Biol Psychiatry 19:1215–1228, 1984

Nakamura Y, Leppert M, O'Connell P, et al: Variable number of tandem repeat (VNTR) markers for human gene mapping. Science 235:1616–1622, 1987

Nassberger L, Traskman-Bendz L: Increased soluble interleukin-2 receptor concentrations in suicide attempters. Acta Psychiatr Scand 88:48–52, 1993

Nemeroff CB, Evans DL: Correlation between the dexamethasone suppression test in depressed patients and clinical response. Am J Psychiatry 141:247–249, 1984

Nemeroff CB, Bissette G, Martin JB, et al: Effect of chronic treatment with thyrotropin-releasing hormone (TRH) or an analog of TRH (linear-beta-alanine TRH) on the hypothalamic-pituitary-thyroid axis. Neuroendocrinology 30:193–199, 1980

Nemeroff CB, Widerlov E, Bissette G, et al: Elevated concentrations of CSF corticotropin-releasing factor-like immunoreactivity in depressed patients. Science 226:1342–1344, 1984

Nemeroff CB, Simon JS, Haggerty JJ, et al: Antithyroid antibodies in depressed patients. Am J Psychiatry 142:840–843, 1985

Nemeroff CB, Owens MJ, Bissette G, et al: Reduced corticotropin-releasing factor (CRF) binding sites in the frontal cortex of suicides. Arch Gen Psychiatry 45:577–579, 1988

Nemeroff CB, Bissette G, Akil H, et al: Neuropeptide concentrations in the cerebrospinal fluid of depressed patients treated with electroconvulsive therapy: corticotropin-releasing factor, beta-endorphin and somatostatin. Br J Psychiatry 158:59–63, 1991a

Nemeroff CB, Knight DL, Krishnan KRR: Reduced platelet [^{3}H]-paroxetine and [^{3}H]-imipramine binding in major depression. Society for Neuroscience Abstracts 17:1472, 1991b

Nemeroff CB, Krishnan KKR, Reed D, et al: Adrenal gland enlargement in major depression: a computed tomographic study. Arch Gen Psychiatry 49:384–387, 1992

Nemeroff CB, Knight DL, Franks J et al: Further studies on platelet serotonin transporter binding in depression. Am J Psychiatry (in press)

Pandey SC, David JM, Schwertz DW, et al: Effect of antidepressants and neuroleptics on phospho-inositide metabolism in human platelets. J Pharmacol Exp Ther 256:1010–1018, 1991

Pandey GN, Sharma RP, Janicak PG, et al: Monoamine oxidase and cortisol response in depression and schizophrenia. Psychiatry Res 44:1–8, 1992

Papez JW: A proposed mechanism of emotion. Archives of Neurology and Psychiatry 38:725–743, 1937

Pardes H, Kauffmann CA, Pincus HA, et al: Genetics and psychiatry: past discoveries, current dilemmas, and future directions. Am J Psychiatry 146:435–443, 1989

Pearlson GD, Rabins PV, Kim WS, et al: Structural brain CT changes and cognitive deficits in elderly depressives with and without reversible dementia. Psychol Med 19:573–584, 1989

Perry EK, Marshall EF, Blessed G, et al: Decreased imipramine binding in the brains of patients with depressive illness. Br J Psychiatry 142:188–192, 1983

Pettito JM, Folds JD, Ozer H, et al: Abnormal diurnal variation in circulating natural killer phenotypes and cytotoxic activity in major depression. Am J Psychiatry 149:694–696, 1992

Petty F: Plasma concentrations of GABA and mood disorders: A blood test for manic depressive disease? Clin Chem 40:296–302, 1994

Petty F, Schlesser MA: Plasma GABA in affective illness. J Affect Disord 3:339–343, 1981

Petty F, Sherman AD: Plasma GABA levels in psychiatric illness. J Affect Disord 6:131–138, 1984

Pitts AF, Kathol RG, Gehris TL, et al: Elevated cerebrospinal fluid corticotropin-releasing hormone and arginine vasopressin in depressed patients with dexamethasone nonsuppression. Society for Neuroscience Abstracts 16:454, 1990

Post RM, Gold P, Rubinow DR, et al: Peptides in cerebrospinal fluid of neuropsychiatric patients: an approach to central nervous system peptide function. Life Sci 31:1–15, 1982

Prange A: The pharmacology and biochemistry of depression. Diseases of the Nervous System 25:217–221, 1964

Prange AJ, Wilson IC, Rabon AM, et al: Enhancement of imipramine antidepressant activity by thyroid hormone. Am J Psychiatry 126:457–469, 1969

Prange AJ Jr, Wilson IC, Lara PP, et al: Effects of thyrotropin-releasing hormone in depression. Lancet 2:999–1002, 1972

Prange AJ Jr, Wilson IC, Lynn CW, et al: L-Tryptophan in mania: contribution to a permissive hypothesis of affective disorders. Arch Gen Psychiatry 30:56–62, 1974

Prange AJ, Loosen PT, Wilson I, et al: The therapeutic use of hormones of the thyroid axis in depression, in Neurobiology of Mood Disorders. Edited by Post CR, Ballenger J. Baltimore, MD, Williams & Wilkins, 1980, pp 311–322

Price RA, Kidd KK, Weissman MM: Early onset (under age 30 years) and panic disorder as markers for etiologic homogenity in major depression. Arch Gen Psychiatry 44:434–440, 1987

Rabins PV, Pearlson GF, Aylward E, et al: Cortical magnetic resonance imaging changes in elderly inpatients with major depression. Am J Psychiatry 148:617–620, 1991

Rao VP, Krishnan KRR, Goli V, et al: Neuroanatomical changes and hypothalamo-pituitary-adrenal axis abnormalities. Biol Psychiatry 26:729–732, 1989

Reame N, Sauder SE, Kelch RP, et al: Pulsatile gonadotropin secretion during the human menstrual cycle: evidence for altered pulse frequency of gonadotropin releasing hormone secretion. J Clin Endocrinol Metab 59:328–337, 1984

Regier DA, Boyd JH, Burke JD Jr, et al: One-month prevalence of mental disorders in the United States: based on five Epidemiologic Catchment Area sites. Arch Gen Psychiatry 45:768–779, 1988

Reus VI, Berlant J, Galante M, et al: Proceedings of the 41th annual meeting of the Society of Biological Psychiatry, Washington, DC, May 1986

Richardson UI, Schonbrunn A: Inhibition of adrenocorticotropin secretion somatostatin in pituitary cells in culture. Endocrinology 108:281–284, 1981

Rimon R, Halonen P: Herpes simplex virus infection and depressive illness. Diseases of the Nervous System 30:338–340, 1969

Risch SC: Growth hormone-releasing factor and growth hormone, in Neuropeptides and Psychiatric Disorders. Edited by Nemeroff CB. Washington, DC, American Psychiatric Press, 1991, pp 93–108

Risch SC, Lewine RJ, Kalin NH, et al: Limbic-hypothalamic-pituitary-adrenal axis activity and ventricular-to-brain ratio in affective illness and schizophrenia. Neuropsychopharmacology 6:95–100, 1992

Ritchie J, Belkin BM, Krishnan KRR, et al: Plasma dexamethasone concentration and the dexamethasone suppression test. Biol Psychiatry 27:159–173, 1990

Robins LN, Helzer JE, Croughan J, et al: National Institute of Mental Health Diagnostic Interview Schedule: its history, characteristics, and validity. Arch Gen Psychiatry 38:381–389, 1981

Roman GC: Senile dementia of the Binswanger type: a vascular form of dementia in the elderly. JAMA 258:1782–1788, 1987

Rosenbaum AH, Maruta T, Schatzberg AF, et al: Toward a biochemical classification of depressive disorders, VII: urinary free cortisol and urinary MHPG in depressions. Am J Psychiatry 140:314–318, 1983

Rosenbaum AH, Schatzberg AF, Bowden CL, et al: MHPG as a predictor of clinical response to fluoxetine: proceedings of the 18th Collegium Internationale Neuro-Psychopharmacologicum Congress, Nice, France. Clin Neuropharmacol 15 (51, part B):209B, 1992

Rothchild AJ, Langlais PJ, Schatzberg AF, et al: Dexamethasone increases plasma free dopamine in man. J Psychiatr Res 18:217–223, 1984

Rothchild AJ, Langlais PJ, Schatzberg AF, et al: The effects of a single dose of dexamethasone on monoamine and metabolite levels in rat brain. Life Sci 36:2491–2501, 1985

Roy A, Pickar D, Paul S, et al: CSF corticotropin-releasing hormone in depressed patients and normal control subjects. Am J Psychiatry 144:641–645, 1987

Roy A, De Jong J, Linnoila M: Cerebrospinal fluid monoamine metabolites and suicidal behavior in depressed patients. Arch Gen Psychiatry 46:609–612, 1989

Royle NJ, Clarkson RE, Wong Z, et al: Clustering of hypervariable minisatellites in the proterminal regions of human autosomes. Genomics 3:352–360, 1988

Rubin RT, Heist K, McGeoy SS, et al: Neuroendocrine aspects of primary endogenous depression, XI: serum melatonin measures in patients and matched controls. Arch Gen Psychiatry 49:558–567, 1992a

Rubin RT, Phillips JJ, Sadow TF, et al: Adrenal gland volume in major depression: increase during the depressive episode and decrease with successful treatment. Proceedings of the annual meeting of the American College of Neuropsychopharmaco-

logy, San Juan, Puerto Rico, December 1992b

Rubinow DR: Cerebrospinal fluid somatostatin and psychiatric illness. Biol Psychiatry 21:341–365, 1986

Rubinow DR, Gold PW, Post RM, et al: CSF somatostatin in affective illness. Arch Gen Psychiatry 40:409–412, 1983

Rubinow DR, Gold PW, Post RM, et al: Somatostatin in patients with affective illness and in normal volunteers, in Neurobiology of Mood Disorders. Edited by Post RM, Ballenger JC. Baltimore, MD, Williams & Wilkins, 1984, pp 369–387

Sachar E, Hellman L, Fukushima D, et al: Cortisol production in depressive illness. Arch Gen Psychiatry 23:289–298, 1970

Sachar EJ, Schalch, DS, Reichlin S, et al: Plasma gonadotrophins in depressive illness: a preliminary report, in Recent Advances in the Psychobiology of the Depressive Illnesses. Edited by Williams TA, Katz MM, Shield JA Jr. Washington, DC, U.S. Department of Health and Welfare, 1972, pp 229–233

Sack DA, James SP, Rosenthal NE, et al: Deficient nocturnal surge of TSH secretion during sleep and sleep deprivation in rapid-cycling bipolar illness. Psychiatry Res 23:179–191, 1988

Samson JA, Gudeman JE, Schatzberg AF, et al: Toward a biochemical classification of depressive disorders, VIII: platelet monoamine oxidase activity in subtypes of depressions. J Psychiatr Res 19:547–555, 1985

Sapru MK, Rao BSSR, Channabasavana SM: Serum dopamine-beta-hydroxylase activity in classical subtypes of depression. Acta Psychiatr Scand 80:474–478, 1989

Schatzberg AF, Mooney JJ: Noradrenergic and cholinergic mechanisms in depressive disorders: implications for future treatment strategies, in Current Practices and Future Developments in the Pharmacotherapy of Mental Disorders. Edited by Meltzer HY, Nerozzi D. New York, Elsevier, 1991, pp 91–97

Schatzberg AF, Rothschild AJ: Serotonin activity in psychotic (delusional) major depression. J Clin Psychiatry 53 (10 suppl):52–55, 1992

Schatzberg AF, Orsulak PJ, Rosenbaum AH, et al: Towards a biochemical classification of depressive disorders, V: biochemical heterogeneity of unipolar depression. Am J Psychiatry 139:471–475, 1982

Schatzberg AF, Rothschild AJ, Bond TC, et al: The

DST in psychotic depression: diagnostic and pathophysiologic implications. Psychopharmacol Bull 20:362–364, 1984

Schatzberg AF, Rothschild AJ, Langlais PJ, et al: A corticosteroid/dopamine hypothesis for psychotic depression and related states. J Psychiatr Res 19:57–64, 1985a

Schatzberg AF, Rothschild AJ, Gerson B, et al: Toward a biochemical classification of depressive disorders, IX: DST results and platelet MAO activity. Br J Psychiatry 146:633–637, 1985b

Schatzberg AF, Rothschild AJ, Langlais PJ, et al: Psychotic and nonpsychotic depressions, II: platelet MAO activity, plasma catecholamines, cortisol, and specific symptoms. Psychiatry Res 20:155–164, 1987

Schatzberg AF, Samson JA, Bloomingdale KL, et al: Toward a biochemical classification of depressive disorders, X: Urinary catecholamines, their metabolites, and D-type scores in subgroups of depressive disorders. Arch Gen Psychiatry 46:260–268, 1989

Schildkraut JJ: The catecholamine hypothesis of affective disorders: a review of supporting evidence. Am J Psychiatry 122:509–522, 1965

Schildkraut JJ, Orsulak PJ, Schatzberg AF, et al: Toward a biochemical classification of depressive disorders, I: differences in urinary excretion of MHPG and other catecholamine metabolites in clinically defined subtypes of depression. Arch Gen Psychiatry 35:1427–1433, 1978a

Schildkraut JJ, Orsulak PJ, LaBrie RA, et al: Toward a biochemical classification of depressive disorders, II: application of multivariate discriminant function analysis to data on urinary catecholamines and metabolites. Arch Gen Psychiatry 35:1436–1439, 1978b

Schildkraut JJ, Orsulak PJ, Schatzberg AF, et al: Possible pathophysiological mechanisms in subtypes of unipolar depressive disorders based on differences in urinary MHPG levels. Psychopharmacol Bull 17:90–91, 1981

Schildkraut JJ, Orsulak PJ, Schatzberg AF, et al: Urinary MHPG in affective disorders, in Neurobiology of Mood Disorders. Edited by Post RM, Ballenger JC. Baltimore, MD, Williams & Wilkins, 1984, pp 519–528

Schilkrut R, Chandra O, Osswald M, et al: Growth hormone during sleep and with thermal stimulation in depressed patients. Neuropsychobiology 1:70–79, 1975

Schlegel S, Maier W, Philipp M, et al: Computed tomography in depression: association between ventricular size and psychopathology. Psychiatry Res 29:221–230, 1989

Schleifer SJ, Keller SE, Meyerson AT, et al: Lymphocyte function in major depressive disorder. Arch Gen Psychiatry 41:484–486, 1984

Schleifer SJ, Keller SE, Siris SG, et al: Depression and immunity: lymphocyte stimulation in ambulatory depressed patients, hospitalized schizophrenic patients, and patients hospitalized for herniorrhaphy. Arch Gen Psychiatry 42:129–133, 1985

Shah SA, Doraiswamy PM, Husain MM, et al: Posterior fossa abnormalities in major depression: a controlled MRI study. Acta Psychiatr Scand 85:474–479, 1992

Sharma RP, Janicak PG, Javaid JI, et al: Platelet MAO inhibition, urinary MHPG, and leucocyte beta-adrenergic receptors in depressed patients treated with phenelzine. Am J Psychiatry 147:1318–1321, 1990

Shopsin B, Gershon S, Goldstein M, et al: Use of synthesis inhibitors in defining a role for biogenic amines during imipramine treatment in depressed patients. Psychopharmacology Communications 1:239–249, 1975

Shopsin B, Friedman E, Gershon S: Parachlorophenylalanine reversal of tranylcypromine effects in depressed outpatients. Arch Gen Psychiatry 33:811–819, 1976

Siever LJ, Uhde TW, Silberman EK, et al: Growth hormone response to clonidine as a probe of noradrenergic receptor responsiveness in affective disorder patients and controls. Psychiatry Res 6:171–183, 1982

Siever LJ, Murphy DL, Slater S, et al: Plasma prolactin change following fenfluramine in depressed patients compared to controls: an evaluation of central serotonergic responsivity in depression. Life Sci 34:1029–1039, 1984

Siever LJ, Trestman RL, Coccaro EF, et al: The growth hormone response to clonidine in acute and remitted depressed male patients. Neuropsychopharmacology 6:165–177, 1992

Sitaram N, Gillin JC, Bunney WE Jr: Cholinergic and catecholaminergic receptor sensitivity in affective illness: strategy and theory, in Neurobiology of Mood Disorders. Edited by Post RM, Ballenger JC. Baltimore, MD, Williams & Wilkins, 1984, pp 519–

528

Solomon GF, Moos RH: Emotions, immunity, and disease: a speculative theoretical integration. Arch Gen Psychiatry 11:657–674, 1964

Souetre E, Salvati E, Wehr TA, et al: Twenty-four hour profiles of body temperature and plasma TSH in bipolar patients during depression and during remission and in normal control subjects. Am J Psychiatry 145:1133–1137, 1988

Southern EM: Detection of specific sequences among DNA fragments separated by gel electrophoresis. J Mol Biol 98:503–517, 1975

Stahl SM, Hauger RL, Rausch JL, et al: Down regulation of serotonin receptor subtypes by nortriptyline and adinazolam in major depressive disorder: Neuroendocrine and platelet markers. Paper presented in part at the 18th Annual Collegium Internationale Neuro-Psychopharmacologicum Congress, Nice, France, June 1992

Stein M, Miller AH, Trestman RL: Depression and the immune system, in Psychoneuroimmunology. Edited by Ader R, Felton DL, Cohen N. New York, Academic Press, 1991, pp 897–930

Stokes PE, Sikes CR: Hypothalamic-pituitary-adrenal axis in affective disorders, in Psychopharmacology: The Third Generation of Progress. Edited by Meltzer HY. New York, Raven, 1987, pp 589–607

Stokes PE, Frazer A, Casper R: Unexpected neuroendocrine-transmitter relationships. Psychopharmacol Bull 17:72–75, 1981

Swann AC, Koslow SH, Katz MM, et al: Lithium carbonate treatment of mania. Arch Gen Psychiatry 44:345–354, 1987

Swann AC, Secunda SK, Stokes PE, et al: Stress, depression and mania; relationship between perceived role of stressful events and clinical and biochemical characteristics. Acta Psychiatr Scand 81:389–397, 1990

Swann AC, Stokes PE, Casper R, et al: Hypothalamic-pituitary-adrenocortical function in mixed and pure mania. Acta Psychiatr Scand 85:270–274, 1992

Swanson LW, Sawchenko PE, Rivier J, et al: Organization of ovine corticotropin-releasing factor immunoreactive cells and fibers in the rat brain: an immunohistochemical study. Neuroendocrinology 36:165–186, 1983

Swayze VW, Andreasen NC, Alliger RJ: Structural brain abnormalities in bipolar affective disorder. Arch Gen Psychiatry 47:1054–1059, 1990

Sweeney D, Nelson C, Bowers M, et al: Delusional versus nondelusional depression: neurochemical differences. Lancet 2:100–101, 1978

Takahashi S, Kondo H, Yoshimura M, et al: Antidepressant effect of thyrotropin-releasing hormone (TRH) and the plasma thyrotropin levels in depression. Folia Psychiatrica et Neurologica Japonica 27:305–314, 1973

Toivola PTK, Gale CC, Goodner CJ, et al: Central alpha-adrenergic regulation of growth hormone and insulin. Hormones 3:192–213, 1972

Traskman L, Asberg M, Bertilsson L, et al: Monoamine metabolites in CSF and suicidal behavior. Arch Gen Psychiatry 10:253–261, 1981

Traskman-Bendz L, Alling C, Oreland L, et al: Prediction of suicidal behavior from biologic tests. J Clin Psychopharmacol 12 (2 suppl):21S–26S, 1992

Tsuang MT, Faraone SV: The Genetics of Mood Disorders. Baltimore, MD, Johns Hopkins University Press, 1990

Unden F, Ljunggren JG, Beck-Friis J, et al: Hypothalamic-pituitary-gonadal axis pulse detection. Am J Physiol 250:E486–E493, 1988

Vale W, Spiess J, Rivier C, et al: Characterization of a 41 residue ovine hypothalamic peptide that stimulates secretion of corticotropin of β-endorphin. Science 213:1394–1397, 1981

Valk J, van der Knaap MS: Magnetic Resonance of Myelin, Myelination, and Myelin Disorders. Berlin, Springer Verlag, 1989

Van Praag HM: Depression, suicide, and the metabolites of serotonin in the brain. J Affect Disord 4:21–29, 1982

Veith RC, Lewis N, Langohr JI, et al: Effect of desipramine on cerebrospinal fluid concentrations of corticotropin-releasing factor in human subjects. Psychiatry Res 46:1–8, 1992

Virkkunen M, Rawlings R, Tokola R, et al: CSF biochemistries, glucose metabolism, and diurnal activity rhythms in alcoholic, violent offenders, fire setters, and healthy volunteers. Arch Gen Psychiatry 51:20–27, 1994

Virkkunen M, Nuutila A, Goodwin FK, et al: Cerebrospinal fluid monoamine metabolite levels in male arsonists. Arch Gen Psychiatry 44:241–247, 1987

Vita A, Saccleti E, Cazzullo C: A CT scan follow-up study of cerebral ventricular size in schizophrenia and major affective disorder. Schizophrenia Res 1:165–166, 1988

Von Bardeleben U, Holsboer F, Stalla GK, et al: Combined administration of human corticotrophin-releasing factor and lysine vasopressin induces escape from dexamethasone suppression in healthy subjects. Life Sci 37:1613–1618, 1985

Watson SJ, Lopez JF, Young EA, et al: Effects of low dose ovine corticotropin-releasing hormone in humans: endocrine relationships and beta-endorphin/beta-lipotropin responses. J Clin Endocrinol Metab 66:10–15, 1986

Weber JL, May PE: Abundant class of human DNA polymorphisms which can be typed using the polymerase chain reaction. Am J Hum Genet 44:388–396, 1989

Weeke A, Weeke J: The 24-hour pattern of serum TSH in patients with endogenous depression. Acta Psychiatr Scand 62:69–74, 1980

Weiss JM, Sundar SK, Becker KJ, et al: Behavioral and neural influences on cellular immune responses: effects of stress and interleukin-1. J Clin Psychiatry 50 (suppl):5, 1989

Weissman MM, Gershon ES, Kidd KK, et al: Psychiatric disorders in the relatives of probands with affective disorders: the Yale University-National Institute of Mental Health Collaborative Study. Arch Gen Psychiatry 41:13–21, 1984

Weissman MM, Merikangas KR, Boyd JH: Epidemiology of affective disorders, in Psychiatry, Vol I. Edited by Michels R, Cavenar JO, Brodie HKH, et al. Philadelphia, PA, JB Lippincott, 1992

Wender PH, Kety SS, Rosenthal D, et al: Psychiatric disorders in the biological and adoptive families of adopted individuals with affective disorders. Arch Gen Psychiatry 43:923–929, 1986

Whalley LJ, Kutcher S, Blackwood DHR, et al: Increased plasma LH in manic-depressive illness: Evidence of a state-independent abnormality. Br J Psychiatry 150:682–684, 1987

Winokur A, Amsterdam J, Caroff S, et al: Variability of hormonal responses to a series of neuroendocrine challenges in depressed patients. Am J Psychiatry 139:39–44, 1982

Wolkowitz OM, Sutton ME, Doran AR, et al: Dexamethasone increases plasma HVA but not MHPG in normal humans. Psychiatry Res 16:101–109, 1985

Wolkowitz OM, Sutton ME, Koulu M et al: Chronic corticosterone administration in rats: behavioral and Biochemical evidence of increased central dopaminergic activity. European Journal of Psychopharmacology 122:329–338, 1986

Wolkowitz OM, Rubinow DR, Breier A, et al: Prednisone decreases CSF somatostatin in healthy humans: implications for neuropsychiatric illness. Life Sci 41:1929–1933, 1987

Woods BT, Yurgelun-Todd D, Benes FM, et al: Progressive ventricular enlargement in schizophrenia: comparison to bipolar affective disorder and correlation with clinical course. Biol Psychiatry 27:341–352, 1990

World Health Organization collaborative study: validity of imipramine platelet binding sites as a biological marker for depression. Pharmacopsychiatry 23:113–117, 1990

World Health Organization: International Statistical Classification of Diseases and Related Health Problems, 10th Revision. Geneva, World Health Organization, 1992

Wynn PC, Aguilera G, Morell J, et al: Properties and regulation of high-affinity pituitary receptors for corticotropin-releasing factor. Biochem Biophys Res Commun 110:602–608, 1983

Wynn PC, Hauger RL, Holmes MC, et al: Brain and pituitary receptors for corticotropin-releasing factor: localization and differential regulation after adrenalectomy. Peptides 5:1077–1084, 1984

Wynn PC, Harwood JP, Catt KJ, et al: Corticotropin-releasing factor (CRF) induces desensitization of the rat pituitary CRF receptor-adenylase cyclase complex. Endocrinology 122:351–358, 1988

Young EA, Watson SJ, Kotun J, et al: Beta-lipotropin-beta-endorphin response to low-dose ovine corticotropin releasing factor in endogenous depression. Arch Gen Psychiatry 47:449–457, 1990

Zis KD, Zis A: Increased adrenal weight in victims of violent suicide. Am J Psychiatry 144:1214–1215, 1987

23

Neurobiology of Schizophrenia

*Michael B. Knable, D.O., Joel E. Kleinman, M.D., Ph.D., and
Daniel R. Weinberger, M.D.*

Schizophrenia is the most common of the so-called "functional psychoses." The emotional and economic costs of this illness, which has a prevalence rate of 1% and which generally begins in late adolescence or early adulthood, are often underestimated. Schizophrenia is characterized by episodes of formal thought disorder, delusions, and hallucinations—the classic "positive symptoms." "Deficit symptoms," such as avolition, flat affect, cognitive problems, and lack of concern for personal hygiene and social conventions, tend to be chronic and resistant to treatment.

Early descriptions of schizophrenia noted familial clusters of the illness. We begin our review with a consideration of the proposed inherited tendency for schizophrenia and the extent to which environmental factors may contribute to the schizophrenic syndrome. Speculation that schizophrenic symptoms result from dysfunction of several brain areas has existed since the disorder was first described. A century of attempts to identify neuropathological correlates of schizophrenia have only recently begun to develop some consensus. We review modern studies using neuropathological and neurochemical techniques, computed tomography (CT), magnetic resonance imaging (MRI), and functional neuroimaging for evidence of altered brain structure and function in schizophrenia.

■ GENETICS AND OBSTETRICAL COMPLICATIONS

Schizophrenia occurs more commonly among family members of affected individuals. However, most cases of schizophrenia occur without an apparent family history, raising the possibility that some cases arise sporadically. Although results from family, twin, and adoption studies provide compelling evidence for a genetic contribution to schizophrenia, the nature of the inherited defect and its degree of penetrance are unknown. Schizophrenia occurs at similar prevalence rates throughout most of the world, despite the diversity of cultural, racial, and socioeconomic groups. This observation also lends weight to the concept of an inherited vulnerability with a relatively stable gene frequency.

Family and twin studies estimate the risk of schizophrenia in first-degree relatives and dizygotic twins of schizophrenic patients to be 10–15 times that of the general population. Many of these studies were performed in Europe at a time when diagnostic criteria for schizophrenia were less stringent than today. Therefore, cases that may now be diagnosed as schizophrenia spectrum disorders or other atypical psychoses may have been included. Recent studies that have attempted to exclude atypical cases postulate a risk for first-degree relatives that is somewhat less than that stated in older studies. (For reviews, see Schulz 1991 and Tsuang et al. 1991.) Monozygotic twins of people with schizophrenia have a concordance rate for schizophrenia of approximately 30%–80%, depending on ascertainment methods (Kendler 1983; McGue 1992; Torrey 1992). Because monozygotic twins do not have concordance rates of 100%, it may be inferred that nongenetic factors also contribute to pathogenesis.

Further support for a genetic vulnerability in schizophrenia comes from two observations in adoption studies: 1) children of schizophrenic mothers who are adopted by nonschizophrenic adults have an increased risk for schizophrenia (Heston 1966; Rosenthal et al. 1975); and 2) children of nonschizophrenic adults who are adopted away and raised by schizophrenic parents do not have an increased risk for schizophrenia (Wender et al. 1977).

Linkage analysis assumes that if a putative disease locus is in close proximity to a known genetic marker, the two segments of genetic material will remain in close proximity after meiosis, even if recombination takes place. Several studies have attempted to "link" a schizophrenic gene to specific chromosomal markers, without reliable success. In 1988, Bassett and colleagues described two family members with gross facial and extremity dysmorphisms and psychosis who were found to have a trisomic portion of chromosome 5 translocated to chromosome 1. In this kindred, two trisomic males and an asymptomatic female carrier of the translocation had temporal lobe atrophy on CT or MRI. One of the trisomic males also had a large cavum septum pellucidum and a cavum vergae (Honer et al. 1992). Sherrington and colleagues (1988) present evidence linking two DNA polymorphisms from chromosome 5 to schizophrenia in five Icelandic and two English pedigrees. Unfortunately, linkage of similar segments of chromosome 5 to the schizophrenic phenotype has not been replicated in a number of other kindreds (Aschauer et al. 1990; Detera-Wadleigh et al. 1989; Hallmayer et al. 1992a; Kaufman et al. 1989; Kennedy et al. 1988; Macciardi et al. 1992; McGuffin et al. 1990; St. Clair et al. 1989).

Linkage analyses of genes for two neurotransmitter receptor proteins have been completed. The gene encoding the serotonin 5-HT$_2$ receptor subtype has been mapped to chromosome 13. Hallmayer and colleagues (1992b) have excluded linkage of the 5-HT$_2$

locus with schizophrenia in a Swedish kindred. Moises and colleagues (1991) have excluded linkage of markers coding for parts of the dopamine D$_2$ receptor and for porphobilinogen deaminase (the deficient enzyme in acute intermittent porphyria) on chromosome 11 to Californian and Swedish pedigrees with schizophrenia.

In genetic association studies, a population with a pathological phenotype is compared to control subjects with regard to the frequency of alleles of known genetic markers. The classical markers are the ABO and Rh blood groups and the human leukocyte antigen (HLA) system. A previously replicated finding of a weak association of paranoid schizophrenia with the HLA-A9 locus (Owen and McGuffin 1991) has not been confirmed by a new study of 33 families (Campion et al. 1992). Crocq and colleagues (1992) have reported that schizophrenic patients have an increased frequency of homozygosity of a polymorphism of the dopamine D$_3$ receptor gene.

It is not entirely surprising that cytogenetic and "candidate-gene" linkage studies have not generated positive results. Molecular biological techniques have been more successfully applied to disorders with known modes of inheritance and clinically homogenous phenotypes. In schizophrenia research, large kindred samples need to be collected to make accurate assessments of inheritance and penetrance, to identify populations at risk for developing the illness, and to examine the role of specific genes. Genetic modeling strategies based on available pedigree data (reviewed by Tsuang et al. 1991) seem to support a complex multifactorial pattern of inheritance rather than a single gene model.

A history of obstetrical complications (OCs) in schizophrenic patients may indicate that an environmental effect is more important than genetic vulnerability in producing psychosis. However, it may be argued that abnormal development of the central nervous system (CNS) based on genetic underpinnings may predispose to OCs. To resolve this controversy, several researchers have tried to determine if OCs were more common in schizophrenic patients who did not have a family history of the disorder. However, it is important to remember that lack of a family history of illness does not rule out a genetic etiology of disease. Several studies support (Lewis and Murray 1987; O'Callaghan et al. 1990) and some refute (McCreadie et al. 1992; Nimgaonkar et al. 1988; Reddy et al. 1990) the proposed relationship between

OCs and theoretically sporadic cases of schizophrenia. Opinion is also divided as to whether a history of OCs is related to ventriculomegaly as measured by CT scan in adult schizophrenic patients (Cannon et al. 1989; Farmer et al. 1987; Lewis and Murray 1987; Nasrallah et al. 1982; Owen et al. 1988; Williams et al. 1985). The proposition that monozygotic twins discordant for schizophrenia might be discriminated by OCs and/or lower than normal birthweight has not been supported in a recent Scandinavian study (Onstad et al. 1992).

Another approach for considering prenatal risk factors in schizophrenia has been the epidemiological analysis of adverse intrauterine events. Several studies have examined the frequency of schizophrenia in offspring born to mothers who were pregnant during documented influenza epidemics. O'Callaghan and colleagues (1991) in the United Kingdom and Mednick and colleagues (1988) in Finland report significantly increased rates of schizophrenia in offspring of mothers who were in their second trimesters of pregnancy during the 1957 influenza A2 pandemic. Kendell and Kemp (1989) found that offspring in their second trimesters of development during the 1957 influenza epidemic in Edinburgh were at increased risk. These authors were not able to demonstrate increased risk when Scottish national data from the 1918 and 1957 epidemics were examined. The findings of Bowler and Torrey (1990) in the United States and those of Done and colleagues in the United Kingdom (1991) do not support a relationship between prenatal exposure to influenza and risk of schizophrenia. Susser and Lin (1992) have described an increased risk of schizophrenia in female offspring exposed to severe food deprivation in their first trimesters of development during the Dutch Hunger Winter of 1944–1945.

■ BRAIN ABNORMALITIES IN SCHIZOPHRENIA

We begin with a discussion of evidence for brain dysfunction in schizophrenia that is observable in the clinic. There is an extensive literature on abnormal clinical neurological signs in schizophrenia. "Soft" neurological signs are not typically ascribable to a focal lesion in the CNS and are thought to reflect disordered motor or sensory function at a complex, integrative level. Soft signs include dysdiadochokinesia, astereognosis, agraphesthesia, mirror phenomena, mild choreiform and tic-like movements, primitive reflexes, and sensory extinction phenomena. "Hard" neurological signs localize lesions to specific tracts, nuclei, nerves, or discrete cortical areas. However, hard signs that occur in isolation from other traditional hard signs may not support the presence of discrete lesions.

Various studies of neurological signs have important methodological differences, but most authors agree on an increased frequency of such signs in schizophrenic patients. Merriam and colleagues (1990) found that neurological signs of prefrontal impairment correlated with deficit symptomatology but not with age, presence of movement disorder, chronicity of illness, or psychological testing. In a study of 16 schizophrenic patients, King and colleagues (1991) found that soft signs correlated with presence of tardive dyskinesia, exposure to neuroleptic drugs, presence of positive and negative symptoms, and cognitive impairment, but not with ventricular size on CT scan. In a larger study that included measures of interrater reliability and factor analyses of related groups of soft signs, Schroder and colleagues (1992) found that the presence of soft signs was correlated with Brief Psychiatric Rating Scale (Overall and Gorham 1962) measures of thought disorder and with third ventricular width as measured by CT scan.

Two studies have supported the observation that neurological signs are more common in the nonpsychiatrically ill and the psychiatrically ill relatives of schizophrenic patients (Kinney et al. 1991; Rossi et al. 1990). Woods and colleagues (1991) report that neurological findings are more common in schizophrenic patients with a family history of psychosis.

Neuropsychological deficits have received increased emphasis in research on schizophrenia. Deficits in attention, memory, and "executive functions" have been observed repeatedly. These deficits implicate primarily prefrontal cortex and medial temporal lobe structures—brain areas in which altered structure and function have been found using the methodologies we describe later in this chapter. Neuropsychological abnormalities in schizophrenia are not thought to be epiphenomena of ongoing psychosis or of medication status and tend to predict long-term disability. (For a review, see Goldberg et al. 1991.)

■ Ventricular Enlargement and Corticosulcal Dilatation

The most widely replicated modern finding in studies of the brains of schizophrenic patients was also one of the earliest published observations. The increased ventricular size and decreased brain volume that were observed by early neuropathologists (Hecker 1871; Vogt and Vogt 1952; Yakovlev et al. 1950) have been replicated in postmortem specimens to which modern diagnostic criteria and quantitative measurement techniques have been applied (Brown et al. 1986; Pakkenberg 1987).

Enlargement of the lateral and third ventricles and cortical sulci have also been demonstrated in a large number of CT scan studies. Despite a number of methodological problems that arise in attempting to measure cerebral structures on CT scan for between-group comparisons (Cleghorn et al. 1991), most studies confirm the presence of ventricular and cortical sulcal enlargement. In a comprehensive review, Shelton and Weinberger (1986) concluded that among the papers they surveyed, lateral ventricular enlargement was found in 75% of the subjects studied, third ventricular enlargement in 83%, and cortical changes in 67%. The proportion of schizophrenic patients with ventricles more than 2 standard deviations larger than the control means has ranged from 3% to 35% (Jernigan 1986). No consistent relationship has been demonstrated between ventricular size in schizophrenic patients and age, duration of neuroleptic exposure, electroconvulsive therapy, or duration of illness (Shelton and Weinberger 1986).

Further evidence against ventriculomegaly as an epiphenomenon is found in the observation of ventriculomegaly in "first-break" schizophrenic patients (Nyback et al. 1982; Schulz et al. 1983; Weinberger et al. 1982) and in affected twins of monozygotic pairs discordant for schizophrenia (Revely et al. 1982; Suddath et al. 1990). Ventricular enlargement also appears to be stable in patients who have been followed prospectively (Illowsky et al. 1988; Sponheim et al. 1991). MRI studies have confirmed the presence of ventricular enlargement (Degreef et al. 1992; Gur et al. 1991; Kelsoe et al. 1988; Suddath et al. 1990; Young et al. 1991; Zipursky et al. 1992).

Clinical correlations of ventriculomegaly in schizophrenic patients include poor premorbid adjustment, cognitive impairment, more negative symptoms, diminished response to neuroleptics, and greater incidence of extrapyramidal movement disorders. However, these findings are contested by some authors. (For reviews, see Cleghorn et al. 1991, Pfefferbaum and Zipursky 1991, and Shelton and Weinberger 1986.)

■ Basal Ganglia

The basal ganglia are a group of functionally and anatomically related subcortical gray matter structures lying in the forebrain and midbrain. The caudate nucleus, claustrum, globus pallidus, putamen, subthalamic nucleus, and substantia nigra are considered parts of the basal ganglia. The nucleus accumbens lies in the anteroventral striatum and is included as part of the basal ganglia in our discussion. Dysfunction of the basal ganglia may contribute to the stereotypies, dyskinesias, catatonia, and possibly to the cognitive deficits seen in schizophrenic patients. Also, abnormalities attributed to limbic, frontal, and temporal cortices can be produced by dysfunction of the rich interconnections between these structures and the basal ganglia.

Traditional neuropathological techniques have been applied to the basal ganglia of schizophrenic patients in a limited number of recent studies and have produced conflicting results. These are summarized in Table 23–1.

It is difficult to generalize from this small group of studies, but several interesting possibilities deserve comment. The putamen and caudate (which compose the neostriatum) and the nucleus accumbens have been reported to have normal volume and area but decreased neuronal diameter. In addition, studies from two different brain collections have revealed decreased volume of the internal segment of the globus pallidus, a finding that was reported in earlier studies (Hopf 1952; Vogt and Vogt 1952). Decreased neuronal diameter in the nucleus accumbens may allow for "hypersensitivity" to normal amounts of nigrostriatal dopamine. Decreased volume of the substantia nigra may indicate that there is a deficiency of afferent striatonigral or corticonigral projections. Such a deficiency could allow for dysregulated nigrostriatal and mesolimbic dopaminergic transmission.

In Table 23–2, the results of MRI volumetric studies of the basal ganglia are presented for comparison with the pathological studies listed above. In general, the results tend to confirm neuropathological find-

Table 23–1. Recent postmortem neuropathologic studies in basal ganglia of schizophrenic subjects

Study	# Subjects/control subjects	Findings
Dom et al. 1981	5 drug-free cases from Vogt collection, 5 control subjects	Decreased cell diameter of Golgi II neurons in neostriatum and nucleus accumbens
Bogerts et al. 1983	6 drug-free cases from Vogt collection, 6 control subjects	Decreased total volume of lateral substantia nigra, decreased neuronal volume in medial substantia nigra
Bogerts et al. 1985	13 drug-free cases from Vogt collection, 9 control subjects	Reduced volume of internal globus pallidus; normal volume of putamen, caudate, and nucleus accumbens
Brown et al. 1986	41/29 (affective disorder control subjects)	No difference in areas of lenticular nuclei or caudate
Pakkenberg 1990	12/12	Reduced total number of neurons in nucleus accumbens with normal neuron numbers in ventral pallidum
Bogerts et al. 1990a	18/21	Decreased volume of internal globus pallidus with normal volumes of external globus pallidus, putamen, caudate, and nucleus accumbens
Heckers et al. 1991	23/23	Increased striatal volume on left, increased volume of globus pallidus on right

Table 23–2. Magnetic resonance imaging (MRI) studies of the basal ganglia in schizophrenia

Study	# Subjects/control subjects	Findings
Kelsoe et al. 1988	24/14	Normal area of caudate, globus pallidus, putamen
Young et al. 1991	31/33	Normal size of caudate; inverse relationship between negative symptom scale and caudate size
Jernigan et al. 1991	42/24	Increased volume of lenticular nucleus. Lenticular size correlates with age at onset
DeLisi et al. 1991	30/15/20*	No difference in caudate or lenticular volume
Swayze et al. 1992	54/48/47**	Enlarged putamen in male subjects bilaterally

* First break patients/chronic patients/neurologic control subjects.
** 48 bipolar patients and 47 control subjects.

ings of normal striatal volume. However, it is interesting to note that two MRI studies (Jernigan et al. 1991; Swayze et al. 1992) and one neuropathological study (Heckers et al. 1991) have found increased size of the neostriatum or its component parts. These findings are seen by the authors as possible evidence of defective pruning of synaptic connections during neuronal development. However, as enlargement of basal ganglia structures has not been seen in recent studies of first-break patients (DeLisi et al. 1991), this finding may represent an artifact of chronic illness, treatment, or measurement technique.

■ Limbic System

The limbic system has been defined in various ways. Generally, a group of interconnected structures in the medial temporal lobe, diencephalon, subcortical gray matter of the forebrain, and septal aspects of the frontal lobe are considered parts of the limbic system. In a broad sense, limbic structures are thought to subserve the integration of sensory input and motoric responses with affective or emotional data. These structures are among the oldest phylogenetic components of the CNS. Areas that are often included in discussion of the limbic system are the hippocampus, the cytoarchitecturally related parahippocampal gyrus, entorhinal and insular cortices, amygdala, septal nuclei, hypothalamus, nucleus accumbens, anterior thalamus, cingulate cortex, and olfactory bulbs.

The most intensive recent neuropathological investigation of postmortem tissue from schizophrenic patients has been focused on the hippocampus and surrounding structures. Table 23–3 lists neuropathological studies of this area, and Table 23–4 presents related data from MRI studies.

These studies strongly implicate medial temporal lobe abnormalities in schizophrenia. The findings of reduced volume of the amygdala, hippocampus, parahippocampal gyrus, and entorhinal cortex have been replicated in most neuropathological and neuroimaging studies. Abnormal cellular orientation and lamination, heterotopic cell groups, and reductions in neuronal size and number that occur in the absence of gliosis suggest prenatal damage to medial temporal lobe areas. Cellular migration from the ventricular surface to the cerebral cortex is essentially complete by the fifth fetal month. Therefore, pathological orchestration of neuronal migration in schizophrenia may occur before this time.

Few studies have used modern diagnostic and neuropathological methods to examine other limbic structures. Two studies of the nucleus basalis of Meynert (Arendt et al. 1983; El-Mallakh et al. 1991) do not demonstrate differences between schizophrenic subjects and control subjects. Benes and colleagues (1986) have reported reduced neuronal density in layer V of cingulate cortex, layer VI of prefrontal cortex, and layer III of motor cortex. These findings were associated with reduced glial numbers and normal neuron-glia ratio and neuronal size. This combination of observations does not support the idea of a degenerative neuronal condition underlying the schizophrenic syndrome.

Several studies noted in Tables 23–3 and 23–4 have reported findings in both the basal ganglia and in mesial temporal structures. Bogerts and colleagues (1985) reported on specimens from the Vogt collection (Vogt and Vogt 1952) that had decreased volume of the internal globus pallidus. These same subjects also had decreased volumes of amygdala, hippocampus, and parahippocampal gyrus. In a later study (1990a), Bogerts and colleagues reproduced the findings of decreased volume of the internal globus pallidus and hippocampus in a new collection. The report by Jernigan and colleagues (1991) regarding decreased medial temporal and orbitofrontal cortical volumes also included the finding of enlarged lenticular nucleus. However, findings by Young and colleagues (1991) of decreased left parahippocampal volume and lack of normal asymmetry in amygdala volume were reported from subjects who had normal

volumes of basal ganglia structures. From these observations, it is difficult to conclude that a reproducible pattern of subcortical anatomical abnormality accompanies anatomical abnormalities in the medial temporal lobe.

■ Neocortex

Little (and inconsistent) research in the literature exists regarding pathology of neocortical areas in schizophrenia. Sporadic reports of reduced cortical thickness and neuronal number have been reported in the older neuropathological literature (Kirch and Weinberger 1986). There have been a few reports of reduced neuronal number and density in the prefrontal regions of the frontal lobes (Benes and Bird 1987; Benes et al. 1986; Colon 1972). MRI reports of decreased temporal lobe volume (Rossi et al. 1991; Suddath et al. 1989, 1990) often do not distinguish between whether decreased volume could be explained solely by hippocampal or by medial temporal cortical thinning. Pathology of lateral temporal neocortex has long been suspected as an origin of positive schizophrenic symptoms and language abnormalities. MRI studies (Barta et al. 1990; Shenton et al. 1992) have found decreased volumes of the superior temporal gyrus. A number of CT and MRI studies that describe generalized reductions in thickness of cerebral cortex suggest that the proposed developmental defect in cortical maturation may not be restricted to medial temporal or frontal neocortex (Pfefferbaum et al. 1988; Weinberger et al. 1979a; Zipursky et al. 1992).

Technological advances in the imaging of brain function have produced the most provocative evidence for dysfunction of neocortex in schizophrenia. Single photon emission computed tomography (SPECT) and positron-emission tomography (PET) have been used to measure regional cerebral blood flow (rCBF) and local cerebral metabolic rate of glucose (LCMRg). These techniques and their merits have been reviewed by Berman and Weinberger (1991). Such studies have not revealed consistent abnormalities in global cerebral metabolism or in lateralization of brain function in schizophrenic patients. Original reports by Ingvar and Franzen (1974a, 1974b) of decreased frontal lobe metabolic activity ("hypofrontality") in schizophrenic patients have been confirmed by some investigators but disputed by others.

Table 23–3. Recent neuropathological studies of the hippocampal region in schizophrenia

Study	Method	# Subjects/ control subjects	Findings
Kovelman and Scheibel 1984	Pyramidal cell orientation and density	10/8	Pyramidal cell disarray in CA_1/CA_2 and prosubiculum/CA_1 interfaces in anterior hippocampus
Bogerts et al. 1985	Volumetric study of 20-μm sections from Vogt collection (left hemisphere only)	13/9	Reduced volume of amygdala, hippocampal formation, parahippocampal gyrus
Brown et al. 1986	Computer assisted determination of area at level of inter-ventricular foramina	41/29*	Enlarged temporal horn of lateral ventricle and reduced thickness of parahippocampal cortex
Roberts et al. 1986	Computer assisted densitometry of GFAP	5/7	No gliosis in left hippocampal area
Jakob and Beckmann 1986	Qualitative histopathology and cell counts	64/10	Abnormal lamination and heterotopic cells in rostral entorhinal and ventral insular cortices; reduced cell counts in insular cortex layers II and III
Colter et al. 1987	Computer assisted determination of cortical area at level of interventricular foramina	17/11[*]	Reduced volume of gyral component of parahippocampal gyrus
Altshuler et al. 1987	Pyramidal cell orientation and density in Yakovlev collection	7/6	No difference between schizophrenic subjects and control subjects; hippocampal disarray correlated with severity of behavioral impairment in schizophrenic subjects
Falkai et al. 1988	Volume and cell counts in ento-rhinal region in Vogt collection	13/11	Neuronal loss and decreased volume of left entorhinal cortex
Christison et al. 1989	Computerized analysis of pyra-midal cell size, shape, and orientation	17/32[**]	Normal hippocampal pyramidal cell size, shape, and orientation in left and right CA_1
Jeste and Lohr 1989	Computer assisted volume and pyramidal cell density of CA_1–CA_4 in Yakovlev collection	13/25[**]	Decreased volume of bilateral anterior and posterior CA_4; decreased pyramidal cell density in bilateral anterior and posterior CA_3/CA_4
Altshuler et al. 1990	Computerized shape analysis and area determinations of single coronal sections at the level of the mammillary bodies	12/17/10[***]	No difference in hippocampal area; reduced parahippocampal area on right; abnormal right hippocampal and parahippocampal shape
Bogerts et al. 1990a	Volume of hippocampal formation	18/21	Decreased volume of right and left hippocampal formation
Arnold et al. 1991	Qualitative histopathology	6/16	Aberrant surface invaginations, lami-nation patterns, heterotopias, and qualitative neuronal loss in entorhinal cortex
Benes et al. 1991	Pyramidal cell disarray, number and size, and camera lucida determination of volume in posterior hippocampus	14/9	No difference in posterior hippocampal volume; reduced number of neurons in CA_1; smaller pyramidal cell neurons CA_1–CA_4
Conrad et al. 1991	Pyramidal cell disarray in right hippocampus	11/7	Increased disarray at CA_1/CA_2 and CA_2/CA_3 interfaces

Note. GFAP = glial fibrillary acidic protein; CA = cornu ammonis.
[*] Control subjects with affective disorders.
[**] Leukotomized and nonschizophrenic control subjects.
[***] Nonschizophrenic and nonschizophrenic suicide control subjects.

Table 23–4.   Recent MRI studies of the hippocampal region in schizophrenia

Study	Method	# Subjects/ control subjects	Findings
DeLisi et al. 1988	Computer assisted volumetric study	24/18	Decreased volume of the anterior amygdalo-hippocampal region bilaterally; decreased volume of right posterior amygdalo-hippocampal region
Suddath et al. 1989	Computer assisted volumetric study	17/17	Decreased volume of bilateral temporal lobe gray matter, especially in region of amygdala and anterior hippocampus
Barta et al. 1990	Computer assisted volumetric study	15/15	Decreased volume of left amygdala, right temporal lobe, and right superior temporal gyrus
Bogerts et al. 1990b	Computer assisted volumetric study	35/25	Decreased volume of left amygdalo-hippocampal region in male first break schizophrenic subjects
Suddath et al. 1990	Computer assisted volumetric study	15/15[*]	Decreased volume of left temporal lobe and of bilateral anterior hippocampus
Rossi et al. 1991	Computer assisted volumetric study	16/10[**]	Reduced bilateral temporal lobe volume
Jernigan et al. 1991	Computer assisted volumetric study	42/24	Reduced volume of cortical areas containing medial temporal lobe and orbitofrontal cortex
Young et al. 1991	Computer assisted volumetric study	31/33	Amygdala smaller on left in control subjects but not in schizophrenic subjects; parahippocampal gyrus smaller on left in schizophrenic subjects but not in control subjects
Shenton et al. 1992	Computer assisted volumetric study	15/15	Decreased volume of gray matter in left anterior amygdalo-hippocampal area, left parahippocampal gyrus, and left superior temporal gyrus

[*] Control subjects are discordant monozygotic twins.
[**] Bipolar control subjects.

Recently, the concept that "hypofrontality" may exist as a state-dependent phenomenon has emerged. When measurements of rCBF during cognitive tasks are performed, schizophrenic patients are consistently hypofrontal. Weinberger and colleagues (1986) demonstrated a lack of activation of dorsolateral prefrontal cortex in schizophrenic patients given an automated version of the Wisconsin Card Sorting Test (WCST; Heaton 1985) during ^{133}Xe rCBF measurement. Physiologic dysfunction of dorsolateral prefrontal cortex (DLPFC) in schizophrenia during the WCST has also been replicated using HMPAO SPECT (Rubin et al. 1991). Relative prefrontal blood flow is correlated with cerebrospinal fluid (CSF) concentrations of homovanillic acid (HVA) and 5-hydroxy-indoleacetic acid (5-HIAA; Weinberger et al. 1988), suggesting that dopaminergic innervation of prefrontal cortex is necessary for normal functional activation. Prefrontal cortical dysfunction may be a discrete abnormality in schizophrenia, because regional differences in cerebral metabolism are not observed during a visual continuous performance vigilance test

(Berman et al. 1986) or during Raven's Progressive Matrices (Raven 1965) (Berman et al. 1988). In studies of monozygotic twins discordant for schizophrenia, diminished activation of the DLPFC during the WCST is invariably associated with the disorder, is not present in unaffected co-twins, is not affected by long-term neuroleptic exposure (Berman et al. 1992), and is correlated with diminished hippocampal volume in the affected twins (Weinberger et al. 1992).

■ **Thalamus and Brain Stem**

Lesch and Bogerts (1984) have described decreased volume of the central nucleus of the thalamus. There is also a report of decreased neuronal numbers in the dorsomedial nucleus of the thalamus (Pakkenberg 1990). These thalamic nuclei deserve further study because of their interconnections with limbic structures and prefrontal cortex. Bogerts and colleagues (1983) have also described decreased size of mesencephalic ventral tegmental cells when schizophrenic subjects are compared with control subjects.

■ Cerebellum

Reduced size of the cerebellar vermis has been described in some schizophrenic patients with CT scanning (Heath et al. 1979; Weinberger et al. 1979b) and in a postmortem study (Weinberger et al. 1980). In an effort to control for vermian atrophy from other causes, Lohr and Jeste (1986) have been unable to replicate this finding in a postmortem sample. Moreover, Weinberger and colleagues (1982) did not observe reduced size of the cerebellar vermis in first-break patients. Taken together, these results suggest that to the extent that cerebellar pathology has been associated with schizophrenia, it is likely to be an epiphenomenon.

■ NEUROCHEMICAL ABNORMALITIES

■ Dopamine

The dopamine hypothesis of schizophrenia has been a major impetus for research for the past 30 years. In the early 1960s, Carlsson and Lindquist (1963) reported that dopamine turnover was increased in laboratory animals given neuroleptics. Subsequently it was shown that the clinical efficacy of neuroleptics was correlated with their ability to displace radioligands from dopamine D_2 receptors (Creese et al. 1976; Seeman et al. 1976). Pharmacological induction of dopamine hyperactivity in laboratory animals produces behavioral alterations that are thought to be similar to the attentional problems seen in schizophrenic patients (Braff and Geyer 1990; Mathysse 1977). In parallel with laboratory investigations, clinicians also observed that psychotic symptoms could be seen in patients exposed to drugs such as amphetamine or L-dopa (Angrist 1973; Ellinwood 1967).

Investigations of dopaminergic function in schizophrenic patients until recently have been constrained by the methodological problems inherent in studies of CSF metabolites and postmortem neurochemical measures. In general, CSF dopamine and HVA levels in schizophrenic patients have not been shown to differ from those of control subjects (Widerlov 1988). In fact, some investigators have found lower than normal levels of CSF HVA in schizophrenic patients that are inversely correlated with the severity of negative symptoms (Bowers 1974; Lindstrom 1985).

Studies of plasma HVA levels have been reviewed by Davis and colleagues (1991). Although some studies have found that plasma HVA levels correlate with severity of symptoms and response to neuroleptic treatment, it should be noted that plasma HVA concentrations are affected substantially by changes in renal clearance, an issue that has not been adequately addressed in these studies. Likewise, the possibility that increased plasma concentrations of HVA in drug-free schizophrenic patients may simply reflect alterations in peripheral autonomic function that accompany psychosis also has been generally disregarded (Potter et al. 1989).

Studies of dopamine and HVA in postmortem brain tissue have yielded inconsistent results (Davis et al. 1991). Three studies have reported increased postmortem dopamine levels. Bird and colleagues (1979a) found increased concentration of dopamine in the nucleus accumbens and anterior perforated substance in schizophrenic patients. Crow and colleagues (1979) found an increased concentration of dopamine that was restricted to the caudate nucleus. Reynolds (1983) described increased dopamine concentrations in the amygdala of schizophrenic patients that was more prominent on the left.

Postmortem studies of dopamine receptor binding in schizophrenic brains have demonstrated an increased number of dopamine D_2 receptors in the caudate, putamen, and nucleus accumbens. These changes have been reported in more than 20 studies (for reviews, see Davis et al. 1991 and Hyde et al. 1991) and would seem to imply that a primary abnormality of the dopamine receptor may underlie dopaminergic dysfunction in schizophrenia. Although chronic neuroleptic treatment is also known to increase the number of dopamine D_2 receptors, a number of studies have reported increased D_2 receptor binding in patients who have been drug free for prolonged periods. (See Hyde et al. 1991 for review.)

Attempts to quantitate D_2 receptor density in vivo with PET have produced inconclusive results. Using ^{11}C-spiperone in 10 drug-naive schizophrenic patients, Wong and colleagues (1986) found increased binding in the caudate nucleus. Two studies using ^{11}C-raclopride have not replicated this finding (Farde et al. 1987, 1990). No group differences between 12 schizophrenic subjects and control subjects could be detected in one study with [76]Br-bromospiperone

(Martinot et al. 1990). Interpretation of these results requires consideration of several problems. First, raclopride has a lower affinity for dopamine receptors than spiperone and may be more easily displaced by endogenous ligand. Second, the studies have used different mathematical models for data analysis—models that are not easily compared. Third, the studies may have used patients with different severity and/or lengths of illness. Dopamine receptor number may be state dependent and may vary under such conditions. Finally, spiperone and bromospiperone bind to serotonergic and adrenergic receptors and may complicate data analysis for this reason.

Fewer studies exist concerning the dopamine D_1 receptor. Interest in this receptor was initially not great, because the clinical efficacy of neuroleptics was not correlated with displacement of ligands from the D_1 receptor. Cross and colleagues (1981) and Seeman and colleagues (1987) have reported that D_1 binding in brains of schizophrenic subjects was not different from that of control subjects. Hess and colleagues (1987) reported decreased D_1 binding in caudate and putamen.

An abnormal functional interaction between D_1 and D_2 receptors in schizophrenia has been suggested by Seeman and colleagues (1989). Pretreatment of striatal homogenates with the D_1 antagonist SCH23390 prevents the ability of dopamine to inhibit binding of the D_2 antagonist raclopride. This D_1–D_2 linkage is present in brain tissue from Parkinson's disease patients but not in schizophrenic patients. A link between the two receptor subtypes is proposed to be mediated by a G protein. This intriguing study has not yet been replicated.

It seems increasingly unlikely that simple hyperdopaminergia can account for the many clinical manifestations of schizophrenia. The mesocortical, mesolimbic, and nigrostriatal dopamine systems differ from one other substantially in their anatomical and functional organizations. (For a review, see Bachneff 1991.) Alterations in these projections may occur in different combinations to produce the variability of the schizophrenic syndrome.

Weinberger (1987) has proposed that many of the negative symptoms of schizophrenia are primarily related to dysfunction of prefrontal cortex and that positive symptoms may reflect disinhibited subcortical dopamine activity as a result of a neocortical abnormality. Damage to the prefrontal cortex in rats

potentiates the behavioral effects of amphetamine (Iversen 1971) and apomorphine (Scatton et al. 1982). Ibotenic acid lesions of medial prefrontal cortex in rats increase behavioral and biochemical evidence of dopamine hyperactivity in the basal ganglia, especially when the animals are stressed (Jaskiw et al. 1990).

Cortical modulation of subcortical dopamine release, in turn, may depend on intact cortical dopaminergic innervation. If mesocortical projections to frontal cortex are damaged with 6-hydroxydopamine in rodents, there is an increase of dopamine turnover and dopamine binding sites in the striatum (Carter and Pycock 1980; Pycock et al. 1980a, 1980b). Thus, cortical hypodopaminergia may play a role in some aspects of the schizophrenic syndrome.

The hypothesis that hypofrontality of schizophrenia may be related to deficient mesocortical dopamine activity is supported by several cerebral blood flow studies. Geraud and colleagues (1987) found that piribedil restored near normal frontal blood flow in drug-free schizophrenic patients selected for "hypofrontality" as measured with ^{133}Xe SPECT. Weinberger and colleagues (1988) found a positive correlation between CSF HVA concentration and prefrontal rCBF during the WCST. Daniel and colleagues (1989) demonstrated improved blood flow to dorsolateral prefrontal cortex during performance of the WCST when six drug-free schizophrenic subjects were administered intravenous apomorphine. A task-specific increase in dorsolateral prefrontal cortical rCBF during the WCST has also been demonstrated in 10 schizophrenic patients maintained on haloperidol after the administration of oral dextroamphetamine (Daniel et al. 1991).

Defective subcortical dopamine transmission may also be altered by aberrant input to dopaminergic neurons from the medial temporal structures that have been implicated in the neuropathological literature on schizophrenia. Ibotenic acid lesions of ventral hippocampus in rats cause increased amphetamine-induced locomotion, increased dopamine concentrations in the nucleus accumbens, and decreased concentrations of dihydrophenylacetic acid (DOPAC) and HVA in the medial prefrontal cortex (Lipska et al. 1992). Thus a medial temporal cortical defect (which has been proposed in schizophrenia) may differentially affect dopamine transmission in subcortical and cortical systems, in a manner consistent with current models of the illness.

Future advances in the study of dopaminergic abnormalities in schizophrenia will likely follow developments in molecular biology. D_3, D_4, and D_5 receptors have now been cloned. The D_3 and D_5 receptors are located primarily in limbic areas of the brain (Sokoloff et al. 1990; Sunahara et al. 1991). Messenger RNA encoding the D_4 receptor is located in frontal cortex, midbrain, and amygdala; it is bound with high affinity by clozapine (Van Tol et al. 1991).

■ Glutamate

The ability of cortical neurons to modulate subcortical dopamine activity is probably dependent on glutamate projections, because glutamate is the dominant neurotransmitter of cerebral cortex. Three principal glutamate receptors have been named for their affinity for the synthetic glutamate analogues N-methyl-D-aspartate (NMDA), quisqualate, or kainate.

Abnormal glutamate transmission has been suspected in schizophrenia for several reasons. Data concerning cortical hypofunction logically imply decreased cortical output. Destruction of cortical glutaminergic fibers increases animals' susceptibility to the behavioral effects of dopaminergic drugs (Scatton et al. 1982). Glutamate normally stimulates the inhibitory neurotransmitter γ-aminobutyric acid (GABA) in the striatum, whereas dopamine inhibits GABA release. Thus, similar behavioral effects could be produced by deficient corticostriatal glutamate activity or excessive mesostriatal dopamine activity (Zukin and Javitt 1991). It has also been shown that the normal phasic depolarization of ventral tegmental neurons is dependent on the presence of NMDA receptor-mediated effects (Johnson et al. 1992).

Glutaminergic system dysfunction in schizophrenia is also predicted by the phencyclidine (PCP) model of psychosis. PCP binds to a receptor located within the ion channel formed by the NMDA receptor complex and prevents the normal neuronal events produced by binding of glutamate to the NMDA receptor. (For a review, see Zukin and Javitt 1991.)

The decreased concentration of glutamate in the CSF of schizophrenic patients reported by Kim and colleagues (1980) has not been replicated by other authors (Gattaz et al. 1982, 1985; Perry 1982). Perry (1982) was unable to demonstrate differences in levels of glutamate measured in six regions of postmortem brain tissue in schizophrenic subjects and control subjects. Toru and colleagues (1988) measured multiple brain areas and found a lower glutamate concentration in the angular gyrus of schizophrenic patients. Using synaptosomal preparations from postmortem schizophrenic brain tissue, Sherman and colleagues have reported on deficient glutamate release with veratridine-induced depolarization (1991a) or on exposure to NMDA or kainic acid (1991b).

The results of glutamate receptor binding studies, summarized in Table 23–5, have been somewhat more consistent.

Although it would be difficult to say that these results can be condensed to form a glutamatergic hypothesis of schizophrenia, they do seem to emphasize the possible complexities of reciprocal interactions between dopaminergic and glutamatergic systems. Decreased binding of glutamate receptor ligands in the hippocampus may imply abnormal cellular development or cell loss in this area. This is supported by the findings of Harrison and colleagues (1991), who have reported a decrease in messenger RNA for the NMDA receptor in the CA_3 region of the hippocampus in postmortem brain tissue from schizophrenic patients. Increased numbers of prefrontal cortical glutamate receptors and glutamate reuptake sites may indicate an abnormally rich glutamategic innervation of prefrontal cortex by other cortical projection neurons. Abnormal elimination of transient synaptic connections during development could explain such a finding. In the basal ganglia, decreased glutamate reuptake sites may indicate a reduction in the number of glutamatergic projections to subcortical areas, with increased MK-801 binding representing a "denervation supersensitivity" phenomenon. Indeed, in all the brain regions mentioned here, it could be argued that abnormalities in glutamate receptor binding do not reflect anything at all about anatomical connections but are purely functional in nature. Future research will determine if glutamate receptor abnormalities in schizophrenia arise as a primary feature of the illness, in response to abnormalities in other neurotransmitter systems, or as an artifact of drug treatments.

■ Serotonin

Early theories implicating serotonin in the pathogenesis of schizophrenia were based on the observation that lysergic acid diethylamide (LSD), an agonist for serotonergic receptors, could produce a psychosis

Table 23–5.   Glutamate receptor binding studies in postmortem schizophrenic brain tissue

Study	Method	# Subjects/ control subjects	Results
Kerwin et al. 1988	^{3}H-kainate and glutamate in hippocampal homogenates	11/9 (Kainate)[*] 10/7 (Glutamate)[*]	Decreased kainate and glutamate binding in left hippocampus
Toru et al. 1988	^{3}H-kainate in homogenates from multiple brain areas	14/10[**]	Increased binding in prefrontal cortex and angular gyrus; negative correlation between ^{3}H-kainate binding and glutamate levels in frontal cortex and thalamus
Kornhuber et al. 1989	^{3}H–MK-801 (PCP binding site ligand) in homogenates from multiple brain areas	10/7[*]	Increased binding in putamen
Deakin et al. 1989	^{3}H-D-aspartate (glutamate reuptake sites) and ^{3}H-kainate in homogenates from seven cortical areas	14/14[*]	Increased binding of both ligands in bilateral orbital frontal cortex; negative correlation of aspartate binding in left polar temporal cortex and dopamine concentration in left amygdala
Kerwin et al. 1990	^{3}H-glutamate (for glutamate and NMDA sites), kainate, CNQX (for quisqualate sites) in medial temporal lobe with autoradiography	8/7[*]	Decreased kainate binding in bilateral CA_4/CA_3 region, DG, PHG, and left CA_2/CA_1; decreased CNQX binding in bilateral CA_4 and left CA_3 regions
Weissman et al. 1991	^{3}H-TCP (for PCP sites) in homogenates of multiple brain regions	44/18[***]	Mild decrease in binding in occipital cortex in schizophrenic subjects and subjects who had committed suicide; no change in putamen
Simpson et al. 1992a	^{3}H-D-aspartate in homogenates of basal ganglia	19/22	Reduced binding in putamen and lateral pallidum
Simpson et al. 1992b	^{3}H-TCP binding in frontal and temporal cortex, hippocampus, and amygdala	13/14	Bilateral increase in binding in orbital frontal cortex

Note.   CA = cornu ammonis; CNQX = 6-cyano-7-nitroquinoxaline-2,3-dione; DG = dentate gyrus; PHG = parahippocampal gyrus; PCP = phencyclidine; TCP = *N*-(1-[2-thienyl]cyclohexyl)piperidine.
[*]On neuroleptics at time of death.
[**]No neuroleptics for 40 days prior to death.
[***]Includes nonpsychotic control subjects who had committed suicide.

with some features similar to that of schizophrenia. Animal studies have provided evidence for modulation of dopamine activity by serotonin (Dickinson and Curzon 1983; Korsgaard et al. 1985). Interest in the serotonin system in schizophrenia has been rekindled, because many atypical neuroleptics (e.g., clozapine, risperidone, ritanserin, setoperone) have 5-HT antagonist properties (Bleich et al. 1988).

There have been few consistently replicated abnormalities of serotonergic neurotransmission in schizophrenia, despite a considerable number of studies. Studies of brain and CSF serotonin and 5-HIAA have produced conflicting results. However, several studies have replicated a correlation between low CSF 5-HIAA and the presence of ventriculomegaly and cortical thinning in schizophrenic patients. (For a review, see Bleich et al. 1988.) Postmortem studies of serotonin receptors have focused mainly on the 5-HT$_2$ receptor subtype. In the nucleus accumbens (Mackay et al. 1978) and striatum (Owen et al. 1981), there is reportedly no difference between schizophrenic subjects and control subjects in 5-HT$_2$

receptor binding. Binding sites in frontal cortex have been reported to be decreased (Arora and Meltzer 1991; Bennett et al. 1979; Laruelle et al. 1993; Mita et al. 1986) or unchanged (Reynolds et al. 1983; Whitaker et al. 1981). Laruelle and colleagues (1993) have also reported increased binding of paroxetine to serotonin reuptake sites in prefrontal cortex.

■ Norepinephrine

The noradrenergic system in schizophrenia has been investigated less intensely than other neurotransmitter systems. The noradrenergic system is implicated in schizophrenia for several reasons. Neuroleptics may produce some therapeutic effects via adrenergic receptors (for a review, see van Kammen 1991). Elevations of plasma and CSF norepinephrine levels have been reported in a number of studies (for a review, see van Kammen and Kelley 1991). Cerebrospinal concentrations of norepinephrine and 3-methoxy-4-hydroxyphenylglycol (MHPG) have been correlated with severity of negative symptoms (Pickar et al. 1990; van Kammen et al. 1990). A few studies have found elevated levels of norepinephrine in limbic areas of postmortem schizophrenic brain tissue (Farley et al. 1978; Kleinman et al. 1982), but conflicting studies also exist (Bird et al. 1979b; Crow et al. 1979). No consistently replicated abnormality of adrenergic receptors has emerged.

■ Peptides and Other Neurochemicals

Cholecystokinin (CCK) is a 33–amino acid peptide that was originally isolated in the gastrointestinal tract. CCK is also present in high concentrations in the brain, coexists with dopamine in mesolimbic neurons, and is thought to act as a neurotransmitter or neuromodulator. Several radioimmunoassay studies have revealed decreased concentrations of CCK in temporal lobe structures of schizophrenic brain (Crow et al. 1982; Ferrier et al. 1985; Roberts et al. 1983). Two other studies did not confirm this finding (Kleinman et al. 1985; Perry et al. 1981).

Farmery and colleagues (1985) reported a 20% decrease in CCK receptor binding in frontal cortex homogenates and a 40% decrease in binding in hippocampal homogenates from postmortem schizophrenic tissue. Using quantitative autoradiography, Kerwin and colleagues (1992) have noted decreased CCK binding sites in the CA_1 region of hippocampus,

subiculum, and parahippocampal gyrus in schizophrenic patients.

Although abnormalities have been reported in acetylcholine, GABA, endogenous opiates, thyrotropin-releasing hormone, somatostatin, neurotensin, substance P, vasoactive intestinal polypeptide, synapsins, and microtubular associated proteins, none of these findings has been consistently replicated.

■ CONCLUSION

Researchers at the beginning of the twentieth century implicated dysfunction of frontal and temporal cortices in psychosis. Recent schizophrenia research has produced findings that support their hypotheses, although the nature and etiology of frontal and temporal lobe dysfunction remains unknown. Although a genetic predisposition to schizophrenia is well established, recent research findings in schizophrenia lead to the conclusion that multifactorial and, in part, environmentally derived insults to the brain probably contribute to the pathology of schizophrenia. Monozygotic twins do not have uniformly high concordance rates for schizophrenia, and the unaffected members of monozygotic twin pairs that are discordant for schizophrenia do not share with their schizophrenic twins the markers of structural brain pathology described in this chapter. In addition, there is some evidence that people with schizophrenia may have an increased incidence of obstetric complications or may have been exposed to viral infections or malnutrition during fetal life that could alter brain development.

As a result of the genetic and environmental factors that may have contributed to the development of schizophrenia, several reproducible structural and physiological abnormalities of the brain can be observed in schizophrenic patients. These include enlargement of the cerebral ventricles, dilatation of cortical sulci, reduction in the size of several anteromedial temporal lobe structures, and hypometabolism of dorsolateral prefrontal cortex during cognitive tasks. Clinical and neuropathological evidence supports the idea that these abnormalities result from a fixed "lesion" that is acquired early in life and that results in a relatively nonprogressive psychotic syndrome. A lack of gliosis in neuropathological studies supports the notion that the neuronal lesions of schizophrenia are acquired before birth.

The onset of psychotic symptoms in adolescence or early adulthood may occur when maturation of a frontotemporolimbic neural network does not occur during a critical period of development.

In light of the structural brain abnormalities observed in schizophrenia, alterations in neurotransmitter function may be regarded as secondary to neuronal loss or altered neuronal development. This hypothesis is supported by the following:

1. Findings in laboratory animals that cortical lesions can differentially effect dopamine neurotransmission in subcortical and in distant cortical areas
2. The correlation between prefrontal rCBF in schizophrenic patients performing cognitive tasks and CSF metabolites of dopamine
3. The correlation between hippocampal size and activation of prefrontal cortical blood flow in schizophrenic patients

However, the possibility exists that primary dysfunction of dopaminergic or other neurotransmitter systems may underlie the schizophrenic syndrome. Future research with better clinical and postmortem samples will be necessary before it can reliably be concluded that increased concentrations of dopamine, altered dopamine receptor function, or alterations in other neurotransmitters occur in schizophrenic patients independently of drug treatment artifacts and structural brain abnormalities.

■ REFERENCES

Altshuler L, Conrad A, Kovelman JA, et al: Hippocampal cell disorientation in schizophrenia: a controlled neurohistologic study of the Yakovlev collection. Arch Gen Psychiatry 44:1094–1098, 1987

Altshuler L, Casanova M, Goldberg T, et al: The hippocampus and parahippocampus in schizophrenic, suicide, and control brains. Arch Gen Psychiatry 47:1029–1034, 1990

Angrist BM, Sathanathan G, Gershon S: Behavioral effects of L-dopa in schizophrenic patients. Psychopharmacologia 31:1–12, 1973

Arendt T, Bigl Y, Arendt A, et al: Loss of neurons in the nucleus basalis of Meynert in Alzheimer's disease, paralysis agitans, and Korsakoff's disease. Acta Neuropathol (Berl) 61:101–108, 1983

Arnold SE, Hyman BT, Van Hoese GW, et al: Some cytoarchitectural abnormalities of the entorhinal cortex in schizophrenia. Arch Gen Psychiatry 48:625–632, 1991

Arora RC, Meltzer HY: Serotonin 2 (5-HT2) receptor binding in the frontal cortex of schizophrenic patients. J Neural Transm Gen Sect 85:19–29, 1991

Aschauer HN, Aschauer-Treiber G, Isenberg KE, et al: No evidence for linkage between chromosome 5 markers and schizophrenia. Hum Hered 40:109–115, 1990

Bachneff SA: Positron emission tomography and magnetic resonance imaging: a review and a local circuit neurons hypo(dys)function hypothesis of schizophrenia. Biol Psychiatry 30:857–886, 1991

Barta PE, Pearlson GD, Powers RE, et al: Auditory hallucinations and smaller superior temporal gyral volume in schizophrenia. Am J Psychiatry 147:1457–1462, 1990

Bassett AS, Jones B, McGullivray B, et al: Partial trisomy chromosome 5 cosegregating with schizophrenia. Lancet 1:799–801, 1988

Benes FM, Bird ED: An analysis of the arrangement of neurons in the cingulate cortex of schizophrenic patients. Arch Gen Psychiatry 44:608–616, 1987

Benes FM, Davidson J, Bird E: Quantitative cytoarchitectural studies of the cerebral cortex of schizophrenics. Arch Gen Psychiatry 43:31–35, 1986

Benes FM, Sorenson I, Bird E: Reduced neuronal size in posterior hippocampus of schizophrenic patients. Schizophr Bull 17:597–608, 1991

Bennett JP, Enna SJ, Bylund DB, et al: Neurotransmitter receptors in frontal cortex of schizophrenics. Arch Gen Psychiatry 36:927–934, 1979

Berman KF, Weinberger DR: Functional localization in the brain in schizophrenia, in American Psychiatric Association Review of Psychiatry, Vol 10. Edited by Tasman A, Goldfinger S. Washington, DC, American Psychiatric Press, 1991, pp 24–59

Berman KF, Zec RF, Weinberger DR: Physiologic dysfunction of dorsolateral prefrontal cortex in schizophrenia, II: role of neuroleptic treatment, attention, and mental effort. Arch Gen Psychiatry 43:126–135, 1986

Berman KF, Illowsky BP, Weinberger DR: Physiologic dysfunction of dorsolateral prefrontal cortex in schizophrenia, IV: further evidence for regional and behavioral specificity. Arch Gen Psychiatry 45:616–622, 1988

Berman KF, Torrey EF, Daniel DG, et al: Regional

cerebral blood flow in monozygotic twins discordant and concordant for schizophrenia. Arch Gen Psychiatry 49:927–934, 1992

Bird ED, Spokes EGS, Iversen LL: Increased dopamine concentrations in limbic areas of brain from patients dying with schizophrenia. Brain 102:347–360, 1979a

Bird ED, Spokes EG, Iversen LL: Brain norepinephrine and dopamine in schizophrenia. Science 204:93–94, 1979b

Bleich A, Brown SL, Kahn R, et al: The role of serotonin in schizophrenia. Schizophr Bull 14:297–315, 1988

Bogerts B, Hantsch J, Herzer M: A morphometric study of the dopamine-containing cell groups in the mesencephalon of normals, Parkinson patients and schizophrenics. Biol Psychiatry 18:951–969, 1983

Bogerts B, Meertz E, Schonfeldt-Bausch R: Basal ganglia and limbic system pathology in schizophrenia. Arch Gen Psychiatry 42:784–791, 1985

Bogerts B, Falkai P, Haupts M, et al: Post-mortem volume measurements of limbic system and basal ganglia structures in chronic schizophrenics. Schizophr Res 3:295–301, 1990a

Bogerts B, Ashtari M, Degreef G, et al: Reduced temporal limbic structure volume on magnetic resonance images in first episode schizophrenia. Psychiatry Res 35:1–13, 1990b

Bowers MB: Cortical dopamine turnover in schizophrenic syndromes. Arch Gen Psychiatry 31:50–54, 1974

Bowler AE, Torrey EF: Influenza and schizophrenia. Arch Gen Psychiatry 47:877, 1990

Braff DL, Geyer MA: Sensorimotor gating and schizophrenia: human and animal model studies. Arch Gen Psychiatry 47:181–188, 1990

Brown R, Colter N, Corsellis JAN, et al: Postmortem evidence of structural brain changes in schizophrenia. Arch Gen Psychiatry 43:36–42, 1986

Campion D, Leboyer M, Hilliaire D, et al: Relationship of HLA to schizophrenia not supported in multiplex families. Psychiatry Res 41:99–105, 1992

Cannon TD, Mednick SA, Parnas J: Genetic and perinatal determinants of structural brain deficits in schizophrenia. Arch Gen Psychiatry 46:883–889, 1989

Carlsson A, Lindquist M: Effect of chlorpromazine or haloperidol on formation of 3-methoxytyramine and normetanephrine in mouse brain. Acta Pharmacol Toxicol 20:140–144, 1963

Carter CJ, Pycock CJ: Behavioral and biochemical effects of dopamine and noradrenaline depletion within medial prefrontal cortex of rat. Brain Res 192:163–176, 1980

Christison GW, Casanova MF, Weinberger DR, et al: A quantitative investigation of hippocampal pyramidal cell size, shape, and variability of orientation in schizophrenia. Arch Gen Psychiatry 46:1027–1032, 1989

Cleghorn JM, Zipursky RB, List SJ: Structural and functional brain imaging in schizophrenia. J Psychiatry Neurosci 16:53–74, 1991

Colon EJ: Quantitative cytoarchitectonics of the human cerebral cortex in schizophrenic dementia. Acta Neuropathol (Berl) 20:1–10, 1972

Colter N, Battal S, Crow TJ, et al: White matter reduction in the parahippocampal gyrus of patients with schizophrenia. Arch Gen Psychiatry 44:1023, 1987

Conrad AJ, Abebe T, Austin R, et al: Hippocampal pyramidal cell disarray in schizophrenia as a bilateral phenomenon. Arch Gen Psychiatry 48:413–417, 1991

Creese I, Burt DR, Snyder SH: Dopamine receptor binding predicts clinical and pharmacological potencies of antischizophrenic drugs. Science 192:481–483, 1976

Crocq MA, Lannfelt L, Mayerova A, et al: Dopamine D3 receptor polymorphism in psychiatric patients. Paper presented at the meeting of the American College of Neuropsychopharmacology, San Juan, PR, December 1992

Cross AJ, Crow TJ, Owen F: ^{3}H-flupenthixol binding in postmortem brains of schizophrenics: evidence for a selective increase in dopamine D2 receptors. Psychopharmacology 74:122–124, 1981

Crow TJ, Baker HF, Cross AJ, et al: Monoamine mechanisms in chronic schizophrenia: postmortem neurochemical findings. Br J Psychiatry 134:249–256, 1979

Crow TJ, Ferrier IN, Johnstone EC, et al: Neuroendocrine aspects of schizophrenia, in Neuropeptides: Basic and Clinical Aspects. Edited by Fink G, Whalley LJ. Edinburgh, Scotland, Churchill-Livingstone, 1982, pp 222–239

Daniel DG, Berman KF, Weinberger DR: The effect of apomorphine on regional cerebral blood flow in schizophrenia. J Neuropsychiatry Clin Neurosci 1:377–384, 1989

Daniel DG, Weinberger DR, Jones DW, et al: The effect of amphetamine on regional cerebral blood flow during cognitive activation in schizophrenia. J Neurosci 11:1907–1917, 1991

Davis KL, Kahn RS, Ko G, et al: Dopamine in schizophrenia: a review and reconceptualization. Am J Psychiatry 148:1474–1486, 1991

Deakin J, Slater P, Simpson M, et al: Frontal cortical and left temporal glutamatergic dysfunction in schizophrenia. J Neurochem 52:1781–1786, 1989

Degreef G, Ashtari M, Bogerts B, et al: Volumes of ventricular system subdivisions measured from magnetic resonance images in first episode schizophrenic patients. Arch Gen Psychiatry 49:531–537, 1992

DeLisi L, Dauphinais ID, Gershon ES: Perinatal complications and reduced size of brain limbic structures in familial schizophrenia. Schizophr Bull 14:185–191, 1988

DeLisi L, Hoff AI, Schwartz JE, et al: Brain morphology in first-episode schizophrenic-like psychotic patients: a quantitative magnetic resonance imaging study. Biol Psychiatry 29:159–175, 1991

Detera-Wadleigh SD, Goldin L, Sherrington R, et al: Exclusion of linkage to 5q11-13 in families with schizophrenia and other psychiatric disorders. Nature 340:391–392, 1989

Dickinson SL, Curzon G: Roles of dopamine and 5-hydroxytryptamine in stereotyped and nonstereotyped behavior. Neuropharmacology 22:805–812, 1983

Dom R, DeSaedeleer J, Bogerts B, et al: Quantitative cytometric analysis of basal ganglia in catatonic schizophrenics, in Biological Psychiatry. Edited by Perris C, Struwe G, Jansson B. Amsterdam, Netherlands, Elsevier, 1981

Done DJ, Johnstone EC, Frith CD, et al: Complications of pregnancy and delivery in relation to psychosis in adult life: data from the British perinatal mortality survey sample. BMJ 302:1576–1580, 1991

Ellinwood EH: Amphetamine psychosis, I: description of the individuals and the process. J Nerv Ment Dis 144:274–283, 1967

El-Mallakh R, Kirch DG, Shelton R, et al: The nucleus basalis of Meynert, senile plaques, and intellectual impairment in schizophrenia. J Neuropsychiatry Clin Neurosci 3:383–386, 1991

Falkai P, Bogerts B, Rozumek M: Limbic pathology in schizophrenia: the entorhinal region. Biol Psychiatry 24:515–521, 1988

Farde L, Wiesel F, Hall H, et al: No D2 receptor in-

crease in PET study of schizophrenia. Arch Gen Psychiatry 44:671, 1987

Farde L, Wiesel FA, Stone-Elander S, et al: D2 dopamine receptors in neuroleptic-naive schizophrenic patients. Arch Gen Psychiatry 47:213–219, 1990

Farley IJ, Price KS, McCullogh E, et al: Norepinephrine in chronic paranoid schizophrenia: above normal levels in limbic forebrain. Science 200:456–458, 1978

Farmer A, Jackson R, McGuffin P, et al: Cerebral ventricular enlargement in chronic schizophrenia: consistencies and contradictions. Br J Psychiatry 150:324–330, 1987

Farmery SM, Owen F, Poulter M, et al: Reduced high affinity cholecystokinin binding in hippocampus and frontal cortex of schizophrenic patients. Life Sci 36:473–477, 1985

Ferrier IN, Crow TJ, Farmery SM, et al: Reduced CCK in the limbic lobe in schizophrenia: a marker for the defect state in schizophrenia. Ann N Y Acad Sci 448:495–500, 1985

Gattaz WF, Gatz D, Beckmann H: Glutamate in schizophrenics and healthy controls. Arch Psychiat Nervenkr 231:221–225, 1982

Gattaz WF, Gasser T, Beckmann H: Multidimensional analysis of the concentration of 17 substances in the CSF of schizophrenics and controls. Biol Psychiatry 20:360–366, 1985

Geraud G, Arne-Bes MC, Guell A, et al: Reversibility of hemodynamic hypofrontality in schizophrenia. J Cereb Blood Flow Metab 7:9–12, 1987

Goldberg TE, Gold JM, Braff DL: Neuropsychological functioning and time-linked information processing in schizophrenia, in American Psychiatric Press Review of Psychiatry, Vol 10. Washington, DC, American Psychiatric Press, 1991, pp 60–78

Gur RE, Mozley D, Resnick SM, et al: Magnetic resonance imaging in schizophrenia, I: volumetric analysis of brain and cerebrospinal fluid. Arch Gen Psychiatry 48:407–412, 1991

Hallmayer J, Maier W, Ackenheil M, et al: Evidence against linkage of schizophrenia to chromosome 5q11-q13 markers in systematically ascertained families. Biol Psychiatry 31:83–94, 1992a

Hallmayer J, Kennedy JL, Wetterberg L, et al: Exclusion of linkage between the serotonin 2 receptor and schizophrenia in a large Swedish kindred. Arch Gen Psychiatry 49:216–219, 1992b

Harrison PJ, McLaughlin D, Kerwin RW: Decreased hippocampal expression of a glutamate receptor gene in schizophrenia. Lancet 1:450–452, 1991

Heath RG, Franklin DE, Schraberg D, et al: Gross pathology of the cerebellum in patients diagnosed and treated as functional psychiatric disorders. J Nerv Ment Dis 167:585–592, 1979

Heaton R: Wisconsin Card Sorting Test. Odessa, TX, Psychological Assessment Resources, 1985

Hecker E: Die Hebephrenie [Hebephrenia]. Archiv für Pathologie, Anatomie, Physiologie und Klinishe Medizin 52:394, 1871

Heckers S, Heinsen H, Heinsen Y, et al: Cortex, white matter, and basal ganglia in schizophrenia: a volumetric postmortem study. Biol Psychiatry 29:556–566, 1991

Hess EJ, Brancha HS, Kleinman JE, et al: Dopamine receptor subtype imbalance in schizophrenia. Life Sci 40:1487–1497, 1987

Heston LL: Psychiatric disorders in foster home reared children of schizophrenic mothers. Br J Psychiatry 112:819–825, 1966

Honer WG, Bassett AS, MacEwan W, et al: Structural brain imaging abnormalities associated with schizophrenia and partial trisomy of chromosome 5. Psychol Med 22:519–524, 1992

Hopf A: Uber histopathologische veranderungen im pallidum und striatum bei schiophrenie. [On histological changes in the pallidum and striatum of schizophrenic patients.] Proceedings of the First International Congress on Neuropathology, Turin, Italy. Rosenberg and Sellier, 3:629–635, 1952

Hyde TM, Casanova MF, Kleinman JE, et al: Neuroanatomical and neurochemical pathology in schizophrenia, in American Psychiatric Press Review of Psychiatry, Vol 10. Edited by Tasman A, Goldfinger SM. Washington, DC, American Psychiatric Press, 1991, pp 7–23

Illowsky BP, Juliano DM, Bigelow LB, et al: Stability of CT scan findings in schizophrenia: results of an 8 year follow-up study. J Neurol Neurosurg Psychiatry 51:209–213, 1988

Ingvar DH, Franzen G: Abnormalities of cerebral blood flow distribution in patients with chronic schizophrenia. Acta Psychiatr Scand 50:425–462, 1974a

Ingvar DH, Franzen G: Distribution of cerebral activity in chronic schizophrenia. Lancet 2:1484–1486, 1974b

Iversen SD: The effect of surgical lesions to frontal cortex and substantia nigra on amphetamine responses in rats. Brain Res 31:295–311, 1971

Jakob H, Beckmann H: Prenatal developmental disturbances in the limbic allocortex in schizophrenics. J Neural Transm Gen Sect 65:303–326, 1986

Jaskiw GE, Karoum F, Weinberger DR: Persistent elevations in dopamine and its metabolites in the nucleus accumbens after mild subchronic stress in rats with ibotenic acid lesions of the medial prefrontal cortex. Brain Res 534:321–323, 1990

Jernigan TL: Anatomical and CT scan studies of psychiatric disorder, in American Handbook of Psychiatry, 2nd Edition, Vol 8: Biological Psychiatry. Edited by Berger PA, Brodie KH. New York, Basic Books, 1986, pp 213–235

Jernigan TL, Zisook S, Heaton RK, et al: Magnetic resonance imaging abnormalities in lenticular nuclei and cerebral cortex in schizophrenia. Arch Gen Psychiatry 48:881–890, 1991

Jeste DV, Lohr JB: Hippocampal pathologic findings in schizophrenia. Arch Gen Psychiatry 46:1019–1024, 1989

Johnson SW, Seutin V, North RA: Burst firing in dopamine neurons induced by N-methyl-D-aspartate: role of electrogenic sodium pump. Science 258:665–667, 1992

Kaufman CA, DeLisi L, Lehner T, et al: Physical mapping, linkage analysis of the putative schizophrenia locus on chromosome 5q. Schizophr Bull 15:441–452, 1989

Kelsoe JR, Cadet JL, Pickar D, et al: Quantitative neuroanatomy in schizophrenia. Arch Gen Psychiatry 45:533–541, 1988

Kendell RE, Kemp IW: Maternal influenza in the etiology of schizophrenia. Arch Gen Psychiatry 46:878–882, 1989

Kendler KS: Overview: a current perspective on twin studies of schizophrenia. Am J Psychiatry 140:1413–1425, 1983

Kennedy J, Giuffra L, Moises H, et al: Evidence against linkage of schizophrenia to markers on chromosome 5 in a northern Swedish pedigree. Nature 336:167–170, 1988

Kerwin RW, Patel S, Meldrum BS, et al: Asymmetrical loss of glutamate receptor subtype in left hippocampus in schizophrenia. Lancet 1:583–584, 1988

Kerwin R, Patel S, Meldrum B: Quantitative autoradiographic analysis of glutamate binding sites in the hippocampal formation in normal and schizophrenic brain post mortem. Neuroscience 39:25–32, 1990

Kerwin R, Robinson P, Stephenson J: Distribution of

CCK binding sites in the human hippocampal formation and their alteration in schizophrenia: a post-mortem autoradiographic study. Psychol Med 22:37–43, 1992

Kim JS, Kornhuber HH, Schmid-Burgk W, et al: Low cerebrospinal fluid glutamate in schizophrenic patients and a new hypothesis on schizophrenia. Neurosci Lett 20:379–382, 1980

King DJ, Wilson A, Cooper SJ, et al: The clinical correlates of neurologic soft signs in chronic schizophrenia. Br J Psychiatry 158:770–775, 1991

Kinney DK, Yurgelun-Todd DA, Woods BT: Hard neurologic signs and psychopathology in relatives of schizophrenic patients. Psychiatry Res 39:45–53, 1991

Kirch DG, Weinberger DR: Anatomical neuropathology in schizophrenia: post-mortem findings, in Handbook of Schizophrenia. Edited by Nasrallah HA, Weinberger DR. Amsterdam, Elsevier, 1986, pp 325–348

Kleinman JE, Karoum F, Rosenblatt JE, et al: Post-mortem neurochemical studies in chronic schizophrenia, in Biological Markers in Psychiatry and Neurology. Edited by Usdin E, Hanin I. New York, Pergamon, 1982

Kleinman JE, Hong J, Iadarola, M et al: Neuropeptides in human brain-postmortem studies. Prog Neuropsychopharmacol Biol Psychiatry 9:91–95, 1985

Kornhuber J, Mack-Burkhardt F, Riedere P, et al: ^{3}H-MK801 binding sites in postmortem brain regions of schizophrenic patients. J Neural Transm Gen Sect 77:231–236, 1989

Korsgaard S, Gerlach J, Christensson E: Behavioral aspects of serotonin-dopamine interaction in the monkey. Eur J Pharmacol 118:245–252, 1985

Kovelman JA, Scheibel AB: A neurohistological correlate of schizophrenia. Biol Psychiatry 19:1601–1621, 1984

Laruelle M, Toti R, Abi-Dargham A, et al: Selective abnormalities of prefrontal serotonergic markers in schizophrenia: a post-mortem study. Arch Gen Psychiatry 50:810–818, 1993

Lesch A, Bogerts B: The diencephalon in schizophrenia: evidence of reduced thickness of the periventricular gray matter. European Archives of Psychiatry and Neurological Sciences 234:212–219, 1984

Lewis SW, Murray RM: Obstetrical complications, neurodevelopmental deviance and risk of schizophrenia. J Psychiatr Res 21:413–422, 1987

Lindstrom LH: Low HVA and normal 5HIAA CSF levels in drug free schizophrenic patients compared to healthy volunteers: correlations to symptomatology and family history. Psychiatry Res 14:265–273, 1985

Lipska BK, Jaskiw GE, Chrapusta S, et al: Ibotenic acid lesions of ventral hippocampus differentially effect dopamine and its metabolites in the nucleus accumbens and prefrontal cortex in rat. Brain Res 585:1–6, 1992

Lohr JB, Jeste DV: Cerebellar pathology in schizophrenia, a neuronometric study. Biol Psychiatry 21:865–875, 1986

Macciardi F, Kennedy JL, Ruocco L, et al: A genetic linkage study of schizophrenia to chromosome 5 markers in a northern Italian population. Biol Psychiatry 31:720–728, 1992

Mackay AVP, Doble A, Bird ED, et al: ^{3}H-Spiperone binding in normal and schizophrenic post-mortem human brain. Life Sci 23:527–532, 1978

Martinot JL, Peron-Magna P, Huret JD, et al: Striatal D2 dopaminergic receptors assessed with positron emission tomography and 76-Br bromospiperone in untreated schizophrenic patients. Am J Psychiatry 147:44–50, 1990

Mathysse S: Role of dopamine in selective attention. Adv Biochem Psychopharmacol 16:667–669, 1977

McCreadie RG, Hall DJ, Berry IJ, et al: The Nithsdale schizophrenia surveys, X: obstetric complications, family history and abnormal movements. Br J Psychiatry 161:799–805, 1992

McGue M: When assessing twin concordance use the probandwise not the pairwise rate. Schizophr Bull 18:171–176, 1992

McGuffin P, Sargeant M, Hetti G, et al: Exclusion of schizophrenia susceptibility gene from chromosome 5q11-q13 region: new data and reanalysis of previous reports. Am J Hum Gen 47:524–535, 1990

Mednick SA, Machon RA, Huttunen MO, et al: Adult schizophrenia following prenatal exposure to an influenza epidemic. Arch Gen Psychiatry 45:189–192, 1988

Merriam AE, Kay SR, Opler LA, et al: Neurologic signs and the positive-negative dimension in schizophrenia. Biol Psychiatry 28:181–192, 1990

Mita T, Hanada S, Nishimo N, et al: Decreased serotonin S2 and increased dopamine D2 receptors in chronic schizophrenics. Biol Psychiatry 21:1407–1414, 1986

Moises HW, Gelernter J, Giuffra LA, et al: No linkage between D2 dopamine receptor gene region and schizophrenia. Arch Gen Psychiatry 48:643–647, 1991

Nasrallah HA, Charles GT, McCalley-Whitters M, et al: Cerebral ventricular enlargement in subtypes of chronic schizophrenia. Arch Gen Psychiatry 39: 774–777, 1982

Nimgaonkar VL, Wessely S, Murray RM: Prevalence of familiality, obstetric complications, and structural brain damage in schizophrenic patients. Br J Psychiatry 153:191–197, 1988

Nyback H, Wiesel FA, Berggren BM: Computed tomography of the brain in patients with acute psychosis and in healthy volunteers. Acta Psychiatr Scand 65:403–414, 1982

O'Callaghan E, Larkin C, Kinsella A, et al: Obstetric complications, the putative familial-sporadic distinction, and tardive dyskinesia in schizophrenia. Br J Psychiatry 157:578–584, 1990

O'Callaghan E, Sham P, Takei N, et al: Schizophrenia after prenatal exposure to 1957 A2 influenza epidemic. Lancet 2:1248–1250, 1991

Onstad S, Skre I, Torgersen S, et al: Birthweight and obstetric complications in schizophrenic twins. Acta Psychiatr Scand 85:70–73, 1992

Overall JE, Gorham DR: The Brief Psychiatric Rating Scale. Psychol Rep 10:799–812, 1962

Owen F, Cross AJ, Crow TJ, et al: Neurotransmitter receptors in brain in schizophrenia. Acta Psychiatr Scand 63:20–28, 1981

Owen MJ, McGuffin P: DNA and classical genetic markers in schizophrenia. Eur Arch Psychiatry Clin Neurosci 240:197–203, 1991

Owen MJ, Lewis SW, Murray RM: Obstetric complications and cerebral abnormalities in schizophrenia. Psychol Med 15:27–41, 1988

Pakkenberg B: Post-mortem study of chronic schizophrenic brains. Br J Psychiatry 151:744–752, 1987

Pakkenberg B: Pronounced reduction of total neuron number in mediodorsal thalamic nucleus and nucleus accumbens in schizophrenics. Arch Gen Psychiatry 47:1023–1028, 1990

Perry RH, Dockray GJ, Dimaline R, et al: Neuropeptides in Alzheimer's disease, depression and schizophrenia. J Neurol Sci 51:465–472, 1981

Perry TL: Normal cerebrospinal fluid and brain glutamate levels in schizophrenia do not support the hypothesis of glutamatergic neuronal dysfunction. Neurosci Lett 28:81–85, 1982

Pfefferbaum A, Zipursky RB: Neuroimaging studies of schizophrenia. Schizophr Res 4:193–208, 1991

Pfefferbaum A, Zipursky RB, Lim KO, et al: Computed tomographic evidence for generalized sulcal and ventricular enlargement in schizophrenia. Arch Gen Psychiatry 45:633–640, 1988

Pickar D, Breier A, Hsiao J, et al: Cerebrospinal fluid and plasma monoamine metabolites and their relation to psychosis. Arch Gen Psychiatry 47:641–648, 1990

Potter WZ, Hsiao JK, Goldman SM: Effects of renal clearance on plasma concentrations of homovanillic acid: methodologic cautions. Arch Gen Psychiatry 46:558–562, 1989

Pycock CJ, Kerwin RW, Carter CJ: Effect of lesions of cortical dopamine terminals on subcortical dopamine in rats. Nature 286:74–77, 1980a

Pycock CJ, Kerwin RW, Carter CJ: Effect of 6-hydroxydopamine lesions of medial prefrontal cortex in rat. J Neurochem 34:91–99, 1980b

Raven JC: Advanced Progressive Matrices, Sets I and II. London, HK Lewis, 1965

Reddy R, Mukherjee S, Schnur DB, et al: History of obstetric complications, family history, and CT scan findings in schizophrenic patients. Schizophr Res 3:311–314, 1990

Reveley AM, Reveley MA, Clifford CA, et al: Cerebral ventricular size in twins discordant for schizophrenia. Lancet 2:540–541, 1982

Reynolds GP: Increased concentration and lateral asymmetry of amygdala dopamine in schizophrenia. Nature 305:527–529, 1983

Reynolds GP, Rossor MN, Iversen LL: Preliminary studies of human cortical 5-HT2 receptors and their involvement in schizophrenia and neuroleptic drug action. J Neural Transm Suppl 18:273–277, 1983

Roberts GW, Ferrier IN, Lee Y, et al: Peptides, the limbic lobe and schizophrenia. Brain Res 288:199–211, 1983

Roberts GW, Colter N, Lofthouse R, et al: Gliosis in schizophrenia. Biol Psychiatry 21:1043–1050, 1986

Rosenthal D, Wender PH, Kety SS, et al: Parent-child relationships and psychopathological disorder in the child. Arch Gen Psychiatry 32:466–476, 1975

Rossi A, De Cataldo S, Di Michele V, et al: Neurologic soft signs in schizophrenia. Br J Psychiatry 157:735–739, 1990

Rossi A, Stratta P, Di Michele V, et al: Temporal lobe structure by magnetic resonance in bipolar affective disorders and schizophrenia. J Affect Disord 21:19–22, 1991

Rubin P, Holm S, Friberg L, et al: Altered modulation of prefrontal and subcortical brain activity in newly diagnosed schizophrenia and schizophreniform disorder. Arch Gen Psychiatry 48:987–995, 1991

Scatton B, Worms P, Lloyd KG, et al: Cortical modulation of striatal function. Brain Res 232:331–343, 1982

Schroder J, Niethammer R, Geider FJ, et al: Neurologic soft signs in schizophrenia. Schizophr Res 6:25–30, 1992

Schulz SC: Genetics of schizophrenia: a status report, in American Psychiatric Press Review of Psychiatry, Vol 10. Edited by Tasman A, Goldfinger SM. Washington, DC, American Psychiatric Press, 1991, pp 79–97

Schulz SC, Koller MM, Kishore PR, et al: Ventricular enlargement in teenage patients with schizophrenia spectrum disorders. Am J Psychiatry 140:1592–1595, 1983

Seeman P, Lee T, Chau-Wong M, et al: Antipsychotic drug doses and neuroleptic/dopamine receptors. Nature 261:717–719, 1976

Seeman P, Bzowej NH, Guan HC, et al: Human brain D1 and D2 dopamine receptors in schizophrenia, Alzheimer's, Parkinson's and Huntington's diseases. Neuropsychopharmacology 1:5–15, 1987

Seeman P, Niznik H, Guan H, et al: Link between D1 and D2 dopamine receptors is reduced in schizophrenia and Huntington diseased brain. Proc Natl Acad Sci U S A 86:10156–10160, 1989

Shelton RC, Weinberger DR: X-ray computerized tomography studies in schizophrenia: a review and synthesis, in Handbook of Schizophrenia, Vol I: The Neurology of Schizophrenia. Edited by Nasrallah HA, Weinberger DR. Amsterdam, Elsevier, 1986, pp 207–250

Shenton ME, Kikinis R, Jolesz FA, et al: Abnormalities of the left temporal lobe and thought disorder in schizophrenia: a quantitative magnetic resonance imaging study. N Engl J Med 327:604–612, 1992

Sherman AD, Davidson AT, Baruah S, et al: Evidence of glutamatergic deficiency in schizophrenia. Neurosci Lett 121:77–80, 1991a

Sherman AD, Hegwood TS, Baruah S, et al: Deficient NMDA-mediated glutamate release from synaptosomes of schizophrenics. Biol Psychiatry 30:1191–1198, 1991b

Sherrington R, Brynjolfsson J, Peturson H, et al : Localization of a susceptibility locus for schizophrenia on chromosome 5. Nature 336:164–167, 1988

Simpson M, Slater P, Royston M, et al: Regionally selective deficits in uptake sites for glutamate and gamma-aminobutyric acid in the basal ganglia in schizophrenia. Psychiatry Res 42:273–282, 1992a

Simpson M, Slater P, Royston M, et al: Alterations in phencyclidine and sigma binding sites in schizophrenic brains. Schizophr Res 6:41–48, 1992b

Sokoloff P, Giros B, Martres M, et al: Molecular cloning and characterization of a novel dopamine receptor (D3) as a target for neuroleptics. Nature 347:146–151, 1990

Sponheim SR, Iacono WG, Beiser M: Stability of ventricular size after the onset of psychosis in schizophrenia. Psychiatry Res 40:21–29, 1991

St. Clair D, Blackwood D, Muir W, et al: No linkage of chromosome 5q11-13 markers to schizophrenia in Scottish families. Nature 339:305–307, 1989

Suddath R, Casanova MF, Goldberg TE, et al: Temporal lobe pathology in schizophrenia: a quantitative magnetic resonance imaging study. Am J Psychiatry 146:464–472, 1989

Suddath R, Christison GW, Torrey EF, et al: Anatomical abnormalities in the brains of monozygotic twins discordant for schizophrenia. N Engl J Med 322:787–794, 1990

Sunahara RK, Guan HC, O'Dowd BF, et al: Cloning of the gene for a human D5 receptor with higher affinity for dopamine than D1. Nature 350:614–619, 1991

Susser ES, Lin SP: Schizophrenia after prenatal exposure to the Dutch Hunger Winter of 1944–1945. Arch Gen Psychiatry 49:983–988, 1992

Swayze VW, Andreasen NC, Alliger RJ, et al: Subcortical and temporal structures in affective disorder and schizophrenia: a magnetic resonance imaging study. Biol Psychiatry 31:21–24, 1992

Torrey EF: Are we overestimating the genetic contribution to schizophrenia? Schizophr Bull 18:159–169, 1992

Toru M, Watanabe S, Shibuya H, et al: Neurotransmitters, receptors and neuropeptides in post-mortem brains of chronic schizophrenic patients. Acta Psychiatr Scand 78:121–137, 1988

Tsuang MT, Gilbertson MW, Faraone SV: The genetics of schizophrenia: current knowledge and future directions. Schizophr Res 4:157–171, 1991

van Kammen D: The biochemical basis of relapse and

drug response in schizophrenia: review and hypothesis. Psychol Med 21:881–895, 1991

van Kammen D, Kelley M: Dopamine and norepinephrine activity in schizophrenia. Schizophr Res 4:173–191, 1991

van Kammen D, Peters J, Yao J, et al: Norepinephrine in acute exacerbations of chronic schizophrenia. Arch Gen Psychiatry 47:161–168, 1990

Van Tol H, Bungow JR, Guan HC, et al: Cloning of the gene for a human dopamine D4 receptor with high affinity for the antipsychotic clozapine. Nature 350:610–614, 1991

Vogt C, Vogt O: Alterations anatomiques de la schizophrenie et d'autres psychoses dites functionelles. [Anatomic alterations of schizophrenia and of other psychoses termed functional.] Proceedings of the First International Congress of Neuropathology. Turin, Italy, Rosenberg and Sellier, 1:515–532, 1952

Weinberger DR: Implications of normal brain development for the pathogenesis of schizophrenia. Arch Gen Psychiatry 44:660–669, 1987

Weinberger DR, Torrey EF, Neophytides AN, et al: Structural abnormalities in the cerebral cortex of chronic schizophrenic patients. Arch Gen Psychiatry 36:935–939, 1979a

Weinberger DR, Kleinman JE, Luchins DJ, et al: Cerebellar atrophy in chronic schizophrenia. Lancet 1:718–719, 1979b

Weinberger DR, Kleinman JE, Luchins DJ, et al: Cerebellar atrophy in schizophrenia: a controlled postmortem study. Am J Psychiatry 137:359–361, 1980

Weinberger DR, DeLisi L, Perman GP, et al: Computed tomography in schizophreniform disorder and other acute psychiatric disorders. Arch Gen Psychiatry 39:778–793, 1982

Weinberger DR, Berman KF, Zec RF: Physiologic dysfunction of dorsolateral prefrontal cortex in schizophrenia, I: regional cerebral blood flow evidence. Arch Gen Psychiatry 43:114–124, 1986

Weinberger DR, Berman KF, Illowsky BP: Physiologic dysfunction of dorsolateral prefrontal cortex in schizophrenia, III: a new cohort and evidence for a monoaminergic mechanism. Arch Gen Psychiatry 45:609–615, 1988

Weinberger DR, Berman KF, Suddath R, et al: Evidence of dysfunction of a prefrontal-limbic network in schizophrenia: a magnetic resonance imaging and regional cerebral blood flow study of discordant monozygotic twins. Am J Psychiatry 149:890–897, 1992

Weissman AD, Casanova MF, Kleinman JE, et al: Selective loss of cerebral cortical sigma but not PCP binding sites in schizophrenia. Biol Psychiatry 29:41–54, 1991

Wender PH, Rosenthal D, Rainer JD, et al: Schizophrenics' adopting parents: psychiatric status. Arch Gen Psychiatry 34:777–784, 1977

Whitaker PM, Crow TJ, Ferrier IN: Tritiated LSD binding in frontal cortex in schizophrenia. Arch Gen Psychiatry 38:278–280, 1981

Widerlov E: A critical appraisal of CSF monoamine metabolite studies in schizophrenia. Ann N Y Acad Sci 537:309–323, 1988

Williams AO, Reveley MA, Kolakowska T, et al: Schizophrenia with good and poor outcome, II: cerebral ventricular size and its clinical significance. Br J Psychiatry 146:239–246, 1985

Woods BT, Kinney DK, Yurgelun-Todd DA: Neurologic "hard" signs and family history of psychosis in schizophrenia. Biol Psychiatry 30:806–816, 1991

Wong DF, Wagner HN, Tune LE, et al: Positron emission tomography reveals elevated D2 dopamine receptors in drug naive schizophrenics. Science 244:1558–1563, 1986

Yakovlev PI, Hamlin H, Sweet WH: Frontal lobotomy neuroanatomical observations. J Neuropathol Exp Neurol 9:250–285, 1950

Young AH, Blackwood DHR, Roxborough H, et al: A magnetic resonance imaging study of schizophrenia: brain structure and clinical symptoms. Br J Psychiatry 158:158–164, 1991

Zipursky RB, Lim KO, Sullivan EV, et al: Widespread cerebral gray matter volume deficits in schizophrenia. Arch Gen Psychiatry 49:195–205, 1992

Zukin SR, Javitt DC: The brain NMDA receptor, psychotomimetic drug effects, and schizophrenia, in American Psychiatric Press Review of Psychiatry, Vol 10. Edited by Tasman A, Goldfinger SM. Washington, DC, American Psychiatric Press, 1991, pp 480–498

Biology of Anxiety Disorders

Murray B. Stein, M.D., and Thomas W. Uhde, M.D.

The 1980s saw a marked surge of interest in anxiety disorders, as evidenced by an explosion of publications in this area. In 1979–1980, 3.0% of the research articles published in the *Archives of General Psychiatry* and the *American Journal of Psychiatry* (psychiatry's two journals with the highest impact factor by Science Citation Indices) were devoted to anxiety and stress-related disorders. By 1989–1990, research articles on anxiety and stress-related disorders accounted for 16.1% of the publications in these two journals (Pincus et al. 1993). This dramatic increase in research has provided us with a wealth of information about biological aspects of the anxiety disorders. In this chapter, we review current neurobiological knowledge of these disorders.

It will be apparent that there is great disparity in the amount of neurobiological research that has been conducted in the various DSM-III-R (American Psychiatric Association 1987) anxiety disorders. Panic disorder (PD) has been the most thoroughly investigated anxiety disorder; accordingly, the largest portion of this chapter is devoted to it. Obsessive-compulsive disorder (OCD) and posttraumatic stress disorder (PTSD) vie for second place in terms of the amount of neurobiological research conducted thus far, with the phobic disorders and generalized anxiety disorder (GAD) coming in a distant third. With the exception of social phobia (SP), the neurobiology of the phobic disorders and GAD are not discussed in this chapter. Interested readers are referred elsewhere for reviews of the biology of simple phobias, GAD, and blood-illness-injury phobias (Hoehn-Saric and McLeod 1993; Marks 1988; Nemiah and Uhde 1989; Uhde and Nemiah 1989).

We have not attempted to provide a comprehensive review of the biology of each anxiety disorder. Such a task is clearly beyond the scope of a single chapter; in fact, an entire book was devoted to the neurobiology of one anxiety disorder (e.g., Ballenger 1990). In addition to limiting our review to a small number of anxiety disorders, we also opted to address mainly those findings with the strongest empirical (and replicable) data bases. We also have drawn attention to a small number of preliminary findings that represent promising avenues of investigation on the neurobiology of anxiety and anxiety disorders.

■ NEUROBIOLOGY OF PD AND AGORAPHOBIA

Until the early 1960s, PD was subsumed under the rubric of different syndromes such as "soldier's heart," "neurocirculatory asthenia," and "cardiac neurosis" (Uhde and Nemiah 1989) and was relegated to backseat status as a minor psychiatric disorder. PD is now known to be a common illness (6-month prevalence is more than 1%; Weissman 1988) with often devastating socioeconomic consequences (e.g., job loss, financial dependence, excessive health care utilization; Markowitz et al. 1989) and psychiatric concerns (e.g., depression, suicide attempts; Weissman et al. 1989). PD is frequently complicated by agoraphobia; therefore, for the purposes of this chapter, panic and agoraphobia are considered as a single diagnostic entity.

Theories regarding the nature and etiology of PD range from the biological to the psychological (Barlow

1988; Reiss 1988; Uhde and Nemiah 1989). Among the anxiety disorders, PD has been the most extensively studied from a biological perspective. However, these research efforts have failed to consistently identify the presence of specific neuroendocrine or other neurobiological correlates of anxiety or panic attacks in patients with PD. Rather than present data within the framework of a single "theory" of PD, in this section we provide an update on current knowledge regarding the familial transmission of PD and present an overview of different hypotheses regarding the pathophysiology of PD, keeping in mind that the PD "syndrome" probably represents a heterogeneous group of different neuropathological diatheses.

■ Heritability of PD

Twin studies in PD uniformly demonstrate a higher concordance rate for monozygotic than dizygotic twins (Torgersen 1990), thereby suggesting (but not proving) a genetic basis for PD. An early study suggested a possible linkage of PD with the α-haptoglobin locus on chromosome 16q22 (Crowe et al. 1987). However, this was not replicated by the same research team with the later addition of more pedigrees (Crowe et al. 1990). More recent investigations (Wang et al. 1992) have used a candidate gene approach in 14 multiplex pedigrees, and found solid evidence *against* linkage between PD and five adrenergic receptor genes. Thus, although a genetic basis

for PD in at least some families is now strongly suspected, linkage to any particular gene has yet to be established.

■ Neurochemical Hypotheses for the Pathophysiology of PD

Early theorists such as Da Costa (1871), impressed by the prominent cardiac symptoms that occur during panic attacks, coined the term *irritable heart syndrome* (for review, see Uhde and Nemiah 1989). An abundance of theories to explain the pathophysiology of PD have since been advanced (Table 24–1), several of which are reviewed here.

Lactate Hypothesis

The lactate hypothesis arose from the clinical observation that chronically anxious patients had decreased exercise tolerance, and it was thus postulated that these subjects had an abnormality in lactate metabolism (Pitts and McClure 1967). It has been consistently demonstrated in subsequent studies that the intravenous (iv) administration of sodium lactate to patients with PD elicits panic attacks in 50%–70% of these individuals but in less than 10% of healthy control subjects (Liebowitz et al. 1984; Pohl et al. 1988). Even though changes in acid-base status (Gorman et al. 1989a, 1990), serum-ionized calcium or phosphate (Fyer et al. 1984; Gorman et al. 1986), intravascular volume, and cerebral blood flow (CBF; Mathew et al. 1989; Reiman et al. 1989) have each been postulated as the mechanism for lactate-induced panic, the avail-

Table 24–1. Neurochemical theories proposed for panic disorder

Substance or system(s) implicated	Suggested reading
Adenosine	Apfeldorf and Shear 1993; Boulenger et al. 1984; Stein et al. 1993a; Uhde 1990
Cholecystokinin	Bradwejn et al. 1990, 1991, 1992; de Montigny 1989; Lydiard et al. 1992
GABA-benzodiazepine	File et al. 1982; Nutt et al. 1990; Roy-Byrne et al. 1990; Zorumski and Isenberg 1991
Isoproterenol	Pohl et al. 1988, 1990
Lactate	Coplan et al. 1992b; Fyer et al. 1984; Gaffney et al. 1988; Gorman et al. 1986, 1988b, 1989a, 1990; Liebowitz et al. 1985; Pitts and McClure 1967
Norepinephrine	Abelson et al. 1992; Cameron et al. 1984, 1990; Charney and Heninger 1986a; Charney et al. 1984, 1987a, 1989; Nesse et al. 1984; Nutt 1989; Rapaport et al. 1989b; Redmond 1979; Schittecatte et al. 1988, 1992; Tancer et al. 1993a; Uhde et al. 1989
Respiratory/CO_2	Gorman et al. 1988a; Gorman et al. 1989b; Gorman and Papp 1990; Griez et al. 1990a, 1990b; Hibbert 1984; Klein 1993; Mathew et al. 1989; Papp et al. 1993; Salkovskis et al. 1986; Woods and Charney 1990
Serotonin	Charney and Heninger 1986b; Charney et al. 1987b; Coplan et al. 1992a; Kahn et al. 1988a, 1988b; Klein et al. 1991; Lesch et al. 1992; Targum and Marshall 1989

able data would suggest that none of these is necessary to its panicogenic properties. In fact, a study (Coplan et al. 1992b) that failed to find alterations in cisternal lactate or carbon dioxide (CO_2) levels following intravenous administration of sodium lactate to nonhuman primates raises serious questions about a direct central nervous system (CNS) effect of lactate. It is possible, however, that lactate may induce secondary changes in acid-base metabolism that affect CNS function.

In contrast, it has been recognized that sodium lactate is a potent respiratory stimulant. The degree to which hyperventilation ensues following lactate administration appears to be a major determinant of who does and does not experience a panic attack following lactate infusion (Gorman et al. 1988b, 1989a). These findings suggest that the mechanism by which lactate induces panic is through its effects on respiratory drive, and they provide a strong rationale for the detailed scrutiny of respiratory function in PD. In fact, the idea that panic attacks may be somehow linked to abnormalities in respiration is among the most compelling theories presently being tested.

Respiratory Hypotheses

A prominent hypothesis, with several variants thereof, proposes that panic attacks are a result of (or at least associated with) abnormalities in respiratory function. Almost all patients with PD complain of shortness of breath or of having trouble breathing during their attacks. As a result, it has been suggested that panic attacks are nothing more than the conglomeration of symptoms that are the direct consequence of chronic hyperventilation (Hibbert 1984), and that respiratory retraining (e.g., conscious modulation of respiratory rate) may be therapeutic (Salkovskis et al. 1986). In fact, voluntary hyperventilation of room air has been shown to reproduce the attacks in 30%–50% of patients with PD (Gorman et al. 1988a; Rapee 1986), suggesting that decrements in carbon dioxide partial pressure (pCO_2) may be important in the pathophysiology of panic in at least a subgroup of individuals.

In apparent contradiction to the findings from hyperventilation studies, the inhalation of CO_2-enriched (5%, 7.5%, or 35%) air—which *raises* pCO_2—provokes panic attacks in an even greater proportion (50%–80%) of patients with PD (Gorman and Papp 1990; Griez et al. 1990a, 1990b; Papp et al.

1993). These findings are consistent with the hypothesis that PD is associated with increased sensitivity in central medullary CO_2 receptors in PD (Gorman et al. 1988a). It is of interest that Mathew and colleagues (1989) found that intravenously administered acetazolamide, an inhibitor of carbonic anhydrase, an agent that putatively causes significant hypercarbia and acidosis, did *not* experience panic attacks at a rate exceeding that of placebo. However, acetazolamide administered to control subjects increases minute volumes and can induce a fall in pCO_2. Gorman and colleagues (1993) also failed to find that acetazolamide stimulates ventilation. Taken together, the observations of Mathew and colleagues, combined with those of the Columbia research team, do not necessarily refute a hypersensitive CO_2 chemoreceptor model of PD.

Several lines of evidence point to a role for respiratory abnormalities in patients with PD, including the possibility that alterations in pCO_2 sensitivity may be an important panicogenic pathway for many patients. Many (if not all) of the stimuli that induce panic (Table 24–1) share an ability to stimulate respiration and/or induce a sense of breathlessness. Klein (1993) has proposed that patients with PD have an abnormally low threshold for sensing impending suffocation, and that panic attacks result from the triggering of a "false suffocation alarm." This hypothesis, appealing because it is rooted in clinical phenomenology and uniquely integrative in nature, will undoubtedly be the subject of considerable scrutiny and much debate in the years to come.

Noradrenergic Hypothesis

Noradrenergic dysfunction in PD has been contemplated by several groups of investigators (Charney and Heninger 1986a; Charney et al. 1984; Nutt 1989; Uhde 1987). One of the major stimuli behind these studies was the work of Redmond and colleagues (Redmond 1979), who demonstrated a relationship between activity of the major noradrenergic site in the brain, the locus ceruleus, and anxiety-like behaviors in primates. Subsequently, researchers have used a variety of experimental techniques in an attempt to demonstrate the presence and importance of noradrenergic dysfunction in PD.

Several groups have used pharmacological probes of the noradrenergic system in this regard. Some but not all research teams showed that patients with PD were behaviorally and cardiovascularly hyperreactive to the anxiogenic effects of orally administered yohimbine (an α_2 antagonist; Charney et al. 1984, 1987a; Uhde et al. 1984a; Gurguis and Uhde 1990), indicating that these patients might have α_2-adrenergic receptor supersensitivity. Some investigators (Charney and Heninger 1986a; Nutt 1989) also found blunted cardiovascular responses to the α_2 agonist clonidine, although this has not always been replicated (Uhde et al. 1989). This finding would actually be suggestive of α_2-adrenergic receptor subsensitivity, rather than supersensitivity as suggested by the yohimbine studies. Charney and Heninger (1986a) proposed the use of the term *dysregulation* to describe this curious state of supersensitivity to an antagonist but subsensitivity to an agonist putatively acting at the same receptor site(s).

To complement the pharmacological challenge studies, investigators turned to the use of presumptive peripheral markers of noradrenergic function. Cameron and colleagues (1984, 1990) have detected reduced density of platelet α_2-adrenergic receptor binding sites, in keeping with the noradrenergic dysregulation hypothesis. Charney and colleagues (1989) failed to find differences in α_2 receptor density between patients with PD and control subjects. However, they did detect reduced basal and stimulated adenylate cyclase levels that could be considered evidence in favor of a postreceptor abnormality, perhaps at the level of the G protein (Manji 1992), in patients with PD. This intriguing finding currently needs replication.

Subnormal or "blunted" growth hormone (GH) responses to clonidine administration have been consistently reported in patients with PD (Abelson et al. 1992; Charney and Heninger 1986a; Nutt 1989; Rapaport et al. 1989a; Tancer et al. 1993a; Uhde et al. 1985, 1986, 1992), with few exceptions (Schittecatte et al. 1988, 1992). The "blunted" GH response to clonidine has usually been attributed to postsynaptic α_2-adrenergic downregulation, and it has accordingly been considered supportive of the noradrenergic hypothesis of panic. However, it must be recognized that the regulation of GH release is complex and includes stimulatory and/or inhibitory inputs from the noradrenergic, cholinergic, dopaminergic, γ-aminobutyric acid (GABA)ergic, and serotonergic systems. Furthermore, GH secretion is directly stimulated by the growth-hormone–releasing factor (GRF) and inhibited both by somatostatin-release inhibiting factor (SRIF) and, via an ultrashort feedback loop, by

GH itself. Thus, we are now faced with the paradox that although a diminished GH response to clonidine is clearly among the best-replicated biological findings in PD, the pathophysiological significance of these findings (particularly with regard to noradrenergic dysfunction) has yet to be fully elucidated (for review, see Uhde et al. 1992).

■ Serotonergic Dysfunction in PD

Serotonin (5-HT) has been alluded to as "a neurotransmitter for all seasons" (van Kammen 1987, p. 1), in reference to the increasing propensity for psychiatric investigators to uncover serotonergic dysfunction in nearly all neuropsychiatric disorders (e.g., depression, schizophrenia, OCD, alcoholism). A more recent addition to the 5-HT rogues' gallery, not surprisingly, is PD (see Coplan et al. 1992a). Although less extensively investigated than the noradrenergic hypothesis in panic and not yet as well replicated as in OCD, a number of studies have provided intriguing indicators that patients with PD may experience an alteration in 5-HT function.

Although failing to find behavioral or neuroendocrine evidence of altered 5-HT function in patients with PD using the indirect 5-HT agonist tryptophan (Charney and Heninger 1986b), Charney and colleagues (1987b) *did* observe that intravenous administration of the direct postsynaptic (primarily) 5-HT receptor agonist m-chlorophenylpiperazine (m-CPP; 0.1 mg/kg) provoked panic attacks not only in 12 of 23 patients with PD, but also in an equal proportion of healthy subjects. Using a lower dose of m-CPP (0.25 mg/kg), Kahn and colleagues (1988a, 1988b) were able to demonstrate exaggerated behavioral (i.e., higher rates of panic induction in patients with PD versus control subjects) and neuroendocrine (i.e., enhanced cortisol release) responsivity to this pharmacological probe, which they interpreted as indicating postsynaptic 5-HT receptor supersensitivity. More recently, Klein and colleagues (1991) also noted m-CPP to be a potent panicogen, and Targum and Marshall (1989) obtained similar findings with the presynaptic 5-HT releaser (i.e., indirect agonist) fenfluramine. Taken together and in the context of the proven efficacy of the selective serotonin reuptake inhibitors (SSRIs) in PD (Chapter 31), these findings strongly suggest that further attention to the 5-HT system (including the use of 5-HT subtype probes; e.g., Lesch et al. 1992) is likely to lead to significant advances in our understanding of the pathophysiology of PD.

■ Adenosinergic Dysfunction

As shown in controlled studies and reviewed by Uhde (1990), patients with PD are known to be hypersensitive to the anxiogenic effects of caffeine (Boulenger et al. 1984). Caffeine's behavioral (including anxiogenic) effects, like those of other methylxanthines, are thought to be attributable to its properties as an antagonist at the receptor level of one of the brain's major neuromodulators, adenosine (Fredholm and Persson 1982). Accordingly, it has been hypothesized that patients with PD might exhibit dysfunction at the level of the adenosine receptor.

Caffeine's ability to enhance taste sensitivity is believed to be due to its antagonist actions at peripheral adenosine receptors within gustatory pathways (Schiffman et al. 1985). Two independent studies found that caffeine lowers the taste threshold for quinine detection to a greater degree in patients with PD than in control subjects (Apfeldorf and Shear 1993; DeMet et al. 1989), thereby lending some credence to an adenosinergic dysfunction model of PD. Accordingly, it was predicted that chronic treatment with an indirect adenosine agonist (dipyridamole) would result in the amelioration of panic symptoms, but this drug has since been proven ineffective in the treatment of PD (Stein et al. 1993a). When subtype-specific (e.g., A1, A2) drugs with good CNS penetrability become available for use in humans, it will be of interest to examine the drugs' efficacy in the treatment of PD.

■ Other Neurobiological Models

As can be seen, there is no shortage of neurobiological models for PD. One might argue that the plethora of models reflects the fact that none of these has been especially satisfactory. Although it is not our intent to burden the reader with an exhaustive list, we would be remiss not to at least draw attention to three additional chemical models that have gained some well-deserved notoriety.

Isoproterenol. The intravenous infusion of the β-adrenergic agonist isoproterenol provokes panic attacks in susceptible individuals at approximately the same rate as sodium lactate (Pohl et al. 1988, 1990). However, when we consider that β-blockers are generally regarded as inefficacious in the treatment of PD, a β-supersensitivity model of PD would appear difficult to support.

Benzodiazepine receptor sensitivity. The unequivocal role for benzodiazepines in the treatment of PD (see Chapter 31), along with the rich preclinical literature on the importance of the GABA-benzodiazepine receptor complex in the mediation of anxiety (File et al. 1982; Zorumski and Isenberg 1991), makes this system a prime candidate for involvement in the pathogenesis of PD. Two groups have independently observed altered benzodiazepine receptor sensitivity in PD (Nutt et al. 1990; Roy-Byrne et al. 1990), as assessed by reduced sensitivity to the benzodiazepine-induced disruption of saccadic eye movements, making this an area of ongoing interest.

Cholecystokinin tetrapeptide. The panicogenic effects of cholecystokinin tetrapeptide (CCK$_4$) (Bradwejn et al. 1990, 1991, 1992; de Montigny 1989) represent an exciting addition to the cadre of known panicogenic agents. Given the intriguing finding that cerebrospinal fluid (CSF) CCK concentrations were lower in 25 patients with PD than in 16 healthy comparison subjects (Lydiard et al. 1992), perhaps reflecting increased CNS CCK-receptor sensitivity in PD, it would appear that investigations of this and related neuropeptides may provide valuable information regarding the neurobiology of panic attacks.

■ Autonomic Dysfunction in PD

PD has been widely hypothesized to be associated with dysfunction of the autonomic nervous system. This is a genuinely attractive hypothesis, given that panic attacks are characterized by the reporting of tachycardia, palpitations, sweating, and trembling, symptoms strongly suggestive of autonomic activation. Although the subjective experience of autonomic-like symptoms in PD is incontestable, objective evidence of autonomic hyperreactivity in PD has been difficult to document in controlled studies.

Ambulatory studies of patients with PD (Woods and Charney 1990) have revealed that panic attacks are not necessarily associated with autonomic activation (i.e., tachycardia or tachypnea). In several well-controlled laboratory studies (Roth et al. 1992; Stein and Asmundson 1994), investigators have been unable to demonstrate autonomic dysfunction in patients with PD. Most researchers would now agree that the resting tachycardia observed in some studies of patients with PD, put forth as evidence in support of autonomic hyperreactivity in these individuals, is an artifact of the experimental situation and is probably attributable to anticipatory anxiety (Hoehn-Saric and McLeod 1993; Roth et al. 1992). Furthermore, some investigators (Asmundson and Stein 1994; Gaffney et al. 1988) have argued that when augmented physiological reactivity *has* been detected in patients with PD, this may simply reflect the poorer cardiovascular fitness of these individuals (J. M. Stein et al. 1992), many of whom restrict their activity because of their agoraphobia and/or their fear of the physical symptoms associated with exertion (Reiss 1988).

Several investigators have argued that although sympathetic hyperfunction has not been convincingly demonstrated in PD, perhaps the autonomic defect is that of vagal hypofunction (George et al. 1989; Yeragani et al. 1990). Here again, the effects of cardiovascular fitness on vagal tone (Goldsmith et al. 1992) must be considered. We recently completed a study of 24 patients with PD and 26 healthy control subjects (with similar habitual levels of aerobic exercise) in which vagal tone was examined across several dynamic tests (e.g., postural change, cold pressor, breathhold, Valsalva maneuver; Stein and Asmundson 1994). We did not find evidence of abnormal vagal tone in the patients with PD in comparison to the control subjects, thereby failing to confirm this hypothesis. At this juncture, then, it is reasonable to conclude that although autonomic activation is a feature of some (but clearly not all) panic attacks, autonomic dysfunction per se is unlikely to play a causative role in the etiopathology of PD.

■ Neuroendocrine Function in PD

Hypothalamic-Pituitary-Adrenal Axis

Although dysfunction within various elements of the hypothalamic-pituitary-adrenal (HPA) axis is a well-established component of the pathophysiology of the affective disorders (Nemeroff 1991; also see Chapter 22), this is not the case for PD. Several studies have observed high rates of dexamethasone nonsuppression or elevated urinary free cortisol (UFC) in patients

with PD, but these have usually been in the context of PD complicated by depression (or, in some studies, severe agoraphobia; reviewed in Stein and Uhde 1990). Adrenocorticotropic hormone (ACTH) responses to corticotropin-releasing hormone (CRH) administration, although abnormally low in depressed patients, are probably normal in nondepressed patients with PD (Rapaport et al. 1989a). Consistent with this finding, Jolkkonen and colleagues (1993) detected normal CSF levels of CRH in their patients with PD.

Hypothalamic-Pituitary-Thyroid Axis

The recognition of abnormal thyroid functioning in some patients with depression led to the investigation of the hypothalamic-pituitary-thyroid (HPT) axis in patients with PD. With few exceptions, a convincing majority of studies has found normal peripheral thyroid hormone levels, normal thyroid hormone end organ responsivity, normal thyroid autoimmune status, and normal thyrotropin (TSH) responses to protirelin (thyrotropin-releasing hormone [TRH]; Stein and Uhde 1993).

■ Sleep in PD

In contrast with the extensive literature on sleep in patients who have affective illness, there have been only a few controlled studies of the sleep of patients with PD (for review, see Uhde 1994). At this juncture, most polysomnographic studies concur that patients with PD have remarkably normal sleep architecture (Mellman and Uhde 1989a; Hauri et al. 1989; Stein et al. 1993b; Uhde 1994); in particular, the absence of shortened rapid eye movement (REM) latency (as seen in depression) is notable. Despite the paucity of sleep architectural abnormalities, it remains to be established whether or not patients with PD exhibit a disturbance in their ability to sustain sleep (Koenigsberg et al. 1992). Such an abnormality, if present, could help explain the occurrence of sleep panic attacks (Mellman and Uhde 1989b). These attacks, which seem to arise preferentially out of the transition between Stages 2 and 3 sleep (Mellman and Uhde 1989a; Uhde 1994), at a time when dreaming is absent and cognitions are at a minimum, provide a compelling argument for the biological (as opposed to psychological) nature of at least some panic attacks. Several groups of investigators are currently attempting to further characterize the pathophysiology of sleep panic in the hope that this will provide clues to the biological basis for waking panic as well.

■ Positron-Emission Tomography Studies in PD

Reiman and colleagues (1984) generated considerable excitement with their positron-emission tomography (PET) finding of abnormal asymmetry of CBF (i.e., left less than right) in lactate-vulnerable patients with PD. This abnormality was seen at rest (or as "at rest" as someone can be with his or her head in a PET scanner) in the nonpanic state. Nordahl and colleagues (1990), using a different PET technique (^{18}F-deoxyglucose) found hippocampal region metabolic asymmetry (also left less than right).

Subsequently, the St. Louis group (Reiman et al. 1989) identified several brain regions—most notably the temporopolar cortex bilaterally, where blood flow increased during a lactate-induced anxiety attack. Unfortunately, this marked increase in temporopolar blood flow was later discovered to be artifactual, actually reflecting increased blood flow to extracranial muscles that occurred during teeth clenching (Drevets et al. 1992). Therefore, though this latter finding has not held up, the finding of hippocampal asymmetric blood flow (and metabolism) seems, for the time being, to be a genuine observation that supports involvement of the limbic lobe in the genesis of panic (Gorman et al. 1989b).

■ Summary of the Biology of PD

The discovery that lactate infusions resulted in panic attacks in susceptible individuals (Pitts and McClure 1967) ushered in a whole era of investigations into the biology of PD. Instead of merely knowing that lactate can induce panic, we now know that a host of other substances (e.g., caffeine, isoproterenol, yohimbine, carbon dioxide, m-CPP, CCK_4, and others (for review, see Uhde et al. 1990) may also do so, although there are exceptions such as TRH and hypoglycemia (Stein and Uhde 1991; Uhde et al. 1984b). Some critics have argued that perhaps there is nothing "biological" at all about the response to this array of panicogens. Rather, each of these substances induces a constellation of physical symptoms that are interpreted by the individual in a way that leads to the experience of panic (Margraf et al. 1986).

Shear and colleagues (1991) have shown that when patients with PD are treated with an effective nonpharmacological modality, cognitive-behavioral therapy (Barlow 1988), they are less vulnerable to lactate-induced panic. These observations provide a powerful impetus for the development of research paradigms that can remove (or at least minimize) the effects of expectancy and cognitions and thus enable us to study the neurobiology of PD in its purest form. Sleep studies (particularly the study of sleep panic attacks) promise to provide us with information concerning autonomic and neurochemical mechanisms that may be involved in the pathophysiology of truly spontaneous panic attacks. Finally, as suggested by Klein (1993), a closer look at the respiratory attributes of various panicogens may illuminate a set of properties requisite for the elicitation of panic.

■ BIOLOGY OF SOCIAL PHOBIA

SP is a disorder marked by the intense fear and/or avoidance of situations in which the individual feels that he or she will be scrutinized by others. In its extreme form, known as the generalized subtype of SP (Gelernter et al. 1992; Heimberg et al. 1993), SP might be considered an extreme form of shyness or even a personality disorder (e.g., avoidant). In its more circumscribed form, known as the discrete or specific subtype of SP, fear and avoidance are limited to one (or perhaps several) phobic situations, most commonly public speaking (Gelernter et al. 1992; Heimberg et al. 1993). It is reasonable to expect that the two subtypes of SP, generalized and discrete, will eventually be shown to be very different from a biological perspective. However, at this juncture, most but not all studies (and these will be highlighted) of the neurobiology of SP have tended to lump these two groups together. This represents a major deficit in the existing literature that we can hope will be addressed by the next generation of studies.

■ Sympathetic Nervous System Function in SP

When placed in social phobic situations (or even in anticipation of such exposure), patients with SP complain of tachycardia, tremor, and blushing—symptoms highly suggestive of adrenergic overactivity. In fact, in some patients, these symptoms are amenable to treatment with β-blockers such as propranolol or atenolol (Liebowitz et al. 1985). These observations have led investigators to test the hypothesis that the sympathetic nervous system (SNS), particularly the β-adrenergic receptor system, might be overactive in patients with SP.

Papp and colleagues (1988) infused intravenous epinephrine (2 µg/kg) into 11 patients with SP. Although eight of the patients noted some anxiety symptoms, none reported that the infusion reproduced the symptoms they experienced in social phobic situations. Possible explanations for this finding include the poor CNS penetrability of intravenous epinephrine, as well as the experimental context that lacked a "performance" or other scrutiny component.

Two groups (Heimberg et al. 1990; Levin et al. 1993) measured cardiovascular responses to a public speaking challenge in patients with SP. Levin and colleagues (1993) failed to find differences in cardiovascular reactivity between patients and control subjects, although (like Heimberg et al. 1990) they noted that the generalized social phobic subjects exhibited *less* cardiovascular activation than the discrete (public speaking) social phobic subjects. These two studies underscore the importance of considering the possibility that these two subgroups may be distinct from a biological perspective.

Peripheral noradrenergic responsivity was recently assessed in 15 patients with SP using a "naturalistic" challenge of the autonomic nervous system, the response to postural (or "orthostatic") change (Stein et al. 1992, 1994). Compared with 20 healthy control subjects, the patients with SP had normal heart rate and blood pressure responses to the postural challenge. In contrast, patients with SP have an exaggerated blood pressure response to the pressor effects of intravenously administered TRH (Tancer et al. 1990b). Most recently, Stein and colleagues (1993c) measured β-adrenoceptor density and affinity on lymphocytes from patients with generalized SP, and found these individuals to be no different from healthy control subjects. At the present time, then, the status of autonomic nervous system functioning in SP remains unresolved.

■ Neuroendocrine Function in SP

Compared with our understanding of neuroendocrine functioning in the depressive disorders or in PD, there is less information about the neuroendocrinology of SP. The team from the National Institute of Mental Health (NIMH; Tancer et al. 1990a) reported normal peripheral thyroid indices and normal thyrotropin responses to TRH in the only study of the HPT axis in SP published so far. Two studies have examined HPA axis function in SP. Uhde and colleagues (1994) reported similar rates of cortisol nonsuppression to dexamethasone in 64 patients with SP (9%) and 30 control subjects (7%). These investigators also observed normal 24-hour UFC levels in the patients with SP, a finding also noted by Potts and colleagues (1991). These observations suggest that HPT and HPA axis functioning are likely to be normal in patients with SP; but again, the generalized versus discrete subtype differences have yet to be examined. Furthermore, more detailed examination of HPA axis functioning using techniques such as corticotropin-releasing factor stimulation, is clearly warranted.

■ Monoaminergic Function in SP

We are aware of only one study that has assessed any aspect of monoaminergic functioning in patients with SP. In this study, Tancer and colleagues (1993b) administered the α_2-agonist clonidine (2 µg/kg iv) to 16 patients with SP and 31 healthy control subjects. They found that the patients with SP displayed a "blunted" (albeit weak) GH response to intravenous clonidine, thereby providing the first putative evidence of noradrenergic dysregulation in this disorder. However, recent findings with oral clonidine failed to find a blunted GH response to clonidine in social phobic patients (M. E. Tancer, M. B. Stein, T. W. Uhde, unpublished data, 1994). As a result, it currently appears that when this neuroendocrine abnormality does occur in patients with SP, it tends to be modest in degree and less consistent than the blunted GH responses found in patients with PD.

■ Summary of the Biology of SP

The neurobiology of SP remains obscure (for review, see Uhde et al. 1991). Given the findings that some patients with SP respond to treatment with monoamine oxidase inhibitors (MAOIs) or SSRIs, the next logical step in this phase of research will be to employ pharmacological probes to examine specific aspects of monoaminergic function (e.g., serotonergic, dopaminergic) in SP. Such studies are currently under way in several laboratories and promise to elucidate the pathophysiology of SP.

■ BIOLOGY OF PTSD

PTSD, the only psychiatric disorder whose definition demands that a particular stressor precede its appearance (Davidson and Foa 1993), serves as the case in point for the myriad ways in which severe, unexpected, and uncontrollable stress may produce a neurobiological disturbance. It has only been in the past decade, and primarily in the past 5 years, that the biology of PTSD has come under scrutiny. Furthermore, although it is understood that PTSD can occur following a variety of different traumatic events (e.g., sexual abuse, criminal victimization, burn injury), the literature on the biology of PTSD in its present state refers almost exclusively to combat-related PTSD. Consequently, our discussion will be limited to that sphere of observation.

■ Psychophysiology of PTSD

A number of studies have documented elevated blood pressure and/or heart rate in combat veterans with PTSD both when they are at rest and when they are exposed to reminders of war (e.g., combat scenes in movies, visualization of combat imagery) (Orr 1990; Pitman et al. 1987, 1990). In addition, several investigators have noted that patients with combat-related PTSD exhibit an exaggerated startle response to loud noises (Butler et al. 1990; Shalev et al. 1992). Orr and Pitman (1993), in an attempt to determine whether the physiological abnormalities characteristic of PTSD could be "faked" (an all too common attribution by those who refuse to believe that PTSD exists), conducted a fascinating study in which they instructed combat veterans without PTSD to attempt to respond as if they *did* have PTSD (e.g., "Try to get yourself worked up"). Most of the veterans were unable to simulate the physiological response patterns of patients with PTSD (Orr and Pitman 1993). Taken together, these observations tentatively confirm that patients with PTSD are autonomically hyperreactive and that this constitutes a core feature of the disorder.

■ Adrenergic Dysfunction in PTSD

In contrast with the robust signs of autonomic hyperfunction arising out of the psychophysiological studies, biochemical evidence for sympathetic hyperfunction has been less clear-cut. Although Kosten and colleagues (1987) found elevated 24-hour

urinary norepinephrine (NE) and epinephrine (E) levels in their patients with PTSD, Pitman and Orr (1990) were unable to replicate this finding. Similarly, McFall and colleagues (1992) found normal resting plasma E and NE levels in patients with PTSD, the latter finding also noted by Blanchard and colleagues (1991). On the other hand, when plasma E or NE responses to stress rather than resting levels are examined, these have so far invariably been reported to be elevated (Blanchard et al. 1991; McFall et al. 1990). Alpha$_2$-adrenergic receptor density on platelets of patients with PTSD has been reported to be reduced, as has coupling between the α_2 receptor and the postreceptor effector systems (Lerer et al. 1987, 1990; Perry et al. 1990), all of which may be secondary to the effects of exposure to elevated catecholamine levels. On the whole, the available data support a role for intermittent (i.e., phasic, but probably not tonic) SNS hyperfunction in the pathophysiology of PTSD.

■ Sleep in PTSD

It should come as no great surprise that patients with PTSD sleep poorly, considering that hyperarousal is a key feature of the disorder. In fact, disrupted sleep is so prominent in patients with PTSD that one author has referred to sleep disturbance as the "hallmark" of PTSD (Ross et al. 1989). Unfortunately, polysomnographic studies in PTSD have been so few and far between (see Ross et al. 1989 and Uhde 1994 for reviews) that it is difficult to draw any definitive conclusions regarding the objectively evaluated sleep of patients with PTSD. In fact, some findings have been entirely unexpected. For example, Dagan and colleagues (1991) recorded increased arousal thresholds from delta sleep in 19 war veterans with PTSD.

Ross and colleagues (1989) have implicated REM dysregulation as a critical factor in the development of both daytime (i.e., flashbacks) and nighttime (i.e., posttraumatic anxiety dreams) symptomatology in PTSD. Given the evidence for adrenergic dysfunction in PTSD (see previous discussion) and in another REM disorder, narcolepsy, it is indeed compelling to want to implicate REM dysfunction in the pathophysiology of PTSD. Although this hypothesis is appealing, data to support it are, unfortunately, lacking. In fact, Mellman and colleagues (1991) reported two cases where symptoms of PTSD and narcolepsy diverged over time. Nonetheless, future studies that attend carefully to the co-occurrence of PTSD and other REM-related disorders such as narcolepsy will undoubtedly cast further light on this potentially important relationship.

■ HPA Axis Functioning in PTSD

There now exists compelling evidence that veterans with combat-related PTSD may have an abnormality in the functioning of their HPA axis (Yehuda et al. 1991a). The evolution and consequences of this hypothetical derangement can be summarized as follows:

A short-term effect of the acute traumatic stressor is believed to be hypercortisolism, the immediate result of which may be hippocampal damage (Sapolsky 1992). Preliminary results from a magnetic resonance imaging (MRI) volumetric study of 22 Vietnam veterans with combat-related PTSD found a 12% reduction in hippocampal volume as compared with 20 healthy control subjects (Bremner et al. 1992). This hippocampal damage may then be manifested in neuropsychological symptoms such as memory deficits, which may eventually be shown to play a role in PTSD.

The longer-term effects of repetitive acute or chronic stress may be somewhat different, however. In this scenario, chronic CRH release (which may occur in PTSD; Smith et al. 1989) may result in an increase in glucocorticoid receptor density (or sensitivity) at the level of the pituitary (Sapolsky 1992). The consequences of such an alteration in glucocorticoid receptors at the pituitary level would be exaggerated or supersensitive negative feedback of ACTH (and, accordingly, cortisol secretion). In fact, there is mounting evidence that this is precisely the state of the HPA axis in patients with combat-related PTSD. These patients have been demonstrated to have increased density of (probably Type II) glucocorticoid receptors on lymphocytes (Yehuda et al. 1991b). As would be predicted from this abnormality, these patients have also been shown to have low levels of 24-hour urinary cortisol excretion (Yehuda et al. 1990) and to exhibit exaggerated suppression of plasma cortisol following dexamethasone administration (Yehuda et al. 1993).

■ Summary of the Biology of PTSD

In contrast with PD, where psychophysiological studies have failed to identify a clear-cut autonomic ab-

normality, studies in PTSD paint a much more lucid portrait of a disorder characterized by phasic sympathetic hyperarousal. Also, in contrast with PD, a role for HPA axis dysfunction in PTSD seems to be emerging. In interpreting these findings, we must be cognizant of several caveats. First, many of the findings (e.g., sympathetic hyperarousal) may be due to depression, which is frequently experienced by patients with PTSD. These findings therefore require replication in nondepressed subjects. Second, most of the patients who have been studied so far have either a current or fairly recent history of substance abuse, and this may account for the findings (e.g., Bremner et al. 1992). It remains to be established whether these findings can be replicated when substance abuse is controlled for. Finally, as we mentioned earlier, the current literature on the biology of PTSD is essentially confined to combat veterans. It will be interesting to learn how these findings will compare with those for PTSD in other populations (e.g., sexual abuse survivors, hurricane victims), which should be the wave of research in the coming decade.

■ BIOLOGY OF OCD

OCD is an excellent example of how new developments in treatment have helped advance the understanding of the pathophysiology of an illness. (It is also probably the only known example of how research in humans has led to an effective treatment for a disease in dogs; Rapoport et al. 1992.) When it became clear that OCD was selectively responsive to antidepressant drugs that potently blocked serotonin reuptake (see Chapter 8), it raised the obvious question "Is there a central serotonergic abnormality in OCD?" The vast majority of research into the neurobiology of OCD has been conducted with this question in mind. The association between OCD and various neurological disorders has also been a focus of study for several research teams.

■ Heritability of OCD

The literature on the heritability of OCD has been reviewed by Black and colleagues (1992). They point out that twin and family studies have failed to demonstrate a specific familial component to OCD, although there is some support for a nonspecific increased risk for anxiety disorders in general among family members of OCD probands. They conclude that although a genetic diathesis for OCD may be present in some individuals, nongenetic factors must also be important. Some authorities speculate that genetic factors may account for more of the variance in the expression of early onset OCD (Bellodi et al. 1992). Interestingly, OCD and Tourette's disorder, which share clinical features in many patients (Green and Pitman 1990), may also be genetically related (Pauls et al. 1991), but this remains to be confirmed.

■ Serotonergic Dysfunction in OCD

Recent neurobiological evidence indicates that central 5-HT dysregulation is a feature of OCD. Several techniques have been used to document the presence of a 5-HT abnormality in OCD. These include the measurement of peripheral markers of (optimistically) central 5-HT function, the measurement of 5-HT breakdown products in the CSF, and (most recently) the administration of 5-HT chemical probes.

■ Peripheral 5-HT Markers in OCD

Serotonin levels in the blood of patients with OCD are, not surprisingly, normal (Flament et al. 1987). Platelet serotonin uptake and binding to platelets of [^{3}H]imipramine have also been examined as putative indices of central 5-HT activity. Studies performed in OCD are summarized in Table 24–2. These studies indicate that affinity for the 5-HT reuptake site is normal in OCD, but leave unanswered the question of whether or not there is a reduced density of 5-HT-reuptake sites in OCD. Given the questionable relationship between platelet and CNS 5-HT-reuptake sites (Moret and Briley 1991), the meaning of these findings is far from clear.

■ CSF Studies in OCD

The 5-HT metabolite 5-hydroxyindoleacetic acid (5-HIAA) has been measured in the CSF of patients with OCD as a potential indicator of central 5-HT turnover. Insel and colleagues (1985) reported a significant increase (30% above control subjects) in CSF 5-HIAA in a small group of patients with OCD ($N = 8$), but this is at odds with an earlier study by Thoren and colleagues (1980) and a more recent report (Lydiard et al. 1990) in which no such differences were found.

Although not a measure of central 5-HT function, it is intriguing that elevated CSF levels of arginine vasopressin (AVP) (Altemus et al. 1992) and somatostatin (Altemus et al. 1993) have been reported in patients with OCD. Although the functional significance of these findings is as yet unknown, these observations serve as the basis for some interesting hypotheses about the role of altered attention and memory in OCD (Altemus et al. 1992).

■ Neuropharmacological Probes of 5-HT Systems in OCD

Zohar and colleagues (1987) were the first to demonstrate that obsessive-compulsive symptoms (OCS) could be transiently exacerbated in some patients with OCD by the oral administration of the 5-HT agonist m-CPP, and that this effect could be blocked by chronic pretreatment with the effective antiobsessional agent clomipramine (Zohar et al. 1988). Since then, the OCS-exacerbating effects of oral m-CPP have been replicated in some studies (Hollander et al. 1988, 1992), but not all (Pigott et al. 1993). To further complicate the issue, intravenous m-CPP appears *not* to possess this property (Charney et al. 1988), although this has also recently been con-

Table 24–2. Studies of [^{3}H]imipramine binding (B_{max} and K_d) and serotonin uptake (V_{max}) in patients with obsessive-compulsive disorder

Study	Control subjects (*n*)	Patients (*n*)	B_{max}	K_d	V_{max}
Insel et al. 1985	12	12	Normal	Normal	Normal
Weizman et al. 1986	18	18	Decreased	Normal	—
Black et al. 1990	22	22	Normal	Normal	—
Bastani et al. 1991	32	20	Decreased	Normal	Normal
Kim et al. 1991	23	24	Normal	Normal	—
Vitiello et al. 1991	16	16	Normal	Normal	Increased
Weizman et al. 1992	9	9	Decreased	Normal	—
Marazziti et al. 1992	17	17	Decreased	Normal	—

tradicted (Pigott et al. 1993). Although these discrepancies may eventually be determined to result from subtle differences between the various protocols used in each study or from heterogeneity within the OCD diagnostic syndrome, other neurotransmitter systems may actually be involved. Even though a putative serotonin agonist (i.e., m-CPP) is being used, and its effects have been reliably blocked with the use of the $5\text{-HT}_1/5\text{-HT}_2$ antagonist metergoline (Pigott et al. 1991), this is no guarantee that serotonergic activation is only the first step in a neurobiological cascade that ultimately results in the generation of OCS. In this regard, several investigators have noted that a role for dopamine must be seriously considered (Goodman et al. 1990; Lemus et al. 1991; McDougle et al. 1990).

■ Neuroimaging and the Neuroanatomy of OCD

Neuroanatomical Considerations

Several different brain lesions in humans have been associated with the appearance of obsessive-compulsive behaviors or outright OCD. Von Economo's encephalitis in the early 1930s was associated with the occurrence of OCD in a number of cases. Swedo and associates (1989a) noted a high prevalence of OCS in patients with Sydenham's chorea as compared to patients with other poststreptococcal illnesses, leading the authors to propose that dysfunction in the striatum may occur in OCD. This hypothesis is greatly strengthened by the finding that OCD shares many clinical characteristics with Tourette's disorder, a disorder strongly believed to involve striatal dysfunction (Shapiro et al. 1988; Green and Pitman 1990). OCD has also been observed in Huntington's disease (Cummings and Cunningham 1992). Taken together, these observations have led to speculation that Tourette's disorder (and other chronic motor tic disorders) and OCD may be etiologically related. In fact, several authorities have proposed that Tourette's disorder and OCD might both be disorders of the striatum, with the precise area of damage within the striatum and the size of the lesion determining clinical symptomatology (Baxter 1990; Goodman et al. 1990; Wise and Rapoport 1989).

This hypothesis could accommodate many of the theories that have preceded it. For example, serotonergic neurotransmission makes up an important component of striatothalamocortical communication (and probably maintains a tonic inhibitory influence on dopamine function in these circuits), raising the possibility that the SSRIs may ameliorate OCS through modulatory effects in these brain regions (Baxter 1990). This theory could also explain the ameliorative effects of psychosurgical interventions that selectively severe fiber bundles interconnecting the orbitofrontal cortex and the dorsomedial and related thalamic nuclei (Modell et al. 1989). In the past few years, direct neuroimaging techniques have become available that have permitted the preliminary testing of some of these theoretical notions.

■ Brain Imaging in OCD

Luxenberg and colleagues (1988) conducted a computed tomography (CT) study in OCD. They found that 10 male patients with childhood-onset OCD had bilaterally reduced caudate volume compared with that of 10 male healthy control subjects. Two MRI studies of OCD have subsequently been published and show mixed results. In the first study (Garber et al. 1989), differences in caudate volume were not detected, but prolonged T_1 relaxation time, possibly indicative of an abnormality in the composition of the tissue, was observed in the frontal white matter as compared to control subjects. In the second study (Kellner et al. 1991), the investigators failed to detect differences between 12 patients with OCD and 12 healthy control subjects on measures of caudate head volume, cingulate thickness, or callosal area.

Techniques such as CT and MRI are only able to assess brain structure, not function. An examination of the literature on other neuropsychiatric disorders such as Parkinson's disease or Huntington's disease reveals that neuroradiologically determinable changes in structure do not occur (or occur only very late in the illness), even though functional indices of regional brain dysfunction are apparent. By analogy, we should not be surprised that the CT and MRI studies have failed to convincingly demonstrate a specific CNS lesion in OCD.

Several investigators have used PET scans to assess brain function in patients with OCD. Three groups—one at UCLA and two at NIMH—have used the ^{18}F-fluorodeoxyglucose (^{18}FDG) method to compare regional cerebral metabolic rates for glucose (CMRg). Baxter and colleagues (1987, 1988) found bilaterally increased CMRg in the caudate of patients with OCD compared with that of healthy control subjects. This group also found increased CMRg in the left orbital region in OCD patients, an effect that was determined to be independent of the presence of major depression in the patients. Nordahl and colleagues (1989) and Swedo and colleagues (1989b) also found increased CMRg in the orbitofrontal region, thereby partially replicating the findings of the Baxter group at UCLA. It is also interesting that both groups noted a tendency toward normalization (i.e., reduction) of orbitofrontal CMRg in OCD patients treated with clomipramine (Benkelfat et al. 1990; Swedo et al. 1992). Baxter and colleagues (1992) also recently reported a reduction in right-sided caudate metabolism in conjunction with response to either fluoxetine or behavior therapy.

■ Summary of the Biology of OCD

In summary, functional brain imaging studies in OCD (including single photon emission computed tomography [SPECT] studies [Machlin et al. 1991; Rubin et al. 1992] that have not been reviewed here) are strongly suggestive of an abnormality in basal ganglia (particularly caudate) and/or orbitofrontal cortical function, which may "normalize" during treatment. Nevertheless, these studies have been hampered by such exceedingly small sample sizes that the cynics among us have a right to wonder whether they will continue to be replicated. Furthermore, as Insel (1992) reminds us in a recent critique of this line of research, we remain remarkably uninformed about how the brain is functioning when patients are actually experiencing OCS, because all studies conducted to date have measured CMRg in the resting state or during a neutral cognitive task. The next phase of neuroimaging research in OCD will certainly need to address this inadequacy, possibly by combining functional neuroimaging techniques with behavioral or pharmacological activation procedures.

■ REFERENCES

Abelson JL, Glitz D, Cameron OG, et al: Endocrine, cardiovascular, and behavioral responses to clonidine in patients with panic disorder. Biol Psychiatry 32:18–25, 1992

Altemus M, Pigott T, Kalogeras KT, et al: Abnormalities in the regulation of vasopressin and corticotropin releasing factor secretion in obsessive-compulsive disorder. Arch Gen Psychiatry 49:9–20, 1992

Altemus M, Pigott T, L'Heureux F, et al: CSF somatostatin in obsessive-compulsive disorder. Am J Psychiatry 150:460–464, 1993

American Psychiatric Association: Diagnostic and Statistical Manual of Mental Disorders, 3rd Edition, Revised. Washington, DC, American Psychiatric Association, 1987

Apfeldorf WJ, Shear MK: Caffeine potentiation of taste in panic disorder. Biol Psychiatry 33:217–219, 1993

Asmundson GJG, Stein MB: Resting cardiovascular measures in patients with panic disorder and social phobia and healthy control subjects: relationship to habitual exercise frequency. Anxiety 1:26–30, 1994

Ballenger JC (ed): Neurobiology of Panic Disorder. New York, Alan R Liss, 1990

Barlow DH: Anxiety and Its Disorders: The Nature and Treatment of Anxiety and Panic. New York, Guilford, 1988

Bastani B, Arora RC, Meltzer HY: Serotonin uptake and imipramine binding in the blood platelets of obsessive-compulsive disorder patients. Biol Psychiatry 30:131–139, 1991

Baxter LR: Brain imaging as a tool in establishing a theory of brain pathology in obsessive compulsive disorder. J Clin Psychiatry 51 (suppl):22–25, 1990

Baxter LR Jr, Phelps ME, Mazziota JC, et al: Local cerebral glucose metabolic rates in obsessive-compulsive disorder: a comparison with rates in unipolar depression and in normal controls. Arch Gen Psychiatry 44:211–218, 1987

Baxter LR, Schwartz JM, Mazziotta JC, et al: Cerebral glucose metabolic rates in non-depressed patients with obsessive-compulsive disorder. Am J Psychiatry 145:1560–1563, 1988

Baxter LR, Schwartz JM, Bergman KS, et al: Caudate glucose metabolic rate changes with both drug and behavior therapy for obsessive-compulsive disorder. Arch Gen Psychiatry 49:681–689, 1992

Bellodi L, Sciuto G, Diaferia G, et al: Psychiatric disorders in the families of patients with obsessive-compulsive disorder. Psychiatry Res 42:111–120, 1992

Benkelfat C, Nordahl TE, Semple WE, et al: Local cerebral glucose metabolic rates in obsessive-compulsive disorder: patients treated with clomipramine. Arch Gen Psychiatry 47:840–848, 1990

Black DW, Kelly M, Myers C, et al: Tritiated imipramine binding in obsessive-compulsive volunteers and psychiatrically normal controls. Biol Psychiatry 27:319–327, 1990

Black DW, Noyes R Jr, Goldstein RB, et al: A family study of obsessive-compulsive disorder. Arch Gen Psychiatry 49:362–368, 1992

Blanchard EB, Kolb LC, Prins A, et al: Changes in plasma norepinephrine to combat-related stimuli among Vietnam veterans with posttraumatic stress disorder. J Nerv Ment Dis 179:371–373, 1991

Boulenger JP, Uhde TW, Wolff EA, et al: Increased sensitivity to caffeine in patients with panic disorders: preliminary evidence. Arch Gen Psychiatry 41:1067–1071, 1984

Bradwejn J, Koszycki D, Meterissian G: Cholecystokinin-tetrapeptide induces panic attacks in patients with panic disorder. Can J Psychiatry 35:83–85, 1990

Bradwejn J, Koszycki D, Meterissian G: Enhanced sensitivity to cholecystokinin-tetrapeptide in panic disorder: clinical and behavioral findings. Arch Gen Psychiatry 48:603–610, 1991

Bradwejn J, Koszycki D, Payeur R, et al: Replication of action of cholecystokinin tetrapeptide in panic disorder: clinical and behavioral findings. Am J Psychiatry 149:962–964, 1992

Bremner JD, Scott TM, Seibyl JP, et al: Neurochemical and neuroanatomical correlates of learning and memory in posttraumatic stress disorder. Paper presented at the 31st annual meeting of the American College of Neuropsychopharmacology, San Juan, PR, December 1992

Butler RW, Braff DL, Rausch J, et al: Physiological evidence of exaggerated startle response in a subgroup of Vietnam veterans with combat-related posttraumatic stress disorder. Am J Psychiatry 147:1308–1312, 1990

Cameron OG, Smith CB, Hollingsworth PJ, et al: Platelet α_2-adrenergic receptor binding and plasma catecholamines: before and during imipramine treatment in patients with panic anxiety. Arch Gen Psychiatry 41:1144–1148, 1984

Cameron OG, Smith CB, Lee MA, et al: Adrenergic function in anxiety disorders: platelet α_2-adrenergic receptor binding, blood pressure, pulse, and plasma catecholamines in panic and generalized anxiety disorder patients and normal subjects. Biol Psychiatry 28:3–20, 1990

Charney DS, Heninger GR: Abnormal regulation of noradrenergic function in panic disorders: effects of clonidine in healthy subjects and patients with agoraphobia and panic disorder. Arch Gen Psychiatry 43:1042–1054, 1986a

Charney DS, Heninger GR: Serotonin function in panic disorders: the effect of intravenous tryptophan in healthy subjects and patients with panic disorder before and during alprazolam treatment. Arch Gen Psychiatry 43:1059–1065, 1986b

Charney DS, Heninger GR, Breier A: Noradrenergic function in panic anxiety: effects of yohimbine in healthy subjects and patients with agoraphobia and panic disorder. Arch Gen Psychiatry 41:751–763, 1984

Charney DS, Woods SW, Goodman WK, et al: Neurobiological mechanisms of panic anxiety: biochemical and behavioral correlates of yohimbine-induced panic attacks. Am J Psychiatry 144:1030–1036, 1987a

Charney DS, Woods SW, Goodman WK, et al: Serotonin function in anxiety, II: effects of the serotonin agonist mCPP in panic disorder patients and healthy subjects. Psychopharmacology 92:14–24, 1987b

Charney DS, Goodman WK, Price LH, et al: Serotonin function in obsessive-compulsive disorder: a comparison of the effects of tryptophan and m-CPP in patients and healthy subjects. Arch Gen Psychiatry 45:177–185, 1988

Charney DS, Innis RB, Duman RS, et al: Platelet α_2-receptor binding and adenylate cyclase activity in panic disorder. Psychopharmacology 98:102–107, 1989

Coplan JD, Gorman JM, Klein DF: Serotonin related functions in panic-anxiety: a critical overview. Neuropsychopharmacology 6:189–200, 1992a

Coplan JD, Sharma R, Rosenblum LA, et al: Effects of sodium lactate infusion on cisternal lactate and carbon dioxide levels in nonhuman subjects. Am J Psychiatry 149:1369–1373, 1992b

Crowe RR, Noyes R, Wilson F, et al: A linkage study of panic disorder. Arch Gen Psychiatry 44:933–937, 1987

Crowe RR, Noyes R Jr, Samuelson S, et al: Close linkage between panic disorder and α-haptoglobin excluded in 10 families. Arch Gen Psychiatry 47:377–380, 1990

Cummings JL, Cunningham K: Obsessive-compulsive disorder in Huntington's disease. Biol Psychiatry

31:263–270, 1992

Da Costa JM: On irritable heart: a clinical study of a form of functional cardiac disorder and its consequences. Am J Med Sci 61:17–52, 1871

Dagan Y, Lavie P, Bleich A: Elevated awakening thresholds in sleep stage 3-4 in war-related posttraumatic stress disorder. Biol Psychiatry 30:618–622, 1991

Davidson JRT, Foa EB (eds): Posttraumatic Stress Disorder: DSM-IV and Beyond. Washington, DC, American Psychiatric Press, 1993

DeMet E, Stein MK, Tran C, et al: Caffeine taste test for panic disorder: adenosine receptor supersensitivity. Psychiatry Res 30:231–242, 1989

de Montigny C: Cholecystokinin tetrapeptide induces panic-like attacks in healthy volunteers: preliminary findings. Arch Gen Psychiatry 46:511–517, 1989

Drevets WC, Videen TQ, MacLeod AK, et al: PET images of blood flow changes during anxiety: correction [letter]. Science 256:1696, 1992

File SE, Lister RG, Nutt DG: The anxiogenic action of benzodiazepine antagonists. Neuropharmacology 21:1033–1037, 1982

Flament MF, Rapaport JL, Murphy DL, et al: Biochemical changes during clomipramine treatment of childhood obsessive-compulsive disorder. Arch Gen Psychiatry 44:219–225, 1987

Fredholm BB, Persson CGA: Xanthine derivatives as adenosine receptor antagonists. Eur J Pharmacol 81:673–676, 1982

Fyer AJ, Gorman JM, Liebowitz MJ, et al: Sodium lactate infusion, panic attacks, and ionized calcium. Biol Psychiatry 19:1437–1447, 1984

Gaffney FA, Benton BJ, Lane LD, et al: Hemodynamic, ventilatory, and biochemical responses of panic patients and normal controls with sodium lactate infusion and spontaneous panic attacks. Arch Gen Psychiatry 45:53–60, 1988

Garber HJ, Ananth JV, Chiu LC, et al: Nuclear magnetic resonance study of obsessive-compulsive disorder. Am J Psychiatry 146:1001–1005, 1989

Gelernter CS, Stein MB, Tancer ME, et al: An examination of syndromal validity and diagnostic subtypes in social phobia and panic disorder. J Clin Psychiatry 53:23–27, 1992

George DT, Nutt DJ, Walker WV, et al: Lactate and hyperventilation substantially attenuate vagal tone in normal volunteers. Arch Gen Psychiatry 46:153–156, 1989

Goldsmith RL, Bigger JT, Steinman RC, et al: Comparison of 24-hour parasympathetic activity in endurance-trained and untrained young men. J Am Coll Cardiol 20:552–558, 1992

Goodman WK, McDougle CJ, Price LH, et al: Beyond the serotonin hypothesis: a role for dopamine in some forms of obsessive-compulsive disorder? J Clin Psychiatry 51 (suppl):36–43, 1990

Gorman JM, Papp LA: Respiratory physiology of panic, in Neurobiology of Panic Disorder. Edited by Ballenger JC. New York, Alan R Liss, 1990, pp 187–203

Gorman JM, Cohen BS, Liebowitz MR, et al: Blood gas changes and hypophosphatemia in lactate-induced panic. Arch Gen Psychiatry 43:1067–1075, 1986

Gorman JM, Fyer MR, Goetz R, et al: Ventilatory physiology of patients with panic disorder. Arch Gen Psychiatry 45:31–39, 1988a

Gorman JM, Goetz RR, Uy J, et al: Hyperventilation occurs during lactate-induced panic. Journal of Anxiety Disorders 2:193–202, 1988b

Gorman JM, Battista D, Goetz RR, et al: A comparison of sodium bicarbonate and sodium lactate infusion in the induction of panic attacks. Arch Gen Psychiatry 46:145–150, 1989a

Gorman J, Liebowitz MR, Fyer AJ, et al: A neuroanatomical hypothesis for panic disorder. Am J Psychiatry 146:148–161, 1989b

Gorman JM, Goetz RR, Dillon D, et al: Sodium D-lactate infusion of panic disorder patients. Neuropsychopharmacology 3:181–189, 1990

Gorman JM, Papp LA, Coplan J, et al: The effect of acetazolamide on ventilation in panic disorder patients. Am J Psychiatry 150:1480–1484, 1993

Green RC, Pitman RK: Tourette Syndrome and obsessive-compulsive disorder, in Obsessive-Compulsive Disorders: Theory and Management, 2nd Edition. Edited by Jenike MA, Baer L, Minichiello WE. Chicago, IL, Year Book Medical, 1990, pp 61–75

Griez E, de Loof C, Pols H, et al: Specific sensitivity of patients with panic attacks to carbon dioxide inhalation. Psychiatry Res 31:193–199, 1990a

Griez E, Zandbergen J, Pols H, et al: Response to 35% CO_2 as a marker of panic in severe anxiety. Am J Psychiatry 145:795–796, 1990b

Gurguis GNM, Uhde TW: Plasma 3-methoxy-4-hydroxy-phenylethylene glycol (MHPG) and growth hormone response to yohimbine in panic disorder patients and normal controls. Psychoneuroendocrinology 15:217–224, 1990

Hauri PJ, Friedman M, Ravaris CL: Sleep in patients with spontaneous panic attacks. Sleep 12:323–337, 1989

Heimberg RG, Hope DA, Dodge CS, et al: DSM-III-R subtypes of social phobia: comparison of generalized social phobics and public speaking phobics. J Nerv Ment Dis 173:172–179, 1990

Heimberg RG, Holt CS, Schneier FR, et al: The issue of subtypes in the diagnosis of social phobia. Journal of Anxiety Disorders 7:249–269, 1993

Hibbert GA: Hyperventilation as a cause of panic attacks. BMJ 288:263–264, 1984

Hoehn-Saric R, McLeod DR: Somatic manifestations of normal and pathological anxiety, in Biology of Anxiety Disorders: Recent Developments. Edited by Hoehn-Saric R, McLeod DR. Washington, DC, American Psychiatric Press, 1993, pp 177–222

Hollander E, Fay B, Cohen R, et al: Serotonergic and noradrenergic sensitivity in obsessive-compulsive disorder: behavioral findings. Am J Psychiatry 145:1015–1017, 1988

Hollander E, DeCaria CM, Nitescu A, et al: Serotonergic function in obsessive-compulsive disorder. Arch Gen Psychiatry 49:21–18, 1992

Insel TR: Toward a neuroanatomy of obsessive-compulsive disorder. Arch Gen Psychiatry 49:739–744, 1992

Insel TR, Mueller EA, Alterman I, et al: Obsessive-compulsive disorder and serotonin: is there a connection? Biol Psychiatry 20:1174–1185, 1985

Jolkkonen J, Lepola U, Bissette, et al: CSF Corticotropin-releasing factor is not affected in panic disorder. Biol Psychiatry 33:136–138, 1993

Kahn RS, Asnis GM, Wetzler S, et al: Neuroendocrine evidence for serotonin receptor hypersensitivity in panic disorder. Psychopharmacology 96:360–364, 1988a

Kahn RS, Wetzler S, van Praag HM, et al: Behavioral indications for serotonin receptor hypersensitivity in panic disorder. Psychiatry Res 25:101–109, 1988b

Kellner CH, Jolley RR, Holgate RC, et al: Brain MRI in obsessive-compulsive disorder. Psychiatry Res 36:45–49, 1991

Kim SW, Dysken MW, Pandey GN, et al: Platelet ^{3}H-imipramine binding sites in obsessive-compulsive behavior. Biol Psychiatry 30:467–474, 1991

Klein DF: False suffocation alarms, spontaneous panics, and related conditions: an integrative hypothesis. Arch Gen Psychiatry 50:306–317, 1993

Klein E, Zohar J, Geraci M, et al: Anxiogenic effects of m-CPP in patients with panic disorder: comparison to caffeine's anxiogenic effects. Biol Psychiatry 30:973–984, 1991

Koenigsberg HW, Pollak CP, Fine J, et al: Lactate sensitivity in sleeping panic disorder patients and healthy controls. Biol Psychiatry 32:539–542, 1992

Kosten TR, Mason JW, Giller EL, et al: Sustained urinary norepinephrine and epinephrine elevation in post-traumatic stress disorder. Psychoneuroendocrinology 12:13–20, 1987

Lemus CZ, Robinson DG, Kronig M, et al: Behavioral responses to a dopaminergic challenge in obsessive-compulsive disorder. Journal of Anxiety Disorders 5:369–373, 1991

Lerer B, Ebstein RP, Shestatsky M, et al: Cyclic AMP signal transduction in post-traumatic stress disorder. Am J Psychiatry 144:1324–1327, 1987

Lerer B, Bleich A, Bennett ER, et al: Platelet adenylate cyclase and phospholipase C activity in posttraumatic stress disorder. Biol Psychiatry 27:735–740, 1990

Lesch KP, Wiesmann M, Hoh A, et al: 5-HT1A receptor-effector system responsivity in panic disorder. Psychopharmacology (Berl) 106:111–117, 1992

Levin AP, Saoud JB, Strauman T, et al: Responses of "generalized" and "discrete" social phobias during public speaking. Journal of Anxiety Disorders 7:207–221, 1993

Liebowitz MR, Fyer AJ, Gorman JM, et al: Lactate provocation of panic attacks, I: clinical and behavioral findings. Arch Gen Psychiatry 41:764–770, 1984

Liebowitz MR, Gorman JM, Fyer AJ, et al: Social phobia: a review of a neglected anxiety disorder. Arch Gen Psychiatry 42:729–736, 1985

Luxenberg JS, Swedo SE, Flament MM, et al: Neuroanatomical abnormalities in obsessive-compulsive disorder detected with quantitative X-ray computed tomography. Am J Psychiatry 145:1089–1093, 1988

Lydiard RB, Ballenger JC, Ellinwood E, et al: CSF monoamine metabolites in obsessive-compulsive disorder. Paper presented at the annual meeting of the American Psychiatric Association, New York, May 1990

Lydiard RB, Ballenger JC, Laraia MT, et al: CSF cholecystokinin concentrations in patients with panic disorder and in normal comparison subjects. Am J Psychiatry 149:691–693, 1992

Machlin SR, Harris GJ, Pearlson GD, et al: Elevated medial-cortical blood blow in obsessive-compulsive patients: a SPECT study. Am J Psychiatry 148:1240–1242, 1991

Manji HK: G proteins: Implications for psychiatry. Am J Psychiatry 149:746–760, 1992

Marazziti D, Hollander E, Lensi P, et al: Peripheral markers of serotonin and dopamine function in obsessive-compulsive disorder. Psychiatry Res 42:41–51, 1992

Margraf J, Ehlers A, Roth W: Sodium lactate infusions and panic attacks: a review and critique. Psychosom Med 48:23–51, 1986

Markowitz JS, Weissman MM, Ouelette R, et al: Quality of life in panic disorder. Arch Gen Psychiatry 46:984–992, 1989

Marks I: Blood-injury phobia: a review. Am J Psychiatry 145:1207–1213, 1988

Mathew RJ, Wilson WH, Tant S: Responses to hypercarbia induced by acetazolamide in panic disorder patients. Am J Psychiatry 146:996–1000, 1989

McDougle CJ, Goodman WK, Price LH, et al: Neuroleptic addition in fluvoxamine-refractory obsessive-compulsive disorder. Am J Psychiatry 147:652–654, 1990

McFall ME, Murburg MM, Ko GN, et al: Autonomic responses to stress in Vietnam combat veterans with posttraumatic stress disorder. Biol Psychiatry 27:1165–1175, 1990

McFall ME, Veith RC, Murburg MM: Basal sympathoadrenal function in posttraumatic stress disorder. Biol Psychiatry 31:1050–1056, 1992

Mellman TA, Uhde TW: Electroencephalographic sleep in panic disorder: a focus on sleep-related panic attacks. Arch Gen Psychiatry 46:178–184, 1989a

Mellman TA, Uhde TW: Sleep panic attacks: new clinical findings and theoretical implications. Am J Psychiatry 146:1204–1207, 1989b

Mellman TA, Ramsay RE, Fitzgerald SG: Divergence of PTSD and narcolepsy associated with military trauma. Journal of Anxiety Disorders 5:267–272, 1991

Modell JG, Mountz JM, Curtis GC, et al: Neurophysiologic dysfunction in basal ganglia/limbic striatal and thalamocortical circuits as a pathogenetic mechanism of obsessive-compulsive disorders. J Neuropsychiatry 1:27–36, 1989

Moret C, Briley M: Platelet ^{3}H-paroxetine binding to the serotonin transporter is insensitive to changes in central serotonergic innervation in the rat. Psychiatry Res 38:97–104, 1991

Nemeroff CB: Corticotropin-releasing factor, in Neuropeptides and Psychiatric Disorders. Edited by Nemeroff CB. Washington, DC, American Psychiatric Press, 1991, pp 75–92

Nemiah JC, Uhde TW: Phobic Disorders, in Comprehensive Textbook of Psychiatry, 5th Edition. Edited by Kaplan HI, Sadock BJ. Baltimore, MD, Williams & Wilkins, 1989, pp 984–1000

Nesse RM, Cameron OG, Curtis GC, et al: Adrenergic function in patients with panic anxiety. Arch Gen Psychiatry 41:771–776, 1984

Nordahl TE, Benkelfat C, Semple WE, et al: Cerebral glucose metabolic rates in obsessive-compulsive disorder. Neuropsychopharmacology 2:23–28, 1989

Nordahl TE, Semple WE, Gross M, et al: Cerebral glucose metabolic differences in patients with panic disorder. Neuropsychopharmacology 3:261–272, 1990

Nutt DJ: Altered central α_2-adrenoceptor sensitivity in panic disorder. Arch Gen Psychiatry 46:165–169, 1989

Nutt DJ, Glue P, Lawson C, et al: Flumazenil provocation of panic attacks: evidence for altered benzodiazepine receptor sensitivity in panic disorder. Arch Gen Psychiatry 47:917–925, 1990

Orr SP: Psychophysiologic studies of posttraumatic stress disorder, in Biological Assessment and Treatment of Posttraumatic Stress Disorder. Washington, DC, American Psychiatric Press, 1990, pp 137–157

Orr SP, Pitman RK: Psychophysiologic assessment of attempts to simulate posttraumatic stress disorder. Biol Psychiatry 33:127–192, 1993

Papp LA, Gorman JM, Liebowitz MR, et al: Epinephrine infusions in patients with social phobia. Am J Psychiatry 145:733–736, 1988

Papp LA, Klein DF, Martinez J, et al: Diagnostic and substance specificity of carbon-dioxide-induced panic. Am J Psychiatry 150:250–257, 1993

Pauls DL, Raymond CL, Stevenson JM, et al: A family study of Gilles de la Tourette syndrome. Am J Human Genet 48:154–163, 1991

Perry BD, Southwick SM, Giller EL: Adrenergic receptor regulation in posttraumatic stress disorder, in

Biological Assessment and Treatment of Posttraumatic Stress Disorder. Edited by Giller EL. Washington, DC, American Psychiatric Press, 1990, pp 87–114

Pigott TA, Zohar J, Hill JL, et al: Metergoline blocks the behavioral and neuroendocrine effects of orally administered m-CPP in patients with OCD. Biol Psychiatry 29:418–426, 1991

Pigott TA, Hill JL, Grady TA, et al: A comparison of the behavioral effects of oral versus intravenous mCPP administration in OCD patients and the effect of metergoline prior to IV mCPP. Biol Psychiatry 33:3–14, 1993

Pincus HA, Henderson B, Blackwood D, et al: Trends in research in two general psychiatric journals in 1969–1990: research on research. Am J Psychiatry 150:135–142, 1993

Pitman RK, Orr SP: 24-hour urinary cortisol and catecholamine excretion in combat-related posttraumatic stress disorder. Biol Psychiatry 27:245–247, 1990

Pitman RK, Orr SP, Forgue DF, et al: Psychophysiologic assessment of posttraumatic stress disorder imagery in Vietnam combat veterans. Arch Gen Psychiatry 44:970–975, 1987

Pitman RK, Orr SP, Forgue DF, et al: Psychophysiologic responses to combat imagery of Vietnam veterans with posttraumatic stress disorder versus other anxiety disorders. J Abnorm Psychol 99:49–54, 1990

Pitts FN Jr, McClure JN: Lactate metabolism in anxiety neurosis. N Engl J Med 277:1329–1336, 1967

Pohl R, Yeragani VK, Balon R, et al: Isoproterenol-induced panic attacks. Biol Psychiatry 24:891–902, 1988

Pohl R, Yeragani VK, Balon R, et al: Isoproterenol-induced panic: a beta-adrenergic model of panic anxiety, in Neurobiology of Panic Disorder. Edited by Ballenger JC. New York, Alan R Liss, 1990, pp 107–120

Potts NL, Davidson JR, Krishnan KR, et al: Levels of urinary free cortisol in social phobia. J Clin Psychiatry 52 (suppl):41–42, 1991

Rapaport MH, Risch SC, Gillin JC, et al: Blunted growth hormone response to peripheral infusions of human growth hormone-releasing factor in patients with panic disorder. Am J Psychiatry 146:92–95, 1989a

Rapaport MH, Risch SC, Golshan S, et al: Neuroendocrine effects of ovine corticotropin-releasing hormone in panic disorder patients. Biol Psychiatry 26:344–348, 1989b

Rapee R: Differential response to hyperventilation in panic disorder and generalized anxiety disorder. J Abnorm Psychol 95:24–28, 1986

Rapoport JL, Ryland DH, Kriete M: Drug treatment of canine acral lick: an animal model of obsessive-compulsive disorder. Arch Gen Psychiatry 49:517–521, 1992

Redmond DE Jr: New and old evidence for the involvement of a brain norepinephrine system in anxiety, in The Phenomenology and Treatment of Anxiety. Edited by Fann WE. New York, Spectrum Press, 1979, pp 153–203

Reiman EM, Raichle ME, Butler FK, et al: A focal brain abnormality in panic disorder, a severe form of anxiety. Nature 310:683–685, 1984

Reiman EM, Raichle ME, Robins E, et al: Neuroanatomical correlates of a lactate-induced panic attack. Arch Gen Psychiatry 46:493–500, 1989

Reiss S: Interoceptive theory of the fear of anxiety. Behav Res Ther 7:84–85, 1988

Ross RJ, Ball WA, Sullivan KA, et al: Sleep disturbance as the hallmark of posttraumatic stress disorder. Am J Psychiatry 146:697–707, 1989

Roth WT, Margraf J, Ehlers A, et al: Stress test reactivity in panic disorder. Arch Gen Psychiatry 49:301–310, 1992

Roy-Byrne PP, Cowley DS, Greenblatt DJ, et al: Reduced benzodiazepine sensitivity in panic disorder. Arch Gen Psychiatry 47:534–538, 1990

Rubin RT, Villanueva-Meyer J, Ananth J, et al: Regional Xenon 133 cerebral blood flow and cerebral technetium 99m HMPAO uptake in unmedicated patients with obsessive-compulsive disorder and matched normal control subjects. Arch Gen Psychiatry 49:695–702, 1992

Salkovskis PM, Jones DR, Clark DM: Respiratory control in the treatment of panic attacks: replication and extension with concurrent measurement of pCO_2. Br J Psychiatry 148:526–532, 1986

Sapolsky RM: Stress, the Aging Brain, and the Mechanisms of Neuron Death. Cambridge, MA, MIT Press, 1992

Schiffman SS, Gill JM, Diaz C: Methylxanthines enhance taste: evidence for modulation of taste by adenosine receptors. Pharmacol Biochem Behav 22:195–203, 1985

Schittecatte M, Charles G, Depauw Y, et al: Growth hormone response to clonidine in panic disorder.

Psychiatry Res 23:147–151, 1988

Schittecatte M, Ansseau M, Charles G, et al: Growth hormone response to clonidine in male patients with panic disorder untreated by antidepressants. Psychol Med 22:1059–1062, 1992

Shalev AY, Orr SP, Peri T, et al: Physiologic responses to loud tones in Israeli patients with posttraumatic stress disorder. Arch Gen Psychiatry 49:870–875, 1992

Shapiro AK, Shapiro ES, Young JG, et al: Gilles de la Tourette Syndrome, 2nd Edition. New York, Raven, 1988

Shear MK, Fyer AJ, Ball G, et al: Vulnerability to sodium lactate in panic disorder patients given cognitive-behavioral therapy. Am J Psychiatry 148:795–797, 1991

Smith MA, Davidson J, Ritchie JC, et al: The corticotropin-releasing hormone test in patients with posttraumatic stress disorder. Biol Psychiatry 26:349–355, 1989

Stein JM, Papp LA, Klein DF, et al: Exercise tolerance testing in panic disorder patients. Biol Psychiatry 32:281–287, 1992

Stein MB, Asmundson GJG: Autonomic function in panic disorder: cardiorespiratory and plasma catecholamine responsivity to multiple challenges of the autonomic nervous system. Biol Psychiatry 36:548–558, 1994

Stein MB, Uhde TW: Panic disorder and major depression: lifetime relationship and biological markers, in Clinical Aspects of Panic Disorder. Edited by Ballenger J. New York, Alan R Liss, 1990, pp 151–168

Stein MB, Uhde TW: Endocrine, cardiovascular, and behavioral effects of intravenous TRH in patients with panic disorder. Arch Gen Psychiatry 48:148–156, 1991

Stein MB, Uhde TW: Thyroid function in anxiety disorders, in The Thyroid Axis and Psychiatric Illness. Edited by Joffe RT, Levitt AJ. Washington, DC, American Psychiatric Press, 1993, pp 255–278

Stein MB, Tancer ME, Uhde TW: Physiologic and plasma norepinephrine responses to orthostasis in patients with panic disorder and social phobia. Arch Gen Psychiatry 49:311–317, 1992

Stein MB, Black B, Uhde TW: Lack of efficacy of the adenosine reuptake inhibitor dipyridamole in the treatment of anxiety disorders. Biol Psychiatry 33:647–650, 1993a

Stein MB, Enns MW, Kryger MH: Sleep in nondepressed patients with panic disorder, II: polysomnographic assessment of sleep architecture and sleep continuity. J Affect Disord 28:1–6, 1993b

Stein MB, Huzel LL, Delaney SM: Lymphocyte β-adrenoceptors in social phobia. Biol Psychiatry 34:45–50, 1993c

Stein MB, Asmundson GJG, Chartier MJ: Autonomic responsivity in generalized social phobia. J Affect Disord 31:211–221, 1994

Swedo SE, Rapoport JL, Cheslow DL, et al: High prevalence of obsessive-compulsive symptoms in patients with Sydenham's chorea. Am J Psychiatry 146:246–249, 1989a

Swedo SE, Schapiro MB, Grady CL, et al: Cerebral glucose metabolism in childhood-onset obsessive-compulsive disorder. Arch Gen Psychiatry 46:518–523, 1989b

Swedo SE, Pietrini P, Leonard HL, et al: Cerebral glucose metabolism in childhood-onset obsessive-compulsive disorder: revisualization during pharmacotherapy. Arch Gen Psychiatry 49:690–694, 1992

Tancer ME, Stein MB, Gelernter CS, et al: The hypothalamic-pituitary-thyroid axis in social phobia. Am J Psychiatry 147:929–933, 1990a

Tancer ME, Stein MB, Uhde TW: Effects of thyrotropin-releasing hormone on blood pressure and heart rate in social phobic and panic patients: a pilot study. Biol Psychiatry 27:781–783, 1990b

Tancer ME, Stein MB, Black B, et al: Blunted growth hormone responses to growth hormone releasing factor and to clonidine in panic disorder. Am J Psychiatry 150:336–337, 1993a

Tancer ME, Stein MB, Uhde TW: Growth hormone response to intravenous clonidine in social phobia: comparison to patients with panic disorder and healthy volunteers. Biol Psychiatry 34:591–595, 1993b

Targum SD, Marshall LE: Fenfluramine provocation of anxiety in patients with panic disorder. Psychiatry Res 28:295–306, 1989

Thoren P, Asberg M, Bertillson L, et al: Clomipramine treatment of obsessive-compulsive disorder, II: biochemical aspects. Arch Gen Psychiatry 37:1289–1294, 1980

Torgersen S: Twin studies in panic disorder, in Neurobiology of Panic Disorder. Edited by Ballenger J. New York, Alan R Liss, 1990, pp 51–58

Uhde TW: Noradrenergic studies in anxiety, in Receptors and Ligands in Psychiatry and Neurology,

Vol 3. Edited by Sen AK, Lee T. London, Cambridge University Press, 1987, pp 375–387

Uhde TW: Caffeine provocation of panic: a focus on biological mechanisms, in Clinical Aspects of Panic Disorder. Edited by Ballenger J. New York, Alan R Liss, 1990, pp 219–242

Uhde TW: The anxiety disorders, in Principles and Practice of Sleep Medicine, 2nd Edition. Edited by Kryger MH, Roth T, Dement W. Philadelphia, PA, WB Saunders, 1994, pp 871–898

Uhde TW, Nemiah JC: Panic and generalized anxiety disorders, in Comprehensive Textbook of Psychiatry, 5th Edition. Edited by Kaplan HI, Sadock BJ. Baltimore, MD, Williams & Wilkins, 1989, pp 952–972

Uhde TW, Boulenger JP, Post RM, et al: Fear and anxiety: relationship to noradrenergic function. Psychopathology 17:8–23, 1984a

Uhde TW, Vittone BJ, Post RM: Glucose tolerance testing in panic disorder. Am J Psychiatry 141:1461–1463, 1984b

Uhde TW, Roy-Byrne PP, Vittone BJ, et al: Phenomenology and neurobiology of panic disorder, in Anxiety and the Anxiety Disorder. Edited by Tuma AH, Maser JD. Hillsdale, NJ, Erlbaum, 1985, pp 557–576

Uhde TW, Vittone BJ, Siever LJ, et al: Blunted growth hormone response to clonidine in panic disorder patients. Biol Psychiatry 21:1077–1081, 1986

Uhde TW, Stein MB, Vittone BJ, et al: Behavioral and physiologic effects of short-term and long-term administration of clonidine in panic disorder. Arch Gen Psychiatry 46:170–177, 1989

Uhde TW, Tancer ME, Gurguis GNM: Chemical models of anxiety: evidence for diagnostic and neurotransmitter specificity. International Review Journal of Psychiatry 2:367–384, 1990

Uhde TW, Tancer ME, Black B, et al: Phenomenology and neurobiology of social phobia: comparison with panic disorder. J Clin Psychiatry 52 (11 suppl):31–40, 1991

Uhde TW, Tancer ME, Rubinow DR, et al: Evidence for hypothalamo-growth hormone dysfunction in panic disorder: profile of growth hormone (GH) responses to clonidine, yohimbine, caffeine, glucose, GRF and TRH in panic disorder patients versus healthy volunteers. Neuropsychopharmacology 6:101–118, 1992

Uhde TW, Tancer ME, Gelernter CS, et al: Normal urinary-free cortisol and post-dexamethasone cortisol in social phobia: comparison to normal controls. J Affect Disord 30:155–161, 1994

van Kammen DP: 5-HT, a neurotransmitter for all seasons? Biol Psychiatry 22:1–3, 1987

Vitiello B, Shimon H, Behar D, et al: Platelet imipramine binding and serotonin uptake in obsessive-compulsive patients. Acta Psychiatr Scand 84:29–32, 1991

Wang ZW, Crowe RR, Noyes R Jr: Adrenergic receptor genes as candidate genes for panic disorder: a linkage study. Am J Psychiatry 149:470–474, 1992

Weissman MM: The epidemiology of panic disorder and agoraphobia, in American Psychiatric Press Review of Psychiatry, Vol 7. Edited by Frances AJ, Hales RE. Washington, DC, American Psychiatric Press, 1988, pp 54–66

Weissman MM, Klerman GL, Markowitz JS, et al: Suicidal ideation and suicide attempts in panic disorder and attacks. N Engl J Med 321:1209–1214, 1989

Weizman A, Carmi M, Hermesh H, et al: High-affinity imipramine binding and serotonin uptake in platelets of eight adolescent and ten adult obsessive-compulsive patients. Am J Psychiatry 143:335–339, 1986

Weizman A, Mandel A, Barber Y, et al: Decreased platelet imipramine binding in Tourette syndrome children with obsessive-compulsive disorder. Biol Psychiatry 31:705–711, 1992

Wise SP, Rapoport JL: Obsessive compulsive disorder: is it basal ganglia dysfunction? in Obsessive-Compulsive Disorder in Children and Adolescents. Edited by Rapoport JL. Washington, DC, American Psychiatric Press, 1989, pp 327–344

Woods SW, Charney DS: Biologic responses to panic anxiety elicited by nonpharmacologic means, in Neurobiology of Panic Disorder. Edited by Ballenger JC. New York, Alan R Liss, 1990, pp 205–217

Yehuda R, Southwick SM, Nussbaum G, et al: Low urinary cortisol excretion in PTSD. J Nerv Ment Dis 178:366–369, 1990

Yehuda R, Lowy MT, Southwick SM, et al: Increased number of glucocorticoid receptor number in posttraumatic stress disorder. Am J Psychiatry 149:499–504, 1991a

Yehuda R, Giller EL, Southwick SM, et al: Hypothalamic-pituitary-adrenal dysfunction in posttraumatic stress disorder. Biol Psychiatry 30:1031–1048, 1991b

Yehuda R, Southwick SM, Krystal JH, et al: Enhanced suppression of cortisol following dexamethasone administration in posttraumatic stress disorder. Am J Psychiatry 150:83–86, 1993

Yeragani VK, Balon R, Pohl R, et al: Decreased R-R variance in panic disorder patients. Acta Psychiatr Scand 81:554–559, 1990

Zohar J, Mueller EA, Insel TR, et al: Serotonergic responsivity in obsessive-compulsive disorder: comparison of patients and healthy controls. Arch Gen Psychiatry 44:946–951, 1987

Zohar J, Insel TR, Zohar-Kadouch RC, et al: Serotonergic responsivity in obsessive-compulsive disorder: effects of chronic clomipramine treatment. Arch Gen Psychiatry 45:167–172, 1988

Zorumski CF, Isenberg KE: Insights into the structure and function of GABA-benzodiazepine receptors: ion channels and psychiatry. Am J Psychiatry 148:162–173, 1991

Biology of Alzheimer's Disease and Animal Models

Donald L. Price, M.D., Lary C. Walker, Ph.D.,
Lee J. Martin, Ph.D., David R. Borchelt, Ph.D.,
Philip C. Wong, Ph.D., and Sangram S. Sisodia, Ph.D.

As more and more people reach old age (Olshansky et al. 1993), there is a significant increase in the prevalence of disorders affecting elderly people. The most common major disability of this age group is impairment in cognitive and memory processes, and Alzheimer's disease (AD) is the most common cause of this problem (Evans et al. 1989; Khachaturian 1985; McKhann et al. 1984). With a prevalence as high as 11% in persons over age 65 years (Bachman et al. 1993; Evans et al. 1989; Pfeffer et al. 1987), AD will affect more than 8 million individuals in the United States by the year 2000. It is therefore imperative to understand the etiologies and pathogeneses of AD and to develop effective treatments.

In this chapter, we examine the clinical features, genetics, risk factors, and brain abnormalities, including those involving vulnerable neuronal systems,

cytoskeletal alterations, and amyloidogenesis, that occur in the brains of people with AD. We then discuss some of the recent advances that have been made in creating animal models of these processes (Price and Sisodia 1994; Price et al. 1992a, 1994).

ALZHEIMER'S DISEASE

Clinical Syndrome

The hallmark of AD (usually appearing in the seventh decade of life) is a decline in cognitive abilities, particularly memory, speed of performance, and problem solving (Khachaturian 1985; McKhann et al. 1984). Patients may show disorders of language, calculation, visuospatial perceptions, judgment, and behavior, as well as evidence of psychoses (Evans et al.

The authors gratefully acknowledge discussions with Drs. Linda C. Cork, Cheryl A. Kitt, John D. Gearhart, Bruce T. Lamb, and Mary Lou Voytko.

This work was supported by grants from the U.S. Public Health Service (NS AG 05146, NS 20471, NS 07179, AG 10480, AG 10491) as well as the American Health Assistance Foundation, the Metropolitan Life Foundation, and The Robert L. and Clara G. Patterson Trust. Drs. Price, Martin, and Borchelt are the recipients of a Leadership and Excellence in Alzheimer's Disease (LEAD) award (AG 07914); Dr. Price received a Javits Neuroscience Investigator Award (NS 10580).

1989; Katzman et al. 1988, 1989; Khachaturian 1985; McKhann et al. 1984). Mental functions and activities of daily living become progressively more impaired. In the late stage, individuals with AD have profound dementia and are mute, incontinent, and bedridden.

Cases of senile dementia are usually classified on the basis of criteria formulated by the NINCDS-ADRDA joint task force (McKhann et al. 1984) as possible, probable, or definite AD. The clinical course of AD may vary considerably, but most patients show declines in mental status, usually at a rate of 3–4 points per year on the Blessed Information-Memory-Concentration test, or the Blessed Dementia Index (Blessed et al. 1968) and 2–3 points per year on the Mini-Mental State Examination (Folstein et al. 1975). Clinical histories, physical examinations, neuropsychological testing, and a variety of diagnostic assessments are used to exclude other causes of dementia and to determine the possibility or probability of a diagnosis of AD (Atack 1989; Khachaturian 1985; McKhann et al. 1984). Neuroimaging studies, including computed tomography (CT) and magnetic resonance imaging (MRI), can identify potentially treatable diseases and disclose abnormalities (particularly in the medial temporal lobe) that may have high predictive value for establishing an accurate diagnosis of AD. Positron-emission tomography (PET) and single photon emission computed tomography (SPECT) techniques show decreased regional glucose metabolism and blood flow in the parietal and temporal lobes, with involvement of other cortical areas at later stages. However, short of the examination of brain biopsy, there are currently no tests that establish the diagnosis of AD in living subjects.

■ Neuronal Systems Vulnerable in AD

Correlative neuropathological-neurochemical studies have shown that clinical symptoms or signs in cases of AD are associated with abnormalities that involve neuronal populations in the hippocampus, neocortex, amygdala, anterior thalamus, basal forebrain cholinergic system, and monoaminergic brain stem systems (i.e., locus ceruleus and raphe complex) (Arnold et al. 1991; Braak and Braak 1991a; D'Amato et al. 1987; De Souza et al. 1986; Hyman et al. 1990; Kemper 1984; Vogels et al. 1990; Whitehouse et al. 1982; Zweig et al. 1988). A characteristic pathology occurs in hippocampus and medial temporal lobe. Pyramidal neurons, particularly those in entorhinal

cortex, CA1 and CA2 (Braak and Braak 1991b; Kemper 1984; Tomlinson et al. 1981), are severely affected in AD. For the most part, these lesions involve glutamatergic systems, which disconnect hippocampus and neocortex. Glutamatergic pyramidal neurons in layers III and V of neocortex (Braak and Braak 1991b; Hardy et al. 1987) are selectively destroyed by the disease process. Also affected are interneurons, some of which use corticotropin-releasing factor (CRF) or somatostatin as transmitters (Beal et al. 1985; Davies et al. 1980; De Souza et al. 1986; Ferrier et al. 1983; Rossor et al. 1980). Levels of somatostatin, somatostatinergic binding sites, and corticotropin-releasing hormone (CRH) are reduced in neocortex (Beal et al. 1985; Davies et al. 1980), whereas binding sites for CRF are increased (De Souza et al. 1986).

Other cortical peptidergic systems do not appear to be altered significantly (Ferrier et al. 1983), but some peptidergic neurons develop neurites associated with senile plaques (Struble et al. 1987). The amygdala is also damaged by disease (Herzog and Kemper 1980; Kemper 1984; Scott et al. 1992). A consistent lesion in AD is degeneration of cholinergic neurons in the medial septum, diagonal band, and nucleus basalis, which provide the principal cholinergic innervation of amygdala, hippocampus, and neocortex of primates (Struble et al. 1986). These cells develop neurofibrillary tangles (NFT) and neurites and, eventually, undergo atrophy and cell death (Arendt et al. 1983; Perry et al. 1982; Vogels et al. 1990; Whitehouse et al. 1982). Reductions occur in levels of acetylcholine as well as the activities of choline acetyltransferase (ChAT) and acetylcholinesterase (Francis et al. 1985; Whitehouse et al. 1986). In hippocampus, with age, there is some decline in ChAT activity; however, in AD, the decrements are very severe. Levels of cortical ChAT activity appear to correlate with the degree of dementia. In some cases of AD, neurons of the anterior nucleus of the thalamus also show evidence of degeneration (Braak and Braak 1991a), and neurites are present in target fields of these cells (e.g., retrosplenial cortex). Neurons of the locus ceruleus and raphe also exhibit perikaryal pathology (i.e., NFT), axons and terminals of these cells may form neurites, and noradrenergic and serotonergic markers may decrease in target fields (Curcio and Kemper 1984; D'Amato et al. 1987; Tomlinson et al. 1981).

The mechanisms that lead to dysfunction and

death of these neurons are not well understood but may involve excitotoxicity (Koh et al. 1990), β-amyloid (Aβ) toxicity (Pike et al. 1991; Price et al. 1992b; Yankner et al. 1989), and the activation of proteases (Saito et al., in press). The principal consequence of all of these lesions is a diminution of synaptic inputs in a variety of brain regions (DeKosky and Scheff 1990; Hamos et al. 1989; Masliah et al. 1989, 1990, 1991a, 1992, 1993; Scheff and Price 1993; Terry et al. 1991).

■ Cytoskeletal Pathology in Neurons

In cases of AD, many affected neurons exhibit NFT, neuropil threads, and neurites. The principal ultrastructural components of these three abnormalities are intracellular accumulations of 15-nm straight filaments and, more importantly, insoluble paired helical filaments (PHF), which are made up principally of abnormally phosphorylated isoforms of tau protein (Arriagada et al. 1992; Goedert 1993; Greenberg and Davies 1990; Lee et al. 1991). Aberrant phosphorylation of tau may promote the formation of the straight filaments that become increasingly modified and cross-linked to form insoluble PHF. Abnormal tau phosphorylation can alter the stability of microtubules, with subsequent effects on intracellular transport, cellular geometry, and neuronal viability. Other NFT-associated epitopes include ubiquitin, microtubule-associated protein-2, neurofilament proteins (particularly phosphorylated epitopes of the 200-kilodalton [kD] protein), and, possibly, the Aβ protein (Cork et al. 1986; Grundke-Iqbal et al. 1986; Kosik et al. 1986; Masters et al. 1985a; Perry et al. 1987).

Neurites, visualized with silver stains, are enlarged neuronal processes containing PHF, 15-nm straight filaments, and various organelles, including mitochondria, membranous inclusions, lysosomes, and, in some cases, synaptic vesicles (Wisniewski and Terry 1973b). Neurites are often enriched in PHF-related epitopes, amyloid precursor protein (APP), ubiquitin, phosphorylated epitopes of neurofilaments, and neurotransmitter markers (Cork et al. 1986, 1990; Cras et al. 1991; Grundke-Iqbal et al. 1986; Kosik et al. 1986; Lee et al. 1991; Martin et al. 1991; Perry et al. 1987). Neuropil threads are altered neuronal processes, predominantly dendrites (Masliah et al. 1992; McKee et al. 1991; Perry et al. 1991). Some of these abnormal processes may represent aberrant sprouts (Masliah et al. 1991b). NFT and

neuropil threads exhibit characteristic distributional patterns over time (Braak and Braak 1991b). For example, NFT involve the transentorhinal region and entorhinal cortex, eventually involving Ammon's horn and isocortex (Braak and Braak 1991b). The severity of these lesions in regions of cerebral cortex appears to correlate with hierarchies of cortical-cortical connections, and nerve cells of association cortices exhibit the greatest vulnerability (Arnold et al. 1991). Because NFT, neurites, and neuropil threads contain similar cytoskeletal constituents, the genesis of these fibrillar inclusions is probably the result of common mechanisms (i.e., aberrant phosphorylation of tau).

■ Amyloidogenesis

A histological hallmark of AD is the presence of senile plaques (Kemper 1984; Khachaturian 1985; McKhann et al. 1984; Probst et al. 1987, 1991). Composed of neurites displayed in proximity to thioflavin S-/Congo red–positive deposits of amyloid, plaques are most common in amygdala, hippocampus, and neocortex (Kemper 1984). Amyloid, consisting of 8-nm extracellular filaments, is composed principally of a unique 4-kD β-peptide, Aβ or β/A4 (Glenner and Wong 1984; Masters et al. 1985a, 1985b), derived from APP (Kang et al. 1987). Aβ represents 14–15 amino acids of the transmembrane domain and 26–28 amino acids of the extracellular domain of APP (Glenner and Wong 1984; Masters et al. 1985a, 1985b). Located on the midportion of the long arm of human chromosome 21 (Kang et al. 1987), the APP gene, encompassing ~400 kilobases (kb) of deoxyribonucleic acid (DNA), gives rise by alternative splicing of APP pre-messenger ribonucleic acid (mRNA) to at least four transcripts that encode Aβ-containing proteins of 695, 714, 751, and 770 amino acids (Kang et al. 1987; Kitaguchi et al. 1988; Ponte et al. 1988). APP-751 and -770 contain a domain that shares homology with the Kunitz class of serine protease inhibitors (KPI) (Kitaguchi et al. 1988; Ponte et al. 1988). Recent studies have shown that APP is a member of a gene family that includes the amyloid precursor-like proteins (APLP) 1 and 2, both of which lack the Aβ domain (Slunt et al. 1994).

In cultured mammalian cells, full-length APP isoforms are modified by the addition of both N- and O-linked carbohydrates and terminal sulfation events (Slunt et al. 1994). A proportion of the synthesized

APP molecules appears at the cell surface, and some of these proteins are cleaved by APP α-secretase at position 16 within Aβ (Esch et al. 1990; Sisodia 1992; Sisodia et al. 1990; Wang et al. 1991) to release the ectodomain of APP, including residues 1–16 of Aβ, into the medium. In vitro and in vivo studies have documented that APP may be processed by alternative pathways (possibly endosomal-lysosomal proteolysis) that result in potentially amyloidogenic C-terminal–containing fragments (Estus et al. 1992; Golde et al. 1992; Haass et al. 1992a; Nordstedt et al. 1991). Moreover, Aβ (4 kD) and a truncated form of Aβ (3 kD) are secreted into the media of cultured cells (including glial cells) and into the cerebrospinal fluid (CSF) (Busciglio et al. 1993; Haass et al. 1992b; Seubert et al. 1992; Shoji et al. 1992).

Transcripts of APP and APLP2 are expressed in most neurons (Koo et al. 1990b; Slunt et al. 1994). In the central nervous system (CNS) of rodents and nonhuman primates, APP (which are present in cell bodies, proximal dendrites, and axons) (Martin et al. 1991) are delivered to axons and terminals via the fast anterograde axonal transport system (Koo et al. 1990a; Martin et al. 1991; Sisodia et al. 1993). Transcripts coding for isoforms with KPI activity are demonstrable in nonneuronal cells. In the peripheral nervous system of rats, holo-APP-695 is the predominant transported isoform (Sisodia et al. 1993). It has been suggested that APP may play roles in synaptic adhesion or interactions (Schubert 1991) and may function as a receptor, possibly coupled to guanine nucleotide-regulated coupling protein G_o (Nishimoto et al. 1993). At present, relatively little is known about the cellular trafficking of APP and the processing of APP at pre- and postsynaptic sites. The distributions and fates of transported APP isoforms in the CNS are not well understood. Significantly, several antibodies elicited against APP epitopes do discriminate between APP and APLP2, suggesting that reports using this reagent to identify APP may need reinterpretation, because the antibodies recognize APLP2 as well.

Although cellular sources of Aβ are not fully understood, neuronal APP appears to be the origin of some Aβ (Koo et al. 1990b; Martin et al. 1991; Probst et al. 1991). Thus, APP-immunoreactive neurites, often decorated or capped by Aβ deposits (Cras et al. 1991; Martin et al. 1991; Probst et al. 1991), are one source of parenchymal amyloid. However, other types of nonneural cells, including astroglia, microglia, and vascular cells, may be critical elements in amyloidogenesis (Frackowiak et al. 1992; Wegiel and Wisniewski 1990; Wisniewski et al. 1991, 1992). A variety of cells may contribute other constituents colocalized in plaques with Aβ, including $α_1$-antichymotrypsin (Abraham et al. 1988, 1989); apolipoprotein E (apoE) (Schmechel et al. 1993; Strittmatter et al. 1993a; Wisniewski and Frangione 1992); and complement components (Johnson et al. 1992).

■ Genetics of AD

The principal identified risk factors for AD are age and genetic influences. Several genetic loci have been linked to disease in early-onset familial AD (FAD). Mutations in APP at position 717 in APP-770 have been identified in 11 early-onset families; in these cases, mutations replace the normally occurring valine residue with either isoleucine, glycine, or phenylalanine (Chartier-Harlin et al. 1991; Goate et al. 1991; Hardy et al. 1991; Mullan et al. 1992). Two related Swedish families with early-onset FAD harbor a double mutation in the APP gene, which results in a substitution of Lys-Met to Asn-Leu at residues 670 and 671 (of APP-770). In addition, a mutation in the APP gene that encodes residue 693 of APP-770, in which a Glu is substituted by Gln, or at residue 692 of APP-770, in which Ala is substituted by Gly, has been linked to disease in two Dutch families with hereditary cerebral hemorrhage with amyloidosis-Dutch (HCHWA-D) (Hendriks et al. 1992; Levy et al. 1990).

In more than 80% of cases of early-onset FAD, a compelling linkage has been demonstrated to markers on chromosome 14 (Schellenberg et al. 1992; St George-Hyslop et al. 1992).

More recently, investigators have identified a genetic locus, thought to be apoE (positioned on the proximal long arm of chromosome 19), which shows linkage to late-onset and sporadic AD (Pericak-Vance et al. 1991; Schmechel et al. 1993; Strittmatter et al. 1993a, 1993b). ApoE, one of 10 apolipoproteins that mediate the metabolism of plasma lipoprotein particles (Breslow 1985), is a 34-kD glycoprotein. It is a principal component of very low- (LDL), intermediate-, and high-density lipoproteins and chylomicrons, which transport cholesterol and other lipids (Mahley 1988). ApoE, which serves as a ligand for receptor-mediated removal of lipoproteins from plasma (through both the LDL receptor and LDL receptor-related protein), is expressed at high levels in liver and brain, and a low level of apoE expression has been reported in virtually all other tissues. In the CNS, apoE is synthesized and secreted by astrocytes (Pitas et al. 1987a) and is upregulated in response to neuronal damage and deafferentation (Ignatius et al. 1986). ApoE is also a major apolipoprotein found in human CSF (Pitas et al. 1987b; Roheim et al. 1979), existing as small spherical and discoidal lipoproteins that transport cholesterol and phospholipids. It is likely that apoE is the major lipid carrier in the CSF.

The three major isoforms of apoE (i.e., apoE2, E3, and E4) are products of three alleles expressed at a single gene locus (Mahley 1988). The molecular basis for the apoE polymorphism is revealed at the level of amino acid sequence where, at codon 112, an arginine is substituted for the normally occurring cysteine. However, in apoE2, an additional cysteine substitution occurs at arginine 158 (Rall et al. 1982). Individuals with one or two copies of the apoE4 allele exhibit an increased risk for late-onset FAD and sporadic AD (Corder et al. 1993; Saunders et al. 1993; Strittmatter et al. 1993a). In patients with late-onset FAD, the E4 allelic frequency is 0.50 compared with 0.16 in age-matched control subjects (Strittmatter et al. 1993a), whereas in sporadic AD, apoE4 shows an allelic frequency of 0.40 (Saunders et al. 1993). In an autopsy series of cases of late-onset AD, there was a significant association between the apoE4 allele with increased parenchymal and vascular Aβ deposits (Schmechel et al. 1993).

ANIMAL MODELS

Aged Nonhuman Primates

Behavioral deficits that occur in aged nonhuman primates closely resemble those that occur in elderly humans (Presty et al. 1987; Rapp and Amaral 1992; Walker et al. 1988b). Our laboratory has behaviorally characterized a colony of rhesus monkeys ages 3–34 (Bachevalier et al. 1991; Presty et al. 1987). Behavioral tasks were chosen on the basis of previous research showing that the successful performance of each task requires the integrity of relatively specific regions of brain. The delayed nonmatching-to-sample task assesses visual object recognition memory. Performance deteriorates when memory is challenged by increasing delay and list length, and impairments in this task are most significant in the

oldest group of monkeys. Because successful performance of the delayed nonmatching-to-sample task depends on the integrity of the parahippocampal gyrus, hippocampus, inferior temporal cortex, ventromedial prefrontal cortex, medial thalamus, and basal forebrain cholinergic system (Aggleton and Mishkin 1983; Zola-Morgan and Squire 1986, 1989), aged monkeys showing deficits in recognition memory are thought to have lesions in one or more of these brain regions.

This cohort of monkeys was also tested on several other tasks, including delayed response (spatial learning), 24-hour concurrent discrimination learning (habit formation), route-following (visuospatial orientation), and a simple visual discrimination task. Declines in short-term memory on the delayed-response task appear when monkeys are in their late teens and early 20s (Bachevalier et al. 1991; Rapp and Amaral 1989). These spatial deficits suggest that abnormalities may exist in the dorsolateral prefrontal cortex and/or dorsal part of the caudate nucleus (Goldman et al. 1971; Passingham 1985). Aged rhesus monkeys are also impaired on a concurrent object discrimination task, which is a measure of habit formation (Bachevalier et al. 1991). This problem has been attributable to abnormalities of the inferior temporal cortex and, possibly, the caudoventral portion of the neostriatum (Mishkin and Appenzeller 1987). Aged monkeys are also less adept at performing a route-following test of visuospatial orientation (Bachevalier et al. 1991). In contrast, tests for simple visual discrimination detect no significant differences between young and old animals.

These behavioral investigations indicate that cognitive and memory deficits in rhesus monkeys appear in the late teens and become more evident in the mid- to late 20s (Bachevalier et al. 1991; Walker et al. 1988b). Impairments in performance of certain spatial abilities occur in some animals in their late teens; however, in other test categories, behavior is not altered until the 20s.

Neuronal Systems Vulnerable in Aged Nonhuman Primates

Aged monkeys exhibit brain abnormalities similar to those that occur in older humans and in individuals with AD (Abraham et al. 1989; Brizzee et al. 1980; Cork et al. 1990; Selkoe et al. 1987; Struble et al. 1982, 1985; Walker et al. 1987, 1988a, 1990; Wisniewski and Terry 1973b). The distributions and severities of the lesions vary among different animals of the same age. Performances on specific behavioral tasks are probably related, in some way yet to be determined, to patterns of these brain abnormalities in individual animals. In addition to neurites and Aβ deposits (see below), alterations occur in specific populations of neurons and in neurotransmitter markers. Prefrontal cortex has been reported to show a reduction in numbers of neurons (Brizzee et al. 1980). Cholinergic neurons are reduced in number in the medial septal nucleus (Stroessner-Johnson et al. 1992); however, the average size of these neurons is increased in aged animals. At caudal levels of the basal forebrain magnocellular complex, this difference is attributable to a disproportionate loss of small- to medium-sized neurons. But at rostral levels, there appears to be a genuine hypertrophy of cholinergic neurons noted only in the brains of behaviorally impaired aged monkeys (Stroessner-Johnson et al. 1992).

In older rhesus monkeys, cholinergic and monoaminergic markers are reduced in some regions of cortex (Beal et al. 1991; Goldman-Rakic and Brown 1981; Wagster et al. 1990; Wenk et al. 1989). ChAT activity is decreased in some regions in the oldest animals, and concentrations of both muscarinic and nicotinic receptor binding sites decline with increasing age (Beal et al. 1991; Wagster et al. 1990; Walker et al. 1988b). The brains of some older monkeys show decreased concentrations of dopamine and norepinephrine in certain regions of cortex (Beal et al. 1991; Goldman-Rakic and Brown 1981; Wenk et al. 1989). These studies suggest that alterations in certain neurotransmitter systems are partly responsible for cognitive impairments in some aged animals.

Cerebral Amyloidogenesis in Aged Monkeys

Aged monkeys (which provide an excellent model to examine alterations in the biology of APP that lead to Aβ amyloidogenesis) develop senile plaques, made up of neurites and deposits of Aβ, that are virtually identical to those that occur in aged humans and in individuals with AD (Abraham et al. 1989; Selkoe et al. 1987; Struble et al. 1985; Walker et al. 1987; Wisniewski and Terry 1973a, 1973b). Early in the third decade of life, rhesus monkeys develop enlarged neurites (i.e., distal axons, nerve terminals, and dendrites) as well as preamyloid deposits in the

parenchyma of cortex (Cork et al. 1990; Selkoe et al. 1987; Struble et al. 1982, 1985; Walker et al. 1988a; Wisniewski and Terry 1973b). These neurites are derived from cholinergic, monoaminergic, serotonergic, γ-aminobutyric acid (GABA)ergic, and peptidergic populations of neurons (Kitt et al. 1984, 1985, 1989; Walker et al. 1985, 1987, 1988a). In individual plaques, neurites may be derived from more than one transmitter-specific system (Walker et al. 1988a).

Neurites accumulate a variety of constituents, including membranous elements, mitochondria (some degenerating), lysosomes, APP, phosphorylated neurofilaments, acetylcholinesterase, transmitter markers, and synaptophysin (Martin et al. 1991). In individual plaques, APP- and synaptophysin-immunoreactive structures are often surrounded by a halo of distorted neuropil that, in adjacent sections, contain Aβ immunoreactivity. The presence of APP-like immunoreactivity in neuronal perikarya, axons, and some neurites within Aβ-containing plaques suggests that neurons (i.e., neurites, dendrites, and degenerating cell bodies) serve as one source for some of the Aβ deposited in the brains of these aged animals. The proximity of Aβ to reactive cells (including astrocytes and microglia) and to vascular elements suggests that several nonneuronal populations of cells participate in the formation of Aβ (Frackowiak et al. 1992; Martin et al. 1991; Masters et al. 1985a; Wisniewski et al. 1992).

Transgenic Mice

Transgenic approaches can directly test whether the overexpression of APP (wild type or mutant) or the expression of Aβ-containing fragments are involved in the pathogenesis of AD-type abnormalities. In the past several years, a variety of groups have attempted to produce mice with Aβ deposits using complementary DNA (cDNA)-based transgenic technologies (Kammesheidt et al. 1992; Kawabata et al. 1991; Lamb et al. 1993; Quon et al. 1991; Sandhu et al. 1991; Wirak et al. 1991). The published research is reviewed below. Unfortunately, although a variety of APP/C-99, -100/Aβ transgenic lines have been developed, with one possible exception (Quon et al. 1991), these animals have not developed the brain abnormalities characteristic of AD (Price and Sisodia 1994; Price et al. 1994). The failure of the initial efforts to generate a satisfactory model of AD may result in part from low levels of transgene expression in these lines of mice. Moreover, no mice with the overexpression of mutated APP have yet been described.

Because the overexpression of APP, as occurs in individuals with Down's syndrome, is thought to lead to the premature deposition of Aβ in the brain (Cork et al. 1990; Giaccone et al. 1989; Glenner and Wong 1984; Masters et al. 1985a, 1985b; Rumble et al. 1989), our colleagues Bruce Lamb and John Gearhart at Johns Hopkins hypothesized that transgenic mice overexpressing APP may mimic the trisomic APP dosage imbalance observed in people with Down's syndrome. Moreover, Lamb and Gearhart suggested that a complete genomic copy would lead to more faithful gene regulation in transgenic mice than have chimeric constructs. To pursue this idea, a yeast artificial chromosome (YAC) carrying the human APP gene that contained an ~650-kb human DNA fragment was identified, purified, and introduced through lipid-mediated transfection into embryonic stem (ES) cells (Lamb et al. 1993). Human APP sequences were stably integrated into ES cell chromosomes and exogenous APP mRNA, and encoded polypeptides were constitutively expressed. These ES cells were used to generate chimeric mice. Subsequent breeding disclosed that the human APP genomic sequences had been transmitted to the mouse germ line and that these sequences were actively transcribed in mouse tissue.

Significantly, the splicing pattern of human APP transcripts in transgenic mouse tissue mirrored the endogenous pattern of alternatively spliced mRNA. Reverse transcriptase-polymerase chain reaction assays, used to assess the relative levels of human and mouse APP mRNA, revealed that human APP mRNA is expressed in brain, heart, kidney, and testes at 80%, 13%, 40%, and 90% of endogenous APP mRNA levels, respectively. Western blot analysis, using an antibody specific for human APP, showed that significant levels of human APP were expressed in the brain, heart, kidney, and testes of this line of transgenic mice. The level of human APP in transgenic mouse brain was ~40% of total APP levels. Immunocytochemical studies with the human APP-specific antibody then disclosed human APP immunoreactivity in neurons in the brains of transgenic mice. These animals have yet to show evidence of AD-type pathology. However, the YAC-ES strategy can be used to introduce modified human APP YAC that encode FAD mutations into the mouse germ line. It can then be determined

whether the presence of these mutations are related directly to the etiology or pathogenesis and brain abnormalities that occur in cases of FAD. Finally, transgenic approaches can be used to introduce into mice the gene encoding human apoE4 and, when identified, the gene on chromosome 14 linked to FAD. These transgenic models will be invaluable in delineating the sequential cellular, biochemical, and molecular pathologies characteristic of AD.

■ CONCLUSION

This review has focused on the neurobiology of AD, emphasizing recent advances. Moreover, we have demonstrated how parallel investigations in humans, aged nonhuman primates, and APP transgenic mice will be critical in defining the relationships between alterations in behavioral performance and neuropathological or biochemical abnormalities in brain. The nonhuman primate is currently very useful for examining the role of age in some of the behavioral and brain abnormalities that resemble those occurring in patients with AD. Transgenic strategies, which have begun to show promise (Lamb et al. 1993; Quon et al. 1991; Sisodia and Price 1992), will be extremely valuable for producing models critical for determining the roles of genetic mechanisms that cause AD-type alterations in behavior and in brain structure and function. Moreover, when transgenic mice with deposits of Aβ become available to researchers, the strategies that have proved valuable in studying aged monkeys can be used in analyzing the mechanisms of pathology in mice. These models are essential if we are to understand the pathogenetic processes in age-associated disease and to test therapeutic approaches designed to improve age-related behavioral deficits in humans with AD.

■ REFERENCES

Abraham CR, Selkoe DJ, Potter H: Immunocytochemical identification of the serine protease inhibitor, α₁-antichymotrypsin, in the brain amyloid deposits of Alzheimer's disease. Cell 52:487–501, 1988

Abraham CR, Selkoe DJ, Potter H, et al: α₁-Antichymotrypsin is present together with the β-protein in monkey brain amyloid deposits.

Neuroscience 32:715–720, 1989

Aggleton JP, Mishkin M: Memory impairments following restricted medial thalamic lesions in monkeys. Exp Brain Res 52:199–209, 1983

Arendt T, Bigl V, Arendt A, et al: Loss of neurons in the nucleus basalis of Meynert in Alzheimer's disease, paralysis agitans, and Korsakoff's disease. Acta Neuropathol (Berl) 61:101–108, 1983

Arnold SE, Hyman BT, Flory J, et al: The topographical and neuroanatomical distribution of neurofibrillary tangles and neuritic plaques in the cerebral cortex of patients with Alzheimer's disease. Cereb Cortex 1:103–116, 1991

Arriagada PV, Growdon JH, Hedley-Whyte ET, et al: Neurofibrillary tangles but not senile plaques parallel duration and severity of Alzheimer's disease. Neurology 42:631–639, 1992

Atack JR: Cerebrospinal fluid neurochemical markers in Alzheimer's disease, in Biological Markers of Alzheimer's Disease. Edited by Boller F, Katzman R, Rascol A, et al. Berlin, Springer-Verlag, 1989, pp 1–160

Bachevalier J, Landis LS, Walker LC, et al: Aged monkeys exhibit behavioral deficits indicative of widespread cerebral dysfunction. Neurobiol Aging 12:99–111, 1991

Bachman DL, Wolf PA, Linn RT, et al: Incidence of dementia and probable Alzheimer's disease in a general population: the Framingham study. Neurology 43:515–519, 1993

Beal MF, Mazurek MF, Tran VT, et al: Reduced numbers of somatostatin receptors in the cerebral cortex in Alzheimer's disease. Science 229:289–291, 1985

Beal MF, Walker LC, Storey E, et al: Neurotransmitters in neocortex of aged rhesus monkeys. Neurobiol Aging 12:407–412, 1991

Blessed G, Tomlinson BE, Roth M: The association between quantitative measures of dementia and of senile changes in the cerebral gray matter of elderly subjects. Br J Psychiatry 144:797–811, 1968

Braak H, Braak E: Alzheimer's disease affects limbic nuclei of the thalamus. Acta Neuropathol (Berl) 81:261–268, 1991a

Braak H, Braak E: Neuropathological staging of Alzheimer-related changes. Acta Neuropathol (Berl) 82:239–259, 1991b

Breslow JL: Human apolipoprotein molecular biology and genetic variation. Annu Rev Biochem 54:699–727, 1985

Brizzee KR, Ordy JM, Bartus RT: Localization of cellular changes within multimodal sensory regions in aged monkey brain: possible implications for age-related cognitive loss. Neurobiol Aging 1:45–52, 1980

Busciglio J, Gabuzda DH, Matsudaira P, et al: Generation of β-amyloid in the secretory pathway in neuronal and nonneuronal cells. Proc Natl Acad Sci U S A 90:2092–2096, 1993

Chartier-Harlin M-C, Crawford F, Houlden H, et al: Early-onset Alzheimer's disease caused by mutations at codon 717 of the β-amyloid precursor protein gene. Nature 353:844–846, 1991

Corder EH, Saunders AM, Strittmatter WJ, et al: Gene dose of apoliprotein-E type 4 allele and the risk of Alzheimer's disease in late onset families. Science 261:921–923, 1993

Cork LC, Sternberger NH, Sternberger LA, et al: Phosphorylated neurofilament antigens in neurofibrillary tangles in Alzheimer's disease. J Neuropathol Exp Neurol 45:56–64, 1986

Cork LC, Masters C, Beyreuther K, et al: Development of senile plaques: relationships of neuronal abnormalities and amyloid deposits. Am J Pathol 137:1383–1392, 1990

Cras P, Kawai M, Lowery D, et al: Senile plaque neurites in Alzheimer disease accumulate amyloid precursor protein. Proc Natl Acad Sci U S A 88:7552–7556, 1991

Curcio CA, Kemper T: Nucleus raphe dorsalis in dementia of the Alzheimer type: neurofibrillary changes and neuronal packing density. J Neuropathol Exp Neurol 43:359–368, 1984

D'Amato RJ, Zweig RM, Whitehouse PJ, et al: Aminergic systems in Alzheimer's disease and Parkinson's disease. Ann Neurol 22:229–236, 1987

Davies P, Katzman R, Terry RD: Reduced somatostatin-like immunoreactivity in cerebral cortex from cases of Alzheimer disease and Alzheimer senile dementa. Nature 288:279–280, 1980

DeKosky ST, Scheff SW: Synapse loss in frontal cortex biopsies in Alzheimer's disease: correlation with cognitive severity. Ann Neurol 27:457–463, 1990

De Souza EB, Whitehouse PJ, Kuhar MJ, et al: Reciprocal changes in corticotropin-releasing factor (CRF)-like immunoreactivity and CRF receptors in cerebral cortex of Alzheimer's disease. Nature 319:593–595, 1986

Esch FS, Keim PS, Beattie EC, et al: Cleavage of amyloid β peptide during constitutive processing of its precursor. Science 248:1122–1124, 1990

Estus S, Golde TE, Kunishita T, et al: Potentially amyloidogenic, carboxyl-terminal derivatives of the amyloid protein precursor. Science 255:726–728, 1992

Evans DA, Funkenstein HH, Albert MS, et al: Prevalence of Alzheimer's disease in a community population of older persons higher than previously reported. JAMA 262:2551–2556, 1989

Ferrier IN, Cross AJ, Johnson JA, et al: Neuropeptides in Alzheimer type dementia. J Neurol Sci 62:159–170, 1983

Folstein MF, Folstein SE, McHugh PR: Mini-Mental State: a practical method for grading the cognitive state of patients for the clinician. J Psychiatr Res 12:189–198, 1975

Frackowiak J, Wisniewski HM, Wegiel J, et al: Ultrastructure of the microglia that phagocytose amyloid and the microglia that produce β-amyloid fibrils. Acta Neuropathol (Berl) 84:225–233, 1992

Francis PT, Palmer AM, Sims NR, et al: Neurochemical studies of early onset Alzheimer's disease: possible influence on treatment. N Engl J Med 313:7–11, 1985

Giaccone G, Tagliavini F, Linoli G, et al: Down patients: extracellular preamyloid deposits precede neuritic degeneration and senile plaques. Neurosci Lett 97:232–238, 1989

Glenner GG, Wong CW: Alzheimer's disease: initial report of the purification and characterization of a novel cerebrovascular amyloid protein. Biochem Biophys Res Commun 120:885–890, 1984

Goate A, Chartier-Harlin MC, Mullan M, et al: Segregation of a missense mutation in the amyloid precursor protein gene with familial Alzheimer's disease. Nature 349:704–706, 1991

Goedert M: Tau protein and the neurofibrillary pathology of Alzheimer's disease. Trends Neurosci 16:460–465, 1993

Golde TE, Estus S, Younkin LH, et al: Processing of the amyloid protein precursor to potentially amyloidogenic derivatives. Science 255:728–730, 1992

Goldman PS, Rosvold HE, Vest B, et al: Analysis of the delayed-alternation deficit produced by dorsolateral prefrontal lesions in the rhesus monkey. Journal of Comparative and Physiological Psychology 77:212–220, 1971

Goldman-Rakic PS, Brown RM: Regional changes of monoamines in cerebral cortex and subcortical structures of aging rhesus monkeys. Neuroscience 6:177–187, 1981

Greenberg SG, Davies P: A preparation of Alzheimer paired helical filaments that displays distinct τ proteins by polyacrylamide gel electrophoresis. Proc Natl Acad Sci U S A 87:5827–5831, 1990

Grundke-Iqbal I, Iqbal K, Quinlan M, et al: Microtubule-associated protein tau: a component of Alzheimer paired helical filaments. J Biol Chem 261:6084–6089, 1986

Haass C, Koo EH, Mellon A, et al: Targeting of cell-surface β-amyloid precursor protein to lysosomes: alternative processing into amyloid-bearing fragments. Nature 357:500–503, 1992a

Haass C, Schlossmacher MG, Hung AY, et al: Amyloid β-peptide is produced by cultured cells during normal metabolism. Nature 359:322–325, 1992b

Hamos JE, DeGennaro LJ, Drachman DA: Synaptic loss in Alzheimer's disease and other dementias. Neurology 39:355–361, 1989

Hardy J, Cowburn R, Barton A, et al: Region-specific loss of glutamate innervation in Alzheimer's disease. Neurosci Lett 73:77–80, 1987

Hardy J, Mullan M, Chartier-Harlin MC, et al: Molecular classification of Alzheimer's disease. Lancet 337:1342–1343, 1991

Hendriks L, van Duijn CM, Cras P, et al: Presenile dementia and cerebral haemorrhage linked to a mutation at codon 692 of the β-amyloid precursor protein gene. Nature Genetics 1:218–221, 1992

Herzog AG, Kemper TL: Amygdaloid changes in aging and dementia. Arch Neurol 37:625–629, 1980

Hyman BT, Van Hoesen GW, Damasio AR: Memory-related neural systems in Alzheimer's disease: an anatomic study. Neurology 40:1721–1730, 1990

Ignatius MJ, Gebicke-Härter PJ, Pate Skene JH, et al: Expression of apolipoprotein E during nerve degeneration and regeneration. Proc Natl Acad Sci U S A 83:1125–1129, 1986

Johnson SA, Lampert-Etchells M, Pasinetti GM, et al: Complement mRNA in the mammalian brain: responses to Alzheimer's disease and experimental brain lesioning. Neurobiol Aging 13:641–648, 1992

Kammesheidt A, Boyce FM, Spanoyannis AF, et al: Deposition of β/A4 immunoreactivity and neuronal pathology in transgenic mice expressing the carboxyterminal fragment of the Alzheimer amyloid precursor in the brain. Proc Natl Acad Sci U S A 89:10857–10861, 1992

Kang J, Lemaire HG, Unterbeck A, et al: The precursor of Alzheimer's disease amyloid A4 protein resembles a cell-surface receptor. Nature 325:733–736, 1987

Katzman R, Terry R, DeTeresa R, et al: Clinical, pathological, and neurochemical changes in dementia: a subgroup with preserved mental status and numerous neocortical plaques. Ann Neurol 23:138–144, 1988

Katzman R, Aronson M, Fuld P, et al: Development of dementing illnesses in an 80-year-old volunteer cohort. Ann Neurol 25:317–324, 1989

Kawabata S, Higgins GA, Gordon JW: Amyloid plaques, neurofibrillary tangles and neuronal loss in brains of transgenic mice overexpressing a C-terminal fragment of human amyloid precursor protein. Nature 354:476–478, 1991

Kemper T: Neuroanatomical and neuropathological changes in normal aging and in dementia. in Clinical Neurology of Aging. Edited by Albert ML. New York, Oxford University Press, 1984, pp 9–52

Khachaturian ZS: Diagnosis of Alzheimer's disease. Arch Neurol 42:1097–1105, 1985

Kitaguchi N, Takahashi Y, Tokushima Y, et al: Novel precursor of Alzheimer's disease amyloid protein shows protease inhibitory activity. Nature 331:530–532, 1988

Kitt CA, Price DL, Struble RG, et al: Evidence for cholinergic neurites in senile plaques. Science 226:1443–1445, 1984

Kitt CA, Struble RG, Cork LC, et al: Catecholaminergic neurites in senile plaques in prefrontal cortex of aged nonhuman primates. Neuroscience 16:691–699, 1985

Kitt CA, Walker LC, Molliver ME, et al: Serotoninergic neurites in senile plaques in cingulate cortex of aged nonhuman primate. Synapse 3:12–18, 1989

Koh JY, Yang LL, Cotman CW: β-amyloid protein increases the vulnerability of cultured cortical neurons to excitotoxic damage. Brain Res 553:315–320, 1990

Koo EH, Sisodia SS, Archer DR, et al: Precursor of amyloid protein in Alzheimer disease undergoes fast anterograde axonal transport. Proc Natl Acad Sci U S A 87:1561–1565, 1990a

Koo EH, Sisodia SS, Cork LC, et al: Differential expression of amyloid precursor protein mRNAs in cases of Alzheimer's disease and in aged nonhuman primates. Neuron 2:97–104, 1990b

Kosik KS, Joachim CL, Selkoe DJ: Microtubule-associated protein τ (tau) is a major antigenic component of paired helical filaments in Alzheimer disease. Proc Natl Acad Sci U S A 83:4044–4048, 1986

Lamb BT, Sisodia SS, Lawler AM, et al: Introduction and expression of the 400 kilobase *precursor amyloid protein* gene in transgenic mice. Nature Genetics 5:22–30, 1993

Lee VMY, Balin BJ, Otvos L Jr, et al: A68: a major subunit of paired helical filaments and derivatized forms of normal tau. Science 251:675–678, 1991

Levy E, Carman MD, Fernandez-Madrid IJ, et al: Mutation of the Alzheimer's disease amyloid gene in hereditary cerebral hemorrhage, Dutch type. Science 248:1124–1126, 1990

Mahley RW: Apolipoprotein E: cholesterol transport protein with expanding role in cell biology. Science 240:622–630, 1988

Martin LJ, Sisodia SS, Koo EH, et al: Amyloid precursor protein in aged nonhuman primates. Proc Natl Acad Sci U S A 88:1461–1465, 1991

Masliah E, Terry RD, DeTeresa RM, et al: Immunohistochemical quantification of the synapse-related protein synaptophysin in Alzheimer disease. Neurosci Lett 103:234–239, 1989

Masliah E, Terry RD, Alford M, et al: Quantitative immunohistochemistry of synaptophysin in human neocortex: an alternative method to estimate density of presynaptic terminals in paraffin sections. J Histochem Cytochem 38:837–844, 1990

Masliah E, Hansen L, Albright T, et al: Immunoelectron microscopic study of synaptic pathology in Alzheimer's disease. Acta Neuropathol (Berl) 81:428–433, 1991a

Masliah E, Mallory M, Hansen L, et al: Patterns of aberrant sprouting in Alzheimer's disease. Neuron 6:729–739, 1991b

Masliah E, Ellisman M, Carragher B, et al: Three-dimensional analysis of the relationship between synaptic pathology and neuropil threads in Alzheimer disease. J Neuropathol Exp Neurol 51:404–414, 1992

Masliah E, Mallory M, Hansen L, et al: Quantitative synaptic alterations in the human neocortex during normal aging. Neurology 43:192–197, 1993

Masters CL, Multhaup G, Simms G, et al: Neuronal origin of a cerebral amyloid: neurofibrillary tangles of Alzheimer's disease contain the same protein as the amyloid of plaque cores and blood vessels. EMBO J 4:2757–2763, 1985a

Masters CL, Simms G, Weinman NA, et al: Amyloid

plaque core protein in Alzheimer disease and Down syndrome. Proc Natl Acad Sci U S A 82:4245–4249, 1985b

McKee AC, Kosik KS, Kowall NW: Neuritic pathology and dementia in Alzheimer's disease. Ann Neurol 30:156–165, 1991

McKhann G, Drachman D, Folstein M, et al: Clinical diagnosis of Alzheimer's disease: report of the NINCDS-ADRDA Work Group under the auspices of Department of Health and Human Services Task Force on Alzheimer's Disease. Neurology 34:939–944, 1984

Mishkin M, Appenzeller T: The anatomy of memory: an inquiry into the roots of human amnesia has shown how deep structures in the brain may interact with perceptual pathways in outer brain layers to transform sensory stimuli into memories. Sci Am 256:80–89, 1987

Mullan M, Crawford F, Axelman K, et al: A pathogenic mutation for probable Alzheimer's disease in the APP gene at the N-terminus of β-amyloid. Nature Genetics 1:345–347, 1992

Nishimoto I, Okamoto T, Matsuura Y, et al: Alzheimer amyloid protein precursor complexes with brain GTP-binding protein G_o. Nature 362:75–79, 1993

Nordstedt C, Gandy SE, Alafuzoff I, et al: Alzheimer β/A4-amyloid precursor protein in human brain: aging associated increases in holoprotein and in a proteolytic fragment. Proc Natl Acad Sci U S A 88:8910–8914, 1991

Olshansky SJ, Carnes BA, Cassel CK: The aging of the human species. Sci Am 268:46–52, 1993

Passingham RE: Memory of monkeys (Macaca mulatta) with lesions in prefrontal cortex. Behav Neurosci 99:3–21, 1985

Pericak-Vance MA, Bebout JL, Gaskell PC Jr, et al: Linkage studies in familial Alzheimer's disease: evidence for chromosome 19 linkage. Am J Hum Genet 48:1034–1050, 1991

Perry G, Friedman R, Shaw G, et al: Ubiquitin is detected in neurofibrillary tangles and senile plaque neurites of Alzheimer disease brains. Proc Natl Acad Sci U S A 84:3033–3036, 1987

Perry G, Kawai M, Tabaton M, et al: Neuropil threads of Alzheimer's disease show a marked alteration of the normal cytoskeleton. J Neurosci 11:1748–1756, 1991

Perry RH, Candy JM, Perry EK, et al: Extensive loss of choline acetyltransferase activity is not reflected by neuronal loss in the nucleus of Meynert in Alzheimer's disease. Neurosci Lett 33:311–315, 1982

Pfeffer RI, Afifi AA, Chance JM: Prevalence of Alzheimer's disease in a retirement community. Am J Epidemiol 125:420–436, 1987

Pike CJ, Walencewicz AJ, Glabe CG, et al: Aggregation-related toxicity of synthetic β-amyloid protein in hippocampal cultures. Eur J Pharmacol 207:367–368, 1991

Pitas RE, Boyles JK, Lee SH, et al: Astrocytes synthesize apolipoprotein E and metabolize apolipoprotein E-containing lipoproteins. Biochim Biophys Acta 917:148–161, 1987a

Pitas RE, Boyles JK, Lee SH, et al: Lipoproteins and their receptors in the central nervous system. J Biol Chem 262:14352–14360, 1987b

Ponte P, Gonzalez-DeWhitt P, Schilling J, et al: A new A4 amyloid mRNA contains a domain homologous to serine proteinase inhibitors. Nature 331:525–532, 1988

Presty SK, Bachevalier J, Walker LC, et al: Age differences in recognition memory of the rhesus monkey (Macaca mulatta). Neurobiol Aging 8:435–440, 1987

Price DL, Sisodia SS: Cellular and molecular biology of Alzheimer's disease and animal models. Annu Rev Med 45:435–446, 1994

Price DL, Borchelt DR, Walker LC, et al: Toxicity of synthetic Aβ peptides and modeling of Alzheimer's disease. Neurobiol Aging 13:623–625, 1992a

Price DL, Martin LJ, Clatterbuck RE, et al: Neuronal degeneration in human diseases and animal models. J Neurobiol 23:1277–1294, 1992b

Price DL, Martin LJ, Sisodia SS, et al: The aged nonhuman primate: a model for the behavioral and brain abnormalities occurring in aged humans, in Alzheimer Disease. Edited by Terry RD, Katzman R, Bick KL. New York, Raven, 1994, pp 231–245

Probst A, Brunnschweiler H, Lautenschlager C, et al: A special type of senile plaque, possibly an initial stage. Acta Neuropathol (Berl) 74:133–141, 1987

Probst A, Langui D, Ipsen S, et al: Deposition of β/A4 protein along neuronal plasma membranes in diffuse senile plaques. Acta Neuropathol (Berl) 83:21–29, 1991

Quon D, Wang Y, Catalano R, et al: Formation of β-amyloid protein deposits in brains of transgenic mice. Nature 352:239–241, 1991

Rall SC, Weisgraber KH, Mahley RW: Human apolipoprotein E: the complete amino acid sequence. J

Biol Chem 257:4171–4178, 1982

Rapp PR, Amaral DG: Evidence for task-dependent memory dysfunction in the aged monkey. J Neurosci 9:3568–3576, 1989

Rapp PR, Amaral DG: Individual differences in the cognitive and neurobiological consequences of normal aging. Trends Neurosci 15:340–345, 1992

Roheim PS, Carey M, Forte T, et al: Apolipoproteins in human cerebrospinal fluid. Proc Natl Acad Sci U S A 76:4646–4649, 1979

Rossor MN, Emson PC, Mountjoy CQ, et al: Reduced amounts of immunoreactive somatostatin in the temporal cortex in senile dementia of Alzheimer type. Neurosci Lett 20:373–377, 1980

Rumble B, Retallack R, Hilbich C, et al: Amyloid A4 protein and its precursor in Down's syndrome and Alzheimer's disease. N Engl J Med 320:1446–1452, 1989

Saito KI, Elce JS, Hamos JE, et al: Widespread activation of calcium-activated neutral proteinase (calpain) in the brain in Alzheimer disease: a potential molecular basis for neuronal degeneration. Proc Natl Acad Sci U S A (in press)

Sandhu FA, Salim M, Zain SB: Expression of the human β-amyloid protein of Alzheimer's disease specifically in the brains of transgenic mice. J Biol Chem 266:21331–21334, 1991

Saunders AM, Strittmatter WJ, Schmechel D, et al: Association of apolipoprotein E allele ε4 with late-onset familial and sporadic Alzheimer's disease. Neurology 43:1467–1472, 1993

Scheff SW, Price DA: Synapse loss in the temporal lobe in Alzheimer's disease. Ann Neurol 33:190–199, 1993

Schellenberg GD, Bird TD, Wijsman EM, et al: Genetic linkage evidence for a familial Alzheimer's disease locus on chomosome 14. Science 258:668–671, 1992

Schmechel DE, Saunders AM, Strittmatter WJ, et al: Increased amyloid β-peptide deposition in cerebral cortex as a consequence of apolipoprotein E genotype in late-onset Alzheimer disease. Proc Natl Acad Sci U S A 90:9649–9653, 1993

Schubert D: The possible role of adhesion in synaptic modification. Trends Neurosci 14:127–130, 1991

Scott SA, DeKosky ST, Sparks DL, et al: Amygdala cell loss and atrophy in Alzheimer's disease. Ann Neurol 32:555–563, 1992

Selkoe DJ, Bell DS, Podlisny MB, et al: Conservation of brain amyloid proteins in aged mammals and humans with Alzheimer's disease. Science 235:873–877, 1987

Seubert P, Vigo-Pelfrey C, Esch F, et al: Isolation and quantification of soluble Alzheimer's β-peptide from biological fluids. Nature 359:325–327, 1992

Shoji M, Golde TE, Ghiso J, et al: Production of the Alzheimer amyloid β protein by normal proteolytic processing. Science 258:126–129, 1992

Sisodia SS: β-amyloid precursor protein cleavage by a membrane-bound protease. Proc Natl Acad Sci U S A 89:6075–6079, 1992

Sisodia SS, Price DL: Amyloidogenesis in Alzheimer's disease: basic biology and animal models. Curr Opin Neurobiol 2:648–652, 1992

Sisodia SS, Koo EH, Beyreuther K, et al: Evidence that β-amyloid protein in Alzheimer's disease is not derived by normal processing. Science 248:492–495, 1990

Sisodia SS, Koo EH, Hoffman PN, et al: Identification and transport of full-length amyloid precursor proteins in rat peripheral nervous system. J Neurosci 13:3136–3142, 1993

Slunt HH, Thinakaran G, von Koch C, et al: Expression of a ubiquitous, cross-reactive homologue of the mouse β-amyloid precursor protein (APP). J Biol Chem 269:2637–2644, 1994

St George-Hyslop P, Haines J, Rogaev E, et al: Genetic evidence for a novel familial Alzheimer's disease locus on chromosome 14. Nature Genetics 2:330–334, 1992

Strittmatter WJ, Saunders AM, Schmechel D, et al: Apolipoprotein E: high-avidity binding to β-amyloid and increased frequency of type 4 allele in late-onset familial Alzheimer disease. Proc Natl Acad Sci U S A 90:1977–1981, 1993a

Strittmatter WJ, Weisgraber KH, Huang DY, et al: Binding of human apolipoprotein E to synthetic amyloid β peptide: isoform-specific effects and implications for late-onset Alzheimer disease. Proc Natl Acad Sci U S A 90:8098–8102, 1993b

Stroessner-Johnson HM, Rapp PR, Amaral DG: Cholinergic cell loss and hypertrophy in the medial septal nucleus of the behaviorally characterized aged rhesus monkey. J Neurosci 12:1936–1944, 1992

Struble RG, Cork LC, Whitehouse PJ, et al: Cholinergic innervation in neuritic plaques. Science 216:413–415, 1982

Struble RG, Price DL Jr, Cork LC, et al: Senile plaques in cortex of aged normal monkeys. Brain Res

361:267–275, 1985

Struble RG, Lehmann J, Mitchell SJ, et al: Basal fore-brain neurons provide major cholinergic innervation of primate neocortex. Neurosci Lett 66:215–220, 1986

Struble RG, Powers RE, Casanova MF, et al: Neuropeptidergic systems in plaques of Alzheimer's disease. J Neuropathol Exp Neurol 46:567–584, 1987

Terry RD, Masliah E, Salmon DP, et al: Physical basis of cognitive alterations in Alzheimer's disease: synapse loss is the major correlate of cognitive impairment. Ann Neurol 30:572–580, 1991

Tomlinson BE, Irving D, Blessed G: Cell loss in the locus coeruleus in senile dementia of Alzheimer type. J Neurol Sci 49:419–428, 1981

Vogels OJM, Broere CAJ, Ter Laak HJ, et al: Cell loss and shrinkage in the nucleus basalis Meynert complex in Alzheimer's disease. Neurobiol Aging 11:3–13, 1990

Wagster MV, Whitehouse PJ, Walker LC, et al: Laminar organization and age-related loss of cholinergic receptors in temporal neocortex of rhesus monkey. J Neurosci 10:2879–2885, 1990

Walker LC, Kitt CA, Struble RG, et al: Glutamic acid decarboxylase-like immunoreactive neurites in senile plaques. Neurosci Lett 59:165–169, 1985

Walker LC, Kitt CA, Schwam E, et al: Senile plaques in aged squirrel monkeys. Neurobiol Aging 8:291–296, 1987

Walker LC, Kitt CA, Cork LC, et al: Multiple transmitter systems contribute neurites to individual senile plaques. J Neuropathol Exp Neurol 47:138–144, 1988a

Walker LC, Kitt CA, Struble RG, et al: The neural basis of memory decline in aged monkeys. Neurobiol Aging 9:657–666, 1988b

Walker LC, Masters C, Beyreuther K, et al: Amyloid in the brains of aged squirrel monkeys. Acta Neuropathol (Berl) 80:381–387, 1990

Wang R, Meschia JF, Cotter RJ, et al: Secretion of the β/A4 amyloid precursor protein: identification of a cleavage site in cultured mammalian cells. J Biol Chem 266:16960–16964, 1991

Wegiel J, Wisniewski HM: The complex of microglial cells and amyloid star in three-dimensional reconstruction. Acta Neuropathol (Berl) 81:116–124, 1990

Wenk GL, Pierce DJ, Struble RG, et al: Age-related changes in multiple neurotransmitter systems in the monkey brain. Neurobiol Aging 10:11–19, 1989

Whitehouse PJ, Price DL, Struble RG, et al: Alzheimer's disease and senile dementia: loss of neurons in the basal forebrain. Science 215:1237–1239, 1982

Whitehouse PJ, Martino AM, Antuono PG, et al: Nicotinic acetylcholine binding sites in Alzheimer's disease. Brain Res 371:146–151, 1986

Wirak DO, Bayney R, Ramabhadran TV, et al: Deposits of amyloid β protein in the central nervous system of transgenic mice. Science 253:323–325, 1991

Wisniewski T, Frangione B: Apolipoprotein E: a pathological chaperone protein in patients with cerebral and systemic amyloid. Neurosci Lett 135:235–238, 1992

Wisniewski HM, Terry RD: Morphology of the aging brain, human and animal. Prog Brain Res 40:167–186, 1973a

Wisniewski HM, Terry RD: Reexamination of the pathogenesis of the senile plaque, in Progress in Neuropathology, Vol II. Edited by Zimmerman HM. New York, Grune and Stratton, 1973b, pp 1–26

Wisniewski HM, Barcikowska M, Kida E: Phagocytosis of β/A4 amyloid fibrils of the neuritic neocortical plaques. Acta Neuropathol (Berl) 81:588–590, 1991

Wisniewski HM, Wegiel J, Wang KC, et al: Ultrastructural studies of the cells forming amyloid in the cortical vessel wall in Alzheimer's disease. Acta Neuropathol (Berl) 84:117–127, 1992

Yankner BA, Dawes LR, Fisher S, et al: Neurotoxicity of a fragment of the amyloid precursor associated with Alzheimer's disease. Science 245:417–420, 1989

Zola-Morgan S, Squire LR: Memory impairment in monkeys following lesions limited to the hippocampus. Behav Neurosci 100:155–160, 1986

Zola-Morgan S, Squire LR, Amaral DG, et al: Lesions of perirhinal and parahippocampal cortex that spare the amygdala and hippocampal formation produce severe memory impairment. J Neurosci 9:4355–4370, 1989

Zweig RM, Ross CA, Hedreen JC, et al: The neuropathology of aminergic nuclei in Alzheimer's disease. Ann Neurol 24:233–242, 1988

26

Biology of Psychoactive Substance Dependence Disorders: Opiates, Cocaine, and Ethanol

Roger E. Meyer, M.D.

■ NOSOLOGICAL CONSIDERATIONS

Psychoactive substance dependence disorders have been defined as a "cluster of cognitive, behavioral, and physiological symptoms that indicate that the person has impaired control of psychoactive substance use and continues use of the substance despite adverse consequences" (DSM-III-R [American Psychiatric Association 1987], p. 166). The symptoms of the dependence syndrome are principally behavioral, as they have been described in DSM-III-R and in ICD-10 (World Health Organization 1992), with a focus on drug-seeking and drug-consuming behaviors. These core symptoms are the same across all categories of substances, recognizing that the physiological symptoms of drug withdrawal may be a part of the syndrome for certain substances (e.g., alcohol and opiates) but less significant for other

substances (e.g., cocaine and other stimulants).

It is possible for patients to manifest tolerance and withdrawal symptoms without manifesting the critical behavioral symptoms of the dependence syndrome. These patients would not be diagnosed as substance dependent according to DSM-III-R or ICD-10. Both ICD-10 and DSM-III-R recognize the persistent risk of relapse in continuing to diagnose substance dependence in individuals who are "currently abstinent" (in the case of ICD-10) or in "full remission" for 6 months or longer (DSM-III-R). ICD-10 notes "evidence that return to substance use after a period of abstinence leads to a more rapid reappearance of other features of the (dependence) syndrome than occurs with non-dependent individuals" (p. 75). In summary, the core dependence syndrome is defined on the basis of drug-seeking behavior that continues despite adverse consequences and that includes a persistent risk of relapse following withdrawal.

Supported in part by grants from the National Institute on Alcohol Abuse and Alcoholism (#P50 AA 03 510-16), the John D. and Catherine T. MacArthur Foundation (#8900078), and the Center for Advanced Study in the Behavioral Sciences (FFRP Fund).

■ ISSUES OF INDIVIDUAL VULNERABILITY AND RISK

Physicians have been intrigued with the causes of addictive disorders for over 200 years (Rush 1791). For most of this century (in the case of illegal drugs) and during Prohibition (in the case of alcohol), public policy derived from the perspective that the problem of addiction and its consequences was largely a function of the "power" of the substance to overwhelm an individual. Efforts to understand addiction focused on the problem of physical dependence and the use of drugs to self-medicate the distressing symptoms of withdrawal (Wikler 1965). Until recently, many psychiatrists focused on addictive disorders as mere epiphenomena—self-medication to treat underlying psychopathology (Meyer 1986b). In the past 15 years, nosologists have attempted to differentiate substance dependence disorders from "substance abuse" (DSM-III [American Psychiatric Association 1980] and DSM-III-R), harmful use (ICD-10), or hazardous use (e.g., "problem drinking").

Although substance use constitutes a risk factor for the development of substance dependence disorders, the latter develops in the context of individual risk factors (e.g., family history, some types of psychopathology, etc.), the environment, and the reinforcing potency (and mode of self-administration) of the drug. In clinical populations of alcoholic individuals, those with antisocial personality disorder report an earlier onset of drinking and a more rapid progression to alcohol dependence than individuals without antisocial personality disorder (Hesselbrock et al. 1986). In countries where per capita alcohol consumption is high (e.g., France), it is less common to find significant comorbid psychopathology among treated alcoholic patients than in countries where per capita alcohol consumption is low (e.g., Taiwan) (Babor et al. 1992; Helzer et al. 1990). As a general rule, psychopathology does not serve as a significant risk factor for substance use (or heavy use) in those cultures or environments where substance use (or heavy use) is normative.

Family history of alcoholism appears to be a risk factor for the development of alcohol dependence on the basis of some still unspecified heritable risk factors (Cotton 1979). Several characteristics identified in sons of alcoholic individuals (e.g., electrophysiological markers and sensitivity to alcohol) have been studied to determine their relationship to the risk of alcohol dependence in these individuals (Begleiter et al. 1984; Schuckit 1984). Behavioral characteristics of children in first- and third-grade classrooms (e.g., shy aggressiveness) suggest an early sign of vulnerability to the later development of alcoholism (Kellam et al. 1983). This may or may not be related to the risk associated with childhood conduct disorder, a risk factor connected with the development of antisocial personality disorder (as well as alcoholism) in adults (Robins 1966), and/or to the heritable Type II subtype of alcoholism associated with a family history of criminality (Cloninger et al. 1981).

In general, research on individual biological and behavioral risk factors associated with alcohol dependence has proceeded much further than efforts to identify individual risk factors related to other types of substance dependence. In contrast, alcohol is a less potent reinforcer in animal models than are opiates or stimulants. Moreover, the route of alcohol self-administration reduces reinforcing potency, whereas intravenous use or smoking of heroin or cocaine enhances reinforcing potency. It is likely that mode of administration is a major risk factor for the development of dependence among users of heroin and cocaine and may be a very significant factor in the rate of progression from use to dependence. At the same time, individual risk factors appear to play some role; "most people who use addictive drugs never come for treatment" because use does not progress to dependence (Jones 1992, p. 109). Further research is clearly needed to identify the biological, psychological, and social characteristics of individuals who progress from drug experimentation to drug dependence. There is a need to identify the biology of risk of drug and alcohol dependence as we begin to clarify the neurobiology of drug reinforcement.

■ BEHAVIORAL NEUROBIOLOGY OF DRUG-SEEKING BEHAVIOR

Of all the diagnostic categories within ICD-10 and DSM-III-R, animal models come closest to specific human disorders in the "drug-seeking behavior" identified as the core element in substance dependence disorders. This section focuses on homologous animal models of opiate, cocaine, and ethanol self-administration, and the biological correlates of this behavior. In general, over the past 30 years, we have gained substantial understanding of drugs as reinforcers. But there are persistent questions regarding the specific "neuroadaptive" changes consequent to chronic drug self-administration that result in human drug dependence, and the persistent risk of relapse following drug withdrawal.

■ Drug Self-Administration Behavior

Weeks (1963) initially developed an animal model of intravenous drug self-administration. Restrained and freely moving rats and monkeys have been chronically catheterized (via intravenous catheter) for study in operant paradigms in which the animals are rewarded with a drug injection consequent to the performance of a task (usually some type of lever-pressing activity). Using this self-administration procedure, researchers have demonstrated that intravenous opiates (Weeks 1963), cocaine (Woods and Schuster 1968), and intragastric ethanol (Yanagita et al. 1969) all serve as reinforcers of operant behavior in monkeys. With the exception of ethanol (see following section), the intravenous self-administration of these drugs will also serve as reinforcers in rats.

Over time, the operant behavior associated with opiate or stimulant self-administration comes under stimulus control; that is, the behavior occurs at those times that the animal has learned that the drug will be "available." Moreover, if the dose per injection is lowered, the animal will increase operant work output to receive more injections (Koob and Bloom 1988). If the dose per injection is increased, operant work output will decrease. When access to opiates or stimulants is limited to several hours per day, animals will maintain a stable level of drug intake within a limited range of doses (Schuster and Thompson 1969). In contrast, under conditions of continuous access, animals will self-administer cocaine to the point of death (Deneau et al. 1969) or will develop substantial tolerance and physical dependence to opiates (Martin et al. 1963). The behavior of monkeys and rats in intravenous opiate, cocaine, and stimulant self-administration paradigms is strikingly homologous to behavioral patterns of human drug dependence (Wise and Bozarth 1987).

■ Animal Models of Alcohol Self-Administration

Although a number of animal models of alcohol consumption have been developed over the past 25 years, there is general consensus that no animal model fully satisfies all of the criteria for an animal model of alcohol dependence. The critical first step in the development of an animal model of alcoholism involves the initiation and maintenance of oral alcohol self-administration; alcohol-related reinforcement must be associated with its pharmacological effects, not its nutritional value. Two conclusions can be derived from a review of the literature on animal models of alcohol consumption: alcohol consumption can be significantly affected by schedules of reinforcement and/or by association with other reinforcers, and alcohol consumption is influenced significantly by pharmacogenetic factors.

Selective breeding of rats that differ in their ethanol-drinking behavior has resulted in at least three groups of rats that strongly differ in their spontaneous drinking or avoidance of alcohol (Eriksson 1971; Li et al. 1987, 1991). The development of these stable traits of preferential alcohol drinking or avoidance has further enabled researchers to examine neurobiological differences in alcohol-preferring (P) rats and nonpreferring (NP) rats. The P rats will drink a 10% ethanol solution in a free-choice paradigm (Li et al. 1987). They will bar press for an ethanol reward in a traditional operant paradigm, they will self-administer ethanol via an intragastric catheter, and they will consume sufficient amounts of alcohol to display physical dependence (Waller et al. 1984). At this juncture, there is good evidence that the P rats consume ethanol for its pharmacological effects, apart from its caloric value (Waller et al. 1984). P rats have lower levels of serotonin in several regions of the central nervous system, and lower levels of both dopamine and serotonin in the nucleus accumbens (NA), when compared with NP rats (Li et al. 1988). The potential significance of these neurochemical data is described in subsequent sections on the neurobiology of drug reinforcement.

Three behavioral paradigms have been developed to initiate alcohol consumption in animals not specifically bred for alcohol preference. Falk and colleagues (1972) induced high levels of alcohol consumption in rats using schedule-induced polydipsia. Unfortunately, alcohol drinking in this paradigm does not appear to be related to the pharmacological effects of ethanol. The sucrose- or saccharine-fading technique pairs sweet taste with alcohol consumption to facilitate initiation of drinking in rats not bred for ethanol preference (Samson 1986). When a stable pattern of consumption has been attained with a 10% ethanol solution, the sweet taste is gradually withdrawn, but the high levels of alcohol consumption continue. In general, the sucrose- or saccharine-fading technique produces stable alcohol-drinking behavior and moderate blood alcohol levels. The persistence of alcohol consumption appears to be related to the pharmacological effects of ethanol. Another technique that has been designed to produce moderate blood alcohol levels is the limited access paradigm in which rats are exposed to alcohol for a limited time (20 minutes) in a novel environment during their light cycle. Blood alcohol levels of 80 mg% have been obtained with this procedure (Gill et al. 1986).

In general, the stability of alcohol-drinking behavior in some of these models permits the analysis of biological correlates of alcohol reinforcement in freely moving animals, as described in the next section. It is now possible to compare the biological correlates of alcohol reinforcement in these paradigms with the mechanisms of stimulant and opiate reinforcement in intravenous drug self-administration paradigms. Additionally, intracerebral drug and alcohol self-administration procedures have provided additional insights on brain mechanisms involved in drug and alcohol reinforcement, as will be described.

■ CONDITIONED PLACE PREFERENCE PARADIGMS

Clinicians have long noted that abstinent patients are more likely to experience "craving" leading to relapse in settings or circumstances previously associated with drug use. Although this has been explained on the basis of several different models of conditioning (see next section), it is curious that these patients purposely reexpose themselves to these high-risk settings despite the contrary advice of their clinicians. It is almost as though the setting previously associated with drug use has been paired to the reinforcing properties of the drug through classical conditioning. In this context, the "place preference" demonstrated

by the abstinent patient is a measure of the reinforcing potency of previous drug experiences. Conditioned place preference paradigms in animals involve an initial determination of spontaneous place preference within a maze or open field. This is followed by the pairing of a drug injection with nonpreferred locations in the maze or open field. By a process of classical conditioning, the animal comes to prefer the setting in which drug administration has occurred. Place preference paradigms have been useful in examining the effects of pharmacological treatments in blocking or enhancing the reinforcing properties of addictive drugs (e.g., Brown et al. 1991).

■ BRAIN STIMULATION REWARD PARADIGMS

Brain stimulation reward (BSR) paradigms build on the observation that animals will press a lever to obtain electrical stimulation in certain brain regions (Olds and Milner 1954). In 1957, Killam and colleagues reported that some substances of abuse increased the response rate for brain stimulation in an operant paradigm. Additionally, they suspected that amphetamine also lowered the threshold of electrical current sufficient to reinforce BSR behavior. In general, the effects of drugs on BSR may vary as a function of whether the investigator is reporting changes in the rate of responding for BSR or changes in the threshold of electrical current that is reinforcing in this paradigm. Moreover, different results may be accounted for by differences in site selection for electrode implantation. The median forebrain bundle (MFB) and the ventral tegmental area (VTA) are the most common sites for electrode placement, although self-stimulation behavior can be elicited from other regions of the brain.

Just as opiates and cocaine are more potent reinforcers than alcohol in drug self-administration paradigms, these drugs also more reliably increase the sensitivity of animals to rewarding electrical brain stimulation. This is manifest most clearly by a decrease in threshold of the electrical impulse required for reinforcement (Kornetsky and Porrino 1992). The effects of ethanol on BSR have been a bit more problematic (e.g., Schaefer and Michael 1987 compared with DeWitte and Bada 1983). Bain and Kornestky (1989) found that response rate was increased and

BSR threshold was lowered only if animals orally self-administered ethanol. Moolten and Kornetsky (1990) replicated this finding in comparing BSR results in animals who self-administered ethanol via intragastric catheter compared with yoked animals receiving ethanol via intragastric catheter in the same dose and time. Only self-administered ethanol reliably lowered BSR thresholds. Lewis (1991) found that low doses (but not higher doses) of ethanol given intraperitoneally reduced BSR thresholds in the ventral noradrenergic bundle (VNB), but not at electrodes placed in the lateral hypothalamus (LH). Kornetsky and colleagues placed electrodes in the MFB at the level of the lateral hypothalamus. The low doses of ethanol administered by Lewis were comparable to doses self-administered by Kornetsky's group and produced motoric stimulation rather than the suppression of motor activity found at higher doses. Lewis's data are also compatible with the psychomotor stimulant theory of addiction proposed by Wise and Bozarth (1987; see next section).

BSR has been used in studies of combined opiate-stimulant administration to demonstrate more profound effects from the drug combination (regarding reinforcing potency) than from the individual drug alone (Kornetsky and Porrino 1992). It has also been used to study the persistent (anhedonic) state following cocaine and other stimulant withdrawal (see next section). Although cocaine or other stimulant drug administration produces a decrease in BSR threshold, the withdrawal state following stimulant administration is characterized by a substantial elevation in BSR threshold (Koob 1992a).

Finally, BSR has been used as a paradigm to investigate the neurochemical basis for drug reinforcement. Kornetsky and Porrino (1992) have reported that naloxone (a narcotic blocking drug) appeared to block or attenuate the threshold lowering effects of a variety of stimulants, when naloxone was administered prior to the stimulant. A dose of 2–4 mg/kg was required for this effect of naloxone, whereas doses as low as 0.25 mg/kg would block the threshold lowering effects of morphine. They also reported that pimozide (0.15 mg/kg) blocked the threshold lowering effects of 2.0 mg/kg of morphine. They concluded that "although the abused psychomotor stimulants and opioids have independent actions that contribute to their reinforcing effects, there are common neuronal substrates for some of the rewarding effects" (p. 74).

There is now substantial evidence linking reward mechanisms in BSR to dopamine systems. Moreover, most investigators would agree that mesolimbic dopamine neurons mediate the reinforcement characteristics of different classes of drugs of abuse, but that other neurotransmitters and receptors play a significant role in the reinforcement properties of opiates and alcohol, for example.

■ CELLULAR AND MOLECULAR MECHANISMS OF DRUG- AND ALCOHOL-SEEKING BEHAVIOR

Given the identical behavioral criteria for substance dependence disorders across drug classes and the evidence of reinforcement associated with most opiate, cocaine, and ethanol self-administration in animals, there is interest in identifying the common cellular and molecular mechanisms that might account for drug-seeking and drug-consuming behaviors across drug classes. As one can imagine, just as animal models of opiate and cocaine self-administration are clearer than the models of alcohol consumption discussed previously, the picture is a bit clearer regarding biological mechanisms of opiate and cocaine reinforcement than for reinforcement mechanisms associated with alcohol.

■ Neurobiology of Stimulant Reinforcement

In 1987, Wise and Bozarth proposed a theory of addiction based on the neurobiology of psychomotor stimulant reinforcement. They argued that

> all addictive drugs have psychomotor stimulant actions, that the stimulant actions of these different drugs have a shared biological mechanism, and that the biological mechanism of these stimulant actions is homologous with the biological mechanisms of positive reinforcement. (p. 469)

They built their model on the theory of reinforcement of Glickman and Schiff (1967), who observed that electrical stimulation of the MFB elicited approach behaviors as well as positive reinforcement. Wise and Bozarth argued that the increased locomotor activity results from activation of the dopaminergic cells of the VTA and substantia nigra, and reinforcement is mediated by effects on dopamine neurons in the VTA and NA.

The evidence for a primary role for dopamine neurons in the reinforcing properties of drugs is strongest in the case of cocaine and other stimulant drugs. Parenteral administration of dopamine receptor antagonists results in increased stimulant self-administration (Yokel and Wise 1975), much as lowering the dose injection of amphetamine or cocaine will result in increased lever pressing for the stimulant drug (see previous discussion). Both D_1 and D_2 receptor subtypes have been implicated in cocaine reinforcement (Koob 1992b). Cocaine binds to the dopamine transporter and effectively blocks dopamine reuptake (Ritz et al. 1987). The model is also supported by data from lesion studies (e.g., Roberts et al. 1980). Drug-naive rats will not learn to self-administer stimulant drugs, and stimulant drug self-administration will be extinguished following lesioning of dopamine neurons in the NA or the VTA with 6-hydroxydopamine. Lesions of the caudate nucleus are relatively ineffective unless accompanied by damage to the NA.

More recently, the model has been supported by data using in vivo microdialysis in the NA. Extracellular dopamine concentrations in the NA are increased by intraperitoneal or intravenously self-administered cocaine and amphetamine (DiChiara and Imperato 1988; Weiss et al. 1992). All of these data, together with studies of BSR, strongly argue for a primary role for dopamine neurons in the biology of stimulant drug reinforcement. From a neuroanatomical perspective, Koob (1992a) notes the relative paucity of data regarding the efferent mechanisms through which the NA may mediate positive reinforcement. Koob suggests that the connection between the NA and the substantia innominata–ventral pallidum may be important in this regard. He also suggests a role for the amygdala system as a mediator of drug reinforcement and reward.

■ Neurobiology of Opiate Reinforcement

It has been known for some time that opiates have primary reinforcing properties that are not dependent on the presence of physical dependence (Schuster and Villareal 1968). Bozarth and Wise (1984) demonstrated the neurobiology of this phenomenon in an apparently unequivocal manner. Drug-naive rats rap-

idly learned to press a lever for microinjections of morphine directly into the VTA. Naloxone challenges failed to elicit the signs of physical dependence in these rats following the morphine injections. Moreover, signs of withdrawal were not seen after long-term morphine infusion in the VTA but were observed after chronic infusion into the periventricular gray region. The data strongly suggested that the pathways mediating opiate reinforcement (e.g., the VTA) were independent of pathways mediating the signs of opiate withdrawal. In addition to the VTA, opiates also act as reinforcers in the NA (Almaric and Koob 1985).

More recently, Koob (1992b) demonstrated that chronic morphine administration results in sensitization of specific brain regions to the effects of direct injections of opiate antagonists. These regions include the NA and the locus ceruleus (LC). Direct placement of a narcotic antagonist in the NA in morphine-dependent rats results in the disruption of food-motivated behaviors and conditioned place aversion. The LC is sensitive to the acute effects of opiates (resulting in a suppression of LC activity), as well as to the effects of opiate withdrawal (characterized by a large increase in LC activity; clonidine suppresses LC activity and is used to treat opiate withdrawal). Thus, it is clear that some neurons are affected both by the acute effects of opiates as well as by opiate withdrawal. The data are consistent with the view that although opiates will serve as reinforcers in the absence of physical dependence, the "motivation" for opiate self-administration is enhanced during opiate withdrawal.

There is evidence that opiate reinforcement involves activation of dopamine neurons, but through a different mechanism than reinforcement associated with stimulant administration. As with stimulants, the parenteral administration of opiates results in an increase in extracellular dopamine concentrations in the NA, as measured by in vivo microdialysis (DiChiara and Imperato 1988; Weiss et al.1992). However, although lesioning of dopamine neurons in the NA (with 6-hydroxydopamine) eliminates stimulant self-administration (as discussed previously), it fails to eliminate opiate self-administration in rats (Koob and Bloom 1988). Opiates may increase the firing rate of dopamine neurons by activating μ-receptors in the VTA and NA producing local disinhibitory effects on the dopamine neurons. Naloxone blocks the effects of opiates on the VTA (Britt and Wise 1983). Koob

(1992a) theorizes that the downstream circuitry from the NA to the substantia innominata–ventral pallidum is important in opiate and stimulant reinforcement.

As was described previously, Wise and Bozarth (1987) have postulated that the reinforcing properties of opiates are mediated by the same mechanisms mediating forward movement and reward for stimulant drugs. For opiates and other depressant drugs, these motoric properties are manifest most clearly at low doses, and subsequent to the development of tolerance to the depressant effects. In contrast to the development of tolerance to the depressant effects of opiates, chronic administration of these drugs results in increased sensitization to their reinforcing properties. Chronic cocaine administration is also characterized by the development of sensitization (reverse tolerance) to the reinforcing properties of the drug. Recent work suggests that chronic opiate and stimulant administration affects gene expression of guanine nucleotide-binding proteins (G proteins) and the cyclic adenosine monophosphate (cAMP) system (see next section). These changes in the molecular biology of second messenger function may be related to the development of sensitization to the reinforcing properties of opiates (and stimulants).

■ Neurobiology of Alcohol Reinforcement

Several lines of evidence suggest that opioid peptides, serotonin, dopamine, and γ-aminobutyric acid (GABA) are all involved in alcohol reinforcement (Koob and Bloom 1988). Pharmacological probes in the context of animal models of ethanol self-administration represent one line of research. Alcohol self-administration is enhanced in association with morphine, whereas narcotic antagonists decrease ethanol drinking (Reid and Hunter 1984). It is unclear whether the effects of narcotic antagonists upon alcohol consumption are more or less specific to alcohol, because narcotic antagonists have a general inhibitory effect on consumatory behavior. Nevertheless, one immediate implication of this experimental work has been the testing of the narcotic antagonist naltrexone in alcohol-dependent human subjects, where it has turned out to be a promising adjunct to behavioral relapse prevention treatment (O'Malley et al. 1992; Volpicelli et al. 1992).

P rats show a relative deficit of serotonin (compared with NP rats; Murphy et al. 1982), and patients with alcoholism show a relative deficit of 5-hydroxyindoleacetic acid (5-HIAA, the principal metabolite of serotonin) in cerebrospinal fluid (CSF) (Ballenger et al. 1979). Low levels of CSF 5-HIAA have also been reported in one group of impulsive individuals who are at high risk for alcoholism (Linnoila et al. 1989). Alcohol increases 5-HIAA levels in NA and other brain regions (suggesting a role for serotonin in alcohol reinforcement; Murphy et al. 1988). Serotonin uptake inhibitors reduce alcohol consumption in animal models and, to a modest degree, in heavy-drinking human subjects (see Naranjo et al. 1987). Paradoxically, the results of a variety of serotonin depletion studies in animal models have failed to establish a consistent finding (summarized by Weiss and Koob 1991). The serotonin story is obviously complex and may become clearer as a result of greater understanding of receptor subtypes and their function. Alcohol may differentially affect one or more receptor subtypes.

A possible role for dopamine in the reinforcing properties of ethanol is suggested by studies of alcohol-preferring rats (P rats versus NP rats), by studies of the effects of dopamine receptor antagonists on alcohol consumption in one of the animal behavioral models (described previously), and by in vivo microdialysis measures of dopamine and/or dopamine metabolites in NA following alcohol administration. Murphy and colleagues (1982) have reported lower levels of dopamine in the NA of P rats compared with that of NP rats. Pfeffer and Samson (1988) have reported that dopamine receptor antagonists reduce operant behavior for alcohol, as well as alcohol consumption, in rats studied in the sucrose-fading procedure. DiChiara and Imperato (1988) reported that intraperitoneal injections of alcohol produced an increase in extraneuronal concentrations of dopamine in the NA, much as injections of other drugs of abuse studied by these investigators.

Not all investigators have observed this effect of alcohol (Vavrousek-Jakuba et al. 1990). However, two groups of investigators have found that alcohol self-administration results in increases in extraneuronal dopamine levels in NA (Vavrousek-Jakuba et al. 1990; Weiss et al. 1992). These results are remarkably similar to the findings of Kornetsky's group on the effects of self-administered ethanol on BSR thresholds (described previously). Weiss and colleagues also found strain differences in dopamine release by self-administered ethanol. Although average ethanol intake and blood alcohol levels were equivalent in

P rats compared with genetically heterogeneous Wistar rats, self-administered ethanol produced a significantly greater increase in dopamine release in the P rats than in the Wistar rats.

Finally, there is some clinical evidence that alcohol is reinforcing in some individuals on the basis of its anxiolytic and intoxicating effects (summarized by Meyer 1986a). There is a good bit of evidence that the anxiolytic effects of alcohol are mediated through its effects on the benzodiazepine (BZ)/GABA receptor. As is described in a later section, in vitro studies of synaptoneurosomes show that alcohol increases chloride flux through the ion channel that is the second messenger of this receptor. Although the mechanism of alcohol's effects is different than for BZs, the net effect—increased chloride flux—is the same. Suzdak and colleagues (1986) have reported that this effect of alcohol was blocked by the BZ partial inverse agonist Ro 15-4513. Of interest to studies on the neurobiology of alcohol reinforcement is the report of Samson and colleagues (1987) that Ro 15-4513 also produced a dose-dependent reduction in alcohol consumption in rats in the sucrose-fading procedure.

■ Neurobiology of Stimulant, Opiate, and Ethanol Reinforcement: Summary

The last decade has been marked by substantial progress in understanding the neurobiology of drug reinforcement. Commencing with robust animal models of intravenous (and later with region-specific intracerebral) opiate and stimulant self-administration (plus several different pharmacogenetic and behavioral models of voluntary oral alcohol consumption), neurobiologists have employed a range of techniques to describe the neurobiological events associated with drug-seeking and -consuming behavior. These range from lesion studies to pharmacological challenge strategies, electrophysiological studies, and in vivo microdialysis methods. The data argue strongly for a major role for dopamine neurons in the NA in the neurobiology of drug and alcohol reinforcement. It is still unclear what changes occur in the NA and its circuits that may account for the high risk of relapse following drug or alcohol withdrawal. The latter would appear to be a problem that is a synergism of two elements: a tendency to use again after a period of abstinence, and (as described in ICD-10) the rapid reinstatement of the elements of the dependence syndrome following the reinitiation of use.

■ BIOBEHAVIORAL THEORIES OF RELAPSE AND RAPID REINSTATEMENT OF DEPENDENCE

Biobehavioral theories that have been invoked to explain relapse and rapid reinstatement of dependence can be grouped into two general categories: conditioning models and homeostatic models. Although conditioning models date back to Pavlov (1926), they were developed most clearly by an American psychiatrist, Abraham Wikler. Conditioning models posit that relapse into drug or alcohol use occurs in those environments or circumstances that have been associated with past drug or alcohol use as a function of Pavlovian conditioning (discussed later in this chapter). Homeostatic models postulate that chronic substance use results in a perturbation of homeostatic mechanisms, such that the addicted individual requires continued use of the substance to maintain homeostasis. The latter is most clearly valid in the context of acute opiate and alcohol withdrawal syndromes (where the preferred drug reverses the symptoms and signs of withdrawal). But the high rate of relapse to opiate, cocaine, and alcohol use in the first 3 to 6 months following withdrawal has suggested the persistence of deficient homeostasis. This has been called "protracted abstinence" (Martin and Jasinski 1969, p. 7). To some extent, both models postulate an antecedent subjective state ("craving," or "desire") that serves as a trigger to drug-seeking behavior, much as hunger serves as a trigger for eating. The models are not mutually exclusive; both may be important in conceptualizing new approaches to treatment (including pharmacotherapy).

■ Conditioning Models of Relapse

Wikler first proposed a conditioning model to explain heroin addiction in 1948. He tested the model in studies of incarcerated addicts at the Addiction Research Center in Lexington, Kentucky, and in experiments in animal models of addicted behavior (Wikler and Pescor 1967; Wikler et al. 1963, 1971). Because he viewed the development of physical dependence as the defining stage of opiate addiction, Wikler believed that, by a process of Pavlovian conditioning, the symptoms and signs of withdrawal (the unconditioned stimulus) are paired to environmental stimuli in the addicted person's home community. Over time, these stimuli elicit withdrawal symptoms that result in relapse to heroin use, when a now drug-free individual returns home after incarceration. Subsequently, Wikler postulated that environmental stimuli could elicit "counteradaptive interoceptive responses" (p. 18)—mirror opposites of the effects of opiates, as individuals anticipated the administration of heroin (Wikler 1974). O'Brien and colleagues (1977) were able to confirm the conditioning of opiate withdrawal symptoms in human subjects, whereas Siegel demonstrated a role for opponent process conditioning in the development of tolerance (summarized by Siegel et al. 1987). Ludwig extended Wikler's theoretical approach to explain relapse to alcohol addiction, linking craving for alcohol by alcoholic patients to conditioned withdrawal symptoms (Ludwig and Wikler 1974).

In addition to evidence of conditioning of the signs and symptoms of abstinence and of opponent process conditioning, there has long been evidence of conditioning of drug effects. Pavlov first noted conditioning of morphine's effects in dogs in 1926. Conditioned place preference represents a behavioral example of the conditioning of the rewarding properties of opiates, stimulants, and alcohol. Meyer and Mirin (1979) demonstrated evidence of conditioned heroin-like effects in drug-free addicted individuals who continued to self-administer heroin (despite pharmacologically effective narcotic blockade) as long as the subjects experienced these conditioned effects. These investigators also observed that "craving" for heroin was highest while subjects anticipated and experienced the conditioned or unconditioned effects of heroin (a priming effect). Priming effects have also been observed in alcoholic individuals (Hodgson et al. 1979; Kaplan et al. 1983; Laberg 1986), and conditioned drug-like effects have been observed in cocaine-dependent subjects (O'Brien et al. 1992).

Stewart and colleagues (1984) postulated that although opponent process conditioning is a parsimonious explanation for the "learned" aspects of tolerance, it is the conditioned drug-like effects that are responsible for relapse. Their model is consistent with the priming effects of low doses of a preferred drug, as well as with data on sensitization suggesting an additive effect when repeated drug use occurs over time in the same environmental setting (Stewart 1992).

As described previously, there is considerable evidence linking the mesolimbic dopamine system (particularly the NA) to the reinforcing properties of stimulants, opiates, and (to some degree) ethanol. Locomotor activity associated with reinforcement has also been linked to the dopaminergic system. There is also some recent direct and indirect evidence linking this system to conditioned drug effects and sensitization. When cocaine or morphine injections are repeatedly paired with specific environmental stimuli, increased locomotor activity is seen in the presence of these stimuli (i.e., in the absence of drug injections; Stewart 1992). Two reports using different methods to assess dopamine release in the NA report dopamine release in association with *anticipated* voluntary alcohol consumption in rats (Vavrousek-Jakuba et al. 1990; Weiss et al. 1992). Shippenberg and colleagues (1992) have presented evidence from lesioning studies that the mesolimbic dopamine system is important for the conditioned reinforcing effects of opiates (conditioned place preference). O'Brien and colleagues (1992) reported dopamine release in NA following saline injections in rats previously exposed to multiple cocaine injections.

If repeated drug exposure only occurs in the presence of specific environmental stimuli, the behavioral sensitization to these drugs is manifested only in the presence of those specific stimuli (Stewart and Vezina 1988). Post and colleagues (1992) have called this context-dependent sensitization. Using in vivo microdialysis, their research group observed significantly increased dopamine release in the NA in animals treated with cocaine who had been previously treated with cocaine in the same environment, compared with control animals exposed to the same amount of cocaine in a different environment or with saline control subjects. These observations provide strong support for the mesolimbic dopamine system in the conditioned components of behavioral sensitization.

If "learning" is an important component to the conditioning of drug effects and sensitization, then it is possible that excitatory amino acids may play some role in the conditioning process. Excitatory amino acids have been implicated in long-term potentiation, which is an important component in learning and memory. Karler and colleagues (1989) reported that systemic injections of MK-801 (a noncompetitive antagonist of *N*-methyl-D-aspartate [NMDA] receptors) blocked the development of sensitization to cocaine and amphetamine. Following up on this work, Stewart and Druhan (1991) found that MK-801 blocked the development of all conditioned amphetamine effects as well as morphine-induced tolerance.

Until recently, conditioning models of addiction have been most useful in conceptualizing clinical approaches to relapse prevention. Clinicians have employed cue exposure techniques in an attempt to extinguish drug-related responses (e.g., Childress et al. 1988). With the development of biological techniques such as regionally specific intracerebral drug administration and in vivo microdialysis, it is possible to examine the neurobiological basis of conditioned drug effects and sensitization. Cador and colleagues (1992) have observed that stress shows cross-sensitization with amphetamine. It is possible that exposure to antecedent stress may amplify the initial effects of stimulant drugs by a process of cross-sensitization, just as environmental stimuli associated with previous episodes of drug use may contribute to sensitization and the risk of relapse.

PERSISTENT ALTERATIONS IN HOMEOSTASIS AND RISK OF RELAPSE

Relapse into heroin, cocaine, and alcohol addiction is most likely to occur in the first 3–6 months of abstinence (e.g., see Meyer 1989), a period that may be characterized by physiological abnormalities, mood disregulation, and a variety of somatic symptoms theoretically linked to the relapse. Meyer (1989) and Kreek (1992a) have suggested that the signs and symptoms of protracted abstinence represent potential targets for pharmacotherapy in the treatment of addiction. The construct should also be useful in applying the tools of molecular neurobiology to relevant animal models of drug or alcohol dependence.

Evidence of Protracted Opiate Abstinence

Martin and Jasinski (1969) described persistent abnormalities in vital signs and neuroendocrine function in heroin-addicted subjects who had been detoxified and had been hospitalized at the Addiction Research Center in Lexington, Kentucky, for 6 months or longer. Prior to the discovery of opiate receptors and endogenous opioid peptides, Dole and Nyswander (1965) postulated that patients addicted to heroin required steady doses of an exogenous opioid to feel "normal." In formulating the rationale for methadone maintenance treatment of heroin addiction, these investigators postulated that, by analogy, methadone was the insulin of those addicted to heroin.

Kreek and colleagues (summarized in Kreek 1992a) have assessed hypothalamic-pituitary reserve using a metyrapone challenge test in patients on methadone maintenance; in drug-free, heroin-addicted individuals during protracted withdrawal; and in control subjects. Metyrapone blocks the final step in the biosynthesis of cortisol in the adrenal cortex and results in increased plasma levels of adrenocorticotropic hormone (ACTH) and β-endorphin. Patients in long-term methadone maintenance were indistinguishable from healthy volunteer subjects. Hyperresponsivity to the metyrapone injection was observed in formerly addicted individuals who were undergoing protracted abstinence (greater than normal increase in ACTH and β-endorphin levels). Opiate administration produced hyporesponsiveness to metyrapone. Subjects on chronic high doses of methadone were tolerant to this effect.

With the discovery of opiate receptors and endogenous opioid peptides, it was anticipated that the development of tolerance and/or physical dependence would be reflected in changes in receptor binding or measurable changes in peptide levels. Although it is now clear that β-endorphin is the most potent ligand for the μ-receptor (which is associated with the reinforcing properties of opiate drugs), tolerance and physical dependence are not clearly associated with changes in receptor binding or total β-endorphin levels. It is possible that tolerance and physical dependence are mediated by more than one neurotransmitter and/or that chronic opiate administration affects gene expression of receptor-related structure and/or function.

Bronstein and colleagues (1990) have reported that pro-opiomelanocortin (POMC) messenger ribonucleic acid (mRNA) levels decline with chronic morphine treatment. Because POMC yields several biologically active peptides, including β-endorphin ACTH, melanocyte-stimulating hormone (MSH), and β-lipotropin, morphine may affect the biosynthesis of β-endorphin. The authors also report that chronic morphine treatment appears to result in preferential production of β-endorphin 1-27 (which functions as an antagonist at the μ-receptor) relative to β-endorphin 1-31 (which functions as an agonist at the μ-receptor). Acute stress also favors the production of β-endorphin 1-27 relative to β-endorphin 1-31. Chronic treatment with naltrexone (a narcotic antagonist) increases the mRNA for POMC and results in an increase in β-endorphin 1-31 relative to β-endorphin 1-27. The work suggests that the POMC system is quite sensitive to the effects of exogenous opiates as well as to acute stress. It would be useful to examine this system in the context of protracted withdrawal, as well as protracted withdrawal in the context of acute stress.

Chronic opiate treatment produces regionally specific changes in gene expression of a number of second messenger functions in brain that are associated with the reinforcing effects of opiates (Beitner-Johnson et al. 1992). Taken together, these changes should result in decreased dopamine synthesis in NA (a prediction that is confirmed by in vivo microdialysis) (Acqua et al. 1992; Brock et al. 1990) and changes in D$_1$ receptor function. Chronic morphine treatment results in a decrease in the phosphorylation state of tyrosine hydroxylase (the rate-limiting enzyme in the synthesis of dopamine) in the NA (Beitner-Johnson et al. 1992). This results in decreased functional activity of the enzyme in NA, whereas there is upregulation (and increased phosphorylation) of the enzyme in the VTA. Chronic morphine treatment also results in a decrease in neurofilament (NF) proteins in dopamine neurons in the VTA (Beitner-Johnson et al. 1992). These effects are regionally specific. The NF proteins form a major component of the cytoskeleton. It is also possible that chronic morphine treatment may alter the structural features of mesolimbic dopamine neurons so as to reduce the ability of these cells to transmit dopamine signals to postsynaptic cells in the NA. The D$_1$ receptor, which uses cAMP as second messenger, is also affected by chronic morphine treatment (Beitner-Johnson et al. 1992). The latter results in decreased levels of G$_i$ protein (the protein that inhibits adenylate cyclase), with increases in adenylate cyclase and cAMP-dependent protein kinase. Identical regionally specific changes in dopamine function occur with chronic cocaine administration (see below). Beitner-Johnson and colleagues (1992) postulate that these changes could result in impairment of the brain's endogenous reward system, with implications for motivation and affect in humans.

The LC is an important mediator of physical dependence upon opiates. Nestler's group reports that chronic morphine treatment results in upregulation of the intracellular cAMP system at multiple levels in the LC (Duman et al. 1988; Nestler et al. 1989). These changes include increased levels of G$_i$ and G$_o$ proteins (alpha subunits), adenylate cyclase, and cAMP-dependent protein kinase, as well as a number of phosphoprotein substrates for the protein kinase in this region. Given the location of these changes, it is possible that the upregulation of the adenylate cyclase system may play a role in the development of tolerance, and physical dependence, as reflected in the activity of the LC neurons. It remains to be seen whether the specific changes in second messenger function in LC and the mesolimbic dopamine system persist beyond the period of chronic opiate administration to account for some of the signs and symptoms of protracted abstinence.

■ Evidence of Protracted Withdrawal Phenomena With Cocaine

In 1986, Gawin and Kleber described the stages and elements of a cocaine abstinence syndrome in a cohort of outpatients in treatment at Yale University. Phase 1 (9 hours to 4 days after the last dose of cocaine) was marked by progression from agitation, depression, anorexia, and high levels of cocaine craving to a later stage of fatigue, exhaustion, hypersomnia, hyperphagia, and the absence of cocaine craving. Phase 2 (1–10 weeks after the last dose of cocaine) was characterized in the first weeks by normal sleep, euthymic mood, low cocaine craving, and low levels of anxiety, with anhedonia, anergia, anxiety, high cocaine craving, and high levels of conditioned craving occurring episodically over the next 2 months. Following this period of "protracted abstinence," subjects still experienced episodic craving and craving in response to specific environmental cues associated with past drug use. The specificity of the stages of cocaine withdrawal has not been confirmed by others (e.g., Weddington et al. 1990).

At this juncture, apart from the acute symptom complex of exhaustion and hyperphagia immediately following binge use of cocaine, there is a relative paucity of data that points clearly to a period of persistent homeostatic dysregulation characteristic of protracted opiate and alcohol withdrawal. Indeed, whereas acute intravenous injections of cocaine produced dose-dependent increases in plasma cortisol concentration (Wilkins et al. 1992), plasma cortisol levels remained normal across 4 weeks of inpatient care in male cocaine-dependent patients (Mendelson et al. 1988). Kreek (1992b) has reported preliminary findings suggesting some abnormalities in hypothalamic-pituitary-adrenal (HPA) function in recently abstinent cocaine-abusing patients. However, systematic studies of HPA function in recently detoxified cocaine-dependent patients using newer challenge strategies (metyrapone or corticotropin-releasing factor [CRF]) have not been performed. Reports of persistent hyperprolactinemia following cocaine withdrawal (Teoh et al. 1990) have not been confirmed by some other investigators (Swartz et al. 1990).

Positron-emission tomography (PET) studies of cerebral metabolism suggest that acute cocaine administration results in a decrease in glucose metabolism, especially in the cerebral cortex, temporal pole, and amygdala (London et al. 1990). Within 1 week of cocaine withdrawal, global cerebral metabolism and regional metabolism in the basal ganglia and orbitofrontal cortex are higher than in control subjects (Volkow et al. 1991). The increased metabolism falls off thereafter in a time-dependent manner, but Volkow and colleagues (1992) report persistent decrements in glucose metabolism in the left and right frontal regions up to 4 months postwithdrawal in more than two-thirds of cocaine users housed on an inpatient unit, compared with control subjects living in the community.

Bauer (1992) has recently reported persistent resting tremor, slowed reaction time, and abnormal electroencephalogram (EEG) responses to a light stimulus in a well-characterized cohort of cocaine-dependent subjects without comorbid psychiatric or addictive disorders. These abnormalities persisted throughout 3 months of monitored abstinence. Herning and colleagues (1992) postulate that some EEG abnormalities observed in abstinent cocaine-dependent subjects (e.g., predominance of beta) are a consequence of enhanced GABA activity. If these abnormalities in motor function and EEG are replicated, it would be important to employ pharmacological challenge strategies to clarify whether the abnormalities are related to residual effects of chronic cocaine on the GABA, dopamine, or another neurotransmitter system.

Gawin and Kleber (1986) initially conceptualized the use of desipramine in the treatment of the anhedonic phase of protracted cocaine withdrawal on the basis of its effects on dopamine reuptake. Pro-

posals to use amantadine and bromocriptine (e.g., Tennant and Sagherian 1987) were similarly based on the hypothesis that the early to middle stages of cocaine withdrawal may be characterized by relative dopamine deficiency. Koob (1992a) has suggested that an animal model for anhedonia is an increase in reward thresholds in BSR. As described previously, acute cocaine administration lowers BSR thresholds, whereas chronic cocaine self-administration results in increased BSR thresholds up to 72 hours following the last administration of cocaine (Koob 1992a). Although desipramine reverses this effect of chronic stimulant administration, the results of desipramine treatment of cocaine-dependent subjects have been inconsistent (Meyer 1992).

As described in the previous section on the molecular neurobiology of chronic opiate administration, chronic cocaine and chronic opiate exposure result in identical changes in gene expression affecting mesolimbic dopamine neurons (Beitner-Johnson et al. 1992). What remains unclear is whether these changes persist and might account for the persistent risk of relapse in drug-free cocaine-dependent (and opiate-dependent) patients. More specifically, it is unclear whether these changes affect responses to stress, to environmental cues associated with past drug use, and to the priming effects of low doses of cocaine (or opiates). Nevertheless, these recent findings offer a potential template to examine possible pharmacotherapy related to molecular mechanisms of drug dependence—treatments that can then be studied in well-designed clinical trials (Meyer 1992).

■ Evidence of Protracted Abstinence to Ethanol

Evidence of symptomatic altered homeostasis following chronic high-dose alcohol consumption is well documented in the clinical and clinical research literature. As with other addictive substances, there is increased probability of relapse in the first 3 months following alcohol withdrawal. Many patients have symptoms of anxiety and depression, even in the absence of a diagnosable Axis I anxiety or mood disorder (summarized by Kranzler and Liebowitz 1985). Insomnia and disturbances in sleep architecture may persist for many months, suggesting the persistence of residual effects of chronic ethanol consumption on circadian rhythm (Gillin et al. 1990). Abnormalities in

HPA axis function (Khan et al. 1984) as well as other endocrine abnormalities (blunted response to TRH; Loosen et al. 1979) have been documented in alcoholic patients up to 4 weeks postwithdrawal. There is persistent impairment of cognitive function, particularly short-term memory, judgment, and visuospatial relations (Becker and Kaplan 1986). Structural brain imaging studies demonstrate increased VBR ratios that recover over time (Carlin et al. 1978), and there are abnormalities in the EEG and evoked potential that return to normal over the first 2–3 weeks of abstinence (Porjesz and Begleiter 1985).

Begleiter and Porjesz (1977; Begleiter et al. 1980) demonstrated a state of latent CNS hyperexcitability that persisted for at least 5 weeks following alcohol withdrawal in rats and monkeys. A challenge dose of ethanol in these animals (up to 37 days postwithdrawal) elicited hyperexcitability in several brain regions: mesencephalic reticular formation, hippocampus, frontal cortex, and posterior association cortex. This reaction could not be elicited in control subjects. The hyperexcitability included characteristics of acute alcohol withdrawal, suggesting that recovering alcoholic patients who resume drinking may trigger withdrawal-like CNS effects, leading to a return to dependent drinking.

Based on the success of methadone maintenance in treating the symptoms and signs of protracted opiate withdrawal, and in preventing illicit use of other opiates, Kissin (1975) proposed that chlordiazepoxide might serve the same functions for ethanol. Although Kissin's reasoning by analogy did not result in a "methadone maintenance-like" treatment for alcoholism (see Meyer 1986a), it is possible that the GABA system may be involved in some aspects of protracted alcohol withdrawal (as it appears to be involved in some aspects of the neuropharmacology of ethanol). Alcohol and BZs have similar acute effects on saccadic eye movements, respiration, mood, and evoked EEG response in human subjects (e.g., Erwin et al. 1986), suggesting a role for the GABA system in the acute effects of ethanol. Both alcohol and BZ agonists markedly potentiate muscimol-stimulated chloride ion flux in rat synaptoneurosomes, albeit via different mechanisms (Mehta and Ticku 1988; Suzdak et al. 1986). With chronic exposure to ethanol, this effect is diminished (Morrow et al. 1991). Cross-tolerance occurs between alcohol and BZs in humans or animal models; BZs remain the treatment of choice in treating acute alcohol with-

drawal. In animal models of alcohol dependence, there is decreased sensitivity to GABAergic agonists and enhanced sensitivity to inverse agonists (Buck and Harris 1990a, 1990b). This same change of sensitivity also occurs with BZ dependence (Little et al. 1988).

Enhanced sensitivity of the receptor to endogenous inverse agonists (and decreased sensitivity to endogenous agonists) could account for the symptoms of anxiety and CNS hyperexcitability during alcohol and BZ withdrawal. Alterations in sensitivity to ethanol and changes in preferential binding (agonist versus inverse agonist) with chronic alcohol administration may be a consequence of changes in gene expression of BZ/GABA receptor subunits. Chronic ethanol administration results in a 40%–50% reduction in α_1 subunit mRNAs in the cerebral cortex of the rat (Morrow et al. 1991) as well as increases in mRNAs for the α_6 subunit and the β_2 subunit (in cerebellum).

As described previously, there is evidence that the effects of ethanol are mediated by more than one neurotransmitter. Glutamate is the major excitatory neurotransmitter in the brain, producing its activation through at least three receptor subtypes (kainate, quisqualate, and NMDA receptors). Inhibition of at least one of these receptors might—along with the effects at the BZ/GABA receptor—contribute to the depressant effects of ethanol. If chronic ethanol treatment results in enhanced glutamate activity, along with diminished agonist sensitivity at the BZ/GABA receptor, this could contribute to the proconvulsant effects of ethanol withdrawal. Indeed, acute ethanol exposure inhibited NMDA activated ion current in in vitro preparations of voltage-clamped rat hippocampal neurons (Lovinger et al. 1989). Quisqualate and kainate receptor subtypes were relatively unaffected by ethanol in these experiments.

In further in vitro studies, Tabakoff's group reported that acute ethanol exposure inhibited calcium flux through the NMDA receptor-gated ion channel (Tabakoff et al. 1991). Chronic ethanol administration in mice resulted in upregulation of the NMDA receptor for at least 8 hours following acute withdrawal (Grant et al. 1990). Withdrawal seizure severity in vivo was reduced by administration of MK-801, an NMDA receptor antagonist (Grant et al. 1990). In contrast, seizure severity was increased, including the production of some lethal seizures, when alcohol-dependent mice were injected with NMDA itself

(Grant et al. 1990). Parenthetically, chronic ethanol exposure also results in an increase in voltage-gated calcium channels (Dolin et al. 1987), and calcium channel antagonists decrease the alcohol withdrawal syndrome in rodents (Little et al. 1986).

Intrinsic to the concept of protracted withdrawal (or abstinence) is the model of a deficit in homeostasis consequent to chronic drug or alcohol use, which is made manifest when the organism is drug- or alcohol-free. Evidence of residual dysfunction is most apparent in association with acute opiate and alcohol withdrawal syndromes. In this situation, homeostasis is restored by drug substitution and controlled detoxification. At another level, evidence of abnormalities of GABA and NMDA receptor sensitivity are most clear during chronic ethanol administration and during acute withdrawal. At this juncture, the most robust evidence of persistent deficits in homeostasis in alcoholic patients comes from clinical studies. Further work is needed to identify persistent residual abnormalities in receptor function that may suggest appropriate pharmacotherapies. In this context, the collection of symptoms and signs of protracted abstinence in alcoholic patients offers an inviting target for clinical trials.

■ SUMMARY AND POSTSCRIPT

Current diagnostic criteria of opiate, stimulant, and alcohol dependence disorders have a high degree of reliability. The development of homologous animal models of opiate and stimulant drug dependence, plus some promising animal behavioral and pharmacogenetic models of alcohol consumption, add the potential dimension of validity to the criteria of these human disorders. The greatest progress on the biology of alcohol, opiate, and stimulant dependence has come in recent years. Building on highly reliable behavioral models, new techniques in neurobiology have enabled investigators to clarify the CNS correlates of drug reinforcement. Much evidence points to the dopamine neurons of the NA and VTA. Although these neurons may form a "final common pathway" for drug reinforcement, it is clear that the effects of different drug classes on these neurons result from different mechanisms. The significance of the findings on the neurobiology of drug reinforcement cannot be overstated.

More recently, neurobiologists have begun to take on the challenge of defining the neurobiological correlates of some of the most important clinical phenomena associated with the dependence syndromes: the tendency to use again after a period of abstinence, and the rapid reinstatement of the elements of the dependence syndrome once drug use has resumed. Two constructs stand from the clinical literature: the role of conditioned cue responsiveness in relapse, and the importance of persistent homeostatic dysregulation following drug/alcohol withdrawal (protracted abstinence). With regard to the latter, if chronic exposure to opiates, cocaine, and alcohol results in changes in gene expression affecting receptor function in behaviorally relevant brain regions, then the clinical reports of patients in treatment (who argue that they "feel normal" when on their drug of choice) seem more compelling.

Neurobiologists would make a major contribution to clinicians if they defined the duration of these changes in gene expression affecting receptor function. Are these changes permanent? Do they respond to acute or chronic treatment with receptor antagonists or other drugs that may modify neurotransmitter, receptor, or second messenger function? Clinical investigators need to describe the symptoms and signs of persistent homeostatic dysregulation more precisely to identify potential targets for pharmacotherapy. This is particularly true for cocaine and stimulant dependence, where the case for "protracted abstinence" has been less well developed than for alcohol or opiates.

Neurobiologists have also begun to pay attention to the neurobiological correlates of the anticipatory state prior to drug-seeking and self-administration behavior. Preliminary results from two laboratories suggest that this anticipatory state (associated with ethanol consumption)—like unconditioned reinforcement—may be associated with dopamine release in the NA. Clinicians have long wondered why their patients returned to environments associated with past drug use despite clinical counseling to the contrary. The preliminary neurobiological data suggest that the effects of these environmental stimuli are similar to the "priming effects" of a low dose of the preferred drug. Indeed, as a consequence of sensitization, the environmental stimuli may enhance the reinforcing properties of the drug use.

Finally, neurobiologists have begun to examine the question of individual and strain differences in vulnerability to drug and alcohol dependence in animal models so as to identify potential risk and/or protective factors that might generalize to human populations (where individual differences are quite significant). Because pharmacogenetic differences in ethanol preference have been significant in developing animal models of alcohol consumption, much more progress has been made in comparing specific neurobiological characteristics of P and NP rats. The issue of individual or strain differences in the reinforcing potency of opiates and cocaine was not explored until relatively recently. Of special interest is the report by Beitner-Johnson and colleagues (1992) comparing the characteristics of mesolimbic dopamine neurons in Fischer and Lewis rats. Lewis rats develop greater degrees of conditioned place preference to parenteral morphine and cocaine compared with Fischer rats. The differences in the molecular neurobiology of mesolimbic dopamine neurons in drug-naive Lewis rats compared with Fischer rats resembled the differences between chronic morphine-treated and chronic cocaine-treated animals (compared with control subjects) in outbred Sprague Dawley rats. These studies suggest that some aspects of vulnerability may be genetically determined.

Other investigators have observed that stress serves to sensitize rats to the reinforcing properties of stimulants (and vice versa), in a process that appears to involve CRF and the HPA axis (Cador et al. 1992). Monkeys reared in isolation spontaneously drink much greater quantities of ethanol than monkeys reared in a normal environment in proximity to their biological mothers (Higley et al. 1991). Environmental factors can seemingly affect gene expression related to CNS function. Over the next few years, neuroscientists will apply tools of increasing sophistication to tease apart the genetic and environmental factors that may contribute to the development of drug and alcohol dependence in homologous animal models of these well-characterized human disorders. As a result of this research, it is highly likely that someday clinicians will have the tools to offer more effective programs of treatment and prevention.

■ REFERENCES

Acqua E, Carboni E, DiChiara G: Profound depression of mesolimbic dopamine release after morphine withdrawal in dependent rats. Eur J Pharmacol 193:133–134, 1992

Almaric M, Koob GF: Low doses of methylnaloxonium in the nucleus accumbens antagonize hyperactivity induced by heroin in the rat. Pharmacol Biochem Behav 23:411–415, 1985

American Psychiatric Association: Diagnostic and Statistical Manual of Mental Disorders, 3rd Edition. Washington, DC, American Psychiatric Association, 1980

American Psychiatric Association: Diagnostic and Statistical Manual of Mental Disorders, 3rd Edition, Revised. Washington, DC, American Psychiatric Association, 1987

Babor TF, Wolfson A, Boivin D, et al: Alcoholism, culture and psychopathology: a comparative study of French, French Canadian, and American alcoholics, in Alcoholism in North America, Europe, and Asia. Edited by Helzer JE, Canino GH. New York, Oxford University Press, 1992, pp 182–195, 1992

Bain GT, Kornetsky C: Ethanol oral self-administration and rewarding brain stimulation. Alcohol 6:499–503, 1989

Ballenger J, Goodwin F, Major L, et al: Alcohol and central serotonin metabolism in man. Arch Gen Psychiatry 36:224–227, 1979

Bauer LO: Neurophysiological aspects of cocaine versus alcohol withdrawal: different syndromes! different treatments? Paper presented at the annual meeting of the American College of Neuropsychopharmacology, San Juan, PR, December 1992

Becker HT, Kaplan RF: Neurophysiological and neuropsychological concomitance of brain dysfunction in alcoholics, in Psychopathology and Addictive Disorders. Edited by Meyer RE. New York, Guilford, 1986, pp 262–292

Begleiter H, Porjesz B: Persistence of brain hyperexcitability following chronic alcoholic exposure in rats. Adv Exp Med Biol 85:209–222, 1977

Begleiter H, DeNoble V, Porjesz B: Protracted brain dysfunction after alcohol withdrawal in monkeys, in Biological Effects of Alcohol. Edited by Begleiter H. New York, Plenum, 1980, pp 231–239

Begleiter H, Porjesz B, Bihari B, et al: Event-related brain potentials in sons of alcoholic fathers. Alcohol Clin Exp Res 7:1493–1496, 1984

Beitner-Johnson D, Guitart X, et al: Common intracellular actions of chronic morphine and cocaine in dopaminergic brain reward regions, in The Neurobiology of Drug and Alcohol Addiction. Edited by Kalivas PW, Sampson HH. Ann N Y Acad Sci

654:70–87, 1992

Bozarth MA, Wise RA: Anatomically distinct opiate receptor fields mediate reward and physical dependence. Science 224:516–517, 1984

Britt MD, Wise RA: Ventral tegmental site of opiate reward: antagonism by a hydrophilic opiate receptor blocker. Brain Res 258:105–108, 1983

Brock JW, Ng JP, Justice JB Jr: Effect of chronic cocaine on dopamine synthesis in the nucleus accumbens as determined by microdialysis with NSD-1015. Neurosci Lett 117:234–239, 1990

Bronstein DM, Prezewlocki R, Akil H: Effects of morphine treatment on pro-opiomelanocortin systems in rat brain. Brain Res 519:102–111, 1990

Brown EE, Finlay JM, Wong JP, et al: Behavioral and neurochemical interactions between cocaine and buprenorphine: implications for the pharmacotherapy of cocaine abuse. J Pharmacol Exp Ther 256:119–126, 1991

Buck KJ, Harris RA: Benzodiazepine agonist and inverse agonist actions on GABAa receptor-operated chloride channels, I: acute effects of ethanol. J Pharmacol Exp Ther 253:706–712, 1990a

Buck KJ, Harris RA: Benzodiazepine agonist and inverse agonist actions on GABAa receptor-operated chloride channels, II: chronic effects of ethanol. J Pharmacol Exp Ther 253:713–719, 1990b

Cador M, Dumas S, Cole BJ, et al: Behavioral sensitization induced by psychostimulants or stress: search for a molecular basis and evidence for a CRF dependent phenomenon, in The Neurobiology of Drug and Alcohol Addiction. Edited by Kalivas PW, Samson HH. Ann N Y Acad Sci 654:416–420, 1992

Carlin PL, Wortzman G, Holgate RC, et al: Reversible cerebral atrophy in recently abstinent chronic alcoholics measured by computerized tomography scans. Science 200:1076–1078, 1978

Childress AR, McLellan AT, Ehrman R, et al: Classically conditioned responses in opioid and cocaine dependence: a roll in relapse, in Learning Factors in Substance Abuse. Edited by Ray BA (DHHS Publ No ADM-88-1576). Rockville, MD, Alcohol, Drug Abuse and Mental Health Administration, 1988, pp 25–43

Cloninger CR, Bohman M, Sigvardsson S: Inheritance of alcohol abuse: cross-fostering analysis of adopted men. Arch Gen Psychiatry 38:861–868, 1981

Cotton NS: The familial incidence of alcoholism: a review. J Stud Alcohol 40:89–116, 1979

Deneau G, Yanagita T, Seavers MH: Self administration of psychoactive substances by the monkey: a measure of psychological dependence. Psychopharmacologia 16:30–48, 1969

DeWitte P, Bada MF: Self-stimulation and alcohol administered orally or intraperitoneally. Exp Neurol 8:675–682, 1983

DiChiara G, Imperato A: Drugs abused by humans preferentially increase synaptic dopamine concentrations in the mesolimbic system of freely moving rats. Proc Natl Acad Sci U S A 85:5274–5278, 1988

Dole VP, Nyswander ME: A medical treatment for diacetylmorphine (heroin) addiction. JAMA 193:646–650, 1965

Dolin S, Little H, Hudspith M: Increased dihydropyridine-sensitive calcium channels in rat brain may underlie ethanol physical dependence. Neuropharmacology 26:275–279, 1987

Duman RS, Tallman JF, Nestler EJ: Acute and chronic opiate-regulation of adenylate cyclase in brain: specific effects in locus ceruleus. J Pharmacol Exp Ther 246:1033–1039, 1988

Eriksson K: Rat strains specially selected for their voluntary alcohol consumption. Annals of Medicine and Experimental Biology Finland 49:67–72, 1971

Erwin CW, Linnoila M, Hartwell J: Effects of buspirone and diazepam, alone and in combination with alcohol, on skill performance and evoked potentials. J Clin Psychopharmacol 6:199–209, 1986

Falk JL, Samson HH, Winger G: Behavioral maintenance of high concentrations of blood-ethanol and physical dependence in the rat. Science 177:811–813, 1972

Gawin FH, Kleber HD: Abstinence symptomatology and psychiatric diagnosis in cocaine abusers. Arch Gen Psychiatry 43:107–113, 1986

Gill K, France C, Amit Z: Voluntary ethanol consumption in rats: an examination of blood/brain ethanol levels and behavior. Alcohol Clin Exp Res 10(4):457–462, 1986

Gillin JC, Smith TL, Irwin M: EEG sleep studies in "pure" primary alcoholism during sub acute withdrawal: relationships to normal controls, age, and other clinical variables. Biol Psychiatry 27:477–488, 1990

Glickman SE, Schiff BB: A biological theory of reinforcement. Psychol Rev 74:81–109, 1967

Grant KA, Valverius P, Hudspith M: Ethanol withdrawal seizures and NMDA receptor complex. Eur J Pharmacol 176:289–296, 1990

Helzer JE, Canino GJ, Yeh E, et al: Alcoholism—North America and Asia: a comparison of population surveys with the diagnostic interview schedule. Arch Gen Psychiatry 47:313–319, 1990

Herning RI, Glover BJ, Guo X, et al: Excessive EEG fast activity in cocaine abusers: pharmacological interventions. Paper presented at the annual meeting of the American College of Psychopharmacology, San Juan, PR, December 1992

Hesselbrock V, Hesselbrock MN, Workman-Daniels KL: The effect of major depression and antisocial personality disorder on alcoholism: course and motivational patterns. J Stud Alcohol 47:207–212, 1986

Higley JD, Hasert MF, Suomi SJ, et al: Nonhuman primate model of alcohol abuse: effects of early experience, personality, and stress on alcohol consumption. Proc Natl Acad Sci U S A 88:7261–7265, 1991

Hodgson R, Rankin H, Stockwell T: Alcohol dependence and the priming effect. Journal of Behavioral Research and Therapy 17:379–387, 1979

Jones RT: What have we learned from nicotine, cocaine, and marijuana about addiction? in Addictive States. Edited by O'Brien CP, Chaffe JH. New York, Raven, 1992, pp 109–122

Kaplan RF, Meyer RE, Stroebel CF: Alcohol dependence and responsivity to an ethanol stimulus as predictors of alcohol consumption. British Journal of Addiction 78:259–267, 1983

Karler R, Calder LD, Chauhry IA: Blockade of "reverse tolerance" to cocaine and amphetamine by MK801. Life Sci 45:599–606, 1989

Kellam SG, Brown CH, Rubin BR, et al: Paths leading to teen-age psychiatric symptoms and substance use: developmental epdemiological studies in Woodlawn, in Childhood Psychopathology and Development. Edited by Guze SB, Earls FJ, Barrett JE. New York, Raven, 1983, pp 17–51

Khan A, Ciraulo DA, Nelson WH, et al: Dexamethasone suppression tests in recently detoxified alcoholics: clinical implications. J Clin Psychopharmacol 4:94–97, 1984

Killam KF, Olds J, Sinclair J: Further studies on the effects of centrally acting drugs on the results of self-stimulation. J Pharmacol Exp Ther 119:157–163, 1957

Kissin B: The use of psychoactive drugs in the long term treatment of chronic alcoholics. Ann N Y Acad Sci 252:385–395, 1975

Koob GF: Neurobiological mechanism in cocaine and opiate dependence, in Addictive States. Edited by O'Brien CP, Jaffe JH. New York, Raven, 1992a, pp 79–92

Koob GF: Neural mechanisms of drug reinforcement, in The Neurobiology of Drug and Alcohol Addiction. Edited by Kalivas PW, Samson HH. Annals of the American Academy of Sciences 654:171–191, 1992b

Koob GF, Bloom FE: Cellular and molecular mechanisms of drug dependence. Science 242:715–723, 1988

Kornetsky C, Porrino L: Brain mechanisms of drug-induced reinforcement, in Addictive States. Edited by O'Brien CP, Jaffe JH. New York, Raven, 1992, pp 59–77

Kranzler H, Liebowitz N: Anxiety and depression in substance abuse: clinical implications. Med Clin North Am 72:867–885, 1985

Kreek MJ: Rational for maintenance pharmacotherapy of opiate dependents, in Addictive States. Edited by O'Brien CP, Jaffe JH. New York, Raven, 1992a, pp 205–230

Kreek MJ: Neuroendocrinology of cocaine abuse. Paper presented at the annual meeting of the American College of Neuropsychopharmacology, San Juan, PR, December 1992b

Laberg JC: Alcohol and expectancies: subjective, psychophysiological, and behavioral responses to alcohol stimuli in severely, moderately, and nondependent drinkers. British Journal of Addiction 81:797–808, 1986

Lewis MJ: Alcohol effects on brain stimulation reward: blood alcohol concentration and site specificity, in Neuropharmacology of Ethanol: New Approaches. Edited by Meyer RE, Koob GF, Lewis MJ, et al. Boston, MA, Birkhauser, 1991, pp 163–178

Li TK, Lumeng L, McBride WJ, et al: Rodent lines selected for factors effecting alcohol consumption. Alcohol Alcohol Suppl 1:91–96, 1987

Li TK, Lumeng L, McBride WJ: Pharmacology of alcohol preference in rodents. Advances in Alcoholism and Substance Abuse 7:73–86, 1988

Li TK, Crabb DW, Lumeng L: Molecular and genetic approaches to understanding alcohol seeking behavior, in Neuropharmacology of Ethanol: New Approaches. Edited by Meyer RE, Koob GF, Lewis

MJ, et al. Boston, MA, Birkhauser, 1991, pp 107–124

Linnoila M, DeJong J, Virkkunen M: Family history of alcoholism in violent offenders and impulsive fire setters. Arch Gen Psychiatry 46:613–616, 1989

Little HJ, Dolin SJ, Halsey MJ: Calcium channel antagonists decrease the ethanol withdrawal syndrome. Life Sci 39:2059–2065, 1986

Little HJ, Gale R, Sellars N, et al: Chronic benzodiazepine treatment increases the effects of the inverse agonist FG 7142. Neuropharmacology 27:383–389, 1988

London EK, Cascella NG, Wong DF, et al: Cocaine-induced reduction of glucose utilization in human brain: a study using positron emission tomography and (fluorine-18)-fluorodeoxyglucose. Arch Gen Psychiatry 47:567–574, 1990

Loosen PT, Prange AJ, Wilson IC: TRH (protireline) in depressed alcoholic men: behavioral changes and endocrine responses. Arch Gen Psychiatry 36:540–547, 1979

Lovinger DM, White G, Weight FF: Ethanol inhibits NMDA-activated ion current in hippocampal neurons. Science 243:1721–1724, 1989

Ludwig AM, Wikler A: Craving and relapse to drink. Quarterly Journal of Studies on Alcohol 35:108–130, 1974

Martin WA, Jasinski DR: Physiological parameters of morphine dependence in man—tolerance, early abstinence and protracted abstinence. J Psychiatr Res 7:7–9, 1969

Martin WR, Winkler A, Eades CG, et al: Tolerance to and physical dependence on morphine in rats. Psychopharmacologia 4:247–260, 1963

Mehta AK, Ticku MK: Ethanol potentiation of gamma amino butyric acid gated chloride channels. J Pharmacol Exp Ther 246:558–564, 1988

Mendelson JH, Teoh SK, Lange U, et al: Anterior pituitary, adrenal, and gonadal hormones during cocaine withdrawal. Am J Psychiatry 145:1094–1098, 1988

Meyer RE: Anxiolytics and the alcoholic patient. J Stud Alcohol 47:269–273, 1986a

Meyer RE: How to understand the relationship between psychopathology and addictive disorders: another example of the chicken and the egg, in Psychopathology and Addictive Disorders. Edited by Meyer RE. New York, Guilford, 1986b, pp 3–16

Meyer RE: Prospects for a rational pharmacotherapy of alcoholism. J Clin Psychiatry 50:403–412, 1989

Meyer RE: New pharmacotherapies for cocaine dependence . . . revisited. Arch Gen Psychiatry 49:900–904, 1992

Meyer RE, Mirin SM: The Heroin Stimulus Implications for a Theory of Addiction. New York, Plenum, 1979

Moolten M, Kornetsky C: Oral self-administration of ethanol and not experimenter administered ethanol facilitates rewarding electrical brain stimulation. Alcohol Clin Exp Res 7:3–9, 1990

Morrow AL, Montpied P, Paul SM: Ethanol and the GABA receptor gated chloride ion channel, in Neuropharmacology of Ethanol: New Approaches. Edited by Meyer RE, Koob GF, Lewis MJ, et al. Boston, MA, Birkhauser, 1991, pp 49–76

Murphy JM, McBride WJ, Luming L, et al: Regional brain levels of monoamines in alcohol-preferring and non-preferring lines of rats. Pharmacol Biochem Behav 16:145–149, 1982

Murphy JM, McBride WJ, Gatto GJ, et al: Effects of acute ethanol administration on monoamine and metabolite content in four brain regions of ethanol-tolerant and non-tolerant alcohol preferring rats. Pharmacol Biochem Behav 29:169–174, 1988

Naranjo C, Sellers EM, Sullivan JT, et al: The serotonin uptake inhibitor citalopram attenuates ethanol intake. Clin Pharmacol Ther 41:266–274, 1987

Nestler EJ, Urdos JJ, Derwilliger R, et al: Regulation of G-proteins by chronic morphine in the rat locus ceruleus. Brain Res 476:230–239, 1989

O'Brien CP, Testa T, O'Brien TJ, et al: Conditioned narcotic withdrawal in human. Science 195:1000–1002, 1977

O'Brien C, Childress AR, McLellan AT, et al: Classical conditioning in drug dependent humans, in The Neurobiology of Drug and Alcohol Addiction. Edited by Kalivas PW, Samson HH. Ann N Y Acad Sci 654:400–415, 1992

Olds J, Milner P: Positive reinforcement produced by electrical stimulation of septal area and other regions of the rat brain. Journal of Comparative Physiological Psychology 47:419–427, 1954

O'Malley SS, Jaffe AJ, Chang G, et al: Naltrexone and coping skills therapy for alcohol dependence: a controlled study. Arch Gen Psychiatry 49:881–887, 1992

Pavlov IP: Conditioned Reflexes. New York, Dover Press, 1926

Pfeffer AO, Samson HH: Haloperidol and apomorphine effects on ethanol reinforcement in free-feeding rats. Pharmacol Biochem Behav 29:343–350, 1988

Porjesz B, Begleiter H: Human brain electrophysiology and alcoholism, in Alcohol and the Brain: Chronic Effects. Edited by Tartar RE, Van Thiel DH. New York, Plenum, 1985, pp 139–182

Post RM, Weiss SRB, Fontana D, et al: Conditioned sensitization to the psychomotor stimulant cocaine, in The Neurobiology of Drug and Alcohol Addiction. Edited by Kalivas PW, Samson HH. Ann N Y Acad Sci 654:386–399, 1992

Reid LD, Hunter GA: Morphine and naloxone modulate intake of ethanol. Alcohol 1:33–37, 1984

Ritz RT, Lamb MC, Oldburg SR, et al: Effects of cocaine on the dopamine transporter. Science 237:1219–1223, 1987

Roberts DCS, Koob GF, Klonoff P, et al: Extinction and recovery of cocaine self-administration following 6-hydroxydopamine lesions of the nucleus accumbens. Pharmacol Biochem Behav 12:781–787, 1980

Robins LN: Deviant Children Grown Up. Baltimore, MD, Williams & Wilkins, 1966

Rush B: An Inquiry Into the Effects of Spirituous Liquors Upon the Human Body and Their Influences Upon the Happiness of Society. Boston, MA, Thomas & Andrews, 1791

Samson HH: Initiation of ethanol reinforcement using a sucrose-substitution procedure in food-and-water-sated rats. Alcohol Clin Exp Res 10(4):436–442, 1986

Samson HH, Tolliver GA, Pfeffer AU, et al: Oral ethanol reinforcement in the rat: effects of the partial inverse benzodiazepine agonist Ro 15-4513. Pharmacol Biochem Behav 27:517–519, 1987

Schaefer GJ, Michael RP: Ethanol and current thresholds for brain self-stimulation in the lateral hypothalamus of the rat. Alcohol 4:209–213, 1987

Schuckit MA: Subjective responses to alcohol in sons of alcoholics and control subjects. Arch Gen Psychiatry 41:879–884, 1984

Schuster CR, Thompson T: Self-administration of and behavioral dependence on drugs. Annual Review of Pharmacology 9:483–502, 1969

Schuster CR, Villareal JE: The Experimental Analysis of Opioid Dependence—Psychopharmacology: A Review of Progress (Public Health Service Publication #1836). Edited by Efron EH. Washington, DC, U.S. Government Printing Office, 1968, pp 811–828

Shippenberg TS, Herz A, Spanagel R: Conditioning of opioid reinforcement: neuroanatomical and neurochemical substrates, in The Neurobiology of Drug and Alcohol Addiction. Edited by Kalivas PW, Sampson HH. Ann N Y Acad Sci 654:347–356, 1992

Siegel S, Hinson RE, Krank MD: Anticipation of pharmacological and non-pharmacological events: classical conditioning and addictive behavior. Journal of Drug Issues 17:83–110, 1987

Stewart J: Neurobiology of conditioning to drugs of abuse, in The Neurobiology of Drug and Alcohol Addiction. Edited by Kalivas PW, Samson HH. Ann N Y Acad Sci 654:335–344, 1992

Stewart J, Druhan JP: The non-competitive MDA antagonist, MK-801 blocks the development of conditioned activity to amphetamine. Society for Neuroscience Abstracts 557:12, 1991

Stewart J, Vezina P: Conditioning and behavioral sensitization, in Sensitization in the Nervous System. Edited by Kalivas PW, Barnes C. Caldwell, NJ, Telford Press, 1988, pp 207–224

Stewart J, deWitt H, Eikelboom R: Role of unconditioned and conditioned drug effects in the self-administration of opiates and stimulants. Psychol Rev 91:251–268, 1984

Suzdak PD, Schwartz RD, Scolnick O, et al: Ethanol stimulates gamma amino butyric acid receptor mediated chloride transport in rat brain synaptoneurosomes. Proc Natl Acad Sci U S A 83:4071–4075, 1986

Suzdak PT, Glowa JR, Crawley JN, et al: A selective imidazobenzodiazepine antagonist of ethanol in the rat. Science 234:1243–1247, 1986

Swartz CM, Breen MD, Leone F: Serum prolactin levels during extended cocaine abstinence. Am J Psychiatry 147:777–779, 1990

Tabakoff B, Rabie CS, Grant KA: Ethanol and NMDA receptor: insights into ethanol pharmacology, in Neuropharmacology of Ethanol: New Approaches. Edited by Meyer RE, Koob GF, Lewis MJ, et al. Boston, MA, Birkhauser, 1991

Tennant FS, Sagherian AA: Double blind comparison of amantadine and bromocriptine for ambulatory withdrawal from cocaine dependence. Arch Intern Med 147:109–112, 1987

Teoh SK, Mendelson JH, Mello NK, et al: Hyperprolactinemia and risk for relapse of cocaine abuse. Biol Psychiatry 28:824–828, 1990

Vavrousek-Jakuba E, Cohen CA, Shoemaker WJ: Ethanol effects of CNS dopamine receptors: in vivo binding following voluntary ethanol intake in rats, in Novel Pharmacological Interventions for Alcoholism. Edited by Naranjo CA, Sellers EM. New York, Springer-Verlag, 1990, pp 372–374

Volkow ND, Fowler JS, Wolf AP, et al: Changes in brain glucose metabolism in cocaine dependence and withdrawal. Am J Psychiatry 148:621–626, 1991

Volkow ND, Hitzemann R, Wang GJ, et al: Long term frontal brain metabolic changes in cocaine abusers. Synapse 11(3):184–190, 1992

Volpicelli JR, Alterman AI, Hayashadi M, et al: Naltrexone in the treatment of alcohol dependence. Arch Gen Psychiatry 49:876–880, 1992

Waller MB, McBride MC, Gatto GJ, et al: Intragastric self infusion of ethanol of the p and np (alcohol preferring and alcohol non-preferring) lines of rats. Science 225:78–80, 1984

Weddington WW, Brown BS, Haertzen CA, et al: Changes in mood, craving, and sleep during short term abstinence reported by male cocaine addicts: a controlled residential study. Arch Gen Psychiatry 47:861–868, 1990

Weeks JR: Experimental morphine addiction: methods for automatic intravenous injections in unrestrained rats. Science 138:143–144, 1963

Weiss F, Koob GF: The neuropharmacology of ethanol self-administration, in Neuropharmacology of Ethanol: New Approaches. Edited by Meyer RE, Koob GF, Lewis MJ, et al. Boston, MA, Birkhauser, 1991, pp 125–162

Weiss F, Herd YL, Ungerstedt U, et al: Neurochemical correlates of cocaine and ethanol self-administration, in The Neurobiology of Drug and Alcohol Addiction. Edited by Kalivas PW, Samson HH. Ann N Y Acad Sci 654:220–241, 1992

Wikler A: Recent progress in research on the neurophysiological basis of morphine addiction. Am J Psychiatry 105:329–338, 1948

Wikler A: Conditioning factors in opiate addiction and relapse, in Narcotics. Edited by Wilmer DM, Kassebaum GG. New York, McGraw-Hill, 1965, pp 85–100

Wikler A: Dynamics of drug dependent: implications of a conditioning theory for research and treatment, in Opiate Addiction: Origins and Treatment. Edited by Fisher S, Freedman AM. Washington, DC, Winston Press, 1974, pp 7–22

Wikler A, Pescor FT: Classical conditioning of morphine abstinence, reinforcement of opioid-drinking behavior and relapse in morphine-addicted rats. Psychopharmacologia 10:255–284, 1967

Wikler A, Martin WR, Pescor FT, et al: Factors regulating oral consumption or an opioid (etonitazine) by morphine-addicted rats. Psychopharmacologia 5:55–76, 1963

Wikler A, Pescor FT, Miller T, et al: Persistent potency of a secondary (conditioned) reinforcer following withdrawal of morphine from physically dependent rats. Psychopharmacologia 20:103–117, 1971

Wilkins J, Gorelick DA, Nademanee K, et al: Hypothalamic-pituitary function during alcohol exposure and withdrawal and cocaine exposure, in Recent Developments in Alcoholism, Vol 10: Alcohol and Cocaine Similarities and Differences. Edited by Galanter M. New York, Plenum, 1992, pp 57–71

Wise RA, Bozarth MA: A psychomotor stimulant theory of addiction. Psychol Rev 94(4):469–492, 1987

Woods JH, Schuster CR: Reinforcement properties of morphine, cocaine, and SPA as a function of unit dose. Int J Addict 3:231–237, 1968

World Health Organization: International Statistical Classification of Diseases and Related Health Problems, Tenth Revision. Geneva, Switzerland, World Health Organization, 1992

Yanagita T, Kiyoshi A, Takahashi S, et al: Self-administration of barbiturates, alcohol (intragastric) and CNS stimulants (intravenous) in monkeys, in National Academy of Sciences–National Research Council Committee on Problems of Drug Dependence. Palo Alto, CA, Stanford University Press, 1969, pp 6039–6051

Yokel RA, Wise RA: Increased lever pressing for amphetamine after pimozide in rats: implications for a dopamine theory of reward. Science 187:547–549, 1975

27

Biology of Eating Disorders

Regina C. Casper, M.D.

Anorexia nervosa and bulimia nervosa form a heterogeneous group of mainly psychiatric disorders. The incidence of anorexia nervosa has slightly risen in recent years (Szmukler et al. 1986), whereas bulimia nervosa has only relatively recently been described as a nosological syndrome (Casper 1983; Russell 1979). There is widespread belief that eating disorders are a product of our society and culture, as indeed they are; but neither disorder is new, and the existence of similar disorders throughout history is well documented (Bell 1985; Ziolko 1976).

The biological changes attending both disorders reflect for the most part the body's adjustment to prolonged undernutrition and to changes in eating pattern; hence, they cannot be considered intrinsic to either disorder. Nevertheless, the biological changes might well play a permissive role in sustaining certain psychopathological mechanisms. Given wide-ranging constitutional differences, individual patients tolerate undernutrition and malnutrition in different ways. But the overriding factor responsible for divergences in the medical status of patients are vast differences in the amount and speed of weight loss, use of laxatives or diuretics, and variations in eating pattern and in the frequency of self-induced vomiting. If treatment succeeds in complete normalization of the eating pattern and of body weight, virtually all physical, metabolic, and endocrine abnormalities normalize as well. However, prolonged emesis, laxative, or diuretic abuse can lead to permanent gastrointestinal, renal, or dental damage.

In this chapter, the physical changes associated with anorexia nervosa are considered separately from those occurring in bulimia nervosa. The adaptation to prolonged starvation and the resulting pathological weight loss in anorexia nervosa of the restricting subtype differs in several ways from the body's adaptation to the frequently encountered emesis and/or cathartic or diuretic abuse in bulimia nervosa, where body weight may fluctuate (sometimes widely) but essentially remains within normal limits. The biological disturbances in the bulimic form of anorexia nervosa can resemble those in either condition.

ANOREXIA NERVOSA

Anorexia nervosa occurs typically in adolescent females, whose profound weight loss is the direct consequence of a long period of reduced food intake, only in exceptional cases related to loss of appetite. The classic attitudinal and behavioral changes—denial of illness, an overriding and irrational fear of becoming overweight, distortions in body image perception, and (often) hypermotility—establish the diagnosis (American Psychiatric Association 1987; Bruch 1973). The starvation process in anorexia nervosa is personally sustained, even though the initial weight loss may not be self-imposed, but may be initiated by loss of appetite because of depression, a physical illness, or religious fasting (Casper and Davis 1977). For the interpretation of the biological changes, it is important to distinguish patients with the restricting subtype who consistently fast from those who also vomit, and from those who fall prey to periodic bouts of overeating and subsequent emesis (Casper et al. 1980a).

■ Bodily Changes

The human body is well equipped to deal with the consequences of temporary starvation and to recover functionally in times of plenty (Keys et al. 1950). Chronic weight loss is better tolerated than acute severe weight loss, and adults seem to adjust more easily to weight loss than children or young adolescents. For adolescents, changes in body weight are calculated as height and weight deviations from the norms published as the Iowa Growth Charts (Jackson and Kelby 1945). Ideal weights derived from the Metropolitan Life Insurance Company generally form the basis for calculating weight loss in adults. The Body Mass Index (BMI; weight in kilograms to height in meters, squared) (Keys et al. 1972) has become popular for standardizing weight loss, because the BMI has a high correlation with skinfold thickness and therefore with body fat mass. The most commonly observed physical changes in anorexia nervosa are listed in Table 27–1.

The starved skeleton-like appearance of the anorexic patient is the result of reduction in subcutaneous fat tissue. The skin acquires a darkish, yellowish color with a rough texture. With advanced emaciation, a lanugo coat of long, silky hair can cover the back, extremities, and cheeks. Not infrequently, petechiae and ecchymoses develop, which are not necessarily associated with thrombocytopenia but may be the result of increased capillary permeability. A decreased core temperature and an inability to adjust to environmental temperature changes have also been reported (Luck and Wakeling 1980; Mecklenburg et al. 1974; Vigersky et al. 1976), similar to the temperature changes reported by Vigersky and colleagues (1977) in young underweight women. Core body temperatures can fall to as low as 93°F, especially in children. Hypothermia and abnormal temperature regulation during starvation and anorexia nervosa seem to be due to a dysregulation in hypothalamic areas.

Heart morphology and function can be profoundly affected in anorexia nervosa and starvation (Schocken et al. 1989). The heart rate can drop below 60 bpm, leading to sinus bradycardia, and can fall as low as 30 bpm in the sleeping state. Hypotension with systolic blood pressures below 70 mm/Hg is common and can be associated with a reduction in cardiac size (Gottdiener et al. 1978). Mitral valve prolapse (despite structurally normal mitral valves) leading to systolic and diastolic ventricular dysfunction is not infrequently recognized on echocardiogram (Myers et al. 1987). In a study of 31 adolescent female and male anorexia nervosa patients who on average had lost 26% of body weight, Fohlin (1977) reported lowered heart and blood volumes and reduced maximal heart rates on exercise compared with children of similar age but normal weight. Loss of body weight alone could not explain the reduced maximal oxygen uptake; hence, hypothermia was thought to have contributed to the lower maximal heart rates. Some patients develop transitory systolic heart murmurs and peripheral edema (Halmi and Falk 1981). It has been recognized that peripheral edema most often

Table 27–1. Physical manifestations in restricting anorexia nervosa

Body weight loss (from 15%–60%) Loss of subcutaneous fat tissue Growth retardation (children)	
Metabolic	Hypothermia Hypometabolism Cold intolerance Carbohydrate intolerance
Central nervous system	Abnormal electroencephalogram Cerebral pseudoatrophy
Gastrointestinal	Delayed gastric emptying Superior mesenteric artery syndrome Constipation
Cardiovascular	Hypotension Bradycardia Arrhythmias Acrocyanosis
Renal	Dehydration Edema Polyuria Nycturia
Hematologic	Anemia (rare) Leukopenia with relative lymphocytosis Thrombocytopenia Bone marrow hypoplasia

occurs as a result of decreased renal perfusion and is not necessarily associated with a reduced plasma protein content or impaired renal function. In patients with anorexia nervosa of the restricting subtype, renal function is preserved despite a reduction in renal concentrating capacity.

Electrocardiographic abnormalities, such sinus bradycardia associated with increased Q-T and QT_c intervals reflect an increased risk for cardiac arrest and ectopic atrial rhythm. Atrioventricular junctional blocks and other forms of arrhythmias have been reported (Powers 1982; Thurston and Marks 1974). For these reasons, the cardiac status of cachectic patients requires careful monitoring, even during refeeding, because congestive heart failure has been reported (Powers 1982).

Morphological brain changes are not uncommon. Brain imaging studies such as computed tomography (CT) reveal enlarged inner and outer cerebrospinal fluid spaces in cases of advanced starvation (Enzmann and Lane 1977; Krieg et al. 1989; Nussbaum et al. 1980; Sein et al. 1981). The nature of this cerebral pseudoatrophy is unclear. It could well be a consequence of reduced intracellular and extracellular water, but it might also be related to the hypercortisolism associated with anorexia nervosa, because pseudoatrophy can be found in Cushing's disease (Heinz et al. 1977).

Sensory perceptual changes, such as changes in taste perception with reduced acuity for sour, salty, and bitter tastes, with sweet taste being the longest preserved, have been documented (Casper et al. 1980b). Such impaired taste perception would be expected to facilitate food avoidance by making meals less palatable. Reduced gastric motility and delayed gastric emptying (Dubois et al. 1979; Saleh and Lebwohl 1980), leading to unpleasant sensations of feeling bloated after eating, are common. Constipation is always present, but patients rarely complain about it.

■ Metabolic Changes

The reduced metabolic rate in anorexia nervosa is the outcome of a reduction in body mass and of a reduction in serum triiodothyronine (T_3) levels (Casper et al. 1991). Depending upon the nature and the severity of the starvation, the metabolic rate can fall to as low as 40% of the normal basal metabolic rate (Vaisman et al. 1988), at which point low T_3 plasma

levels and reduced thyroxine (T_4) plasma levels are the rule. Fasting hypoglycemia (Mecklenburg et al. 1974) and increased lipid mobilization reflected in elevated free fatty acid levels (Casper et al. 1988a) and β-hydroxybutyric acid levels (Pirke et al. 1985) have been documented in patients with anorexia nervosa. Other functional metabolic changes include glucose intolerance similar to that reported in cases of total starvation (Unger et al. 1963), with an abnormal rise in postabsorptive plasma glucose levels and a slow decline (Casper et al. 1977). Flat glucose plasma levels following glucose ingestion are most likely because of malabsorption. Impaired glucose tolerance is rarely the result of low circulating insulin levels. Instead, increased insulin receptor binding capacity has been reported in the cachectic state of anorexia nervosa (Wachslicht-Rodbard et al. 1979). Insulin receptor binding capacity normalized with weight restoration and a normal food intake. No correlation between circulating insulin levels and insulin binding was observed.

Table 27–2 illustrates the metabolic and hormonal factors that may have a bearing on the outcome of the glucose tolerance test in anorexia nervosa of either the restricting or bulimic subtype.

With weight gain, glucose tolerance has been shown to normalize (Casper et al. 1988a). Hypercarotenemia is not only the result of excessive ingestion of foods containing carotene, but, not unlike the frequently observed hypercholesterolemia, mostly consisting of low-density lipoproteins, it results from

Table 27–2. Factors influencing glucose metabolism in anorexia nervosa

Low insulin plasma levels Increased insulin binding to receptors on erythrocytes and monocytes	
Increased glucocorticoids and human growth hormone (HGH)	Malabsorption oral versus intravenous route
Glucose tolerance and intolerance in anorexia nervosa	
Dietary carbohydrate deficiency	Excessive exercising Hypokalemia
	Increased free fatty acids (FFAs) and ketoacids
Increased gastric inhibitory peptides Increased pancreatic polypeptides	

reduced enzymatic degradation and metabolic clearance. Therefore, treatment to reduce plasma cholesterol levels would not consist in reducing the intake of dietary fat. Instead, highly caloric meals ought to be encouraged to achieve a positive metabolic balance that will promptly lower plasma cholesterol levels.

Hematological changes such as mild anemia and moderate to severe leukopenia, often associated with relative lymphocytosis, seem to be the result of reversible bone marrow hypoplasia with increase in the mucopolysaccaride content in bone marrow (Mant and Faragher 1972). Interestingly, clinical observations do not support an increased susceptibility to infection in anorexia nervosa, even in patients with lymphopenia, except in advanced chronic cases (Bowers and Eckert 1978).

Levels of serum proteins remain generally within the low-normal range, and hypoalbuminemia generally indicates protracted and severe undernutrition (Casper et al. 1980b). Serum transferrin levels—measured directly or calculated from measurements of total iron-binding capacity (TIBC)—reflect protein deficiency much earlier than total protein albumin levels, because of their shorter half-life. Transferrin levels are almost always reduced in patients with anorexia nervosa.

■ Sleep Changes

Insomnia and a reduction in sleep time with early morning awakening is common in underweight and malnourished anorexia nervosa patients, but few patients ever complain about sleep disturbances. In fact, anorexia nervosa patients who awake early feel animated and vigorous, and they commonly engage in activities such as exercise or housecleaning.

Polysomnographic studies have reported significant reductions in sleep efficiency, total sleep time, and amount of slow wave sleep (SWS) (Kupfer and Bulik 1984; Lauer et al. 1988; Levy et al. 1987, 1988; Neil et al. 1980). Several studies noted reduced rapid eye movement (REM) latency (Katz et al. 1984; Lauer et al. 1990; Neil et al. 1980), an abnormality that has been considered specific for depression. Indeed, Katz and colleagues (1984) found a significant negative correlation between scores on the Hamilton Rating Scale for Depression (Hamilton 1960) and REM latency. This is unlike the study by Walsh and colleagues (1985), who failed to find an association between depressive symptoms and REM latency, but reported shorter REM latency in anorexia nervosa patients with concurrent depressive disorders.

Several factors that have been shown to influence sleep (e.g., age, chronicity, nutrition) need to be considered for interpreting sleep changes in anorexia nervosa. Sleep studies have rarely recorded the typical adolescent anorexia nervosa patient. The patients most often recorded were treatment-refractory patients in their twenties, but even in those, the relatively young age might have prevented the full spectrum of sleep abnormalities characteristic for depression to come into play. On the other hand, treatment-refractory patients are more likely to have comorbid disorders that could account for some of the associated sleep disturbances. Food deprivation alone affects sleep in animals (McFayden et al. 1973) and in humans (Karacan et al. 1973). Consistent with this nutritional deficiency theory, once anorexia nervosa patients gain weight, they show significant increases in total sleep, SWS, and REM sleep (Crisp et al. 1971; Evans 1983; Levy et al. 1987), albeit some studies have failed to observe a correlation between the amount of body weight and sleep variables (Lauer et al. 1990). Without comparisons to similarly underweight or undernourished age-matched control groups, the abnormal sleep findings in anorexia nervosa remain difficult to interpret.

■ Adaptation of the Neuroendocrine System in Anorexia Nervosa

The conceptualization of anorexia nervosa as an endocrine disorder by Simmonds (1914) led to a wealth of studies describing hormonal deficiencies, presumably all the result of pituitary insufficiency. Currently, there is consensus that pituitary function overall is not impaired in anorexia nervosa (Dreyfus and Mamou 1947; Garfinkel et al. 1975; Scheithauer et al. 1988). Most of the adaptive regulatory changes seem to originate from functional changes in and/or above the hypothalamus. Factors associated with anorexia nervosa that alone or in combination have been shown to bring about changes in hormone levels include the following:

1. Pathological body weight loss.
2. A reduced caloric intake, insufficient for weight maintenance.
3. Selective food intake leading to different kinds of

malnutrition or undernutrition. For example, a vegetarian diet or a diet consisting exclusively of cereals and bread may result in amino acid, trace element, or vitamin deficiencies, depending on individual habits and preferences.

4. Abnormal patterns of eating with gorging and emesis (anorexia nervosa, bulimic subtype).

5. As yet unknown factors that could turn out to be specific to anorexia nervosa.

The first three of these factors far outweigh the others in their contribution to the dysregulation of endocrine systems.

■ The Hypothalamic-Pituitary-Adrenal (HPA) Axis

Early reports of reduced urinary excretion of 17-ketosteroids were taken as a sign of pituitary-adrenal insufficiency in anorexia nervosa (Perloff et al. 1954). However, ketosteroids are poor indicators of adrenal function, because both gonadal and adrenal steroid hormones contribute to urinary ketosteroid excretion. In fact, the daily cortisol production rate in absolute terms and expressed as a function of body mass and body surface area has been found to be significantly increased in anorexia nervosa (Boyar et al. 1977; Walsh et al. 1978). Thus, urinary free cortisol is elevated in anorexia nervosa patients relative to nonanorexic control subjects (Boyar et al. 1977). Higher than normal resting plasma cortisol levels (yet normal levels of cortisol-binding globulin with reduced affinity), an increase in the number of secretory episodes and the time spent in secretory activity, as well as flattening of the normal diurnal secretory rhythm, are all common (Casper et al. 1979; Doerr et al. 1980; Fichter et al. 1986; Walsh et al. 1978). A reduced metabolic clearance rate, which prolongs the half-life of plasma cortisol as well as by alterations in steroid metabolic pathways, contributes to the increase in circulating cortisol plasma levels. Aside from weight loss, motor hyperactivity (Casper et al. 1991) and emotional distress may be involved in the activation of the HPA axis. The contribution of a coexisting depression to the HPA changes is difficult to establish, unless the patient is in metabolic balance and has regained at least 10%–15% of body weight (Doerr et al. 1980).

Studies by Gold and colleagues (1986) suggest that the hyperactivity of the adrenal cortex in an-

orexia nervosa might be related to increased secretion of corticotropin-releasing hormone (CRH); indeed, CRH levels have been reported to be elevated (Glowa and Gold 1991; Hotta et al. 1991). The anorexiant effects of CRH could well facilitate food abstention in anorexia nervosa, although tolerance seems to develop following repeated CRH exposure (Krahn et al. 1990). Interestingly, Gold and colleagues (1986) reported a significantly reduced net adrenocorticotropic hormone (ACTH) response to CRH, but normal baseline ACTH plasma levels in anorexia nervosa patients with the highest cortisol levels. Following some weight gain, the ACTH response to CRH continued to be markedly attenuated; but when their weight was fully restored to normal, anorexia nervosa patients demonstrated a normal ACTH response as well as a normal ACTH-to-cortisol ratio upon stimulation with CRH. The data suggest that the basal hypercortisolism in anorexia nervosa is related to a regulatory defect at or above the hypothalamic level and that with full weight recovery, eucortisolism is reestablished in the majority of patients.

The dexamethasone (DM) suppression test lacks specificity for anorexia nervosa, because most of the changes can be attributed to starvation. When DM, a highly potent synthetic corticosteroid, is given at 11 P.M. to block production of CRH and release of ACTH and cortisol, severely underweight and malnourished anorexia nervosa patients invariably fail to show the DM-induced suppression of cortisol secretion the next morning or the next afternoon (Gerner and Gwirtsman 1981). Following weight gain and in positive caloric balance, most patients suppress morning and afternoon plasma cortisol levels after DM administration to less than 5 mg/dl. Although depressed patients and patients with other psychiatric disorders may also show escape from DM suppression, no consistent relationship in acute anorexia nervosa has been found between depressive symptoms or a diagnosis of depressive disorder and DM suppression. Herpertz-Dahlman and Remschmidt (1990) have suggested that the DM suppression test might be of prognostic value and predict relapse in anorexia nervosa. From a clinical point of view, regular body weight measurements would seem more convenient for predicting relapse than repeated DM suppression tests.

Reduced caloric intake and weight loss clearly play a major role in this escape from DM suppression. Fasting, weight loss, and protein-calorie malnutrition can each cause alterations in the HPA axis in animals (Scapagnini et al. 1971) and control subjects that resemble those seen in patients with anorexia nervosa. Fichter and colleagues (1986) have subjected healthy subjects to 3 weeks of total food abstinence and reported a rise in 24-hour plasma cortisol levels, with an attenuated circadian pattern of cortisol release associated with a greater number of secretory episodes and a prolonged half-life of plasma cortisol. Half of the DM suppression tests performed in the fasting state showed insufficient suppression after administration of 1.5 mg DM, but DM suppression normalized with weight regain.

Because cortisol stimulates gluconeogenesis, the increased cortisol levels would be expected to play a role in maintaining adequate blood glucose concentrations. Elevated cortisol levels also have been shown to inhibit thyroid-stimulating hormone (TSH) release and thus decrease T_4 and consequently T_3 production. The decreased T_3 production in turn has been shown to lead to changes in metabolic pathways of cortisol, with an increase in the ratio of tetrahydrocortisol to tetrahydrocortisone (Boyar and Bradlow 1977; Zumoff et al. 1983).

■ The Hypothalamic-Pituitary-Gonadal (HPG) Axis

Primary or secondary amenorrhea in females and impotence in males are considered diagnostic for anorexia nervosa (American Psychiatric Association 1987). Secondary amenorrhea is associated with markedly reduced estradiol and absent progesterone plasma levels. Largely depending upon the degree of weight loss, a regression from the adult diurnal and nocturnal plasma luteinizing hormone (LH) pattern occurs with reactivation of the typical mid- and prepubertal LH pattern and ultimately the continuous low LH plasma levels of early puberty (Boyar et al. 1974; Katz et al. 1978; Pirke et al. 1979). Thus patients, whose weight loss exceeds 45% of body weight, invariably display the low sleep-dependent LH secretion pattern reminiscent of prepuberty.

The pituitary responsiveness can be tested through administration of synthetic gonadatropin-releasing hormones (GnRH) at different degrees of body weight loss. The blunted LH and less consistently blunted follicle stimulating hormone (FSH) responses (Sherman and Halmi 1977) to GnRH typical of prepuberty suggest a hypothalamic or supra-

hypothalamic defect. Pulsatile GnRH administration can restore ovarian activity even in anorexia nervosa patients who are markedly underweight (Guisti et al. 1988). Following a substantial weight gain to about 70% of ideal body weight, anorexia nervosa patients can display not only normal but also occasionally excessive LH release following GnRH bolus injections (Beumont et al. 1976).

The same transitory supersensitivity of the pituitary gonadotrophs occurs during normal puberty. At about 80%–90% of ideal body weight normal pituitary-gonadal responsiveness can be restored (Ferrari et al. 1989), but individuals vary substantially regarding the timing of normalization. As weight restoration proceeds, the diurnal and nocturnal LH plasma levels undergo anew the maturational pubertal release pattern, with sequential changes in ovarian activity. Thus, the restitutive changes observed in anorexia nervosa mimic the normal sequential changes during puberty. Normal cyclical LH release and menstrual function can resume after months following weight recovery, but more often several years pass before menstrual function is restored. The mechanism for the impaired GnRH secretion is unclear. The observation that naloxone infusion can restore LH pulses suggests endogenous opioid overactivity (Brambilla et al. 1991), although secretory changes in melatonin may well contribute (Ferrari et al. 1989).

The processes leading up to normal pubertal maturation are insufficiently understood. A theory proposed by Frisch and Revelle (1970) is relevant to anorexia nervosa. Frisch (1985) suggested that a certain amount of accumulated body fat was necessary to initiate puberty and that reproductive function depended on an optimal amount of body fat. Although this theory is still being debated, it would explain changes in reproductive function in anorexia nervosa patients and in athletes for whom excessive exercise might have increased muscle mass at the expense of body fat. However, this theory does not easily explain the frequently observed menstrual function changes in bulimia nervosa patients whose body fat mass shows little change.

Numerous studies have shown a drop in birth rate during famine or times of food scarcity, underlining the importance of an adequate food supply for reproductive function (Wade and Schneider 1992; Wilmsen 1982). In view of the menstrual changes reported under conditions of starvation, the notion that the secondary amenorrhea in anorexia nervosa reflects a primary hypothalamic deficit remains an unconfirmed hypothesis. The phenomenon of psychogenic amenorrhea, for example, suggests that stress might well play a role in early-onset amenorrhea (Nillius 1978) as might alterations in the diet (e.g., a vegetarian diet; Goldin et al. 1982) and excessive exercise (Brooks et al. 1984; Dale et al. 1979; Frisch et al. 1980). Furthermore, large individual variations exist in the stability of the HPG axis.

Prolonged amenorrhea with low plasma estradiol levels has been associated with low bone density (Rigotti et al. 1984; Szmukler et al. 1985). This finding raises two as yet unanswered questions about the need for estrogen replacement in young, normally active underweight girls or women and the long-term consequences of low plasma estradiol and possible risks associated with reduced bone density (Ettinger et al. 1985). In anorexia nervosa patients, estradiol metabolism is shifted toward an increased production of 2-hydroxyestrone (2-OH estrone) at the expense of estriol (Fishman et al. 1975). Remarkably, this increase in the catechol estrogens and the decrease in estriol formation have been reported in hyperthyroidism rather than hypothyroidism (Fishman et al. 1976). This greater formation of 2-OH estrone has two effects: 1) 2-OH estrone has a high binding capacity for estrogen receptors, but little biological activity; and 2) 2-OH estrone inhibits tyrosine hydroxylase and catechol-O-methyltransferase (COMT), two enzymes important for the synthesis and disposition of catecholamines. These two mechanisms can reduce the biological activity of estradiol even further.

Nevertheless, the commonly observed physical activity (Casper et al. 1991) may well counteract the reduction in bone density, and no controlled studies exist that have demonstrated an increase in bone density with estradiol administration. To the contrary, the risks of estradiol administration to the not fully grown adolescent patient may well exceed its benefits. Plasma testosterone levels have been reported in the normal range (Casper et al. 1979). Boyar and Bradlow (1977) have demonstrated (as in clinical hypothyroidism) a decrease in 5-α-reductase activity, which leads to diminished androsterone production at the expense of the β-route leading to etiocholanolone. Etiocholanolone has little androgen-like activity but tends to be pyrogenic. This enzymatic shift can be reversed by acute T_3 administration (Boyar and Bradlow 1977).

■ The Hypothalamic-Pituitary-Thyroid (HPT) Axis

The hypometabolic adaptation to starvation is achieved not so much by changes in thyroid glandular function that is overall unaffected with normal total T_4 plasma levels, but by reduced peripheral conversion of T_4 to T_3. About 80%–90% of T_3 derives from extrathyroidal conversion of T_4. Moreover, within days of severe undernutrition with carbohydrate deprivation, the peripheral deiodination of T_4 to T_3 is shunted into the inactive form, reverse T_3, which reduces T_3 levels further (Vagenakis et al. 1975). This change may represent another protective mechanism during the catabolic state. In patients with anorexia nervosa, T_3 serum levels can drop to as low as half of those of nonanorexic control subjects (Moshang and Utiger 1977; Moshang et al. 1975). Dialyzable free T_4 levels have been found to remain in the normal range. This low T_3 state contributes to symptoms such as constipation, dry skin and hair, bradycardia, cold intolerance, hypercarotenemia, and hypercholesterolemia, as well as to the decreased resting metabolic rate. Hypothyroidism is ruled out by normal TSH serum levels in the presence of low serum T_3; instead, a readjustment of the pituitary set point of TSH release seems to take place. Similar changes in the HPT axis, termed the euthyroid-sick syndrome, have been seen in other forms of malnutrition and in patients with severe nonthyroidal illnesses (Bermuder et al. 1975). Low T_3 plasma levels help conserve muscular tissue during sickness and starvation. Exogenous administration of T_3 leads to an increase in nitrogen excretion in starvation and in anorexia nervosa patients (Gardner et al. 1979; Leslie et al. 1978).

Thus, it is not surprising that the administration of thyrotropin-releasing hormone (TRH) results in quantitatively normal and occasionally slightly delayed TSH release (Casper and Frohman 1982; Kiriike et al. 1986; Leslie et al. 1978; Miyai et al. 1975). During weight gain, temporary rises of T_3 into the hyperthyroid range and exaggerated TSH responses can be observed (Casper and Frohman 1982; Moore and Mills 1979).

■ Human Growth Hormone (HGH)

Basal growth hormone (HGH) levels have been found slightly or markedly elevated in acutely starving anorexia nervosa patients (Casper et al. 1977). Growth hormone release is stimulated by other forms of undernutrition (Alvarez et al. 1972; Pimstone et al. 1967) and even by short-term fasting, and will normalize promptly with refeeding, especially with ingestion of carbohydrates. The presence of normal or elevated plasma growth hormone and cortisol levels distinguishes anorexia nervosa from hypopituitarism. Paradoxical growth hormone release has been reported by Macaron and colleagues (1978) in response to TRH administration and by Casper and colleagues (1977) to glucose administration. Under normal conditions, growth hormone secretion is augmented during SWS onset early during the night. This association can be disturbed in patients with anorexia nervosa in whom nocturnal growth hormone surges have been found to be prolonged or decreased in amplitude (Kalucy et al. 1976). Both hormones are protective counterregulatory hormones that stimulate gluconeogenesis in response to the threat of hypoglycemia with undernutrition. Growth hormone also stimulates the mobilization of fatty acids from fat tissue and seems to play a synergistic role with sex steroids during the adolescent growth spurt in conjunction with somatomedin (Phillips and Vassilopoulou-Sellin 1980).

■ Arginine Vasopressin

In response to osmotic challenge tests, patients with anorexia nervosa have been shown to have erratically high or reduced vasopressin responses consistent with partial diabetes insipidus, resulting in mild polyuria (Gold et al. 1983). In response to water deprivation, patients often do not sufficiently concentrate urine but respond normally when given vasopressin. Thus, most patients do have a relative but not an absolute deficiency of vasopressin secretion, which can also be observed after fasting (Drenick 1977). Even intermittent decreases in vasopressin may cause polyuria despite episodic high levels. With weight improvement, the instability of the vasopressin response can persist in some patients. However, in a study by Gold and colleagues (1983), most weight-improved patients were found to have normal vasopressin responses to sodium loading.

■ Prolactin

Prolactin is one of the few hormones that shows little, if any, alteration during the course of anorexia nervosa or in malnutrition (Beumont et al. 1974; Casper and Frohman 1982; Ferrari et al. 1990; Isaacs et al. 1980; Kiriike et al. 1986; Mecklenburg et al. 1974; Wakeling et al. 1979). Given that pituitary lactotrophs reflect central nervous system (CNS) dopaminergic tone, the normal prolactin plasma levels would argue against a dopamine deficiency theory of anorexia nervosa. Most investigators have found normal plasma prolactin secretion patterns in response to TRH administration, although some have observed elevated levels (Travaglini et al. 1976) or found a temporary delay in peak prolactin responses (Vigersky et al. 1976).

■ Melatonin

Melatonin, produced by the pineal gland, is an important neuromodulator of reproductive function. In various mammalian species, melatonin has been shown to inhibit gonadal development and function (Rivest 1987). Changes in the circadian pattern of melatonin may modulate pubertal development and ovarian cyclicity.

The reports on the circadian rhythm of melatonin in anorexia nervosa are somewhat conflicting. Ferrari and colleagues (1989, 1990) have reported a similar albeit significantly higher circadian profile of plasma melatonin in anorexia nervosa patients as in control subjects, with an increased ratio between day and night melatonin levels and abnormal daytime secretory peaks of melatonin. By contrast, Kennedy and colleagues (1991) have reported similar melatonin plasma levels in underweight or weight-improved patients and healthy control subjects; however, there was a tendency for the patients with the lowest weight to have the highest nocturnal melatonin levels. Thus, increases in melatonin levels and the persistence of melatonin secretion during the day might contribute to the inhibition of pituitary-gonadal function in anorexia nervosa patients.

■ ANOREXIA NERVOSA–BULIMIC SUBTYPE AND BULIMIA NERVOSA

The starvation-induced changes in anorexia nervosa of the bulimic subtype and in bulimia nervosa resemble in many ways those seen in anorexia nervosa of the restricting subtype. The additional binge-eating and self-induced vomiting and/or diuretic and laxative abuse produce a new set of medical complications listed in Table 27–3.

■ Physical Changes

Despite generally normal body weight in bulimia nervosa, these patients can nevertheless undergo large body weight fluctuations as a result of episodic fasting followed by periods of overeating. Binge-eating can cause acute gastric dilatation and, in rare cases, gastric rupture (Backett 1985; Saul et al. 1981). Repeated vomiting has been found to lead to erosion of dental enamel, esophagitis, Mallory-Weiss syndrome, and (rarely) esophageal rupture. Salivary gland enlargement is common, with the parotid glands most frequently affected, resulting in a "chipmunk" appearance, but its mechanism is unclear. It could be related to excess saliva production, rapid overeating, repeated vomiting, excess use of chewing gum, or alkalosis. Parotid biopsies have revealed normal hyperplastic tissue (Levin et al. 1980; Walsh et al. 1982), although pancreatitis has been reported (Marano and Sangree 1984; Zerbe 1992). Salivary

Table 27–3. Physical manifestations in bulimia nervosa (and in anorexia nervosa, bulimic subtype)

Body weight fluctuations (2–50 lbs.) Parotid enlargement Dehydration	
Metabolic	Hypothermia Hypometabolism Hypokalemia Hypochloremic alkalosis
Central nervous system	Abnormal electroencephalogram
Orogastrointestinal	Dental enamel erosion Swelling of salivary glands Esophagitis Mallory-Weiss tears Gastric dilation Gastric rupture Diarrhea
Cardiovascular	Electrocardiogram changes Arrhythmias Cardiac arrest
Renal	Dehydration Alkalosis Renal calculi Renal insufficiency
Pulmonary	Aspiration pneumonia

gland enlargement can be associated with elevated serum amylase levels, which need to be distinguished from elevated serum amylase levels in pancreatitis through isoenzyme assay, although Cox and colleagues (1983) have also reported pancreatic abnormalities in bulimia nervosa patients. In patients who abuse alcohol or drugs, vomiting during semiconscious states might lead to aspiration or aspiration pneumonia that can cause death.

■ Metabolic Changes

The intermittent caloric deprivation in bulimia nervosa patients has been shown to elevate levels of free fatty acids and β-hydroxybutyric acid in plasma, suggesting excess lipid mobilization as a result of caloric malnutrition (Pirke et al. 1985). A serious and potentially life-threatening metabolic complication is hypokalemia. Potassium depletion is most often a result of emesis and/or laxative or diuretic abuse (Elkinton and Huth 1958; Wallace et al. 1968; Warren and Steinberg 1979). Because the potassium concentration of gastric fluid is fairly low, only a small portion of the potassium depletion is probably the result of potassium loss from gastric fluid or saliva, as a result of the loss of hydrochloric acid from gastric fluid through vomiting. Most of the potassium loss is because of a rise in renal potassium excretion secondary to metabolic alkalosis.

On the other hand, hypokalemia can result from significant intestinal potassium loss through chronic diarrhea following laxative abuse. Moderate to severe hypokalemia leads to weakness in skeletal and smooth muscle; more dangerous are cardiac conduction abnormalities, arrhythmia, and (ultimately) cardiac arrest. Chronic metabolic alkalosis can be associated with hypokalemic nephropathy and occasionally simulate Bartter's syndrome, characterized by hypokalemic alkalosis, hyperaldosteronism, and hyperplasia of the renal juxtaglomerular apparatus. Urinary chloride levels distinguish this condition from Bartter's syndrome. Not infrequently, it will be necessary to prescribe potassium supplements for bulimia nervosa patients, with dosage adjustments dependent on the frequency of vomiting. The orthostatic hypotension can be worsened by a reduction in plasma volume caused by significant electrolyte imbalances and intermittent dehydration as a result of vomiting. A serious renal complication, aside from renal calculi, can be renal failure.

Green and Rau (1974) were the first to report electroencephalogram (EEG) abnormalities in bulimia nervosa, the most common abnormality being a paroxysmal 14- and 6-per-second spike pattern. This pattern, however, can also be observed in non-bulimic adolescents (Maulsby 1979). It is therefore not surprising that Mitchell and colleagues (1983) reported normal EEG recordings in more than 80% of older bulimia nervosa patients. Hoffman and colleagues (1990) reported magnetic resonance imaging (MRI) changes, and Hagman and colleagues (1990) demonstrated differences in the activation of various brain regions between bulimia nervosa patients and control subjects based on positron-emission tomography (PET) scanning. Interestingly, Hagman and colleagues (1990) also found a positive correlation between the severity of the dynamic PET changes and the severity of the bulimia, suggesting a metabolic component. The significance of the PET changes for the functional brain activity remains unclear.

Sleep Changes

Bulimia nervosa patients show less significant disruptions in sleep continuity than do anorexia nervosa patients (Levy et al. 1987; Waller et al. 1989; Walsh et al. 1985), and most studies found their REM latency to be indistinguishable from that of control subjects (Levy et al. 1988; Walsh et al. 1985). The increased incidence of drug abuse, alcoholism, and affective disorder that can affect sleep parameters needs to be monitored for evaluating sleep parameters in bulimia nervosa patients. The phenomena of sleepwalking and sleep-related eating in bulimia nervosa doubtlessly deserve more systematic investigation (Guirgis 1986; Gupta 1991).

Neuroendocrine Changes

Far fewer endocrine investigations have been performed in bulimia nervosa than in anorexia nervosa. Some bulimia nervosa patients shows endocrine changes; others do not (Mitchell et al. 1983; Wetzin et al. 1991). Dietary restriction and abnormal eating very likely play a role, because few hormonal abnormalities are observed when food intake becomes more normal (Casper et al. 1988b). For instance, Kiyohara and colleagues (1987) documented abnormal eating patterns in all bulimia nervosa patients

who displayed abnormal TSH responses to TRH. Similarly, in most patients, normal peak glucose and insulin levels after oral glucose administration have been reported (Blouin et al. 1991; Casper et al 1988b; Mitchell and Bantle 1983; Weingarten et al. 1988). In normal weight bulimic women, insulin responses after intravenous glucose administration were in the normal range (Coiro et al. 1992), but cortisol levels remained unchanged and HGH levels showed a rise instead of a fall. Somatostatin levels have generally found to be normal (Kaye et al. 1988). Oligomenorrhea or menstrual irregularities seem to somewhat exceed the rates observed in nonbulimic women (Pirke et al. 1987a; Stewart et al. 1987), and abnormalities in LH release have been reported (Pirke et al. 1987b).

Patients with bulimia nervosa show more often DM-nonsuppression than would be expected, given their seemingly normal body weight (Gwirtsman et al. 1983; Hudson et al. 1982, 1983; Levy and Dixon 1987; Walsh et al. 1987), but comorbid pathology that was not ruled out in most studies may have contributed to the findings. On the other hand, Walsh and colleagues (1987) measured 24-hour cortisol secretion patterns and cortisol release upon ACTH stimulation in symptomatic bulimia nervosa patients and found a normal cortisol secretion pattern and normal cortisol increase following ACTH. Similarly, Gold and colleagues (1986) reported normal ACTH levels following CRH administration in bulimia nervosa patients of normal weight.

CONCLUSION

The prolonged and severe caloric restriction and the resultant catabolic state that characterizes anorexia nervosa bring about innumerable biological changes. In fact, the restricting subtype of anorexia nervosa, with its profound and pathological weight loss, can be considered a model of long-term starvation without attendant organic illness. Anorexia nervosa provides a wealth of information about the physiological, metabolic, and endocrine consequences of varying degrees of undernutrition and malnutrition.

Follow-up studies suggest that if the fasting anorexia nervosa patient is restored to a weight appropriate for age and height and eats normal caloric and nutritional meals, then full biological recovery with normalization of all metabolic and endocrine parameters is likely. A potential problem that will require further study is whether undernutrition in early adolescence affects long-term skeletal growth.

In the case of bulimia nervosa, where episodic caloric deficiency (mostly as a result of emesis) can result in a puzzling array of generally moderate but sometimes life-threatening physiological, metabolic, and neuroendocrine disturbances, permanent physical damage has been reported. Such injury is invariably the result of vomiting behavior and abuse of laxatives or diuretics and other noxious substances (e.g., ipecac use can lead to cardiomyopathy).

Various efforts have been made to sort out the biological differences between eating disorders and depressive disorders. The remarkable similarities between the HPA axis abnormalities in anorexia nervosa and depressive disorder will require more careful examination against the background of either malnutrition and weight loss in depressive disorders or of a comorbid affective disorder in anorexia nervosa before a common underlying mechanism can be postulated. The overlap in the HPA axis disturbances between the two disorders should not detract from obvious differences in the clinical picture. For instance, early morning awakening (typically observed in both conditions) can easily distinguish the two, given the marked differences in mood and energy level. This is because patients with anorexia nervosa usually awaken refreshed and full of vigor, as opposed to depressed patients, who typically dwell on morbid worries and feel lethargic in the morning. Lethargy in the presence of abnormally low plasma cortisol levels would be highly suggestive of Addison's disease.

The thyroid axis is another system that can be used to distinguish the two disorders. The recently developed supersensitive TSH assays give normally low TSH plasma levels in anorexia nervosa, indicating a "euthyroid sick syndrome," whereas elevated TSH levels would be suggestive of hypothyroidism that may or may not be associated with depressive symptoms.

In the eating disorders, then, nutritional deficits and changes in body composition (more specifically, differences in the severity and duration of weight loss), eating pattern, dietary composition, comorbidity, age, or treatment status account for most of the variance in the biological findings. Unless more homogeneous populations can be investigated with superb experimental control of all these confounding variables, it would seem premature to assign etiological significance to any of the recorded biological changes.

■ REFERENCES

Alvarez LC, Dimas CO, Catro A, et al: Growth hormone in malnutrition. J Clin Endocrinol Metab 34:400–409, 1972

American Psychiatric Association: Diagnostic and Statistical Manual of Mental Disorders, 3rd Edition, Revised. Washington, DC, American Psychiatric Association, 1987

Backett SA: Acute pancreatitis and gastric dilation in a patient with anorexia nervosa. Postgrad Med J 61:39–40, 1985

Bell RM: Holy Anorexia. Chicago, IL, University of Chicago Press, 1985

Bermuder F, Surks MI, Oppenheimer JH: High incidence of decreased serum triiodothyronine concentration in patients with nonthyroidal disease. J Clin Endocrinol Metab 41:27–31, 1975

Beumont PJV, Freisen HG, Gelder MG, et al: Plasma prolactin and luteinizing hormone levels in anorexia nervosa. Psychol Med 4:219–221, 1974

Beumont PJV, George GCW, Pimstone BL, et al: Body weight and the pituitary response to hypothalamic-releasing hormones in patients with anorexia nervosa. J Clin Endocrinol Metab 40:221–227, 1976

Blouin AG, Blouin JH, Braaten JT, et al: Physiological and psychological responses to a glucose challenge in bulimia. International Journal of Eating Disorders 10:285–296, 1991

Bowers TK, Eckert E: Leukopenia in anorexia nervosa: lack of increased risk of infection. Arch Intern Med 138:1520–1523, 1978

Boyar RM, Bradlow HL: Studies of testosterone metabolism in anorexia nervosa, in Anorexia Nervosa. Edited by Vigersky RA. New York, Raven, 1977, pp 271–276

Boyar RM, Katz J, Finkelstein JW, et al: Anorexia nervosa: immaturity of the 24-hour luteinizing hormone secretory pattern. N Engl J Med 291:861–865, 1974

Boyar RM, Hellman LD, Roffwarg HP, et al: Cortisol secretion and metabolism in anorexia nervosa. N Engl J Med 296:190–193, 1977

Brambilla F, Ferrari E, Petraglia F, et al: Peripheral

opioid secretory pattern in anorexia nervosa. Psychiatry Res 39:115–127, 1991

Brooks SM, Sanborn CF, Albrecht BH, et al: Diet in athletic amenorrhoea [letter]. Lancet 1:559–560, 1984

Bruch H: Eating Disorders. New York, Basic Books, 1973

Casper RC: On the emergence of bulimia nervosa as a syndrome: a historical view. International Journal of Eating Disorders 2:3–16, 1983

Casper RC, Davis JM: On the course of anorexia nervosa. Am J Psychiatry 134:974–978, 1977

Casper RC, Frohman LA: Delayed TSH release in anorexia nervosa following injection of thyrotropin releasing hormone (TRH). Psychoneuroendocrinology 7:59–68, 1982

Casper RC, Davis JM, Pandey GN: The effect of nutritional status and weight changes on hypothalamic function tests in anorexia nervosa, in Anorexia Nervosa. Edited by Vigersky RA. New York, Raven, 1977, pp 137–147

Casper RC, Chatterton RT Jr, Davis M: Alterations in serum cortisol and its binding characteristics in anorexia nervosa. J Clin Endocrinol 49:406–411, 1979

Casper RC, Eckert ED, Halmi KA, et al: Bulimia: its incidence and clinical importance in patients with anorexia nervosa. Arch Gen Psychiatry 37:1030–1035, 1980a

Casper RC, Kirschner B, Sandstead HH, et al: An evaluation of trace metals, vitamins, and taste function in anorexia nervosa. Am J Clin Nutr 33:1801–1808, 1980b

Casper RC, Pandey GN, Jaspan JB, et al: Eating attitudes and glucose tolerance in anorexia nervosa patients at 8-year followup compared to control subjects. Psychiatry Res 25:283–299, 1988a

Casper RC, Pandey GN, Jaspan JB, et al: Hormone and metabolite plasma levels after oral glucose in bulimia and healthy controls. Biol Psychiatry 24:663–674, 1988b

Casper RC, Schoeller DA, Kushner R, et al: Total daily energy expenditure and activity level in anorexia nervosa. Am J Clin Nutr 53:1143–1150, 1991

Coiro V, Volpi R, Marchesi C, et al: Abnormal growth hormone and cortisol, but not thyroid-stimulating hormone, responses to an intravenous glucose tolerance test in normal-weight, bulimic women. Psychoneuroendocrinology 17:639–645, 1992

Cox KL, Cannon RA, Ament ME, et al: Biochemical and ultrasound abnormalities of the pancreas in anorexia nervosa. Dig Dis Sci 28:255–229, 1983

Crisp AH, Stonehill E, Fenton GW: The relationship between sleep, nutrition and mood: a study of patients with anorexia nervosa. Postgrad Med J 47:207–213, 1971

Dale D, Gerlach DH, Wilhite AL: Menstrual dysfunction in distance runners. Obstet Gynecol 54:47–53, 1979

Doerr P, Fichter M, Pirke KM, et al: Relationship between weight gain and hypothalamic pituitary adrenal function in patients with anorexia nervosa. Journal of Steroid Biochemistry 13:529–537, 1980

Drenick H: Role of vasopressin and prolactin in abnormal salt and water metabolism of obese patients before and after fasting and during refeeding. Metabolism 26:309–317, 1977

Dreyfus G, Mamou H: Cachéxie cérebro-hypophysaire d'origine fonctionnelle et à évolution mortelle sans altérations histologiques à l'autopsie. [Cachexia of central hypophyseal origin leading to death without histological changes at autopsy.] Ann Endocrinol (Paris) 8:540–544, 1947

Dubois A, Gross HA, Ebert MH, et al: Altered gastric emptying and secretion in primary anorexia nervosa. Gastroenterology 77:319–323, 1979

Elkinton JR, Huth EJ: Body fluid abnormalities in anorexia nervosa and undernutrition. Metabolism 5:376–403, 1958

Enzmann DR, Lane B: Cranial computer tomography findings in anorexia nervosa. J Comput Assist Tomogr 1:410–414, 1977

Ettinger B, Genant HK, Cann CE: Long-term estrogen replacement therapy prevents bone loss and fractures. Ann Intern Med 102:319–324, 1985

Evans FJ: Sleep, eating, and weight disorders, in Eating and Weight Disorders. Edited by Richard K. New York, Springer, 1983, pp 147–178

Ferrari E, Foppa S, Bossolo PA, et al: Melatonin and pituitary-gonadal function in disorders of eating behavior. Journal of Pineal Research 7:115–124, 1989

Ferrari E, Fraschini F, Brambilla F: Hormonal circadian rhythms in eating disorders. Biol Psychiatry 27:1007–1020, 1990

Fichter M, Pirke KM, Holsboer F: Weight loss causes neuroendocrine disturbances: experimental study in healthy starving subjects. Psychiatry Res 17:61–72, 1986

Fishman J, Boyar RM, Hellman L: Influence of body weight on estradiol metabolism in young women.

J Clin Endocrinol Metab 41:989–991, 1975

Fishman J, Hellman L, Zumoff B, et al: Effect of thyroid on hydroxylation of estrogen in man. Journal of Clinical Endocrinology 25:365–376, 1976

Fohlin L: Body composition, cardiovascular and renal function in adolescent patients with anorexia nervosa. Acta Paediatr Suppl 268:1–20, 1977

Frisch RL: Fatness, menarche, and female fertility. Perspect Biol Med 28:611–633, 1985

Frisch RL, Revelle R: Height and weight at menarche and a hypothesis of critical body weights and adolescent events. Science 169:397–398, 1970

Frisch RL, Wyshak G, Vincent L: Delayed menarche and amenorrhea in ballet dancers. N Engl J Med 303:17–19, 1980

Garfinkel PE, Brown GH, Stancer HC, et al: Hypothalamic-pituitary function in anorexia nervosa. Arch Gen Psychiatry 32:739–744, 1975

Gardner DF, Kaplan MM, Stanley CA, et al: Effect of triiodothyronine replacement on the metabolic and pituitary responses to starvation. N Engl J Med 300:579–584, 1979

Gerner RH, Gwirtsman HE: Abnormalities of dexamethasone suppression test and urinary MHPG in anorexia nervosa. Am J Psychiatry 138:650–653, 1981

Glowa JR, Gold PW: Corticotropin releasing hormone produced profound anorexigenic effects in the rhesus monkey. Neuropeptides 18:55–61, 1991

Gold PW, Kaye W, Robertson GL, et al: Abnormalities in plasma and cerebrospinal fluid arginine vasopressin in patients with anorexia nervosa. N Engl J Med 308:1117–1123, 1983

Gold PW, Gwirtsman H, Avgerinos PC, et al: Abnormal hypothalamic-pituitary-adrenal function in anorexia nervosa: pathophysiologic mechanisms in underweight and weight-corrected patients. N Engl J Med 314:1335–1342, 1986

Goldin BR, Adlercrentz H, Gorbach SL: Estrogen excretion patterns and plasma levels in vegetarian and omnivorous women. N Engl J Med 307:1542–1547, 1982

Gottdiener JS, Gross HA, Henry WL, et al: Effects of self-induced starvation on cardiac size and function in anorexia nervosa. Circulation 58:426–433, 1978

Green RS, Rau JH: Treatment of compulsive eating disturbances with anticonvulsant medication. Am J Psychiatry 131:428–432, 1974

Guirguis WR: Sleepwalking as a symptom of bulimia. BMJ 293:587–588, 1986

Guisti M, Torre R, Traverso L: Endogenous opioid blockade and gonadotropin secretion: role of pulsatile luteinizing hormone-releasing hormone administration in anorexia nerovsa and weight loss amenorrhea. Fertil Steril 49:797–801, 1988

Gupta MA: Sleep-related eating in bulimia nervosa—an underreported parasomnia disorder. Sleep Research 20:182, 1991

Gwirtsman HE, Roy-Byrne P, Yager J, et al: Neuroendocrine abnormalities in bulimia. Am J Psychiatry 140:559–563, 1983

Hagman JO, Buchsbaum MS, Wer JG, et al: Comparison of regional brain metabolism in bulimia nervosa and affective disorder assessed with positron emission tomography. J Affect Disord 19:153–162, 1990

Halmi KA, Falk JR: Common physiological changes in anorexia nervosa. International Journal of Eating Disorders 1:16–27, 1981

Hamilton M: A rating scale for depression. J Neurol Neurosurg Psychiatry 23:56–62, 1960

Heinz ER, Martinez J, Haenggeli A: Reversibility of cerebral atrophy in anorexia nervosa and Cushing's syndrome. J Comput Assist Tomogr 1:415–418, 1977

Herpertz-Dahlman B, Remschmidt H: The prognostic value of the dexamethasone suppression test for the course of anorexia nervosa—comparison with depressive diseases. Z Kinder Jugendpsychiatr 18:5–11, 1990

Hoffman GW, Ellinwood EH, Rockwell WJK, et al: Cerebral atrophy and T1 measured by magnetic resonance imaging in bulimia. Biol Psychiatry 27:116–119, 1990

Hotta M, Shibasaki T, Yamauchi N, et al: The effects of chronic central administration of corticotropin-releasing factor on food intake, body weight, and hypothalamic-pituitary-adrenocortical hormones. Life Sci 48:1483–1491, 1991

Hudson JI, Laffer PS, Pope HG: Bulimia related to affective disorder by family history and response to the DST. Am J Psychiatry 139:685–687, 1982

Hudson JI, Pope HG, Jonas JM, et al: HPA axis hyperactivity in bulimia. Psychiatry Res 8:111–117, 1983

Isaacs, AJ, Leslie D, Gomez J, et al: The effect of weight gain on gonadotrophins and prolactin in anorexia nervosa. Acta Endocrinol (Copenh) 94:145–150, 1980

Jackson RL, Kelby AG: Growth charts for use in pediatric practice. J Pediatr 27:215–229, 1945

Kalucy RC, Crisp AH, Chard T, et al: Nocturnal hormonal profiles in massive obesity, anorexia nervosa and normal females. J Psychosom Res 20:595–604, 1976

Karacan I, Rosenbloom AL, Londono JH, et al: The effect of acute fasting on sleep and the sleep-growth hormone response. Psychosomatics 14:33–37, 1973

Katz JL, Boyar R, Roffwarg H, et al: Weight and circadian luteinizing hormone secretory pattern in anorexia nervosa. Psychosom Med 40:549–567, 1978

Katz JL, Kuperberg A, Pollack CP, et al: Is there a relationship between eating disorder and affective disorder? New evidence from sleep recordings. Am J Psychiatry 141:753–759, 1984

Kaye WH, Rubinow D, Gwirtsman HE, et al: CSF somatostatin in anorexia nervosa and bulimia: relationship to the hypothalamic-pituitary-adrenal cortical axis. Psychoneuroendocrinology 13:265–272, 1988

Kennedy SH, Brown GM, McVey G, et al: Pineal and adrenal function before and after refeeding in anorexia nervosa. Biol Psychiatry 30:216–224, 1991

Keys A, Brozek J, Henschel A, et al: The Biology of Human Starvation. Minneapolis, MN, University of Minnesota Press, 1950

Keys A, Fidanza F, Karvonan MJ, et al: Indices of relative weight and obesity. Journal of Chronic Disease 25:329–343, 1972

Kiyohara K, Tamai H, Karibe C, et al: Serum thyrotropin (TSH) responses to thyrotropin-releasing hormone (TRH) in patients with anorexia nervosa and bulimia: influence of changes in body weight and eating disorders. Psychoneuroendocrinology 12:21–28, 1987

Kiriike N, Nishiwaki S, Izumiya Y, et al: Thyrotropin, prolactin and growth hormone responses to thyrotropin-releasing hormone in anorexia nervosa and bulimia. Biol Psychiatry 21:167–176, 1986

Krahn DD, Gosnell BA, Majchrzak MG: The anorectic effects of CRH and restraint stress decrease with repeated exposures. Biol Psychiatry 27:1094–1102, 1990

Krieg JC, Lauer C, Leinsinger G, et al: Brain morphology and regional cerebral blood flow in anorexia nervosa. Biol Psychiatry 25:1041–1048, 1989

Kupfer DJ, Bulik CM: Sleeping and waking EEG in anorexia nervosa, in The Psychobiology of Anorexia Nervosa. Edited by Pirke KM, Ploog D. Berlin, Springer-Verlag, 1984, pp 73–86

Lauer CJ, Zulley J, Krieg JC, et al: EEG sleep and the cholinergic REM induction test in anorexic and bulimic patients. Psychiatry Res 26:171–181, 1988

Lauer CJ, Krieg JC, Riemann D, et al: A polysomnographic study in young psychiatric inpatients: major depression, anorexia nervosa, bulimia nervosa. J Affect Disord 18:235–245, 1990

Leslie RD, Isaacs AJ, Gomez J, et al: Hypothalamo-pituitary-thyroid function in anorexia nervosa: influence of weight gain. BMJ 2:526–528, 1978

Levin PA, Falko JM, Dixon K, et al: Benign parotid enlargement in bulimia. Ann Intern Med 93:827–829, 1980

Levy AB, Dixon KN: DST in bulimia without endogenous depression. Biol Psychiatry 22:783–786, 1987

Levy AB, Dixon KN, Schmidt H: REM and delta sleep in anorexia nervosa and bulimia. Psychiatry Res 20:189–197, 1987

Levy AB, Dixon KN, Schmidt H: Sleep architecture in anorexia nervosa and bulimia. Biol Psychiatry 23:99–101, 1988

Luck P, Wakeling A: Altered thresholds for thermoregulatory sweating and vasodilation in anorexia nervosa. BMJ 281:906–908, 1980

Macaron C, Wilber JF, Green O, et al: Studies of growth hormone, (GH), thyrotrophin (TSH) and prolactin (PRL) secretion in anorexia nervosa. Psychoneuroendocrinology 3:181–185, 1978

Mant MJ, Faragher BS: The haematology of anorexia nervosa. Br J Haematol 23:737–749, 1972

Marano AR, Sangree MH: Acute pancreatitis associated with bulimia. J Clin Gastroenterol 6:245–248, 1984

Maulsby RL: EEG patterns of uncertain diagnostic significance, in Current Practice of Clinical Electroencephalography. Edited by Klass DW, Daly DD. New York, Raven, 1979

McFayden UM, Oswald I, Lewis SA: Starvation and human slow-wave sleep. J Appl Physiol 35:391–394, 1973

Mecklenburg RS, Loriaux DL, Thompson RH, et al: Hypothalamic dysfunction in patients with anorexia nervosa. Medicine (Baltimore) 53:147–159, 1974

Mitchell JE, Bantle JP: Metabolic and endocrine investigations in women of normal weight with the bulimia syndrome. Biol Psychiatry 18:355–364, 1983

Mitchell JE, Hosfield W, Pyle RL: EEG findings in patients with the bulimia syndrome. International Journal of Eating Disorders 2:17–23, 1983

Miyai K, Yamamoto T, Axukizawa M, et al: Serum thyroid hormones and thyrotropin in anorexia nervosa. J Clin Endocrinol Metab 40:334–338, 1975

Moore R, Mills H: Serum T_3 and T_4 levels in patients with anorexia nervosa showing transient hyperthyroidism during weight gain. Clin Endocrinol (Oxf) 10:433–439, 1979

Moshang T, Utiger RD: Low triiodothyronine euthyroidism in anorexia nervosa, in Anorexia Nervosa. Edited by Vigersky RA. New York, Raven, 1977, pp 263–270

Moshang T Jr, Parks JS, Balsor L, et al: Low serum triiodothyronine in patients with anorexia nervosa. J Clin Endocrinol Metab 40:470–473, 1975

Myers DG, Starke H, Pearson PH, et al: Leaflet to left ventricular size disproportion and prolapse of a structurally normal mitral valve in anorexia nervosa. Am J Cardiol 60:911–914, 1987

Neil JF, Merikangas JR, Foster FG, et al: Waking and all-night sleep EEG's in anorexia nervosa. Clin Electroencephalogr 11:9–15, 1980

Nillius SJ: Psycho-pathology of weight-related amenorrhea, in Advances in Gynaecological Endocrinology. Edited by Jacobs HS. London, Royal College of Obstetrics and Gynaecologists, 1978, pp 118–130

Nussbaum M, Shenker IR, Marc J, et al: Cerebral atrophy in anorexia nervosa. J Pediatr 96:867–869, 1980

Perloff WH, Lasche EM, Nodine JH, et al: The starvation state and functional hypopituitarism. JAMA 155:1307–1313, 1954

Phillips LS, Vassilopoulou-Sellin R: Somatomedins. N Engl J Med 312:438–446, 1980

Pimstone BL, Barbezat G, Hansen JPL, et al: Growth hormone and protein-calorie malnutrition. Lancet 2:1333–1334, 1967

Pirke KM, Fichter MM, Lund R, et al: Twenty-four hour sleep wake pattern of plasma LH in patients with anorexia nervosa. Acta Endocrinol 92:193–204, 1979

Pirke KM, Pahl J, Schweiger U, et al: Metabolic and endocrine indices of starvation in bulimia: a comparison with anorexia nervosa. Psychiatry Res 15:33–39, 1985

Pirke KM, Fichter MM, Chlond C, et al: Disturbances of the menstrual cycle in bulimia nervosa. Clin Endocrinol (Oxf) 27:245–251, 1987a

Pirke KM, Fichter MM, Schweiger V, et al: Gonadotropin secretion pattern in bulimia nervosa. International Journal of Eating Disorders 6:655–661, 1987b

Powers PS: Heart failure during treatment of anorexia nervosa. Am J Psychiatry 139:1167–1170, 1982

Rigotti NA, Nussbaum SR, Herzog DB, et al: Osteoporosis in women with anorexia nervosa. N Engl J Med 311:1601–1606, 1984

Rivest RW: The female rat as a model describing patterns of pulsatile LH secretion during puberty and their control by melatonin. Gynecol Endocrinol 1:279–293, 1987

Russell GFM: Bulimia nervosa: an ominous variant of anorexia nervosa. Psychol Med 9:429–448, 1979

Saleh JW, Lebwohl P: Metoclopramide-induced gastric emptying in patients with anorexia nervosa. Am J Gastroenterol 74:127–132, 1980

Saul SH, Dekker A, Watson CG: Acute gastric dilation with infarction and perforation. Gut 22:978–983, 1981

Scapagnini U, Moberg GP, Van Loon GR, et al: Relation of the brain 5-hydroxytryptamine content to the diurnal variation in plasma corticosterone in the rat. Neuroendocrinology 7:90–96, 1971

Scheithauer BW, Kovacs KT, Jariwala LK, et al: Anorexia nervosa: an immunohistochemical study of the pituitary gland. Mayo Clin Proc 63:23–28, 1988

Schocken DD, Holloway JD, Powers PS: Weight loss and the heart: effects of anorexia nervosa and starvation. Arch Intern Med 149:877–881, 1989

Sein P, Searson S, Nicol AR: Anorexia nervosa and pseudo-atrophy of the brain. Br J Psychiatry 139:257–258, 1981

Sherman BM, Halmi KA: Effect of nutritional rehabilitation on hypothalamic-pituitary function in anorexia nervosa, in Anorexia Nervosa. Edited by Vigersky RA. New York, Raven, 1977, pp 211–223

Simmonds M: Ueber Hypophysisschwund mit toedlichem Ausgang. [About atrophy of the pituitary gland leading to death.] Dtsch Med Wochenschr 40:322, 1914

Stewart DE, Raskin J, Garfinkel PE, et al: Anorexia nervosa, bulimia and pregnancy. Am J Obstet Gynecol 157:1194–1198, 1987

Szmukler GI, Brown SW, Parsons V, et al: Premature loss of bone in chronic anorexia nervosa. BMJ 290:26–27, 1985

Szmukler G, McCance C, McCrone L, et al: Anorexia nervosa: a psychiatric case register study from Aberdeen. Psychol Med 16:49–58, 1986

Thurston J, Marks P: Electrocardiographic abnormalities in patients with anorexia nervosa. Br Heart J 36:719–723, 1974

Travaglini P, Beck-Peccoz P, Ferrari C, et al: Some aspects of hypothalamic-pituitary function in patients with anorexia nervosa. Acta Endocrinol (Copenh) 81:252–262, 1976

Unger RH, Eisentraut AM, Madison LL: The effects of total starvation upon the levels of circulating glucagon and insulin in man. J Clin Invest 42:1031–1039, 1963

Vagenakis AG, Portnay GI, Burger A, et al: Diversion of peripheral thyroxine metabolism from activating to inactivating pathways during complete fasting. J Clin Endocrinol Metab 41:191–194, 1975

Vaisman N, Rossi MF, Goldberg E, et al: Energy expenditure and body composition in patients with anorexia nervosa. J Pediatr 113:919–924, 1988

Vigersky RA, Loriaux DL, Andersen AE, et al: Delayed pituitary hormone response to LRF TRF in patients with anorexia nervosa and with secondary amenorrhea associated with simple weight loss. J Clin Endocrinol Metab 43:898–900, 1976

Vigersky RA, Andersen AE, Thompson RH, et al: Hypothalamic dysfunction in secondary amenorrhea associated with simple weight loss. N Engl J Med 296:1141–1145, 1977

Wachslicht-Rodbard H, Gross HA, Rodbard D, et al: Increased insulin binding to erythrocytes in anorexia nervosa. N Engl J Med 300:882–887, 1979

Wade GN, Schneider JE: Metabolic fuels and reproduction in female mammals. Neurosci Biobehav Rev 16:235–272, 1992

Wakeling A, DeSouza VA, Gore MBR, et al: Amenorrhea, body weight and serum hormone concentration, with particular reference to prolactin and thyroid hormones in anorexia nervosa. Psychol Med 9:265–272, 1979

Wallace M, Richards P, Chesser E, et al: Persistent alkalosis and hypokalaemia caused by surreptitious vomiting. Q J Med 37:577–588, 1968

Waller DA, Hardy BW, Pole R, et al: Sleep EEG in bulimic, depressed, and normal subjects. Biol Psychiatry 25:661–664, 1989

Walsh BT, Katz JK, Levin J, et al: Adrenal activity in anorexia nervosa. Psychosom Med 40:499, 1978

Walsh BT, Croft CB, Katz JA: Anorexia nervosa and salivary gland enlargement. Int J Psychiatry Med 11:255–261, 1982

Walsh BT, Goetz R, Roose SP, et al: EEG-monitored sleep in anorexia nervosa and bulimia. Biol Psychiatry 20:947–956, 1985

Walsh BT, Roose SP, Katz JL, et al: Hypothalamic-pituitary-adrenal-cortical activity in anorexia nervosa and bulimia. Psychoneuroendocrinology 12:131–140, 1987

Warren SE, Steinberg SM: Acid-base and electrolyte disturbances in anorexia nervosa. Am J Psychiatry 136:415–418, 1979

Weingarten HP, Hendler P, Rodin J: Metabolism and endocrine secretion in response to a test meal in normal weight bulimic women. Psychosom Med 50:273–285, 1988

Wetzin TE, McConaha, C, McKee M, et al: Circadian patterns of cortisol, prolactin, and growth hormonal secretion during bingeing and vomiting in normal weight bulimic patients. Biol Psychiatry 30:37–40, 1991

Wilmsen EN: Studies in diet, nutrition, and fertility among a group of Kalahari Bushmen in Botswana. Social Science Information 21:95–125, 1982

Zerbe KJ: Recurrent pancreatitis presenting as fever of unknown origin in a recovering bulimic. International Journal of Eating Disorders 12:337–340, 1992

Ziolko HU: Hyperorexia nervosa. Psychotherapie, Medizinische Psychologie 26:10–12, 1976

Zumoff B, Walsh BT, Katz JL, et al: Subnormal plasma dehydroisoandrosterone to cortisol ratio in anorexia nervosa: a second hormonal parameter of ontogenic regression. J Clin Endocrinol Metab 56:668–672, 1983

Psychopharmacological Treatment

Donald F. Klein, M.D., Section Editor

28

Treatment of Depression

*Dennis S. Charney, M.D., Helen L. Miller, M.D.,
Julio Licinio, M.D., and Ronald Salomon, M.D.*

The effectiveness of pharmacological treatment of depressed patients compares very favorably with the drug treatment of chronic medical disorders such as hypertension and diabetes. The spectrum of available antidepressant drugs permits the clinician to choose a specific antidepressant drug based on depressive subtype and coexisting medical conditions. For patients who do not respond to the initial antidepressant drug prescribed, a range of options exist for subsequent drug treatment approaches. In this chapter, we review the clinical strategies involved in the drug treatment of depressed patients, including initial medical and psychiatric evaluation, acute and maintenance antidepressant treatment, and therapeutic approaches to the treatment-refractory depressed patient.

■ HISTORICAL BACKGROUND

The most dramatic and fundamental discoveries in the pharmacotherapy of psychiatric disorders took place in the two decades after World War II. After witnessing the great progress made in the pharmacology of medical disorders, with the advent of chemotherapy for tuberculosis, syphilis, and other major medical disorders, research psychiatrists were committed to discovery of drugs that would cure (or at least ameliorate) psychiatric disorders. Major breakthroughs occurred with the observation that lithium was useful for manic states (Cade 1949) and when chlorpromazine was shown to be highly effective for psychotic symptoms (Delay and Deniker 1952).

In the early 1950s, several investigators noted that iproniazid, initially used to treat tuberculosis, caused an elevation of mood in some patients (Crane 1956). In the United States, Kline and colleagues started to use iproniazid in depressed patients. According to Kline, his original impetus to try iproniazid for treatment of depression was further supported not only by these clinical data, but also by the effects of that drug on laboratory animals, causing hyperalertness and hyperactivity. The clinical efficacy of iproniazid in the treatment of depression was quickly established (Kline 1970; Loomer et al. 1957, 1958). Consequently, other irreversible monoamine oxidase inhibitors (MAOIs) were synthesized, found to be effective for depression, and approved for general use. After about 5 years of widespread use, the highly effective MAOIs became increasingly less popular in the treatment of depression due to their side-effect profile, particularly the cardiovascular responses following tyramine ingestion. Recently, reversible selective MAOIs have been introduced in Europe and South America, exhibiting a favorable side-effect profile with reduced tyramine sensitivity. The future availability of those compounds in the United States may enhance the interest of the psychiatric clinicians in this class of antidepressants.

At approximately the same time iproniazid was reported to be an antidepressant, in Switzerland Roland Kuhn was testing the tricyclic compound G 22355 (imipramine) in the treatment of psychiatric patients (Kuhn 1958). Kuhn observed that imipramine, though lacking antipsychotic properties, improved depressed mood in some schizophrenic patients. Subsequently, imipramine was tested in depressed patients and documented as an effective antidepressant (Kuhn 1970a, 1970b, 1989). The mechanism of action underlying imipramine's antidepressant properties was not initially known. Subsequently, it was determined that the ability of imipramine to inhibit the reuptake of norepinephrine and serotonin (5-HT) was related to its antidepressant activity (Carlsson et al. 1968; Glowinski and Axelrod 1964). This discovery facilitated the development of other tricyclic antidepressants (TCAs) that inhibited monoamine reuptake.

Based on the therapeutic properties of the MAOIs and TCAs and the monoamine hypothesis of depression, a search began in the 1970s for drugs that would selectively enhance the function of one of the monoamine systems, rather than all three. A specific and potent dopamine reuptake inhibitor, nomifensine, was synthesized and used with success in the treatment of depression; however, hematological side effects (i.e., hemolytic anemia) have precluded its wide use. It is noteworthy that nomifensine was effective in some depressed patients for whom other antidepressants were not helpful.

The search for drugs acting specifically at the level of one monoamine system also led to the development of compounds with primary actions on the 5-HT system. Fluoxetine was the first available selective serotonin reuptake inhibitor (SSRI) to be marketed for the treatment of depression (Beasley et al. 1991, 1992). Subsequently, two other SSRIs, sertraline (Amin et al. 1989) and paroxetine (Rickels et al. 1992), have been developed and approved for use in treating depression. Most recently, venlafaxine, an antidepressant with potent effects on inhibiting both norepinephrine and serotonin reuptake, has been marketed in the United States. Large-scale clinical experience with venlafaxine is needed before its specific role in the treatment of depression can be delineated.

PHARMACOTHERAPY OF THE ACUTE DEPRESSIVE EPISODE

Early recognition and treatment of depressive illness may have important implications for treatment responsiveness. Studies of the instantaneous probabilities of recovery indicate the longer the patient is ill, the lower the chances are of recovering. The shorter the episode of depression prior to initiating treatment, the higher the chances of recovery are and the lower the impairment in social and vocational adjustment will be (Keller et al. 1982a, 1982b; Lavori et al. 1984).

Medical Evaluation

The initial evaluation of patients presenting with depressive symptoms should include a careful medical history and physical examination and appropriate laboratory testing. Consideration must be given to the possible existence of physical illnesses that may present as depression or have depression as an associated symptom. Medical conditions that should be considered when evaluating the depressed patients are listed in Table 28–1. In some cases, treatment of the underlying medical condition is sufficient to eliminate depressive symptoms. However, in many cases, depressive symptoms will persist, necessitating the use of antidepressant drugs. Drug-induced depression will occasionally be encountered. The drug classes listed in Table 28–2 have been associated with depressive symptoms. The patient's medication should be reviewed and drugs that are less centrally active substituted when possible.

Another rationale for a comprehensive medical assessment is that the identification of specific medical disorders will influence the choice of antidepressant drugs. The blockade of neurotransmitter receptors by antidepressant drugs is related to numerous side effects of antidepressant drugs and drug-drug interactions. Knowledge of these pharmacological features of antidepressant drugs are therefore important in the selection of antidepressant drugs for the patient with depression and a coexisting major medical disorder. Table 28–3 summarizes the relationship between specific receptors and antidepressant-induced side effects. The antidepressants with the highest and lowest affinity for these receptors are listed (Richelson 1991; Richelson and Nelson 1984). Antidepressant drug recommendations based on the co-occurrence with specific medical disorders are reviewed later in this chapter (Table 28–4 [Richelson 1989]).

Table 28–1. Medical conditions associated with depressive symptoms

Endocrine disorders	Nutritional deficiencies
Hypothyroid	Folate
Hyperthyroid	Vitamin B_{12}
Cushing's disease	Pyridoxine (B_6)
Addison's disease	Riboflavin (B_2)
Hyperparathyroidism	Thiamine (B_1)
Hypoparathyroidism	Iron
Hypoglycemia	
Pheochromocytoma	
Carcinoid	
Ovarian failure	
Testicular failure	
Infectious diseases	**Neurological disorders**
Syphilis	Alzheimer's disease
Mononucleosis	Multiple sclerosis
Hepatitis	Parkinson's disease
AIDS	Head trauma
Tuberculosis	Narcolepsy
Influenza	Brain tumors
Encephalitis	Wilson's disease
Lyme disease	
Cancer	**Cardiovascular disease**
Pancreatic cancer	Cardiomyopathy
Lung cancer	Cerebral ischemia
	Congestive heart failure
	Myocardial infarction

Table 28–2. Classes of drugs associated with depressive symptoms

Drugs of abuse	Gastrointestinal drugs
Phencyclidine	Cimetidine
Marijuana	
Amphetamines	
Cocaine	**Cytotoxic agents**
Opiates	
Sedative-hypnotics	
Alcohol	**Corticosteroids**
Antihypertensive drugs	**Oral contraceptives**
Reserpine	
Propranolol	
Methyldopa	
Guanethidine	
Clonidine	

Cardiovascular disease. The SSRIs (fluoxetine, sertraline, paroxetine) and bupropion are preferred in patients with heart conduction disease, orthostatic hypotension, ventricular arrhythmias, and/or ischemic heart disease. These drugs have little or no effect on heart rate, heart rhythm, or blood pressure. Although the SSRIs have not been systematically evaluated in patients with cardiovascular disease, they do not prolong either the P-R or QRS intervals or cause orthostatic hypotension as TCAs do. No serious cardiovascular side effects have been reported with SSRIs, except for several cases of severe sinus node slowing (Buff et al. 1991; Ellison et al. 1990; Feder 1991; Glassman et al. 1993).

There has been one investigation of bupropion in depressed patients with severe heart disease (Roose et al. 1991). Bupropion was found to be free of effects on heart conduction or contractility. Neither SSRIs nor bupropion have yet been carefully investigated in patients with arrhythmias and heart failure (Glassman and Preud'homme 1993).

The TCAs have been used safely in patients with preexisting cardiac disease for many years, but these drugs should generally be avoided as first-choice antidepressants in these patients. The effects of TCAs to slow intraventricular conduction, as reflected in the increased QRS, P-R, and QT_c intervals on the electrocardiogram, may pose a risk to patients with prolonged conduction times or heart block and patients maintained on quinidine or other Type 1 antiarrhythmics. The orthostatic hypotension and rebound tachycardia produced by TCAs is a risk to patients with congestive heart failure, particularly those with left ventricular impairment, and in patients taking drugs such as diuretics or vasodilators (Glassman and Preud'homme 1993).

Until recently, it had been suggested that certain preexisting arrhythmias would benefit from TCA treatment because, at therapeutic plasma concentrations, TCAs suppress arrhythmias and their cardiac effects are similar to Class I antiarrhythmic drugs (Glassman and Bigger 1981; Glassman et al. 1987; Rawling and Fozzard 1979; Weld and Bigger 1980). However, several recent multicenter studies have shown that Class I antiarrhythmic drugs are associated with increased mortality when administered to patients with ventricular arrhythmias following myocardial infarction (Cardiac Arrhythmia Suppression Trial Investigators 1989; Cardiac Arrhythmia Suppression Trial II Investigators 1992; Horowitz et al. 1987;

Table 28–3.   Relationship between blockade of neurotransmitter receptors and antidepressant-induced side effects

Receptor subtype	Side effects	*Receptor affinity			
		High		Low	
Histamine-1 receptor	Sedation	Doxepine	++++	SSRIs	±
	Weight gain	Trimipramine	++++	Bupropion	±
	Hypotension	Amitriptyline	+++	Trazodone	+
	Potentiation of CNS depressants	Maprotiline	+++	Desipramine	+
				Nortriptyline	+
Muscarinic receptors	Dry mouth	Amitriptyline	+++	Bupropion	0
	Blurred vision	Clomipramine	+++	Trazodone	0
	Urinary retention	Protriptyline	+++	SSRIs	±
	Constipation			Nortriptyline	+
	Memory dysfunction			Desipramine	+
	Tachycardia				
α₁ receptors	Postural hypotension	Doxepine	++++	Bupropion	±
	Reflex tachycardia	Trimipramine	++++	SSRIs	±
	Potentiation of antihypertensive	Trazodone	++++		
	effects of prazosin	Amoxapine	+++		
α₂ receptors	Blockade of antihypertensive	Trazodone	++	Bupropion	0
	effects of clonidine, alpha-	Trimipramine	++	SSRIs	+
	methyldopa, guanfacine	Amitriptyline	++		
5-HT₂ receptors	Ejaculatory dysfunction	Amoxapine	++++	Bupropion	0
		Trazodone	+++	SSRIs	±
	Hypotension	Doxepine	++	Desipramine	±
	Alleviation of migraine	Amitriptyline	++		

Note.   0 = no affinity; ± = negligible affinity; + = weak affinity; ++ = moderate affinity; +++ = high affinity; ++++ = very high affinity.
*Drugs with higher receptor affinity are associated with a greater frequency of receptor-mediated side effects.
Source.   Adapted from Richelson 1991.

Morganroth and Goin 1991; Pratt et al. 1990). There is also documentation that these antiarrhythmic drugs may also carry a mortality risk when used in patients with atrial fibrillation (Coplen et al. 1990; Falk 1989; Selzer and Wray 1964). Class I antiarrhythmic drugs are sodium channel blockers. TCAs have Class I antiarrhythmic properties. Thus, Glassman and colleagues (1993) have suggested that TCAs may have similar mortality risks when used in depressed patients with a recent myocardial infarction and, perhaps, in a wider range of cardiac disease. It has been hypothesized that the risk of using Class I antiarrhythmias increases proportionately with the severity of ischemic heart disease (Bigger 1990; Echt et al. 1991).

Neurological disease.   Desipramine, MAOIs, and SSRIs are preferred for depressed patients with seizure disorders or for patients at risk for seizures due to predisposing factors such as head trauma, multiple central nervous system (CNS) medications, and substance abuse. These drugs lower the seizure threshold less than other antidepressant drugs. Three antidepressant drugs—maprotiline, clomipramine, and bupropion—should be particularly avoided in these patients at risk for seizures (Jick et al. 1983; Settle 1992; Trimble 1978). Maprotiline causes an increased incidence of seizures with rapid dose escalation and higher doses (Dessain et al. 1987). Clomipramine has been reported to have a high seizure risk (Peck et al. 1983; Trimble 1978). Bupropion should be avoided in seizure disorder patients because in doses higher than 300 mg daily it has an observed seizure rate approximately twice that observed with most other antidepressants (Davidson 1989; Johnston et al. 1991).

Depression is a common sequelae following stroke, occurring in an estimated 30% of cases. The

Table 28–4. Antidepressant drugs of choice for depressed patients with comorbid medical disorders

Comorbid disorder	Drugs of choice
Cardiovascular	
Congestive heart failure or ischemic heart disease Conduction disturbance Tachycardia Orthostatic hypotension	For each of these conditions the SSRIs (fluoxetine, sertraline, or paroxetine) or bupropion are preferred. Of the tricyclic antidepressants, nortriptyline or desipramine are best.
Neurological	
Seizure disorder	Desipramine, MAOIs, SSRIs (avoid bupropion, clomipramine, maprotiline)
Organic brain syndrome	SSRIs, bupropion, trazodone
Migraine headaches	Amitriptyline, trazodone, amoxapine, doxepine
Parkinson's disease	Amitriptyline, doxepine, SSRIs (avoid amoxapine)
Chronic pain	SSRIs, amitriptyline, doxepine
Stroke	SSRIs
Gastrointestinal	
Peptic ulcer disease	Doxepine, trimipramine
Chronic diarrhea	Doxepine, trimipramine, amitriptyline
Chronic constipation	SSRIs, bupropion, trazodone
Sexual dysfunction	
Erectile failure	Bupropion
Anorgasmia	Bupropion, desipramine
Ophthalmological disease	
Angle closure glaucoma	SSRIs, bupropion, trazadone

Source. Adapted from Richelson 1989.

SSRIs may be safer in treatment of these patients because of their lower incidence of cardiovascular side effects and lack of anticholinergic properties.

Confusion in patients with organic brain syndromes can be exacerbated by anticholinergic effects of antidepressant drugs. Therefore, drugs such as SSRIs, trazodone, maprotiline, amoxapine, bupropion, and desipramine, are indicated in those patients. These agents should also be used in patients with other conditions that may worsen due to cholinergic receptor blockade, such as neurogenic bladder and prostate disease.

There is recent evidence that migraine headaches may be effectively treated with serotonin receptor antagonists, particularly the 5-HT$_{1D}$ receptor antagonist sumatriptan (Humphrey 1992). Therefore, antidepressant drugs such as amoxapine and trazodone,

with high affinity for 5-HT receptors, may be useful for depressed patients with migraine.

Depression occurs in approximately 50% of patients with Parkinson's disease. There is evidence of reduced 5-HT function in parkinsonian patients with depression (Mayeux et al. 1984). It is possible SSRIs may be particularly helpful in these patients. The anticholinergic effects of antidepressants such as amitriptyline and doxepin reduce the motor deficits of Parkinson's disease. Amoxapine should be avoided because of its dopamine receptor blocking actions.

Cancer. An estimated 25% of patients with cancer report clinically significant depressive symptoms. Antidepressant drugs should be chosen based on cancer-related somatic problems. Patients experiencing significant weight loss and reduced appetite may benefit from antidepressant TCAs that increase appetite and produce weight gain. On the other hand, the anticholinergic effects of TCAs may be contraindicated in cancer patients recovering from abdominal surgery or stomatitis. SSRIs, bupropion, or trazodone, should be used in these patients.

Allergic disease. Antidepressant drugs such as doxepin, trimipramine, amitriptyline, and maprotiline, which have strong antihistamine properties, are indicated for depressed patients with severe allergic disorders such as dermatologic allergies and idiopathic pruritus.

Gastrointestinal disease. Depressed patients with peptic ulcer disease may particularly benefit from trimipramine and doxepin because of their strong anticholinergic and histamine-2 (H_2) antagonist properties. Drugs with potent anticholinergic effects should be avoided in treatment of depressed patients with chronic constipation. Conversely, these drugs may be useful for depressed patients with chronic diarrhea.

Sexual dysfunction. Erectile impotence may be due to a variety of medical conditions generally related to endocrine, drug, local, neurological, and vascular causes (McConnell and Wilson 1991). TCAs and MAOIs have been demonstrated to reduce erectile function and are therefore contraindicated in patients with erectile impotence (Segraves 1992). In contrast, bupropion does not produce erectile dysfunction and, when used in patients with a history of TCA-induced erectile failure, normal function is restored (Gardner and Johnston 1985).

Inability to ejaculate, greatly delayed ejaculation, and anorgasmia have been reported with TCAs, MAOIs, and SSRIs (Segraves 1992). Bupropion is also not associated with these side effects and is the drug of choice for patients prone to the development of these symptoms (Gardner and Johnston 1985).

Ophthalmic disease. Antidepressant drugs with little or no anticholinergic effects should be used in depressed patients with angle-closure glaucoma.

■ Psychiatric Evaluation

The initial psychiatric evaluation of the depressed patient should focus on the determination of whether other psychiatric disorders coexist with the depression and the assessment of depression disorder subtype. The existence of comorbid psychiatric disorders will influence the choice of antidepressant. For example, SSRIs are the drug of choice for patients with comorbid depression and obsessive-compulsive disorder (OCD) patients (Goodman et al. 1990). Further, there is preliminary evidence that the SSRIs may be indicated for patients with posttraumatic stress disorder (PTSD [Nagy et al. 1993]) and for obese patients (Marcus et al. 1990). MAOIs may be the most effective agent for depressed patients with panic disorder (Sheehan et al. 1983a). There is evidence (discussed in greater detail later in this chapter) that specific depressive subtypes (i.e., atypical depression, delusional depression, bipolar depression) respond preferentially to specific antidepressant agents.

■ FACTORS INFLUENCING THE ANTIDEPRESSANT DRUG OF CHOICE

■ Symptomatic Predictors of Antidepressant Response

Most studies indicate that depressed patients with melancholia characterized by key symptoms—pervasive anhedonia, nonreactivity of mood, diurnal variation, early morning awakening, guilt, and psychomotor change—respond better to TCAs than do patients with nonmelancholic depression (Paykel 1972; Raskin and Crook 1976; Simpson et al. 1976). Of the individual symptoms, psychomotor retardation, loss of interest, and anhedonia are the best prognostic indicators (Downing and Rickels 1973; Hollister and Overall 1965; Overall et al. 1966; Paykel 1972; Raskin and Crook 1976; Simpson et al. 1976). In contrast, sleep and appetite disturbances are not predictive of antidepressant response (for review, see Joyce and Paykel 1989). It is noteworthy, however, that TCAs are superior to placebo in patients with nonmelancholic depression (Quitkin et al. 1989).

There is consistent evidence that depressed patients with an associated personality disorder or narcissistic, hypochondriacal, or histrionic personality traits respond less well to TCAs (Bielski and Friedel 1976; Hirschfeld et al. 1986; Paykel 1979; Pfohl et al. 1984; Shawcross and Tyrer 1985). MAOIs may be helpful for these patients.

Depressions of longer duration appear to be less likely to respond to antidepressants (Keller et al. 1984). The chance of responding to antidepressants is reduced with each recurrence (Cassano et al. 1983; Keller et al. 1986). Both dysthymia (Keller et al. 1982a, 1982b, 1983) and depressions secondary to medical disorders or other psychiatric conditions, have been associated with less favorable outcome (Keller et al. 1983, 1984).

■ Neurobiological Predictors

A large number of research studies have attempted to identify neurobiological predictors of antidepressant response (Joyce and Paykel 1989). The results of these investigations have generally been disappointing. The hypothesis suggesting the existence of norepinephrine- and serotonin-deficient depressive subtypes has not been confirmed. Further, characterization of the depression by levels of the norepinephrine metabolite 3-methoxy-4-hydroxyphenylglycol (MHPG) or the serotonin metabolite 5-hydroxyindoleacetic acid (5-HIAA) has not found to be of practical use in the selection of antidepressant drugs. Most studies have demonstrated that a low urinary MHPG level is associated with therapeutic responses to imipramine (Beckmann and Goodwin 1975; Fawcett et al. 1972; Janicak et al. 1986; Maas et al. 1972, 1982; Rosenbaum et al. 1980; Schatzberg et al. 1980). A similar relationship has been identified between low urinary MHPG and therapeutic responses to nortriptyline (Hollister et al. 1980) and maprotiline (Schatzberg et al. 1980, 1981). However, the variability in these studies is too high for the findings to be clinically useful. There is no correlation between urinary MHPG levels and therapeutic responses to amitriptyline (Beckmann and Goodwin 1975; Coppen et al. 1979; Gaertner et al. 1982; Maas et al. 1982; Spiker et al. 1980). Preliminary data suggest that low cerebrospinal fluid (CSF) 5-HIAA relates to therapeutic responses to zimeldine (Aberg-Wistedt et al. 1981), clomipramine (VanPraag 1977), imipramine (Goodwin et al. 1973), and nortriptyline (Asberg et al. 1973).

The ratio of serum tryptophan (the amino acid precursor of serotonin) to large neutral amino acids have been found to have modest value (25% of the variance) in predicting clinical response to amitriptyline, clomipramine, and paroxetine (Møller et al. 1983, 1990). The ratio of tyrosine (the amino acid precursor to norepinephrine and dopamine) to large neutral amino acids may relate to nortriptyline (Møller et al. 1985) and maprotiline (Møller et al. 1986) responses.

A series of investigations have evaluated the possibility that the effect of single doses of a stimulant drug (e.g., amphetamine, methylphenidate) on mood is predictive of antidepressant response. Mood elevation following stimulant administration has been found to be associated with a therapeutic response to imipramine (Brown and Brawley 1983; Sabelli et al. 1983; van Kammen and Murphy 1978) and desipramine (Ettigi et al. 1983; Sabelli et al. 1983; Spar and LaRue 1985). An absent or dysphoric mood response following stimulant administration has been proposed to predict therapeutic responses to amitriptyline (Brown and Brawley 1983; Sabelli et al. 1983; Spar and LaRue 1985) and nortriptyline (Sabelli et al. 1983). Similar to the studies involving urinary MHPG and amino acid ratios, the high variability in the findings limits therapeutic application.

One of most consistently documented neuroendocrine abnormalities in depressive illness is the blunted suppression of cortisol after dexamethasone administration (Carroll 1982). This abnormality usually normalizes during successful antidepressant treatment (Greden et al. 1983; Holsboer et al. 1982), and failure to normalize is associated with poor outcome and early relapse (Greden et al. 1983; Targum 1984). However, the lack of cortisol suppression by dexamethasone is not associated with a greater likelihood of responding to antidepressant treatment in general (Brown and Shuey 1980; Gitlin and Gerner 1986; Gitlin et al. 1984; Greden et al. 1983; McLeod et al. 1970; Peselow and Fieve 1982) or to specific antidepressant drugs (Brown and Qualls 1981; Fraser 1983; Gitlin and Gerner 1986; Greden et al. 1981). It has been suggested, however, that this neuroendocrine dysfunction is associated with lack of placebo or psychotherapy response and the need for antidepressant drug or electroconvulsive therapy (ECT [Peselow et al. 1986; Rush 1983]).

Shortened rapid eye movement latency is a well-documented sleep abnormality in patients with depression. Preliminary data indicate that a reduced rapid eye movement latency is associated with poor placebo response (Coble et al. 1979) and positive response to TCAs (Coble et al. 1979; Hochli et al. 1986; Kupfer et al. 1976, 1980; Svendsen and Christensen 1981).

■ DEPRESSIVE SUBTYPES AND ANTIDEPRESSANT RESPONSE (Table 28–5)

■ Unipolar Major Depression

An extensive review of overall efficacy of antidepressant drug treatment in uncomplicated unipolar major depression indicates that approximately 65% of patients treated with antidepressants improve compared with 30% on placebo (Davis 1985). To date, no antidepressant drug stands out as having better efficacy. Therefore, the initial choice of an antidepressant drug for a patient with unipolar major depression, with or without melancholia, depends on the associated medical conditions and the drug-induced side effects.

The discovery of the TCAs represented a major breakthrough in clinical psychiatry. The efficacy of this class of antidepressant compound for moderate and severe depression is unquestioned. Although the use of these medications as a first-choice agent is still appropriate in many cases, these compounds are being used less often because of the availability of newer antidepressant drugs with less adverse side-effect profiles and less lethality with overdose. As noted previously, there are certain comorbid medical conditions in which TCAs may especially be indicated in depressed patients. Purchase price may be a factor to consider when selecting an antidepressant, because the generic TCAs are much less expensive than the SSRIs and bupropion.

The availability of the SSRIs has provided another therapeutic option for the clinician. In fact, fluoxetine—the first of the SSRIs to be made available—is the most widely used antidepressant in the United States. These agents are appropriate first-choice antidepressant drugs because of their broad spectrum efficacy, favorable side-effect profile, and lack of lethality with overdose. The SSRIs are effective in psychiatric disorders that frequently occur in combination with depression. For example, the SSRIs have therapeutic efficacy in treatment of OCD and PTSD, conditions for which TCAs (except clomipramine) are generally ineffective. It should be noted that the SSRIs have adverse side effects that may need to be attended to, such as headache, tremor, nausea, diarrhea, insomnia, agitation, and nervousness. Sexual dysfunction (particularly anorgasmia in men and

Table 28–5.   Treatments of choice for depressive subtypes

Major depression

All antidepressants of equal efficacy

Choice of antidepressant based upon side effects, comorbid medical conditions, family history of drug treatment response, previous response to antidepressant drugs

Atypical depression

Monoamine oxidase inhibitors (MAOIs) demonstrate superior efficacy to tricyclic antidepressants (TCAs)

Selective serotonin reuptake inhibitors (SSRIs) need further study

Delusional depression

Antidepressant drug alone is usually ineffective

Antidepressant and antipsychotic combination effective in many patients

Electroconvulsive therapy probably the most effective treatment

Bipolar depression

All antidepressant drugs may produce mania or hypomania. Bupropion may be least likely

MAOIs may be more effective than TCAs

Bipolar depression may be more responsive to lithium than unipolar depression

Lithium-MAOI and lithium-carbamazepine combinations may be effective for refractory patients

Dysthymic disorder

Antidepressant efficacy may be reduced compared with major depression

MAOIs may be more effective than TCAs

SSRIs need further study

Geriatric depression

Drug of choice based largely on side-effect profile

Low or absent anticholinergic properties—desipramine, nortriptyline, SSRIs, bupropion

Reduced cardiovascular adverse effects—desipramine, nortriptyline, SSRIs, bupropion

Generally use lower doses

Comorbid psychiatric disorders

Panic disorder—bupropion and trazodone not effective

Obsessive-compulsive disorder—SSRIs drugs of choice

Eating disorders—SSRIs may be the drugs of choice

women) and ejaculatory disturbances are more common with these drugs than TCAs. In addition, paroxetine, sertraline, and fluoxetine inhibit cytochrome P_{450} enzymes, thereby reducing the metabolism of drugs such as warfarin, phenytoin, and digoxin, which are metabolized by this system (Bergstrom et al. 1992; Crewe et al. 1992).

Bupropion is an antidepressant with different neurochemical properties than those of other available antidepressant drugs. It has weak effects on noradrenergic and serotonin reuptake, and its dopamine-enhancing actions are sufficiently weak to make it an unlikely mechanism of action. Bupropion is equal in efficacy to the TCAs and SSRIs for major depression. There is anecdotal evidence that bupropion may be useful for patients with bipolar disorder, particularly for maintenance prophylaxis (Haykal and Akiskal 1990; Shopsin 1983; Wright et al. 1985). Bupropion is generally well tolerated, with fewer side effects than TCAs. It fails to cause sedation, weight gain, sexual dysfunction, or anticholinergic effects and has minimal cardiovascular toxicity and low lethality with overdose. A therapeutic disadvantage is that bupropion is not effective for treatment of panic disorder and OCD (Sheehan et al. 1983b).

MAOIs (e.g., tranylcypromine, phenelzine, isocarboxazid) are extremely effective antidepressant agents. As described later in this chapter, they may be superior to other antidepressants in the treatment of atypical depression (Liebowitz et al. 1988). In addition, they are also effective for treatment of panic disorder (Sheehan et al. 1983b), PTSD (Kosten et al. 1991), social phobia (Liebowitz et al. 1986), and bulimia (Walsh et al. 1984). The factor limiting the use of the MAOIs is their side-effect profile. The available MAOIs are irreversible inhibitors of the enzyme monoamine oxidase. Patients must avoid foods containing tyramine, because the inability of peripheral MAO to metabolize tyramine may lead to hypertension and (rarely) cerebral hemorrhage or death (Cooper 1989). Other MAOI side effects include weight gain, orthostatic hypotension, delayed ejaculation, and the spectrum of anticholinergic signs and symptoms.

A relatively new development is the forthcoming availability of short-acting reversible inhibitors, such as brofaromine and moclobemide. These drugs are less vulnerable to the tyramine reaction and often have fewer side effects. Several preliminary treatment trials indicate these drugs may have a similar therapeutic spectrum of action as reversible MAOIs (Lecrubier and Guelfi 1990).

Trazodone is an antidepressant that is distinguished biochemically from the TCAs, SSRIs, and MAOIs. It has moderate 5-HT reuptake inhibition properties but is also a postsynaptic 5-HT receptor antagonist. Its principal metabolite m-chlorophenyl-piperazine (m-CPP) is a nonselective 5-HT receptor agonist. Controlled trials indicate trazodone is similar in efficacy to other antidepressants. However, it is not particularly useful for treating panic disorder (Charney et al. 1986), and there is no evidence that it is effective for treating OCD. Its side-effect profile is notable for a lack of anticholinergic effects and low lethality with overdose. Its principal adverse effects are sedation, lightheadedness, confusion, orthostatic hypotension, nausea, and (in rare cases) priapism.

■ Atypical Depression

There is now a general consensus that a nonmelancholic atypical depressive syndrome exists that responds preferentially to MAOIs (Liebowitz et al. 1988; Quitkin et al. 1990, 1991). Patients with this syndrome generally meet criteria for major depression but also have excessive mood reactivity (i.e., complete, transient remission from depressed mood due to positive environmental factors) and one or more of the associated features of overeating, oversleeping, or extreme fatigue, and chronic oversensitivity to rejection (Liebowitz et al. 1988; F. Quitkin, personal communication, June 1993). In comparison to TCAs, the MAOIs have superior efficacy for these symptoms associated with atypical depression, as well as borderline and labile personality and self-rated interpersonal sensitivity (Liebowitz et al. 1988).

In considering the initial antidepressant drug trial in atypical depression, the clinician must balance the greater response to MAOIs (i.e., phenelzine) against its greater side effect risk. It is appropriate to use MAOIs as a first-choice treatment in this disorder. Alternatively, because some patients with atypical depression will respond to SSRIs (F. Quitkin, personal communication, June 1993), these drugs may be tested first.

■ Delusional Depression

Considerable data from descriptive, neurobiological, and treatment response investigations suggest delusional depression is a distinct subtype of depressive illness (see Joyce and Paykel 1989 for review). The evidence is convincing that delusional depressive patients have a poorer response to TCAs than nondelusional depressed patients. The recommended drug treatment for delusional depression is a combination of antidepressant and antipsychotic drugs

(Charney and Nelson 1981; Nelson and Bowers 1978; Spiker et al. 1985). Most clinicians suggest initiating treatment with an antipsychotic drug until psychotic symptoms are under control before adding the antidepressant drug to the regimen. The antipsychotic dose is generally less than that required to treat the psychotic symptoms associated with schizophrenia. The antipsychotic drug will elevate antidepressant blood levels necessitating lower antidepressant drug doses and, when appropriate, monitoring blood levels. There is no evidence that specific antidepressant or antipsychotic drugs are more effective in delusional depression.

■ Bipolar Depression

The concept that bipolar and unipolar affective disorders are distinct entities is based on family studies, a variety of biological studies, clinical characteristics, course of illness, and treatment response (see Joyce and Paykel 1989 for review). When treating a bipolar patient in the depressed phase of his or her disorder, the clinician must treat the patient's depressive state but avoid eliciting a manic episode. Most studies indicate that essentially all antidepressant drugs can induce mania in bipolar patients (Bunney 1977; Prien et al. 1973).

There is some evidence bipolar depressive patients are more likely to have an antidepressant response to lithium than unipolar depressed patients (Baron et al. 1975; Goodwin et al. 1972; Himmelhoch et al. 1972; Mendels et al. 1979; Noyes et al. 1974). There are anecdotal reports that bipolar depressive patients may be more responsive to phenelzine and to lithium and tranylcypromine (Himmelhoch et al. 1972) than TCAs. In some bipolar depressed patients refractory to standard treatment, carbamazepine alone or carbamazepine plus lithium is effective (Post 1991).

■ Dysthymic Disorder

Dysthymia was first recognized as a disorder in 1980, with the publication of DSM-III (American Psychiatric Association 1980). The inclusion of dysthymic disorder with the affective disorders represents a significant theoretical shift and led to new ways of thinking about the etiology and treatment of the illness (Kocsis and Frances 1987). Dysthymia is generally conceptualized as an illness with an insidious onset, beginning at an early age. Dysthymia and major depression may occur simultaneously in some subjects. The coexistence of dysthymia with a major depressive episode is referred to as double depression (Keller et al. 1983). This background is important when reviewing the dysthymia literature, because it has not been as well characterized as other affective disorders and the biology and treatment of dysthymic disorder are not well understood.

Dysthymic disorder appears to respond to a variety of antidepressant agents, including TCAs, MAOIs, and SSRIs (Howland 1991; Rosenthal et al. 1992). Data suggest that MAOIs may be superior to TCAs in the treatment of this disorder, but this question is unresolved. Interpretation of treatment studies is complicated by the variability of diagnostic criteria used; by the high incidence of comorbidity of dysthymia with other illness (especially major depression); and by the lumping together of both patients with dysthymia and those with major depression in investigations of other depressive subtypes, such as atypical depression. There is also overlap between dysthymia and atypical depression in that both illnesses tend to be chronic. Moreover, there is a paucity of double-blind placebo-controlled treatment trials.

Some theoretical issues cloud research into treatment of dysthymia, particularly the degree that it is distinct from major depression as opposed to a varying expression of the same illness. For example, although the concept of a double depression is a useful one, it is not clear that a person with both dysthymia and major depression in fact has two illnesses, as opposed to a single illness varying in severity over time (Garvey et al. 1989). Further research is needed, both to clarify the diagnostic classification of dysthymia and to compare comparative efficacy of antidepressant agents in the treatment of this illness. However, despite the paucity of double-blind placebo-controlled treatment trials, it has been well demonstrated that dysthymic disorder responds to antidepressant medication. The risks of nontreatment should be emphasized. Studies have found that most subjects with dysthymic disorder go on to develop major depression. Patients with double depression that recover from an episode of major depression but continue with dysthymic symptoms are at greater risk for relapse into major depression. The risk of relapse increases the longer the episode of dysthymia continues (Keller et al. 1992).

■ Geriatric Depression

Depression in the geriatric population (over age 65) constitutes a major public health problem and is often underdiagnosed and undertreated (National Institutes of Health Consensus Development Panel 1992). This is due in part to the insidious nature of depression in elderly people. In contrast to a young adult's presentation, depressed mood in an elderly person may be less prominent than other depressive symptoms such as changes in appetite, sleep, loss of interest, anergia, and social withdrawal—changes that themselves may appear to be "due to" aging and attendant medical problems.

Although relatively few controlled studies of antidepressant efficacy have been conducted in depressed patients over age 60, most antidepressants are believed to be equally efficacious for geriatric depression (see Salzman 1993 for review). Very little is known about antidepressant efficacy in very old depressed patients (those over age 85).

The risk of adverse drug side effects is increased in elderly people for several reasons. Elderly patients are more likely to have concomitant medical disorders, to be more sensitive to drug side effects, and to be taking other medications, thereby increasing drug-drug interactions. In addition, drugs are excreted more slowly and metabolized less efficiently in elderly people. Therefore, therapeutic drug monitoring of drug levels is especially indicated in older depressed patients. Antidepressant drugs should be initiated at low doses and increased very gradually (Neshkes and Jarvik 1987).

The efficacy studies involving TCAs favor nortriptyline and desipramine, because they are less likely to produce orthostatic hypotension (which can lead to falls and fractures) and have fewer anticholinergic, cardiovascular, and sedative adverse effects. Monitoring of plasma levels of desipramine and nortriptyline and electrocardiograms will facilitate effective and safe use (Reynolds et al. 1992; Salzman 1993).

The SSRIs may be particularly effective for elderly patients. The low incidence of cardiovascular side effects and lack of anticholinergic properties offer advantages over most other antidepressant classes (Altamura et al. 1989; Cohn et al. 1990; Dunner et al. 1992). As with the TCAs, the SSRIs should be initiated at low doses (fluoxetine, 5 mg; sertraline, 12.5 mg; paroxetine, 10 mg) and increased slowly as needed. The shorter half-lives of sertraline and paroxetine suggest these drugs may be more appropriate than fluoxetine for use in treating elderly patients.

Bupropion has been demonstrated to be as efficacious for elderly patients as other antidepressant drugs (Branconnier et al. 1983; Kane et al. 1983). Similar to SSRIs, it does not produce anticholinergic side effects or orthostatic hypotension. The activating effects of bupropion may be a disadvantage for some individuals. As more experience is gained with bupropion in treating elderly patients, it may emerge as one of the drugs of choice for this population.

Trazodone with its sedative properties and lack of anticholinergic effects may offer advantages to elderly depressed patients who are agitated. However, trazodone may cause orthostatic hypotension and cardiac arrhythmias, thus limiting its usefulness in treating elderly patients.

Although not widely prescribed for elderly patients, the MAOIs (especially phenelzine) have been found to be effective and safe for the treatment of geriatric depression. In low doses, psychomotor stimulants may improve depressed mood, loss of interest, and anergia in some elderly individuals.

ECT is extremely effective in the treatment of depression in elderly patients. When the depression is very severe or is accompanied by delusions, ECT is the treatment of choice. A limitation of the use of ECT is that relapse after effective ECT is common, and usually alternative maintenance treatment is needed (Sackeim et al. 1990). Another disadvantage of ECT for elderly patients is the probability of a transient post-ECT confusion is elevated. Use of unilateral treatments with a brief pulse current to reduce confusion after the procedure may be helpful (Kramer 1987).

■ DURATION OF TREATMENT

Many patients with depressive illness are prone to relapse if antidepressant treatment is not continued. Data indicate that 50% or more of patients experiencing an episode of depression will eventually experience a recurrence (Angst 1990; Lee and Murray 1988). The continuation of TCA for 6 months after resolution of depressive symptoms reduces the relapse rate by over 50% compared with placebo (Prien and Kupfer 1986). These data have led to the recommendation that pharmacological treatment for a first episode of depression should continue for 6 months after a patient's symptoms have responded to an antidepressant medication.

Patients with recurrent major depression require longer-term antidepressant drug maintenance. The advice concerning the duration of antidepressant treatment provided by the 1985 National Institute of Mental Health (NIMH) Consensus Development Conference on the pharmacological prevention of depressive recurrences remains useful: "Duration of treatment must be determined on an individual basis depending upon the previous pattern of episodes, degree of impairment produced, the adverse consequences of a new recurrence, and the patient's ability to tolerate the drug" (p. 473).

This recommendation is helpful on a generic basis, but it needs to be more specific to be of practical use for the clinician. Unfortunately, there is a scarcity of long-term clinical trials designed to develop guidelines for chronic antidepressant drug use. Most of the available data are based on studies of 1-year antidepressant drug maintenance. TCAs, MAOIs, and SSRIs have all been shown to reduce relapse rates by more than 50% during this time period compared with placebo (Doogan and Caillard 1992; Eric 1991; Georgotas et al. 1989; Montgomery et al. 1988, 1991). In addition, it has been shown that patients maintained on imipramine on full-dosage for 3 years had a 20% relapse rate versus an 80% relapse on placebo (Frank et al. 1990). Only one controlled study has evaluated the efficacy of an antidepressant beyond 3 years. An extension of the original 3-year maintenance study of imipramine to 5 years revealed that imipramine continued to have a clinically significant prophylactic effect (Kupfer et al. 1992).

These studies strongly indicate the continued efficacy of full-dose antidepressant therapy in preventing relapse over a period of several years. The clinical implications of this work suggest that patients who have recovered from an initial depressive episode or prior depressive episodes spaced far apart (i.e., greater than 5 years) should be maintained on that antidepressant for 6 months to 1 year. However, patients with prior depressive episodes occurring less than 3 years apart should probably be maintained on antidepressants at full dosage for at least 3 and probably up to 5 years. Patients with frequent recurrent depressive episodes may require lifetime treatment with antidepressants.

Discontinuation of antidepressant drug maintenance therapy should be done with a slow taper. It is also helpful to involve a significant other, friend, or close family member to help the patient monitor for the return of symptoms and, if necessary, alert the treating clinician.

■ THERAPEUTIC MONITORING OF ANTIDEPRESSANT BLOOD LEVELS

Therapeutic plasma levels have only been established for imipramine, desipramine, and nortriptyline (American Psychiatric Association Task Force Report 1985). However, information is available regarding other antidepressants for which blood levels may be useful in the treatment of refractory patients or for elderly depressed patients to determine whether drug dosage may be adequate (see Preskorn 1989 and Preskorn and Fast 1991 for review).

Pharmacokinetic studies indicate that individuals vary greatly in the absorption, distribution, and excretion of antidepressants, suggesting some patients will require monitoring of plasma levels to determine optimal drug dosage. Therapeutic antidepressant drug monitoring (TDM) may therefore enhance the safe and efficacious use of antidepressants. TDM may aid in determining compliance. It is well known that a substantial number of patients do not take their medications as prescribed. Noncompliance or partial compliance may reduce response to treatment because of wide fluctuations in plasma levels.

For some antidepressant drugs, TDM enables the clinician to maximize therapeutic dosage. Most studies have shown that there is an association between the plasma levels of nortriptyline, imipramine, and desipramine and clinical efficacy (Glassman et al. 1977; Nelson et al. 1982; Risch et al. 1979). The available evidence suggests a curvilinear relationship between nortriptyline plasma levels and antidepressant efficacy, with maximal therapeutic efficacy achieved with levels of 50–175 ng/ml. Thus, if the nortriptyline plasma level is less than 50 ng/ml, the dose should be raised, and if it is greater than 175 ng/ml, the nortriptyline dose should be lowered. The evidence for imipramine supports a linear relationship between plasma levels of imipramine plus desipramine (to which imipramine is metabolized) and clinical response. A similar relationship has been identified between desipramine plasma levels and therapeutic efficacy. Therefore, raising serum levels of imipramine and desipramine above a threshold value by increasing drug doses may convert nonresponders into responders. For example, in one study, 10 desipramine-resistant depressive patients improved when dosage was adjusted to raise desipramine plasma concentration to 125 ng/ml or above (Nelson et al. 1982). Most investigations support a more limited role for the plasma levels of antidepressants other than nortriptyline, imipramine, or desipramine. In these cases, a plasma level determination might be useful when abnormal metabolism or poor compliance is suspected. Less established documentation is available for antidepressant drugs such as amitriptyline, doxepin, trimipramine, protriptyline, amoxapine, maprotiline, trazodone, bupropion, and fluoxetine (Preskorn and Fast 1991).

Monitoring of antidepressant drug levels may also help the clinician avoid drug toxicity. For certain antidepressant drugs, a relationship exists between plasma concentration and toxicity. There are data indicating the effect of TCAs on cardiac function (i.e., delayed intraventricular conduction and rhythm disturbances) and on brain neuronal activity (i.e., seizures, delirium) are concentration dependent (Preskorn 1989). The same may be true for other antidepressants such as bupropion that exhibit a dose-dependent increase in drug-induced seizures (Preskorn 1991). The SSRIs may not require TDM, because relationships to clinical response or adverse effects have not been identified.

Therapeutic antidepressant drug monitoring may assist in the evaluation of drug-drug interactions. A number of pharmacological agents, which are commonly coadministered with antidepressants, may alter steady-state antidepressant drug levels. For example, drugs that stimulate the hepatic microsomal enzyme system (e.g., anticonvulsants, barbiturates, chronic alcohol use, glutethimide, chloral hydrate, nicotine, oral contraceptives) will lower drug levels of most antidepressant drugs. On the other hand, TCA antidepressant drug levels are increased by neuroleptic drugs and stimulants that inhibit hepatic metabolism. Coadministration of fluoxetine and TCAs increase TCA blood levels due to hepatic metabolism inhibition via cytochrome P_{450}-2D6 (Bergstrom et al. 1992). Sertraline and paroxetine have similar inhibitory effects on cytochrome P_{450}-2D6 (Crewe et al. 1992), but clinical experience with these drugs in combination with TCAs is limited. Inhibition of cytochrome P_{450}-2D6 will also raise levels of anticonvulsants, neuroleptics, certain antiarrthymic drugs, and β-adrenergic blocking drugs. Dosage adjustments of these drugs may be needed in patients receiving SSRIs.

◼ ANTIDEPRESSANT DRUGS AND SUICIDE

As noted, there is excellent evidence that antidepressant drugs are extremely effective in both acute treatment of depression and in preventing recurrence. However, the ability of antidepressant drugs to reduce the incidence of suicide in depressed patients remains to be established. Some data suggest that SSRIs may be more effective than standard antidepressants in decreasing suicidal ideation, but these data are preliminary and inconsistent. This issue has been a great concern for clinicians and patients because of the suggestion that the SSRI fluoxetine may precipitate or exacerbate suicidal ideation or behavior (Beasley et al. 1991; Mann and Kapur 1991; Power and Cowen 1992; Teicher et al. 1990).

Several reviews have examined the data relevant to the question of whether antidepressant pharmacotherapy is associated with the emergence of suicidal ideation and behavior. These studies indicate that although suicidal ideation may rarely emerge during antidepressant treatment in depressed patients, these responses occur with essentially all types of antidepressant drugs, and a causal relationship to antidepressant drugs has not been established. Further, the emergence or intensification of suicidal ideation and behavior with antidepressant drugs is not limited to patients with primary depression. It appears that patients with a history of impulsive-aggressive behavior may be particularly prone to these effects (Mann and Kapur 1991; Power and Cowen 1992).

The conclusions of Mann and Kapur (1991) are appropriate in this context.

> Clinicians should be aware that emergence or intensification of suicidal ideation of behavior in patients receiving antidepressant treatment has been reported in patients with various psychiatric diagnoses and has not been proven to be associated with any specific type of antide-

pressant. Whether certain antidepressants precipitate or aggravate suicidal ideation in a small, vulnerable subpopulation of psychiatric patients who require antidepressants is uncertain. In practice, whatever the antidepressant medication, the clinician should always monitor the patient to assess the severity of depression and suicidal ideation, aggressive ideational behavior, agitation, and akathisia. (p. 1032)

It is possible that the frequency of suicidal ideation or behavior is more frequent in patients who are nonresponsive, have unrecognized akathisia, and have attempted suicide previously. Patients should be informed of this rare adverse reaction and must be instructed to immediately contact their clinician should these symptoms occur (Mann and Kapur 1991).

■ APPROACHES TO TREATMENT OF REFRACTORY DEPRESSION

Despite the well-documented effectiveness of antidepressant drugs, a significant proportion of the depressed patient population does not respond adequately to treatment, estimates typically ranging from 10% to 30%. Given the relatively high prevalence of depression, this means a substantial number of patients are not adequately responding to treatment (Nierenberg et al. 1991).

For the purposes of this discussion, we have used a definition that has a lower threshold than that generally used in clinical practice. Refractory depression is defined as an episode of major depression, not secondary to a medical or drug-induced condition, which fails to respond (or to maintain a response) to an adequate trial of an antidepressant drug of established efficacy. An adequate trial is defined as 6 weeks of treatment with the antidepressant at a dosage considered therapeutic.

Once it has been established that a patient is resistant to an antidepressant, several options are available to the treating clinician: maximizing the trial of that same antidepressant; changing to a different antidepressant; or selecting a drug combination or nonpharmacological treatment, such as ECT (Table 28–6).

Table 28–6. Therapeutic options for treatment-refractory depressed patients

Treatment	Efficacy	Replicability
Lithium augmentation of antidepressant drugs	+++	+++
Electroconvulsive therapy	+++	+++
Thyroid (T₃) augmentation of antidepressant drugs	++–+++	++
Desipramine and fluoxetine	++–+++	+
Stimulant augmentation of antidepressant drugs	+–++	++
TCA and MAOI combination	+	++
High dose MAOI	++	+
Estrogen	0–+	++

Note. Efficacy was rated as follows: 0, ineffective; +, slightly effective; ++, moderately effective; +++, very effective. Replication refers to the extent to which the efficacy of the treatment has been investigated; it was rated as follows: +, open studies and/or only one controlled study conducted; ++, several controlled studies conducted but further investigation indicated for complete evaluation; +++, highly replicated and consistent degree of efficacy reported.

■ Maximizing the Antidepressant Drug Trial

When a patient fails to respond to an antidepressant, a clinician may maximize the response to that same antidepressant by increasing its dose and/or the duration of the trial. Measuring the plasma levels of certain antidepressants may help determine if a dosage adjustment is needed. There is evidence that a substantial percentage (85%) of the MAO enzyme must be inhibited to produce therapeutic responses. Some patients fail to respond to conventional doses of MAOIs because of inadequate inhibition of MAO. There are reports from studies that were not placebo controlled that higher than conventional doses of tranylcypromine (90–200 mg/day) may be a safe and effective treatment for refractory depression (Amsterdam 1991).

■ Changing the Antidepressant Drug

When a patient does not respond to an adequate antidepressant trial, the clinician frequently decides to change to a different antidepressant. The choice of the next antidepressant should involve those considerations ordinarily included in the initial selection of an antidepressant, such as side-effect profile, past antidepressant trial responses, family history of antidepressant responses, course of illness, premorbid personality, and depressive subtype.

Another method that has been advocated in choosing an antidepressant is consideration of its neuropharmacological properties. For example, if a patient has not responded to an adequate trial with fluoxetine (a potent blocker of serotonin reuptake), a trial with desipramine (a potent blocker of norepinephrine reuptake) is indicated. This rationale has become a basis for a common clinical practice, but its validity has not been confirmed in systematic clinical trials (Nolen et al. 1988). There is some evidence that two SSRIs, fluoxetine (Beasley et al. 1990) and fluvoxamine (Delgado et al. 1988), may be effective in some patients in whom treatment with TCAs was unsuccessful.

Treatment with MAOIs may be useful for depressed patients who have failed to respond to TCAs such as imipramine. In a recently completed double-blind crossover trial, phenelzine was found to be effective in approximately two-thirds of patients who failed to respond to imipramine (McGrath et al. 1993). These patients were chronically depressed, nonmelancholic, mood-reactive depressed patients with many symptoms characteristic of atypical depression. In another double-blind crossover study, 75% of a group of anergic bipolar depressed patients had failed treatment with imipramine, but therapeutic responses to tranylcypromine occurred in many patients (Thase et al. 1992). This work was consistent with previous open-label trials in a similar patient population (Himmelhoch et al. 1991). Thus, these results suggest that many depressed patients characterized by anergia, psychomotor retardation, and symptoms of atypical depression will have therapeutic responses to MAOIs despite previous treatment resistance to TCAs.

ANTIDEPRESSANT DRUG COMBINATIONS

Tricyclic and Monoamine Oxidase Inhibitor Antidepressants

The rationale for combining a TCA with an MAOI was based on the monoamine deficiency hypothesis of depression. The combined ability of TCAs to inhibit presynaptic reuptake of biogenic amines and MAOIs to reduce metabolic breakdown of biogenic amines, theoretically results in increased neurotransmitter in the synapse.

Most initial reports of combined TCA-MAOI therapy in the treatment of refractory depression were encouraging. However, most of these studies employed open designs in which there were no placebo control or comparison treatment groups (Pande et al. 1991; Razani et al. 1983; Schmauss et al. 1988; White and Simpson 1981). To date, no controlled study has demonstrated an advantage in efficacy in the combination of a TCA and an MAOI compared with either agent given alone. Most of the research supporting this combination approach in refractory depression come from open clinical trials and anecdotal reports. On the other hand, despite early alarm about adverse side effects associated with this combination, the relative safety of this approach has been substantiated provided certain guidelines are adhered to (Pande et al. 1991). There may be an occasional patient who benefits from this treatment approach (Tyrer and Murphy 1990).

Desipramine and Fluoxctine Combination

Several uncontrolled studies have found that when fluoxetine and desipramine are used in combination, they have a synergistic effect. In several cases when desipramine was added to fluoxetine, the patients showed rapid improvement. These patients had previously been unresponsive to fluoxetine or desipramine alone (Eisen 1989). A case series of 30 treatment-refractory depressed patients reported an 87% response rate to a combination of fluoxetine and non-MAOI antidepressants (Weilburg et al. 1989). Further, preliminary data suggested a more rapid antidepressant response in depressed patients treated with fluoxetine and desipramine in combination than in patients treated with desipramine alone (Nelson et al. 1990). There are many anecdotal reports of the efficacy of this combination in treatment-refractory patients, and the combination is widely used in clinical practice. However, double-blind placebo-controlled studies are needed to document the efficacy of this treatment combination.

Antidepressant and Stimulant Combinations

The combination of a TCA and methylphenidate is usually mentioned as a treatment approach to refractory depression. However, to our knowledge, there are no studies of its efficacy that utilize a comparison treatment group. In the most frequently cited report, 7 treatment-refractory patients with psychotic depression were give 20-mg doses of methylphenidate in addition to an imipramine regimen. Five of the seven patients experienced rapid and robust improvements (Wharton et al. 1971). However, the clinical improvement may have been due to methylphenidate-induced increases in imipramine plasma levels. In a single case report, there was robust and rapid resolution of a patient's intractable depression when methylphenidate was added to ongoing desipramine treatment. There was no concomitant change in plasma desipramine level (Drimmer et al. 1983).

A report on clinical experience with a combination of either pemoline or dextroamphetamine and an MAOI in 32 depressed patients who were severely treatment refractory indicated the combination was safe and effective (Fawcett et al. 1991). Six patients became manic ($n = 1$) or hypomanic ($n = 5$). This treatment approach may be a viable option for severely ill patients.

■ LITHIUM AUGMENTATION OF ANTIDEPRESSANT ACTION

Unlike many pharmacological approaches to the treatment of refractory depressed patients, the investigations of the efficacy of lithium when added to a chronic antidepressant regimen were initiated because of a specific hypothesis that was based on preclinical neurobiological research (DeMontigny et al. 1981, 1983; Heninger et al. 1983). DeMontigny hypothesized that lithium's ability to increase presynaptic transmission of serotonin would potentiate TCA-induced postsynaptic serotonergic supersensitivity, resulting in enhanced efficacy of transmission in the brain serotonergic system. Although other mechanisms for the lithium effectiveness are possible, the discovery of this treatment approach represents the potential impact that a hypothesis generated from basic neuroscience research can have on the development and implementation of new treatment strategies.

There are very strong data from more than 20 investigations supporting the effectiveness of adding lithium carbonate to ongoing antidepressant treatment in treatment-refractory depressed patients

(Austin et al. 1991; Charney et al. 1991; Kramlinger and Post 1989). It has not been determined if starting an antidepressant and lithium concomitantly is equally efficacious in treating refractory depression. Similarly, it is not known whether the lithium-antidepressant combination is necessary for preventing relapse and, if not, which agent should be used alone for prophylaxis. Preliminary observations indicate the effectiveness of lithium augmentation is sustained and reduces the relapse rate—particularly in patients who had an acute, marked response to lithium augmentation (Nierenberg et al. 1990).

The earliest reports of lithium augmentation found that patients who failed to respond to standard treatment with antidepressants experienced dramatic improvements in depressive symptomatology within 48–72 hours following the addition of lithium (DeMontigny et al. 1981). Subsequent controlled investigations have revealed a more variable response to lithium. Approximately 25% of patients who respond to lithium augmentation will exhibit dramatic responses within a week of adding lithium. More commonly the response is gradual, with a response latency of up to 3 weeks.

The overall response rate of patients with treatment-refractory depression is approximately 50%, with patients with nonpsychotic melancholic depression or bipolar depression most likely to respond. However, many depressed patients with nonmelancholic depression or delusional depression also respond to lithium augmentation. Lithium appears to be effective when added to all classes of antidepressant drugs, including carbamazepine. There is no evidence supporting any superiority of one antidepressant type when lithium is added.

A controlled fixed-dose lithium investigation has recently been conducted to determine proper lithium dose. This study and clinical experience suggest lithium should be used in the typical fashion, titrating doses to a lithium level of 0.5–0.8 mEq/L (Stein and Bernadt 1993).

■ LITHIUM AND MONOAMINE OXIDASE INHIBITORS

Shortly after the introduction of lithium carbonate into the United States for the treatment of bipolar disorders, two reports (Himmelhoch et al. 1972; Zall

1971) were published on using lithium and an MAOI together. The rationale seemed less to do with biological theory and more to do with a growing awareness that lithium alone was not always effective in the acute treatment of bipolar depression. In these open uncontrolled trials, an MAOI was added to ongoing lithium administration in a total of 24 lithium-resistant subjects. Most had already failed to respond to TCAs alone. Nineteen out of 24 experienced substantial improvement after the MAOI was added. In a more recent investigation, 11 of 12 well-defined refractory unipolar depressed patients who had not responded to other lithium-antidepressant combinations were successfully treated when tranylcypromine was added to lithium (Price et al. 1985).

The robustness of the responses reported suggests that the lithium-MAOI combination may be a potent antidepressant treatment appropriate for use in treatment-refractory patients. Nevertheless, double-blind placebo-controlled clinical trials are needed to confirm these results. In addition, further investigation should help clarify if the sequence in which an MAOI and lithium are combined affects efficacy (Nelson and Byck 1982).

■ THYROID HORMONES AND ANTIDEPRESSANT DRUGS

In 1963, Prange reported a case of hyperthyroidism in which imipramine seemed to induce a toxic reaction. Based on this clinical observation and the preclinical evidence that thyroid hormone enhances adrenergic receptor sensitivity, Prange reasoned that modest amounts of triiodothyronine (T_3) might accelerate imipramine's antidepressant activity without producing toxicity. In a placebo-controlled study of 20 depressed (but not treatment-refractory) patients, a more rapid onset of antidepressant action was observed in the imipramine-T_3 group compared with the imipramine-placebo group (Prange et al. 1969). Several other studies also found that a T_3-TCA combination provided a more rapid relief of symptoms than a TCA alone. There was a general trend in these studies for women to respond better than men.

These favorable reports of T_3's effect on the rate of TCA response stimulated investigation into the efficacy of the T_3-TCA combination in refractory depression. Open studies (Banki 1975; Earle 1969;

Ogura et al. 1974; Schwartz et al. 1984; Tsutsui et al. 1979) showed that when T_3 was added to TCAs for treatment-refractory depressed patients, there was a favorable outcome in about two-thirds of the cases. The significance of any conclusion drawn from these studies is weakened by several methodological flaws, including the absence of standardized diagnostic and treatment response rating criteria and a nonblind design. The results of controlled studies are less consistent. Two studies demonstrated antidepressant effects of T_3 augmentation (Goodwin et al. 1982; Joffe and Singer 1991), whereas two other investigations did not (Gitlin et al. 1987). However, a recent placebo-controlled comparison of lithium and T_3 augmentation of TCAs in treatment-refractory patients with unipolar depression found both of these agents to be equal in efficacy and superior to placebo (Joffe et al. 1993). The effectiveness of thyroid augmentation is not related to varying degrees of subclinical hypothyroidism in depressed patients.

■ ESTROGEN

In the 1930s, a number of reports were published on the use of estrogen in depression occurring around the time of menopause. The rationale for the choice of estrogen for treatment was the premise that symptoms (including depression) occurring in the menopause were the result of decreasing hormone levels. The findings of these studies were inconsistent, ranging from conclusions that estrogen had no proven value to assertions that it was a specific treatment for involutional melancholia. A more recent investigation failed to demonstrate an antidepressant effect of estrogen in perimenopausal patients (Coope 1981). However, a double-blind placebo-controlled study used much higher doses of conjugated estrogen (Premarin at doses of up to 25 mg daily) in pre- and postmenopausal treatment-refractory depressed patients. A significant improvement in depression ratings was observed, but not complete remission in the estrogen-treated patients (Klaiber et al. 1979). There was no significant association of estrogen response with menopausal status. Citing the catecholamine deficiency hypothesis of depression, the authors speculated that estrogen might exert an antidepressant action by augmenting central noradrenergic activity. However, preclinical studies indicate the effect of estrogen on brain 5-HT function may mediate some of its actions on depressed mood (Fischette et al. 1984).

There are few published reports of combined antidepressant-estrogen treatment. In studies comparing imipramine plus estrogen with imipramine alone, the combination demonstrated no clear advantage (Oppenheim 1984; Prange 1972; Shapira et al. 1985). Several case reports suggest possible beneficial effects of adding contraceptives to antidepressants for treatment of refractory depression (Sherwin 1991).

Currently there are not enough data to support an estrogen trial early in the course of treatment for patients with treatment-refractory depression. An advantage to an antidepressant-estrogen combination has yet to be demonstrated. In addition, the side effects resulting from long-term estrogen administration to pre- and postmenopausal depressed women have not been definitively determined.

■ ELECTROCONVULSIVE THERAPY

As previously discussed, most investigations suggest that ECT is of equal or superior efficacy to that of TCAs or MAOIs in the treatment of severe depression. A possible exception is that ECT is not effective for treating atypical depression. The results from several different centers indicate ECT is often effective in cases of depressions unresponsive to TCA treatment (Avery and Winokur 1977; Devanand et al. 1991). For example, in the British Cooperative Study, there was a 50% response rate with ECT in those patients who did not improve on imipramine (Clinical Psychiatry Committee of the British Medical Research Council 1965). Similarly, in another study, 6 out of 9 amitriptyline nonresponders improved with ECT (Browne and Kreeger 1963). In a study of 153 endogenously depressed patients who were imipramine nonresponders, 120 (or 78%) responded to ECT (Avery and Lubrano 1979). When Paul and colleagues (1981) reviewed their experience with ECT in intractably and seriously depressed patients over an 8-year period at NIMH, they found that only 1 of 9 patients failed to respond favorably.

ECT is particularly indicated in patients with psychotic depression. Major depression with psychotic features appears to be relatively resistant to single-agent antidepressant treatment compared with major depression without psychotic features. There is substantial improvement in efficacy when a conventional antidepressant is combined with an antipsychotic in the treatment of delusional depression. In one study, when an antipsychotic and TCA were administered together in a delusionally depressed sample, the total drug response rate was 70% compared with 22% for a single agent (Charney et al. 1981). Nevertheless, seven of the eight who had inadequate responses to the antipsychotic-TCA treatment did respond to ECT. For most patients with psychotic depression, ECT or the TCA-antipsychotic combination is the treatment of choice.

■ MISCELLANEOUS APPROACHES

The depression treatment literature is rich with a variety of other pharmacological and nonpharmacological approaches. However, their efficacy in refractory depression has not been sufficiently studied to warrant detailed inclusion in this review. Pharmacological approaches of interest include the use of S-adenosylmethionine (Rosenbaum et al. 1990) and steroid suppression therapy (Murphy et al. 1991). Examples of innovative nonpharmacological approaches for depressed patients with hypothesized biological rhythm disturbances include sleep deprivation and bright-light treatment (Levitt et al. 1991).

■ THE FUTURE OF DRUG TREATMENT FOR DEPRESSIVE ILLNESS

The clinician now has an impressive drug armamentarium from which to treat depressive illness. Most patients with severe depressive illness will have good therapeutic responses to antidepressant drugs, with an acceptable degree of unwanted adverse side effects. Furthermore, a variety of effective drug treatment approaches have been developed to effectively treat most patients who do not respond to the initial antidepressant drug used.

However, there remain important deficits in knowledge relevant to the pharmacological treatment of depression. There is a dearth of descriptive and biological markers capable of identifying subtypes of depressive illness characterized by therapeutic responses to specific antidepressants. The mechanisms of action of antidepressant drugs have not been established. This limits the discovery of new, more effective, rapid-acting antidepressant drugs.

It is likely that the future development of antidepressant drugs will move beyond drugs whose therapeutic properties relate to monoamine reuptake or metabolism inhibition. Drugs with specific actions on monoamine receptor subtypes are being synthesized and tested in treatment of depressed patients. Psychopharmaceutical research will focus less on the monoamine systems because of recent data suggesting these systems may not be primary in the pathophysiology of depression. Further understanding of the effects of antidepressant drug action at sites distal to receptor recognition sites may provide new approaches for developing new classes of antidepressant drugs.

■ REFERENCES

Aberg-Wistedt A, Jostell KG, Ross SB, et al: Effects of zimelidine and desipramine on serotonin and noradrenaline uptake mechanisms in relation to plasma concentrations and to therapeutic effects during treatment of depression. Psychopharmacology (Berl) 74:297–305, 1981

Altamura AC, DeNovelis F, Guercetti G, et al: Fluoxetine compared with amitriptyline in elderly depression: a controlled clinical trial. Int J Clin Pharmacol Res 9:391–396, 1989

American Psychiatric Association: Diagnostic and Statistical Manual of Mental Disorders, 3rd Edition. Washington, DC, American Psychiatric Association, 1980

American Psychiatric Association Task Force Report: Tricyclic antidepressants: blood level measurements and clinical outcome. Am J Psychiatry 142:155–182, 1985

Amin M, Lehmann H, Mirmiran J: A double-blind, placebo-controlled dose-finding study with sertraline. Psychopharmacol Bull 25:164–167, 1989

Amsterdam JD: Use of high dose tranylcypromine in resistant depression, in Advances in Neuropsychiatry and Psychopharmacology, Vol 2: Refractory Depression. Edited by Amsterdam JD. New York, Raven, 1991, pp 123–130

Angst J: Natural history and epidemiology of depression, in Results of Community Studies in Prediction and Treatment of Recurrent Depression. Edited by Cobb J, Goeting N. Southampton, England, Duphar Medical Relations, 1990

Asberg M, Bertilsson L, Tuck D, et al: Indoleamine metabolites in cerebrospinal fluid of depressed patients before and during treatment with nortriptyline. Clin Pharmacol Ther 14:277–286, 1973

Austin MP, Souza FG, Goodwin GM: Lithium augmentation in antidepressant-resistant patients: a quantitative analysis. Br J Psychiatry 159:510–514, 1991

Avery D, Lubrano A: Depression treated with imipramine and ECT: the DeCardis study reconsidered. Am J Psychiatry 136:559–562, 1979

Avery D, Winokur G: The efficacy of electroconvulsive therapy and antidepressants in depression. Biol Psychiatry 12:507–524, 1977

Banki CM: Triiodothyronine in the treatment of depression. Orv Hetil 116:2543–2546, 1975

Baron M, Gershon ES, Rudy V, et al: Lithium carbonate response in depression: Prediction by unipolar/bipolar illness, average-evoked response, catechol-O-methyltransferase, and family history. Arch Gen Psychiatry 32:1107–1111, 1975

Beasley CM Jr, Sayler ME, Cunningham GE, et al: Fluoxetine in tricyclic refractory major depressive disorder. J Affect Disord 20:193–200, 1990

Beasley CM Jr, Dornseif BE, Bosomworth JC, et al: Fluoxetine and suicide: a meta-analysis of controlled trials of treatment for depression. BMJ 303:685–692, 1991

Beasley CM, Masica DN, Potvin JH: Fluoxetine: a review of receptor and functional effects and their clinical implications. Psychopharmacology (Berl) 107:1–10, 1992

Beckmann H, Goodwin FK: Antidepressant response to tricyclics and urinary MHPG in unipolar patients. Arch Gen Psychiatry 32:17–21, 1975

Bergstrom RF, Peyton AL, Lemberger L: Quantification and mechanism of the fluoxetine and tricyclic antidepressant interaction. Clin Pharmacol Ther 51(3):239–248, 1992

Bielski RJ, Friedel RO: Prediction of tricyclic antidepressant response: a critical review. Arch Gen Psychiatry 33:1479–1489, 1976

Bigger JT Jr: Implications of the Cardiac Arrhythmia Suppression Trial for antiarrhythmic drug treatment. Am J Cardiol 65:3D–10D, 1990

Branconnier RJ, Cole JO, Ghazvinian S, et al: Clinical pharmacology of bupropion and imipramine in elderly depressives. J Clin Psychiatry 44 (5, sec 2):130–133, 1983

Brown P, Brawley P: Dexamethasone suppression test and mood response to methylphenidate in primary depression. Am J Psychiatry 140:990–993, 1983

Brown WA, Qualls CB: Pituitary-adrenal disinhibition in depression: marker of a subtype with characteristic clinical features and response to treatment. Psychiatry Res 4:115–128, 1981

Brown WA, Shuey I: Response to dexamethasone and subtype of depression. Arch Gen Psychiatry 37:747–751, 1980

Browne MW, Kreeger LC: A clinical trial of amitriptyline in depressive patients. Br J Psychiatry 109:692–694, 1963

Buff DD, Brenner R, Kirtane SS, et al: Dysrhythmia associated with fluoxetine treatment in an elderly patient with cardiac disease. J Clin Psychiatry 52:174–176, 1991

Bunney WE: The switch process in manic-depressive psychosis. Ann Intern Med 87:319–335, 1977

Cade JFJ: Lithium salts in the treatment of psychotic excitement. Med J Aust 36:349–352, 1949

Cardiac Arrhythmia Suppression Trial (CAST) Investigators: Preliminary report: effect of encainide and flecainide on mortality in a randomized trial of arrhythmia suppression after myocardial infarction. N Engl J Med 321:406–412, 1989

Cardiac Arrhythmia Suppression Trial II Investigators: Effect of the antiarrhythmic agent moricizine on survival after myocardial infarction. N Engl J Med 327:227–233, 1992

Carlsson A, Fuxe K, Ungerstedt U: The effect of imipramine on central 5-hydroxytryptamine neurons. J Pharm Pharmacol 20:150–151, 1968

Carroll BJ: The dexamethasone suppression test for melancholia. Br J Psychiatry 140:292–304, 1982

Cassano GB, Maggini C, Akiskal HS: Short-term, subchronic, and chronic sequelae of affective disorders. Psychiatr Clin North Am 6:55–67, 1983

Charney DS, Nelson JC: Delusional and nondelusional unipolar depression: further evidence for distinct subtypes. Am J Psychiatry 138:328–333, 1981

Charney DS, Woods SW, Goodman WK, et al: Drug treatment of panic disorder: the comparative efficacy of imipramine, alprazolam and trazodone. J Clin Psychiatry 47:580–585, 1986

Charney DS, Delgado PL, Southwick SM, et al: Current hypotheses of the mechanism of antidepressant treatments: implications for the treatment of refractory depression, in Advances in Neuropsychiatry and Psychopharmacology, Vol 2: Refrac-

tory Depression. Edited by Amsterdam JD. New York, Raven, 1991, pp 23–40

Clinical Psychiatry Committee of the British Medical Research Council: Clinical trial of the treatment of depressive illness. British Medical Journal 1:881–886, 1965

Coble PA, Kupfer DJ, Spiker DG, et al: EEG sleep in primary depression: a longitudinal placebo study. J Affect Disord 1:131–138, 1979

Cohn CK, Shrivastava R, Mendels J, et al: Double-blind, multicenter comparison of sertraline and amitriptyline in elderly depressed patients. J Clin Psychiatry 51 (12, suppl B):28–33, 1990

Coope J: Is estrogen therapy effective in the treatment of menopausal depression? J R Coll Gen Pract 31:134–140, 1981

Cooper AJ: Tyramine and irreversible monoamine oxidase inhibitors in clinical practice. Br J Psychiatry 155 (suppl 6):38–45, 1989

Coplen SE, Antman EM, Berlin JA, et al: Efficacy and safety of quinidine therapy for maintenance of sinus rhythm after cardioversion: a metaanalysis of randomized control trials. Circulation 82:1106–1116, 1990

Coppen A, Rama Rao VA, Ruthven CRJ, et al: Urinary 4-hydroxy-3-methoxyphenylglycol is not a predictor for clinical response to amitriptyline in depressive illness. Psychopharmacology (Berl) 64:95–97, 1979

Crane GE: The psychiatric side-effects of iproniazid. Am J Psychiatry 112:494–501, 1956

Crewe HK, Lennard MS, Tucker GT, et al: The effect of selective serotonin re-uptake inhibitors on cytochrome P4502D6 (CYP2D6) activity in human liver microsomes. Br J Pharmacol 34:262–265, 1992

Davidson J: Seizures and bupropion: a review. J Clin Psychiatry 50:256–261, 1989

Davis JM: Antidepressant drugs in Comprehensive Textbook of Psychiatry, Vol 4, 4th Edition. Edited by Kaplan HI, Saddock BJ. Baltimore, MD, Williams & Wilkins, 1985

Delay J, Deniker P: Trente-huit cas de psychoses traitées par la cure prolongée et continue de 4560 RP. Le Congrès des Medicins Alienistes et Neurologistes de France, Vol 50. In Compte redu du Congrès. Paris, Masson et Cie, 1952

Delgado PL, Price LH, Charney DS, et al: Efficacy of fluvoxamine in treatment-refractory depression. J Affect Disord 15:55–60, 1988

DeMontigny CF, Grunberg AF, Deschenes JP: Lithium

induces rapid relief of depression in tricyclic antidepressant drug non-responders. Br J Psychiatry 138:252–256, 1981

DeMontigny CF, Ceurnoyer G, Morissette R, et al: Lithium carbonate addition in tricyclic antidepressant-resistant unipolar depression. Arch Gen Psychiatry 40:1327–1334, 1983

Dessain EC, Schatzberg AF, Woods BT, et al: Maprotiline treatment in depression. Arch Gen Psychiatry 43:86–90, 1987

Devanand DP, Sacheim HA, Prudic J: Electroconvulsive therapy in the treatment-resistant patient. Psychiatr Clin North Am 14(4):905–923, 1991

Doogan DP, Caillard V: Sertraline in the prevention of depression. Br J Psychiatry 160:217–222, 1992

Downing RW, Rickels K: Predictors of response to amitriptyline and placebo in three outpatient treatment settings. J Nerv Ment Dis 156:109–129, 1973

Drimmer EJ, Gitlin MJ, Gwirtouran HE: Desipramine and methylphenidate combination treatment of depression: case report. Am J Psychiatry 140:241–242, 1983

Dunner DL, Cohn JB, Walshe TI, et al: Two combined, multicenter double-blind studies of paroxetine and doxepin in geriatric patients with major depression. J Clin Psychiatry 53 (2 suppl): 57–60, 1992

Earle BV: Thyroid hormone and tricyclic antidepressants in resistant depressions. Am J Psychiatry 126:1667–1669, 1969

Echt DS, Liebson PR, Mitchell LB, et al: Mortality and morbidity in patients receiving encainide, flecainide, or placebo: the Cardiac Arrhythmia Suppression Trial. N Engl J Med 324:781–788, 1991

Eisen A: Fluoxetine and desipramine: a strategy for augmenting antidepressant response. Pharmacopsychiatry 22:272–273, 1989

Ellison JM, Milofsky JE, Ely E: Fluoxetine-induced bradycardia and syncope in two patients. J Clin Psychiatry 51:385–386, 1990

Eric L: A prospective, double-blind, comparative, multicentre study of paroxetine and placebo in preventing recurrent major depressive episodes. Biol Psychiatry 29 (suppl 11):254S–255S, 1991

Ettigi PG, Hayes PE, Narasimhacharr N, et al: d-Amphetamine response and dexamethasone suppression test as predictors of treatment outcome in unipolar depression. Biol Psychiatry 18:499–504, 1983

Falk RH: Flecainide-induced ventricular tachycardia and fibrillation in patients treated for atrial fibrillation. Ann Intern Med 111:107–111, 1989

Fawcett J, Maas JW, Dekirmenjian H: Depression and MHPG excretion: response to dextroamphetamine and tricyclic antidepressants. Arch Gen Psychiatry 26:246–251, 1972

Fawcett J, Kravitz HM, Sajecka JM, et al: CNS stimulant potentiation of monoamine oxidase inhibitors in treatment-refractory depression. J Clin Psychopharmacol 11:127–132, 1991

Feder R: Bradycardia and syncope induced by fluoxetine. J Clin Psychiatry 52:139, 1991

Fischette CT, Biegon A, McEwen: Sex steroid modulation of the serotonin behavioral syndrome. Life Sci 35:1197–1206, 1984

Frank E, Kupfer DJ, Perel JM, et al: Three-year outcomes for maintenance therapies in recurrent depression. Arch Gen Psychiatry 47:1093–1099, 1990

Fraser AR: Choice of anti-depressant based on test. Am J Psychiatry 140:786–787, 1983

Gaertner HJ, Kreuter F, Scharck G: Do urinary MHPG and plasma drug levels correlate with response to amitriptyline therapy? Psychopharmacology (Berl) 76:236–239, 1982

Gardner EA, Johnston JA: Bupropion: an antidepressant without sexual pathophysiological action. J Clin Psychopharmacol 5:24–29, 1985

Garvey MJ, Cook BL, Tollefson GD, et al: Antidepressant response in chronic major depression. Compr Psychiatry 30(3):214–217, 1989

Georgotas A, McCue RE, Cooper TB: A placebo controlled comparison of nortriptyline and phenelzine in maintenance therapy of elderly depressed patients. Arch Gen Psychiatry 46:783–786, 1989

Gitlin MJ, Gerner RH: The dexamethasone suppression test and response to somatic treatment: a review. J Clin Psychiatry 47:16–21, 1986

Gitlin MJ, Gwirtsman H, Fairbanks L, et al: Dexamethasone suppression test and treatment response. J Clin Psychiatry 45:387–389, 1984

Gitlin MJ, Weiner H, Fairbanks L: Failure of T_3 to potentiate tricyclic antidepressant response. J Affect Disord 13:267–272, 1987

Glassman AH, Bigger JT Jr: Cardiovascular effects of therapeutic doses of tricyclic antidepressants: a review. Arch Gen Psychiatry 38:815–820, 1981

Glassman AH, Preud'homme XA: Review of the cardiovascular effects of heterocyclic antidepressants. J Clin Psychiatry 54 (2 suppl):16–22, 1993

Glassman AH, Perel JM, Shostak M, et al: Clinical implications of imipramine plasma levels for depressive illness. Arch Gen Psychiatry 34:197–204, 1977

Glassman AH, Roose 5P, Giardina EGV, et al: Cardiovascular effects of tricyclic antidepressants, in Psychopharmacology: The Third Generation of Progress. Edited by Meltzer HY. New York, Raven, 1987, pp 1437–1442

Glassman AH, Roose SP, Bigger JT Jr: The safety of tricyclic antidepressants in cardiac patients: risk-benefit reconsidered. JAMA 269:2673–2675, 1993

Glowinski J, Axelrod J: Inhibition of uptake of tritiated-noradrenaline in the intact rat brain by imipramine and structurally related compounds. Nature 204:1318–1319, 1964

Goodman WK, Price LH, Delgado PL, et al: Specificity of serotonin reuptake inhibitors in the treatment of obsessive-compulsive disorder: comparison of fluvoxamine and desipramine. Arch Gen Psychiatry 47:577–585, 1990

Goodwin FK, Murphy DL, Dunner DL, et al: Lithium response in unipolar versus bipolar depression. Am J Psychiatry 129:44–47, 1972

Goodwin FK, Post RM, Murphy DL: Cerebrospinal fluid amine metabolites and therapies for depression. Program of the Scientific Proceedings of the annual meeting of the American Psychiatric Association, pp 24–25, 1973

Goodwin FK, Prange AJ, Post RM, et al: Potentiation of antidepressant effects by L-tri-iodothyranine in tricyclic nonresponders. Am J Psychiatry 139:34–38, 1982

Greden JF, Kronfol Z, Gardner R, et al: Dexamethasone suppression test and selection of antidepressant medications. J Affect Disord 3:389–396, 1981

Greden JF, Gardner R, King D: Dexamethasone suppression tests in anti-depressant treatment of melancholia: the process of normalization and test-retest reproducibility. Arch Gen Psychiatry 40:493–500, 1983

Haykal RF, Akiskal HS: Bupropion as a promising approach to rapidly cycling bipolar II patients. J Clin Psychiatry 51:450–455, 1990

Heninger GR, Charney DS, Sternberg DE: Lithium carbonate augmentation of antidepressant treatment: an effective prescription for treatment-refractory depression. Arch Gen Psychiatry 40:1335–1342, 1983

Himmelhoch JM, Detre T, Kupfer DJ, et al: Treatment of previously intractable depressions with tranylcypromine and lithium. J Nerv Ment Dis 155:216–220, 1972

Himmelhoch JM, Thase ME, Mallinger AG, et al: Tranylcypromine versus imipramine in anergic bipolar depression. Am J Psychiatry 148:910–916, 1991

Hirschfeld RMA, Klerman GL, Andreasen NC, et al: Psycho-social predictors of chronicity in depressed patients. Br J Psychiatry 148:648–654, 1986

Hochli D, Riemann D, Zulley J, et al: Initial REM sleep suppression by clomipramine: a prognostic tool for treatment response in patients with a major depressive disorder. Biol Psychiatry 21:1217–1220, 1986

Hollister LE, Overall JE: Reflections on the specificity of action of antidepressants. Psychosomatics 6:361–365, 1965

Hollister LE, Davis KL, Berger PA: Subtypes of depression based on excretion of MHPG and response to nortriptyline. Arch Gen Psychiatry 37:1107–1110, 1980

Holsboer F, Liebl R, Hofschuster E: Repeated dexamethasone suppression test during depressive illness: normalization of test result compared with clinical improvement. J Affect Disord 4:93–101, 1982

Horowitz LN, Zipes DP, Bigger JT Jr, et al: Proarrhythmia, arrhythmogenesis or aggravation of arrhythmia—a status report. Am J Cardiol 59:54E–56E, 1987

Howland RH: Pharmacotherapy of dysthymia: a review. J Clin Psychopharmacol 11(2):83–92, 1991

Humphrey P: 5-Hydroxytryptamine receptors and drug discovery, in Serotonin Receptor Subtypes: Pharmacological Significance and Clinical Implications (International Academic and Biomedical Drug Research, Vol 1). Edited by Langer SZ, Brunello N, Racagni G, et al. Basel, Switzerland, Karger, 1992, pp 129–139

Janicak PG, Davis JM, Chan C, et al: Failure of urinary MHPG levels to predict treatment response in patients with unipolar depression. Am J Psychiatry 143:1398–1402, 1986

Jick H, Dinan BJ, Hunter JR, et al: Tricyclic antidepressants and convulsions. J Clin Psychopharmacol 3:182–185, 1983

Joffe RT, Singer W: Thyroid hormone potentiation of antidepressants in Advances in Neuropsychiatry and Psychopharmacology, Vol 2: Refractory Depression. Edited by Amsterdam JD. New York, Raven, 1991, pp 185–190

Joffe RT, Singer W, Levitt AJ, et al: A placebo-controlled comparison of lithium and triiodothyronine augmentation of tricyclic antidepressants in unipolar refractory depression. Arch Gen Psychiatry 50:387–393, 1993

Johnston JA, Lineberry CG, Ascher JA, et al: A 102-center prospective study of seizure in association with bupropion. J Clin Psychiatry 52:450–456, 1991

Joyce PR, Paykel ES: Predictors of drug response in depression. Arch Gen Psychiatry 46:89–99, 1989

Kane JM, Cole K, Sarantakos S, et al: Safety and efficacy of bupropion in elderly patients: preliminary observations. J Clin Psychiatry 44 (5, sec 2):134–136, 1983

Keller MB, Shapiro RW, Lavori PW, et al: Recovery in major depressive disorder: analysis with the life table and regression models. Arch Gen Psychiatry 39:905–910, 1982a

Keller MB, Shapiro RW, Lavori PW, et al: Relapse in major depressive disorder: analysis with the life table. Arch Gen Psychiatry 39:911–915, 1982b

Keller MB, Lavori W, Endicott J, et al: "Double depression": two year follow-up. Am J Psychiatry 140:289–694, 1983

Keller MB, Klerman GL, Lavori PW, et al: Long-term outcome of episodes of major depression: Clinical and public health significance. JAMA 252:788–792, 1984

Keller MB, Lavori PW, Rice J, et al: The persistent risk of chronicity in recurrent episodes of nonbipolar major depressive disorder: a prospective follow-up. Am J Psychiatry 143:24–28, 1986

Keller MB, Lavori PW, Mueller TI, et al: Time to recovery, chronicity, and levels of psychopathology in major depression: a 5-year prospective follow-up of 431 subjects. Arch Gen Psychiatry 49:809–816, 1992

Klaiber EL, Bouerman DM, Vogel W, et al: Estrogen therapy for severe persistent depression in women. Arch Gen Psychiatry 36:550–554, 1979

Kline NS: Monoamine oxidase inhibitors: an unfinished picaresque tale, in Discoveries in Biological Psychiatry. Edited by Ayd FJ, Blackwell B. Philadelphia, PA, JB Lippincott, 1970, pp 194–204

Kocsis JH, Frances AJ: A critical discussion of DSM-III Dysthymic Disorder. Am J Psychiatry 144:1534–1542, 1987

Kosten TR, Frank JB, Dan E, et al: Pharmacotherapy for posttraumatic stress disorder using phenelzine or imipramine. J Nerv Ment Dis 179:366–370, 1991

Kramer BA: Electroconvulsive therapy use in geriatric depression. J Nerv Ment Dis 175:233–235, 1987

Kramlinger KG, Post RM: The addition of lithium to carbamazepine: antidepressant efficacy in treatment-resistant depression. Arch Gen Psychiatry 46:794–800, 1989

Kuhn R: The treatment of depressive states with G22355 (imipramine) hydrochloride. Am J Psychiatry 115:459–464, 1958

Kuhn R: The imipramine story in Discoveries in Biological Psychiatry. Edited by Ayd FJ, Blackwell B. Philadelphia, PA, JB Lippincott, 1970a, pp 205–217

Kuhn R: Foreword, in Tofranil® (Imipramine). Berne, Switzerland, Verlag Stamplfi, 1970b, pp vi–vii

Kuhn R: The discovery of modern antidepressants. Psychiatr J Univ Ottawa 14:249–252, 1989

Kupfer DJ, Foster FG, Reich L, et al: EEG sleep changes as predictors in depression. Am J Psychiatry 133:622–626, 1976

Kupfer DJ, Spiker DG, Coble PA, et al: Depression, EEG sleep, and clinical response. Compr Psychiatry 21:212–220, 1980

Kupfer DJ, Frank E, Perel JM, et al: Five-year outcome for maintenance therapies in recurrent depression. Arch Gen Psychiatry 49:769–773, 1992

Lavori PW, Keller MB, Klerman GL: Relapse in affective disorders: a reanalysis of the literature using life table methods. J Psychiatr Res 18:13–21, 1984

Lecrubier Y, Guelfi JD: Efficacy of reversible inhibitors of monoamine oxidase-A in various forms of depression. Acta Psychiatr Scand 360:18–23, 1990

Lee AS, Murray AM: The long term outcome of Maudsley depressives. Br J Psychiatry 153:741–751, 1988

Levitt AJ, Joffe RT, Kennedy SH: Bright light augmentation in antidepressant nonresponders. J Clin Psychiatry 52:336–337, 1991

Liebowitz MR, Fyer AJ, Gorman JM, et al: Phenelzine in social phobia. J Clin Psychopharmacol 6:93–98, 1986

Liebowitz MR, Quitkin FM, Stewart JW, et al: Antidepressant specificity in atypical depression. Arch Gen Psychiatry 45:129–137, 1988

Loomer HP, Saunders JC, Kline NS: Iproniazid, an amine oxidase inhibitor, as an example of a psychic energizer. Congressional Record 1382–1390, 1957

Loomer HP, Saunders JC, Kline NS: A clinical and pharmaco-dynamic evaluation of iproniazid as a psychic energizer (Psychiatric Research Report No

8). Washington, DC, American Psychiatric Association, 1958, pp 129–141

Maas JW, Fawcett JA, Dekirmenjian H: Catecholamine metabolism, depressive illness, and drug response. Arch Gen Psychiatry 26:252–262, 1972

Maas JW, Kocsis JH, Bowden CL, et al: Pretreatment neurotransmitter metabolites and response to imipramine or amitriptyline treatment. Psychol Med 12:37–43, 1982

Mann JJ, Kapur S: The emergence of suicidal ideation and behavior during antidepressant pharmacotherapy. Arch Gen Psychiatry 48:1027–1033, 1991

Marcus MD, Wing RR, Ewing L, et al: A double blind, placebo-controlled trial of fluoxetine plus behavior modification in the treatment of obese binge-eaters and non-binge eaters. Am J Psychiatry 147:876–881, 1990

Mayeux R, Stern Y, Cote L, et al: Altered serotonin metabolism in depressed patients with Parkinson's disease. Neurology 34:642–646, 1984

McConnell JD, Wilson JDD: Impotence, in Harrison's Principles of Internal Medicine. Edited by Wilson JD, Braunwald E, Isselbagher KJ, et al. New York, McGraw-Hill, 1991, pp 296–299

McGrath PJ, Stewart JW, Nunes EV, et al: A double-blind crossover trial of imipramine and phenelzine for outpatients with treatment-refractory depression. Am J Psychiatry 150:118–123, 1993

McLeod WR, Carroll B, Davies B: Hypothalamic dysfunction and antidepressant drugs. British Medical Journal 2:480–481, 1970

Mendels J, Ramsey TA, Dyson WL, et al: Lithium as an antidepressant. Arch Gen Psychiatry 36:845–846, 1979

Møller SE, Honore P, Larsen OB: Tryptophan and tyrosine ratios to neutral amino acids in endogenous depression: relation to antidepressant response to amitriptyline and lithium/L-tryptophan. J Affect Disord 5:67–79, 1983

Møller SE, Odum K, Kirk L, et al: Plasma tyrosine/neutral amino acid ratio correlated with clinical response to nortriptyline in endogenously depressed patients. J Affect Disord 9:223–229, 1985

Møller SE, de Beurs P, Timmerman L, et al: Plasma tryptophan and tyrosine ratios to competing amino acids in relation to antidepressant response to citalopram and maprotiline. Psychopharmacology (Berl) 88:96–110, 1986

Møller SE, Bech P, Bjerrum H, et al: Plasma ratio tryptophan/neutral amino acids in relation to clinical response to paroxetine and clomipramine in patients with major depression. J Affect Disord 18:59–66, 1990

Montgomery SA, Dufour H, Brion S, et al: The prophylactic efficacy of fluoxetine in unipolar depression. Br J Psychiatry 153 (suppl 3):69–76, 1988

Montgomery SA, Doogan DP, Burnside R: The influence of different relapse criteria on the assessment of long-term efficacy of sertraline. Int Clin Psychopharmacol 6 (suppl 2):37–46, 1991

Morganroth J, Goin JE: Quinidine-related mortality in the short-to-medium-term treatment of ventricular arrhythmias: a meta-analysis. Circulation 84:1977–1983, 1991

Murphy BE, Dhar V, Ghadirian AM, et al: Response to steroid suppression in major depression resistant to antidepressant therapy. J Clin Psychopharmacol 11:121–126, 1991

Nagy LM, Morgan CA Ill, Southwick SM, et al: Open prospective trial of fluoxetine for posttraumatic stress disorder. J Clin Psychopharmacol 13:107–113, 1993

National Institutes of Health Consensus Development Panel on Depression in Late Life: Diagnosis and treatment of depression in late life (NIH consensus conference). JAMA 268:1018–1024, 1992

Nelson JC, Bowers MB: Delusional unipolar depression: description and drug response. Arch Gen Psychiatry 35:1321–1328, 1978

Nelson CJ, Byck R: Rapid response to lithium in phenelzine non-responders. Br J Psychiatry 141:85–86, 1982

Nelson JC, Jatlow P, Quinlan DM, et al: Desipramine plasma concentration and antidepressant response. Arch Gen Psychiatry 39:1419–1422, 1982

Nelson JC, Mazure CM, Bowers MB, et al: Rapid antidepressant effect of desipramine plus fluoxetine. New Research Program and Abstracts of the annual meeting of the American Psychiatric Association, May 1990, NR 454

Neshkes RE, Jarvik LF: Affective disorders in the elderly. Annu Rev Med 38:445–456, 1987

Nierenberg AA, Price LH, Charney DS: After lithium augmentation: a retrospective follow-up of patients with antidepressant-refractory depression. J Affect Disord 18(3):167–175, 1990

Nierenberg AA, Keck PE Jr, Samson J, et al: Methodological considerations for the study of treatment-resistant depression, in Advances in

Neuropsychiatry and Psychopharmacology, Vol 2: Refractory Depression. Edited by Amsterdam JD. New York, Raven, 1991, pp 1–12

Nolen WA, van de Putte JJ, Dijken WA, et al: Treatment strategy in depression, I: non-tricyclic and selective reuptake inhibitors in resistant depression: a double-blind partial crossover study on the effects of oxaprotiline and fluvoxamine. Acta Psychiatr Scand 78:668–675, 1988

Noyes R, Dempsey GM, Blum A, et al: Lithium treatment of depression. Compr Psychiatry 15:187–193, 1974

Ogura C, Okuma T, Uchida Y, et al: Combined thyroid (triiodothyronine)-tricyclic antidepressant treatment in depressive states. Folia Psychiatrica et Neurologica Japonica 28:179–186, 1974

Oppenheim G: Rapid mood cycling with estrogen: implications for therapy. J Clin Psychiatry 45:34–35, 1984

Overall JE, Hollister LE, Johnson M, et al: Nosology of depression and differential response to drugs. JAMA 195:946–948, 1966

Pande AC, Calarco MM, Grunhaus LJ: Combined MAOI-TCA treatment in refractory depression, in Advances in Neuropsychiatry and Psychopharmacology, Vol 2: Refractory Depression. Edited by Amsterdam JD. New York, Raven, 1991, pp 115–122

Paul SM, Extein I, Call HM, et al: Use of ECT with treatment-resistant depressed patients at the NIMH. Am J Psychiatry 134:486–489, 1981

Paykel ES: Depressive typologies and response to amitriptyline. Br J Psychiatry 120:147–156, 1972

Paykel ES: Predictors of treatment response, in Psychopharmacology of Affective Disorders. Edited by Paykel ES, Coppen A. Oxford, England, Oxford University Press, 1979, pp 193–220

Peck AW, Stern WC, Watkinson C: Incidence of seizures during treatment with tricyclic antidepressant drugs and bupropion. J Clin Psychiatry 44 (5, sec 2):197–201, 1983

Peselow ED, Fieve RR: Dexamethasone suppression test and response to antidepressants in depressed outpatients. N Engl J Med 307:1216–1217, 1982

Peselow ED, Loutin A, Wolkin A, et al: The dexamethasone suppression test and response to placebo. J Clin Psychopharmacol 6:286–291, 1986

Pfohl B, Stangl D, Zimmerman M: The implications of DSM-III personality disorders for patients with major depression. J Affect Disord 7:309–318, 1984

Post RM: Anticonvulsants as adjuncts or alternatives to lithium in refractory bipolar illness, in Advances in Neuropsychiatry and Psychopharmacology, Vol 2: Refractory Depression. Edited by Amsterdam JD. New York, Raven, 1991, pp 155–165

Power AC, Cowen PJ: Fluoxetine and suicidal behaviour: some clinical and theoretical aspects of a controversy. Br J Psychiatry 161:735–741, 1992

Prange AJ: Paroxysmal auricular tachycardia apparently resulting from combined thyroid-imipramine treatment. Am J Psychiatry 119:994–995, 1963

Prange AJ: Estrogen may well affect response to antidepressant. JAMA 219:143–144, 1972

Prange AJ, Wilson IC, Rabon AM, et al: Enhancement of imipramine antidepressant activity by thyroid hormone. Am J Psychiatry 126:457–469, 1969

Pratt GM, Brater DC, Harrell FE Jr, et al: Clinical and regulatory implications of the Cardiac Arrhythmia Suppression Trial. Am J Cardiol 65:103–105, 1990

Preskorn SH: Tricyclic antidepressants: the whys and hows of therapeutic drug monitoring. J Clin Psychiatry 50 (7, suppl):34–42, 1989

Preskorn SH: Should bupropion dosage be adjusted based upon therapeutic drug monitoring? Psychopharmacol Bull 27(4):637–643, 1991

Preskorn SH, Fast GA: Therapeutic drug monitoring for antidepressants: efficacy, safety, and cost effectiveness. J Clin Psychiatry 52 (6 suppl):23–33, 1991

Price LH, Gharney DS, Heninger GR: Efficacy of lithium-tranylcypromine treatment in refractory depression. Am J Psychiatry 142:619–623, 1985

Prien RF, Kupfer DJ: Continuation drug therapy for major depressive episodes: how long should it be maintained? Am J Psychiatry 143:18–23, 1986

Prien RF, Klett J, Caffey EM: Lithium carbonate and imipramine in prevention of affective episodes. Arch Gen Psychiatry 29:420–425, 1973

Quitkin FM, McGrath P, Liebowitz MR, et al: Monoamine oxidase inhibitors in bipolar endogenous depressives. J Clin Psychopharmacol 1:70–74, 1989

Quitkin FM, McGrath PJ, Stewart JW, et al: Atypical depression, panic attacks, and response to imipramine and phenelzine. Arch Gen Psychiatry 47:935–941, 1990

Quitkin FM, Harrison W, Stewart JW, et al: Response to phenelzine and imipramine in placebo nonresponders with atypical depression. Arch Gen Psychiatry 48:319–323, 1991

Raskin A, Crook TA: The endogenous-neurotic distinction as a predictor of response to antidepressant drugs. Psychol Med 6:59–70, 1976

Rawling DA, Fozzard HA: Effects of imipramine on cellular electrophysiological properties of cardiac Purkinje fibers. J Pharmacol Exp Ther 209:371–375, 1979

Razani J, White KL, White J, et al: The safety and efficacy of combined amitriptyline and tranylcypromine antidepressant treatment: a controlled trial. Arch Gen Psychiatry 40:657–661, 1983

Reynolds CF III, Frank E, Perel JM, et al: Combined pharmacotherapy and psychotherapy in the acute and continuation treatment of elderly patients with recurrent major depression: a preliminary report. Am J Psychiatry 149:1687–1692, 1992

Richelson E: Antidepressants: pharmacology and clinical use, in Treatments of Psychiatric Disorders: A Task Force Report of the American Psychiatric Association. Chaired by Karasu TB. Washington, DC, American Psychiatric Association, 1989

Richelson E: Side effects of old and new generation antidepressants: a pharmacologic framework. J Clin Psychiatry 9:13–19, 1991

Richelson E, Nelson A: Antagonism by antidepressants of neurotransmitter receptors of normal human brain in vitro. J Pharmacol Exp Ther 230:94–102, 1984

Rickels K, Amsterdam J, Clary C, et al: The efficacy and safety of paroxetine compared with placebo in outpatients with major depression. J Clin Psychiatry 53 (suppl):30–32, 1992

Risch SC, Huey LY, Janowsky DS: Plasma levels of tricyclic antidepressants and clinical efficacy: review of the literature—parts I and II. J Clin Psychiatry 40:4–16 and 58–69, 1979

Roose SP, Palack GW, Glassman AH, et al: Cardiovascular effects of bupropion in depressed patients with heart disease. Am J Psychiatry 148:512–516, 1991

Rosenbaum AH, Schatzberg AF, Maruta T, et al: MHPG as a predictor of antidepressant response to imipramine and maprotiline. Am J Psychiatry 137:1090–1092, 1980

Rosenbaum JF, Fava M, Falk WE, et al: The antidepressant potential of oral S-adenosyl-L-methionine. Acta Psychiatr Scand 81:432–436, 1990

Rosenthal J, Hemlock C, Hellerstein DJ, et al: A preliminary study of serotonergic antidepressants in treatment of dysthymia. Prog Neuropsychopharmacol Biol Psychiatry 16:933–941, 1992

Rush AJ: Cognitive therapy of depression: rationale, techniques and efficacy. Psychiatr Clin North Am 6:105–127, 1983

Sabelli HC, Fawcett J, Javaid JJ, et al: The methylphenidate test for differentiating desipramine responsive from nortriptyline responsive depression. Am J Psychiatry 140:212–214, 1983

Sackeim HA, Prudic J, Devanand DP, et al: The impact of medication resistance and continuation pharmacotherapy on relapse following response to electroconvulsive therapy in major depression. J Clin Psychopharmacol 10:96–104, 1990

Salzman C: Pharmacologic treatment of depression in the elderly. J Clin Psychiatry 54 (2 suppl):23–28, 1993

Schatzberg AF, Orsulak PJ, Rosenbaum AH, et al: Toward a biochemical classification of depressive disorders, IV: pretreatment urinary MHPG levels as predictors of antidepressant response to imipramine. Communications in Psychopharmacology 4:441–445, 1980

Schatzberg AF, Rosenbaum AH, Orsulak PJ: Toward a biochemical classification of depressive disorders, III: pretreatment urinary MHPG levels as predictors of response to treatment with maprotiline. Psychopharmacology (Berl) 75:34–38, 1981

Schmauss M, Kapfhammer HP, Meyer P, et al: Combined MAO-inhibitor and tri-(tetra) cyclic antidepressant treatment in therapy resistant depression. Prog Neuropsychopharmacol Biol Psychiatry 12:523–532, 1988

Schwartz G, Halaris A, Baxter L: Normal thyroid function in desipramine nonresponders compared to responders by the addition of L-tri-iodothyronine. Am J Psychiatry 141:1614–1616, 1984

Segraves RT: Sexual dysfunction complicating the treatment of depression. J Clin Psychiatry 10:75–83, 1992

Selzer A, Wray HW: Quinidine syncope: paroxysmal ventricular fibrillations occurring during treatment of chronic atrial arrhythmias. Circulation 30:17–26, 1964

Settle EC Jr: Antidepressant side effects: issues and options. J Clin Psychiatry 10:48–61, 1992

Shapira B, Oppenheim G, Zohar J, et al: Lack of efficacy of estrogen supplementation to imipramine in resistant female depressives. Biol Psychiatry 20:576–579, 1985

Shawcross CR, Tyrer P: Influence of personality on response to monoamine oxidase inhibitors and tricyclic antidepressants. J Psychiatr Res 19:557–562, 1985

Sheehan DV, Ballenger J, Jacobsen G: Treatment of endogenous anxiety with phobic, hysterical and hypochondriacal symptoms. Arch Gen Psychiatry 40:125–138, 1983a

Sheehan DV, Davidson J, Manschreck T, et al: Lack of efficacy of a new antidepressant (bupropion) in the treatment of panic disorder with phobias. J Clin Pharmacol 3:28–31, 1983b

Sherwin BB: Estrogen and refractory depression, in Advances in Neuropsychiatry and Psychopharmacology, Vol 2: Refractory Depression. Edited by Amsterdam JD. New York, Raven, 1991, pp 209–218

Shopsin B: Bupropion's prophylactic efficacy in bipolar affective illness. J Clin Psychiatry 44 (5, sec 2):163–169, 1983

Simpson GM, Lee HL, Cuche Z, et al: Two doses of imipramine in hospitalized endogenous and neurotic depressions. Arch Gen Psychiatry 33:1093–1102, 1976

Spar JA, LaRue A: Acute response to methylphenidate as a predictor of outcome of treatment with TCAs in the elderly. J Clin Psychiatry 46:466–469, 1985

Spiker DG, Edwards D, Hanin I, et al: Urinary MHPG and clinical response to amitriptyline in depressed patients. Am J Psychiatry 137:1183–1187, 1980

Spiker DD, Weiss JC, Dealy RS, et al: The pharmacological treatment of delusional depression. Am J Psychiatry 142:430–436, 1985

Stein G, Bernadt M: Lithium augmentation therapy in tricyclic-resistant depression: a controlled trial using lithium in low and normal doses. Br J Psychiatry 162:634–640, 1993

Svendsen K, Christensen PDG: Duration of REM sleep latency as predictor of effect of antidepressant therapy. Acta Psychiatr Scand 64:238–243, 1981

Targum SD: Persistent neuroendocrine dysregulation in major depressive disorder: a marker for early relapse. Biol Psychiatry 19:305–318, 1984

Teicher MH, Glod C, Cole JO: Emergence of intense suicidal preoccupation during fluoxetine treatment. Am J Psychiatry 147:207–210, 1990

Thase ME, Mallinger AD, McKnight D, et al: Treatment of imipramine-resistant recurrent depression, IV: a double-blind crossover study of tranylcypromine for anergic bipolar depression. Am J Psychiatry 149:195–198, 1992

Trimble MR: Nonmonoamine oxidase inhibitor antidepressants and epilepsy: a review. Epilepsia 19:241–250, 1978

Tsutsui S, Yamazaki Y, Namba T, et al: Combined therapy of T_3 and antidepressants in depression. J Int Med Res 7:138–146, 1979

Tyrer P, Murphy S: Efficacy of combined antidepressant therapy in resistant neurotic disorder. Br J Psychiatry 156:115–118, 1990

van Kammen DP, Murphy DL: Prediction of imipramine antidepressant response by a one day d-amphetamine trial. Am J Psychiatry 135:1179–1184, 1978

VanPraag HM: New evidence of serotonin deficient depressions. Neuropsychobiology 3:56–63, 1977

Walsh BT, Stewart JW, Roose SP, et al: Treatment of bulimia with phenelzine: a double-blind, placebo-controlled study. Arch Gen Psychiatry 41:1105–1109, 1984

Weilburg JB, Rosenbaum JF, Biederman J, et al: Fluoxetine added to non-MAOI antidepressants converts nonresponders to responders: a preliminary report. J Clin Psychiatry 50:447–449, 1989

Weld FM, Bigger JT Jr: Electrophysiological effects of imipramine on ovine cardiac Purkinje and ventricular muscle fibers. Circ Res 46:167–175, 1980

Wharton RN, Perel JM, Dayton PG, et al: A potential clinical use for methylphenidate (Ritalin) with tricyclic antidepressants. Am J Psychiatry 127:1619–1625, 1971

White K, Simpson G: Combined MAOI-tricyclic antidepressant treatment: a reevaluation. J Clin Psychopharmacol 1:264–282, 1981

Wright D, Galloway L, Kim J, et al: Bupropion in the long-term treatment of cyclic mood disorders: mood stabilizing effects. J Clin Psychiatry 46:22–25, 1985

Zall H: Lithium carbonate and isocarboxazid: an effective drug approach in severe depressions. Am J Psychiatry 127:136–139, 1971

29

Treatment of Bipolar Disorder

Charles L. Bowden, M.D.

■ RATIONALE FOR TREATMENT

Bipolar disorder is unique among psychiatric diseases in the multiple factors associated with it that influence treatment strategies. It is chronic, recurrent, severely impairing, and usually present from adolescence or early adulthood, thus spanning the most vocationally productive years and the years of childbearing. Many of the treatments for bipolar disorder have established efficacy and provide not only symptomatic control but excellent social and vocational function. These benefits are not simply achieved in most cases because of complexities of the disease and its treatments. The subsyndromal variations of bipolar disorder—both based on symptom constellation and illness course—have major differences in prognosis and require different treatment strategies.

Bipolar disorder has been difficult to study because of the wide fluctuations in mood state intrinsic to the disease, the numerous factors that can confound treatment effects, and the impaired insight and psychotic function of patients during severe points of illness. These factors are addressed in turn here, with the intent of providing guidelines both for overall treatment strategy and for handling details and special problems that arise on an individual case basis.

■ SYMPTOMATIC AND ILLNESS COURSE FEATURES AFFECTING PHARMACOTHERAPY

■ Acute Mania and Hypomania

Although certain epidemiological differences appear to distinguish hypomania from mania, efficacy of treatments has not appeared to differ (Davis 1976). Also, many of the undesirable sequelae or concomitants of the illness (e.g., substance abuse, suicide risk) appear to be equivalent in the two groups. Thus, although most studies of treatments have been with bipolar I patients, the recommendations here are intended for both groups, with the caveat that experimental data from bipolar II patients are limited. A major difference between mania and hypomania affecting treatment is that hypomania is much more likely to escape detection by the psychiatrist and to be rationalized as healthy function by the patient. Both factors thus increase the possibility of incorrect diagnosis and of poor compliance with treatment.

A small percentage of patients have only manic or hypomanic episodes. Although these patients have been little studied with regard to treatment, standard antimanic regimens (both for acute and maintenance treatment) are generally instituted, without use of antidepressant medication.

■ Acute Depression

The present criteria for diagnosis of depression in bipolar disorder require a major depressive episode. This is in part based on evidence that the symptom profile and severity of the depressed bipolar patient are relatively similar to that of the patient with major depression (Katz et al. 1982). This poses problems that may result in incorrect diagnosis and therefore inappropriate treatment. Depressive episodes in bipolar patients are generally shorter than in patients with major depression. This is most evident in rapid-cycling patients. The brevity of a hypomanic or depressive episode may result in failure to recognize a patient as bipolar or as experiencing a depressive episode.

The frequency of certain symptoms differs in bipolar patients compared with unipolar patients. Hypersomnia and psychomotor retardation are more common in bipolar depression, and anxiety and agitation are less common (Beigel and Murphy 1971; Katz et al. 1982). Patients with atypical unipolar depression also frequently have hypersomnia and psychomotor retardation, but they have prominent anxiety as well. As many as 25% of bipolar patients may have three or four depressive episodes before their first manic episode (Angst 1985; Angst et al. 1978). If the clinician does not recognize a bipolar pattern, this may result in prolonged treatment of the patient with antidepressants, with the attendant risks of precipitating manic episodes and increasing cycle frequency. Attention to several factors during assessment may reduce such erroneous diagnostic classification. The younger the patient at the first episode of depression, the greater the likelihood of an underlying bipolar disorder (Carson and Stover 1978). The more frequent and the greater the number of depressive episodes, the greater the likelihood of bipolar disorder (Goodwin and Jamison 1990). The more frequently either bipolar depression or major depression has occurred in a patient's relatives, the more likely that his or her illness is bipolar disorder.

■ Severity of Illness

Severity of bipolar episodes varies both qualitatively and quantitatively. Cyclothymia is thought by most authorities to be linked to (or a mild form of) bipolar disorder, although the question has been little studied (Akiskal et al. 1979). A decision to try medications indicated for bipolar disorder is thus largely made on the plausible basis that the patient senses that he or she has substantial dysfunction from the mood instability.

Approximately half of all manic patients will exhibit psychotic symptoms. Patients with psychotic features have responded less well to lithium in some but not all studies (Goodwin and Jamison 1990). Unconfirmed reports suggest that valproate and carbamazepine may be relatively more effective in more severely ill manic patients.

Patients who move from a depressive episode directly into a manic episode respond less well to standard lithium therapy than those who characteristically move from depression to euthymia (Grof et al. 1987).

■ Subsyndromal Variations

Mixed mania. Since 1980, strong evidence has been published for syndromal variations that have important treatment implications. Mixed or dysphoric manic patients respond less well both to acute and chronic treatment with lithium (Keller et al. 1986; Prien et al. 1988; Swann et al. 1986). Suggestive evidence of relatively favorable response to valproate or carbamazepine needs to be followed by randomized, blinded studies (Calabrese and Delucchi 1990; Post et al. 1987). Additional features that may aid in identifying such patients include older age at first onset of illness, fewer episodes per unit of time, and no family history of mood disorder.

Pure or classical mania. Patients whose symptoms are principally along the behavioral dimensions of elevated mood, elation, grandiosity, increased activity, and reduced need for sleep constitute the group that responds best to acute treatment with lithium (Keller et al. 1986; Swann et al. 1986). It is not well established whether this advantage holds for maintenance-phase outcome. Additional features that may aid in identifying these patients include early first onset of illness and positive family history for mood disorders.

Rapid cycling. Patients with a greater frequency of episodes have quite low response rates to lithium both during acute and prophylactic treatment (Dunner and Fieve 1974; Dunner et al. 1976a, 1976b). Currently rapid cycling is defined as 4 or more episodes of any combination of depression or mania during a 12-month period. Much remains to be clarified about this group of patients. For example, it is unclear whether most rapid-cycling patients do so over the full course of their illness or, conversely, do so only for limited periods, perhaps principally secondary to exposure to mood-destabilizing agents.

Comorbid Substance Abuse

Patients with concurrent substance abuse (including alcoholism) respond less well to standard bipolar disorder regimens. It is important that the substance abuse be eliminated through direct intervention. Concurrent attention to the bipolar illness is warranted. Some substance abuse appears to be an effort either to extend manic symptoms or to alleviate dysphoric symptoms of the disorder, and it may resolve with alleviation of the manic or depressive episode. Because more than half of both bipolar I and II patients have concurrent substance abuse conditions, close attention to this during evaluation or at times of breakthrough episodes is important (Reiger et al. 1988).

Secondary Bipolar Disorders

A wide range of medical disorders results in disturbance of mood, either concurrently or as sequelae of the medical disorder. When possible, treatment should concurrently be aimed at the primary disorder. Patients with secondary bipolar disorders tend to have mixed symptomatology and to have more manic than depressed episodes. Lithium is relatively ineffective in treatment of these conditions. Uncontrolled studies suggest more favorable responses with carbamazepine or valproate (Kahn et al. 1988).

PHARMACOTHERAPIES

General Principles of Drug Treatment

Life charting. Life charting has a special role in bipolar disorder management. Because of the fluctuating mood states and varying symptom presentations requiring changing medication regimens, as well as the nearly uniform long-term treatment required, it can be difficult to glean drug treatment–clinical response relationships from the traditional medical record with progress notes. Life charting offers a graphically succinct means of capturing several domains of treatment and response on one sheet.

Many of the benefits of life charting directly affect drug therapy. Partial response patterns, evidence of antidepressant-induced rapid cycling, gradual loss of efficacy, and evidence for the effectiveness of non-drug therapies such as bright lights are among the potential benefits of this approach. Life charting is relatively labor intensive and requires regular updating. Patients' active participation in developing a life chart is desirable (Post et al. 1988).

Optimizing sleep. Benzodiazepines often relieve insomnia and related agitation and restlessness. Their adjunctive use is particularly important early in treatment, before the mood stabilizer has become effective, and as needed to regularize sleep during maintenance treatment. Although standard doses of any benzodiazepine may be helpful, two drugs warrant special consideration. Lorazepam has the advantage of parental administration to the patient unable or unwilling to take oral medication. Clonazepam has a long duration of action, thus reducing the need for frequent dosing and producing consistent sedation both at night and (if needed) during the day. Additionally, clonazepam (one of a small number of drugs that is metabolized by nitro reduction) is not pharmacokinetically altered by enzyme inducers such as carbamazepine or enzyme inhibitors such as fluoxetine.

Eliminating mood destabilizers. Many bipolar patients are exquisitely sensitive to chemical agents that may destabilize mood (Goodwin and Jamison 1990). The clinician should inquire about such medication or substance use and, when warranted, couple this with toxicological screening. Although antidepressants are the most important group in this regard, some patients are destabilized by a panoply of substances, such as mild quantities of alcohol, topical steroids, medications for glaucoma, or mild use of stimulant drugs.

Combining drug therapies. Empirical evidence reveals that the majority of bipolar patients in maintenance treatment receive a combination of drugs rather than monotherapy. Although some of this is attributable to failure to discontinue a medication that is no longer needed, most authorities believe that combined drug therapy is needed to achieve the best possible clinical response in a substantial number of patients.

Combined drug therapy is of two types. The first is concurrent use of two or more mood-stabilizing drugs. Reports have been published on the effectiveness and good tolerance of all such combinations (Kramlinger and Post 1989). More caution should be exercised in combining valproate and carbamazepine. Carbamazepine may increase the percentage of a potentially hepatotoxic valproate metabolite (Ketter et al. 1992). There is extensive evidence that most hepatotoxic consequences of valproate are limited to young children. The second type of combined therapy is a mood-stabilizing agent plus one or more adjunctive drugs. These will generally be limited to concurrent benzodiazepines, neuroleptics, and/or antidepressants.

In considering the addition of a second or third drug to a therapeutic regimen, the psychiatrist first needs to ascertain that the first drug has been tried in adequate dosage over a reasonable time and that the drug is well tolerated. Next, he or she needs to choose a drug that has a different pharmacodynamic mechanism than the current drug. This would rule out use of two tricyclic antidepressants (TCAs), for example. The pharmacokinetic properties of the drugs need to be understood. With the exception of the enzyme-inducing effects of carbamazepine, most drugs either have no effects on other drug metabolism or inhibit hepatic microsomal oxidation, potentially increasing plasma concentrations of oxidatively metabolized drugs. The potential for additive adverse effects has to be considered. For example, both lithium and valproate may induce an intention tremor. At present, there is no evidence that would suggest a different dosage range for drugs used in combination than for the same drug used in monotherapy. It is plausible, although not explicitly studied, that somewhat smaller dosages might be employed when two drugs are used concurrently.

If improvement occurs after addition of the second drug, consideration should be given to gradual tapering of the dosage of the first drug, as no other procedure ensures that the improvement is tied to the two drugs in combination rather than the second drug alone. Combined drug therapy warrants closer monitoring for adverse effects and greater utilization of plasma concentration monitoring to ensure that drug concentrations have not strayed outside the ranges generally deemed safe and effective.

Whereas combined drug therapy with two or more mood stabilizers is likely to be indefinite, the default expectation for addition of an adjunctive medication should be that the drug will be tapered shortly after the target symptoms that led to its use are alleviated. Unless these symptoms recur during the taper, the medication should be discontinued.

As it is unlikely that conclusive, large-scale experimental studies of combined drug therapies will be conducted, it is important that the psychiatrist see these therapeutic efforts as near experiments. For practical purposes, this means changing only one drug variable at a time, documenting the symptoms carefully, and using life charts to graphically depict the patient's response to different therapeutic regimens. The patient needs to understand the rationale for the combined drug therapy and any risks associated with drug interactions.

■ Acute Mania and Hypomania

Lithium. Lithium, valproate, and carbamazepine have relatively well-established efficacy in acute mania. Only lithium is approved by the U.S. Food and Drug Administration for this indication, and it has the advantage of more than 20 years of general use. Lithium is most likely to be effective in patients with pure manic symptomatology (i.e., elation and grandiosity) but not dysphoric features (Himmelhoch and Garfinkel 1986; Himmelhoch et al. 1991; Prien et al. 1984, 1988; Secunda et al. 1985). Response rates in these patients may be as high as 90%. By way of contrast, lithium is effective much less often in patients with mixed mania (Prien et al. 1988; Secunda et al. 1985) or rapid cycling (Dunner and Fieve 1974). More severely ill and psychotically manic patients may also respond less well to lithium. Lithium is generally poorly tolerated in elderly patients, with cognitive and gastrointestinal adverse effects especially prominent (Shulman et al. 1987).

The recently completed first study of lithium in treating patients with acute mania was a double-blind, parallel-group, placebo-controlled research effort. Forty-nine percent of the patients had a moderate or better response within 3 weeks of vigorous lithium treatment, but without any use of neuroleptic. This represents a highly and clinically significant difference over placebo. Thirty-one percent of patients were actually worse at last assessment. Dropout rates and adverse events were somewhat higher in patients treated with lithium than in those treated with valproate (Bowden et al. 1994).

Given the accumulated experience with lithium and its established prophylactic efficacy, clinicians will initially treat most manic patients with lithium. The time to initial (albeit not full) response is generally 7 to 14 days for those patients who are successfully treated with lithium. However, initial improvement may not commence sooner than the third or fourth week for some patients. Because of the often disruptive and dangerous behavior of the acutely manic patient, adjunctive medications are often required during this lag period. Lithium plasma concentrations required for acutely manic patients are often somewhat higher than needed for maintenance therapy. Although a loading-dose strategy does not appear to be effective, dosage should be increased as rapidly as tolerated until either the patient responds or a plasma level of 1.2–1.4 mEq/L is reached. Although lithium has numerous serious adverse effects, most of these will not be problematic during treatment of acute episodes. Those that occur commonly with acute treatment are gastrointestinal irritation, tremor, metallic taste, and cognitive dulling.

Valproate. In a recent double-blind, parallel-group study in hospitalized acutely manic patients, valproate and lithium were equally effective, and both were significantly better than placebo (Bowden et al. 1994). Significant improvement with valproate was present from the fifth day of treatment. Dropout rates, particularly for reasons of adverse effects, were lower in valproate than lithium treated subjects. The symptoms that showed the earliest and most robust response to valproate were largely those comprising the primary manic syndrome: elevated mood, reduced need for sleep, and excessive activity. Those symptom areas (e.g., accelerated speech, poor judgment), which are elevated in mania but not specific thereto, were less responsive to either drug.

The quality and scope of double-blind placebo-controlled studies of valproate effectiveness in acute mania is better than that for lithium. Both of the placebo-controlled studies have shown highly clinically significant clinical superiority of valproate over placebo (Bowden et al. 1994; Pope et al. 1991). Open studies suggest that valproate may be as effective in treatment of patients with mixed mania as in those with pure mania, and in rapid-cycling patients

(Calabrese and Delucchi 1990).

Valproate can be administered in a loading dose of 20 mg/kg. Although well tolerated, it is not established that this strategy speeds response. The side effects of valproate most likely to occur during acute treatment include gastrointestinal irritation, tremor, sedation, and cognitive dulling.

Carbamazepine. Carbamazepine has many characteristics similar to valproate. The effectiveness of both drugs in mania was initially serendipitously observed by practicing physicians. This fact has contributed to the unusual way in which both drugs have been studied. In particular, no industry-sponsored placebo-controlled studies have been done with carbamazepine. The one placebo-controlled study was a crossover design with 19 patients that did not allow comparison of relative efficacy. Nevertheless, more than a dozen controlled studies indicate response rates comparable to lithium and valproate (Post et al. 1988). One of the two parallel-group comparisons with lithium found a lower response rate in carbamazepine than lithium (Lerer et al. 1987). The other, composed of a relatively treatment-refractory sample, reported only a 33% response rate for both drugs (Small et al. 1991).

Comparisons with neuroleptics have shown equivalent response rates, whereas lithium was generally superior to neuroleptics in controlled trials (Goodwin and Jamison 1990). Carbamazepine was more effective in treatment of patients with mixed mania than in those with pure mania. It may be as effective in more severe, psychotic, and rapid-cycling patients as in patients with pure mania (Post et al. 1989).

Carbamazepine requires cautious initial administration. A starting dose of 200 mg bid with gradual increase to levels above 4 µg/ml will often avoid or reduce sedation, cognitive dulling, diplopia, gastrointestinal irritability, and psychomotor slowing, which otherwise are relatively frequent early adverse effects. Carbamazepine causes hepatic enzyme induction that is generally clinically identifiable starting around the fourth to the eighth week of treatment. This complicates management, requiring relatively frequent plasma level measurement and dosage increase to bring the patient back into the range at which initial response occurred. Similarly, any other oxidatively metabolized medication will likely require an increased dosage. In the case of oral contraceptives, the uncertainty of contraceptive effectiveness given the lower drug level warrants use of another mode of contraception. Rashes are relatively common and can include severe hemorrhagic responses (e.g., Stevens-Johnson syndrome) that require prompt discontinuation. Regular monitoring of white blood cell and platelet count is important, although the relatively common 20%–30% reduction in granulocyte count and platelet count warrants more frequent monitoring, not discontinuation of the medication.

No fixed dose–type studies that would be needed to determine whether there are plasma level–response relationships have been conducted with either valproate or carbamazepine. The available data suggest only rough relationships of plasma concentration to response. Therefore, for both drugs, dosage should be increased as tolerated until response is obtained or a valproate concentration of approximately 120 µg/ml or a carbamazepine concentration of 12 µg/ml is achieved. Despite the lack of strong plasma level–response guidelines, plasma concentration monitoring every 2 to 3 months is still warranted. This ensures that the concentration is not moving upward or downward despite a stable dosage, serves as a check on compliance, and establishes that the patient is within the concentration range at which a positive initial response occurred.

There are several clinical circumstances that warrant initiation of treatment of acute mania with either valproate or carbamazepine, rather than lithium. Given the chronic, recurrent nature of bipolar disorder, the psychiatrist will often have information regarding any prior poor response to or toleration of lithium. Patients with psoriasis, impaired renal function, acne, and thyroid disorders may be more safely treated with valproate or carbamazepine. Elderly patients are particularly sensitive to the cognitive effects of lithium and generally tolerate valproate or carbamazepine better. Given the equivalent efficacy of valproate and lithium and the somewhat better tolerability and the lower risk of serious adverse effects from valproate, valproate may warrant consideration for initial mood stabilization. Such a decision needs also to weigh the less adequate studies on valproate's long-term effectiveness. No direct comparisons of the effectiveness of carbamazepine and valproate have been conducted. Adverse cognitive effects and serious toxicities appear to be more common with carbamazepine than valproate, and pharmacokinetic complexities make treatment implementation more complex with carbamazepine than valproate.

Other Antimanic Agents

Verapamil. A small number of manic patients have been reported to respond to verapamil (Dubovsky et al. 1986). These results are suggestive and warrant further study of calcium channel blockers. Verapamil would seem an unlikely candidate, because of its relatively low lipophilicity. By contrast, nimodipine and nifedipine are quite lipophilic (Brunet et al. 1990). Clonidine has been found no better than placebo in a small, well-designed, double-blind parallel-group study (Janicak et al. 1989).

Acute Depression

Direct experimental data about drug efficacy in bipolar depression is inadequate. Only one double-blind randomized parallel-group, placebo-controlled study of bipolar patients has been conducted (Cohn et al. 1989). The consequence of this is that recommendations for treatment of bipolar depression are based largely on data that are either outdated, derived from research on a different disease (i.e., major depression), or both. The response rate of bipolar and unipolar depressed patients to TCAs appears to be similar (Koslow et al. 1983). Bipolar depression specifically characterized by anergia is more responsive to monoamine oxidase inhibitors (MAOIs) than to TCAs (Himmelhoch et al. 1991). More than half of bipolar depressed patients who failed to respond to imipramine subsequently respond to tranylcypromine. Initial dosages and patterns of dosage escalation and dosage ranges do not differ from that for major depression. With the exception of the risks of mood destabilization (expressed as either hypomania, rapid cycling, or both), the side-effect profile does not differ.

Because of their favorable side-effect profile, selective serotonin reuptake inhibitors (SSRIs) are promising agents for bipolar depression. Positive results have been reported with fluoxetine and paroxetine. Fluoxetine was superior to placebo and nonsignificantly better than imipramine in one placebo-controlled study (Cohn et al. 1989). There were fewer side effects in the patients treated with fluoxetine than in those treated with imipramine. Bupropion has also been reported as effective in a small open study (Shopsin 1983).

There are insufficient data to conclude that one class of drugs is more effective than others in treatment of bipolar depression. Given the greater likelihood of cognitive impairment, autonomic overstimulation, hypotension, sedation, and weight gain, as well as the potential lethality in suicide attempts associated with all TCAs, I have a general preference for SSRIs as first-choice agents for treatment of acute bipolar depression. Among the SSRIs, the long half-life of fluoxetine is a potential disadvantage, because plasma level would not drop by 50% for approximately 1 month after discontinuing the drug if the patient developed hypomania.

If the patient is unresponsive to one of these agents, is intolerant to them, or has a medical contraindication to their use, electroconvulsive therapy (ECT) may be implemented. ECT has been reported superior to TCAs in bipolar depression, although the studies have substantial methodological limitations (Goodwin and Jamison 1990).

Several studies—only one of which was prospective and controlled—indicate that all of the above classes of antidepressants can either precipitate manic or (more often) hypomanic episodes, or destabilize the course of illness, resulting in a rapid-cycling course (Prien et al. 1984; Wehr and Goodwin 1987). The frequency of development of drug-induced mania is not established, although studies suggest that it may be around 20% of bipolar patients (Himmelhoch et al. 1991). The few studies that have not reported this adverse effect have tended to exclude the very subjects who would be at risk for mood destabilization (Kupfer et al. 1988; Lewis and Winokur 1982). Furthermore, concurrent lithium does not consistently prevent the development of manic episodes (Quitkin et al. 1981). As this area of risk with current antidepressants has become better understood, the recommendation for use of antidepressants in bipolar disorder has changed to that of limiting them to administration during depressive episodes. Thus, once the patient is free of the symptoms of depression, the dose should be tapered over a period of several weeks and then discontinued. A small percentage of bipolar patients (mostly women) will have a preponderance of depressive rather than manic episodes. These may require maintenance use of an antidepressant.

Mood-stabilizing agents have also been tried for treatment of acute bipolar depression. Although most studies of lithium have shown superiority over placebo or equivalence to TCAs, methodological problems limit generalizability. Most of these studies included unipolar patients, lacked placebo control subjects, or both (Worrall et al. 1979). The one study that compared lithium, imipramine, and placebo in bipolar depressed patients found both imipramine and lithium superior to placebo, with imipramine somewhat more effective than lithium (Fieve et al. 1968). Additionally, improvement in depressive symptoms in patients treated with lithium was often not evident for 3–4 weeks.

Prophylactic studies uniformly indicate that lithium is much more effective in reducing the frequency of manic relapses than of depressive relapses. Thus despite the experimental data, there is little current support for use of lithium to treat acute depressive episodes. Additionally, most bipolar patients experiencing a depressed episode will already be taking lithium. Uncontrolled studies with carbamazepine and valproate suggest that each is less effective in relieving depression than mania (Calabrese and Delucchi 1990; Post et al. 1989).

■ Maintenance Treatment

Although authorities discuss the relative merits of committing a newly diagnosed patient to maintenance treatment, this is warranted in all but a few exceptional cases. Bipolar disorder is in nearly all instances recurrent and chronic, with no tendency for the patient to mature out of the disease. Single episodes of mania are rare. Furthermore, the risks of not treating prophylactically include the disease's suicide rate of approximately 15%, the strong likelihood of recurrent episodes, and the serious social and vocational morbidity associated with the illness.

Post and colleagues (1992) presented suggestive evidence that discontinuation of lithium may lead to drug-induced treatment refractoriness, wherein previously effective treatments lose their effectiveness on readministration. Exceptions to this recommendation for maintenance treatment include the patient in whom toxic precipitants of a manic episode have confounded the diagnostic picture (i.e., what appears as mania may represent a toxic psychosis rather than a first bipolar episode). A person who spontaneously remits after a first, brief, apparent manic episode would not warrant initiation of maintenance treatment.

Lithium. Maintenance phase studies of lithium's superiority over placebo are substantially more conclusive for maintenance treatment than for acute treatment, with early studies showing approximately a 2:1 superiority of lithium over placebo (Baastrup et al. 1970; Davis 1976). Lithium discontinuation is followed by a high rate of relapse, with most new episodes being of manic rather than depressed type (Suppes et al. 1992).

Although no placebo-controlled maintenance treatment studies of lithium's effectiveness have been conducted in more than 20 years, recent studies indicate that a substantial number of patients have inadequate responses to lithium therapy. A naturalistic follow-up of outpatients with bipolar disorder found that the outcome was no better for patients maintained on lithium than for those on no medication (Harrow et al. 1990). Even among patients with an initial successful response to lithium for 2 years, only about half continued to do unequivocally well in subsequent years (Maj et al. 1989). Additionally, the mortality in patients treated with lithium for long periods did not differ from those not treated (Vestergaard and Aagaard 1991).

Part of the poor response over time may have to do with inadequate dosing. Gelenberg and colleagues (1989) found that relapse rates were higher among patients maintained at plasma levels of 0.4–0.6 mEq/L than among patients maintained at 0.8–1.0 mEq/L. The difference in relapse rates were only for manic episodes—suggesting, as do most studies, that lithium's prophylactic benefits are largely against new manic or hypomanic episodes. Additionally, the differences held only for patients with one or two prior episodes and thus cannot be generalized to patients with frequent episodes (Gelenberg et al. 1989).

Lithium dosing for maintenance therapy is analogous to that for acute mania. However, somewhat lower dosage may be required than for acute mania (probably linked to increased lithium clearance rates tied to increased renal blood flow) during some manic episodes. Lithium's side effects are much more problematic during maintenance therapy than acute therapy. Additional problems unlikely to occur during acute treatment include weight gain, acne, thyroid abnormalities, polydipsia, and polyuria. The group of side effects most likely to cause poor compliance or discontinuation of lithium are those on the central nervous system. These include impaired cognition, impaired short-term memory, poor coordina-

tion, muscular weakness, and lethargy (Jamison et al. 1979). In monitoring for these side effects, it is important to assess thyroid function approximately every 6 months. This is because of the high frequency of hypothyroidism during lithium treatment, and the potential for hypothyroidism to then compromise the patient's clinical response.

The combination of a relatively low percentage of patients with good long-term outcomes, the frequency and functional severity of side effects, and lithium's very narrow therapeutic index have stimulated studies of alternative mood stabilizers.

Valproate. Whereas high-quality studies of valproate have been conducted in subjects with acute mania, only open trials have been conducted for maintenance-phase therapy. The best conceived and executed of these found that prophylactic effectiveness was high for patients entering the study during a pure or mixed manic episode, and was good for patients with rapid cycling. Patients entering during a depressive episode fared much less well (Calabrese and Delucchi 1990).

Valproate's dosage and plasma levels appear to be the same for maintenance phase as for acute treatment. As with lithium, additional side effects will need to be considered. Transient hair loss may occur after several weeks of therapy. Increased appetite and weight gain may occur, in what is probably a dose-dependent response. Although cognitive dulling can occur, it appears to be dose related, and generally manageable by adjustment of timing of valproate dosage, or reduction of dosage. Although increased hepatic enzymes have been reported, the recent double-blind study of divalproex sodium in the treatment of acute mania did not indicate any trends for increase in hepatic enzymes (Bowden et al. 1994).

Carbamazepine. Carbamazepine has also been inadequately studied in maintenance phase treatment. Lusznat and colleagues (1988) found no significant differences between lithium and carbamazepine among patients treated for up to a year, although a larger percentage of carbamazepine-treated patients relapsed during treatment. Small and colleagues (1991) reported a trend favoring lithium over carbamazepine in the long-term maintenance phase treatment of initially hospitalized, treatment-refractory manic patients. Carbamazepine was inferior to lithium in a random assignment study without concomitant medication (Lerer et al. 1987). Another small study found carbamazepine superior to placebo; however, nearly all patients received supplemental neuroleptics (Goncalves and Stoll 1985). This and the Lerer study suggest (albeit without much data) that antipsychotic medication may be needed when carbamazepine is used.

Retrospective analyses suggest that at least half of bipolar patients initially responding to carbamazepine will relapse over a 3- to 4-year period (Frankenburg et al. 1988; Post et al. 1990). Although not encouraging, these results should not be viewed pessimistically in light of the similar long-term results reported from the analogous studies of lithium summarized previously. Definitive studies require an experimental design and prospective, randomized, double-blind, and generally placebo-controlled procedures, the sum of which are difficult to execute in bipolar patients.

Dosing approaches for carbamazepine require some modification during the second through the sixth month of treatment. Sometime during this period, most patients undergo hepatic enzyme induction, thus requiring a consequent increase in carbamazepine dose to return the patient to the plasma level that was initially effective. In addition to the acute phase side effects, several additional side effects require monitoring during maintenance phase treatment. Hematological and hepatic function require monitoring. Hyponatremia may be clinically significant, particularly in older patients. Carbamazepine not only lowers its own levels but also those of all oxidatively metabolized drugs (Jann et al. 1985; Kahn et al. 1990). Careful inquiry as to continued efficacy of such other drugs, and use of drug level monitoring (when available), will ward off most problems of this type.

Adjunctive treatments. Thyroid supplementation of lithium therapy has been reported effective in alleviating rapid-cycling symptomatology in a small, open trial (Bauer and Whybrow 1990). Although hypermetabolic doses were used, authorities differ on the merits of such a high-dose strategy, because of the potential for adverse effects such as tachycardia and bone demineralization with elevated thyroid function (Lehmke et al. 1992).

The indications for benzodiazepines and neuroleptics are the same in maintenance treatment as in acute treatment. The principle difference is that the risk of tardive dyskinesia from neuroleptic therapy is, for practical purposes, limited to chronic treatment. Unless gradual withdrawal of the neuroleptic results in an exacerbation of delusional, hallucinatory, or severely aggressive behavior not otherwise controlled without neuroleptics, the medication should be discontinued. As with other psychotic conditions, even those patients requiring long-term neuroleptic medication can often be gradually reduced in dosage, thereby reducing side-effect burden and risk.

Open trials have suggested that otherwise treatment refractory bipolar patients may improve and maintain their recovery with clozapine treatment (McElroy et al. 1991). The dosage range used has been 25–90 mg/day. Initially, only low dosages are characteristically well tolerated, and dosage escalation must often be accomplished slowly (McElroy et al. 1991). Given the potential for agranulocytosis from both carbamazepine and clozapine, the two drugs should not be used together.

■ SOURCES OF NEW INFORMATION

The study of bipolar disorder is an exciting one, with numerous studies under way that hold promise of improving clinical care. This rapid pace of new information can make it difficult for the psychiatrist or other mental health professional to keep up. The journals *Depression* and *The Journal of Affective Disorders* publish articles relevant to the topic. In terms of drug effects, *The Journal of Clinical Psychopharmacology*, *The Journal of Clinical Psychiatry*, *The American Journal of Psychiatry*, and *Neuropsychopharmacology* each have substantial offerings on the topic. Finally, the major work *Manic Depressive Illness* (1990) by Goodwin and Jamison contains a wealth of factual information and integrative assessments about the drug therapy of bipolar disorder.

■ REFERENCES

Akiskal HS, Khani MK, Scott-Strauss A: Cyclothymic temperamental disorders. Psychiatr Clin North Am 2:527–554, 1979

Angst J: Switch from depression to mania: a record study over decades between 1920 and 1982. Psychopathology 18:140–154, 1985

Angst J, Felder W, Stassen HH: The course of affective disorders, I: change of diagnosis of monopolar, unipolar, and bipolar illness. Archiv für Psychiatrie und Nervenkrankheiten 226:57–64, 1978

Baastrup PC, Poulsen JC, Schou M, et al: Prophylactic lithium: double-blind discontinuation in manic-depressive and recurrent-depressive disorders. Lancet 2:326–330, 1970

Bauer MS, Whybrow PC: Rapid cycling bipolar affective disorder, II: treatment of refractory rapid cycling with high-dose levothyroxine: a preliminary study. Arch Gen Psychiatry 47:435–440, 1990

Beigel A, Murphy DL: Assessing clinical characteristics of the manic state. Am J Psychiatry 128:688–694, 1971

Bowden CL, Brugger AM, Swann AC, et al: Efficacy of divalproex vs lithium and placebo in the treatment of mania. JAMA 271:918–924, 1994

Brunet G, Cerlick B, Robert P, et al: Open trial of a calcium antagonist, nimodipine, in acute mania. Clin Neuropharmacol 13:22, 1990

Calabrese JR, Delucchi GA: Spectrum of efficacy of valproate in 55 patients with rapid-cycling bipolar disorder. Am J Psychiatry 147:431–434, 1990

Carson G, Stover M: Affective disorders in adolescence: issues in misdiagnosis. J Clin Psychiatry 39:59–66, 1978

Cohn JB, Collins G, Ashbrook E, et al: A comparison of fluoxetine, imipramine, and placebo in patients with bipolar depressive disorder. Int Clin Psychopharmacol 4:313–322, 1989

Davis JM: Overview: maintenance therapy in psychiatry, II: affective disorders. Am J Psychiatry 133:1–13, 1976

Dubovsky SI, Franks RD, Allen S, et al: Calcium antagonists in mania: a double blind study of verapamil. Psychiatry Res 18:309–320, 1986

Dunner DL, Fieve RR: Clinical factors in lithium carbonate prophylaxis failure. Arch Gen Psychiatry 30:229–233, 1974

Dunner DL, Dwyer T, Fieve RR: Depressive symptoms in patients with unipolar and bipolar affective disorder. Compr Psychiatry 17:447–451, 1976a

Dunner DL, Fleiss JL, Fieve RR: The course of development of mania in patients with recurrent depression. Am J Psychiatry 133:905–908, 1976b

Fieve RR, Platman SR, Plutchik RR: The use of lithium in affective disorders, I: acute endogenous depression. Am J Psychiatry 125:487–491, 1968

Frankenburg FR, Tohen M, Cohen BM, et al: Long-term response to carbamazepine: a retrospective study. J Clin Psychopharmacol 8:130–132, 1988

Gelenberg AJ, Kane JM, Keller MB, et al: Comparison of standard and low serum levels of lithium for maintenance treatment of bipolar disorder. N Engl J Med 321:1489–1493, 1989

Goncalves N, Stoll KD: Carbam pin bei manischen syndromen: eine kontrollierte doppel blind studie. [Carbamazepine in manic syndromes: a controlled double-blind study.] Nervenerzt 56:43–47, 1985

Goodwin FK, Jamison KR: Manic-Depressive Illness. New York, Oxford University Press, 1990

Grof E, Haag M, Grof P, et al: Lithium response and the sequence of episode polarities: preliminary report on a Hamilton sample. Prog Neuropsychopharmacol Biol Psychiatry 11:199–203, 1987

Harrow M, Goldberg JF, Grossman LS, et al: Outcome in manic disorders: a naturalistic follow-up study. Arch Gen Psychiatry 47:665–671, 1990

Himmelhoch JM, Garfinkel ME: Sources of lithium resistance in mixed mania. Psychopharmacol Bull 22:613–620, 1986

Himmelhoch JM, Thase MF, Mallinger AG, et al: Tranylcypromine versus imipramine in anergic bipolar depression. Am J Psychiatry 148:910–916, 1991

Jamison KR, Gerner RH, Goodwin FK: Patient and physician attitudes toward lithium: relationship to compliance. Arch Gen Psychiatry 36:866–869, 1979

Janicak PG, Sharma RP, Easton M, et al: A double-blind, placebo-controlled trial of clonidine in the treatment of acute mania. Psychopharmacol Bull 25:243–245, 1989

Jann MW, Ereshefsky L, Saklad SR, et al: Effects of carbamazepine on plasma haloperidol levels. J Clin Psychopharmacol 5:106–109, 1985

Kahn D, Stevenson E, Douglas CJ: Effect of sodium valproate in three patients with organic brain syndromes. Am J Psychiatry 145:101–111, 1988

Kahn EM, Schulz SC, Perel JM, et al: Change in haloperidol level due to carbamazepine—a complicating factor in combined medication for schizophrenia. J Clin Psychopharmacol 10:54–57, 1990

Katz MM, Robins E, Croughan J, et al: Behavioral measurement and drug response characteristics of unipolar and bipolar depression. Psychol Med 12:25–36, 1982

Keller MB, Lavori PW, Coryell W, et al: Differential

outcome of pure manic, mixed/cycling, and pure depressive episodes in patients with bipolar illness. JAMA 255:3138–3142, 1986

Ketter TA, Pazzaglia P, Post RM: Synergy of carbamazepine and valproic acid in affective illness: case report and review of literature. J Clin Psychopharmacol 12:276–282, 1992

Koslow SH, Maas JW, Bowden CL, et al: CSF and urinary biogenic amines and metabolites in depression and mania: a controlled, univariate analysis. Arch Gen Psychiatry 40:999–1010, 1983

Kramlinger KG, Post RM: The addition of lithium carbonate to carbamazepine: antidepressant efficacy in treatment-resistant depression. Arch Gen Psychiatry 46:794–800, 1989

Kupfer DJ, Carpenter LL, Frank E: Possible role of antidepressants in precipitating mania and hypomania in recurrent depression. Am J Psychiatry 145:804–808, 1988

Lehmke J, Bogner U, Felsenberg D, et al: Determination of bone mineral density by quantitative computed tomography and single photon absorptiometry in subclinical hyperthyroidism: a risk of early osteopaenia in post-menopausal women. Clin Endocrinol (Oxf) 36:511–517, 1992

Lerer B, Moore N, Meyendorff E, et al: Carbamazepine versus lithium in mania: a double-blind study. J Clin Psychiatry 48:89–93, 1987

Lewis JL, Winokur G: The induction of mania: a natural history study with controls. Arch Gen Psychiatry 39:303–306, 1982

Lusznat R, Murphy DP, Nunn CMH: Carbamazepine vs lithium in the treatment and prophylaxis of mania. Br J Psychiatry 153:198–204, 1988

Maj M, Priozzi R, Kemali D: Long-term outcome of lithium prophylaxis in patients initially classified as complete responders. Psychopharmacology 98:535–538, 1989

McElroy SL, Keck PE, Pope HG, et al: Correlates of antimanic response to valproate. Psychopharmacol Bull 27:127–133, 1991

Pope HG, Jr, McElroy SL, Keck PE, Jr, et al: Valproate in the treatment of acute mania: a placebo-controlled study. Arch Gen Psychiatry 48:62–68, 1991

Post RM, Uhde TW, Roy-Byrne PP, et al: Correlates of antimanic response to carbamazepine. Psychiatry Res 21:71–83, 1987

Post RM, Roy-Byrne PP, Uhde TW: Graphic representation of the life course of illness in patients with affective disorder. Am J Psychiatry 145:844–848, 1988

Post RM, Rubinow DR, Uhde TW, et al: Dysphoric mania: Clinical and biological correlates. Arch Gen Psychiatry 46:353–358, 1989

Post RM, Leverich GS, Rosoff AS, et al: Carbamazepine prophylaxis in refractory affective disorders: a focus on long-term follow-up. J Clin Psychopharmacol 10:318–327, 1990

Post RM, Leverich GS, Altsuler L, et al: Lithium-discontinuation-induced refractoriness: preliminary observations. Am J Psychiatry 149:1727–1729, 1992

Prien RF, Kupfer DJ, Mansky PA, et al: Drug therapy in the prevention of recurrences in unipolar and bipolar affective disorders: report of the NIMH Collaborative Study Group comparing lithium carbonate, imipramine, and a lithium carbonate-imipramine combination. Arch Gen Psychiatry 41:1096–1104, 1984

Prien RF, Himmelhoch JM, Kupfer DJ: Treatment of mixed mania. J Affect Disord 15:9–15, 1988

Quitkin FM, Kane J, Rifkin A, et al: Prophylactic lithium carbonate with and without imipramine for bipolar I patients: a double-blind study. Arch Gen Psychiatry 38:902–907, 1981

Reiger DA, Boyd JH, Burke JD, Jr, et al: One-month prevalence of mental disorders in the United States: based on five Epidemiological Catchment Area sites. Arch Gen Psychiatry 45:977–986, 1988

Secunda S, Katz MM, Swann A, et al: Mania: diagnosis, state measurement and prediction of treatment response. J Affect Disord 8:113–121, 1985

Shopsin B: Bupropion's prophylactic efficacy in bipolar affective illness. J Clin Psychiatry 44:163–169, 1983

Shulman KI, Mackenzie S, Hardy B: The clinical use of lithium carbonate in old age: a review. Prog Neuropsychopharmacol Biol Psychiatry 11:159–164, 1987

Small JG, Klapper MH, Milstein V, et al: Carbamazepine compared with lithium in the treatment of mania. Arch Gen Psychiatry 48:915–921, 1991

Suppes T, McElroy SL, Gilbert J, et al: Clozapine in the treatment of dysphoric mania. Biol Psychiatry 32:270–280, 1992

Swann AC, Secunda SK, Katz MM, et al: Lithium treatment of mania: clinical characteristics, specificity of symptom change, and outcome. Psychiatry Res 18:127–141, 1986

Vestergaard P, Aagaard J: Five-year mortality in lithium-treated manic-depressive patients. J Affect Disord 21:33–38, 1991

Wehr TA, Goodwin FK: Can antidepressants cause mania and worsen the course of affective illness? Am J Psychiatry 144:1403–1411, 1987

Worrall EP, Moody JP, Peet M, et al: Controlled studies of the acute antidepressant effects of lithium. Br J Psychiatry 135:255–262, 1979

30

Treatment of Schizophrenia

Peter F. Buckley, M.D., and Herbert Y. Meltzer, M.D.

■ ASSESSMENT FOR TREATMENT

The contemporary concept of schizophrenia represents a distillation of multiple clinical perspectives. These include the Kraepelinian concept of chronicity of illness and progressive deterioration with prominence of "positive" symptoms (i.e., delusions, hallucinations, disordered thought processes, disorganized behavior); the Bleulerian perspective highlighting the "splitting" or disorganization of thought processes and affective loss; and the Schneiderian concept, which emphasizes distinct phenomenological features (i.e., "first-rank symptoms"). All three concepts, plus empirical observations, have contributed to a standard set of diagnostic criteria for schizophrenia. A summary of DSM-IV (American Psychiatric Association 1994) criteria for schizophrenia is given in Table 30–1.

Because psychotic symptoms are common features of a wide range of functional and organic brain disorders, the diagnosis of schizophrenia rests upon the recognition of a characteristic constellation of symptoms and signs—most critically, the evaluation for and positive exclusion of other disorders. It is therefore essential to do a careful history (including collateral history), a thorough physical examination, and laboratory tests to rule out physical illness or drug-induced psychosis. In practice, however, the most common sources of diagnostic confusion are other functional disorders, including acute mania or psychotic depression, delusional disorders, or schizotypal personality disorder, as well as psychomimetic drug abuse (e.g., phencyclidine, lysergic acid diethylamide [LSD], marijuana, and cocaine).

In recent years, different symptom complexes have received attention in an effort to clarify the concept of schizophrenia and treatment responsivity. Crow (1980) proposed a Type I–Type II model of schizophrenia. The Type I syndrome was characterized by more florid positive symptomatology and good response to neuroleptic treatment; the Type II syndrome, thought to reflect an underlying structural brain abnormality, had predominantly negative symptomatology and was relatively refractory to conventional neuroleptic treatment. Although this positive-negative distinction among symptoms was intuitively appealing, it has proved to be an oversimplification that does not conform to clinical realities. The major problems with this model have been discussed in detail elsewhere (Meltzer 1985). Most patients have both positive and negative symptoms.

The research reported was supported in part by USPHS MH 41684, and grants from the Elisabeth Severance Prentiss, John Pascal Sawyer, and Laureate Foundations. Dr. Meltzer is the recipient of a USPHS Research Career Scientist Award MH 47808. The authors thank Diane Mack for her secretarial assistance.

Table 30–1.   Summary of diagnostic criteria for schizophrenia from *Diagnostic and Statistical Manual of Mental Disorders, 4th Edition* (DSM-IV)

A. One month's or longer duration of at least two:
  1. Delusions
  2. Hallucinations
  3. Disorganized speech (e.g., frequent derailment or intolerance)
  4. Grossly disorganized or catatonic behavior
  5. Negative symptoms (e.g., affective flattening, alogia, avolition)

B. Deterioration in psychosocial function or failure to attain expected function.

C. Duration: continuous signs of illness for ≥ 6 months; period must include at least 1 month of symptoms that meet criterion A (i.e., active phase symptoms), and may include periods of prodromal or residual symptoms. During prodromal or residual periods, illness may manifest by only negative symptoms or ≥ two symptoms listed in criterion A present in attenuated form (e.g., odd beliefs, unusual perceptual experiences).

D. Schizoaffective and Mood Disorder Exclusion: Schizoaffective Disorder and Mood Disorder with Psychotic features have been ruled out since 1) no major depressive or manic episodes occurred concurrently with active phase symptoms; or 2) if mood episodes occurred during active phase symptoms, their total duration was brief relative to the duration of active and residual periods.

E. Substance/General Medical Condition Exclusion: not due to the direct effects of a substance (e.g., drugs of abuse, medication) or a general medical condition.

Subtypes
  1. Paranoid—prominence of persecutory or grandiose delusions or hallucinations
  2. Catatonic—symptoms of stupor, rigidity, negativism, excitement or posturing
  3. Disorganized—absence of systematized delusions; marked incoherence; inappropriate or silly affect
  4. Undifferentiated—prominent delusions and hallucinations accompanied by incoherence and grossly disorganized behavior
  5. Residual—mainly emphasize negative symptoms of schizophrenia; absence of florid psychosis

Source. Adapted from American Psychiatric Association 1994.

There is no robust relationship between symptoms and enlarged ventricles. In general, anhedonia, apathy, blunted affect, and poverty of speech are considered to be negative symptoms, whereas delusions and hallucinations clearly represent positive symptoms of the illness. Inappropriate affect, bizarre behavior, or some aspects of thought disorder are best considered positive symptoms but have also been construed less often as negative symptoms (Andreasen et al. 1990; McGlashan and Fenton 1992).

More recent studies have attempted to clarify and further refine the positive/negative symptom distinction (Andreasen et al. 1990; Liddle 1987; Thompson and Meltzer 1993). They suggest that three symptom complexes may be identified: 1) positive symptoms (reality distortion); 2) negative symptoms (psychomotor poverty syndrome); and 3) symptoms of disorganization (disorganization syndrome). The proposition that distinct neuroanatomical networks might underlie each symptom complex is supported by research on cerebral blood flow. The reality distortion syndrome was associated with hyperperfusion in the left parahippocampal region, whereas negative symptoms were related to a relative hypoperfusion in the left dorsolateral prefrontal cortex. In contrast, the disorganization symptom complex was associated with hypoperfusion in the right ventral prefrontal cortex. This heuristic work has yet to be replicated.

Other efforts to determine the nature of negative symptoms in schizophrenia represent a further, and complementary, line of inquiry. Because negative symptoms of schizophrenia may be difficult to distinguish from either depression or extrapyramidal side effects (EPS) of antipsychotic medication (Barnes et al. 1989; Carpenter 1987, 1994), the concept of "primary" (i.e., enduring) and "secondary" (i.e., mood-, medication-, or social disability–related) negative symptoms has gained credence (Table 30–2).

Carpenter (1987, 1994) has suggested that primary negative symptoms represent a distinct "deficit" subtype of schizophrenia that, although less amenable to antipsychotic medication, may nevertheless hold important implications for the targeting of specific symptoms for pharmacological and psychosocial treatments.

The interrelationships between symptoms over time and their relative responsivity to neuroleptic treatment are less clear. Many classifications have been based on cross-sectional assessments and have failed to account for the potential variability in each symptom complex over time (Breier et al. 1991; Fenton and McGlashan 1991; Kay and Singh 1989). This has important implications for the predictive value of positive and negative symptoms. In the Chestnut Lodge Longitudinal Study of 187 schizophrenic patients, negative symptoms were less com-

Table 30–2. Primary negative symptoms and the diagnostic criteria for the deficit syndrome of schizophrenia

1. At least two of the following six negative symptoms must be present:
   a) Restricted affect
   b) Diminished emotional range
   c) Poverty of speech
   d) Curbing of interests
   e) Diminished sense of purpose
   f) Diminished social drive

2. Some combination of two or more of the negative symptoms listed above have been present for the preceding 12 months and always were present during periods of clinical stability (including chronic psychotic states). These symptoms may or may not be detectable during transient episodes of acute psychotic disorganization or decompensation.

3. The negative symptoms above are primary (i.e., not secondary to factors other than the disease process). Such factors include:
   a) Anxiety
   b) Drug effect
   c) Suspiciousness (and other psychotic symptoms)
   d) Mental retardation
   e) Depression

4. The patient meets DSM-III-R criteria for schizophrenia.

Source. Kirkpatrick et al. 1989.

mon than positive symptoms initially and fluctuated early in the illness (Fenton and McGlashan 1991). However, over time these symptoms became more stable and were ultimately more reliable predictors of outcome. Those patients with negative symptoms tended to have a more insidious onset of illness with poorer outcome. This was particularly true of patients who showed a rapid increase in negative symptomatology early in the course of their illness. The National Institute of Mental Health (NIMH) follow-up study conducted by Breier and colleagues (1991) yielded similar findings. Conversely, positive symptoms are generally thought to predict good outcome (Bartko et al. 1990).

The relative ineffectiveness of conventional neuroleptics on relieving negative symptoms, as shown in some of the earlier treatment studies, represented a core aspect of Crow's Type I–Type II dichotomy (for extensive review, see Meltzer et al. 1986). However, many studies did show some modest improvement in negative symptoms. These were largely in

studies of chronic patients with acute exacerbations, so that in some instances improvement in negative symptoms may have been a consequence of improvement in positive symptoms (Meltzer et al. 1986; Opler et al. 1994). Negative symptoms have been shown to respond to treatment with conventional antipsychotics (for review, see Meltzer et al. 1986). Current evidence suggests that negative symptoms are more remediable with clozapine treatment than with conventional antipsychotics (Breier et al. 1994; Kane et al. 1988). In the multicenter study, neuroleptic-refractory patients treated with clozapine showed significant improvement on the anergia subscale of the Brief Psychiatric Rating Scale (BPRS) (Overall and Gorham 1962) compared with patients receiving chlorpromazine (Kane et al. 1988). In an outpatient study involving less severely ill patients, a comparable response in negative symptoms was seen in the clozapine-treated group, whereas negative symptoms worsened in the haloperidol-treated group (Breier et al. 1994). The relative impact on typical and atypical antipsychotics on negative symptoms is an issue of considerable current interest, particularly with the development of newer antipsychotics. However, this is a complex and controversial issue that calls for further research.

Greater attention has also been paid to the detection and significance of depressive symptoms in schizophrenia and their pharmacological management (Siris 1991). Approximately half of schizophrenia patients will experience a significant depressive episode during the course of their illness (most commonly following a relapse—so-called postpsychotic depression). Detection of depressive illness in schizophrenia is important, because depression is a notable risk factor for suicide; approximately 7%–10% of schizophrenia patients ultimately commit suicide (Roy 1982). However, the use of adjunctive antidepressant medication is not routinely advocated but should be instituted when a patient's depressed mood is severe, persistent, or associated with suicidal thoughts (Siris 1991). A more recent study of depression in schizophrenia indicated that not only was depressive symptomatology ameliorated with adjunctive antidepressant medication, but the duration of acute psychotic relapse was also shortened (Siris et al. 1994).

Finally, the relevance of substance abuse in the presentation and treatment outcome of schizophrenia has received much attention recently (Buckley et al.

1994; Mueser et al. 1990). Although estimates vary widely (more frequently with false negatives), conservative estimates suggest that 25%–50% of schizophrenic patients abuse alcohol or illicit drugs at some stage during their illness (Buckley et al. 1994). With the development of dual diagnosis treatment programs, the evaluation and effective management of such patients has become a critical concern. Moreover, substance abuse is closely associated with and often sustains medication noncompliance (Mueser et al. 1990; Weiden et al. 1991). Thus, the extent and pattern of substance abuse (if any) should constitute an important aspect of the evaluation process, with regard to both the clarification of diagnosis and to the development of an individualized treatment plan.

Although the assessment and ultimate diagnosis of schizophrenia remains a clinical concern, a number of widely used scheduled interviews and research rating scales are available to augment and objectify this evaluation. The requirements for strict objective determination of symptomatology may vary according to the treatment setting. Nevertheless, some of these scales are readily adopted into routine clinical evaluation and may provide valuable information that could help the selection of appropriate pharmacological treatments and the subsequent measurement of their efficacy. The BPRS is perhaps the most commonly used rating scale in clinical and research assessment of psychotic disorders. It measures a broad range of symptoms, including delusions, hallucinations, conceptual disorganization, affect, depressed mood, and psychic anxiety. Indeed, the widespread popularity of the BPRS may stem from the fact that it samples aspects of clinical judgment routinely evaluated by the physician. It is not a detailed scale of behavioral measurement. A 20% decrease in total BPRS score is used in some studies as a clinically significant measure of treatment response in cases of treatment-refractory schizophrenia (Kane et al. 1988; also see later section on "Assessment of Response"), but this is too limited an objective for first-break schizophrenia patients (Lieberman et al. 1993). Details on other commonly used scales for the assessment of schizophrenia are given in Tables 30–3 and 30–4.

These rating scales are of particular utility when assessing patients who have had a number of relapses of schizophrenia and who require further pharmacological management. In these cases, a thorough evaluation of the patients' disability should en-

Table 30–3. Instruments used in the evaluation of schizophrenia

Diagnostic/structured interview schedules	Comments
Schedule for Affective Disorders and Schizophrenia (SADS; Endicott and Spitzer 1978)	Formal interview taking 1½–2 hours; versions include SADS-L (Lifetime) and SADS-C (Change); covers a broad range of symptoms
Diagnostic Interview Schedule (DIS; Robbins et al. 1979)	Developed for epidemiological use; less detailed than other schedules for schizophrenia
Structured Clinical Interview for DSM-III (SCID; Spitzer et al. 1985)	Designed to show DSM-III diagnoses; SCID-P (psychosis) version for schizophrenia research
Comprehensive Assessment of Symptoms and History (CASH; Andreasen et al. 1992)	Designed to evaluate major psychoses; covers positive and negative symptoms, past history, premorbid function, and cognitive functioning

compass psychosocial, vocational, and side effects of treatment and other measures (in addition to psychopathological ones) in an attempt to achieve a multidimensional perspective of treatment responsivity (Meltzer 1992a). Moreover, a detailed history of all previous neuroleptic treatments (e.g., dosages, duration, side effects) is essential in planning future pharmacological treatment strategies. These concepts are elaborated on in the section "Assessment of Response."

■ SELECTION OF TREATMENT

Neuroleptic drugs are traditionally the first-line treatment of schizophrenia and have been used unless patients develop intolerable side effects (e.g., severe parkinsonism or tardive dyskinesia [TD]) or demonstrate minimal response. As we will discuss, risperidone might be considered as a first-line drug. There are numerous classes of antipsychotic drugs and, within each class, usually more than one agent. Agents available in the United States and information on their dose ranges, haloperidol equivalences, and galenic forms are given in Table 30–5.

The conventional antipsychotic drugs are believed to act through a similar mechanism of action—

Table 30–4. Instruments used in the evaluation of schizophrenia

Rating scales	Comments
Brief Psychiatric Rating Scale (BPRS; Overall and Gorham 1962)	18-item version covers broad range of symptoms; most commonly used scale in psychopharmacological research in schizophrenia
Scale for Assessment of Positive Symptoms (SAPS; Andreasen 1984)	Provides detailed ratings for types of hallucinations, delusions, bizarre behavior, and formal thought disorder
Scale for Assessment of Negative Symptoms (SANS; Andreasen 1983)	Evaluates alogia, affective blunting, avolition (i.e., apathy, anhedonia), asociality, attentional impairment
Positive and Negative Syndrome Scale (PANSS; Kay et al. 1987)	Comprehensive scale covering positive, negative, and general psychopathology items
Deficit Syndrome Scale (Kirkpatrick et al. 1989)	Differentiates negative symptoms of schizophrenia from secondary causes (e.g., depression, drug-related)
Quality of Life Scale (QLS; Heinrichs et al. 1984)	21-item scale detailing psychosocial functioning in interpersonal relationships, motivation and future expectations, and activities of daily living
Global Assessment Scale (GAS; Endicott et al. 1976)	Records highest level of functioning (i.e., symptoms, vocational, psychosocial) during last year and current episode of illness

that is, decreasing dopaminergic activity by initial blockade of D_2-type dopamine (DA) receptors and subsequent development (over days to weeks) of blockade of the firing of ventral tegmental area (VTA) and nigrostriatal DA neurons, or so-called depolarization inactivation (Bunney et al. 1987). The inactivation of the VTA neurons may be the basis for the antipsychotic action, whereas the effect on the striatum contributes to EPS and also possibly to the development of TD. This hypothesis is undoubtedly an oversimplification. These drugs also have variable affinities for binding to other neurotransmitter receptors, including serotonergic, histaminergic, adrenergic, muscarinic, γ-aminobutyric acid (GABA)ergic,

and glutamatergic receptors. It is likely that these effects account more for the side-effect profile than the clinical efficacy of individual neuroleptics. Because of the similarity in their fundamental mechanism of action, it is not surprising that these agents show little difference in efficacy in clinical practice (Baldessarini et al. 1988). The mechanism of action of the newer antipsychotics such as clozapine and risperidone may be through an antagonism of a combination of different subtypes of serotonin and DA receptors (Meltzer 1992b), although once again these agents have more widespread pharmacological effects (Meltzer and Nash 1991; Roth et al. 1994).

Up to 70%–90% of patients with schizophrenia and other psychotic disorders will have clinically significant amelioration of their psychosis when treated with an adequate dosage of these agents for a sufficient time. However, many of these patients remain impaired, especially with negative symptoms. In general, the lowest dosages of the dose ranges listed in Table 30–5 should be employed, especially for maintenance treatment. Higher doses definitely produce more severe EPS. It may be 4–6 weeks before an antipsychotic effect is achieved in some patients. There is no robust evidence that higher doses of neuroleptics speed the antipsychotic effect. Augmenting low-dose neuroleptic treatment with benzodiazepines for agitation and chloral hydrate for sleep may facilitate the management of acutely psychotic patients without the need to use high-dose neuroleptics. Maintenance doses of neuroleptics may be in the range of 5 mg haloperidol equivalent per day.

The choice of which drug to use is based on various considerations. In general, low-potency drugs (i.e., those in which the dosage range is up to or greater than 300 mg/day—chlorpromazine, mesoridazine, chlorprothixene, and thioridazine) are more sedative and more hypotensive than high-potency agents such as haloperidol and fluphenazine. These agents, in turn, produce more EPS than the low-potency agents. Thus, highly agitated and excited patients may be better candidates for agents such as parenteral chlorpromazine. If there is minimal need for sedation and no evidence from history of drug response to expect unusual sensitivity to EPS, high-potency agents such as haloperidol and fluphenazine are generally prescribed. However, if a patient develops an acute dystonic reaction or akathisia, he or she is likely to become noncompliant.

Table 30–5.   Available antipsychotic drugs, dosage, and dosage forms

	Dosage range[a]	Parenteral dosage	Galenic forms
Phenothiazines			
Acetophenazine maleate (Tindal)	40–120	—	Oral
Chlorpromazine hydrochloride (Thorazine)	200–800	25–50	Oral, liquid injection, suppository
Fluphenazine hydrochloride fluphenazine decanoate (Prolixin-D) fluphenazine enanthate (Prolixin-E)	2–60	1.25–2.5 12.5–50 q 1–4 weeks	Oral, liquid, injection
Mesoridazine besylate (Serentil)	75–300	25	Oral, liquid, injection
Perphenazine (Trilafon)	8–32	5–10	Oral, liquid, injection
Thioridazine hydrochloride (Mellaril)	150–800		Oral, liquid, injection
Trifluoperazine hydrochloride (Stelazine)	5–20	1–2	Oral, liquid, injection
Triflupromazine hydrochloride (Vesprin)		20–60	Injection
Butyrophenone			
Haloperidol decanoate (Haldol)	5–30 40–100 25–100 q 1–4 weeks	5–10 haloperidol-D	Oral, injection
Dibenzodiazepine			
Clozapine (Clozaril)	100–900	—	Oral
Dibenzoxapine			
Loxapine succinate (Loxitane)	40–100	25	Oral, liquid, injection
Indole			
Molindone hydrochloride (Moban)	50–225		Oral, injection
Diphenylbutylpiperidine			
Pimozide (Orap)	2–6		Oral
Thioxanthenes			
Chlorprothixene (Taractan)	50–400	25–50	Oral, liquid, injection
Thiothixene hydrochloride (Navane)	5–30	2–4	Oral, liquid, injection
Benzisoxazole			
Risperidone (Risperdal)	4–8		Oral

[a] The dosage ranges are representative of the effective doses that are generally used in clinical practice.

Switching from a high-potency agent to a medium-potency (e.g., trifluoperazine) or low-potency drug (thioridazine) may be helpful in some cases.

Risperidone is a benzisoxazole compound that was approved for use in the United States in 1994. It shares with clozapine (discussed later) potent serotonergic ($5-HT_{2A}$) receptor antagonism relative to weak dopamine (DA_2) receptor blockade. Like clozapine, risperidone also produces antagonism of α-adrenergic and histamine receptors. Unlike clozapine, it stimulates prolactin secretion (even at lower doses) and may cause galactorrhea in females. Risperidone also has an active metabolite, 9-hydroxyrisperidone, which has a much longer half-life than risperidone ($T\frac{1}{2} = 22$ hours versus

3.6 hours, respectively). For most white patients, the active metabolic moiety is mainly the 9-hydroxy compound.

In multinational and United States multicenter trials of typical schizophrenic patients, risperidone, at doses of 4–8 mg/day, has been reported to have greater efficacy and to produce fewer EPS than haloperidol (Borison et al. 1992; Chouinard et al. 1993).

The United States multicenter trial involved 20 centers in the United States and 6 in Canada. The Canadian data are already published in full (Chouinard et al. 1993) and, overall, they mirror the findings of the larger study. In this latter study, 523 patients were randomized to receive haloperidol (20 mg/day), risperidone (2, 6, 10, or 16 mg/day), or placebo for the duration of an 8-week double-blind trial (Chouinard et al. 1993; Marder and Meibach 1994). Efficacy measures included the Positive and Negative Syndrome Scale (PANSS) (Kay et al. 1987) and the Clinical Global Impression Scale (CGI) (Guy 1976). The risperidone group showed significant improvement relative to the placebo group in PANSS total score by the end of the first week of treatment, whereas total PANSS scores for the haloperidol group were significantly better than for the placebo group in the fourth week. Risperidone in daily doses of 6 mg and 16 mg was more effective than either haloperidol or placebo, with 6 mg risperidone proving superior to placebo and haloperidol for both the positive *and* negative subscales of the PANSS.

In this and other studies, the moderate dosage (6 mg/day) proved to be the optimum trade-off between clinical efficacy and the emergence of EPS and other side effects (Chouinard et al. 1993; Marder and Meibach 1994). Risperidone can suppress the symptoms of TD, but it is not known if it is superior to typical neuroleptics in this regard (Chouinard et al. 1993). Whether it produces a lower incidence of TD is unknown. Although lower ratings for TD during treatment with risperidone has been observed in the multicenter trials, the brief duration of these studies does not support a claim for an antidyskinetic effect with risperidone. Larger, prospective long-term trials will be needed to adequately address this important issue.

At higher doses, risperidone's advantages over haloperidol are less evident, possibly because of excessive DA receptor blockade. Like clozapine, risperidone is associated with seizures and sedation. Side effects include sedation, akathisia, hypotension, weight gain, and difficulty with concentration (Borison et al. 1992); tolerability of risperidone is, however, quite good.

Risperidone is indicated for patients who have a history of developing EPS on current agents, even thioridazine, the typical antipsychotic that causes the least EPS. No long-acting or parenteral form is currently available. It is not yet known if risperidone will be as effective as clozapine in the treatment of neuroleptic-refractory schizophrenia. Thus far, no direct comparison between risperidone and clozapine in treatment-refractory schizophrenia has been reported. In the absence of such data, switching patients' medication from clozapine to risperidone should be done with caution.

Remoxipride

Remoxipride is a substituted benzamide that has been reported to produce fewer EPS than comparable doses of haloperidol. It is a selective D_2 DA receptor antagonist similar to sulpiride, an agent that has been used extensively in Europe since the 1960s. In multicenter trials, remoxipride failed to demonstrate superior clinical efficacy over standard neuroleptics (Lewander et al. 1992). However, it does possess a more favorable side-effect profile, with lesser propensity to produce EPS or sedation. It should therefore be useful in treating patients for whom compliance because of EPS and sedation with low-potency drugs such as thioridazine is a problem. However, it has recently been reported to be associated with aplastic anemia in about 1 in 10,000 treated patients. For this reason, remoxipride has been withdrawn from general use throughout the world. In the absence of new data on its risk of causing aplastic anemia, it is unlikely to be approved for use in the United States.

Electroconvulsive Therapy

The other major form of somatic treatment for schizophrenia is electroconvulsive therapy (ECT) (Hertman 1992). The advent of neuroleptics has led to the infrequent use of ECT today. However, a short course of ECT (e.g., 6–12 treatments) may sometimes be useful as an adjunctive treatment to neuroleptic drugs for patients with limited response to neuroleptic treatment (Sajatovic and Meltzer 1993). Excited catatonia and severe agitation should ordinarily be treated with antipsychotics, benzodiazepines or mood stabilizers, seclusion, and physical restraint; but if these fail, ECT might prove effective.

In practice, the rapid response to ECT that occurs in patients with severe catatonia may avert secondary complications of dehydration and the like. For this reason, catatonia remains an important clinical indication for the use of ECT in schizophrenia (Dodwell and Goldberg 1989). There is no systematic evidence that maintenance ECT can prevent relapse in schizophrenia even when it is effective in the acute stage.

Psychosocial Treatments

Although neuroleptics are the mainstay of treatment, there is also a range of important nonpharmacological treatments for schizophrenia (Bellack and Mueser

1993; Keith et al. 1991). These are aimed at supporting the patient, fostering independent living skills, and improving psychosocial functioning. They also contribute to better compliance with medication. The involvement of key relatives or other significant figures in the patient's life is a key component of psychosocial treatments (Bellack and Mueser 1993). Important aspects of such treatments include individual supportive psychotherapy, group supportive psychotherapy, group educative psychotherapy, family supportive psychotherapy, family educative psychotherapy, social skills training, cognitive rehabilitation, vocational training, and crisis management.

The concept of expressed emotion (EE) is particularly relevant to these approaches. This concept measures the negative or intrusive attitudes that relatives express about the patient and several outcome studies have indicated the predictive value EE in relapse of schizophrenia (for review, see Kavanagh 1992). However, alternative plausible perspectives of EE argue that high expressed emotion (HEE) within the family may be a direct consequence of the patient's refractory illness. In this view, the modern concept of EE is merely a reinvention of earlier social theories that laid the blame for schizophrenia firmly on the relatives (Lefley 1992). Summarizing the results of 34 studies of EE and relapse, Kavanagh (1992) has estimated that over the first 9–12 months of follow-up, a relapse rate of 21% is observed for patients from low-EE families, as opposed to a relapse rate of 48% among those from high-EE families. Within the second year, these relapse rates rise to 27% and 66% for low-EE and high-EE groups, respectively (Kavanagh 1992).

Consistent with this EE hypothesis, skills-oriented or educative family interventions (aimed at reducing EE) have been shown in some but by no means all studies to significantly improve the course of schizophrenia when compared with routine or individual treatments (Hogarty et al. 1986, 1988, 1991; Kavanagh 1992; Keith et al. 1991; Lam 1991). Summarizing the results of 11 treatment studies that preselected for HEE, Kavanagh (1992) reported that relapse rates over the first 9 months ran at 10% for family intervention groups, compared with 48% for routine or individual treatment. Over a 2-year period, relapse rates of 33% and 71% are observed for each group, perhaps suggesting a clear benefit from a more intensive aftercare educational program involving the patient's relatives. However, the more recent studies of Hogarty and colleagues (1986, 1988, 1991) and the NIMH Treatment Strategies in Schizophrenia (TSS) (Keith et al. 1991; Schooler et al. 1993) exemplify the methodological difficulties with this research and its relatively poor treatment outcome when strictly compared with medication treatment. In the Hogarty team's series of studies (Hogarty et al. 1986, 1988, 1991), social skills training—either alone or in combination with medication treatment—was compared with family psychoeducation and with routine outpatient pharmacotherapy. By the end of the 2-year evaluation period, there was no difference in relapse rates or hospitalization between any of these groups, specifically with no additional advantage shown in the combined skills therapy–pharmacotherapy group.

Similar results are now also beginning to emerge from the TSS (Schooler et al. 1993). These studies temper the initial enthusiasm for psychosocial and family intervention strategies. They suggest that any effect derived from treatment is likely to be mediated through support for the patient or through improved coping with the illness, rather than by ameliorating some core characteristic or pathophysiological attribute of schizophrenia. Indeed, the lack of association of HEE with other clinical and psychophysiological variables (e.g., arousal, attention) suggests that such psychosocial treatments do not have a fundamental positive effect on the disorder (Kavanagh 1992; Lefley 1992).

Moreover, this research has generally been conducted on well-motivated and treatment-compliant families; accordingly, it is probably not generalizable. Even within such samples, there are high nonattendance rates over time, which further limit the applicability of the findings (Hogarty et al. 1991). These difficulties most likely reflect wider problems that this research has not addressed adequately—namely the adverse social factors (e.g., poor housing, education) that mitigate against treatment for families and patients (Bachrach 1992). These wider social issues in the rehabilitation of chronically mentally ill people clearly require close attention if patients are to be expected to comply with treatment regimens (Bachrach 1992; Munich and Lang 1993). Moreover, adverse social factors are intrinsically related to substance abuse comorbidity and medication noncompliance. A multifaceted approach (currently undefined) is therefore needed to minimize the negative influences of these factors on course of illness.

■ INITIATION OF TREATMENT

In general, neuroleptics are best commenced at a low dosage (5–10 mg/day haloperidol equivalent) and gradually titrated upward according to the clinical requirements. The patient (and his or her family, if possible) should first be given an explanation of the need and rationale of treatment and of potential side effects, particularly the early risk of an acute dystonic reaction. Because such reactions are distressing and are directly related to the dose and rate of incremental increase in neuroleptic dosage (Casey 1991), this is another reason for initiating treatment conservatively. Formerly, high doses of neuroleptics were given parenterally over the first few days of treatment—so-called rapid neuroleptization—in the erroneous belief that this would be more effective and also shorten the duration of the acute psychosis (Baldessarini et al. 1988). This practice is no longer advocated. The use of higher dosage (greater than 40 mg haloperidol equivalents) for the acute treatment of schizophrenia is also no more efficacious than prescribing neuroleptics at a more moderate dose (15–20 mg haloperidol equivalents) (Kane and Marder 1993; Rifkin et al. 1990). It is also noteworthy that, for the patient who has relapsed because of noncompliance, simply reinstating medication at the previous dosage may be effective. Indeed, compliance may continue to be a problem even in the hospital, in which case medication can be given in liquid form. Alternatively, it may be advisable to begin the patient directly on depot neuroleptic treatment (Glazer and Kane 1992).

Perhaps the most important aspect of the acute treatment of schizophrenia is to allow an adequate trial of any given agent. The initial sedative and anxiolytic effects of antipsychotic drugs occur shortly after treatment begins, but the actual antipsychotic response is often delayed, highly variable between patients, and may take at least 6 weeks to occur. Indeed, the median time to remission in a recent study was 11 weeks (Lieberman et al. 1993). Accordingly, premature discontinuation of a drug or substitution with an alternative class of neuroleptic is inadvisable and may result in subsequent confusion as to which treatment was actually effective.

For the same reasons, polypharmacy should generally be avoided. In particular, there is no justification for the concomitant use of a parenteral and an oral antipsychotic drug unless the patient's treatment is being converted to the regular use of intramuscular neuroleptic. In some instances, particularly when agitation is a prominent feature, the adjunctive use of benzodiazepines may be helpful (Wolkowitz and Pickar 1991). It should also be recognized that these agents may augment the response to the neuroleptic (see section on "Neuroleptic Resistance"). However, benzodiazapines should be used judiciously in the management of symptoms in acutely psychotic patients, as they may cause disinhibition and contribute to the emergence of aggressive behavior in these patients (Corrigan et al. 1993).

■ ASSESSMENT OF RESPONSE

There are two important facts to bear in mind when assessing response to neuroleptic treatment. First, for those who have been on neuroleptics and have shown a particular time-course or pattern of treatment response, a similar response will likely be seen in any later episode (Kolakowska et al. 1985). Although this may be a useful clinical rule of thumb, it is certainly not invariable. Both earlier and more recent research has indicated that some patients appear to show a progressively poorer response to neuroleptics with each successive relapse (Loebel et al. 1993). Second, the time-course of response to treatment shows wide interindividual variation. In a study of 70 first-episode schizophrenic patients (Lieberman et al. 1993), the mean and median times to remission were 36 weeks and 11 weeks, respectively. By the end of the first year of treatment, 83% of this sample had shown a response to treatment.

The criterion of adequacy of response is critical to any assessment of treatment efficacy. If the threshold is set high, such as a return to the highest level of premorbid functioning (perhaps an appropriate, albeit unrealistic, expectation in most cases) (Meltzer 1990, 1992c), then neuroleptic treatment failure is correspondingly manifest. If the criterion is solely that of symptomatic relief (i.e., resolution of positive symptoms), then the equally debilitating effects of negative symptomatology and secondary handicaps of the illness may not be taken sufficiently into account. At best, the assessment of treatment response should be judged along a multidimensional continuum (Meltzer 1992a) that emphasizes many potentially independent facets of the illness (Table 30–6).

Table 30–6. Important measures of outcome in the treatment of schizophrenia

Psychopathology	Quality of life
Cognitive function	Family burden
Extrapyramidal symptoms	Cost of illness
Social function	Compliance
Independent living	

This broadening of the concept of treatment response imposes the need to have a prior comprehensive baseline evaluation of functioning and also to measure response in multiple areas, not just psychopathology.

Some of the scales alluded to earlier (Tables 30–3 and 30–4) are of importance in objectifying treatment response. The BPRS is particularly relevant because it is reliable, easy to use, and sensitive to changes in symptoms (Overall and Gorham 1988). In recent years, the criterion of a 20% decrease in BPRS total score has become a widely accepted index of treatment response (Kane et al. 1988). Although this may serve as a useful measure of response, it is important to note that some patients who may attain such a criterion (e.g., from a baseline BPRS of 68 to 43) will still exhibit substantial impairment. Other measures also become important. For instance, the Quality of Life Scale (Heinrichs et al. 1984) provides an evaluation of other equally pertinent aspects of function that need to be considered in assessing treatment response. These measures include the extent of interpersonal involvement, the capacity for independent living, and the motivation and direction toward vocational activity. Improvement on any of these measures may be clinically significant and, significantly, may occur independently of other measures, including psychopathology (Goldberg et al. 1987; Meltzer 1992a).

■ CONTINUATION, MAINTENANCE, AND MONITORING

More than 30 years of research and clinical experience attest to the efficacy of maintenance neuroleptic treatment in reducing relapses in patients with schizophrenia. However, this benefit must be weighed against the cumulative risk of TD and the distressing effects of continued EPS. These opposing concerns have shaped contemporary research and

clinical practice to determine the lowest effective dose for treatment. Recent fixed-dose studies indicate that continued neuroleptic treatment at a moderate dose range (e.g., 12.5–25 mg fluphenazine decanoate every 2 weeks) confers the most clinical benefit with an "acceptable" trade-off with EPS (Levinson et al. 1990; Rifkin et al. 1990; Van Putten et al. 1990). Levinson and colleagues (1990) reported no overall greater clinical improvement with higher doses of oral fluphenazine (i.e., 10, 20, or 30 mg/day) but an associated increase in EPS. However, among those patients who responded by an excess of 40% on symptomatic ratings, a strong correlation between increasing neuroleptic dosage and clinical response was observed.

In contrast, Rifkin and colleagues (1990) noted no difference in either clinical response or side-effect profile between 87 schizophrenic patients who were randomized to receive 10 mg, 30 mg, or 80 mg of haloperidol qd for 6 weeks. In a further fixed-dose study among 80 schizophrenic patients receiving either 5 mg, 10 mg, or 20 mg of haloperidol qd for 4 weeks (Van Putten et al. 1990), the significant symptomatic improvement observed in the patient group taking the highest dose was tempered by higher measures of withdrawal and akinesia, and also by the fact that 33% left the hospital against medical advice (versus 4% of patients in the low-dose group). Overall, these studies suggest that during short-term treatment, moderate dosage strategies appear most efficacious and have the optimum risk-benefit profile.

The wider interindividual variation in clinical response to neuroleptics, coupled with increased understanding of the pharmacokinetics of neuroleptic drugs, have prompted much research interest in the determination of neuroleptic plasma levels. It is believed that this will aid treatment dosage strategies and lead to individualized treatments (Van Putten et al. 1991). Unfortunately, this optimism has not been supported by research. Earlier studies (reviewed by Van Putten et al. 1991) had suggested the existence of a curvilinear relationship between plasma levels of some neuroleptics and therapeutic response—a "therapeutic window"—with both low and high plasma levels resulting in less successful treatment. Van Putten and colleagues (1991) have proposed that, based on their studies, the therapeutic window for haloperidol is 5–12 ng/ml. Currently, however, the clinical utility of plasma levels for standard neuroleptics remains largely confined to assessing medication compliance or helping to differentiate between neuroleptic toxicity and worsening of psychosis.

A number of studies have sought to define the most appropriate minimum dosage for effective maintenance treatment in schizophrenia (Hogarty et al. 1988; Kane et al. 1985; Marder et al. 1984, 1987). These studies have indicated that marked reductions in neuroleptic medication (i.e., up to 90% in Kane et al. 1985) may be achieved in stable schizophrenic patients who are carefully monitored. In a 1-year study of 125 schizophrenic patients receiving fluphenazine decanoate at dosages of 12.5–50 mg, 1.5–10 mg, or 1.25–5 mg every 2 weeks (Kane et al. 1985), the comparable relapse rates were 7%, 24%, and 56%, respectively. Patients who relapsed while on low-dose treatment were frequently restabilized with a temporary increase in dosage and generally did not require hospitalization. Studies by Marder and colleagues (1984, 1987) used different definitions of relapse and showed similar rates of relapse between a low dose group and a standard dose group at 1-year follow-up. However, by the second year, 69% of patients in the 5-mg fluphenazine decanoate group had had an exacerbation of symptoms, compared with 35% of patients in the 25-mg fluphenazine decanoate group. When a more stringent definition of "relapse" was applied, rates of 44% and 31%, respectively, were observed.

The results of the study by Hogarty and colleagues (1988) suggested a similar pattern, with patients who were receiving lower dosages also showing better social adjustment. In summary, these findings suggest that, for those patients who are clinically stable, there may be some benefit from lower neuroleptic dosage in maintenance treatment. Notably, however, this is also associated with a somewhat higher risk of relapse, albeit that such relapses are less severe and are frequently managed without recourse to hospitalization. Obviously, such strategies are not applicable to patients who have relapsed previously with dose reduction, or for those patients whose behavior (e.g., suicidal or violent) would preclude trying this approach.

The importance of ensuring compliance with treatment in schizophrenic patients cannot be overstated. Noncompliance rates are notoriously variable, which also partially reflects important methodological issues (Weiden et al. 1991), and rates as high as 50% have been recorded (Weiden et al. 1991). Factors associated with poor compliance include persistent psychotic symptoms (especially persecutory or grandiose delusions), poor insight and denial of illness, dissatisfaction with care providers, acute EPS, and poor social support. Efforts may be made to remediate many of these factors. However, the utility of long-acting depot neuroleptic preparations should not be overlooked. Many patients with previously poor compliance and recurrent psychosis do very well with this treatment regimen (Glazer and Kane 1992).

The use of community detention to achieve compulsory medication compliance represents a further, but more controversial, approach to the management of neuroleptic noncompliance (Fennell 1991; Wear and Brahms 1991). However, there are insufficient data to evaluate the long-term effectiveness of this strategy, which is obviously complicated by legal and ethical concerns.

■ MANAGEMENT OF SIDE EFFECTS

Side effects of treatment with conventional neuroleptics are common (Ayd 1961; Casey 1991; Chakos et al. 1992) and are the chief reason for poor treatment compliance (Van Putten 1974; Weiden et al. 1991). Common side effects are outlined in Tables 30–7 and 30–8.

■ Neuromuscular Side Effects

The main neuromuscular side effects include acute dyskinesia, parkinsonism, and akathisia (collectively termed EPS), TD, and neuroleptic malignant syndrome (NMS). Ayd (1961) reported on the incidence of side effects in more than 3,000 patients evaluated for up to 6 years and noted that 38% of patients showed EPS—2% had dystonia, 15% parkinsonism, and 21% had akathisia. In a prospective study of 70 first-episode schizophrenic patients (Chakos et al. 1992), 38% of patients showed no EPS, whereas 38% had one form of EPS, 21% two forms, and 3% all three forms of EPS. Parkinsonism was observed in 34% of patients, acute dystonia in 36%, and akathisia in 18%.

Table 30–7. Side effects of conventional neuroleptic drugs

Type	Characteristics	Prevalence	Risk factors	Management
Acute dystonia	Oculogyric crises, dysarthria, acute neck truncal spasms	2%–90%	Young males, high-potency neuroleptics	Dosage reduction, or change drug class; anticholinergic administration (benztropine 2 mg im/po)
Parkinsonism	Tremor; cog-wheel rigidity, bradykinesia	2%–90%	Dose-related	Dose reduction, anticholinergic administration
Akathisia	Subjective and objective motor restlessness	35%	Dose-related; low serum iron status?	Dose reduction or change drug class; benzodiazepines (diazepam 2 mg tid); β-blocker (propranolol 10–40 mg bid)
Tardive dyskinesia	Involuntary choreic or athetoid movements, orofacial and peripheral	5%–50%	Female gender, age, brain disease; concomitant anti-parkinsonian treatments? history of previous extrapyramidal side effects; affective symptoms	Reduce or stop neuroleptic; vitamin E 400–1,200 mg; benzodiazepines; β-blocker; GABAergic drug (Depakote 400–1,000 mg); clozapine
Seizures	Grand mal, myoclonic	0.1%	Dosage, epileptogenic tendency	Dosage reduction, concomitant anticonvulsant drug (Depakote 400–1,000 mg)
Neuroleptic malignant syndrome	Pyrexia, muscle rigidity, autonomic instability, clouding of consciousness, elevated creatine phosphokinase	0.1%–1%	High, rapid neuroleptic dosing; agitation	Rule out other medical conditions; stop neuroleptic; supportive measures; dopamine agonist (bromocriptine 15–30 mg); muscle relaxant (dantrolene 100–400 mg)

Table 30–8. Side effects of conventional neuroleptic drugs

Type	Characteristics	Prevalence	Management
Sedation	Tolerance develops over time	~ 70%	Lower dosage; change to nonsedating drug; add L-dopa or methylphenidate
Weight gain		15%–20%	Practical measures
Hypotension	Antiadrenergic effect	10%–30%	Dosage reduction; different class
Anticholinergic effects	Cognitive impairment, blurred vision, dry mouth, constipation, sexual dysfunction	~ 60%	Dosage reduction; different class
Hormonal	Elevated prolactin, reduced testosterone	Variable	Treatment of breast abscess if develops; add bromocriptine, dosage reduction, different class
Jaundice	Cholestatic	< 0.1%	Investigate for other causes; change drug
Marrow toxicity	Agranulocytosis	< 0.1%	Consult with hematologist; stop neuroleptic
Retinitis pigmentosa		Low	Avoid high doses of thioridazine

■ Acute Dystonic Reactions

Acute dystonic reactions typically occur within the first 4 days of neuroleptic treatment and are more common in young male patients who are receiving high-potency neuroleptics (Casey 1991). These reactions are characterized by sustained, involuntary muscular spasm, most often involving the facial, head, or neck muscles. Examples include spasm of masticatory muscles (trismus), obicularis oculi (blepharospasm), oculogyric crises (i.e., fixed upward gazing of the eyes), torticollis, dysarthria, and dysphagia. Such spasms are painful and very distressing and may go undetected or misinterpreted by staff. The exact pathophysiological mechanism underlying acute dystonia is unclear. It is thought to be the result of either an acute hypodopaminergic state in the basal ganglia due to neuroleptic blockade of DA receptors or, alternatively, a relative imbalance between neuroleptic-induced elevation in presynaptic DA turnover and postsynaptic receptor blockade.

Treatment of acute dystonia is swiftly effective with parenteral anticholinergics (e.g., benztropine 2 mg im) or antihistaminics (e.g., diphenhydramine 50 mg im). If this does not relieve the dystonia, then a further administration after about 40 minutes will be necessary. Anticholinergic drugs are generally administered for a week or more thereafter. If there is a recurrence, then the neuroleptic dosage should be reduced or changed to a lower-potency agent. When acute dystonic reactions occur, they must be recorded carefully in the clinical records so that anticholinergic drugs will be given prophylactically later and the offending neuroleptic drug avoided. Some advocate the widespread prophylactic use of anticholinergics to avoid the development of EPS. But the greater risk of anticholinergic toxicity and the apparent increased risk for TD associated with this strategy suggest that a more conservative, individualized use of concomitant anticholinergic therapy is more appropriate (Boodhood and Sandler 1991). This is, however, an area of controversy. In a series of papers, Lavin and Rifkin (1991a, 1991b) reviewed controlled studies on the prophylactic and long-term use of anticholinergics and concluded that the benefits outweighed the attendant risks. They advocated the regular use of anticholinergics because of the highly detrimental effects of acute EPS on subsequent medication compliance.

■ Parkinsonism

Parkinsonism is similar to idiopathic parkinson's disease, consisting of tremor, rigidity, and bradykinesia. It appears to be a direct (dose-related) consequence of DA receptor blockade in the nigrostriatal pathway (Casey 1991). These symptoms generally emerge after a few days of neuroleptic treatment and are more common in older patients. Up to 60% of patients may show one or more of the features of parkinsonism. Detection of parkinsonism is important, because it is readily treated with the addition of an anticholinergic drug. Amantadine and deprenyl are ineffective in the treatment of neuroleptic-induced parkinsonism (Casey 1993). Also, bradykinesia may be misinterpreted as either depressed mood or anergia. In extreme cases, parkinsonian rigidity may be mistaken for catatonia or NMS (Buckley et al. 1991).

■ Akathisia

Akathisia is a syndrome of subjective and objective motor restlessness associated with neuroleptic treatment. Patients experience anxiety, inner restlessness, an inability to stand still, and constant pacing (Adler et al. 1989). It may be very distressing for them and is a chief cause of neuroleptic noncompliance (Van Putten 1974; Weiden et al. 1991). Akathisia is often overlooked or misperceived as anxiety or worsening of psychosis. Its pathophysiology is the least understood of the acute EPS and does not appear to solely reflect nigrostriatal DA receptor blockade. Alterations in iron metabolism may be a predisposing factor for akathisia (Barnes et al. 1992). Anticholinergic drugs are not useful in its treatment, but the addition of a β-blocker (e.g., propranolol 20 mg bid) or a benzodiazepine (e.g., diazepam 2 mg tid) may be more effective (Adler et al. 1989). Neuroleptic dosage reduction or substitution of a lower-potency-antipsychotic drug are other alternatives for the management of akathisia. Prescribing thioridazine may also be useful.

■ Tardive Movement Disorder

Tardive dyskinesia and tardive dystonia are serious, potentially irreversible side effects of long-term neuroleptic treatment characterized by the late appearance of choreiform or athetoid movements of body regions, particularly the orofacial and truncal regions (Barnes 1990; Casey 1991; Waddington et al., in press). Although neuroleptic dosage and duration of treatment have been implicated as risk factors, their association with TD is inconsistent (Barnes et al. 1990). Advancing age, female gender, affective disorders, and evidence of organic brain impairment have been variously implicated as risk factors for TD (Waddington et al., in press), although it is impossible to clinically predict the later emergence of TD in individual patients. Diabetes is also established as a risk factor (Woerner et al. 1993). Acute EPS have also been associated specifically with vulnerability to TD (Barnes 1990).

Although no single theory adequately accounts for the manifestation of TD, the notion of supersensitivity of nigrostriatal DA receptors following chronic exposure to neuroleptics remains a heuristic view of the pathophysiology of TD (Casey 1991, 1993). However, this role is unlikely to be primary. Modulatory effects of other neurotransmitter systems such as the GABAergic or noradrenergic ones are also considered important and are partially supported by animal and clinical studies (Casey 1991; Gerlach and Casey 1988). Current management strategies for TD reflect these theories. First, the risk of TD may be minimized by using the lowest effective dose of neuroleptic for the shortest duration of time, clinical circumstances permitting. Discontinuation of neuroleptics alone results in a 50% improvement in TD by 3 months in more than one-third of patients, with further improvement over time (Glazer et al. 1990).

Both dopaminergic and DA-depleting agents have been tried in TD, but results are at very best inconsistent (Feltner and Hertzman 1993). GABAergic drugs (e.g., gamma-vinyl GABA), adrenergic drugs (e.g., pindolol, gamma-linoleic acid), calcium channel blockers (e.g., nifedipine, verapamil), and clonazepam have all been used with limited success in the treatment of TD (Feltner and Hertzman 1993). More recently, vitamin E has been advocated as an effective treatment on the basis of theories of oxidation and free radical processes in the development of TD (Adler et al. 1993; Feltner and Hertzman 1993). The efficacy of vitamin E (α-tocopherol) in the treatment of TD—a known antioxidant that might protect against damage to nerve cell membranes—remains controversial. Two earlier studies indicated therapeutic benefit for vitamin E in 4-week treatment periods of patients with moderate to severe TD (Elkashef et al. 1990; Lohr et al. 1987). Subsequent reports were less convincing, although a well-conducted treatment study over 8–12 weeks showed a prominent effect of vitamin E on TD (i.e., 32.5% improvement after vitamin E versus 3.0% worsening after placebo) (Adler et al. 1993). This effect was most pronounced in patients with a short duration (< 5 years) of TD.

Thus, though further studies are needed, the potential utility of vitamin E in TD is noteworthy, particularly as this agent is without side effects. Presently, clozapine is the best treatment option for moderate to severe, persistent TD (Lieberman et al. 1991; Meltzer and Luchins 1984). Clozapine has as yet not been directly implicated to induce TD and may even actively ameliorate it. In a prospective study of TD in 30 clozapine-treated schizophrenic patients, 16 patients showed a 50% or greater reduction in TD. This effect was most marked in patients with severe TD and dystonia (Lieberman et al. 1991).

■ Neuroleptic Malignant Syndrome

NMS is an uncommon (i.e., incidence < 0.9%) and potentially fatal complication of neuroleptic treatment. It is characterized by the development of fever, rigidity, autonomic instability, altered consciousness, and (of poor diagnostic specificity) elevated creatine kinase (CK) activity (Meltzer 1973) and raised white blood cell (WBC) count in the absence of any other medical condition that might explain these symptoms (Kellam 1990; Rosebush and Stuart 1989). Rapid increases in dosage of neuroleptic drugs, parenteral administration, agitation, and diagnosis of affective disorder are all risk factors for the development of NMS (Kellam 1990). NMS may develop after removal of antiparkinsonian agents. The pathophysiology of NMS is thought to involve acute dopaminergic blockade in the hypothalamus and/or basal ganglia. When NMS is suspected, the patient should have a thorough physical examination and organic and septic workup to rule out other causes. If no other causes are evident, then immediate cessation of neuroleptics (and lithium, if it is being administered) and provision of full supportive measures are recommended. DA agonists (e.g., bromocriptine 30 mg/day) and muscle relaxants (e.g., dantrolene 400 mg/day) should be given as adjunctive therapy.

There is reason to believe that more specific muscle relaxant analogues of dantrolene will soon be available for use in NMS (Shader and Greenblatt 1992). ECT may also be given to manage acute psychotic symptoms during NMS (Hermesh et al. 1987). The risk of recurrence on reexposure to neuroleptics—approximately 30% of patients have a recurrence of NMS—may be minimized by delaying rechallenge by 2 weeks post-NMS and by using a neuroleptic of an alternative class (Rosebush et al. 1989). Clozapine is not the specifically recommended agent of first choice in rechallenge (Buckley and Meltzer 1993). However, if NMS recurs in a patient on typical neuroleptic drugs, clozapine should be given.

■ Other Side Effects

Other adverse effects of standard antipsychotic medication are, in general, of lesser morbidity, but they may be distressing for patients and may limit the choice and ultimate dosage of neuroleptic.

Standard neuroleptic drugs lower the seizure threshold. A history of epilepsy or organic brain impairment is a risk factor for the development of seizures on neuroleptics. However, seizures are uncommon during treatment. Most patients experience some sedative effect while on neuroleptics. This is more commonly associated with low-potency agents that possess prominent antiadrenergic and antimuscarinic effects (e.g., mesoridazine). Tolerance usually develops, though if sedation persists, multiple daily regimens, neuroleptic dose reduction, or substitution are worthwhile management strategies.

Hypotension is a frequent cardiovascular side effect, attributable to α_1-antiadrenergic effects and more commonly seen with low-potency agents. Tachycardia may also be observed, as may nonspecific T wave changes on electrocardiogram (ECG), which result from atropine-like effects on the myocardium. Other common anticholinergic adverse effects include blurred vision, worsening of glaucoma in patients with narrow-angle glaucoma, dry mouth, reduced gastrointestinal motility, urinary hesitancy, and impotence. Anticholinergic toxicity, ranging from subtle memory impairment to delirium, may result from concomitant use of anticholinergic drugs; elderly patients are particularly prone to this problem. These adverse effects may be avoided by careful clinical observation and judicious management of neuroleptic dosage and any concomitant medications.

Hyperprolactinemia is the chief endocrine side effect of standard neuroleptics and is a direct consequence of blockade of pituitary DA receptors (Meltzer and Fang 1976). This accounts for amenorrhea in female patients and for galactorrhea, which may occasionally result in a breast abscess. These drugs may also reduce urinary concentrations of estrogen and progesterone.

Leukocytosis, eosinophilia, or leukopenia may occur with standard neuroleptic treatment. However, agranulocytosis occurs in only 1 in 2,000 patients receiving standard neuroleptics.

Neuroleptics uncommonly induce hepatitis with a cholestatic pattern, which is generally self-limiting and resolves with brief cessation of treatment. Dermatological reactions, hypersensitivity urticaria, photosensitivity, or slate-gray hyperpigmentation occur in less than 5% of patients receiving standard neuroleptics. These effects are managed conservatively with dermatological consultation, as necessary. Pigmentation retinopathy has been described in patients receiving doses of thioridazine above 1,000 mg/day. Low doses of thioridazine are therefore advocated in long-term maintenance therapy.

It is also important to recognize that adverse effects can also occur from interactions with other drugs (Goff and Baldesarrini 1993). These may result from alterations in the metabolism of neuroleptics (e.g., carbamazepine induces the hepatic microsomal system that metabolizes haloperidol, thereby leading to lowering of plasma levels), or additive toxic effects (e.g., combined anticholinergic effects with concomitant use of tricyclic antidepressant medications). Patients need to be alerted to these potential adverse effects. Commonly prescribed drugs that interact with antipsychotics are given in Table 30–9.

■ DISCONTINUATION

Realistic concerns regarding the long-term morbidity associated with maintenance neuroleptic treatment raise the issue of when and how to discontinue treatment. The acknowledged prognostic features indicating a favorable outcome in schizophrenia—female gender, late onset of illness, acute onset with clear precipitating factor, florid presentation, good premorbid adjustment—obviously need to be taken into account in determining an individual patient's suitability for discontinuation of neuroleptics. Unfortunately, other information as to which patients are more likely to relapse on discontinuation is scant. Apart from the use of biochemical predictors (i.e., response to methylphenidate challenge), it is not possible to readily predict subsequent relapse (Lieberman et al. 1987).

The targeted or intermittent maintenance strategy has been attempted to reduce relapse in stable patients who are selected to discontinue treatment. This strategy relies heavily on the patient's and family's ability to recognize prodromal symptoms of relapse: anxiety, irritability, sleep disturbance, perceptual aberrations, oddity of behavior, and paranoid ideas of reference. Also, intensive psychosocial and educative support is necessary. Unfortunately, the initial optimism engendered by earlier studies (Carpenter et al. 1987; Herz et al. 1982) has not been maintained after further study (Carpenter et al. 1990; Herz et al. 1991; Jolley et al. 1989, 1990). This indicated that not only do patients on targeted strategies fare significantly worse in terms of relapse, but these patients also show only modest reductions in overall side effects when compared with those who are continued on conventional maintenance treatment.

The 1- and 2-year outcome reports of Jolley and colleagues (1989, 1990) exemplify the problems associated with this intermittent treatment strategy. Fifty-four patients, randomized to receive either active intramuscular neuroleptic treatment or placebo, were followed intensively for 2 years. Both groups received brief courses of oral neuroleptics when prodromal symptoms or relapse occurred. At 1 year, the intermittent treatment group showed equal relapse and prodromal rates with better overall functioning. But by the end of the second year, only 50% of the patients receiving target treatment had survived the 2-year period without hospitalization, compared with a survival rate of more than 90% in the group that received continuous treatment. In addition, prolonged relapses and episodes of prodromal symptoms were more frequent in the intermittent treatment group. This group had lower rates of treatment side effects but did not show an overall advantage in psychosocial functioning from this strategy.

These results, and the similar findings of Herz and colleagues (1991), suggest that the decision to discontinue treatment must be individualized for

Table 30–9. Commonly observed drug interactions with antipsychotics

Effect	Agents
Raise conventional neuroleptic plasma levels	Anxiolytics, antidepressants
Raise clozapine plasma levels	Valproate
Lower conventional neuroleptic plasma levels	Carbamazepine, cimetidine, phenytoin, tobacco
Lower clozapine plasma levels	Tobacco
Sedation	Anxiolytics, anticonvulsants, alcohol, antidepressants, antihypertensives
Hypotension	Antihypertensives, antidepressants
Agranulocytosis	Carbamazepine with clozapine
Delirium, neurotoxicity	Anticholinergics, antidepressants, disulfiram, lithium

each patient whose illness has remained stabilized on medication for a prolonged period. This decision must carefully weigh the risk-benefit ratio of neuroleptic treatment or discontinuation in such circumstances.

■ NEUROLEPTIC RESISTANCE

Conservative estimates suggest that some 15%–30% of patients have a schizophrenic illness that is refractory to conventional neuroleptic treatments (Kane et al. 1988; Meltzer 1992c). Because this figure is based largely on symptomatic measures of response and does not take into account broader yet equally important measures (i.e., vocational attainment, quality of life), it is likely that the true estimate of neuroleptic resistance may be even greater. Moreover, it is these patients who mainly account for the staggering economic burden of schizophrenia, the high rates of hospitalization, and the high prevalence of suicidal behavior.

These patients are notoriously difficult to treat. By definition, they have failed to experience sufficient response from previous neuroleptic treatments and often present with moderate to severe persistent psychopathology that is poorly controlled by medication. Indeed, by the time of evaluation, the medication regimens are often complicated with the use of multiple psychotropics and with significant distressing side effects, such as akathisia or TD.

The first principle in the management of such patients is to obtain a thorough baseline evaluation. This should encompass assessment of symptoms, social function, capacity to work, extent of support systems, and presence of side effects of treatment. Ideally, this should be done while the patient is in a drug-free state. In practice, however, this is only possible infrequently. The severity of the patient's illness, concerns about further deterioration during untreated psychosis (Loebel et al. 1992), and pragmatic issues of hospitalization and utilization review mitigate against a drug-free evaluation. A detailed chronology of past neuroleptic treatments and response is essential and is best corroborated by obtaining any previous hospital records that are available (Meltzer 1992c). If there is doubt, then a 6-week trial (or longer) of a standard neuroleptic should be given and, ideally, the response objectified using some of the rating scales discussed previously.

■ The Role of Clozapine

Clozapine, a dibenzodiazepine, is now the primary treatment option for treatment-refractory schizophrenia (Kane et al. 1988; Meltzer 1992a, 1992c). It was withdrawn from study in the United States following the death of eight Finnish patients from clozapine-related agranulocytosis in 1975. Clozapine remained of interest, however, because during a period of restricted use in Europe and the United States between 1975 and 1985, it was noted that clozapine was superior to typical neuroleptics with regard to TD and EPS, and, possibly, efficacy. In a study that was pivotal to the reintroduction of clozapine into the United States, 270 neuroleptic-refractory and 22 neuroleptic-intolerant patients were randomized to receive either clozapine or chlorpromazine plus benztropine (Kane et al. 1988). By the end of the 6-week trial, 30% of the clozapine-treated subjects were classified as responders (a final BPRS Total Score ≤ 36 and a CGI score of mild), compared with just 4% of patients who received the conventional antipsychotic. Improvements were noted in the clozapine-treated group in both positive and negative symptoms beginning at 1 and 2 weeks, respectively. Subsequently, clozapine was found to decrease symptoms of disorganization (Meltzer 1992c). Although 30% of patients respond within 6 weeks of treatment, it is important to stress that improvement in psychopathology on clozapine may take 6–12 months to achieve (Meltzer et al. 1990); a trial of clozapine of just 6 weeks is therefore insufficient. Moreover, improvements in one domain of outcome may occur independently of another (Meltzer 1992a).

Patients need a careful evaluation before beginning treatment with clozapine (Meltzer 1992c). A full blood count, liver function tests, and ECG are advisable both to rule out medical conditions that may complicate treatment and also to establish baseline laboratory results. Clozapine can usually be given to patients with a previous history of agranulocytosis or blood dyscrasia due to other drugs, but increased surveillance is desirable, especially during the first 6 months of treatment.

Clozapine treatment should begin gradually at an initial dose of 12.5 mg/day, increasing the dosage on alternate days in increments of 25 mg, up to 100 mg. Thereafter, incremental rises should be by 50 mg on alternate days until a dose of 400–450 mg/day is achieved. The optimum dose is determined mainly by clinical response and also by tolerance of side effects (discussed later). If the response is insufficient, then the dosage can be increased to 900 mg/day, bearing in mind that an effective response may be delayed and time-dependent. If the dosage exceeds the usual range and the patient continues to show a disappointing response to clozapine, determination of clozapine plasma levels may be a useful guide to management (Hasegawa et al. 1993; Perry et al. 1991). In contrast to the lack of clinical guidance of plasma levels of conventional antipsychotics in routine treatment (see section on "Continuation, Maintenance, and Monitoring"), a plasma clozapine level of greater than 370 ng/ml has been consistently shown to predict good response to clozapine treatment (Hasagawa et al. 1993). This rationale can then be utilized as an approach for either incremental dosage strategies or assisting augmentation strategies in clozapine therapy (P. F. Buckley, M. Hasegawa, P. Cole, C. Lys, and H. Y. Meltzer, unpublished data, June 1994).

In general, clozapine is best given as monotherapy from the start. If this is not clinically feasible, then the medication should be simplified so that the patient is receiving a single neuroleptic such as haloperidol (in oral form only). Patients should be withdrawn from typical neuroleptic drugs as the dose of clozapine is increased to 450 mg/day. Benzodiazepines should be avoided because of the risk (based mainly on case reports) of respiratory depression with concomitant use of clozapine and benzodiazepines during the initial phases of treatment.

Important side effects of clozapine and their management are highlighted in Table 30–10. The most serious of these is agranulocytosis, which is reported to occur in 1%–2% of patients receiving clozapine (Krupp and Barnes 1992) and is the reason why all clozapine-treated patients in the United States require a weekly monitoring of their WBC. The peak risk period for developing agranulocytosis is in the first 18 weeks of treatment; as yet, there are no clinical predictors as to which patients are likely to develop this side effect. Evidence from some recent evaluations of United States data on weekly WBC estimations from patients treated with clozapine suggests that this close monitoring is associated with a low rate of agranulocytosis (0.8% of patients receiving clozapine). This has also provided preliminary evidence that increasing age and female gender may be risk factors for the development of clozapine-related agranulocytosis (Alvir et al. 1993). For patients who show an abrupt or marked fall in WBC count or whose WBC falls between 3,500/mm^3 to 3,000/mm^3, the WBC should be checked twice weekly. If the WBC falls to below 3,000/mm^3 but not less than 2,000/mm^3, then therapy should be interrupted and WBC monitored daily. A WBC of less than 2,000 or absolute neutrophil count less than 1,000/mm^3 are indications for immediate cessation of clozapine. When the WBC falls to less than 150 or absolute neutrophil count reaches 500/mm^3, then clozapine therapy should never be resumed.

Agranulocytosis is an indication for hospitalization with the institution of reverse isolation. A full septic workup is mandatory, and the prophylactic use of antibiotics is often advisable. If the onset of infec-

Table 30–10. Side effects of clozapine

Side effect	Incidence	Action
Agranulocytosis	0.8%	Monitor white blood cell count (WBC) weekly; if WBC < 2,000, stop clozapine; hospitalize; treat infection aggressively; never give clozapine again
Seizures	3%, dose-related	Decrease clozapine; add phenytoin or valproate
Sedation	40%, dose-related	Give maximum dosage at night; reduce dose
Hypersalivation	31%	Benztropine or clonidine may help
Tachycardia	> 25%	Treat if > 140 or symptomatic; add low dose of β-blocker
Hypertension	9%	Monitor; add β-blocker if blood pressure high or persistent
Hypotension	9%	Monitor; encourage fluid intake; alter dosage regimen
Dizziness	20%	Tolerance often develops; monitor; alter dosage regimen
Constipation	14%	Laxative, if required
Weight gain	Variable, > 3%	Reduce food intake; exercise
Nausea	5%	Supportive measures

tion precedes the cessation of clozapine, then the mortality rate associated with agranulocytosis may be quite high. The use of one of the known granulocyte-stimulating factors will help to restore normal bone marrow production (Gerson and Meltzer 1992; Lieberman and Alvir 1992).

Major motor seizures occur at a rate of approximately 3% at 300 mg/day and 6% at 600 mg/day of clozapine (Sajatovic and Meltzer, in press). Myoclonus occurs less frequently. These effects are not a cause for discontinuation of clozapine; rather, they should be treated either by a reduction in the clozapine dosage or the addition of an anticonvulsant agent. Valproic acid is usually effective but may increase clozapine levels. Carbamazepine should be avoided because of the risk of agranulocytosis, but if it is absolutely necessary for seizure control, it can be given.

The other main side effects of clozapine are cardiovascular effects, sedation, weight gain, and hypersalivation. The chief cardiovascular effects are orthostatic hypotension, tachycardia, and ECG changes. In general, these effects are seen early in treatment, are short-lived, and seldom result in discontinuation of clozapine. They are best managed by careful monitoring of vital signs, alterations in clozapine dosage (i.e., transient reduction in dose or dose administered in a tid regimen), and with a cardiology consultation if difficulties persist. Sedation is less serious but a common and distressing side effect. It is generally observed early in treatment, and tolerance develops over time. Alterations in the dosage regimen are usually effective although, in severe cases, the addition of methylphenidate or L-dopa may be warranted (H. Y. Meltzer, unpublished data, June 1994). Weight gain is another distressing side effect, with reported rates varying from 13% (Povlsen et al. 1985) to 83% (Cohen et al. 1990). Simple strategies including dietary advice, exercise, and monitoring are usually effective. Hypersalivation generally occurs at night, again often at the initial phases of treatment. If this becomes troublesome or persistent, the addition of benztropine or clonidine (an α_1 receptor agonist) will usually relieve this side effect.

Some patients cannot tolerate clozapine or even refuse to try this drug. In addition, many financial and political constraints influence the availability of clozapine for treatment-refractory patients. In these circumstances, the use of the more traditional neuroleptic augmentation strategies is advisable.

Some of the most commonly used augmenting agents and their relative indications are given in Table 30–11.

In general, the effects of these drugs when added to neuroleptics are not dramatic and do not generalize across patient samples (Christison et al. 1991; Meltzer 1992c), so the choice as to which agent to use is still unclear. The initial optimism for the efficacy of lithium augmentation does not appear to be justified (Schulz et al. 1990). Moreover, lithium therapy needs to be closely monitored to avoid neurotoxicity associated with concomitant neuroleptic treatment and the potentially accentuated risk of NMS. More recent interest has focused on the use of serotonin agonists and antagonists, with some preliminary findings showing encouraging benefits in treating both persistent positive and negative symptoms (Goff et al. 1991; Silver and Nasser 1992). Benzodiazepines have also been shown to be helpful in ameliorating persistent psychotic symptoms in some patients (Meltzer 1992c; Wolkowitz and Pickar 1991). However, these effects are at best modest and must be weighed against the adverse effects of these agents. There is also the potential for rebound psychotic and anxiety symptoms, particularly those associated with the later withdrawal of high-potency triazolobenzodiazepines such as alprazolam. When negative symptoms predominate, L-dopa or bromocriptine to accentuate dopaminergic activity may be useful, although this strategy may also be associated with a risk of precipitating a relapse of positive symptoms.

Anticonvulsants (specifically carbamazepine) appear to be ineffective as a primary treatment for schizophrenia (Carpenter et al. 1991), but they may be of use in persistently psychotic patients who manifest impulsive or violent behavior (Meltzer 1992c).

Table 30–11. Neuroleptic augmentation strategies in treatment-refractory schizophrenia

Symptom	Adjunctive treatment
Persistent positive symptoms	Lithium, anticonvulsants, electroconvulsive therapy
Persistent negative symptoms	L-dopa, bromocriptine, benzodiazepine
Depressive symptoms	Antidepressants, lithium
Hypomania	Lithium
Anxiety	Benzodiazepine
Aggression	Anticonvulsants

Patients who have EEG abnormalities or episodic dyscontrol behaviors may also benefit from adjunctive anticonvulsant therapy. There is also a very extensive literature, previously well reviewed (Christison et al. 1991; Meltzer 1992c), on the use of opioid drugs, β-blockers, calcium channel blockers, and neuropeptide analogues in treatment-refractory schizophrenia. With the possible exception of propranolol, there is as yet little evidence to support the use of these agents.

Finally, the role of ECT in the treatment of persistently psychotic patients has recently come under renewed scrutiny (Sajatovic and Meltzer 1993). Maintenance ECT may be of value in the management of treatment-refractory patients and can result in reduction of positive symptoms and rates of rehospitalization (Sajatovic and Meltzer 1993). However, ECT needs to be given at least monthly.

■ CONCLUSION

Although the neurobiological basis of neuroleptic responsivity in schizophrenia remains obscure, significant advances have been made in defining appropriate treatment strategies for patients with this disorder. A detailed and multifaceted assessment is the cornerstone of any proposed treatment. At present, there are only modest differences between individual classes of neuroleptics used in the treatment of acute episodes of schizophrenia. For long-term maintenance treatment, neuroleptics are the mainstay. Psychosocial rehabilitation programs may also be offered to prevent relapse and improve function, although much research is still needed in this area.

Discontinuation of neuroleptics is a realistic option for only a small minority of patients and, based on current evidence, it is unclear how such patients may be suitably selected. Clozapine is now the treatment of choice in the treatment of neuroleptic-nonresponsive schizophrenia and has demonstrated efficacy in a wide range of outcome measures. The role of alternative treatments for neuroleptic-nonresponsive illness (including neuroleptic augmentation strategies or adjunctive ECT) is now less clear. These agents are probably best reserved for patients who either refuse or cannot tolerate clozapine treatment. The advent of clozapine and other new antipsychotics offers encouragement and optimism not only for the treatment of schizophrenia.

Significantly, these agents also provide a neurobiological framework upon which to explore the nature of schizophrenia itself.

■ REFERENCES

Adler LA, Angrist B, Reiter S, et al: Neuroleptic-induced akathisia: a review. Psychopharmacology 97:1–11, 1989

Adler LA, Peselow E, Rotrosen J, et al: Vitamin E treatment of tardive dyskinesia. Am J Psychiatry 150:1405–1407, 1993

Alvir JMJ, Lieberman JA, Safferman AZ, et al: Clozapine-induced agranulocytosis incidence and risk factors in the United States. N Engl J Med 329:162–167, 1993

American Psychiatric Association: Diagnostic and Statistical Manual of Mental Disorders, 4th Edition. Washington, DC, American Psychiatric Association, 1994

Andreasen NC: The Scale for the Assessment of Negative Symptoms (SANS). University of Iowa, Iowa City, IA, 1983

Andreasen NC: The Scale for the Assessment of Positive Symptoms (SAPS). University of Iowa, Iowa City, IA, 1984

Andreasen NC, Flam M, Swayze VW, et al: Positive and negative symptoms of schizophrenia. Arch Gen Psychiatry 47:615–621, 1990

Andreasen NC, Flam M, Arndt S: The Comprehensive Assessment of Symptoms and History (CASH): an instrument for assessing diagnosis and psychopathology. Arch Gen Psychiatry 49:615–623, 1992

Ayd FJ: A summary of drug-induced extrapyramidal reactions. JAMA 175:1054–1060, 1961

Bachrach LL: Psychosocial rehabilitation and psychiatry in the care of long-term patients. Am J Psychiatry 149:1455–1463, 1992

Baldessarini RJ, Cohen BM, Teicher MH: Significance of neuroleptic dose and plasma level in the pharmacological treatment of psychoses. Arch Gen Psychiatry 45:79–91, 1988

Barnes TRE: Movement disorder associated with antipsychotic drugs: the tardive syndromes. International Review of Psychiatry 2:355–366, 1990

Barnes TRE, Liddle PF, Curson DA, et al: Negative symptoms, tardive dyskinesia, and depression in chronic schizophrenia. Br J Psychiatry 155:99–103, 1989

Barnes TRE, Halstead SM, Liddle PF: Relationship between iron status and chronic akathisia in an inpatient population with chronic schizophrenia. Br J Psychiatry 161:791–796, 1992

Bartko G, Frecska E, Horvath S, et al: Predicting neuroleptic response from a combination of multilevel variables in acute schizophrenic patients. Acta Psychiatr Scand 82:408–412, 1990

Bellack AS, Mueser KT: Psychosocial treatment of schizophrenia. Schizophr Bull 19:317–336, 1993

Boodhood JA, Sandler WM: Anticholinergic antiparkinsonian drugs in psychiatry. Br J Hosp Med 46:167–169, 1991

Borison RL, Diamond BI, Pathiraja AP, et al: Clinical overview of risperidone, in Novel Antipsychotics. Edited by Meltzer HY. New York, Raven, 1992, pp 233–240

Breier A, Schreiber JL, Dyer J, et al: National Institute of Mental Health Longitudinal Study of Schizophrenia. Arch Gen Psychiatry 48:239–246, 1991

Breier A, Buchanan RW, Kirkpatrick B, et al: Effects of clozapine on positive and negative symptoms in outpatients with schizophrenia. Am J Psychiatry 151:20–26, 1994

Buckley PF, Meltzer HY: Clozapine and NMS. Br J Psychiatry 162:556, 1993

Buckley PF, Cannon M, Larkin C: Abuse of neuroleptic drugs. British Journal of Addiction 86:789–790, 1991

Buckley PF, Way L, Meltzer HY: Substance abuse among patients with treatment resistant schizophrenia: characteristics and implications for clozapine therapy. Am J Psychiatry 151:154–159, 1994

Bunney BS, Sesack SR, Silva NL: Midbrain dopaminergic systems: neurophysiology and electrophysiological pharmacology, in Psychopharmacology: The Third Generation of Progress. Edited by Meltzer HY. New York, Raven, 1987, pp 113–126

Carpenter WT: The phenomenology and course of schizophrenia: treatment implications, in Psychopharmacology: The Third Generation of Progress. Edited by Meltzer HY. New York, Raven, 1987, pp 1121–1128

Carpenter WT: The deficit syndrome. Am J Psychiatry 151:327, 1994

Carpenter WT Jr, Heinrichs DW, Hanlon TE: A comparative trial of pharmacologic strategies in schizophrenia. Am J Psychiatry 144:1466–1470, 1987

Carpenter WT, Hanlon TE, Heinrichs DW, et al: Continuous versus targeted medication in schizophrenic outpatients; outcome results. Am J Psychiatry 147:1138–1148, 1990

Carpenter WT, Kurz R, Kirkpatrick HB, et al: Carbamazepine maintenance treatment in outpatient schizophrenics. Arch Gen Psychiatry 48:69–72, 1991

Casey DE: Neuroleptic drug-induced extrapyramidal syndromes and tardive dyskinesia. Schizophr Res 4:109–120, 1991

Casey DE: Neuroleptic-induced acute extrapyramidal syndromes and tardive dyskinesia. Psychopharmacology (Berl) 16:589–610, 1993

Chakos MH, Mayerhoff DI, Loebel AD, et al: Incidence and correlates of acute extrapyramidal symptoms in first episode of schizophrenia. Psychopharmacol Bull 28:81–86, 1992

Chouinard G, Jones B, Remington G, et al: A Canadian multicenter placebo-controlled study of fixed doses of risperidone and haloperidol in the treatment of chronic schizophrenic patients. J Clin Psychopharmacol 13:25–40, 1993

Christison GW, Kirch DJ, Wyatt RJ: When symptoms persist: choosing among alternative somatic treatments for schizophrenia. Schizophr Bull 17:217–245, 1991

Cohen S, Chiles J, McNaughton A: Weight gain associated with clozapine. Am J Psychiatry 147:503–504, 1990

Corrigan PW, Yudofsky SC, Silver JM: Pharmacological and behavioral treatments for aggressive psychiatric inpatients. Hosp Community Psychiatry 44:125–133, 1993

Crow TJ: Schizophrenia: more than one molecular process. British Medical Journal 280:66–68, 1980

Dodwell D, Goldberg D: A study of factors associated with response to electroconvulsive therapy in patients with schizophrenic symptoms. Br J Psychiatry 154:635–639, 1989

Elkashef AM, Ruskin PE, Bacher N, et al: Vitamin E in the treatment of tardive dyskinesia. Am J Psychiatry 147:505–506, 1990

Endicott J, Spitzer RL: A diagnostic interview: the Schedule for Affective Disorders and Schizophrenia. Arch Gen Psychiatry 35:837–844, 1978

Endicott J, Spitzer RL, Fleiss JL: The Global Assessment Scale: a procedure for measuring overall severity of psychiatric disturbance. Arch Gen Psychiatry 33:766–771, 1976

Feltner DE, Hertzman M: Progress in the treatment of tardive dyskinesia: theory and practice. Hosp

Community Psychiatry 44:25–34, 1993

Fennell PWH: Arrest or injection? do we need them? Journal of Forensic Psychiatry 2:153–166, 1991

Fenton WS, McGlashan TH: Natural history of schizophrenia subtypes, II: positive and negative symptoms and long-term course. Arch Gen Psychiatry 48:978–985, 1991

Gerlach J, Casey DE: Tardive dyskinesia. Acta Psychiatr Scand 77:369–378, 1988

Gerson SL, Meltzer HY: Mechanisms of clozapine-induced agranulocytosis. Drug Saf 7:17–25, 1992

Glazer WM, Kane JM: Depot neuroleptic therapy: an underutilized treatment option. J Clin Psychiatry 53:426–433, 1992

Glazer WM, Morgenstein H, Schooler N, et al: Predictors of improvement in tardive dyskinesia following discontinuation of neuroleptic medication. Br J Psychiatry 157:585–592, 1990

Goff DC, Baldessarini RJ: Drug interactions with antipsychotic agents. J Clin Psychopharmacol 13:57–65, 1993

Goff DC, Midha KK, Brotman AW, et al: An open trial of buspirone added to neuroleptics in schizophrenic patients. J Clin Psychopharmacol 11:193–197, 1991

Goldberg TE, Weinberger DR, Berman KF, et al: Further evidence of dementia of the prefrontal type in schizophrenia? Arch Gen Psychiatry 44:1008–1014, 1987

Guy W (ed): ECDEU Assessment Manual for Psychopharmacology (DHEW Publ No ADM-76-338). Washington, DC, U.S. Government Printing Office, 1976

Hasegawa M, Guitierrez-Esteinou R, Way L, et al: Relationship between clinical efficacy and clozapine plasma concentrations in schizophrenia: effect of smoking. J Clin Psychopharmacol 13:383–390, 1993

Heinrichs DW, Hanlon ET, Carpenter WT Jr: The Quality of Life Scale: an instrument for rating the deficit syndrome. Schizophr Bull 10:388–398, 1984

Hermesh H, Aizenburg D, Weizman A: A successful electroconvulsive treatment of neuroleptic malignant syndrome. Acta Psychiatr Scand 75:237–239, 1987

Hertman M: ECT and neuroleptics as primary treatments for schizophrenia. Biol Psychiatry 31:217–220, 1992

Herz MI, Szymanski HV, Simon JC: Intermittent medication for stable schizophrenic outpatients: an alternative to maintenance medication. Am J Psychiatry 139:918–922, 1982

Herz MI, Glazer WM, Mostert MA, et al: Intermittent vs maintenance medication in schizophrenia: two-year results. Arch Gen Psychiatry 48:333–339, 1991

Hogarty GE, Anderson CM, Reiss DJ, et al: Family psychoeducation, social skills training, and maintenance chemotherapy in the aftercare treatment of schizophrenia, I: one-year effects of a controlled study on relapse and expressed emotion. Arch Gen Psychiatry 43:633–642, 1986

Hogarty GE, McEvoy JP, Munetz M, et al: Familial and environmental/personal indicators in the course of schizophrenia research group: dose of fluphenazine, familial expressed emotion, and outcome in schizophrenia. Arch Gen Psychiatry 45:797–805, 1988

Hogarty GE, Anderson CM, Reiss DJ, et al: Family psychoeducation, social skills training, and maintenance chemotherapy in the aftercare treatment of schizophrenia, II: two-year effects of a controlled study on relapse and adjustment. Arch Gen Psychiatry 48:340–347, 1991

Jolley AG, Hirsch SR, McRink A, et al: Trial of brief intermittent neuroleptic prophylaxis for selected schizophrenic outpatients: clinical outcome at one year. BMJ 298:985–990, 1989

Jolley AG, Hirsch SR, Morrison E, et al: Trial of brief intermittent neuroleptic prophylaxis for selected schizophrenic outpatients: clinical outcome at two years. BMJ 301:837–847, 1990

Kane J, Marder SR: Psychopharmacologic treatment of schizophrenia. Schizophr Bull 19:287–302, 1993

Kane JM, Rifkin A, Woerner M, et al: High dose versus low dose strategies in the treatment of schizophrenia. Psychopharmacol Bull 21:533–537, 1985

Kane JM, Honigfeld G, Singer J, et al: Clozapine for the treatment-resistant schizophrenic: a double-blind comparison with chlorpromazine. Arch Gen Psychiatry 45:789–796, 1988

Kavanagh DJ: Recent developments in expressed emotion and schizophrenia. Br J Psychiatry 160:601–609, 1992

Kay SR, Singh MM: The positive-negative distinction in drug-free schizophrenic patients: stability, response to neuroleptics, and prognostic significance. Arch Gen Psychiatry 46:711–718, 1989

Kay SR, Fisz Bein A, Opler LA: The Positive and Negative Syndrome Scale (PANSS) for schizophrenia. Schizophr Bull 13:261–276, 1987

Keith SJ, Matthews SM, Schooler NR: Psychosocial treatment of schizophrenia: a review of psycho-educational family approaches, in Schizophrenia Research. Edited by Tamminga CA, Schulz SC. New York, Raven, 1991, pp 247–254

Kellam AMP: The (frequently) neuroleptic malignant syndrome. Br J Psychiatry 157:169–173, 1990

Kirkpatrick B, Buchanan RW, McKenney PD: Schedule for the deficit syndrome: an instrument for research in schizophrenia. Psychiatry Res 30:119–123, 1989

Kolakowska T, Williams AO, Ardern M, et al: Schizophrenia with good and poor outcome. Br J Psychiatry 146:229–246, 1985

Krupp P, Barnes P: Clozapine-associated agranulocytosis: risk and aetiology. Br J Psychiatry 160 (suppl 7):38–40, 1992

Lam DH: Psychosocial family intervention in schizophrenia: a review of empirical studies. Psychol Med 21:423–441, 1991

Lavin M, Rifkin A: Prophylactic antiparkinson drug use, I: initial prophylaxis and prevention of extrapyramidal side effects. J Clin Pharmacol 31:763–768, 1991a

Lavin M, Rifkin A: Prophylactic antiparkinson drug use, II: withdrawal after long-term maintenance therapy. J Clin Pharmacol 31:769–777, 1991b

Lefley HP: Expressed emotion: conceptual, clinical, and social policy issues. Hosp Community Psychiatry 43:591–595, 1992

Levinson DF, Simpson GM, Singh H, et al: Fluphenazine dose, clinical response and extrapyramidal symptoms during acute treatment. Arch Gen Psychiatry 47:761–768, 1990

Lewander T, Uppfeldt G, Köhler C, et al: Remoxipride and raclopride: pharmacological background and clinical outcome, in Novel Antipsychotics. Edited by Meltzer HY. New York, Raven, 1992, pp 67–78

Liddle PF: Syndromes of chronic schizophrenia. Br J Psychiatry 151:145–151, 1987

Lieberman JA, Alvir JMJ: A report of clozapine induced agranulocytosis in the United States: incidence and risk factors. Drug Saf 7 (suppl):1–2, 1992

Lieberman JA, Kane JM, Alvir JMJ: Provocative tests with psychostimulant drugs in schizophrenia. Psychopharmacology (Berl) 91:415–433, 1987

Lieberman JA, Saltz BL, Johns CA, et al: The effects of clozapine on tardive dyskinesia. Br J Psychiatry 158:503–510, 1991

Lieberman JA, Jody D, Geisler S, et al: Time course and biological predictors of treatment response in first episode schizophrenia. Arch Gen Psychiatry 50:369–376, 1993

Loebel AD, Lieberman JA, Alvir JMJ, et al: Duration of psychosis and outcome in first episode schizophrenia. Am J Psychiatry 149:1183–1188, 1992

Loebel AD, Lieberman JA, Alvir JMJ, et al: Consistency of treatment response across successive psychotic episodes in recent-onset schizophrenia. Schizophr Res 8:243, 1993

Lohr JB, Cadet JL, Lohr MA, et al: Alpha-tocopherol in tardive dyskinesia. Lancet 1:913–934, 1987

Marder SR, Meibach RC: Risperidone in the treatment of schizophrenia. Am J Psychiatry 151:825–835, 1994

Marder SR, Van Putten T, Mintz J, et al: Costs and benefits of two doses of fluphenazine. Arch Gen Psychiatry 41:1025–1029, 1984

Marder SR, Van Putten T, Mintz J, et al: Low and conventional dose maintenance therapy with fluphenazine decanoate: two year outcome. Arch Gen Psychiatry 44:510–517, 1987

McGlashan TH, Fenton WS: The positive/negative distinction in schizophrenia: review of natural history validators. Arch Gen Psychiatry 49:63–72, 1992

Meltzer HY: Rigidity, hyperpyrexia and coma following fluphenazine enanthate. Psychopharmacologia 29:337–346, 1973

Meltzer HY: Dopamine and negative symptoms in schizophrenia: critique of the Type I-Type II hypothesis, in Controversies in Schizophrenia: Changes and Constancies. Edited by Alpert M. New York, Guilford, 1985, pp 110–136

Meltzer HY: Commentary: defining treatment refractoriness in schizophrenia. Schizophr Bull 16:563–565, 1990

Meltzer HY: Dimensions of outcome with clozapine. Br J Psychiatry 160:36–43, 1992a

Meltzer HY: The mechanism of action of clozapine in relation to its clinical advantage, in Novel Antipsychotic Drugs. Edited by Meltzer HY. New York, Raven, 1992b, pp 1–13

Meltzer HY: Treatment of the neuroleptic-nonresponsive schizophrenic patient. Schizophr Bull 18(3)515–542, 1992c

Meltzer HY, Fang VS: Effect of neuroleptics on serum prolactin in schizophrenic patients. Arch Gen Psychiatry 33:279–286, 1976

Meltzer HY, Luchins DJ: Effect of clozapine in severe tardive dyskinesia: a case report. J Clin Psychopharmacol 4:286–287, 1984

Meltzer HY, Nash JF: Effects of antipsychotic drugs on serotonin receptors. Pharmacol Rev 43:587–604, 1991

Meltzer HY, Sommers AA, Luchins DJ: The effect of neuroleptics and other psychotropic drugs on negative symptoms in schizophrenia. J Clin Psychopharmacol 6:329–338, 1986

Meltzer HY, Burnett S, Bastani B, et al: Effect of six months of clozapine treatment on the quality of life of chronic schizophrenic patients. Hosp Community Psychiatry 41:892–897, 1990

Mueser KT, Yarnold PR, Levinson DF, et al: Prevalence of substance abuse in schizophrenia: demographic and clinical correlates. Schizophr Bull 16:31–53, 1990

Munich RL, Lang E: The boundaries of psychiatric rehabilitation. Hosp Community Psychiatry 44:661–666, 1993

Opler LA, Albert D, Ramirez PM: Psychopharmacologic treatment of negative schizophrenic symptoms. Compr Psychiatry 35:16–28, 1994

Overall JE, Gorham DR: The Brief Psychiatric Rating Scale. Psychol Rep 10:799–812, 1962

Overall JE, Gorham DR: Reliability of the BPRS. Psychopharmacol Bull 26:18–24, 1988

Perry PJ, Miller DD, Arndt S, et al: Clozapine and norclozapine plasma concentrations and clinical response of treatment-refractory schizophrenic patients. Am J Psychiatry 148:231–235, 1991

Povlsen UJ, Noring U, Fog T, et al: Tolerability and therapeutic effect of clozapine: a retrospective investigation of 216 patients treated with clozapine for up to 12 years. Acta Psychiatr Scand 71:176–185, 1985

Rifkin A, Doddi S, Karajgi B, et al: Dosage of haloperidol for schizophrenia. Arch Gen Psychiatry 48:166–170, 1990

Robbins L, Helzer J, Croughan J, et al: The National Institute of Mental Health Diagnostic Interview Schedule. Rockville, MD, National Institute of Mental Health, 1979

Rosebush P, Stuart T: A prospective analysis of 24 episodes of neuroleptic malignant syndrome. Am J Psychiatry 146:717–725, 1989

Rosebush PI, Stuart TD, Gelenberg AJ: Twenty neuroleptic rechallenges after neuroleptic malignant syndrome in 15 patients. J Clin Psychiatry 50:295–298, 1989

Roth BL, Craigo SC, Choudhary MS, et al: Binding of typical and atypical antipsychotic agents to 5-hydroxytryptamine$_6$ (5-HT$_6$) and 5-hydroxytryptamine$_7$ (5-HT$_7$) receptors. J Pharmacol Exp Ther 268:1403–1410, 1994

Roy A: Suicide in chronic schizophrenia. Br J Psychiatry 141:171–177, 1982

Sajatovic M, Meltzer HY: The effect of short-term electroconvulsive treatment plus neuroleptics in treatment-resistant schizophrenia and schizoaffective disorder. Convulsive Therapy 9(3):167–175, 1993

Sajatovic M, Meltzer HY: Clozapine-induced myoclonus and generalized seizures: relation to serotonin. Br J Psychiatry (in press)

Schooler NR, Keith SJ, Severe JB, et al: Treatment strategies in schizophrenia: effects of dosage reduction and family management on outcome. Schizophr Res 9:260, 1993

Schulz SC, Kahn EM, Baker RW, et al: Lithium and carbamazepine augmentation in treatment refractory schizophrenia, in The Neuroleptic-Nonresponsive Patient: Characterization and Treatment. Edited by Angrist B, Schulz SC. Washington, DC, American Psychiatric Press, 1990, pp 109–136

Shader RD, Greenblatt DJ: A possible new approach to the treatment of the Neuroleptic Malignant Syndrome. J Clin Psychopharmacol 12:155, 1992

Silver H, Nasser A: Fluvoxamine improves negative symptoms in treated chronic schizophrenia: an add-on double-blind, placebo-controlled study. Biol Psychiatry 31:698–704, 1992

Siris SG: Diagnosis of secondary depression in schizophrenia. Schizophr Bull 17:75–98, 1991

Siris SG, Bermanzohn PC, Mason SE, et al: Maintenance imipramine therapy for secondary depression in schizophrenia: a controlled trial. Arch Gen Psychiatry 51:109–115, 1994

Spitzer RL, Williams JBV, Gibbon M: Structured clinical interview for DSM III-R (SCID, 7.1.85 review). New York, New York State Psychiatric Institute, Biometrics Research Department, 1985 [722 West 168th Street, New York, NY 10037]

Thompson PA, Meltzer HY: Positive, negative, and disorganisation factors from the Schedule for Affective Disorders and Schizophrenia and the Present State Examination. Br J Psychiatry 163:344–351, 1993

Van Putten T: Why do schizophrenic patients refuse to take their drugs? Arch Gen Psychiatry 31:67–72, 1974

Van Putten T, Marder SR, Mintz J: A controlled dose comparison of haloperidol in newly admitted schizophrenic patients. Arch Gen Psychiatry 47:754–758, 1990

Van Putten T, Marder SR, Wirshing WC, et al: Neuroleptic plasma levels. Schizophr Bull 17:197–216, 1991

Waddington JL, O'Callaghan E, Buckley PF, et al: Vulnerability of the tardive dyskinesia in schizophrenia: an exploration of individual patient factors, in Neuroleptic-Induced Movement Disorders: A Comprehensive Survey. Edited by Yassa R, Jeste D, Nair NPV. Cambridge, England, Cambridge University Press (in press)

Wear AN, Brahms D: To treat or not to treat: illegal, ethical and therapeutic implications of treatment refusal. J Med Ethics 17:131–135, 1991

Weiden PJ, Dixon L, Frances A, et al: Neuroleptic noncompliance in schizophrenia, in Schizophrenia Research. Edited by Tamminga CA, Schulz SC. New York, Raven, 1991, pp 285–296

Woerner MG, Saltz BL, Kane JM, et al: Diabetes and the development of tardive dyskinesia. Am J Psychiatry 150:966–968, 1993

Wolkowitz OM, Pickar D: Benzodiazepines in the treatment of schizophrenia: a review and reappraisal. Am J Psychiatry 48:714–726, 1991

31

Treatment of Anxiety Disorders

C. Barr Taylor, M.D.

The psychopharmacological treatment of panic and other anxiety disorders has changed dramatically in the past 10 years. The changes in treatment were enhanced by the publication of the *Diagnostic and Statistical Manual of Mental Disorders, Third Edition* (DSM-III; American Psychiatric Association 1980), which allowed for uniform diagnoses—by the evidence from epidemiology of the high prevalence of these disorders, by the development of new pharmacological and cognitive therapies, and by a general increase in research in this area. Even 10 years ago, the customary psychopharmacological treatment in the United States was to use benzodiazepines for treatment of most anxiety disorders. Now a variety of agents have been shown to be effective. The psychological treatment of anxiety disorders has also expanded and been better integrated into the pharmacological treatment (Taylor and Arnow 1988).

PANIC DISORDER

Panic disorder (with and without phobic avoidance) is the most common anxiety disorder, occurring in 2%–6% of the population (Myers et al. 1984). The target symptoms of panic disorder include panic attacks, anticipatory and generalized anxiety, avoidance (agoraphobia), and (to varying degrees) worry, somatic symptoms, and even obsessions. Panic disorder is a long-term disorder, with frequent relapses, changes in symptomatology, and comorbidity. Of the latter, depression and alcohol use and abuse are particularly relevant when considering which psy-

chopharmacological agents should be used. The psychopharmacological treatment of panic disorder can be conceptualized as occurring in two phases, short- and long-term, with much more being known about the former than the latter.

■ Short-Term, Acute Treatment

The short-term goals of psychopharmacological treatment are symptom relief and initiation of psychological therapies. Many patients achieve relief of the target symptoms and improvement in work, family, and social functioning within 8 weeks of treatment with combinations of psychological therapy and pharmacotherapy.

Antidepressants

Antidepressants should be considered as the first line of treatment for patients with panic disorder, especially if depression is present. Of all the antidepressants, imipramine has been used the longest and has been most extensively investigated. The benefits of imipramine for reducing the frequency of panic attacks were first noted more than 30 years ago by Klein and Fink (1962), and a number of studies since have substantiated its benefits. The largest study involved 1,168 patients in 14 countries and compared imipramine, alprazolam, and placebo (Cross-National Collaborative Panic Study 1992). At the end of the study, the effects of the two active drugs were similar to each other, and both were superior to placebo for most outcome measures. Surprisingly, there were no differences between the active treatments and placebo in the number of panic attacks per week at

8 weeks. The mean daily dose of imipramine was 155 mg; a higher dose may be needed for some patients. The results of this study were confounded by the large dropout rates in the placebo group (44%) and the imipramine group (30%), both of which were significantly higher than the dropout rate of the alprazolam group (17%). Although the data suggest a drug treatment effect, the strong placebo effect cannot be ignored (Marks et al. 1992). Table 31–1 shows the advantages and disadvantages of tricyclic antidepressants (TCAs) for anxiety disorders.

Imipramine should be started at doses of 25–50 mg and gradually increased. Most patients achieve a therapeutic benefit at 150–250 mg, although it can be increased to 300 mg. Therapeutic effects are usually achieved with plasma imipramine plus desipramine levels of a 100–150-mg/ml range (Ballenger 1991; Mavissakalian et al. 1984). About 25% of panic disorder patients begun on imipramine demonstrate what has been called an "activation response" characterized by flushing of the skin, a feeling of restlessness, sweating, palpitations, and other symptoms. Most patients find these symptoms intolerable. In such patients, imipramine can be reduced to very low doses (10 mg) and increased gradually.

The dropout rate in published studies of imipramine is high. As noted previously, 30% of the patients dropped out from the Cross-National Collaborative Panic Study (1992). In a review of longer-term treatment with imipramine, 84% of patients were found to have experienced side effects (Noyes et al. 1989). Of the total study population, side effects were present but not distressing in 34% of patients, distressing but tolerable in 23% of patients, very distressing in 10% of patients, and intolerable in 17% of patients. Thirty-four percent of patients gained weight. Many of these side effects can be handled by

a reduction in dosage, but the high percentage of side effects suggests a major limitation of the use of imipramine.

Desipramine would theoretically work as well as imipramine because it is the main metabolite of imipramine. However, imipramine may be more serotonergic than desipramine, which may give it greater efficacy, assuming that the serotonin system is important in panic disorder. In European studies, clomipramine has been shown to be effective for treatment of panic (Amin et al. 1977). Amitriptyline and nortriptyline may also be effective, but fewer and less well-designed studies are available (Ballenger 1986). Trazodone has been shown to be less effective than imipramine or alprazolam (Charney et al. 1986). Bupropion, an atypical antidepressant, and maprotiline, a noradrenaline uptake inhibitor, do not appear to be effective (Den Boer and Westenberg 1988; Sheehan et al. 1983).

Monoamine oxidase inhibitors (MAOIs) are also effective antipanic and antiphobic agents (Table 31–2). Of the three available MAOIs, phenelzine has been studied most extensively and has been shown to be as efficacious as imipramine. Isocarboxazid and tranylcypromine are probably also effective. Recently, so-called reversible and selective MAOIs with serotonin reuptake inhibitory properties have been developed. In comparison with irreversible nonselective MAOIs, such drugs have reduced tyramine-potentiating effects. The efficacy of these agents for panic disorder is now being evaluated in clinical trials.

The 5-hydroxyindoleacetic acid (5-HIAA) reuptake inhibitors (e.g., fluoxetine, sertraline, paroxetine, and fluvoxamine) may prove to be effective

---

Table 31–1. Advantages and disadvantages of tricyclic antidepressants for anxiety disorders

Advantages	Disadvantages
Single daily dose	Delayed onset of action
Antidepressant	Activation syndrome
Generics available	Side effects
Well-studied	Anticholinergic
	Orthostatic hypotension
	Weight gain
	? Blood pressure increase
	Overdosage

Table 31–2. Advantages and disadvantages of classic monoamine oxidase inhibitors (MAOIs) for anxiety disorders

Advantages	Disadvantages
Single daily dose	Delayed onset of action
Antidepressant	Diet or hypertensive crises
Generics available	Hyperpyrexic reactions
	Insomnia
	Side effects
	Anticholinergic
	Orthostatic hypotension
	Weight gain
	Overdosage

antipanic agents. There is increasing evidence of the role of serotonin (5-HT) in anxiety disorders (Coplan et al. 1992). A few small sample and uncontrolled studies have suggested that these agents may reduce frequency of panic attacks (Schneier et al. 1990). For instance, 60 patients with panic disorder were randomized to 8 weeks fluvoxamine (150 mg) or ritanserin (a specific 5-HT$_2$ receptor antagonist). Fluvoxamine was associated with a significant decrease in panic attacks and avoidance; ritanserin was ineffective (Den Boer and Westenberg 1990). Black and colleagues (1993) randomized 75 patients with moderate to severe panic disorder to 8 weeks of fluvoxamine, cognitive therapy, or placebo. Fluvoxamine produced a significant reduction in clinical anxiety in clinicians' ratings of global improvement in panic attack frequency and significantly reduced disability compared with placebo. Fluvoxamine also was superior to cognitive therapy on many of the measures. Controlled clinical trials of several 5-HIAA drugs are now under way. These agents may prove to be the drug of choice for panic disorder (Table 31–3). Anxious patients sometimes require a lower initial dose, at least of fluoxetine.

Benzodiazepines

Benzodiazepines are effective for reducing panic attack, phobic behavior, and anticipatory anxiety. Of the many benzodiazepines, alprazolam has been most extensively studied, with the results of two large cross-national trials reported (Ballenger et al. 1988; Cross-National Collaborative Panic Study 1992). In the first large multicenter trial, 526 patients were randomized to alprazolam or placebo. Of these, 86% of the alprazolam subjects completed the trial, compared with only 50% of the placebo subjects. At the primary comparison point (week 4 of the study), 82% of the subjects receiving alprazolam were considered moderately improved or better versus 42% of the pla-

cebo group. At that point, 50% of the alprazolam group versus 28% of placebo subjects were free of panic attacks. For those subjects who completed the trial, there was no significant difference in total number of panic attacks or in disability ratings between alprazolam or placebo, although the former were much less fearful and avoidant than the latter.

As noted previously, in the Cross-National Collaborative Panic Study, Phase 2, which compared imipramine and alprazolam with placebo, there was a significant placebo effect, particularly for frequency of panic attacks. However, there was also a high placebo dropout rate: only 56% of the placebo patients completed the study, compared with 70% of the patients treated with imipramine and 83% of those treated with alprazolam. The high placebo dropout rate makes it difficult to detect differences between the active medications and placebo. The placebo subjects who dropped out did so largely because they were not improving; the placebo patients who remained were presumably a bias sample.

Schweizer and colleagues (1993) randomized 106 patients with panic disorder into an acute 8-week treatment phase followed by 6 months of maintenance treatment. Significantly more patients treated with alprazolam than with imipramine or placebo remained in therapy and experienced panic attack and phobia relief during the acute treatment phase. Of note, 11% of the panic patients, 41% of the imipramine patients, and 57% of the placebo patients dropped out. During the maintenance phase, neither tolerance nor daily dose increase of alprazolam was observed, and the patients maintained their treatment gains. The weight of evidence suggests that alprazolam is an effective antipanic and antiphobic agent, at least as long as it is being used.

Benzodiazepines are probably equally effective at comparable doses. For example, diazepam is roughly one-tenth as effective as alprazolam; if given at doses of 20–60 mg, it appears to be as effective as alprazolam (Dunner et al. 1986). However, at those doses, diazepam causes relatively more sedation than alprazolam, and this side effect may limit its usefulness. Clonazepam has also been shown to be effective. It is as potent as alprazolam and has the advantage of a longer half-life. At the end of one trial, 50%, 46%, and 14% of subjects on clonazepam, alprazolam, and placebo, respectively, were free of panic attacks (Tesar et al. 1991). The mean dose of clonazepam was 2.5 mg (maximum dose was 6 mg).

Table 31–3. Advantages and disadvantages of 5-HIAA–reuptake inhibitors for anxiety disorders

Advantages	Disadvantages
Single daily dose	Delayed onset of action
Antidepressant	Few well-controlled studies
No dependence or withdrawal	Side effects
	Insomnia
	Irritability

Lorazepam (mean daily dose of 7 mg) was as effective as alprazolam in one study (Schweizer et al. 1990).

The choice of a benzodiazepine, then, depends on potency, half-life, and evidence of effectiveness from clinical studies. Although effective, alprazolam has the disadvantage of a short half-life. Thus, frequent dosing may be necessary; some patients complain of breakthrough anxiety, either in the morning or between doses. A sustained release pill is now being evaluated that may reduce this problem. Alprazolam should be initiated at 0.25–0.5 mg tid. Doses should be increased every 4 to 6 days as needed and tolerated. Clonazepam should be initiated at 0.5 tablet per day, and then increased every 3 to 5 days to therapeutic goals. Some investigators recommend that the medication should be increased until the patient is symptom free. However, one study found no relationship between dose and outcome. In a study of alprazolam, 13 out of 14 patients with a serum level of 15–77 ng/ml, achieved with doses of 1–6 mg/day, reached zero panic attacks at the end of the study (Wincor et al. 1991). A study of alprazolam at 2 mg or 6 mg compared with placebo found only a few statistically significant differences between the two groups, and both were better than placebo (Lydiard et al. 1992). Furthermore, higher doses require longer withdrawal.

Benzodiazepines should also be used cautiously in elderly patients. Elderly people have altered pharmacokinetics and pharmacodynamics, concomitant illness, reduced compliance, and increased sensitivity to drugs (Salzman 1990). Older patients may be more sensitive to dependence, rebound, and memory impairment. They are more likely to exhibit increased sedation, an increased tendency toward falls, psychomotor dyscoordination, and decreased concentration. Among the drugs with a short half-life, high-potency compounds (e.g., lorazepam, alprazolam) may be more toxic than low-potency compounds (e.g., oxazepam) in elderly patients.

Benzodiazepines have a number of disadvantages over antidepressants (Table 31–4). They often produce sedation, increase the effects of alcohol, can produce dyscoordination, and are associated with dependence and withdrawal (Busto et al. 1986). Benzodiazepine withdrawal occurs even after only 4–8 weeks of use. Moreover, studies suggest that withdrawal-like phenomena can be precipitated by benzodiazepine receptor antagonists after as little as

1 day of benzodiazepine administration (Spealman 1986).

If benzodiazepines have been used for a few weeks or more, then a careful plan of discontinuation is needed. Patients can have severe panic attacks during the rebound. With a rapid dosage taper, rebound occurred in 35% of patients in the Cross-National Trial (Pecknold et al. 1988). Withdrawal syndrome can be sufficiently severe to cause epileptic seizures, confusion, and psychotic symptoms (Noyes et al. 1986; Owen and Tyrer 1983; Taylor and Arnow 1988). For most patients, withdrawal symptoms are more diffuse, including anxiety, panic, tremor, muscle twitching, perceptual disturbances, and depersonalization (Busto et al. 1986; Owen and Tyrer 1983; Taylor and Arnow 1988). Possibly because of these side effects, many patients are reluctant to stop the benzodiazepines. Rickels and colleagues (1993) attempted to withdraw 27 patients who had been on alprazolam for 6 months or longer. Of these, only 17 were withdrawn. One year later, 8 of 9 patients who were not able to withdraw were still taking medication, and 8 of 17 of those who had stopped had resumed taking medication.

Benzodiazepines should be withdrawn gradually (Noyes et al. 1988), perhaps over 4 months. With a slow, flexible taper, Pecknold (1988) found no rebound and only 7% of patients had clinically significant withdrawal symptoms. Benzodiazepine doses should be reduced more slowly at the end of the taper (Rickels et al. 1990). In withdrawing patients from alprazolam, it may be easier to switch patients to clonazepam, because clonazepam can be given in fewer doses (Patterson 1990).

Upon discontinuation of benzodiazepines, some patients seem to have a rebound of anxiety, which is a different phenomenon than withdrawal. Withdrawal represents the return of neurochemical systems to baseline levels and may include new

Table 31–4. Advantages and disadvantages of benzodiazepines for anxiety disorders

Advantages	Disadvantages
Rapid onset	Dependence and withdrawal
Well-tolerated	Sedation
Generics available	Interactions with alcohol
Few drug-drug interactions	Impair motor coordination
Little effect on cardio-vascular status	Short-term memory impairment

symptoms, such as seizures. Rebound is usually defined as an occurrence of a previously existing symptom at a greater-than-pretreatment level during the discontinuation period (Ballenger 1992). Withdrawal is often associated with weakness and insomnia, two symptoms that are not present in most nondepressed anxious patients. Previous discontinuous exposure to benzodiazepines might sensitize patients to subsequent withdrawal effects (Rickels et al. 1990). Withdrawal symptoms are usually less severe than the initial anxiety symptoms. They are usually significantly reduced by the end of the first week of withdrawal and are mostly gone by the end of the second postdiscontinuation week. Thus, symptoms that persist 3 weeks after patients have been off medication usually represent either a return of the original anxiety or the continuation of anxiety that has not been adequately treated.

Previous drug or alcohol abuse is a risk factor for dependence and increased use of benzodiazepines (Haskell et al. 1986; Lennane 1986). Such a history is not an absolute contraindication to their use, but benzodiazepines should be used with particular caution in this population. When considering benzodiazepine use with chronically anxious patients, the patient's diagnosis should be documented, his or her status and medication carefully monitored and documented, and other forms of therapy applied concurrently.

Other Medications

Buspirone, which may have antianxiety properties, does not appear to be effective for panic disorder (Sheehan et al. 1990). Neuroleptics are generally not useful because of their acute and long-term toxicity, and they may even exacerbate panic symptoms.

Concomitant Psychotherapy

Cognitive-behavioral approaches have been shown to significantly reduce panic attacks and avoidance and have been the most extensively evaluated (Barlow 1988, 1990; Shear et al. 1991a, 1991b; Taylor and Arnow 1988; Welkowitz et al. 1991; Zinbarg et al. 1992). Other psychological therapies have also been shown to be effective, at least in small sample studies (Arnow et al. 1988; Ost 1988). The combination of cognitive therapy with behavior therapy for avoidance is a relatively recent development (Taylor and Arnow 1988) and seems to have enhanced the outcome in patients with panic but relatively little avoid-

ance. The proper application of cognitive-behavioral therapy requires a careful analysis of the patient's individual cognitions and behaviors, practice of alternative cognitions, and exposure to the feared situations (usually in a gradual fashion), with attention to generalization and maintenance of treatment. Most cognitive therapy interventions require at least 12–18 hours of treatment spaced over 3–6 months with follow-up sessions to deal with relapse.

As mentioned previously, Black and colleagues (1993) compared fluvoxamine, cognitive therapy, and placebo and found that fluvoxamine was superior to cognitive therapy on many of the ratings, whereas cognitive therapy was not superior to fluvoxamine on any rating. Furthermore, fluvoxamine produced improvement earlier than cognitive therapy. Although the cognitive therapy seemed to be properly conducted, it was less effective than has been reported with other studies. Klosko and colleagues (1990) compared alprazolam and behavior therapy in the treatment of panic disorder. Patients were randomized to cognitive therapy, alprazolam, or placebo, or they became waiting-list control subjects. The cognitive therapy group was significantly more effective than placebo and waiting-list conditions on most measures; the alprazolam group was not significantly different from cognitive therapy or placebo. It appears that both medication and cognitive-behavioral therapy are effective for reducing symptoms and disability associated with panic disorder.

Several studies have found that imipramine combined with cognitive-behavioral therapy works better than either alone (Telch et al. 1985). However, Marks and Swinson (1990) found no advantage for alprazolam combined with exposure therapy, and Klosko and colleagues (1990) have argued that benzodiazepines may impede the effects of behavior therapy. A large National Institute of Mental Health trial is now under way to clarify the relative contributions of cognitive-behavioral therapy and imipramine for panic disorder.

In our experience, thoughtful integration of cognitive-behavioral therapy and pharmacotherapy produces an optimal outcome (Taylor and Arnow 1988). For instance, many patients require some medication before they are able to undertake intensive exposure therapy. Psychological interventions can facilitate withdrawal of medication and prepare patients for long-term treatment.

■ Long-Term Treatment

Panic disorder is a chronic, long-term condition, and the length of pharmacological treatment remains controversial. Most of the studies reported above have only focused on short-term outcomes. Current clinical practice generally involves a trial of 3–6 months of an effective medication. More controversial is continued therapy for an additional 6–12 months or longer. We do know that relapse rates are very high after the medication has been discontinued. Depending on the medication, concomitant psychological treatment, the length of follow-up, and the criteria, relapse rates of 20%–80% have been reported (Ballenger 1992). With medication alone, probably less than one-half of patients remain well after medication has been discontinued for 6 months or longer. Ballenger (1992) has argued that the medications that are shown to be effective have few adverse physical effects; therefore, the length of treatment should be based only on questions of effectiveness.

In several series of panic disorder patients, there was no evidence of patients developing an abusive pattern during long-term use of benzodiazepines to treat panic disorder symptoms (Rifkin et al. 1989). The evidence that patients with depression (another long-term therapy) do much better with maintenance medication should also be considered (Kupfer et al. 1992). In light of the controversies surrounding long-term medication use, and because the medication may no longer be effective, it is good practice to have patients undergo a routine discontinuation of the medication after 6 months to a year, especially if they are on benzodiazepines. Patients should remain off the medication for at least a month before being restarted on it, to give adequate time for adjustment following discontinuation.

Cognitive-behavioral therapy interventions prepare patients for possible relapses by suggesting that they should do the following: prepare for, and even expect, relapses; practice the cognitive-behavioral techniques that they have used if relapse occurs; and seek help immediately if they are not able to accept the relapse symptoms or experience a return of avoidance, increased disability, or impairment. The medication previously prescribed is usually reinstated if it was successful, or a new medication is prescribed if it might have an advantage over the old medication.

■ GENERALIZED ANXIETY DISORDER

Generalized anxiety disorder (GAD), like panic disorder, is common, occurring in at least 2%–3% of the population (Weissman et al. 1978). The main features of GAD are chronic cognitive, behavioral, symptomatic, and physiological symptoms of hyperarousal and anxiety. GAD commonly occurs with other anxiety disorders and depression, and the latter should always be entertained when symptoms of GAD are present. When depression or panic disorder are present, they should be treated first.

Benzodiazepines have been the mainstay of treatment for patients with GAD. Benzodiazepines are effective in the short run for reducing symptoms of GAD. Different types of benzodiazepines at equivalent doses are equally effective for generalized anxiety, and the agent used should be chosen on the basis of potency, half-life, and side effects.

The issues discussed previously regarding the use of benzodiazepines with panic disorder apply to GAD. In 1980, after reviewing studies on benzodiazepine effects, the British Medical Association concluded that the effects of such drugs do not persist beyond 3–4 months (Committee on the Review of Medicine 1980). However, other experts have argued that benzodiazepines are effective for much longer. For instance, Haskell and colleagues (1986) studied 194 patients with a history of diazepam use. The patients on long-term diazepam treatment were as symptomatic as patients presenting for anxiety treatment. Yet 158 of the 194 had tried to stop at some time and, of these, 142 reported the reemergence of anxiety symptoms. However, the patients believed that they were deriving benefit from treatment.

Rickels and colleagues (1991) followed 123 patients who had participated in a benzodiazepine discontinuation program. At follow-up, a mean of 2.9 years later, 55 (45%) of the patients were not taking benzodiazepines. Discontinuing chronic benzodiazepine use did not result in significant worsening of anxious or depressive symptoms. Of these, 25% still had substantial levels of anxiety. The study provides more evidence that GAD is chronic or recurrent and may benefit from long-term treatment. However, the use of benzodiazepines for long-term treatment remains controversial. Having patients discontinue benzodiazepines allows for adequate reassessment and institution of new treatments (Rickels et al. 1991).

The problems with benzodiazepines have created an intensive search for alternative agents effective in reducing symptoms of GAD. Buspirone, an azaperone derivative and a 5-HT$_{1A}$ partial agonist, has been shown to be as effective as benzodiazepines and significantly better than placebo in controlled clinical trials (Goldberg and Finnerty 1979; Napoliello 1986; Rickels et al. 1982; Wheatley 1982) at doses of 20–40 mg. In these trials, improvement continued from pretreatment through the fourth week of treatment and paralleled but was somewhat slower than that of the benzodiazepines (Rickels et al. 1990).

In a 40-month follow-up of 34 patients participating in a comparison of buspirone and clorazepate, 30% of the patients treated with clorazepate were still taking a benzodiazepine regularly, and 25% were taking them on an as-needed basis, but none of those treated with buspirone were still receiving medication (Sussman 1993). This suggests that buspirone can be discontinued more easily than benzodiazepines. Buspirone produces less drowsiness, psychomotor impairment, and alcohol potentiation and has less potential for addiction or abuse compared with benzodiazepines. Buspirone has slow onset (its major drawback) and does not have anticonvulsive effects. A comparison between alprazolam and buspirone found both to be equally effective for GAD and superior to placebo (Enkelmann 1991). The buspirone group had a higher dropout rate than alprazolam (36% versus 13%). Buspirone seems to be most helpful in treating anxious patients who do not demand immediate relief of symptoms, including patients who have taken benzodiazepines (Rickels 1990). A meta-analysis of GAD treatment studies found that diazepam had a somewhat greater effect than buspirone (Cox et al. 1992). Some researchers add buspirone to reduce rebound symptoms during patients' discontinuation from benzodiazepines (Udelman and Udelman 1990). Buspirone will not block the potential serious withdrawal effects of benzodiazepines and should not be used instead of a gradual benzodiazepine withdrawal.

An important and perhaps overlooked finding is that imipramine may have anxiolytic effects (Hoehn-Saric et al. 1988; Kahn et al. 1986; McLeod et al. 1990). Imipramine had a significant effect on reducing anticipatory anxiety in the cross-national alprazolam and imipramine trial, but the effect was only significantly different by the eighth week of treatment. Lower doses than used for treatment of panic disorder are often effective. Treatment effectiveness may not occur until patients have been on medication for a month or longer.

Studies of serotonin reuptake blockers are under way, and these medications may prove to have significant antianxiety effects. Clomipramine has been shown to be effective in at least one uncontrolled study (Wingerson et al. 1992).

A number of new antianxiety agents are being developed. The partial benzodiazepine receptor agonists bretazenil and abecarnil have been shown to have some antianxiety effects (Ballenger et al. 1992; Haefely et al. 1992). These newer agents may have the advantages of benzodiazepines, such as less risk of physical dependence. However, it is still too early to know how useful they will be in treating anxiety disorders.

The cognitive-behavioral treatment of GAD has been less well evaluated than that of panic disorder. A combination of relaxation and related techniques aimed at decreasing hyperarousal—cognitive-behavioral therapy, skills training and coping, and alteration in life-style factors, as appropriate—are often beneficial (Kabat-Zinn et al. 1992; Taylor 1978; Taylor and Arnow 1988), but long-term controlled studies are lacking. Traditional psychodynamic therapies are often effective in alleviating symptoms of chronic anxiety.

■ SOCIAL PHOBIA

Social phobia is a common, disabling, and often unrecognized anxiety disorder, occurring in about 1%–2% of the population (Myers et al. 1984). Although social phobia shares many features of panic disorder and often occurs with it, it has separate phenomenological features. For instance, the five most common fears of people with social phobia are speaking before a group, eating in public, writing in public, using public lavatories, and being stared at or the center of attention; the five most common fears of panic disorder are driving or traveling, stores, crowds, restaurants, and elevators (Uhde et al. 1991). People with social phobia do not have spontaneous panic attacks and don't panic when they are alone or asleep. Fear of negative evaluation is the critical cognitive feature of social phobia. Many people with social phobia also have avoidant personality disorder, characterized by chronic patterns of shyness and avoidance. Social phobia is often quite disabling and results in extreme anxiety, avoidance, work and social impairment, depression, and substance abuse (Liebowitz et al. 1985).

The pharmacological treatment of social phobia has lagged behind the treatment of other anxiety disorders. Most of the pharmacological studies are small in scale and uncontrolled. High-potency benzodiazepines, particularly alprazolam and clonazepam, have been reported to produce improvement in symptoms of social phobia (Lydiard et al. 1988; Reiter et al. 1990). For instance, in an uncontrolled study of 26 patients (most of whom had other diagnoses and had received various previous treatments), 85% of patients showed moderate to significant improvement at doses of clonazepam of 0.5–5.0 mg/day, with the mean dose being 2.1 (Davidson et al. 1991).

Liebowitz and colleagues (1988) decided to use MAOIs to treat social phobia after observing that MAOIs are of use in a variety of phobias and reduce excessive interpersonal sensitivity in patients with atypical depression. Because such sensitivity to criticism is typical of people with social phobia, it made sense to determine if an MAOI would be effective for this condition. In a sample of 74 patients, phenelzine was superior to both atenolol and placebo with no significant differences between the latter two agents (Liebowitz et al. 1992). There is also evidence that moclobemide, an experimental reversible inhibitor of MAO, may also be effective for social phobia (Liebowitz et al. 1991; Versiani et al. 1992). In a controlled trial with 45 patients randomized to phenelzine, alprazolam, or placebo for 23 weeks, all 3 groups demonstrated improvement, and there were no differences in self-reported data (Uhde et al. 1991). However, subjects who had been treated with alprazolam or phenelzine did better on a clinician-rated work and social disability scale. After a 4-week drug-free period, the phenelzine-treated group remained significantly improved compared with the placebo group on this measure, but the alprazolam group did not differ from placebo.

β-blockers have also been used in treatment of social phobia, with mixed results. For performance anxiety, β-blockers have been shown to benefit activities such as pistol shooting, bowling, playing stringed instruments, and public speaking (Liebowitz et al. 1991). Doses of propranolol of 10–40 mg before

such performances can often reduce fear. The early β-blocker studies focused on performance anxiety, and this subgroup of people with social phobia may respond differently from individuals with generalized social fears. As noted previously, Liebowitz and colleagues found that atenolol had no effect on treatment of social phobia. A small controlled trial found no effects of propranolol and placebo in patients receiving behavioral treatment (Falloon et al. 1981).

Uncontrolled trials have also found some benefits from buspirone in social phobia in doses up to 60 mg/day (Liebowitz et al. 1991). Buspirone had no effect on exposure therapy in a controlled clinical trial (Clark and Agras 1991). Fluoxetine has also been reported to be effective in case reports (Black et al. 1992). Further controlled trials of both drugs are needed.

As with panic disorder, cognitive-behavioral therapy is an appropriate adjunctive treatment to psychopharmacology. A major line of basic research in behavioral therapy has been devoted to one type of social phobia—that of speech phobia. This research has led to a number of treatment approaches including systematic desensitization, social skills training, imaginal flooding, applied relaxation training, graduated exposure, anxiety management, and a variety of cognitive-restructuring procedures (i.e., self-instructional training, rational-emotive therapy, and cognitive-behavioral group therapy; Liebowitz et al. 1985). These approaches are often effective, at least for the more circumscribed phobias (Heimberg and Barlow 1991).

Several studies have found that pharmacological treatments did not improve outcome over cognitive-behavioral therapy alone. For instance, concomitant use of buspirone did not improve outcome of exposure therapy with performance phobia, or propranolol did not improve outcome with social skills training (Clark and Agras 1991; Stravynksi et al. 1982). This is not surprising, because buspirone has not been shown to be an effective medication for social phobia. In another study, cognitive-behavioral treatment programs were compared with treatment by phenelzine, alprazolam, or placebo for subjects with social phobia (Gelernter et al. 1991). All patients improved in all groups. Patients treated with phenelzine plus self-exposure showed greater improvement than other groups did in a measure of trait anxiety. On one fear measure, patients treated with cognitive-behavioral group therapy showed additional improvement from the posttest to follow-up assessment, whereas patients treated with alprazolam plus exposure showed deterioration in this measure. Comparative studies are needed before the relative benefits of psychopharmacological and psychological treatments alone and in combination are known.

■ OBSESSIVE-COMPULSIVE DISORDER

Obsessive-compulsive disorder (OCD) is much more common than formerly thought, with a 6-month point prevalence of 1%–2% and a lifetime prevalence of 2%–3% (Myers et al. 1984; Robins et al. 1984). Until recently, therapists treating OCD patients were often frustrated by the lack of effective treatments. Now, with the availability of clomipramine in this country and the development of many new psychopharmacological agents, many patients can have some relief from their symptoms.

Clomipramine is the drug of choice for the treatment of OCD. Case reports of the value of clomipramine appeared more than 20 years ago. Since then, its effectiveness has been confirmed in a number of double-blind trials in OCD (Goodman et al. 1992). At the end of one large trial, obsessive and compulsive symptoms had decreased 35%–42% on the Yale-Brown Obsessive-Compulsive Scale (Kim et al. 1990), the standard instrument for measuring improvement, compared to 2%–5% in placebo groups (Clomipramine Collaborative Study Group 1991). Significant improvement was generally not apparent until after about 6 weeks of clomipramine treatment, with doses up to 300 mg. Fewer than 20% of patients discontinued clomipramine prematurely because of side effects. Although few studies have compared clomipramine to other antidepressants, a consistent pattern seems to emerge. Drugs that are less potent blockers of serotonin reuptake than clomipramine are generally ineffective in treatment of OCD. For instance, clomipramine was shown to be more effective than nortriptyline (Thoren et al. 1980) or desipramine (Leonard et al. 1988).

The effectiveness of clomipramine has led the way to the study of newer, potent selective serotonin reuptake inhibitors (SSRIs) for treating OCD. There are now at least four SSRIs in various phases of study: fluvoxamine, fluoxetine, sertraline, and paroxetine.

Thus far, only the results of small-scale studies have been reported. In both single-blind and controlled studies, fluvoxamine (up to 300 mg/day) has been shown effective in reducing obsessive-compulsive symptoms (Goodman et al. 1989; Perse et al. 1988). Clinically meaningful improvement often did not occur until about 6 to 8 weeks of treatment.

Fluoxetine has also been shown to be effective, at least in a 12-week open trial. Fluoxetine was gradually increased as tolerated to a maximum mean daily dose of about 75 mg (Jenike et al. 1989). It was not clear from the trial if patients would respond at lower doses if given more time. A preliminary fixed-dose study comparing 10 weeks of single daily doses of 20 mg, 40 mg, or 60 mg of fluoxetine with placebo did not find a clear-cut advantage of the 40- or 60-mg doses over the 20-mg dose (Wheadon 1991). Fluoxetine has also been shown to be superior to desipramine (Goodman et al. 1990). Sertraline has also been studied in at least one double-blind trial. The magnitude of the drug effect in this trial was less than that typically observed in clomipramine and fluvoxamine studies, perhaps because of higher-than-expected placebo response and a relatively short drug treatment—8 weeks (Chouinard et al. 1990). Fluoxetine has recently received U.S. Food and Drug Administration approval for treating OCD.

If patients do not respond to one SSRI at adequate doses, then another should be tried. If a patient shows a partial response, then it may be appropriate to begin a combined treatment. At this point in the history of OCD, combined treatments are largely based on case reports and single-case design, rather than rigorous studies (Jefferson, in press). Currently recommended strategies add agents to ongoing SSRI therapy that may modify serotonergic function, such as buspirone, lithium, or fenfluramine. In an open-label study, Hollander and colleagues (1990) reported that the addition of the serotonin releaser and reuptake blocker fenfluramine to ongoing treatment with various SSRIs led to improvement in OCD symptoms in 6 of 7 patients. The use of lithium to treat OCD has been more equivocal. One study reported improvement in OCD with 3 of 4 patients treated with fluoxetine and lithium, but no effective treatment was found with 16 patients who had demonstrated a partial response to clomipramine (Pigott et al. 1991). Only 3 of 30 patients improved when lithium was added to fluvoxamine-refractory patients (McDougle et al. 1991).

Buspirone has been studied in treatment-refractory OCD patients. The results have been mixed; some studies show a benefit and others show none (Goodman et al. 1992). Interestingly, a small study found that buspirone alone was equal in efficacy to clomipramine (Pato et al. 1991). Buspirone might be added for patients on SSRIs who are anxious.

Before the advent of the SSRI drugs, neuroleptics were used to treat OCD, often to little effect. However, in carefully selected patients, neuroleptics may be of use, particularly if the patient has tics (such as Tourette's disorder), delusions, or personality disorder (Goodman et al. 1992). The clinician should be wary about exposing patients to the risk of chronic neuroleptic treatment.

Clonazepam has been used with OCD to some effect (Hewlett et al. 1990). Trazodone has been shown to potentiate fluoxetine in patients with depression (Nierenberg et al. 1992) and may be useful as an adjunct to fluoxetine, but it does not seem to be effective by itself (Pigott et al. 1992).

The length of psychopharmacological treatment for OCD remains an unsolved problem. OCD is a chronic illness, and patients will probably require medication indefinitely. Relapse after discontinuation of medications is likely (e.g., Pato et al. 1988).

Behavioral treatments may provide a better long-term result than psychopharmacological ones. Forty-seven percent ($n = 16$) of 34 patients who had been treated 6 years earlier with exposure therapy for 3 or 6 weeks and with clomipramine or placebo for 36 weeks remained much improved (O'Sullivan et al. 1991). The few patients who were taking TCAs at follow-up assessment were no more improved than those who were medication free or were taking other drugs, and the patients given clomipramine during treatment were no more improved at follow-up than their placebo-taking counterparts. The study suggests that psychopharmacology treatment might enhance psychological therapies. However, one study found no benefit of adding imipramine to exposure therapy (Foa et al. 1992).

POSTTRAUMATIC STRESS DISORDER

Posttraumatic stress disorder (PTSD) has a lifetime prevalence of at least 1% (Helzer et al. 1987). The psychopharmacological treatment of PTSD is only in its early research stages and is reviewed only briefly here.

Open studies of TCAs have found some benefit with some PTSD symptoms for various TCAs (Burstein 1984; Falcon et al. 1985; Kauffman et al. 1987), but controlled trials have not substantiated the benefits suggested in the open trials. For instance, a double-blind placebo-controlled trial of amitriptyline (average dose = 169 mg/day) found improvement on ratings of the Hamilton Rating Scale for Depression (Hamilton 1960) by 8 weeks for 42 veterans with PTSD (Davidson et al. 1987). However, 64% of the patients who received amitriptyline and 72% of the patients who received placebo still met the diagnostic criteria for PTSD after treatment. In a double-blind placebo-controlled crossover study, desipramine at dosages up to 200 mg for a maximum of 4 weeks had no significant effect on PTSD symptomatology (Reist et al. 1989). Unfortunately, these controlled trials do not substantiate the benefits suggested in the open trials.

MAOIs have also been shown to be effective in open trials (Davidson et al. 1987; Hogben and Cornfield 1981; Shen and Park 1983; Van der Kolk 1983). An 8-week, double-blind, randomized comparison of imipramine (average dose = 240 mg/day), phenelzine (average dose = 71 mg/day), and placebo was conducted with 34 veterans (Frank et al. 1988). Patients in both active-drug groups improved especially for the symptoms of nightmares, flashbacks, and intrusive recollections, but no change was observed for symptoms of avoidance. Overall, the patients who received phenelzine had greater improvement (but not significantly so) than those patients who received imipramine.

Inhibitors of adrenergic activity (e.g., propranolol, clonidine) have also been used with some success. However, these medications seem to have been more effective in combination with TCAs (Kinzie and Leung 1989).

Many other medications have been tried in the treatment of PTSD. On the assumption that kindling plays an important pathophysiological role in PTSD, agents that reduce kindling (e.g., carbamazepine, lithium, valproate) have been tried. Carbamazepine was successful in reducing aggressive outbursts and anger in veterans with PTSD (Lipper et al. 1986; Wolf et al. 1988). Lithium, which affects multiple neurotransmitter systems, has been effective in open-label studies of relatively few patients (Bunney et al. 1987; Kitchner and Greenstein 1985). In an open clinical trial, 10 of 16 Vietnam veterans showed significant improvement after treatment with valproate (Fesler 1991). Benzodiazepines may improve some symptoms but have been associated with an increase in anger (Feldman 1987). There have been no published reports on the use of SSRIs.

After reviewing the psychopharmacological studies of PTSD, Silver and colleagues (1990) concluded that the positive symptoms of PTSD (e.g., reexperiencing of the event and increased arousal) often respond to medication, whereas negative symptoms (e.g., avoidance and withdrawal) respond poorly. When there is no comorbid condition, antidepressant medications seem to be the initial drug of choice. Both TCAs and MAOIs appear effective. β-blockers should be considered in treatment of patients with persistent symptoms of autonomic arousal if there are no medical contraindications. Medications that have been shown to possess antiaggressive properties can be used in patients who have extreme anger or irritability.

■ CONCLUSION

Psychopharmacological treatment can reduce the symptoms and disability of most patients with anxiety disorders. Perhaps the most impressive recent treatment advance in this area is the discovery that many anxiety disorders can be effectively treated with SSRIs. The demonstration that clomipramine and fluoxetine can help patients with OCD provides new hope for those who have this once difficult to treat disorder.

■ REFERENCES

American Psychiatric Association: Diagnostic and Statistical Manual of Mental Disorders, 3rd Edition. Washington, DC, American Psychiatric Association, 1980

Amin MM, Ban TA, Pecknold JC, et al: Clomipramine (Anafranil) and behaviour therapy in obsessive-compulsive and phobic disorders. J Int Med Res 5 (suppl 5):33–37, 1977

Arnow BA, Taylor CB, Agras WS, et al: Enhancing agoraphobia treatment outcome by changing cou-

ple communication patterns. Behavior Therapy 16:452–467, 1988

Ballenger JC: Pharmacotherapy of the panic disorders. J Clin Psychiatry 47 (6, suppl):27–32, 1986

Ballenger JC: Long-term pharmacologic treatment of panic disorder. J Clin Psychiatry 2 (suppl):18–23, 1991

Ballenger JC: Medication discontinuation in panic disorder. J Clin Psychiatry 53 (suppl 3):26–31, 1992

Ballenger JC, Burrows G, DuPont R, et al: Alprazolam in panic disorder and agoraphobia—results from a multicenter trial, I: efficacy in short-term treatment. Arch Gen Psychiatry 45:413–422, 1988

Ballenger JC, McDonald S, Noyes R Jr, et al: The first double-blind, placebo-controlled trial of a partial benzodiazepine agonist, abecarnil (ZK 112-119), in generalized anxiety disorder. Adv Biochem Psychopharmacol 47:431–437, 1992

Barlow DH: Anxiety and its Disorders. New York, Guilford, 1988

Barlow DH: Long-term outcome for patients with panic disorder treated with cognitive/behavioral treatment. J Clin Psychiatry 51 (suppl):17–23, 1990

Black B, Uhde TW, Tancer ME: Fluoxetine for the treatment of social phobia. J Clin Psychopharmacol 12:293–295, 1992

Black D, Wesner R, Bowers W, et al: A comparison of fluvoxamine, cognitive therapy, and placebo in the treatment of panic disorder. Arch Gen Psychiatry 50:44–50, 1993

Bunney WE Jr, Garland-Bunney GL: Mechanisms of action of lithium in affective illness: basic and clinical implications, in Psychopharmacology: The Third Generation of Progress. Edited by Meltzer HY. New York, Raven, 1987, pp 533–565

Burstein A: Treatment of post-traumatic stress disorder with imipramine. Psychosomatics 25:681–687, 1984

Busto U, Sellers EM, Naranjo CA, et al: Withdrawal reaction after long-term therapeutic use of benzodiazepines. N Engl J Med 315:854–659, 1986

Charney DS, Woods SW, Goodman WK, et al: Drug treatment of panic disorder: the comparative efficacy of imipramine, alprazolam, and trazodone. J Clin Psychiatry 47:580–586, 1986

Chouinard G, Goodman W, Greist J, et al: Obsessive-compulsive disorder—treatment with sertraline: a multicenter study. Psychopharmacol Bull 26:279–284, 1990

Clark DB, Agras WS: The assessment and treatment

of performance anxiety in musicians. Am J Psychiatry 148:598–605, 1991

Clomipramine Collaborative Study Group: Clomipramine in the treatment of patients with obsessive-compulsive disorder. Arch Gen Psychiatry 48:730–738, 1991

Committee on the Review of Medicine: Systematic review of the benzodiazepines. BMJ 1:910–912, 1980

Coplan JD, Gorman JM, Klein DF: Serotonin related functions in panic-anxiety: a critical overview. Neuropsychopharmacology 6:189–200, 1992

Cox BJ, Swinson RP, Lee PS: Meta-analysis of anxiety disorder treatment studies [letter]. J Clin Psychopharmacol 12:300–301, 1992

Cross-National Collaborative Panic Study, Second Phase Investigators: Drug treatment of panic disorder: comparative efficacy of alprazolam, imipramine, and placebo. Br J Psychiatry 160:191–202, 1992

Davidson J, Walker JI, Kilts C: A pilot study of phenelzine in the treatment of post-traumatic stress disorder. Br J Psychiatry 150:252–255, 1987

Davidson JRT, Ford SM, Smith RD, et al: Long-term treatment of social phobia with clonazepam. J Clin Psychiatry 52 (11, suppl):16–20, 1991

Den Boer JA, Westenberg HG: Effect of a serotonin and noradrenaline uptake inhibitor in panic disorder: a double-blind comparative study with fluvoxamine and maprotiline. Int Clin Psychopharmacol 3(1):59–74, 1988

Den Boer JA, Westenberg HG: Serotonin function in panic disorder: a double blind placebo controlled study with fluvoxamine and ritanserin. Psychopharmacology (Berl) 102:85–94, 1990

Dunner DL, Ishiki D, Avery DH, et al: Effect of alprazolam and diazepam on anxiety and panic attacks in panic disorder: a controlled study. J Clin Psychiatry 47:458–460, 1986

Enkelmann R: Alprazolam versus buspirone in the treatment of outpatients with generalized anxiety disorder. Psychopharmacology (Berl) 105:428–432, 1991

Falcon S, Ryan C, Chamberlain K, et al: Tricyclics: possible treatment for posttraumatic stress disorder. J Clin Psychiatry 46:385–388, 1985

Falloon IR, Lloyd GG, Harpin RE: The treatment of social phobia; real-life rehearsal with non-professional therapists. J Nerv Ment Dis 169:180–184, 1981

Feldman TB: Alprazolam in the treatment of posttraumatic stress disorder [letter]. J Clin Psychiatry 48:216–217, 1987

Fesler FA: Valproate in combat-related posttraumatic stress disorder. J Clin Psychiatry 52:361–364, 1991

Foa EB, Kozak MJ, Steketee GS, et al: Treatment of depressive and obsessive-compulsive symptoms in OCD by imipramine and behavioral therapy. Br J Clin Psychol 31:279–292, 1992

Frank JB, Kosten TR, Giller EL Jr, et al: A randomized clinical trial of phenelzine and imipramine for posttraumatic stress disorder. Am J Psychiatry 145:1289–1291, 1988

Gelernter CS, Uhde TW, Cimbolic P, et al: Cognitive-behavioral and pharmacological treatments for social phobia: a controlled study. Arch Gen Psychiatry 48:938–945, 1991

Goldberg HL, Finnerty RJ: The comparative efficacy of buspirone and diazepam in the treatment of anxiety. Am J Psychiatry 136:1184–1187, 1979

Goodman WK, Price LH, Rasmussen SA, et al: The efficacy of fluvoxamine in obsessive compulsive disorder: a double-blind comparison with placebo. Arch Gen Psychiatry 46:36–44, 1989

Goodman WK, Price LH, Delgado PL, et al: Specificity of serotonin reuptake inhibitors in the treatment of obsessive-compulsive disorder: comparison of fluvoxamine and desipramine. Arch Gen Psychiatry 47:577–585, 1990

Goodman WK, McDougle CJ, Price LH: Pharmacotherapy of obsessive compulsive disorder. J Clin Psychiatry 53 (4, suppl):29–37, 1992

Haefely W, Facklam M, Schoch P, et al: Partial agonists of benzodiazepine receptors for the treatment of epilepsy, sleep, and anxiety disorders, in GABAergic Synaptic Transmission. Edited by Biggio G, Concas A, Costa E. New York, Raven, 1992, pp 379–394

Hamilton M: A rating scale for depression. J Neurol Neurosurg Psychiatry 23:56–62, 1960

Haskell D, Cole JO, Schniebolk S, et al: A survey of diazepam patients. Psychopharmacol Bull 22:434–438, 1986

Heimberg RG, Barlow DH: New developments in cognitive-behavioral therapy for social phobia. J Clin Psychiatry 52 (11, suppl):21–30, 1991

Helzer JE, Robins LN, McEvoy L: Post-traumatic stress disorder in the general population: findings of the Epidemiological Catchment Area Survey. N Engl J Med 317:1630–1634, 1987

Hewlett WA, Vinogradov S, Agras WS: Clonazepam

treatment of obsessions and compulsions. J Clin Psychiatry 51:158–161, 1990

Hoehn-Saric R, McLeod DR, Zimmerli WD: Differential effects of alprazolam and imipramine in generalized anxiety disorder: somatic versus psychiatric symptoms. J Clin Psychiatry 49:293–301, 1988

Hogben GL, Cornfield RB: Treatment of traumatic war neurosis with phenelzine. Arch Gen Psychiatry 38:440–445, 1981

Hollander E, DeCaria CM, Schneier FR, et al: Fenfluramine augmentation of serotonin reuptake blockade antiobsessional treatment. J Clin Psychiatry 51:119–123, 1990

Jefferson JW: Pharmacologic augmentation strategies for treatment-resistant obsessive-compulsive disorder, in Obsessive-Compulsive Disorder: Its Nature and Treatment. Edited by Greist JH, Jefferson JW. Washington, DC, American Psychiatric Press (in press)

Jenike MA, Buttolph L, Baer L, et al: Open trial of fluoxetine in obsessive-compulsive disorder. Am J Psychiatry 146:909–911, 1989

Kabat-Zinn J, Massion AO, Kristeller J, et al: Effectiveness of a meditation-based stress reduction program in the treatment of anxiety disorders. Am J Psychiatry 149:936–943, 1992

Kahn RJ, McNair DM, Lipman RS, et al: Imipramine and chlordiazepoxide in depression and anxiety disorders, II: efficacy in anxious outpatients. Arch Gen Psychiatry 43:79–95, 1986

Kauffman CD, Reist C, Djenderedijan A, et al: Biological markers of affective disorders and post-traumatic stress disorder: a pilot study with desipramine. J Clin Psychiatry 48:366–367, 1987

Kim SW, Dysken MW, Kuskowski M: The Yale-Brown Obsessive-Compulsive Scale: a reliability and validity scale. Psychiatry Res 34:99–106, 1990

Kinzie JD, Leung P: Clonidine in Cambodian patients with posttraumatic stress disorder. J Nerv Ment Dis 177:546–550, 1989

Kitchner I, Greenstein R: Low dose lithium carbonate in the treatment of posttraumatic stress disorder: brief communication. Mil Med 150:378–381, 1985

Klein DF, Fink M: Psychiatric reaction patterns to imipramine. Am J Psychiatry 119:4324–4338, 1962

Klosko J, Barlow D, Tassinari R, et al: A comparison of alprazolam and behavior therapy in treatment of panic disorder. J Consult Clin Psychol 58(1):77–84, 1990

Kupfer DJ, Frank E, Perel JM, et al: Five-year outcome for maintenance therapies in recurrent depression. Arch Gen Psychiatry 49:769–773, 1992

Lennane KJ: Treatment of benzodiazepine dependence. Med J Aust 144:594–597, 1986

Leonard H, Swedo S, Coffey M, et al: Clomipramine vs. desipramine in childhood obsessive-compulsive disorder. Psychopharmacol Bull 24:43–45, 1988

Liebowitz MR, Gorman JM, Fyer AJ, et al: Social phobia: review of a neglected anxiety disorder. Arch Gen Psychiatry 42:729–736, 1985

Liebowitz MR, Gorman JM, Fyer AJ, et al: Pharmacotherapy of social phobia: an interim report of a placebo-controlled comparisons of phenelzine and atenolol. J Clin Psychiatry 49:252–257, 1988

Liebowitz MR, Schneier FR, Hollander E, et al: Treatment of social phobia with drugs other than benzodiazepines. J Clin Psychiatry 52 (11, suppl): 10–15, 1991

Liebowitz MR, Schneier F, Campeas R, et al: Phenelzine vs. atenolol in social phobia: a placebo-controlled comparison. Arch Gen Psychiatry 49:290–300, 1992

Lipper S, Davidson JR, Grady TA, et al: Preliminary study of carbamazepine in post-traumatic stress disorder. Psychosomatics 27:849–854, 1986

Lydiard RB, Laraia MT, Howell EF, et al: Alprazolam in the treatment of social phobia. J Clin Psychiatry 49:17–19, 1988

Lydiard RB, Lesser IM, Ballenger JC, et al: A fixed-dose study of alprazolam 2 mg, alprazolam 6 mg, and placebo in panic disorder. J Clin Psychopharmacol 12:96–103, 1992

Marks IM, Swinson RP: Alprazolam and exposure for panic disorder with agoraphobia: summary of London/Toronto results. J Psychiatr Res 24:100–101, 1990

Marks I, Greist J, Basoglu M, et al: Comment on the second phase of the Cross-National Collaborative Panic Study. Br J Psychiatry 160:202–205, 1992

Mavissakalian M, Perel J, Michelson L: The relationship of plasma imipramine and N-desmethylimipramine to improvement in agoraphobia. J Clin Psychopharmacol 4:36–40, 1984

McDougle CJ, Price LH, Goodman WK, et al: A controlled trial of lithium augmentation in fluvoxamine-refractory obsessive-compulsive disorder: lack of efficacy. J Clin Psychopharmacol 11:175–184, 1991

McLeod DR, Hoehn-Saric R, Zimmerli WD, et al: Treatment effects of alprazolam and imipramine: physiological versus subjective changes in patients with generalized anxiety disorder. Biol Psychiatry 28:849–861, 1990

Myers JK, Weissman MM, Tischler GL, et al: Six-month prevalence of psychiatric disorders in three communities: 1980–1982. Arch Gen Psychiatry 41:959–967, 1984

Napoliello MJ: An interim multicentre report on 7,677 anxious geriatric out-patients treated with buspirone. Br J Clin Pract 40:71–73, 1986

Nierenberg AA, Cole JO, Glass L: Possible trazodone potentiation of fluoxetine: a case series. J Clin Psychiatry 53:83–85, 1992

Noyes R Jr, Perry PJ, Crowe R, et al: Seizures following the withdrawal of alprazolam. J Nerv Ment Dis 174:50–52, 1986

Noyes R, Garvey MJ, Cook B, et al: Benzodiazepine withdrawal: a review of the evidence. J Clin Psychiatry 49:382–389, 1988

Noyes R, Garvey MJ, Cook BL, et al: Problems with tricyclic antidepressant use in patients with panic disorder or agoraphobia: results of a naturalistic follow-up study. J Clin Psychiatry 50:163–169, 1989

Ost LG: Applied relaxation vs progressive relaxation in the treatment of panic disorder. Behav Res Ther 26(1):13–22, 1988

O'Sullivan G, Noshirvani H, Marks I, et al: Six-year follow-up after exposure and clomipramine therapy for obsessive compulsive disorder. J Clin Psychiatry 52:150–155, 1991

Owen RT, Tyrer P: Benzodiazepine dependence: a review of the evidence. Drugs 25:385–398, 1983

Pato MT, Zohar-Kadouch R, Zohar J, et al: Return of symptoms after discontinuation of clomipramine in patients with obsessive-compulsive disorder. Am J Psychiatry 145:1521–1525, 1988

Pato MT, Pigott TA, Hill JL, et al: Controlled comparison of buspirone and clomipramine in obsessive-compulsive disorder. Am J Psychiatry 148:127–129, 1991

Patterson JF: Withdrawal from alprazolam dependency using clonazepam: clinical observations. J Clin Psychiatry 51 (suppl):47–49, 1990

Pecknold JC, Swinson RP, Krich K, et al: Alprazolam in panic disorder and agoraphobia: results from a multicenter trial, III: discontinuation effects. Arch Gen Psychiatry 45:429–436, 1988

Perse TL, Greist JH, Jefferson JW, et al: Fluvoxamine treatment of obsessive-compulsive disorder. Am J Psychiatry 144:1543–1548, 1988

Pigott TA, Pato MT, L'Heureux F, et al: A controlled comparison of adjuvant lithium carbonate or thyroid hormone in clomipramine-treated patients with obsessive-compulsive disorder. J Clin Psychopharmacol 11:242–248, 1991

Pigott TA, L'Heureux F, Rubenstein CS, et al: A double-blind, placebo controlled study of trazodone in patients with obsessive-compulsive disorder. J Clin Psychopharmacol 12:156–162, 1992

Reist C, Kauffmann CD, Haier RJ, et al: A controlled trial of desipramine in 18 men with posttraumatic stress disorder. Am J Psychiatry 146:513–516, 1989

Reiter SR, Pollack MH, Rosenbaum JF, et al: Clonazepam for the treatment of social phobia. J Clin Psychiatry 51:470–472, 1990

Rickels K: Buspirone in clinical practice. J Clin Psychiatry 51 (suppl):51–54, 1990

Rickels K, Weisman K, Norstad N, et al: Buspirone and diazepam in anxiety: a controlled study. J Clin Psychiatry 43:81–86, 1982

Rickels K, Schweizer E, Case WG, et al: Long-term therapeutic use of benzodiazepines, I: effects of abrupt discontinuation. Arch Gen Psychiatry 47:899–907, 1990

Rickels K, Case WG, Schweizer E, et al: Long-term benzodiazepine users 3 years after participation in a discontinuation program. Am J Psychiatry 148:757–761, 1991

Rickels K, Schweizer E, Weiss S, et al: Maintenance drug treatment for panic disorder, II: short- and long-term outcome after drug taper. Arch Gen Psychiatry 50:61–68, 1993

Rifkin A, Doddi S, Karajgi B, et al: Benzodiazepine use and abuse by patients at outpatient clinics. Am J Psychiatry 146:1331–1332, 1989

Robins LN, Helzer JE, Weissman MM, et al: Lifetime prevalence of specific psychiatric disorders in three sites. Arch Gen Psychiatry 412:958–967, 1984

Salzman C: Anxiety in the elderly: treatment strategies. J Clin Psychiatry 51 (suppl):18–21, 1990

Schneier FR, Liebowitz MR, Davies SO, et al: Fluoxetine in panic disorder. J Clin Psychopharmacol 10:119–121, 1990

Schweizer E, Pohl R, Balon R, et al: Lorazepam vs. alprazolam in the treatment of panic disorder. Pharmacopsychiatry 23(2):90–93, 1990

Schweizer E, Rickels K, Weiss S, et al: Maintenance drug treatment of panic disorder, I: results of a prospective, placebo-controlled comparison of alprazolam and imipramine. Arch Gen Psychiatry 50:51–60, 1993

Shear MK, Ball G, Fitzpatrick M, et al: Cognitive-behavioral treatment for panic: An open study. J Nerv Ment Dis 179:468–472, 1991a

Shear MK, Fyer AJ, Ball G, et al: Vulnerability to sodium lactate in panic disorder patients given cognitive-behavioral therapy. Am J Psychiatry 148:795–797, 1991b

Sheehan DV, Davidson J, Manschreck TC, et al: Lack of efficacy of a new antidepressant (bupropion) in the treatment of panic disorder with phobias. J Clin Psychopharmacol 3:23–31, 1983

Sheehan DV, Raj AB, Sheehan KH, et al: Is buspirone effective for panic disorder? J Clin Psychopharmacol 10:3–11, 1990

Shen WW, Park S: The use of monoamine oxidase inhibitors in the treatment of traumatic war neurosis: case report. Mil Med 148:430–431, 1983

Silver JM, Sandberg DP, Hales RE: New Approaches in the pharmacotherapy of post-traumatic stress disorder. J Clin Psychiatry 51 (10, suppl):33–38, 1990

Spealman RD: Disruption of schedule-controlled behavior by Ro 15-1788 one day after acute treatment with benzodiazepines. Psychopharmacology (Berl) 88:398–400, 1986

Stravynski A, Marks I, Yule W: Social skills problems in neurotic outpatients: social skills training with and without cognitive modification. Arch Gen Psychiatry 39:1378–1385, 1982

Sussman N: Treating anxiety while minimizing abuse and dependence. J Clin Psychiatry 54 (suppl 5):44–51, 1993

Taylor CB: Relaxation Training and Related Techniques, in Behavior Modification: Principles and Clinical Applications. Edited by Agras WS. Boston, MA, Little, Brown, 1978, pp 134–162

Taylor CB, Arnow B: The Nature and Treatment of Anxiety Disorders. New York, Free Press, 1988

Telch MJ, Agras WS, Taylor CB, et al: Combined pharmacological and behavioral treatment for agoraphobia. Behav Res Ther 23:325–335, 1985

Tesar GE, Rosenbaum JF, Pollack MH, et al: Double-blind, placebo-controlled comparison of clonazepam and alprazolam for panic disorder. J Clin Psychiatry 52:69–76, 1991

Thoren P, Asberg M, Cronholm B, et al: Clomipramine treatment of obsessive-compulsive disorder, I: a controlled clinical trial. Arch Gen Psychiatry 37:1281–1285, 1980

Udelman HD, Udelman DL: Concurrent use of buspirone in anxious patients during withdrawal from alprazolam therapy. J Clin Psychiatry 51 (suppl):46–50, 1990

Uhde TW, Tancer ME, Black B, et al: Phenomenology and neurobiology of social phobia: comparison with panic disorder. J Clin Psychiatry 52 (11, suppl):31–40, 1991

Van der Kolk BA: Psychopharmacological issues in posttraumatic stress disorder. Hosp Community Psychiatry 34:683–691, 1983

Versiani M, Nardi AE, Mundim FD, et al: Pharmacotherapy of social phobia: a controlled study with moclobemide and phenelzine. Br J Psychiatry 161:353–360, 1992

Weissman MM, Myers JK, Harding PS: Psychiatric disorders in a U.S. urban community. Am J Psychiatry 135:459–462, 1978

Welkowitz LA, Papp LA, Cloitre M, et al: Cognitive-behavior therapy for panic disorder delivered by psychopharmacologically oriented clinicians. J Nerv Ment Dis 179:473–477, 1991

Wheadon DE: Placebo controlled multi-center trial of fluoxetine in OCD. Paper presented at the 5th World Congress of Biological Psychiatry, Florence, Italy, June 12, 1991

Wheatley D: Buspirone: multicenter efficacy study. J Clin Psychiatry 43:92–94, 1982

Wincor MZ, Munjack DJ, Palmer R: Alprazolam levels and response in panic disorder: preliminary results. J Clin Psychopharmacol 11:48–51, 1991

Wingerson D, Nguyen C, Roy-Byrne PP: Clomipramine treatment for generalized anxiety disorder [letter]. J Clin Psychopharmacol 12:214–215, 1992

Wolf ME, Alavi A, Mosnaim AD: Posttraumatic stress disorder in Vietnam veterans: clinical and EEG findings; possible therapeutic effects of carbamazepine. Biol Psychiatry 23:642–644, 1988

Zinbarg RT, Barlow DH, Brown JA, et al: Cognitive-behavioral approaches to the nature and treatment of anxiety disorders. Annu Rev Psychol 43:235–267, 1992

32

Treatment of Alzheimer's Disease and Other Dementias

Murray A. Raskind, M.D.

Alzheimer's disease (AD) is the most common disorder causing dementia in later life, afflicting at least 2 million people in the United States. As in all disorders causing dementia, the primary symptoms of AD are acquired impairment of memory and other intellectual functions. AD is specifically characterized by insidious onset, gradual but inexorable progression, and development of fluent aphasia and apraxia as the disease progresses into its later stages. In addition to these primary cognitive and neurological deficits, AD is characterized by noncognitive behavioral problems (Wragg and Jeste 1989). These noncognitive problems are highly prevalent in AD and in other late-life disorders causing dementia and are the most common cause of eventual inability to remain with caregivers in the community. The most troublesome of these noncognitive behavioral problems are disruptive agitated behaviors, such as physical and verbal aggressive behaviors, uncooperativeness with activities necessary for personal hygiene and safety, wandering, delusions and hallucinations, and motoric hyperactivity.

In this chapter, I review the evidence for efficacy of psychopharmacological approaches to the management of these disruptive agitated behaviors in AD and other disorders causing dementia. I also review the management of depression (or depressive signs and symptoms) complicating AD and other disorders

causing dementia. The chapter's focus is on the results of placebo-controlled studies evaluating psychopharmacological therapies. But because well-designed placebo-controlled studies are scarce (despite the extensive use of a wide variety of psychotropic medications to control agitated disruptive behaviors in AD), data from studies that are not placebo controlled but are nevertheless informative are also presented.

■ PREVALENCE OF PSYCHOTROPIC DRUG USE IN DISORDERS CAUSING DEMENTIA

Disruptive behaviors occur in at least 40% of patients with AD during the course of their illness (Reisberg et al. 1987), and the true prevalence is probably even higher. Most of these AD patients (as well as patients with other disorders causing dementia who manifest disruptive behaviors) are prescribed psychotropic medications of one type or another as a part of their treatment regimens (Salzman 1987). The epidemiology of disruptive behaviors and psychotropic drug prescribing patterns in nursing home settings has been well studied. In a random sample of 50 residents of a proprietary nursing home, Rovner and colleagues (1986) documented noncognitive behavioral problems in the majority of patients ($n = 38$). Among the 40% ($n = 20$) of patients with 5 or more behavioral problems, the most frequently reported were disruptiveness, restlessness, noisiness, and aggressive behaviors.

With this high prevalence of noncognitive behaviors complicating the management of patients with AD and other disorders causing dementia, it is not surprising that the use of psychotropic medications in long-term care facilities is common. Beers and colleagues (1988) reviewed psychotropic medication use in intermediate care facility residents in the state of Massachusetts. To ensure that the homes represented typical geriatric facilities rather than those caring for deinstitutionalized mental hospital patients, homes were not studied if they had admitted more than 20% of their residents from inpatient psychiatric hospitals. These investigators found that more than half of all elderly residents were receiving a psychotropic medication. Twenty-six percent were receiving antipsychotic medication, and 28% were receiving sedative-hypnotics (primarily benzodiazepines and sedating antihistamines).

Buck (1988) examined the administration of psychotropic medications to Medicaid recipients residing continuously in nursing homes in Illinois. Of these residents, 60% received at least one psychotropic medication during the year. The antipsychotic drugs haloperidol and thioridazine and the benzodiazepine flurazepam were the most frequently prescribed medications. Avorn and colleagues (1989) surveyed a random sample of 55 rest homes in Massachusetts and found that more than half of the residents were taking at least one psychoactive medication. Antipsychotic medications were being administered to 39% of patients. In a follow-up investigation, they studied 837 residents in 44 rest homes with particularly high levels of antipsychotic drug use. For approximately half of these residents, there was no evidence of participation by a physician in decisions about their psychiatric status during the year of the study.

A study by Garrard and colleagues (1992) suggests that the stereotype of the "neglected psychotropic drug user" in nursing homes may be simplistic and overstated. In this longitudinal study of psychotropic drug use in a cohort of elderly nursing home residents ($N = 5,752$, mean age = 83) that included predominantly patients with late-onset dementia necessitating nursing home placement, the subjects' drug use was examined upon admission, 3 months later, and either at discharge or at end of study. At each admission, 17% of the cohort ($n = 996$) were receiving antipsychotic medications, but this antipsychotic drug use was not a static phenomenon. Twenty-four percent of the subjects ($n = 243$) had discontinued antipsychotics at 3 months. Of those subjects not receiving antipsychotics at admission, 5% ($n = 229$) were receiving antipsychotics at 3 months. Benzodiazepines were used by 21% of subjects ($n = 1,204$) on admission. However, the number of residents using benzodiazepines had dropped to 15% ($n = 885$) 3 months later and continued to be 15% at discharge. In fact, twice as many residents were taken off benzodiazepines as started on them following admission to the nursing home. This important study suggests that health care practitioners are attempting to use some guidelines to determine the appropriateness of the prescription of one or another psychotropic medication to patients with dementia. Unfortunately, health care practitioners are hampered by the lack of a broad data base from well-designed placebo-controlled studies providing guidelines for the rational use of psychotropic medications in behaviorally disturbed dementia patients. An overriding theme of this chapter is that such studies clearly need to be performed before behaviorally disturbed patients with dementia can be managed optimally.

■ ANTIPSYCHOTIC DRUGS

The antipsychotic drugs are widely prescribed to patients with AD and other disorders causing dementia that are complicated by disruptive behaviors (Harrington et al. 1992). The rationale for the use of these drugs in such patients is at least partially based on phenomenological similarities to signs and symptoms seen in schizophrenia and other "functional" disorders, in which antipsychotic drugs have clearly been demonstrated effective in nonelderly patients. It is true that delusions and hallucinations are common in AD (Wragg and Jeste 1989). Cummings and colleagues (1987) reported that persecutory delusions occurred in 30% of patients with AD and in 40% of patients with multi-infarct dementia. Hallucinations were frequent but somewhat less common in this study. However, it should be emphasized that psychotic behaviors in AD—particularly delusions—are often qualitatively different from those that complicate schizophrenia.

In AD, as well as in other disorders causing dementia, the most common delusions are relatively unelaborated paranoid beliefs such as that money or property has been stolen. Systematized complex delusions and grandiose delusions are uncommon in these disorders. In fact, delusions in AD often appear to be based on the underlying memory deficits. For example, the AD patient forgets where he or she has placed an item and then assumes that it has been stolen. Or, when an article of clothing discarded many years earlier cannot be located, the patient not unreasonably assumes that it has been taken. AD patients often stubbornly insist in a delusion-like manner that long-deceased people remain alive and can become distraught when these same individuals cannot be contacted. Although these beliefs in theft, in deceased people continuing to exist, or in the spouse being an impostor may meet formal criteria for delusions, they are in many ways unlike the delusions of schizophrenia for which the antipsychotic drugs have proved so effective. These phenomenological differences between psychotic features of AD and the psychotic features of schizophrenia may explain why the following review of treatment outcome studies suggests that the antipsychotic drugs are less effective in AD patients with psychotic features than they are in schizophrenic patients.

It should also be mentioned that nonpsychotic disruptive behaviors are commonly treated with antipsychotic medications. Motor restlessness, aggressive verbal and physical outbursts, persistent pacing, and uncooperativeness often coexist with delusions and/or hallucinations or are assumed (rightly or wrongly) in some manner to be related to an underlying psychotic process that is difficult to evaluate because of aphasic or other communication disturbances. Therefore, AD patients in trials of antipsychotics may not already have strictly defined psychotic symptoms.

Because the adverse effects of antipsychotic drugs, particularly extrapyramidal effects, can be very troubling for the elderly dementia patient (Devanand et al. 1989), the clinician should carefully weigh risks versus benefits before prescribing antipsychotic drugs for delusions and hallucinations that are not bothersome either to the patient or to caregivers. In these instances, the potential adverse effects of antipsychotic medications such as decreased mobility and excessive sedation may complicate management more than they improve the patient's quality of life. On the other hand, a number of studies have demonstrated that psychotic symptoms in AD are associated with more rapid cognitive deterioration (Drevets and Rubin 1989; Jeste et al. 1992; Lopez et al. 1991; Stern et al. 1987). Careful treatment outcome studies are needed to clarify whether pharmacological control of psychotic symptoms might modify disease progression.

Clinical outcome trials of antipsychotic drug therapy in dementia patients with disruptive behaviors are more numerous than for any other class of psychotropic medication. Even so, there are relatively few placebo-controlled studies providing interpretable data. Furthermore, many of the studies performed before the introduction of DSM-III (American Psychiatric Association 1980) use somewhat confusing diagnostic nomenclature and occasionally use the term "psychotic" to connote severe dementia rather than the presence of delusions and/or hallucinations. Also, these earlier studies were frequently performed in state hospital populations of chronic stay patients and included both patients with degenerative neurological disorders and patients with chronic schizophrenia who had grown old.

In one of these early studies, chlorpromazine was compared with placebo in a double-blind crossover design that included 29 patients with the diagnosis of dementia (Seager 1955). Global ratings of disturbed behaviors favored chlorpromazine over placebo, but sedation and falls were more common in the chlorpromazine group. Acetophenazine was compared with placebo in 14 patients with the diagnosis of dementia and with associated hyperactive behaviors such as assaultiveness, nocturnal wandering, irritability, hyperexcitability, and "abnormal fear" (Hamilton and Bennett 1962a). Improvement of these hyperactive behaviors was greater in the acetophenazine group than in the placebo group, but excessive sedation was a major adverse effect of acetophenazine.

Haloperidol was compared with placebo in 18 dementia patients (mean age = 72) for the control of agitation, overactivity, and hostility (Sugerman et al. 1964). Significant differences favoring haloperidol compared with placebo were noted in ratings of hallucinations, restlessness, and uncooperativeness. The haloperidol group had a substantial number of subjects who developed unsteady gait and/or pseudoparkinsonian signs. In this study, the best response to haloperidol occurred in the patients who were most severely agitated prior to randomization.

In contrast to these three studies (Hamilton and Bennett 1962a; Seager 1955; Sugerman et al. 1964), other studies performed prior to the introduction of DSM-III failed to demonstrate an advantage for antipsychotic medications compared with placebo in dementia patients. A common feature of these studies is the absence of target signs and symptoms (e.g., hallucinations, delusions, severe agitation, and severe hyperactivity) that responded better to antipsychotic medication than to placebo in the three studies described previously. Trifluoperazine was compared with placebo in 27 patients with severe dementia whose mean age was 71 (Hamilton and Bennett 1962b). In this study, target symptoms were apathy, withdrawal, and cognitive and behavioral deterioration (e.g., incontinence, loss of ambulation, and severe disorientation). Trifluoperazine was no more effective than placebo in this study, and the antipsychotic drug induced sedation and parkinsonian signs and symptoms in most of the patients on active medication.

Thiothixene was compared with placebo in a study of dementia patients in whom the target symptoms were primarily cognitive deficits (Rada and Kellner 1976). Global improvement was noted equally in the thiothixene and placebo groups. Thirteen of 22 patients receiving thiothixene were rated as at least minimally globally improved. Similarly, 11 of 20 patients in the placebo group were rated as at least minimally globally improved. The apparent placebo response in this study is of interest and has also been demonstrated in some of the more recent placebo-controlled trials of antipsychotic medications in dementia patients. These are described later in this chapter.

Several studies have been performed since the introduction of DSM-III and DSM-III-R (American Psychiatric Association 1987). In these studies, the use of explicit diagnostic criteria for primary degenerative dementia of the Alzheimer's type and multi-infarct dementia increases confidence that elderly patients with chronic schizophrenia and other chronic psychotic psychiatric disorders beginning in early life have been excluded from the study populations. In addition, these studies have required that either psychotic symptoms (i.e., delusions and hallucinations) or disruptive nonpsychotic behaviors be present as target symptoms.

In the only study to have been carried out in a typical community nursing home in elderly patients (mean age = 83) who met criteria for either AD or multi-infarct dementia and who had psychotic or nonpsychotic disruptive behaviors, thioridazine and loxapine were compared with placebo (Barnes et al. 1982). Improvement was significantly greater on either active drug than on placebo for Brief Psychiatric Rating Scale (BPRS) (Overall and Gorham 1962) ratings of excitement and uncooperativeness. However, suspiciousness and hostility improved both with active drug and with placebo, and the differences between active drug and placebo responses were not statistically significant. Only one-third of the patients in the study overall were rated as either moderately or markedly improved on a clinical global impression of change scale. These results suggest limited efficacy for antipsychotic drugs in a population of behaviorally disturbed and very old dementia patients, a population carefully evaluated to exclude people with chronic schizophrenia persisting into late life. These results also reinforce the need for placebo control of drug outcome studies in late-life dementia patients with AD or other late-onset disorders causing dementia.

In another placebo-controlled study, haloperidol and loxapine were compared with placebo in 64 older subjects (mean age = 73) who were inpatients at a large state psychiatric hospital (Petrie et al. 1982). In this study, diagnoses included AD and multi-infarct dementia. Active antipsychotic medications were significantly more effective than placebo for treating suspiciousness, hallucinatory behavior, excitement, hostility, and uncooperativeness. Global ratings of improvement, however, were similar to those found by Barnes and colleagues (1982). Thirty-two percent of loxapine patients and 35% of haloperidol patients were rated as moderately or markedly improved compared with 9% of patients who had been randomized to the placebo conditions.

The global improvement rates for active drug in both the Barnes and colleagues (1982) and the Petrie and colleagues (1982) studies were significantly greater than for placebo, but substantially lower than those usually reported for nonelderly patients treated with antipsychotic medications for schizophrenia. In addition, both of these studies found a high prevalence of parkinsonian signs and symptoms in the active medication groups. In a small but informative study, Devanand and colleagues (1989) compared haloperidol to placebo in a crossover study of nine outpatients who met diagnostic criteria for probable AD and who had clear psychotic behaviors (delusions and hallucinations). Eight of the nine subjects also had nonpsychotic disruptive behaviors. In this study, haloperidol was clearly and statistically significantly superior to placebo, but cognitive function worsened during active drug treatment and extrapyramidal adverse effects limited the improvement in quality of life achieved by subjects in the haloperidol condition. In contrast to all other studies of antipsychotic drugs in dementia patients, these investigators carefully selected patients who had psychotic signs and symptoms complicating AD. Their results suggest that antipsychotic drugs may be most effective in dementia patients whose noncognitive behavioral disturbances most closely resemble the classic psychotic signs and symptoms of schizophrenia. However, their study also pointed out the limiting effect of drug-induced parkinsonian symptoms on the efficacy of haloperidol in this population.

A meta-analysis of studies evaluating antipsychotic drugs in behaviorally disturbed dementia patients (Schneider et al. 1990) concluded that antipsychotic drugs are significantly more effective than placebo in this population, but the effect size is small and no single antipsychotic drug appeared better than another. The question of long-term antipsychotic drug maintenance was recently addressed by an antipsychotic drug discontinuation study in behaviorally disturbed dementia patients who appeared to have benefited from antipsychotic medications and had then been maintained on them chronically. Risse and colleagues (1987) substituted placebo for maintenance antipsychotic medication in nine male dementia patients (mean age = 65) who had symptomatically improved after treatment with antipsychotic medication for the control of agitated behaviors and had been maintained on antipsychotic medication for at least 90 days. At the end of the 6-week substitution period, only one patient had developed disruptive behavior severe enough to warrant reinstitution of antipsychotic medication. Of the remaining eight patients, one was rated as more agitated, two were unchanged, and five actually were rated as less agitated. These results support periodic trials of antipsychotic medication discontinuation even in patients who appear initially to have benefited from antipsychotic medication treatment in the past.

DRUGS WITH PHARMACOLOGICAL EFFECTS ON SEROTONIN SYSTEMS

The presence of a serotonergic deficiency in AD as manifested by decreased concentrations of the serotonin metabolite 5-hydroxyindoleacetic acid (5-HIAA) in postmortem brain tissue and in cerebrospinal fluid (Blenow et al. 1991; Hardy et al. 1985) provides some rationale for the use of drugs that affect serotonergic systems in the treatment of behavioral disturbances in AD. Clinical trials of two such drugs—the serotonin reuptake blocker trazodone and the serotonin partial agonist buspirone—are reviewed here. The reader should be cautioned that interpretability of these studies is limited by their anecdotal nature and uncontrolled designs.

Simpson and Foster (1986) treated four older dementia patients whose symptomatology was complicated by disruptive behaviors with trazodone. Trazodone was introduced after therapy with antipsychotic drugs had been ineffective. Two subjects met criteria for AD and two for probable alcoholic dementia. All four patients were men in their 60s, and none had signs and symptoms suggestive of an underlying depressive disorder. In doses of trazodone ranging from 200–500 mg daily, the drug anecdotally decreased agitation, combative behavior, and violent outbursts.

In a similar study, Pinner and Rich (1988) treated seven dementia patients with trazodone for symptomatic aggressive behavior. Patients were in their 50s and 60s and had a variety of dementia diagnoses, including AD, dementia following head trauma, alcoholic dementia, and combined schizophrenia and AD. Three of these seven patients (all of whom had failed to show a therapeutic response to prior treatment with antipsychotic drugs) demonstrated a marked decrease in aggressive behavior following 4 to 6 weeks of trazodone treatment at 200–300 mg qd. Three other patients had no response, and one patient was unable to take the drug for more than 11 days because of unspecified adverse effects. An advantage of trazodone compared with antipsychotics that supports further evaluation of this compound in the treatment of AD patients with disruptive behaviors is its lack of extrapyramidal adverse effects. Although trazodone is sedating and can produce orthostatic hypotension (as well as rarely producing priapism), it appears to have been well tolerated in the anecdotal reports in the literature.

Buspirone, an apparent 5-HT$_{1A}$ agonist, has an even more benign adverse-effect profile than trazodone. Colenda (1988) reported a 74-year-old woman with AD who manifested agitated behaviors including constant rocking, angry outbursts, and oppositional behavior, and who had failed to respond therapeutically to haloperidol. After a 2-month course of buspirone at 45 mg qd, marked improvement in the patient's agitated behaviors was noted. Tiller and colleagues (1988) reported a similarly positive response to buspirone (15 mg qd) in a patient with multi-infarct dementia complicated by agitated behaviors. Sakauye and colleagues (1993) recently reported an open-label study of buspirone in 10 patients with AD complicated by agitated behaviors. At doses of buspirone of 30–40 mg qd, there was a modest but significant overall reduction (22%) on the Cohen-Mansfield Agitated Behavior Scale (Cohen-Mansfield et al. 1989). There was substantial variability in response, with four patients apparently demonstrating marked declines in disruptive behaviors, three patients showing minimal or no change, and two with slight elevations in ratings of agitated behaviors. Without a placebo-controlled design, these reports are difficult to interpret; but given the relatively low toxicity of buspirone, the drug appears to merit further investigation.

■ ANTIMANIC DRUGS

The effectiveness of antimanic drugs for the hyperactivity, aggressive behaviors, and temper outbursts seen in patients in the manic phase of bipolar disorder has prompted trials of these drugs for treatment of agitated disruptive behaviors in patients with AD or other disorders causing dementia. As with the drugs acting on serotonergic systems, information on the antimanic drugs in dementia patients with disruptive behaviors is anecdotal in nature. In an open study of carbamazepine (Marin and Greenwald 1989), two AD patients and one multi-infarct dementia patient who had failed to respond to haloperidol for treatment of combative agitated behaviors appeared to improve markedly within 2 weeks of carbamazepine at doses ranging from 100–300 mg qd.

In a more extensive open study of carbamazepine in AD patients who had failed to respond to

antipsychotic drugs (Gleason and Schneider 1990), five of nine patients showed clinical improvement in their symptoms as rated by the BPRS. Particular symptomatic improvement in responders was noted for hostility, agitation, and uncooperativeness. Ataxia and confusion occurred in two of the patients whose agitated behaviors had improved with carbamazepine therapy. These adverse effects resolved with dose reduction. The mean dose of carbamazepine in this study was 480 mg qd, and the mean plasma level achieved was 6.5 μg/ml. Tempering these enthusiastic but uncontrolled open studies is an earlier study in which 19 elderly dementia patients were prescribed carbamazepine (100–300 mg qd) or placebo in a crossover design (Chambers et al. 1982). No overall benefit from carbamazepine was detected for the target symptoms of wandering, overactivity, and restlessness, but the low doses of carbamazepine prescribed may have limited the possible detection of efficacy.

The anticonvulsant and antimanic drug sodium valproate was evaluated in an open-label study in 4 patients with AD complicated by disruptive agitated behaviors but who were without clear psychotic signs or symptoms (Mellow et al. 1993). Sodium valproate was prescribed for periods of 1 to 3 months at doses ranging from 500 mg bid to 500 mg tid. Substantial behavioral improvement was observed in 2 of the 4 patients, and no adverse effects were noted. Lithium, the classic antimanic drug, has also been evaluated in open studies in dementia patients with disruptive behaviors. Holton and George (1985) prescribed a low dose of lithium (250 mg qd) for 4 weeks to 10 such patients who ranged in age from 72 to 85. Disruptive behaviors were not improved during the 4-week open lithium trial, but the low dose of lithium prescribed may have been outside a potential therapeutic range.

■ BENZODIAZEPINES

The use of benzodiazepines in dementia patients with disturbed behaviors was reviewed by Stern and colleagues (1991). Several placebo-controlled studies of benzodiazepines were performed in the 1960s and 1970s. Although specific subject diagnoses are difficult to determine, these studies probably included mostly patients with AD and other disorders causing dementia.

Sanders (1965) compared oxazepam with placebo in elderly (mean age = 81) "emotionally disturbed" patients. Although oxazepam was superior to placebo after 6 weeks of treatment, there was no difference between the placebo-treated and oxazepam-treated patients at the end of the 8-week treatment period. Agitation and anxiety were symptoms that showed the most favorable response to active treatment. These data suggest that tolerance to the benzodiazepine may have developed by the end of the treatment protocol.

Thioridazine and diazepam were compared in a nonplacebo-controlled comparison study for the control of behavioral symptoms associated with "senility" (Kirven and Montero 1973). Although both drugs were associated with symptomatic improvement, there was a trend in favor of thioridazine. As with the Sanders (1965) study, the data suggested that tolerance may have developed to the benzodiazepine by the end of the treatment protocol. In both of these studies, psychotic symptoms such as delusions and/or hallucinations were not specifically rated.

In another study (Coccaro et al. 1990), the efficacy of an antipsychotic drug (haloperidol), a benzodiazepine (oxazepam), and a sedating antihistamine (diphenhydramine) were compared for the treatment of agitated behaviors in a group of elderly institutionalized patients, most of whom met criteria for AD. The patients' mean age was 75, and target signs and symptoms included tension, excitement, verbal aggressiveness, physical aggressiveness, pacing, fidgeting, and increased motor activity. These behaviors decreased in all treatment groups over the 8-week period, but there was no differential response to the three psychotropic drugs. There was a trend for modestly greater improvement with diphenhydramine and haloperidol than with oxazepam. Because this study lacked a placebo group, the investigators acknowledged that the modest improvements in objective ratings of behavioral problems may have been due to factors other than drug treatment. This study is of interest because it suggests that sedation (a common effect of these otherwise markedly different drugs) may have been the factor producing improvement. This study also does not provide evidence favoring benzodiazepines for the treatment of behaviorally disturbed dementia patients, given that oxazepam appeared to be even less effective than the other two drugs.

■ PRACTICAL MANAGEMENT OF DISRUPTIVE BEHAVIORS IN AD AND OTHER DISORDERS CAUSING DEMENTIA

The available data base suggests that antipsychotic drugs should still be the first agents tried for the management of disruptive behaviors. However, the magnitude of effect is modest and dramatic treatment responses are rare. Before antipsychotic medications are instituted, it is prudent for the clinician to evaluate the general medical condition of the patient to rule out a general medical etiology for disruptive behaviors (e.g., pain, thyrotoxicosis) or an adverse effect of some nonpsychotropic medication (e.g., theophylline, L-dopa). Environmental and behavioral approaches also should be instituted where possible. For example, the pacing behavior of patients in the middle stages of AD is best treated by providing a secure environment in which patients can get up and walk around at any time of the day or night. Pacing appears unresponsive to psychotropic medication treatment, and akathisia from antipsychotic medications can exacerbate pacing. Although research evaluating the efficacy of behavioral approaches to disruptive behaviors is limited (Teri et al. 1992), collaboration with a clinical psychologist or other mental health professional knowledgeable in behavioral techniques can prove rewarding.

It appears that the closer the disruptive behaviors of the AD patient resemble the psychotic signs and symptoms seen in schizophrenia, the more effective antipsychotic drugs will be. Clinical experience suggests that the choice of a particular antipsychotic drug should be based on the tolerability of the adverse effects of a given agent by the patient to whom it will be prescribed. Haloperidol and other high-potency drugs are more likely to produce parkinsonian signs and symptoms than a low-potency antipsychotic drug such as thioridazine. However, thioridazine and other low-potency drugs are more likely to produce anticholinergic adverse effects (e.g., urinary retention, constipation, dry mouth, blurred vision, central anticholinergic delirium), orthostatic hypotension, and excess sedation. As an example, haloperidol would be a reasonable first choice of medication for the elderly male patient with prostatic hypertrophy and no parkinsonian-like motor signs such as bradykinesia or rigidity. However, because rigidity is common in the later stages of AD, a patient with such rigidity might better tolerate a lower-potency drug such as thioridazine.

All drugs should be started at a low but constantly prescribed dose, such as 1 mg of haloperidol or 25 mg of thioridazine qd. Because the therapeutic action of these drugs may not be immediately apparent, the dose should be increased gradually, perhaps every week if the desired therapeutic effect has not been achieved and adverse effects are either not present or are well tolerated. As the dose increases, clinical experience suggests that in the more frail elderly patient, dividing the total dose into a tid regimen may avoid excessive peak plasma drug concentrations that could potentially increase acute adverse effects such as orthostatic hypotension. Divided dosing does, however, increase demands on caregivers and nursing personnel. In the very elderly patient with AD or another disorder causing dementia, a dose of haloperidol higher than 3 mg qd or thioridazine greater than 75 mg qd often is poorly tolerated. On the other hand, the less common early-onset patient who is in his or her 50s or 60s and whose general medical condition is sound may both tolerate and need higher doses of antipsychotic medication for adequate management of disruptive agitated behaviors.

As should be apparent from this review of clinical outcome trials of psychotropic drugs other than antipsychotics for disruptive behaviors in AD and other disorders causing dementia, there are no well-established guidelines for choosing a psychotropic medication for patients in whom antipsychotic drugs are either ineffective or poorly tolerated. Buspirone at a starting dose of 5 mg tid but with gradual increases up to 15 mg tid has the advantage of a relatively benign adverse-effect profile. Trazodone starting at 50 mg qd with gradual increases to 50 or 100 mg tid may also be effective, but orthostatic hypotension or excessive sedation may complicate the use of trazodone in some patients. Violent behavior may respond to carbamazepine or valproate. These drugs are reasonably well tolerated, although sedation and ataxia can occur. Short half-life benzodiazepines may be useful if subjective anxiety is prominent or can be reasonably inferred from the patient's behavioral problems. However, the benzodiazepines have a high incidence of ataxia and excessive sedation and can impair cognitive function in elderly patients (Sunderland et al. 1989). Further-

more, tolerance to the therapeutic antianxiety or anti-agitation effects of the benzodiazepines is common.

■ DEPRESSION COMPLICATING AD AND OTHER DISORDERS CAUSING DEMENTIA

Because depression per se can impair cognitive function (Cohen et al. 1982), the recognition and effective treatment of depression complicating a disorder causing dementia offers the potential for both improving mood and maximizing the patient's cognitive abilities. However, the recognition of a true depressive disorder in the patient with AD or another illness causing dementia can be difficult. The overlap of signs and symptoms between depression and dementia can make diagnosis of depression in the dementia patient confusing. Common to both disorders are apathy, sleep disturbances, loss of interest in previously interesting activities, and changes in psychomotor activity. Even with these diagnostic difficulties, a number of studies have found a high prevalence of depressive signs and symptoms in AD (Reifler et al. 1986; Rovner et al. 1986). It has also been demonstrated that depressive signs and symptoms in AD patients are associated with added functional impairment (Pearson et al. 1989).

Although anecdotal reports suggest that antidepressant drugs are effective for the treatment of depression complicating AD and other disorders causing dementia (Jenike 1985), only one placebo-controlled study has actually addressed the question of efficacy in these patients. Reifler and colleagues (1989) compared imipramine with placebo in a double-blind outcome study for the treatment of major depressive episode complicating AD. Subjects in this study met both DSM-III-R criteria for primary degenerative dementia of the Alzheimer's type and DSM-III-R criteria for major depressive episode. Patients were still living in the community but were in the middle stages of AD (mean Mini-Mental State Examination [Folstein et al. 1975] score = 17) and had depression of mild to moderate severity (mean Hamilton Rating Scale for Depression [Hamilton 1960] score = 19). Patients were prescribed imipramine (mean dose = 83 mg qd; mean plasma level of imipramine plus desmethyl imipramine = 116 ng/ml) or placebo for 8 weeks. Substantial and highly significant improvement in depressive signs and symptoms was documented in both the imipramine and the placebo groups, but the amount of improvement in both groups was almost identical. This study suggests that patients with AD who manifest mild to moderate degrees of depressive symptomatology respond to antidepressant interventions but the behavioral and environmental components of such interventions are important.

Because Reifler and colleagues (1989) did not include patients with severe depression in their study, their results are only applicable to patients with mild to moderate dementia and with a modest amount of depressive symptomatology. However, it is the latter type of patient who accounts for the bulk of depressive signs and symptoms complicating AD. Interpretation of this study is also complicated, because the emergence of adverse effects limited the amount of imipramine prescribed. A higher dose of imipramine might have been even more effective than the substantial placebo group. Tricyclic antidepressants also have been evaluated in a placebo-controlled study of depression (both major depressive episode and dysthymia) complicating stroke. It is likely that a substantial proportion of the subjects in this study had at least mild multi-infarct dementia. In this study (Lipsey et al. 1984), nortriptyline was more effective than placebo for depressive signs and symptoms. More placebo-controlled studies of antidepressants for the treatment of depression complicating disorders causing dementia are clearly needed.

■ CONCLUSION

Further studies are necessary to provide rational guidelines for the psychopharmacological management of noncognitive behavioral problems complicating AD and other disorders causing dementia. Extrapolations from the large body of psychotherapeutic drug outcome studies in younger patients with such diseases as schizophrenia and depression starting in adolescence or middle age often are not relevant to elderly dementia patients who are behaviorally disturbed. Careful evaluations of newer antipsychotic agents with minimal extrapyramidal toxicity such as clozapine and respiridone may improve the applicability of the general class of antipsychotic drugs for behaviorally disturbed dementia patients. Placebo-controlled outcome studies of

drugs such as buspirone and trazodone can establish or refute the hints of efficacy derived from anecdotal reports. The antimanic drugs, particularly carbamazepine and sodium valproate, also deserve careful evaluations in well-designed clinical trials. Careful attention to accurate phenomenological description of specific types of behavioral problems may help to establish therapeutic specificity of a drug for a given behavioral problem. Such studies are currently under way.

■ REFERENCES

American Psychiatric Association: Diagnostic and Statistical Manual of Mental Disorders, 3rd Edition. Washington, DC, American Psychiatric Association, 1980

American Psychiatric Association: Diagnostic and Statistical Manual of Mental Disorders, 3rd Edition, Revised. Washington, DC, American Psychiatric Association, 1987

Avorn J, Dreyer P, Connelly MA, et al: Use of psychoactive medication and the quality of care in rest homes. N Engl J Med 320:227–232, 1989

Barnes R, Veith R, Okimoto J, et al: Efficacy of antipsychotic medications in behaviorally disturbed dementia patients. Am J Psychiatry 139:1170–1174, 1982

Beers M, Avorn J, Soumerai SB, et al: Psychoactive medication use in intermediate-care facility residents. JAMA 260:3016–3020, 1988

Blenow KAJ, Wallin A, Gottfries CG, et al: Significance of decreased lumbar CSF levels of HVA and 5-HIAA in Alzheimer's disease. Neurobiol Aging 13:107–113, 1991

Buck JA: Psychotropic drug practice in nursing homes. J Am Geriatr Soc 36:409–418, 1988

Chambers CA, Bain J, Rosbottom R, et al: Carbamazepine in senile dementia and overactivity—a placebo controlled double blind trial. IRCS Journal of Medical Science 10:505–506, 1982

Coccaro EF, Kramer E, Zemishlany Z, et al. Pharmacologic treatment of noncognitive behavioral disturbances in elderly demented patients. Am J Psychiatry 147:1640–1656, 1990

Cohen RM, Weingartner HW, Smallberg A, et al: Effort and cognition in depression. Arch Gen Psychiatry 39:593–597, 1982

Cohen-Mansfield J, Marx MS, Rosenthal AS: A description of agitation in a nursing home. J Gerontol 44:77–84, 1989

Colenda CC: Buspirone in treatment of agitated demented patient. Lancet 1:1169, 1988

Cummings JL, Miller B, Hill MA, et al: Neuropsychiatric aspects of multi-infarct dementia and dementia of the Alzheimer type. Arch Neurol 44:389–393, 1987

Devanand DP, Sackheim HA, Brown RP, et al: A pilot study of haloperidol treatment of psychosis and behavioral disturbance in Alzheimer's disease. Arch Neurol 46:854–857, 1989

Drevets WC, Rubin E: Psychotic symptoms and the longitudinal course of senile dementia of the Alzheimer type. Biol Psychiatry 25:39–48, 1989

Folstein MF, Folstein SE, McHugh PR: Mini-Mental State: a practical method for grading the cognitive state of patients for the clinician. J Psychiatr Res 12:189–198, 1975

Garrard J, Dunham T, Makris L, et al: Longitudinal study of psychotropic drug use by elderly nursing home residents. J Gerontol 47:M183–M188, 1992

Gleason RP, Schneider LS: Carbamazepine treatment of agitation in Alzheimer's outpatients refractory to neuroleptics. J Clin Psychiatry 51:115–118, 1990

Hamilton LD, Bennett JL: Acetophenazine for hyperactive geriatric patients. Geriatrics 17:596–601, 1962a

Hamilton LD, Bennett JL: The use of trifluoperazine in geriatric patients with chronic brain syndrome. J Am Geriatr Soc 10:140–147, 1962b

Hamilton M: A rating scale for depression. J Neurol Neurosurg Psychiatry 23:56–62, 1960

Hardy J, Adolfsson R, Alafuzoff I, et al: Review: transmitter deficits in Alzheimer's disease. Neurochem Int 7:545–563, 1985

Harrington C, Tompkins C, Curtis M, et al: Psychotropic drug use in long-term care facilities: a review of the literature. Gerontologist 32:822–833, 1992

Holton A, George K: The use of lithium in severely demented patients with behavioral disturbance. Br J Psychiatry 146:99–100, 1985

Jenike MA: MAO inhibitors as treatment for depressed patients with primary degenerative dementia (Alzheimer's disease). Am J Psychiatry 142:763–764, 1985

Jeste DV, Wragg RE, Salmon DP, et al: Cognitive deficits with Alzheimer's disease with and without delusions. Am J Psychiatry 149:184–189, 1992

Kirven LE, Montero EF: Comparison of thioridazine and diazepam in the control of nonpsychotic symptoms associated with senility: double-blind study. J Am Geriatr Soc 21:546–551, 1973

Lipsey JR, Pearlson GD, Robinson RG, et al: Nortriptyline treatment of post-stroke depression: a double blind study. Lancet 1:297–300, 1984

Lopez OL, Becker JT, Brenner RP, et al: Alzheimer's disease with delusions and hallucinations: neuropsychological and electroencephalographs correlates. Neurology 41:906–912, 1991

Marin DB, Greenwald BS: Carbamazepine for aggressive agitation in demented patients. Am J Psychiatry 146:805, 1989

Mellow AM, Solano-Lopez C, Davis S: Sodium valproate in the treatment of behavioral disturbance in dementia. J Geriatr Psychiatry Neurol 6:28–32, 1993

Overall JE, Gorham DR: The Brief Psychiatric Rating Scale. Psychol Rep 10:799–812, 1962

Pearson JL, Teri L, Reifler BV, et al: Functional status and cognitive impairment in Alzheimer's disease patients with and without depression. J Am Geriatr Soc 37:1117–1121, 1989

Petrie WM, Ban TA, Berney S, et al: Loxapine in psychogeriatrics: a placebo- and standard-controlled clinical investigation. J Clin Psychopharmacol 2:122–126, 1982

Pinner E, Rich CL: Effects of trazodone on aggressive behavior in seven patients with organic mental disorders. Am J Psychiatry 145:1295–1296, 1988

Rada RT, Kellner R: Thiothixene in the treatment of geriatric patients with chronic organic brain syndrome. J Am Geriatr Soc 24:105–107, 1976

Reifler BV, Larson E, Teri L, et al: Dementia of Alzheimer's type and depression. J Am Geriatr Soc 34:855–859, 1986

Reifler BV, Teri L, Raskind M, et al: Double-blind trial of imipramine in Alzheimer's disease patients with and without depression. Am J Psychiatry 146:45–49, 1989

Reisberg B, Borenstein J, Salob SP, et al: Behavioral symptoms in Alzheimer's disease: phenomenology and treatment. J Clin Psychiatry 48 (5, suppl):9–15, 1987

Risse SC, Cubberly L, Lampe TH, et al: Acute effects of neuroleptic withdrawal in elderly dementia patients. Journal of Geriatric Drug Therapy 2:65–67, 1987

Rovner BW, Kafonek S, Filipp L, et al: Prevalence of

mental illness in a community nursing home. Am J Psychiatry 143:1446–1449, 1986

Sakauye KM, Camp CJ, Ford PA: Effects of buspirone on agitation associated with dementia. Am J Geriatr Psychiatry 1:82–84, 1993

Salzman C: Treatment of the elderly agitated patient. J Clin Psychiatry 48 (5, suppl):19–22, 1987

Sanders JF: Evaluation of oxazepam and placebo in emotionally disturbed aged patients. Geriatrics 20:739–746, 1965

Schneider LS, Pollock VE, Lyness SA: A metaanalysis of controlled trials of neuroleptic treatment in dementia. J Am Geriatr Soc 38:553–563, 1990

Seager CP: Chlorpromazine in treatment of elderly psychotic women. British Medical Journal 1:882–885, 1955

Simpson DM, Foster D: Improvement in organically disturbed behavior with trazodone treatment. J Clin Psychiatry 47:191–193, 1986

Stern RG, Duffelmeyer ME, Zemishlani Z, et al: The use of benzodiazepines in the management of behavioral symptoms in dementia patients. Psychiatr Clin North Am 14:375–384, 1991

Stern Y, Mayeux R, Sano M, et al: Predictions of disease course in patients with probable Alzheimer's disease. Neurology 37:1649–1653, 1987

Sugerman AA, Williams BH, Adlerstein AM: Haloperidol in the psychiatric disorders of old age. Am J Psychiatry 120:1190–1192, 1964

Sunderland T, Weingartner T, Cohen RM, et al: Low-dose oral lorazpam administration in Alzheimer subjects and age-matched controls. Psychopharmacology (Berl) 99:129–133, 1989

Teri L, Rabins P, Whitehouse P, et al: Management of behavior disturbance in Alzheimer disease: current knowledge and future directions. Alzheimer Dis Assoc Disord 6:77–88, 1992

Tiller JW, Dakis JA, Shaw JM: Short-term buspirone treatment in disinhibition with dementia. Lancet 2:510, 1988

Wragg RE, Jeste DV: Overview of depression and psychosis in Alzheimer's disease. Am J Psychiatry 146:577–587, 1989

Treatment of Childhood and Adolescent Disorders

Mina K. Dulcan, M.D., Joel D. Bregman, M.D.,
Elizabeth B. Weller, M.D., and Ronald A. Weller, M.D.

■ SPECIAL ISSUES IN THE PSYCHOPHARMACOLOGICAL TREATMENT OF CHILDREN AND ADOLESCENTS

In this chapter, we examine how psychopharmacology for children and adolescents differs from that for adults. (Detailed discussions of specific drugs can be found in Section II of this textbook.) For disorders and their treatment that are similar in youths and adults, the reader should refer to other chapters in this section. This chapter includes the treatment of disorders that occur in both adults and children that are not covered in other chapters of this text, such as attention-deficit hyperactivity disorder (ADHD), mental retardation, and autistic disorder. Whenever possible, DSM-III-R or DSM-IV terminology (American Psychiatric Association 1987, 1994) is used. Unfortunately, many drug studies conducted with children and adolescents have used other diagnostic categories, and it is difficult to know how well the results hold for contemporary diagnoses.

■ Evaluation

The evaluation of a young person is complicated by the interaction of psychopathology with the child's environment and with developmental processes. An interview with at least one parent or adult caretaker is essential. Information from teachers is desirable in all cases and indispensable in ADHD. Standardized rating scales are useful (Achenbach 1991). A recent medical history and physical examination are necessary, with laboratory follow-up as indicated. A drug screen or pregnancy test may be required. Whenever a student's functioning in school is impaired, psychoeducational testing (including, at a minimum, intelligence quotient [IQ] and academic achievement tests) should be obtained. Additional testing for learning disabilities may be needed.

■ Treatment Planning

Psychiatric diagnosis, specific target symptoms, and the strengths and weaknesses of the patient, the family, the school, and the community all enter into the choice of intervention strategies. The child and his or her parents (as appropriate) are included in a discussion of treatment options, available resources, parent and child motivation, potential risks and benefits of each intervention, and the risks of no treatment. Psychopharmacology as a sole treatment is rarely satisfactory for young persons. Most cases require one or more additional interventions to address remaining symptoms, such as parent guidance or training in behavior modification; modification of school program; and individual, family, and group psychotherapy.

■ Ethical Issues

The careful clinician attempts to balance the risks of medication, the risks of the untreated disorder, and the expected benefits of medication relative to other treatments. Clinical experience with the use of a psychotropic drug in adults should generally be substantial before that drug is used to treat children and adolescents. Because pharmaceutical houses rarely undertake the expense and trouble of testing drugs in children and adolescents, the U.S. Food and Drug Administration (FDA) guidelines as published in the *Physicians' Desk Reference* (PDR) cannot be relied upon for appropriate indications, age ranges, or doses.

Children and adolescents are under the supervision of adults. These adults may misinterpret a youngster's response to the environment as indicating either a need for medication or improvement because of a medication. Many adults seek to use drugs to control or eliminate troublesome behavior, instead of investigating the family or institutional dynamics that may be provoking and maintaining such behavior or implementing more time-consuming, difficult, and expensive therapeutic or behavioral management strategies. At times, the most appropriate response to a behavioral problem is a behavior modification program or a change in classroom placement or teaching strategy, not the initiation of a medication or an increase in dosage. This is particularly the case when there is evidence that the disturbance is localized to the classroom situation, when it seems to be a reaction to a change in teachers or to a particular teacher's tactics in dealing with the child, or when the child has a learning disability. Consent for drug treatment of children and adolescents is a complex issue (Popper 1987). The age at which a young person can give informed consent varies from state to state, but "assent" to medication use is considered possible to obtain from a patient who is over age 7 (Popper 1987). When prescribing for indications that are "unapproved" by the FDA, it may be prudent to inform the family of this, as well as of existing evidence for safe and effective use (Appler and McMann 1989). Published information sheets to supplement educational discussion with the physician regarding specific medications are now available (Dulcan 1992). Small group teaching (Knight et al. 1990) or a medication manual (Bastiaens 1992; Bastiaens and Bastiaens 1993) may be useful in educating young patients about their medications.

■ The Meaning of Medication

Emanative effects are indirect and inadvertent cognitive and social (i.e., nonpharmacological) consequences of prescribing a drug. These can be positive or negative and may influence the child's self-esteem or attributions of the source of problems and their solution (Henker and Whalen 1980) or the parent's or teacher's view of the child (Amirkhan 1982).

A placebo response is common in children with ADHD, depression, Tourette's disorder, or autism. This is not surprising, given children's suggestibility, the power of adult influence, the "magical thinking" that is normal in young children, and the natural waxing and waning of symptoms. Occasionally, the expectations about drug efficacy that parents, teacher, and child may have might be so significant that a blind placebo trial is required, even in the clinical setting. Examples include initiating stimulant medication or determining if a chronically administered drug continues to be required and effective or is no longer needed, is ineffective, or is even exacerbating the condition (Doherty et al. 1987; Fine and Jewesson 1989; McBride 1988; Ullmann and Sleator 1986; Varley and Trupin 1983).

■ Measurement of Outcome

The physician must specify target symptoms and obtain affective, behavioral, and physical baseline and posttreatment data. Side effects that are tolerable in adults may be unacceptable in the long-term treatment of children. Children's cognitive limitations in identifying and reporting physical symptoms or changes in mood require a skilled clinician to detect drug-induced changes. Therapeutic and side effects can be assessed by interviews and rating scales for patient, parent, and other adults such as teachers and nurses (in an inpatient setting) (Garvey et al. 1991), direct observation by the clinician, physical examination, and (where appropriate) laboratory or psychometric tests evaluating attention or learning (Barkley 1990; Conners 1985; Gadow and Swanson 1985).

■ Compliance

Faithful adherence to a prescribed regimen requires the cooperation of one or both parents, the child, and often additional caretakers and school personnel. Pediatric medications may be incorrectly used because of parental factors such as lack of perceived need for drug, carelessness, inability to afford medication, misunderstanding of instructions, complex schedules of administration (Briant 1978), and family dynamics. Both developmental and psychopathological factors may impede the patient's cooperation. Even in intensively monitored protocols, missed doses and unilateral discontinuation by a parent (even when the child has responded positively) are common (Brown et al. 1987; Firestone 1982). Recent media attention to alleged inappropriate use of medications, especially Ritalin and Prozac, has made families and some teachers highly resistant to pharmacotherapy.

Many children cannot or will not swallow pills. Some drugs are available in elixir form (Geller et al. 1992) or can be dissolved in juice. If necessary, a behavior modification program may be implemented to shape pill-swallowing behavior (Pelco et al. 1987).

■ Developmental Toxicology

Developmental toxicology refers to the unique or especially severe side effects resulting from interaction between a drug and a patient's physical, cognitive, or emotional development. Interference with learning in school or with the development of social relationships within the family or with peers can have lasting effects. Behavioral toxicity (i.e., negative effects on mood, behavior, or learning) often develops before physical side effects are observed, especially in young children (Campbell et al. 1985).

■ Metabolism and Kinetics

Dosage may be determined empirically or by extrapolation from adult doses according to weight or age. Unfortunately, dosage studies in children are rare. Few data exist on the parameters that determine pharmacokinetics in children (Briant 1978). Young children absorb some drugs more rapidly than adults, leading to higher peak levels (Jatlow 1987). Some children may require divided doses to minimize fluctuations in blood level (particularly for tricyclic antidepressants), although more frequent doses may reduce medication compliance. Age-related factors that may influence distribution include uptake by actively growing tissue and proportional size of organs and tissue masses. In children, drugs such as lithium (which are primarily distributed in body water) have a proportionally larger volume of distribution and therefore lower concentration (Jatlow 1987). By

age 1, glomerular filtration rate and renal tubular mechanisms for secretion reach adult levels. Hepatic enzyme activity develops early, and rate of drug metabolism is related to liver size. Prepubertal children have relatively large livers and may require a larger dose per kilogram of body weight of drugs that are primarily metabolized by the liver (Briant 1978).

The rate of hepatic drug transformation often decreases abruptly toward adult levels around puberty, requiring careful clinical monitoring (Jatlow 1987). The pubertal increase in gonadal hormones may be a factor (Ryan et al. 1986). Proportion of fat, which serves as a reservoir for lipid-soluble compounds, increases during the first year of life, followed by a gradual loss until the pubertal increase (in girls) (Briant 1978).

■ ATTENTION-DEFICIT HYPERACTIVITY DISORDER

■ Assessment for Treatment

We refer to ADHD in this section, although much of the research discussed here used a variety of other diagnostic terms. Parent interviews and standardized rating scales are the core of the assessment process (Achenbach 1991; Barkley 1990). The interview with a child or adolescent who might have ADHD may or may not be helpful in diagnosis. Some children and most adolescents with ADHD are able to pay attention and maintain behavioral control while in the office setting. Few have insight into their own difficulties or are willing or able to report them accurately. School information, such as the Teacher Report Form of the Child Behavior Checklist (Achenbach 1991), is essential. Psychoeducational testing is indicated to assess possible low IQ or specific developmental disorders (i.e., learning disabilities) that may be masquerading as ADHD or may coexist with ADHD. Achievement testing helps in educational planning. Sensory deficits and medical or social etiologies of poor attention must be ruled out.

■ Selection of Treatment

The number and variety of symptoms in many youngsters with ADHD and the limitations of existing interventions often require multimodal treatment (Satterfield et al. 1987; Whalen and Henker 1991).

Parent education and training in techniques of behavior management are virtually always needed. Specific developmental disorders (learning disabilities) or lags in achievement because of inattention are frequent and require tutoring or special class placement. Social skills deficits may respond to group therapy. Because raising a child with ADHD exacerbates family discord, family therapy may be essential if medication or behavior modification are to be effective.

Behavior modification is able to address symptoms that stimulants do not, although it is more expensive. Many parents find behavior management training more difficult to sustain than pharmacotherapy (Firestone et al. 1981), but some may prefer behavioral therapy to medical treatment (Thurston 1981). Targeted behavioral interventions are effective in the short term in improving behavior, social skills, and academic performance (Ayllon and Rosenbaum 1977; Dubey et al. 1983; Mash and Dalby 1979) but are less useful in reducing inattention, hyperactivity, or impulsivity (Abikoff and Gittelman 1984). Time-limited interventions, however, do not typically produce long-lasting behavior change in children with ADHD. Hyperactive children often require both instruction to remedy deficits in social or academic skills and contingency management to induce them to use the skills (Pelham and Bender 1982).

For many youngsters with ADHD, neither stimulant medication nor behavioral therapy alone is sufficient to normalize behavior and academic performance (DuPaul and Rapport 1993). There are nonresponders to each intervention. Although children without ADHD can detect medication-induced improvement in the behavior of hyperactive children (Whalen et al. 1987), the social skills or peer ratings of popularity of hyperactive children rarely improve to the level of their nonhyperactive peers with stimulant treatment alone (Ullmann and Sleator 1985; Whalen et al. 1989). Some studies have found intensive behavior modification and methylphenidate to have additive effects in children who were partial responders to either intervention, in many cases yielding performance indistinguishable from that of nonhyperactive peers (Gittelman et al. 1980; Pelham and Bender 1982; Pelham and Murphy 1986; Pelham et al. 1980, 1986).

The decision to medicate is based on the presence of inattention, impulsivity, and often hyperactivity that are not due to another treatable cause and that are persistent and sufficiently severe to cause

functional impairment at school, and usually also at home and with peers. The child's parents must be willing to monitor medication and to attend appointments.

It is difficult to predict whether an individual patient with ADHD will respond to a specific medication. Neurological soft signs, electroencephalogram (EEG), or neurochemical measures do not appear to be useful predictors of stimulant responsivity (Halperin et al. 1986; Zametkin et al. 1986). Reduced response to stimulants in youths with ADHD who have comorbid anxiety is controversial (Livingston et al. 1992; Pliszka 1989).

Stimulants. In most circumstances, a stimulant drug is the first pharmacological choice for a patient with ADHD. Although drug abuse does not result from properly monitored prescribed stimulants (and abuse of methylphenidate or pemoline is exceedingly rare in any event), caution may be indicated in the presence of conduct disorder or preexisting chemical dependency. If the risk of drug abuse by the patient or the patient's peers or family is high, pemoline, desipramine (DMI), or clonidine may be preferable to methylphenidate or dextroamphetamine.

In preschool children, stimulant efficacy is more variable and the rate of side effects is higher, especially sadness, irritability, clinginess, insomnia, and anorexia (Barkley 1988; Cohen et al. 1981; Conners 1975; Schleifer et al. 1975). Stimulants should be used in this age group in more severe cases or when parent training and placement in a highly structured, well-staffed preschool program have been unsuccessful or are not possible. However, stimulants can reduce oppositional and aggressive behavior and increase on-task behavior in preschoolers, especially when used together with a contingency management program (Speltz et al. 1987).

Stimulants are effective in the treatment of adolescents with cognitive and/or behavioral symptoms of ADHD (Brown and Sexson 1989; Evans and Pelham 1991; Klorman et al. 1990). Contrary to popular belief, youngsters who are positive responders as children do not automatically require a change in drug at puberty. Newly diagnosed adolescents may be started on a stimulant. In addition, anecdotal reports indicate that stimulants improve academic performance in some children who have attention deficits without hyperactivity (Famularo and Fenton 1987).

Clonidine. Clonidine is useful in modulating mood and activity level and improving cooperation and frustration tolerance in a subgroup of children with ADHD, especially those who are very highly aroused, hyperactive, impulsive, defiant, irritable, explosive, and labile (Hunt et al. 1990). Although clonidine has no direct effect on attention, it may be used alone in children with a personal or family history of tics or those who are nonresponders or negative responders to stimulants. It is most useful in combination with a stimulant when stimulant response is only partial or when stimulant dose is limited by side effects (Hunt et al. 1991). The combination may allow a lower dose of stimulant medication (Hunt et al. 1991). Clonidine often improves ability to fall asleep, whether insomnia is due to ADHD overarousal, oppositional refusal to go to bed, or stimulant effect or rebound (Brown and Gammon 1992).

Tricyclic antidepressants. A tricyclic antidepressant (TCA) may be used to treat ADHD if stimulants are contraindicated because of tics, Tourette's disorder (Riddle et al. 1988), or risk of the patient or a parent abusing or selling drugs. A TCA may be indicated if stimulants are ineffective, or if side effects (especially tics, dysphoria, weight loss, or severe rebound) are unacceptable. These drugs may be considered first if family history and patient symptoms strongly suggest comorbid anxiety or depression (Kutcher et al. 1992). Although depressive symptoms in children with ADHD have not been found to differentially predict positive outcome of TCA treatment, a TCA may decrease depressive symptoms in youngsters with ADHD and avoids the risk of stimulant-induced dysphoria (Biederman et al. 1989a). The longer duration of action does not require a dose at school and minimizes rebound effects. Drawbacks include the inconvenience and expense of electrocardiogram (ECG) monitoring, serious potential cardiac side effects (especially in prepubertal children), and the danger of accidental or intentional overdose. There have been several case reports of sudden death in prepubertal children taking DMI (Riddle et al. 1993), but a causal relationship has not been demonstrated.

Improvement in ADHD symptoms resulting from use of TCAs exceeds the effects of placebo but is less dramatic than stimulant effects (Pliszka 1987). TCAs result in minimal improvement but no impairment on cognitive tests (Biederman et al. 1989a; Donnelly et al. 1986; Rapport et al. 1993). DMI or nortriptyline is preferable to amitriptyline or imipramine because of fewer anticholinergic side effects and longer maintenance of therapeutic effect (Biederman et al. 1989a; Rapoport et al. 1985; Wilens et al. 1993). The use of TCAs in young patients is discussed in the following section on depression.

Bupropion. Bupropion, taken in doses up to approximately 6 mg/kg (divided into two daily doses), may improve behavior and possibly cognitive performance of children with ADHD and conduct disorder (Casat et al. 1989; Clay et al. 1988; Simeon et al. 1986). Bupropion use is described in the section on aggression.

■ Assessment of Response

Multiple outcome measures are essential. The direction and magnitude of effects in various domains (i.e., cognitive, behavioral, social) is typically inconsistent. A given dose of medication often produces improvement in some areas but no change or worsening in others. Data from a patient's parents and teachers on behavior and academic performance before initiating stimulant medication and at regular intervals during treatment are essential (Barkley et al. 1988). The CAP (Child Attention Problems) Rating Scale (Barkley 1990) is a brief teacher rating scale derived from the Teacher Report Form of the Child Behavior Checklist (Achenbach 1991) that is convenient to use weekly (Tables 33–1 and 33–2). In the absence of any intervention, rating scale scores tend to decline from the first administration to the second, and then rise with frequent repeated administration (Diamond and Deane 1988). Observational measures (Barkley et al. 1988), computerized tests of attention and vigilance (Barkley 1990; Conners 1985; Swanson 1985), and measures of academic productivity and accuracy (Gadow and Swanson 1985; Pelham 1985) may also be useful in assessing drug effect.

■ Stimulants

This category of drugs includes methylphenidate (Ritalin), dextroamphetamine (Dexedrine), and magnesium pemoline (Cylert).

Initiation of treatment. The physician should explicitly debunk common myths about stimulant treatment. Stimulants do not have a paradoxical sedative action, they do not cause drug abuse, and they may be indicated and effective after puberty.

There are no predictors of which drugs will be best for a particular child. Methylphenidate is the most commonly used and best studied. It may be more effective in reducing motor activity (Borcherding et al. 1989). Dextroamphetamine is less expensive but it is not included in many formularies. Its disadvantages include negative attitudes of pharmacists (including some who are unwilling to stock it), possible greater risk of growth retardation, and higher potential for abuse. A substantial number of children respond to one stimulant but not another (Elia et al. 1991).

Longer-acting preparations of methylphenidate

(Ritalin Sustained Release [SR]) and dextroamphetamine (Dexedrine Spansule) are appealing when the duration of action of the standard formulations is very short (2½–3 hours), if there is severe rebound, or if administering medication every 4 hours (or at school) is inconvenient, stigmatizing, or impossible. For some children, Ritalin SR is less reliable and less effective than two doses of the standard preparation, although SR works better for a few children. Onset of action may be delayed up to 2 hours and may be more variable from day to day (Pelham et al. 1987). On the other hand, Dexedrine Spansule appears to have more consistent results than standard methylphenidate and to be more effective for some children (Pelham et al. 1990). It also has a greater range of available doses (see Table 33–3). Excessively high

---

Table 33–1. Child Attention Problems (CAP) Rating Scale

Child's Name: _____ Child's Age: _____

Today's Date: _____ Child's Sex: Male [ ] Female [ ]

Filled Out By: _____

Below is a list of items that describes pupils. For each item that describes the pupil **now or within the past week,** check whether the item is **Not True, Somewhat or Sometimes True,** or **Very or Often True.** Please check all items as well as you can, even if some do not seem to apply to this pupil.

	Not true	Somewhat or sometimes true	Very or often true
1. Fails to finish things he/she starts	[ ]	[ ]	[ ]
2. Can't concentrate, can't pay attention for long	[ ]	[ ]	[ ]
3. Can't sit still, restless, or hyperactive	[ ]	[ ]	[ ]
4. Fidgets	[ ]	[ ]	[ ]
5. Daydreams or gets lost in his/her thoughts	[ ]	[ ]	[ ]
6. Impulsive or acts without thinking	[ ]	[ ]	[ ]
7. Difficulty following directions	[ ]	[ ]	[ ]
8. Talks out of turn	[ ]	[ ]	[ ]
9. Messy work	[ ]	[ ]	[ ]
10. Inattentive, easily distracted	[ ]	[ ]	[ ]
11. Talks too much	[ ]	[ ]	[ ]
12. Fails to carry out assigned tasks	[ ]	[ ]	[ ]

Please feel free to write any comments about the pupil's work or behavior in the last week.

Source. Reprinted with permission of Craig Edelbrock, Ph.D.

doses may result if a child chews an SR tablet or spansule instead of swallowing it.

Magnesium pemoline may be administered once a day and has the least abuse potential of the stimulants. However, its absorption and metabolism vary widely, and some children need twice daily doses. Pemoline appears to have both immediate and delayed action (Pelham et al. 1990). The half-life increases with chronic administration (Sallee et al. 1985). Possible pemoline-induced chemical hepatitis (Nehra et al. 1990), although rare, requires monitoring of liver enzymes, and (along with the higher incidence of involuntary movements) limits the usefulness of pemoline.

Table 33–2. Child Attention Problems (CAP) Rating Scale scoring

Each of the 12 items is scored 0, 1, or 2.

Total score = sum of the scores on all items

Subscores:

Inattention: Sum of scores on items 1, 2, 5, 7, 9, 10, and 12

Overactivity: Sum of scores on items 3, 4, 6, 8, and 11

Scores recommended as the upper limit of the normal range (93rd percentile):

	Boys	Girls
Inattention	9	7
Overactivity	6	5
Total Score	15	11

Source. Reprinted with permission of Craig Edelbrock, Ph.D.

Stimulant medication should be initiated with a low dose, and titrated every week or two, within the recommended range, according to response and side effects, using body weight as a rough guide (see Table 33–3). Preschool children or patients with attention-deficit disorder without hyperactivity may benefit from and better tolerate lower doses. Starting with only a morning dose may be useful in assessing drug effect, by comparing morning and afternoon school performance. The need for an after school dose or medication on weekends is individually determined by target symptoms.

Continuation, maintenance, and monitoring. The clinician should work closely with parents on dose adjustments and obtain regular reports from teachers and annual academic testing. The child should not be responsible for his or her own medication. These youngsters are impulsive and forgetful at best, and most dislike the idea of taking medication, even when they can talk about its positive effects and cannot identify any side effects. They will often avoid, "forget," or refuse medication outright.

Management of side effects. Most side effects are similar for all stimulants (see Table 33–4). Giving medication after meals minimizes anorexia without impeding absorption. Insomnia may be because of the drug effect, a rebound effect, or a preexisting sleep problem. Stimulants may either worsen or improve irritable mood (Gadow 1992). Black male ad-

Table 33–3. Clinical use of stimulant medications

	Methylphenidate (Ritalin)	Dextroamphetamine (Dexedrine)	Pemoline (Cylert)
How supplied (mg)	5, 10, 20 Sustained release 20	5, 10 Elixir (5 mg/5 ml) Spansule 5, 10, 15	18.75, 37.5, 75
Single-dose range (mg/kg/dose)	0.3–0.7	0.15–0.5	0.5–2.5
Daily dose range (mg/day)	10–60	5–40	37.5–112.5
Usual starting dose (mg)	5–10 qd or bid	2.5 or 5 qd or bid	18.75 or 37.5 qd
Maintenance number of doses per day	2–4	2–4	1–2
Monitor	Pulse Blood pressure Weight Height Dysphoria Tics	Pulse Blood pressure Weight Height Dysphoria Tics	Pulse Blood pressure Weight Height Dysphoria Tics Liver function

Source. Adapted with permission from Dulcan and Popper 1991.

olescents may be at risk for mild chronically elevated blood pressure on stimulants (Brown and Sexson 1989), but other cardiovascular side effects are exceedingly rare (Safer 1992).

Table 33–4.   Side effects of stimulant medications

Common initial side effects (try dose reduction)

Anorexia

Weight loss

Irritability

Abdominal pain

Headaches

Emotional oversensitivity, easy crying

Less common side effects

Insomnia

Dysphoria (especially at higher doses)

Decreased social interest

Impaired cognitive test performance (especially at very high doses)

Less than expected weight gain

Rebound overactivity and irritability (as dose wears off)

Anxiety

Nervous habits (e.g., picking at skin, pulling hair)

Withdrawal effects

Insomnia

Rebound attention-deficit hyperactivity disorder (ADHD) symptoms

Depression (rare)

Hypersensitivity rash, conjunctivitis, or hives

Rare but potentially serious side effects

Motor tics

Tourette's disorder

Depression

Growth retardation

Tachycardia

Hypertension

Psychosis with hallucinations

Stereotyped activities or compulsions

Side effects reported with pemoline only

Choreiform movements

Dyskinesias

Night terrors

Lip licking or biting

Chemical hepatitis (elevated serum glutamic-oxaloacetic transaminase [SGOT] and serum glutamic-pyruvic transaminase [SGPT], jaundice, epigastric pain) (very rare) (Patterson 1984)

Source. Adapted with permission from Dulcan and Popper 1991.

Although stimulant-induced growth retardation has been a concern, the decrease in expected weight gain is small, despite statistical significance. The effect on height is rarely clinically significant. The magnitude is dose related and appears to be greater with dextroamphetamine than with methylphenidate or pemoline (Greenhill 1981). The mechanism is not through effects on growth hormone (Greenhill 1981). Tolerance to this effect has been reported. Medication-free summers (if clinically appropriate) may facilitate height or weight normalization (Klein et al. 1988). A study of young adults treated in childhood with methylphenidate showed no decrement in final height (Klein and Mannuzza 1988).

Rebound effects consisting of increased excitability, activity, talkativeness, irritability, and insomnia beginning 3–15 hours after a dose may be seen daily, or for up to several days after sudden withdrawal of high daily doses of stimulants. This may resemble a worsening of the original symptoms (Zahn et al. 1980).

Attention is required to avoid possible lowering of the child's self-esteem and self-efficacy, stigmatization by peers, and dependence by parents and teachers on medication rather than making needed changes in the environment (Whalen and Henker 1991). Both patients and relevant adults can be instructed that medication enables the youngster to accomplish what he or she wishes to do; it does not "make" him or her do anything. Children and adolescents should be given full credit for improvement and helped to take an appropriate amount of responsibility for problems that arise. A useful analogy is the assistance provided by leg braces or eyeglasses.

There is no evidence that stimulants produce a decrease in the seizure threshold. In contrast to popular lay belief, taking stimulants prescribed for ADHD does not result in addiction.

Discontinuation.   If symptoms are not severe outside of the school setting, the young person should have an annual drug-free trial in the summer of at least 2 weeks, and longer if possible. If school behavior and academic performance are stable, a carefully monitored trial off medication during the school year (but *not* at the beginning) will provide data on whether medication is still needed.

Treatment resistance.   Stimulant tolerance is reported anecdotally, but noncompliance should be the first possibility considered when medication appears to have become ineffective. Decreased drug effect may also be because of an increase in the patient's weight or a reaction to a change at home or school. Lower efficacy of a generic preparation is another possibility. True tolerance may be more likely with the long-acting formulations (Birmaher et al. 1989). If it occurs, another of the stimulants may be substituted.

If both methylphenidate and dextroamphetamine in appropriate doses are ineffective, several strategies are possible. More intensive psychosocial treatment is often indicated. An innovative strategy for cases that are difficult to manage is the combination of short-acting and longer-acting stimulant medications (Fitzpatrick et al. 1992). If a stimulant is partially effective, it may be combined with clonidine. A TCA trial is often successful in stimulant nonresponders. Bupropion would be a possibility if other drugs failed. Anecdotal data suggest the use of fluoxetine, alone or in combination with methylphenidate (Gammon and Brown 1993).

■ Clonidine

Initiation of treatment. Baseline blood pressure and pulse should be measured and an ECG and laboratory blood studies (especially fasting glucose) obtained before starting clonidine. Clonidine is initiated at a low dose of 0.05 mg (one-half of the smallest manufactured tablet) at bedtime. This converts the side effect of initial sedation into a benefit. An alternate strategy is to begin with 0.025 mg qid.

Continuation, maintenance, and monitoring. The dose of clonidine is titrated gradually over several weeks to 0.15–0.30 mg/day (0.003–0.01 mg/kg/day) in three or four divided doses. Very young children (ages 5–7) may require lower initial and maintenance doses. The transdermal form (skin patch) may improve compliance and reduce variability in blood levels. It lasts only 5 days in children (compared with 7 days in adults) (Hunt et al. 1990). Once the daily dose is determined using pills, an equivalent size patch may be substituted (0.1, 0.2, or 0.3 mg/day). The patch may be cut to adjust the dose. It should be noted that patches do not adhere well in hot, humid climates.

Clonidine has a slow onset of therapeutic action, in part because of the gradual dose increase needed to minimize side effects, and perhaps also because of the time required for receptor downregulation (Hunt et al. 1991). Significant clinical response is not seen for as long as a month, and maximal effect may be delayed for several more months.

Management of side effects. Clonidine's most troublesome side effect is sedation, although it tends to decrease after several weeks. Dry mouth, nausea, and photophobia have been reported, with hypotension and dizziness possible at high doses. The skin patch often causes local pruritic dermatitis. Depression may occur, most often in patients with a personal or family history of depressive symptoms (Hunt et al. 1991). Glucose tolerance may decrease, especially in those at risk for diabetes.

Discontinuation. When clonidine is discontinued, it should be tapered rather than stopped suddenly. This is necessary to avoid a withdrawal syndrome consisting of increased motor restlessness, headache, agitation, and elevated blood pressure and pulse rate (Leckman et al. 1986).

■ Tricyclic Antidepressants

When treating ADHD, DMI or imipramine is begun with 10 or 25 mg qd and increased weekly to a maximum dose of 5 mg/kg/day (divided tid in children). Plasma levels do not predict efficacy. Some patients respond to a daily dose as low as 2 mg/kg. Nortriptyline is started at 10 or 25 mg/day and may be increased as tolerated until clinical effect or 4.5 mg/kg/day (mean 2 mg/kg/day) (given in two divided doses) is reached. It is possible that the serum level (50 to 150 ng/ml) may relate to therapeutic response (Wilens et al. 1993). The use of TCAs in treating children and adolescents is discussed in the next section.

A cautionary note should be added here: the combination of imipramine and methylphenidate has been associated with a syndrome of confusion, affective lability, marked aggression, and severe agitation that disappeared when the medications were discontinued (Grob and Coyle 1986). The mechanism may be methylphenidate's interference with hepatic metabolism of imipramine, resulting in a longer half-life and elevated blood levels.

MOOD DISORDERS

Bipolar Disorders

Assessment for treatment. Historically, mania has been underdiagnosed in children and adolescents (Weller et al. 1986a). Many clinicians still are not aware of the existence of mania in children and adolescents or do not encounter it often enough to fully master its assessment and treatment. Referral of such patients to centers that specialize in childhood mood disorders may be considered. Clinical assessment should be done by talking to the child and the parents together and then individually. When assessing the child, it is important to ask age-specific questions that cover the DSM-IV criteria. Useful instruments include the Diagnostic Interview for Children and Adolescents Revised (DICA-R) (Reich and Welner 1988) and the Schedule for Affective Disorder and Schizophrenia for School-Age Children (KIDDIE-SADS) (Chambers et al. 1985). Unfortunately, both instruments are somewhat cumbersome. The DICA-R can be used by a well-trained psychometrician; however, the KIDDIE-SADS requires a child and adolescent clinician with additional training in the interview. The DICA-R often gives a false positive for mania in a child who has conduct disorder or ADHD. Manic children can be distinguished from children with ADHD by their higher score on the Mania Rating Scale (MRS) (Fristad et al. 1992). Children with ADHD scored 0 to 12, whereas manic children received scores of 14 to 39. The widely used Conners Parent and Conners Teacher Rating Scales (Goyette et al. 1978) do not distinguish between ADHD and mania. A careful history can differentiate the manic child from a child with hyperactivity or conduct disorder. In mania, a cyclic history is more common; symptoms are more chronic in conduct disorder or ADHD. Family psychiatric history may also be useful.

Medical conditions such as multiple sclerosis, seizure disorders, and brain tumors that may mimic mania must be ruled out. As in any child or adolescent with a first episode of psychosis, a magnetic resonance imaging (MRI) or computed tomography (CT) scan should be considered as part of a baseline workup for a manic youth. The medical evaluation should include routine blood studies, including complete blood count (CBC) with differential, electrolytes, thyroid function tests, blood urea nitrogen (BUN), creatinine, and creatinine clearance. A baseline ECG is advisable, because manic children often become depressed and may need TCAs in addition to mood-stabilizing medications.

Selection of treatment. Despite the lack of published double-blind placebo-controlled studies conducted with bipolar children and adolescents, many clinicians use mood-stabilizing medications in an effort to help their patients with this potentially devastating illness. Extrapolation is necessary from the successful psychopharmacological treatment of adults with bipolar disorder.

Lithium carbonate is the drug most commonly used to stabilize mood in children (Weller et al. 1986b). Although manic children and adolescents treated with lithium may become easier to redirect, the more dramatic response to lithium observed in adult manic patients does not occur as often. Manic youngsters with preadolescent onset of psychopathology have a poorer response to lithium than those with adolescent-onset mania without prepubertal psychopathology (Strober et al. 1988). In a study that used lithium to treat aggressive children and adolescents, positive responders had mood symptoms, a family history of mood disorders, and/or lithium-responsive relatives (Youngerman and Canino 1978).

Because the degree of symptom abatement with lithium is often disappointing, other medications such as carbamazepine (Tegretol) have been tried, although there are no double-blind placebo-controlled studies with bipolar children and adolescents. (The use of carbamazepine is discussed in the section on the treatment of aggression.) Some child and adolescent psychiatrists are using valproic acid, although there are no double-blind placebo-controlled studies proving its efficacy in children.

Consent from parents or guardians and assent from the patient should be obtained before starting a child or adolescent on a mood-stabilizing medication. It should be made clear to the responsible adult that data substantiating the efficacy of treating children and adolescents with mania or hypomania with these agents are limited; data are mostly from open studies or anecdotal reports.

Assessment of response. Treatment response in bipolar youths is best evaluated by experienced clinicians. The MRS can be used to assess response—

total scores decrease with successful treatment. In adolescents, the Beigel-Murphy Scale (Beigel et al. 1971) can also be used.

■ Lithium

Initiation of treatment. In the past, many physicians would start a child on 300 mg of lithium for several weeks and slowly increase it to 900 mg/day. Using a weight-based dosage guide for prepubertal children, therapeutic levels can be safely attained in a much shorter time (Weller et al. 1986b). Lithium has a half-life of approximately 24 hours. Thus, it can be given once a day. However, some patients have gastrointestinal problems when they take a single dose at bedtime. For that reason, lithium is usually given bid or tid with meals to minimize gastrointestinal upset. More frequent doses may reduce compliance. There have been no systematic studies in children comparing the efficacy and side effects of different dosing regimens. In general, the blood level should not exceed 1.4 mEq/L. Peak serum levels will occur within 1–2 hours after ingestion. Steady-state serum levels are achieved after 5 days. Blood should be drawn for a serum level 8–12 hours after ingesting the last evening dose and before the first morning dose. For children, an 8 A.M. sampling time is most commonly used. Some clinicians suggest that higher lithium levels can be used in preschool-aged children. However, data supporting the safety and efficacy of this practice have not been published.

Although lithium comes in different forms, in our practice (E. B. W. and R. W.) we have found little advantage to using compounds other than lithium carbonate, which has reliable serum levels as well as reasonable cost.

Continuation, maintenance, and monitoring. A child or adolescent being treated with lithium carbonate should have a medical checkup at least once a month to ensure that the lithium is tolerated well and to monitor compliance. Although in the acute manic phase serum levels up to 1.4 mEq/L are tolerated well, clinical experience suggests that maintenance levels can be lower (i.e., 0.6–1.2 mEq/L). Although it is theoretically possible to substitute saliva levels of lithium for serum levels, this has not yet become common in clinical practice (Weller et al. 1987). BUN and creatinine should be periodically checked, because lithium may cause alterations in kidney

function. Lithium may produce goiter and/or hypothyroidism; therefore, a thyroid-stimulating hormone (TSH) test should be obtained every 4–6 months.

Management of side effects. Lithium is well tolerated by most children and adolescents. The most common side effects in children (i.e., tremor, weight gain, accentuation of preexisting enuresis, polyuria, polydypsia, and polyphagia) (Weller et al. 1986b) rarely require discontinuation of lithium. Lithium carbonate deposits in the bones, but whether this has any significant impact on a growing child whose epiphyseal plate is not closed is unknown. However, lithium has not been reported to interfere with the growth of children. The impact of lithium on cognitive functioning in children has not been studied in detail. Hypokalemia is a very rare side effect. It can be managed by feeding children two bananas, two large carrots, two cups of skim milk, half a honeydew melon, or an avocado daily. This may be preferable to giving potassium tablets that can further irritate the gastrointestinal tract and usually have a taste that children dislike. When a child is taking lithium carbonate, the patient and the family should be taught to be especially cautious when the patient develops physical illness with fever, vomiting, or diarrhea, uses rigorous dieting to lose weight, or takes diuretics or nonsteroidal anti-inflammatory agents. Any of these situations should immediately be brought to the psychiatrist's attention. Lithium should be discontinued while a patient has fever, vomiting, or diarrhea.

Discontinuation. Gradual tapering off of medication is recommended. The patient should be followed closely after discontinuing medication and should be checked for signs of relapse to mania or for symptoms of depression so that episodes can be treated early and hospitalization avoided. The kindling hypothesis suggests special caution regarding discontinuation of mood stabilizers.

There are no studies that address the issue of how long lithium should be continued once started. A naturalistic study (Strober et al. 1990) found that adolescents who discontinued their lithium were three times more likely to relapse compared with those who continued the medication. Most relapses were within the first year after cessation of treatment. Once lithium is started, it seems advisable to continue it for at least 6 months and preferably a year.

Generalizing from studies of lithium termination in adults, even longer duration of treatment might be considered.

■ Valproic Acid

Initiation of treatment. Valproic acid can cause hepatotoxicity, although this is extremely rare in patients over age 10; the greatest risk is for patients less than 3 years old. Thus, baseline liver function tests are necessary before starting treatment (Trimble 1990). The half-life of valproic acid is 8–15 hours. Steady-state plasma levels can therefore be measured after 3–5 days on a fixed dose.

Valproic acid is available in tablets, capsules (Depakene 250 mg), and elixir of 250 mg/5 ml (16-oz. bottles). Depakote, an enteric coated tablet formulation of valproic acid available in 125-, 250-, and 500-mg sizes, is recommended to avoid gastrointestinal side effects.

Valproic acid should be started at a dose of 250 mg qd and increased by 250 mg every 4 days (not to exceed 60 mg/kg/day). Therapeutic levels are 50–120 ng/ml. However, the plasma levels are not as useful as for lithium and carbamazepine.

Continuation, maintenance, and monitoring. Liver function tests should be done periodically.

Management of side effects. Side effects of valproate include nausea, vomiting, anorexia, lethargy, and abdominal pain, although these may be minimized by starting with a low dose and titrating up slowly. Hepatotoxicity is possible, but when valproate is discontinued, recovery of liver enzymes occurs within several weeks. A very rare complication of valproate treatment of children and adolescents is (potentially fatal) pancreatitis (Trimble 1990). However, most patients who experience this are taking multiple anticonvulsants. Neutropenia and thrombocytopenia as well as macrocytic anemia have been reported in valproate-treated patients.

Treatment resistance. If mania is treatment-resistant, several options can be discussed. However, it should always be remembered that although such strategies have been employed in adults, there are few if any studies of their efficacy in children and adolescents.

A possible strategy is the addition of an antipsychotic agent, most commonly haloperidol. Despite an isolated report of complications from the simultaneous use of haloperidol and lithium in some adult patients, most tolerate this combination fairly well. Clinical experience (E. B. W.) suggests that the use of haloperidol should be considered in treating patients with psychotic mania, in manic patients with obsessive-compulsive disorder (OCD) traits and frequent rumination, and in manic patients whose mania is comorbid with psychiatric diagnoses that would respond to haloperidol, such as Tourette's disorder.

Clinicians have used carbamazepine in the treatment of dysphoric or treatment-resistant mania in adults. Recently its use for similar indications in children has been considered, despite the lack of published data regarding its efficacy. (The use of carbamazepine is discussed in the section on the treatment of aggression.)

Valproic acid has been increasingly used to treat lithium-resistant adult manic patients. Some clinicians have advocated using valproate even before a trial of lithium and/or carbamazepine.

Other medications that have occasionally been used in treatment-resistant mania include clonazepam, lorazepam, clonidine, verapamil, propranolol, and physostigmine. Electroconvulsive therapy has occasionally been used in treatment-resistant manic teenagers. Because of a lack of data or even clinical experience with most of these treatments in children and adolescents (except for occasional anecdotal cases), the reader is referred to the chapter on the treatment of mania in adults (Chapter 29).

■ Depression

For many years, depression was not recognized in children and adolescents. Recognition of mood disorders in this age group during the last 20 years has resulted in increased interest in diagnosing and treating depression in young patients (Weller and Weller 1990). It is clear that the successful pharmacological treatment of mood disorders in children and adolescents awaits well-designed multicenter double-blind placebo-controlled studies. The importance of working with schools and parents by educating them about the illness should not be underestimated. Also, individual and/or group therapies may address social deficits that cannot be helped with medication alone.

Assessment for treatment. An assessment using DSM-IV criteria should be done by the clinician, including meeting with the parents, interviewing the child, and obtaining information from the child's school. Because most children with mood disorders have a family history of such disorders, it is important that parental illness not be permitted to color the reporting of psychopathology in the child. However, the child and a parent may be simultaneously depressed. Reports from school, where the teacher can be an objective observer of the child's behavior in comparison with that of other children, can be a very important part of the evaluation. Although teacher evaluations may be more difficult to obtain for high school students who change classes every hour, information from the school is still valuable. For example, the most disturbed youths often come to the attention of the school counselor, the school nurse, or the principal because of poor attendance or declining academic performance.

In addition to using the diagnostic interviews discussed in the section on mania in this chapter, the assessment of a depressed child or adolescent should include the Child Depression Rating Scale, Revised (CDRS-R) (Poznanski et al. 1985), which is similar to the Hamilton Rating Scale for Depression (Hamilton 1967). Self-assessment is also very important. In children, the Child Depression Inventory (CDI) (Kovacs 1985) is frequently used. However, children often do not reveal much about themselves because they can determine the "normal" response and answer accordingly. In one study, the CDI did not differentiate children with depression from those with conduct disorder (Fristad et al. 1988). In adolescents, the Beck Depression Inventory (Beck et al. 1961) can be used.

The proper role of the laboratory assessment of depression is controversial. This is particularly true of the dexamethasone suppression test (DST), which has been the most widely studied test in children and adolescents (Weller and Weller 1988). The DST is positive in approximately 50% of prepubertal depressed children and 40% of depressed adolescents. In a study of hospitalized children, the DST was positive in 70% of depressed subjects (Weller et al. 1984). Normalization of DST with treatment has been reported in a small group of depressed children (Weller et al. 1986c).

To perform the DST, 0.5 mg dexamethasone is given to prepubertal children and 1 mg to adolescents at 11 P.M. Plasma cortisol levels are measured at 4 P.M. and 11 P.M. the next day. If the cortisol level is greater than or equal to 5 ng/ml, cortisol is nonsuppressed and the DST is considered positive. A positive DST is most frequently observed in hospitalized, suicidal, or so-called "endogenously depressed" children and adolescents.

Selection of treatment. TCAs have been the most studied medications in the treatment of depression in children and adolescents. In open studies, 75% of patients treated with antidepressants have responded positively (Weller and Weller 1990). However, when double-blind placebo-controlled studies are considered, only one study demonstrated an advantage of imipramine over placebo (Preskorn et al. 1987). In this study of a small sample of hospitalized prepubertal children, dexamethasone nonsuppression and comorbid anxiety symptoms were associated with a positive response to imipramine. In adolescents, no double-blind study shows the efficacy of TCAs over placebo. More double-blind placebo-controlled studies with larger sample sizes are needed to clearly determine the efficacy of TCAs in the treatment of depressed children and adolescents.

In recent years, a new class of antidepressants, the selective serotonin reuptake inhibitors (SSRIs), have been introduced. These new antidepressants include fluoxetine (Prozac), sertraline (Zoloft), and paroxetine (Paxil).

One published study of fluoxetine in depressed children and adolescents who did not respond to TCAs reported improvement among these subjects (Joshi et al. 1989). Although several open trials had given researchers hope, preliminary findings from double-blind placebo-controlled multicenter studies do not seem very promising (Consortium on Mood Disorders in Children and Adolescents 1993). When used, fluoxetine is started with 20 mg/day or less. Most patients do not need more than 40 mg qd. Some clinicians are also giving it on an every-other-day basis. (The use of fluoxetine is discussed in the section on OCD.) It should be kept in mind that these medications are new, and their long-term effects on growing children are unknown. Their advantages over TCAs include the absence of cardiac side effects and relative safety in overdose.

Additional agents (including monoamine oxidase inhibitors [MAOIs]) are discussed in the section on treatment resistance.

Assessment of response. To fully assess response to medication, input from the child, parents, and the school should be obtained. Both the CDI and the Beck Depression Inventory can be used to assess changes in symptomatology. The CDRS-R can combine input from clinician, child, parent, and teacher.

Initiation of treatment. Before initiating treatment with a TCA, a complete physical examination should be done. Also, it should be determined if there is a history of any cardiac problems (especially arrhythmias and conduction defects) in the child or the family. Any history of sudden death in the family should also be fully evaluated. DMI has been linked to sudden death in several prepubertal children, although causality remains controversial. An ECG should be performed before initiating treatment. If abnormalities are seen in a routine ECG, an ECG with a rhythm strip should be obtained and interpreted by a pediatric cardiologist. A CBC with differential, BUN, creatinine, creatinine clearance, and thyroid function tests are recommended as part of a baseline laboratory evaluation; approximately 20%–30% of depressed children and adolescents develop bipolar disorder on follow-up and may require mood-stabilizing medications.

Treatment should be initiated with a small dose of the TCA and gradually increased. Some experts believe that plasma level monitoring may be helpful in determining optimum dose (if a laboratory that measures TCAs reliably is available) (Preskorn et al. 1988), although this is controversial. TCAs have long half-lives; hence, once-a-day dosing is adequate for antidepressant effect. However, if comorbid ADHD is present, a thrice-daily regimen may be preferred. For imipramine, the daily dose should not exceed 5 mg/kg or 200 mg, whichever is smaller. Equivalent doses for other TCAs should be used. Most studies of TCAs have used imipramine and nortriptyline; there have been few studies using amitriptyline. Serial ECGs are recommended when the daily dose is above 3 mg/kg because of the potential for arrhythmias. Table 33–5 lists titration parameters.

Continuation, maintenance, and monitoring. Once response to the antidepressant has occurred (after approximately 3–8 weeks), the medication should be continued for a period of 4–6 months. Throughout this period, the clinician should continue to monitor side effects and response. Monitoring the

Table 33–5. Guidelines for the use of tricyclic antidepressants for the treatment of depression and attention-deficit hyperactivity disorder (ADHD) in children and adolescents

Electrocardiogram and vital sign limits to titration: reduce dose or discontinue drug if reached

	Age 10 or younger	Age 11 or older
P-R interval (sec)	0.18	0.21
QRS interval (sec)	0.12	0.12
	150% of baseline	150% of baseline
QTc interval (sec)	0.48	0.48
Sustained resting heart rate (bpm)	110	110
Routine heart rate (bpm)	130	130
Chronic blood pressure (mmHg)	130/85	140/85
Resting blood pressure (mmHg)	140/90	150/95

Source. N. Ryan, personal communication, May 1993.

medication with plasma levels is recommended by some to assure compliance and avoid toxicity (Preskorn et al. 1988), although this is controversial. Periodic ECGs should be obtained if the dose exceeds 3 mg/kg/day.

Management of side effects. The most common side effects of TCAs are dry mouth, tremor, constipation, and tachycardia. Drowsiness and dizziness sometimes occur with initiation of treatment. However, with proper instruction in how to manage transient postural hypotension, most children tolerate this side effect and adjust to it. Dry mouth can usually be managed by instructing the patient to chew sugarless gum or wax, or to sip water or diet drinks. These techniques will help keep the mouth moist while minimizing the risk of dental cavities and weight gain. In extreme cases that do not respond to these measures, xerolube mouthwash can be used. If a TCA-induced tremor becomes intolerable, decreasing the dosage should be considered. If constipation is a problem, a high fiber diet and increased liquids are helpful. Bedtime snacks of popcorn are fun for children and provide good roughage. In the occasional situation where a stool softener is needed, Colace (200 mg at bedtime) can be used. If ECG changes appear, alternatives include decreasing the dose or switching to another antidepressant.

Discontinuation. After a child or adolescent has been asymptomatic for 4–6 months, stopping the medication should be considered. It is not advisable to stop the medication when a child or adolescent is confronting stressful life events (e.g., starting school, a parental divorce, or moving to a different town). Currently some clinicians are keeping their young patients on TCAs chronically, especially when a patient has had multiple episodes of unipolar depression.

Discontinuation of antidepressants should not be done abruptly, to avoid a flu-like withdrawal syndrome of malaise, aches, and nausea, as well as depressive symptoms (Petti and Law 1981). Tapering off the medication gradually is recommended, especially if the patient has been taking it for a long time.

Treatment resistance. Ryan and colleagues (1988a) and Strober and colleagues (1992) have reported some success in open-label studies using lithium augmentation in adolescents who have not responded or have had only a partial response to antidepressants. Some researchers (E. B. W. and R. W.) have also had some success in using lithium augmentation in prepubertal children with residual symptoms of depression after antidepressant treatment. Lithium augmentation is especially helpful in children with a family history of bipolar illness or those with comorbid aggressive conduct disorder. Although there are no empirical guidelines regarding the optimum blood level in lithium augmentation, lithium serum levels should not exceed 1.0 mEq/L.

MAOIs have rarely been used to treat children and adolescents because the required dietary restrictions present problems for this age group. However, most children and adolescents do not mind being deprived of chopped chicken liver, Chianti, aged cheese, or anchovies. Children and adolescents are most likely to get in trouble by impulsively gorging themselves on chocolate or on pepperoni and sausage pizza. Ryan and colleagues (1988b) have successfully used MAOIs to treat teenagers who did not respond to TCAs. We (E. B. W. and R. W.) have used MAOIs to treat prepubertal children who are unresponsive to TCAs and lithium in cases where both the child and the family were reliable and responsible.

■ SCHIZOPHRENIA

■ Assessment for Treatment

Target symptoms should be identified. Before beginning medication, a complete physical examination and baseline laboratory workup (including CBC with differential, liver profile, and urinalysis) should be done.

■ Selection of Treatment

The cornerstone of treatment is an intensive and comprehensive school-based program that may include a highly structured environment, supportive reality-based individual psychotherapy, and family psychoeducational treatment. Hospitalization and/or long-term residential treatment may be needed. Medication may be essential if positive psychotic symptoms (e.g., delusions or hallucinations) cause significant impairment or interfere with other interventions.

A variety of neuroleptics appear to have modest efficacy in children and adolescents (Teicher and Glod 1990; Whitaker and Rao 1992). In general, however, young schizophrenic patients are less responsive to pharmacotherapy than adults and continue to have substantial impairment, even if the more florid symptoms such as hallucinations, anxiety, and agitation abate (Campbell et al. 1985). Clinical experience suggests that an antihistamine such as diphenhydramine may be useful if a patient's sleep is severely disturbed.

■ Assessment of Response

Full efficacy may require several weeks to appear. Parent and teacher reports are essential, in addition to self-report in adolescents.

■ Initiation of Treatment

Doses must be titrated with careful attention to positive and negative effects. Age, weight, and severity of symptoms do not provide clear dose guidelines. The initial dose should be very low, with gradual increments, no more than once or twice a week. Children metabolize these drugs more rapidly than adults but also require lower plasma levels for efficacy (Teicher and Glod 1990). Older adolescents with schizophrenia may require doses of neuroleptics in the adult range. Young adolescents fall in between, and doses must be empirically determined.

■ Continuation, Maintenance, and Monitoring

Antipsychotic drugs are highly lipophilic. Chlorpromazine has been demonstrated to have a lower plasma concentration in children than adults after the same weight-adjusted dose (Rivera-Calimlim et al. 1979). However, the magnitude of the difference exceeds that expected from the small proportional excess of adipose tissue in children compared with adults. This is probably because of children's increased efficiency of hepatic biotransformation (Jatlow 1987). Developmental changes in protein binding may be influential as well. Although a single daily dose (usually at bedtime) is generally preferred, divided doses may be used during titration (especially in hospitalized patients) to minimize side effects and permit finer dose adjustments.

■ Management of Side Effects

Acute extrapyramidal side effects (EPS), including dystonic reactions, parkinsonian tremor and rigidity, drooling, and akathisia, occur as in adults. Laryngeal dystonia is potentially fatal. Acute dystonia may be treated with oral or intramuscular diphenhydramine 25 or 50 mg, or benztropine 0.5 to 2.0 mg. When medication is initiated for an outpatient, a responsible adult should be instructed to watch for a dystonic reaction and given a supply of medication to give the child if needed. Adolescent boys seem to be more vulnerable to acute dystonic reactions than adult patients, so the physician may be more inclined to use prophylactic antiparkinsonian medication. Clinical experience suggests that children do not respond well to anticholinergics, and reduction of neuroleptic dose is therefore preferable (Campbell et al. 1985). For treatment or prevention of parkinsonian symptoms, adolescents may be given benztropine, 1–2 mg/day, in divided doses. Chronic parkinsonian symptoms are often drastically underrecognized by clinicians (Richardson et al. 1991). The neuromuscular consequences may impair performance of age-appropriate activities, and the subjective effects may lead to noncompliance with medication. Akathisia may be especially difficult to identify in very young patients or those with limited verbal ability.

Tardive dyskinesia (TD) has been documented in children and adolescents after as brief a period of treatment as 5 months (Herskowitz 1987), and it may appear even during periods of constant medication dose. Before being placed on a neuroleptic and periodically thereafter, each patient should have a careful examination for abnormal movements, using a scale such as the Abnormal Involuntary Movement Scale (AIMS) (Munetz and Benjamin 1988). Parents and patients (if they are able) should receive regular explanations of the risk of movement disorders. Concerns regarding the development of TD in long-term use and the prominence of negative symptoms in young schizophrenic patients suggest that clozapine may prove to be useful (Birmaher et al. 1992; Teicher and Glod 1990).

Potentially fatal neuroleptic malignant syndrome has been reported in children and adolescents (Latz and McCracken 1992; Steingard et al. 1992).

Weight gain may be problematic in the long-term use of the low-potency neuroleptics. Abnormal laboratory findings seem to be less often reported in studies with children than with adults, but the clinician should be alert to the possibility, especially of agranulocytosis or hepatic dysfunction. If an acute febrile illness or easy bruising occurs, medication should be withheld and CBC with differential and liver enzymes should be determined (Campbell et al. 1985). Children may be at greater risk of neuroleptic-induced seizures than adults, because of their immature nervous systems and the very high prevalence of abnormal EEGs in seriously disturbed children (Teicher and Glod 1990).

Of particular concern is behavioral toxicity, manifested as worsening of preexisting symptoms or development of new symptoms such as hyper- or hypoactivity, irritability, apathy, withdrawal, stereotypies, tics, or hallucinations (Campbell et al. 1985). Children and adolescents are more sensitive to cognitive dulling and sedation that interfere with the ability to benefit from school resulting from low-potency antipsychotic drugs (e.g., chlorpromazine, thioridazine) (Campbell et al. 1985; Realmuto et al. 1984).

Anticholinergic side effects are unusual. Miscellaneous side effects include abdominal pain, enuresis (Realmuto et al. 1984), photosensitivity, and various neuroendocrine effects that may be especially distressing to adolescents.

For a more detailed discussion of neuroleptic

side effects and their management, see Whitaker and Rao (1992).

■ Discontinuation

Withdrawal dyskinesias, which are usually transient but potentially irreversible, are seen in 8%–51% of neuroleptic-treated children and adolescents (Campbell et al. 1985). Other withdrawal-emergent symptoms include nausea, vomiting, loss of appetite, diaphoresis, and hyperactivity (Gualtieri and Hawk 1980). A variety of behavioral symptoms may appear up to several weeks after neuroleptic withdrawal and persist for as long as 8 weeks (Gualtieri et al. 1984). These must be distinguished from a return of manifestations of the original disorder. A prolonged drug-free trial may be indicated, if possible, to ascertain if neuroleptics are truly needed.

■ Treatment Resistance

Neuroleptic resistance is common in young schizophrenic patients. Two or three different classes of drug may be tried, with clozapine as a possibility (Birmaher et al. 1992; Blanz and Schmidt 1993). Common therapeutic errors leading to the perception of treatment resistance include incorrect diagnosis, subtherapeutic or excessive medication doses, premature changes in medication before efficacy can appear, failure to monitor target symptoms or patient compliance, hasty or irrational polypharmacy, and failure to provide psychosocial therapies (McClellan and Werry 1992).

■ AGGRESSION

■ Assessment for Treatment

Many aggressive patients carry a primary or secondary diagnosis of conduct disorder. When aggression is secondary to another psychiatric diagnosis, such as depression (increased irritability), mania (psychosis, irritability), schizophrenia (paranoid delusions or hallucinations), pervasive developmental disorder, or substance abuse, the primary disorder is the appropriate focus of treatment.

Adults such as parents, teachers, juvenile justice authorities, and child care and nursing staff are quick to report verbal or physical aggression and demand its elimination. The physician's first duty is to perform a careful evaluation, seeking primary psychiatric disorders. There is a high frequency of brain damage in patients with violent conduct disorders. A focused history may disclose symptoms suggestive of temporal lobe, psychomotor, or complex partial seizures (Lewis et al. 1982).

The youth's environment must be considered in detail, because aggression is often a response to the dynamics or reinforcement structure of a family, school, neighborhood, group home, or inpatient unit. Psychodynamic, systems, and behavioral theories may all be useful in understanding the conditions that precipitate and maintain aggressive behavior and in reducing its frequency and severity. Parents and school personnel are likely to be unsophisticated regarding behavior modification, and they may require strong encouragement to institute appropriate contingency management programs. The clinician should guard against being persuaded to use medication alone when a clinical evaluation suggests that other interventions instead of or in addition to medication would be more appropriate (e.g., aggression secondary to frustration at overly high academic demands or in response to peer bullying). On the other hand, there are times when a chemical restraint is preferable to a physical restraint and may facilitate other forms of treatment or permit the child's placement in a less restrictive environment.

■ Selection of Treatment

A variety of classes of medication may be prescribed in an attempt to reduce aggression. If the aggression is impulsive and the youth also has a diagnosis of ADHD, the first choice is a stimulant. In children with ADHD who are positive responders to stimulants, oppositional defiant behavior and aggression are reduced, along with improvements in activity level and attention (Amery et al. 1984; Hinshaw et al. 1989; Klorman et al. 1989; Murphy et al. 1992; Whalen et al. 1987). Although stimulants have been suggested for the treatment of conduct disorder without ADHD, there are as yet no data to support this strategy.

Patients with severe impulsive aggression with emotional lability and irritability who have an abnormal EEG or a strong clinical suggestion of episodic phenomena may deserve a trial of carbamazepine, although deliberate aggression is rarely part of a frank seizure (Evans et al. 1987). Preliminary data suggest efficacy in children with severe explosive aggression, even in the absence of neurological findings (Kafantaris et al. 1992). Valproic acid has been used, but there are no systematic data on its efficacy.

β-adrenergic blockers may be useful in treating patients with otherwise uncontrollable rage reactions and impulsive aggression, especially those with evidence of organicity (Kuperman and Stewart 1987; Williams et al. 1982). However, evidence of organicity does not appear to be a prerequisite for efficacy (Grizenko and Vida 1988).

Historically, neuroleptics have been used to control aggression. In view of the risk of cognitive dulling and TD, neuroleptics should be low on the list of medication options. Studies of hospitalized severely aggressive children ages 6–12 have demonstrated the short-term efficacy of haloperidol (1–6 mg qd or 0.04–0.21 mg/kg/day), thioridazine (mean 170 mg/day), and molindone (mean 26.8 mg/day) compared with placebo in reducing (though not eliminating) aggression, hostility, negativism, and explosiveness (Campbell et al. 1985; Greenhill et al. 1985). (The use of neuroleptics in children and adolescents is discussed in the previous section on schizophrenia.)

Lithium may be considered in the treatment of children and adolescents with severe aggression, especially when it is impulsive and accompanied by explosive affect and poor self-control (Campbell et al. 1984; Platt et al. 1984). The presence in an aggressive child or adolescent of a family history of bipolar mood disorder (especially if lithium-responsive) may suggest a lithium trial before considering other pharmacological options. (The use of lithium in children and adolescents is described in the section on mood disorders.)

One pilot study found bupropion reduced symptoms of conduct disorder, whether or not ADHD was also present (Simeon et al. 1986). Trazodone may be useful in decreasing aggression in children and adolescents with disruptive behavior disorders (Ghaziuddin and Alessi 1992). Clonidine may reduce aggression even in the absence of ADHD (Kemph et al. 1993). (See the section on ADHD regarding the use of clonidine.)

■ Assessment of Response

Careful documentation of precipitants, severity, frequency, and targets of aggression is necessary for evaluating efficacy of treatment. An instrument such as the Overt Aggression Scale (Yudofsky et al. 1986) can facilitate this process.

■ Carbamazepine

Initiation of treatment. Baseline hemoglobin, hematocrit, CBC with differential, white blood cell (WBC) count, platelet count, and liver functions should be measured before starting a child on carbamazepine.

The initial dose is 100 mg daily, with food. Children eliminate carbamazepine more rapidly than adults (Jatlow 1987). Plasma levels (drawn approximately 12 hours after the last dose) are crucial, because dosage calculated by weight correlates poorly with plasma concentration. The half-life is approximately 9 hours. Titration is gradual (increased weekly by 100 mg/day), guided by plasma levels, to a usual plateau of 8–12 mEq/ml. The usual daily dose range is 10–50 mg/kg, divided into three doses for children and two for older adolescents. Autoinduction of hepatic enzymes may lead to declining plasma concentration (especially in the first 6 weeks) requiring periodic increases in dose. Carbamazepine lowers the plasma levels of neuroleptics, imipramine, and valproic acid.

Continuation, maintenance, and monitoring. The degree of ongoing laboratory monitoring necessary is controversial. A conservative recommendation includes CBC and liver function studies weekly for the first 4 weeks, monthly for 4 months, and every 3 months thereafter (Silverstein et al. 1983). A more modest regimen is CBC (with differential and platelet count), serum iron, BUN, and creatinine after the first month, and every 3–6 months thereafter (Trimble 1990). Tests should always be ordered if a rash, sore throat, fever, malaise, lethargy, weakness, vomiting, increased urinary frequency, anorexia, jaundice, easy bruising, bleeding, or mouth ulcers develop. If the neutrophil count drops below 1,000 or hepatitis occurs, the drug should be stopped (Silverstein et al. 1983).

Side effects. The most common adverse effects of carbamazepine are drowsiness, nausea, rash, diplopia, nystagmus, and reversible dose-related leukopenia. Other side effects include vomiting, vertigo, ataxia, tics, muscle cramps, exacerbation of seizures, rare blood dyscrasias, hepatotoxicity, severe skin reactions (e.g., Stevens-Johnson syndrome or systemic lupus-like syndrome), and inappropriate secretion of antidiuretic hormone (which in rare cases leads to acute renal failure) (Evans et al. 1987; Trimble 1990). Teratogenic effects have been demonstrated. Adverse behavioral reactions (e.g., extreme irritability, agitation, insomnia, obsessive thinking, hallucinations, delirium, psychosis, paranoia, hyperactivity, aggression, and mania) may be seen during the first 1–4 weeks of treatment (Evans et al. 1987; Herskowitz 1987; Pleak et al. 1988).

■ β-Adrenergic Blockers

The most clinical experience has been obtained with propranolol. Pindolol and nadolol have been suggested as alternatives with fewer side effects and longer half-lives, but they have not been tested in children. (See Connor 1993 for an extensive review.)

Initiation of treatment. The premedication workup should include a recent history and physical examination, with particular attention to medical contraindications: asthma, diabetes, bradycardia, heart block, cardiac failure, or hypothyroidism. Fasting blood sugar and a glucose tolerance test may be indicated if there is risk of diabetes. An ECG may be considered.

In children and adolescents, the initial dose of propranolol is 10 mg tid, increasing by 10–20 mg every 3–4 days, monitoring pulse and blood pressure (minimum pulse 50, blood pressure 80/50). The standard daily dose range is 10–120 mg for children and 20–300 mg for adolescents, divided into three doses (2–8 mg/kg/day) (Coffey 1990). The short elimination half-life in children (2–4 hours) may necessitate four daily doses. Dose is titrated to clinical effect or side effects. Maximum improvement at a given dose may not be seen for up to 12 weeks. When propranolol or pindolol are used together with chlorpromazine or thioridazine (but not haloperidol), blood levels of both drugs are elevated.

Side effects. Side effects are generally the same in children as in adults. Tiredness, mild hypotension, and bradycardia are the most common.

Discontinuation. β-Blockers should be tapered gradually to avoid rebound hypertension and tachycardia.

■ Bupropion

Bupropion is administered in two or three daily doses, beginning with a dose of 50 mg/day or 3 mg/kg/day, with titration over 2 weeks to a maximum of 250 mg/day or 6 mg/kg/day, whichever is less. The most serious potential side effect is a decrease in the seizure threshold. Other side effects in children include skin rash, perioral edema, nausea, increased appetite, and agitation. Exacerbation of tics (Spencer et al. 1993) or hypomania is possible.

■ Trazodone

The dose used in the few reported cases has been 75 mg/day (mean 0.35 mg/kg/day) (Ghaziuddin and Alessi 1992). Reported side effects in youths include mild sedation and increased penile erections. Priapism is possible.

■ Treatment Resistance

If aggression is not reduced at the highest appropriate drug dose, a different class of drug should be considered. A closer look at the family and school environment is indicated, with initiation of more intensive psychosocial treatment, perhaps including hospitalization.

■ ANXIETY DISORDERS

■ Separation Anxiety Disorder (SAD)

Assessment for treatment. In SAD, cognitive, affective, somatic, or behavioral symptoms appear in response to genuine or fantasied separation from attachment figures. Common presenting problems are school refusal or insomnia. The differential diagnosis of school avoidance (formerly called "school phobia") includes medical illness, realistic fear of something at school (e.g., bullies or a punitive teacher), simple phobia, social phobia, agoraphobia, mood disorder, schizophrenia, truancy (secondary to conduct or oppositional defiant disorder), or substance abuse. Certain medications, such as propranolol (prescribed for headache) or haloperidol (prescribed for Tourette's disorder) may produce symptoms of separation anxiety and school refusal.

Selection of treatment. Psychological interventions such as family therapy, collaboration with school personnel, and behavior modification using contingencies and systematic desensitization are primary (American Academy of Child and Adolescent Psychiatry 1993). If a parent's anxiety or mood disorder is causing difficulty for him or her in separating from the child, then the parent should also receive direct psychiatric treatment (possibly including medication) as well as guidance in child management. Medication for the child or adolescent may be useful as an adjunct if psychosocial treatment is ineffective after 3–4 weeks.

The efficacy of imipramine in SAD is controversial (Bernstein et al. 1990; Klein et al. 1992). Benzodiazepines may be used in the short-term treatment of children with severe anticipatory anxiety. There are suggestions that alprazolam (0.03 mg/kg or 0.5–6.0 mg/day) may be useful in the treatment of SAD or "school refusal" (Bernstein et al. 1990; Kutcher et al. 1992).

Assessment of response. Response is measured behaviorally (e.g., return to school, ability to sleep alone) and by asking the child questions about subjective distress.

Imipramine. For children with school avoidance, one source suggests a recommended maximum dose of imipramine of 125 mg/day (McDaniel 1986). The starting dose for children age 6–8 is 10 mg at bedtime and for older children, 25 mg at bedtime. The dose may be increased by 10–50 mg per week, depending on the age of the child. Children with SAD only may respond at 25–50 mg/day, but those with school avoidance require at least 75 mg/day. Some require a higher dose for complete response. If youngsters are going to respond to imipramine treatment, they usually do so completely within 6–8 weeks. Medication is continued at least another 8 weeks and then gradually withdrawn. (See the section on mood disorders for more detail on the use of imipramine.)

■ Overanxious Disorder and Generalized Anxiety Disorder

Assessment for treatment. Children with overanxious disorder or generalized anxiety disorder have a variety of worries, almost always including unrealistic worry about future events. Children with overanxious disorder often appear shy, self-doubting, and self-deprecating and have multiple somatic complaints. They may show habit disturbances, such as nail-biting, hair-pulling, or thumb-sucking.

Selection of treatment. A variety of treatment modalities are typically used, although systematic data exist only for behavioral interventions. Behavioral methods include relaxation, desensitization by progressive exposure or through imagination, and contingent reinforcement of approach to feared objects or situations. Psychotherapy is often oriented toward promoting psychological individuation and autonomy in the child and family. Cognitive therapy is directed at changing self-defeating and pessimistic attitudes. Assertiveness training can be helpful, especially in a group setting. Treatment of any parental anxiety disorder is important.

Controlled drug studies of children who have only anxiety disorders are lacking. Benzodiazepines may be used in the short-term treatment of children with severe anticipatory anxiety. Although an open trial of alprazolam (0.5–1.5 mg/day) for children with avoidant and overanxious disorders was promising (Simeon and Ferguson 1987), a double-blind study did not find that alprazolam was superior to placebo in the context of an intensive treatment program (Simeon et al. 1992). Efficacy may have been limited by low doses and the short duration of treatment. Antihistamines are commonly prescribed, although no empirical data exist regarding their use. Anecdotal data suggest the efficacy of buspirone (15–30 mg/day) in the treatment of adolescents with overanxious disorder (Kranzler 1988; Kutcher et al. 1992).

Assessment of response. Both parental behavioral reports and patient ratings of anxiety in target domains are useful.

■ Benzodiazepines

Initiation of treatment. Infants and children absorb diazepam faster and metabolize it more quickly than adults (Simeon and Ferguson 1985). The usual daily dose ranges for children and adolescents are lorazepam 0.25–6.0 mg, diazepam 1–20 mg, and alprazolam 0.25–4.0 mg. The dosage schedule depends on age (i.e., more frequent dosing in children) and the specific drug (Coffey 1990; Kutcher et al. 1992).

Continuation, maintenance, and monitoring. Generally, these drugs should be used for relatively brief periods.

Management of side effects. In addition to the risks of substance abuse and physical or psychological dependence, side effects include sedation, cognitive dulling, ataxia, confusion, and emotional lability. Paradoxical or disinhibition reactions may occur, manifested by acute excitation, irritability, increased anxiety, hallucinations, increased aggression and hostility, rage reactions, insomnia, euphoria, and/or incoordination (Coffey 1990; Reiter and Kutcher 1991; Simeon and Ferguson 1985).

Discontinuation. When treatment with benzodiazepines is being discontinued, the dose needs to be tapered gradually to avoid withdrawal seizures or rebound anxiety.

■ Antihistamines

Initiation of treatment. The initial dose of diphenhydramine or hydroxyzine in children and adolescents is 10–25 mg/day. Either drug is titrated gradually up to a maximum of 200–300 mg/day (5 mg/kg/day) (Coffey 1990).

Side effects. The most common side effects are dizziness and oversedation. Some children become paradoxically agitated. Occasionally incoordination, blurred vision, dry mouth, nausea, abdominal pain, or agitation may occur. At high doses, the seizure threshold is lowered. Leukopenia and agranulocytosis are extremely rare. Antihistamines have been reported to cause acute dystonic reactions, tics, and possibly (with chronic administration) TD. They should not be prescribed to asthmatic individuals, because anticholinergic effects dry the mucous membranes.

■ Buspirone

Tentative guidelines for children and adolescents suggest a starting dose of 2.5–5.0 mg daily, increasing to three times a day over 2–3 days (Kutcher et al. 1992). The dose may be increased gradually to a maximum of 20 mg/day in children and 60 mg/day in adolescents, in three divided doses (0.3–0.6 mg/kg/day). The therapeutic effects may be delayed for 1–2 weeks after reaching the proper dose, with maximal effects not seen for an additional 2 weeks (Coffey 1990).

Reported adverse effects with buspirone in adults include insomnia, dizziness, anxiety, nausea, headache, restlessness, agitation, depression, and confusion (Coffey 1990). Clinical experience with children and adolescents is limited.

Buspirone can be discontinued relatively rapidly (i.e., in 4 days) (Kutcher et al. 1992).

■ Obsessive-Compulsive Disorder

Assessment for treatment. OCD is a chronic and often disabling disorder in childhood and adolescence. Lifetime prevalence in older adolescents is 1.9% (Flament et al. 1988). Between one-third and one-half of adult patients with OCD report onset of the disorder early in life. The clinical manifestations of OCD are similar at all ages, although in children rituals are more common than obsessions (Rapoport et al. 1992).

Selection of treatment. Medication is the mainstay of OCD treatment. Behavior modification techniques are less well developed, more difficult to implement, and largely untested compared with those for adults. Family and individual psychotherapy may be useful for residual symptoms that do not respond to pharmacotherapy.

Double-blind placebo-controlled studies of clomipramine (CMI) in youths have reported a 35%–75% reduction in OCD symptoms in 60% of subjects, independent of depression (DeVeaugh-Geiss et al. 1992; Flament et al. 1985; Leonard et al. 1989). Plasma levels of CMI and its metabolites correlated with the presence of side effects but not with clinical response. Efficacy appears to be specific for serotonin reuptake blockade, because DMI failed to reduce OCD symptomatology.

Both open and double-blind placebo-controlled studies of fluoxetine (20–80 mg/day) alone or in combination with low doses of CMI have reported moderate to marked improvement in OCD symptomatology, including reductions of more than 50% in the level of functional impairment (Riddle et al. 1990, 1992; Simeon et al. 1990). Approximately half of subjects are responders, regardless of the presence of Tourette's disorder.

Assessment of response. The Leyton Obsessional Inventory-Child Version (Berg et al. 1988) or the Children's Version of the Yale-Brown Obsessive Compulsive Scale (Goodman et al. 1989) may be used to quantify symptom severity.

Clomipramine. A starting dose of CMI 25 mg qd has been recommended with increases of 25–50 mg qd every 4–7 days. The maximum recommended dose is 3 mg/kg/day, up to 200 mg/day. Response is delayed for 10 days to 2 weeks (as in the treatment of depression), unlike the immediate response seen in the treatment of ADHD or enuresis (Rapoport 1986).

Children's experience is similar to adults, including tremor, fatigue, anticholinergic effects, dizziness, and sweating. Dose-dependent paranoia and aggression have been reported in two case studies. Cardiovascular monitoring (see Table 33–5) is necessary, given the potential for tachycardia, hypertension (and rarely, hypotension), and arrhythmias related to the use of TCAs in children.

Fluoxetine. Fluoxetine is begun at a dose of 5–20 mg/day, usually in the morning. Although early reports cited higher doses, clinical experience suggests that relatively few youths require a dose greater than 20 mg/day for the treatment of OCD. Dose adjustments may require alternate-day regimens, the use of the liquid formulation, or dissolving medication in juice and dispensing aliquots.

Although there are relatively few somatic side effects in children (anorexia, weight loss, headaches, nausea, vomiting, tremor), behavioral toxicity is common, perhaps related to akathisia. Symptoms include restlessness, insomnia, social disinhibition, agitation (Riddle et al. 1990/1991), and mania (Venkataraman et al. 1992). Suicidal ideation, self-destructive behavior, aggression, and psychotic symptoms have also been reported, although many children with these symptoms had preexisting risk factors for the development of these clinical features (King et al. 1991).

Treatment typically is required for years. Relapse is common when fluoxetine is discontinued (Leonard et al. 1991).

Strategies developed for the treatment of treatment-resistant adults with OCD are largely untested in children and adolescents.

■ Panic Disorder

Assessment for treatment. Recent reports have documented both panic disorder and agoraphobia in children and adolescents (Ballenger et al. 1989). The diagnostic criteria and physical symptom profile are the same as in adults. Cognitive immaturity may preclude anticipatory anxiety or the characteristic cognitions during an attack (i.e., fear of dying, going crazy, or doing something uncontrolled) (Nelles and Barlow 1988).

Selection of treatment. Case reports suggest alprazolam (0.25–2.5 mg/day divided tid or qid) or imipramine may be effective (Ballenger et al. 1989; Biederman 1987; Kutcher et al. 1992). Clonazepam efficacy (1–4 mg/day divided bid or tid) is supported by preliminary controlled data (Reiter et al. 1992). The benzodiazepines can cause disinhibition and angry outbursts (Reiter and Kutcher 1991). Other medications that have been used in adults (e.g., SSRIs) may be considered. Doses used are typically conservative to avoid sedation that would impede the patient's academic learning. Supportive and educational individual and family psychotherapy may be useful.

■ Posttraumatic Stress Disorder

Assessment for treatment. Although the diagnostic criteria for posttraumatic stress disorder are essentially the same at all ages, the symptoms in children differ in some ways from those seen in adults (Terr 1987). Immediate effects of trauma include fear of separation from parent(s), of death, and of further fear, leading to withdrawal from new experiences. Perceptual distortions occur (most commonly in time sense and in vision) but auditory, touch, and olfactory misperceptions have been described. In children, reexperiencing the event is likely to occur in the form of nightmares, daydreams, and/or repetitive, potentially dangerous reenactment in symbolic play or in actual behavior, rather than in intrusive flashbacks. A variety of fears develop, including fear of repetition of the experience and of other situations that may involve separation or danger or may remind the child of the event. Children may experience somatic symptoms, such as headaches and stomachaches. Increased arousal in children is most often manifested as sleep disturbances, which may add to functional impairment in other areas (Pynoos et al. 1987). Regression and guilt are common.

Key items in the assessment include preexisting stressors, previous loss, anxiety or depression, the nature and degree of exposure to the threat, and life changes secondary to the stressor itself.

Selection of treatment. Controlled trials of any treatments are lacking. Individual insight-oriented play and verbal individual or group psychotherapy have been used most often. Systematic desensitization of specific trauma-related fears may be useful in conjunction with other interventions. Supportive therapy for parents and siblings can deal with trauma experienced by family members and thus reduce contagion. Parents may require therapeutic attention for their own posttraumatic stress disorder symptoms and/or to help them deal appropriately with their child's symptoms and reenactment.

The use of psychotropic medication to treat posttraumatic stress disorder in children has not been systematically evaluated. Anecdotal reports suggest that propranolol may be effective in the treatment of agitated, hyperaroused children and adolescents with posttraumatic stress disorder (Famularo et al. 1988). Initial doses used were 0.8 mg/kg/day, divided into three doses, with titration to 2.5 mg/kg/day, unless limited by hypotension, bradycardia, or sedation.

■ Anxiety in the Medical Setting

Pain, unfamiliar surroundings and people, frightening procedures, separation from parents, and fears of disability or death predictably cause anxiety in medically ill children. Psychosocial interventions should be given first priority. If, despite these efforts, anxiety is severe or interferes with medical care, diphenhydramine (25–100 mg/dose), hydroxyzine (25–100 mg/dose), diazepam (1–15 mg/dose), or alprazolam (0.003–0.025 mg/kg/dose) (Coffey 1986; Pfefferbaum et al. 1987) may be considered for short periods or immediately before procedures. Hydroxyzine, methylated tricyclics (e.g., amitriptyline, doxepin, and imipramine), and the phenothiazines perphenazine and fluphenazine may be used to potentiate analgesics (Lacouture et al. 1984).

■ TOURETTE'S DISORDER

■ Assessment for Treatment

Tourette's disorder, or syndrome (TS), is a chronic motor *and* vocal tic disorder with a duration of more than 1 year, an onset during childhood or adolescence, and a prevalence of 0.03%–1.6%. The tics wax and wane over time and vary in complexity from simple movements or vocalizations (e.g., eye blinks, coughs) to complex, seemingly purposeful behaviors or verbalizations (e.g., facial expressions, coprolalia) (Cohen et al. 1992). Genetic studies suggest that TS is an autosomal dominant condition with incomplete, gender-specific penetrance and variable expression (Pauls and Leckman 1986). Linkage studies point to a clinical spectrum that includes TS proper, chronic tic disorder (CTD), OCD, and probably transient tic disorder (TTD). TS is complicated by OCD in 40% of cases. Although about half of children with TS referred for treatment have attention-deficit disorders, a genetic association with TS appears unlikely (Pauls et al. 1986).

■ Selection of Treatment

The treatment of TS and associated conditions should be comprehensive and directed toward fostering adaptive development and improving overall functioning rather than simply reducing tic symptoms. Psychopharmacological treatment can be quite effective. Careful monitoring for several months before starting medication is possible, because TS is a chronic disorder and not usually an emergency. This permits establishing a baseline of symptoms and assessing the need for psychological and educational interventions.

Studies have focused primarily on blockade of dopamine D_2 and α-adrenergic receptors, because hypersensitivity of these neurochemical systems has been hypothesized to underlie TS. Dopamine antagonists have been the mainstay of treatment and are effective in 60%–70% of cases, reducing tic symptoms by approximately 60%–70% (Regeur et al. 1986; Shapiro and Shapiro 1984; Shapiro et al. 1989). Haloperidol is typically effective in doses of 0.5–6.0 mg qd and pimozide (also a calcium channel blocker) in doses of 1–10 mg qd. Double-blind placebo-controlled crossover studies demonstrated on standardized assessments that tics decreased 65% with haloperidol and 60% with pimozide, versus 43% with placebo (Shapiro and Shapiro 1984; Shapiro et al. 1989). Other dopamine antagonists have been reported to be effective in open clinical trials, including fluphenazine and piquindone.

Alternative medications have been sought because of the neuroleptics' troublesome side-effect profile. The efficacy of the α-adrenergic agonist clonidine is controversial. Some studies report a 35%–50% reduction in tic and behavioral symptomatology in a substantial minority of patients (Leckman et al. 1991), whereas other studies report no benefit (Goetz et al. 1987). Vocal tics and associated behavioral manifestations such as impulsivity, restlessness, and inattention are the most responsive symptoms. OCD symptoms do not improve.

Preliminary reports regarding the use of calcium channel blockers and opioid antagonists have been promising, although findings have been inconsistent (Micheli et al. 1990). In addition, anticholinergic stimulation through the use of nicotine gum has been reported to augment the efficacy of neuroleptics.

Several studies have focused on the treatment of comorbid neuropsychiatric conditions that frequently complicate TS. Fluoxetine has been reported to significantly reduce OCD symptomatology among the more than one-half of TS patients who also manifest OCD (Riddle et al. 1990). Tic frequency and severity are unaffected. CMI has also been advocated for the treatment of patients with TS and OCD, taken with or without a neuroleptic (Cohen et al. 1992).

The treatment of comorbid ADHD symptomatology is complicated and controversial. Stimulant medications have been reported to exacerbate or precipitate tics in as many as half of children with TS (see Robertson and Eapen 1992 for review). They also have been reported to cause no change in or to actually reduce tics among children with TS. However, until additional well-controlled studies are completed, the use of stimulants in TS should be approached carefully. Clonidine or DMI (alone or in combination with neuroleptics; Cohen et al. 1992) have been suggested as useful treatments for children with TS and comorbid ADHD. Some clinicians advocate the combination of a neuroleptic and a stimulant (with careful monitoring). Depression is common among children and adults with TS. If pharmacological treatment is elected, an antidepressant may be used in conjunction with clonidine or a neuroleptic.

■ Assessment of Response

The natural waxing and waning course of TS makes evaluation of medication efficacy difficult. A variety of symptom rating scales may be used to quantify the number and severity of tics as well as the patient's school and social impairment (Walkup et al. 1992).

■ Neuroleptics

Initiation of treatment. Initial dose of haloperidol is 0.5 mg/day. It may be slowly increased up to 1–3 mg/day, divided in twice-daily doses (Cohen et al. 1992). Pimozide, which may be given in a single daily dose, is started at 1 mg/day and may be gradually increased to a maximum of 6–10 mg/day (0.2 mg/kg).

Management of side effects. Neuroleptic side effects in children include akathisia, sedation, lethargy, feeling like a "zombie," intellectual dulling, weight gain, anxiety, irritability, dysphoria, parkinsonian symptoms, and TD (Cohen et al. 1992). In patients with TS, it may be especially difficult to distinguish medication-induced movements from those characteristic of the disorder. Dysphoria and school avoidance have also been reported (Mikkelsen et al. 1981). The side-effect profiles of haloperidol and pimozide are generally similar, although pimozide may cause less sedation and EPS. At a maximum dose of 0.3 mg/kg/day (or 20 mg/day), pimozide does not adversely affect cardiovascular functioning (Shapiro et al. 1989). QTc intervals lengthen, but remain within the normal range. ECGs should be monitored before and during pimozide treatment.

Discontinuation. When haloperidol (and sometimes pimozide) is withdrawn, a severe exacerbation of symptoms may last for up to several months.

■ Clonidine

Initiation of treatment. A gradual increase in dosage to a maximum of approximately 5 μg/kg/day (or 0.25 mg qd) is recommended. (See the section on ADHD for further discussion.)

Management of side effects. Clonidine is generally well tolerated. Among youths with TS, 90% of subjects experienced transient sedation, whereas one-third to one-half reported dry mouth, dizziness, and irritability (Goetz et al. 1987; Leckman et al. 1991).

Discontinuation. If clonidine is to be discontinued, a gradual taper is recommended to avoid rebound tic symptoms and elevations in blood pressure and pulse.

■ AUTISTIC DISORDERS

■ Assessment for Treatment

Autism is a developmental disorder of early onset that involves significant deficits in social reciprocity, pragmatic (social) communication, and the range and nature of preferred interests and activities. Autism differs from mental retardation in that there are qualitative deviations of development, not simply delays.

■ Selection of Treatment

Virtually all of the psychotropic medications have been tried in clinical practice to ameliorate the developmental deficits and behavioral difficulties associated with autism. Unfortunately, no medication has yet been identified that fundamentally changes its core social and linguistic features. However, medications can often reduce the frequency and intensity of associated behavioral disturbances, which include hyperactivity, agitation, mood instability, aggression, self-injury, and stereotypy. Several neurochemical systems have been implicated in the etiology of the social and behavioral manifestations of the disorder, including the dopaminergic, serotonergic, and endogenous opioid systems.

Neuroleptics such as haloperidol, trifluoperazine, or pimozide result in behavioral improvement in most cases. For example, haloperidol has been evaluated in a series of elegant placebo-controlled studies involving well over 100 autistic children (Anderson et al. 1984, 1989; Campbell et al. 1978). In doses of 0.5–4.0 mg/day, haloperidol significantly reduced hyperactivity, stereotypy, and withdrawal, without adversely affecting cognitive performance. In addition, haloperidol improved discrimination learning and language acquisition when used in combination with positive reinforcement and behavioral interventions (Campbell et al. 1982).

The use of neuroleptics is covered in the section on schizophrenia. It is important to give a trial of sufficient length to determine if the drug is efficacious, barring serious side effects requiring immediate discontinuation. If the drug appears to be helpful, it should be continued for at least several months. Although few short-term side effects occur, prospective studies have indicated that withdrawal dyskinesias develop in 25%–30% of children, leading to concern regarding the potential for development of TD. The more sedating neuroleptics such as chlorpromazine cause excessive sedation without significant clinical improvement. At 3- to 6-month intervals, the drug should be discontinued so that the child may be observed for withdrawal dyskinesias and to determine if the drug is still necessary. Some children may have physical withdrawal symptoms or a rebound phenomenon consisting of worsening of behavior for up to 8 weeks after the medication is stopped (Campbell et al. 1985).

Results of controlled studies of fenfluramine (involving about 200 subjects) are mixed (see Aman and Kern 1989). Clinical benefit was reported in about half of the studies for one-third of the subjects. Responsive symptoms included hyperactivity, stereotypy, and withdrawal. There were no consistent improvements in learning, IQ, or language. Side effects were common and included weight loss, irritability, and sedation. Neurotoxicity has been reported in animals but not in humans.

Methylphenidate may reduce target symptoms of inattention, impulsivity, and overactivity in some higher-functioning children and adolescents with autistic disorder (Birmaher et al. 1988; Strayhorn et al. 1988). However, stimulants may increase internal preoccupation, withdrawal, and stereotypy.

The opioid antagonists have received preliminary study in autism because of their possible involvement in attachment behavior and suggestions that endogenous opioid levels may be abnormal in some autistic individuals. Several controlled, acute-dose trials of naltrexone found modest improvements in activity level and attention. A longer-term controlled study reported improvements in activity level, withdrawal, and communication on global assessments but not on more systematic measures (Campbell et al. 1990). No significant side effects have been reported, although reversible hepatic inflammation may occur at higher doses.

Several other medications have received preliminary study. Two small controlled trials of clonidine reported modest reductions in hyperactivity, overstimulation, and irritability (Frankhauser et al. 1992). The SSRIs have attracted attention because of the frequent occurrence of compulsive, ritualistic behavior among autistic individuals. One small controlled study of CMI (Gordon et al. 1992) and several case reports of CMI, fluoxetine, and fluvoxamine suggest improvement in compulsive behavior, withdrawal, and irritability. Lithium has been reported to reduce symptomatology among autistic individuals who manifest cyclic mood disturbances. Finally, several case reports suggest that β-blockers, buspirone, and trazodone may reduce agitation and explosive outbursts in some autistic individuals (Ratey et al. 1987).

■ ENURESIS

■ Assessment for Treatment

Functional enuresis is diagnosed when the frequency of medically unexplained urinary incontinence exceeds developmental (i.e., age-specific) expected norms. Enuresis is strongly familial, especially in males. Neurodevelopmental delays are common in enuretic boys, whereas frequent physiological causes of diurnal enuresis in girls include vaginal reflux of urine, "giggle incontinence," and urgency incontinence. Enuresis is occasionally caused by psychiatric disorders. Anxious children may experience urinary frequency, resulting in daytime incontinence if toilet facilities are not readily available, or if the child is fearful of certain bathrooms. In oppositional defiant disorder, refusal to use the toilet may be part of the child's battle for control. Many children with ADHD wait until the last minute to urinate, then lose continence on the way to the bathroom. Secondary enuresis may be related to stress, trauma, or a psychosocial or developmental crisis.

Before starting any treatment of enuresis, baseline measures of frequency of wetting should be obtained.

■ Selection of Treatment

For younger children with nocturnal enuresis, the most useful strategy is to minimize secondary symptoms by discouraging parents from punishing or ridiculing the child while awaiting spontaneous

remission with maturation. For older children who are motivated to stop bedwetting, a monitoring and reward procedure may be effective. "Bladder training" exercises may be helpful. If these simple interventions are unsuccessful, a urine alarm combined with behavior modification is recommended. Children may need treatment of comorbid psychopathology and management of psychosocial stressors before they are motivated to participate in or are responsive to behavioral techniques.

Low doses of a TCA or desmopressin acetate (DDAVP) can be helpful if behavioral interventions are ineffective, if there is associated mood or anxiety disorder (for TCAs), or for special occasions (e.g., overnight camp). However, behavioral treatments are the first choice, because they avoid medication side effects and are longer lasting.

All of the TCAs have been found to be equally effective in the treatment of nocturnal enuresis. The mechanism remains unclear, but it does not seem to be by altering sleep architecture, by treating depression, or through peripheral anticholinergic activity. In 80% of patients, TCAs reduce the frequency of bedwetting within the first week. Total remission, however, occurs in relatively few patients. Wetting returns when the drug is discontinued.

■ Assessment of Response

Daily charts are used to monitor progress.

■ Tricyclic Antidepressants

Initiation of treatment. Much lower doses of TCAs are needed to treat enuresis than for the treatment of depression. As a result, baseline and periodic ECGs are not necessary. Imipramine is started at 10–25 mg at bedtime and increased in 10- to 25-mg increments weekly to 50 mg (75 mg in preadolescents), if necessary. Maximum dose is 2.5 mg/kg/day (Ryan 1990). At these doses, side effects are rare.

Treatment resistance. Tolerance to TCAs may develop, requiring a dose increase. For some children, TCAs lose their effect entirely.

■ Desmopressin

DDAVP is an analogue of antidiuretic hormone administered as a nasal spray to treat nocturnal enuresis. Onset of action is rapid (i.e., several days) and side effects are negligible (e.g., rare nasal mucosa dryness or irritation, and headache) in patients with normal electrolyte regulation. DDAVP acts by increasing water absorption in the kidneys, thereby reducing the volume of urine. Evening fluid restriction is advised to avoid hyponatremia (possibly resulting in seizures) (Beach et al. 1992). A major drawback of DDAVP is its expense: $100–$240 per month. Few patients become completely dry, and relapse occurs when medication is stopped (Klauber 1989). The usual dose is 10–40 µg intranasally at bedtime. The likelihood of relapse may be decreased by tapering the drug slowly.

■ Discontinuation

Because enuresis has a high spontaneous remission rate, children and adolescents on chronic medication should have a drug-free trial at least every 6 months.

■ SLEEP DISORDERS

■ Insomnia

Assessment for treatment. Chronic childhood insomnia is much more frequent in children with psychiatric disorders. What parents report as the child's insomnia is often related to behavioral or habit problems in settling for the night, especially in children with ADHD, oppositional defiant disorder, or SAD. Difficulty falling asleep, sleep continuity disturbance, and/or early morning awakening can be secondary to depression, psychosis, or separation anxiety. A decreased need for sleep can be a symptom of mania. Insomnia may also be secondary to caffeine or to prescribed or over-the-counter medication (e.g., phenobarbital, theophylline, decongestants, or stimulants) or to substance abuse. A detailed sleep diary is needed before initiating any treatment. Sleep laboratory studies may be useful in complex cases.

Selection of treatment. The first step in treating insomnia is treatment of any primary psychiatric disorder. To address true insomnia, parents or adolescents are taught to remove environmental factors interfering with sleep and to develop a bedtime routine, which may include the use of a transitional object or a night-light. Behavioral treatment removes the secondary gain of parental attention for night wakening and provides positive reinforcement for appropriate sleep behavior, or at least for staying quietly in the child's own room. Older children and adolescents may benefit from hypnosis or systematic instruction in relaxation techniques. Short-term medication may give parents a respite to regain enough energy to pursue other solutions.

Many children respond with paradoxical agitation to sedatives. Hypnotic medications are not recommended for chronic use. Chloral hydrate (500–1,000 mg) or an antihistamine (see above) such as diphenhydramine (1 mg/kg at bedtime) (Russo et al. 1976) or hydroxyzine may be indicated for short-term use in a crisis or for severe insomnia that has not responded to psychological interventions (Coffey 1986). If there is extreme fear or anxiety, a short-acting benzodiazepine such as triazolam may be used briefly.

■ Sleep Terror Disorder (Pavor Nocturnus) and Sleepwalking Disorder (Somnambulism)

Assessment for treatment. Episodes of sleep terror typically occur during the first third of the night, in non-REM sleep Stages 3 and 4, lasting 1–10 minutes. The child appears terrified, screams, stares, has dilated pupils, sweats, and has rapid pulse and hyperventilation. He or she is agitated and confused and cannot be comforted. When alert, the child most commonly has no memory of the episode. Return to sleep is rapid when the episode is over, with complete amnesia in the morning. Stress, exhaustion, or a febrile illness may increase frequency. In children, there is no typically associated psychopathology. A variety of sedative, neuroleptic, and antidepressant medications, alone or in combination, have been reported to cause night terrors and/or somnambulism (Nino-Murcia and Dement 1987).

Somnambulism is characterized by repeated episodes of arising from bed and engaging in motor activities while still asleep. Episodes (which last a few minutes to half an hour) typically occur 1–3 hours after falling asleep, during Stage 3 and 4 delta (non-REM) sleep. The child or adolescent engages in perseverative, stereotyped movements (e.g., picking at blankets), which may progress to walking and other complex behaviors. He or she is difficult to waken, and coordination is poor. Speech, when present, is usually incomprehensible. The youngster may awaken and be confused, may return to bed, or may lie down somewhere else and continue sleeping. Morning amnesia is typical. Sleepwalking is often seen in children who had night terrors when younger. Likelihood of sleepwalking is increased when the child is overtired or under stress.

Selection of treatment. For both pavor nocturnus and somnambulism, restricting fluids before bedtime may avoid episodes that are triggered by a full bladder (Nino-Murcia and Dement 1987). Most cases of both disorders respond to support and education while waiting for the child to outgrow the problem. Parents of sleepwalkers should be guided to remove hazards in the environment, and they may need to lock the child's door. Medication (i.e., low-dose imipramine or diazepam at bedtime) is used if the episodes are frequent, dangerous, severely disrupting the family, or interfering with daytime functioning (Nino-Murcia and Dement 1987; Pesikoff and Davis 1971). Imipramine may be given at a dose of 10–50 mg (depending on weight) at bedtime.

■ EMOTIONAL AND BEHAVIORAL SYMPTOMS IN MENTALLY RETARDED CHILDREN

■ Assessment for Treatment

Mental retardation (MR) is a developmental condition that includes subaverage intellectual functioning, impairments in adaptive behavior, and an onset during the developmental period. As such, MR is not amenable to pharmacological treatment. Most people with MR do not exhibit emotional and behavioral difficulties. If such difficulties do occur, the clinician should conduct a thorough assessment, with the goal of identifying a psychiatric disorder and/or psychosocial stressors responsible for the symptoms, and then develop a *comprehensive* treatment plan. To improve the validity and reliability of psychiatric diagnosis, standardized assessment instruments can be used, including the Beck Depression Inventory, the CDI, the Aberrant Behavior Checklist (Aman et al. 1985), or the Psychopathology Instrument for Mentally Re-

tarded Adults (Aman et al. 1986), among others (Sturmey et al. 1991).

Community-based epidemiological studies indicate that the prevalence of psychiatric disorders among people with MR is higher than in the general population (Gillberg et al. 1986). The full range of psychopathology is present, including disruptive behavior disorders, anxiety disorders, mood disorders, and schizophrenia.

■ Selection of Treatment

Psychotropic medications can play an important role in the treatment of psychiatric disorders affecting individuals with MR (Aman and Singh 1988; Bregman 1991).

About 10%–20% of children with MR manifest ADHD. Recent, well-controlled studies involving more than 100 subjects indicate that methylphenidate significantly reduces hyperactivity, impulsivity, and inattention, and improves performance on laboratory measures of attention and memory (Handen et al. 1990, 1992). Responders (i.e., 60%–75% of those studied) tend to have milder cognitive deficits and to be free from disorders such as autism and schizophrenia. Children with MR may be particularly prone to side effects such as irritability, withdrawal, stereotypy, and overinclusive attention.

Schizophrenia affects 1%–2% of the mentally retarded population. Neuroleptic medications appear to be as efficacious among patients with MR as they are among those in the general population (Menolascino et al. 1986).

Major and minor depression is common among mentally retarded individuals, and case reports document the efficacy of antidepressants. However, double-blind studies are greatly needed. Mood-stabilizing agents (e.g., lithium carbonate, anticonvulsants) have received preliminary study for the treatment of bipolar disorder and aggressive behavior among individuals with MR. For example, clinical reports and two placebo-controlled trials found lithium to be useful for reducing the frequency and severity of affective cycles and of aggressive and self-injurious behavior in as many as two-thirds to three-quarters of patients (Craft et al. 1987).

Most medication studies that have targeted the treatment of destructive behavior and stereotypy in patients with MR have not considered psychiatric diagnosis. Psychotropic medications of various classes have been tried, with widely inconsistent results. The neuroleptics have received the most extensive study. Some reports have been very favorable; however, several well-controlled studies have been discouraging. Recent data suggest that D_1 dopamine receptor supersensitivity may underlie some forms of self-injurious behavior and preliminary studies of mixed D_1/D_2 receptor antagonists have been encouraging. Definitive results must await controlled studies. The use of neuroleptics for these behavioral difficulties must be weighed against their potential side effects, which include impairment in cognitive performance and the development of akathisia or TD (affecting 15%–35% of MR patients receiving chronic neuroleptic treatment). Low-potency neuroleptics may actually increase aggression.

Medications that enhance serotonergic activity have been reported to decrease destructive behavior. These medications include lithium, buspirone, trazodone, and fluoxetine. However, only lithium has been evaluated in controlled studies. The endogenous opioid system has been implicated in at least some forms of self-injury and stereotypy. Preliminary studies (some well controlled) of the opioid antagonists naloxone and naltrexone have reported favorable results; however, others have not. Some investigators have suggested that heightened noradrenergic activity may result in hyperarousal and lead to explosive, destructive behavior. Several open clinical trials have reported that β-blockers such as propranolol are effective in some cases (Ratey et al. 1987). Although benzodiazepines and other sedative-hypnotics are often prescribed for the treatment of destructive behavior among people with MR, exacerbation of aggression and self-injurious behavior and paradoxical excitement may occur. Buspirone has been suggested as an alternative anxiolytic for patients with MR (Ratey et al. 1991).

■ CONCLUSION

When used carefully, psychopharmacological agents can be powerful components of the therapeutic armamentarium used to treat children and adolescents. However, far more empirical work is required to identify and document optimal treatments, both pharmacological and psychotherapeutic.

■ REFERENCES

Abikoff H, Gittelman R: Does behavior therapy normalize the classroom behavior of hyperactive children? Arch Gen Psychiatry 41:449–454, 1984

Achenbach TM: Integrative Guide for the 1991 CBCL/4–18, YSR, and TRF profiles. Burlington, VT, University of Vermont Department of Psychiatry, 1991

Aman M, Kern R: Review of fenfluramine in the treatment of the developmental disabilities. J Am Acad Child Adolesc Psychiatry 28:549–565, 1989

Aman MG, Singh NN (eds): Psychopharmacology of the Developmental Disabilities. New York, Springer-Verlag, 1988

Aman MG, Singh NN, Stewart AW, et al: The Aberrant Behavior Checklist: a behavior rating scale for the assessment of treatment effects. American Journal of Mental Deficiency 89:485–491, 1985

Aman MG, Watson JE, Singh NN, et al: Psychometric and demographic characteristics of the Psychopathology Instrument for Mentally Retarded Adults. Psychopharmacol Bull 22:1072–1076, 1986

American Academy of Child and Adolescent Psychiatry: Practice parameters for the assessment and treatment of anxiety disorders. J Am Acad Child Adolesc Psychiatry 32:1089–1098, 1993

American Psychiatric Association: Diagnostic and Statistical Manual of Mental Disorders, 3rd Edition, Revised. Washington, DC, American Psychiatric Association, 1987

American Psychiatric Association: Diagnostic and Statistical Manual of Mental Disorders, 4th Edition. Washington, DC, American Psychiatric Association, 1994

Amery B, Minichiello MD, Brown GL: Aggression in hyperactive boys: response to d-amphetamine. J Am Acad Child Adolesc Psychiatry 23:291–294, 1984

Amirkhan J: Expectancies and attributions for hyperactive and medicated hyperactive students. J Abnorm Child Psychol 10:265–276, 1982

Anderson LT, Campbell M, Grega DM, et al: Haloperidol in the treatment of infantile autism: effects on learning and behavioral symptoms. Am J Psychiatry 141:1195–1202, 1984

Anderson LT, Campbell M, Adams P, et al: The effects of haloperidol on discrimination learning and behavioral symptoms in autistic children. J Autism Dev Disord 19:227–239, 1989

Appler WD, McMann GL: "Off-label" uses of approved drugs: limits on physicians' prescribing behavior. J Clin Psychopharmacol 9:368–370, 1989

Ayllon T, Rosenbaum MS: The behavioral treatment of disruption and hyperactivity in school settings, in Advances in Clinical Child Psychology, Vol 2. Edited by Lahey BB, Kazdin AE. New York, Plenum, 1977, pp 83–118

Ballenger JC, Carek DJ, Steele JJ, et al: Three cases of panic disorder with agoraphobia in children. Am J Psychiatry 146:922–924, 1989

Barkley RA: The effects of methylphenidate on the interactions of preschool ADHD children with their mothers. J Am Acad Child Adolesc Psychiatry 27:336–341, 1988

Barkley RA: Attention Deficit Hyperactivity Disorder: A Handbook for Diagnosis and Treatment. New York, Guilford, 1990

Barkley RA, Fischer M, Newby RF, et al: Development of a multimethod clinical protocol for assessing stimulant drug response in children with attention deficit disorder. Journal of Clinical Child Psychology 17:14–24, 1988

Bastiaens L: The impact of an intensive educational program on knowledge, attitudes, and side effects of psychotropic medications among adolescent inpatients. Journal of Child and Adolescent Psychopharmacology 2:249–258, 1992

Bastiaens L, Bastiaens DK: A manual of psychiatric medications for teenagers. Journal of Child and Adolescent Psychopharmacology 3:M1–M59, 1993

Beach PS, Beach RE, Smith LR: Hyponatremic seizures in a child treated with desmopressin to control enuresis: a rational approach to fluid intake. Clin Pediatr (Phila) 31:566–569, 1992

Beck AT, Ward CH, Mendelson M, et al: An inventory for measuring depression. Arch Gen Psychiatry 4:561–571, 1961

Beigel A, Murphy DL, Bunney WE Jr: The Manic-State Rating Scale. Arch Gen Psychiatry 25:256–262, 1971

Berg CZ, Whitaker A, Davies M, et al: The survey form of the Leyton Obsessional Inventory-Child Version: norms from an epidemiological study. J Am Acad Child Adolesc Psychiatry 27:759–763, 1988

Bernstein GA, Garfinkel BD, Borchardt CM: Comparative studies of pharmacotherapy for school re-fusal. J Am Acad Child Adolesc Psychiatry 29:773–781, 1990

Biederman J: Clonazepam in the treatment of prepubertal children with panic-like symptoms. J Clin Psychiatry 48 (suppl):38–41, 1987

Biederman J, Baldessarini RJ, Wright V, et al: A double-blind placebo controlled study of desipramine in the treatment of ADD, I: efficacy. J Am Acad Child Adolesc Psychiatry 28:777–784, 1989a

Biederman J, Baldessarini RJ, Wright V, et al: A double-blind placebo controlled study of desipramine in the treatment of ADD, II: serum drug levels and cardiovascular findings. J Am Acad Child Adolesc Psychiatry 28:903–911, 1989b

Birmaher B, Quintana H, Greenhill LL: Methylphenidate treatment of hyperactive autistic children. J Am Acad Child Adolesc Psychiatry 27:248–251, 1988

Birmaher B, Greenhill L, Cooper T, et al: Sustained release methylphenidate: pharmacokinetic studies in ADHD males. J Am Acad Child Adolesc Psychiatry 28:768–772, 1989

Birmaher B, Baker R, Kapur S, et al: Clozapine for the treatment of adolescents with schizophrenia. J Am Acad Child Adolesc Psychiatry 31:160–164, 1992

Blanz B, Schmidt MH: Clozapine for schizophrenia [letter]. J Am Acad Child Adolesc Psychiatry 32:223, 1993

Borcherding GB, Keysor CS, Cooper TB, et al: Differential effects of methylphenidate and dextro-amphetamine on the motor activity level of hyperactive children. Neuropsychopharmacology 2:255–263, 1989

Bregman JD: Current developments in the understanding of mental retardation, part II: psychopathology. J Am Acad Child Adolesc Psychiatry 30:861–872, 1991

Briant RH: An introduction to clinical pharmacology, in Pediatric Psychopharmacology: The Use of Behavior Modifying Drugs in Children. Edited by Werry JS. New York, Brunner/Mazel, 1978, pp 3–28

Brown RT, Sexson SB: Effects of methylphenidate on cardiovascular responses in attention deficit hyperactivity disordered adolescents. J Adolesc Health 10:179–183, 1989

Brown RT, Borden KA, Wynne ME, et al: Compliance with pharmacological and cognitive treatments for attention deficit disorder. J Am Acad Child Adolesc Psychiatry 26:521–526, 1987

Brown TE, Gammon GD: ADHD-associated difficulties falling asleep and awakening: clonidine and methylphenidate treatments. Paper presented at the annual meeting of the American Academy of Child and Adolescent Psychiatry, Washington, DC, October 1992

Campbell M, Anderson LT, Meier M, et al: A comparison of haloperidol, behavior therapy, and their interaction in autistic children. J Am Acad Child Psychiatry 17:640–655, 1978

Campbell M, Anderson LT, Small AM, et al: The effects of haloperidol on learning and behavior in autistic children. J Autism Dev Disord 12:167–175, 1982

Campbell M, Small AM, Green WH, et al: Behavioral efficacy of haloperidol and lithium carbonate. Arch Gen Psychiatry 41:650–656, 1984

Campbell M, Green WH, Deutsch SI (eds): Child and Adolescent Psychopharmacology. Beverly Hills, CA, Sage, 1985

Campbell M, Anderson LT, Small AM, et al: Naltrexone in autistic children: a double-blind and placebo-controlled study. Psychopharmacol Bull 26:130–135, 1990

Casat CD, Pleasants DZ, Schroeder DH, et al: Bupropion in children with attention deficit disorder. Psychopharmacol Bull 25:198–201, 1989

Chambers WJ, Puig-Antich J, Hirsch MT, et al: The assessment of affective disorders in children and adolescents by structured interview. Arch Gen Psychiatry 42:696–702, 1985

Clay TH, Gualtieri T, Evans RW, et al: Clinical and neuropsychological effects of the novel antidepressant bupropion. Psychopharmacol Bull 24:143–148, 1988

Coffey BJ: Therapeutics III: pharmacotherapy, in Manual of Clinical Child Psychiatry. Edited by Robson KS. Washington, DC, American Psychiatric Press, 1986, pp 149–184

Coffey BJ: Anxiolytics for children and adolescents: traditional and new drugs. Journal of Child and Adolescent Psychopharmacology 1:57–83, 1990

Cohen D, Riddle M, Leckman J: Pharmacotherapy of Tourette's syndrome and associated disorders. Psychiatr Clin North Am 15:109–129, 1992

Cohen NJ, Sullivan J, Minde K, et al: Evaluation of the relative effectiveness of methylphenidate and cognitive behavior modification in the treatment of kindergarten-aged hyperactive children. J Abnorm Child Psychol 9:43–54, 1981

Conners CK: Controlled trial of methylphenidate in preschool children with minimal brain dysfunction. International Journal of Mental Health 4:61–74, 1975

Conners CK: The computerized continuous performance test. Psychopharmacol Bull 21:891–892, 1985

Connor DF: Beta blockers for aggression: a review of the pediatric experience. Journal of Child and Adolescent Psychopharmacology 3:99–114, 1993

Consortium on Mood Disorders in Children and Adolescents, Toronto, Ontario, September 1993

Craft M, Ismail IA, Krishnamurti D, et al: Lithium in the treatment of aggression in mentally handicapped patients: a double-blind trial. Br J Psychiatry 150:685–689, 1987

DeVeaugh-Geiss J, Moroz G, Biederman J, et al: Clomipramine hydrochloride in childhood and adolescent obsessive compulsive disorder: multicenter trial. J Am Acad Child Adolesc Psychiatry 31:45–49, 1992

Diamond JM, Deane FP: Conners Teacher's Questionnaire: Is frequent administration clinically useful? Paper presented at annual meeting of the American Academy of Child and Adolescent Psychiatry, Seattle, WA, October 1988

Doherty M, Gordon A, Brown J, et al: Placebo substitution during medication reductions: controlling for expectancies. Paper presented at the annual meeting of the American Academy of Child and Adolescent Psychiatry, October 1987

Donnelly M, Zametkin AJ, Rapoport JL, et al: Treatment of childhood hyperactivity with desipramine: plasma drug concentration, cardiovascular effects, plasma and urinary catecholamine levels, and clinical response. Clin Pharmacol Ther 39:72–81, 1986

Dubey DR, O'Leary SG, Kaufman KF: Training parents of hyperactive children in child management: a comparative outcome study. J Abnorm Child Psychol 11:229–246, 1983

Dulcan MK: Information for parents and youth on psychotropic medications. Journal of Child and Adolescent Psychopharmacology 2:81–101, 1992

Dulcan MK, Popper CW: Stimulants, in Concise Guide to Child and Adolescent Psychiatry. Washington, DC, American Psychiatric Press, 1991, pp 188–195

DuPaul GJ, Rapport MD: Does methylphenidate normalize the classroom performance of children with attention deficit disorder? J Am Acad Child Adolesc

Psychiatry 32:190–198, 1993

Elia J, Borcherding BG, Rapoport JL, et al: Methylphenidate and dextroamphetamine treatments of hyperactivity: are there true nonresponders? Psychiatry Res 36:141–155, 1991

Evans RW, Clay TH, Gualtieri CT: Carbamazepine in pediatric psychiatry. Journal of the American Academy of Child Psychiatry 26:2–8, 1987

Evans SW, Pelham WE: Psychostimulant effects on academic and behavioral measures for ADHD junior high school students in a lecture format classroom. J Abnorm Child Psychol 19:537–552, 1991

Famularo R, Fenton T: The effect of methylphenidate on school grades in children with attention deficit disorder without hyperactivity. J Clin Psychiatry 48:112–114, 1987

Famularo R, Kinscherff R, Fenton T: Propranolol treatment for childhood posttraumatic stress disorder, acute type. Am J Dis Child 142:1244–1247, 1988

Fine S, Jewesson B: Active drug placebo trial of methylphenidate: a clinical service for children with an attention deficit disorder. Can J Psychiatry 34:447–449, 1989

Firestone P: Factors associated with children's adherence to stimulant medication. Am J Orthopsychiatry 52:447–457, 1982

Firestone P, Kelly MJ, Goodman JT, et al: Differential effects of parent training and stimulant medication with hyperactives: a progress report. J Am Acad Child Adolesc Psychiatry 20:135–147, 1981

Fitzpatrick PA, Klorman F, Brumaghim JT, et al: Effects of sustained-release and standard preparations of methylphenidate on attention deficit disorder. J Am Acad Child Adolesc Psychiatry 31:226–234, 1992

Flament MF, Rapoport JL, Berg CZ, et al: Clomipramine treatment of childhood obsessive-compulsive disorder. Arch Gen Psychiatry 42:977–983, 1985

Flament MF, Whitaker A, Rapoport JL, et al: Obsessive compulsive disorder in adolescence. J Am Acad Child Adolesc Psychiatry 27:764–771, 1988

Frankhauser M, Karumanchi V, German M, et al: A double-blind, placebo-controlled study of the efficacy of transdermal clonidine in autism. J Clin Psychiatry 53:77–82, 1992

Fristad MA, Weller EB, Weller RA, et al: Self-report vs. biological markers in assessment of childhood depression. J Affect Disord 15:339–345, 1988

Fristad MA, Weller EB, Weller RA: The mania rating scale: can it be used in children? a preliminary report. J Am Acad Child Adolesc Psychiatry 31:252–257, 1992

Gadow KD: Pediatric psychopharmacology: a review of recent research. J Child Psychol Psychiatry 33:153–195, 1992

Gadow KD, Swanson HL: Assessing drug effects on academic performance. Psychopharmacol Bull 21:877–886, 1985

Gammon GD, Brown TE: Fluoxetine and methylphenidate in combination for treatment of attention deficit disorder and comorbid depressive disorder. Journal of Child and Adolescent Psychopharmacology 3:1–10, 1993

Garvey CA, Gross D, Freeman L: Assessing psychotropic medication side effects among children: a reliability study. Journal of Clinical Psychiatric Nursing 4:127–131, 1991

Geller JL, Gaulin BD, Barreira PJ: A practitioner's guide to use of psychotropic medication in liquid form. Hosp Community Psychiatry 43:969–971, 1992

Ghaziuddin N, Alessi NE: An open clinical trial of trazodone in aggressive children. Journal of Child and Adolescent Psychopharmacology 2:291–297, 1992

Gillberg C, Persson E, Grufman M, et al: Psychiatric disorders in mildly and severely mentally retarded urban children and adolescents: epidemiological aspects. Br J Psychiatry 149:68–74, 1986

Gittelman R, Abikoff H, Pollack E, et al: A controlled trial of behavior modification and methylphenidate in hyperactive children, in Hyperactive Children: The Social Ecology of Identification and Treatment. Edited by Whalen CK, Henker B. New York, Academic Press, 1980, pp 221–243

Goetz CG, Tanner CM, Wilson RS, et al: Clonidine and Gilles de la Tourette's syndrome: double-blind study using objective rating methods. Ann Neurol 21:307–310, 1987

Goodman WK, Price LH, Rasmussen SA, et al: The Yale-Brown Obsessive Compulsive Scale, I: development, use, and reliability. Arch Gen Psychiatry 46:1006–1011, 1989

Gordon C, Rapoport J, Hamburger S, et al: Differential response of seven subjects with autistic disorder to clomipramine and desipramine. Am J Psychiatry 149:363–366, 1992

Goyette CH, Conners CK, Ulrich RF: Normative data

on revised Conners Parent and Teacher Rating Scales. J Abnorm Child Psychol 6:221–236, 1978

Greenhill LL: Stimulant-related growth inhibition in children: a review, in Strategic Interventions for Hyperactive Children. Edited by Gittleman M. New York, ME Sharpe, 1981, pp 39–63

Greenhill LL, Solomon M, Pleak R, et al: Molindone hydrochloride treatment of hospitalized children with conduct disorder. J Clin Psychiatry 46:20–25, 1985

Grizenko N, Vida S: Propranolol treatment of episodic dyscontrol and aggressive behavior in children. Can J Psychiatry 33:776–778, 1988

Grob CS, Coyle JT: Suspected adverse methylphenidate-imipramine interactions in children. Developmental and Behavioral Pediatrics 7:265–267, 1986

Gualtieri CT, Hawk B: Tardive dyskinesia and other drug-induced movement disorders among handicapped children and youth. Applied Research in Mental Retardation 1:55–69, 1980

Gualtieri CT, Quade D, Hicks RE, et al: Tardive dyskinesia and other clinical consequences of neuroleptic treatment in children and adolescents. Am J Psychiatry 141:20–23, 1984

Halperin JM, Gittelman R, Katz S, et al: Relationship between stimulant effect, electroencephalogram, and clinical neurological findings in hyperactive children. J Am Acad Child Adolesc Psychiatry 25:820–825, 1986

Hamilton M: Development of a rating scale for primary depressive illness. British Journal of Social and Clinical Psychology 6:278–296, 1967

Handen B, Breaux A, Janosky J, et al: Effects and noneffects of methylphenidate in children with mental retardation and ADHD. J Am Acad Child Adolesc Psychiatry 31:455–461, 1992

Handen BL, Breaux AM, Gosling A, et al: Efficacy of Ritalin among mentally retarded children with ADHD. Pediatrics 86:922–930, 1990

Henker B, Whalen CK: The many messages of medication: hyperactive children's perceptions and attributions, in The Ecosystem of the "Sick" Child. Edited by Salzinger S, Antrobus J, Glick J. New York, Academic Press, 1980, pp 141–166

Herskowitz J: Developmental toxicology, in Psychiatric Pharmacosciences of Children and Adolescents. Edited by Popper C. Washington, DC, American Psychiatric Press, 1987, pp 81–123

Hinshaw SP, Henker B, Whalen CK, et al: Aggressive, prosocial, and nonsocial behavior in hyperactive boys: dose effects of methylphenidate in naturalistic settings. J Consult Clin Psychol 57:636–643, 1989

Hunt RD, Capper S, O'Connell P: Clonidine in child and adolescent psychiatry. Journal of Child and Adolescent Psychopharmacology 1:87–102, 1990

Hunt RD, Lau S, Ryu J: Alternative therapies for ADHD, in Ritalin: Theory and Patient Management. Edited by Greenhill LL, Osman BB. New York, Mary Ann Liebert, Inc, 1991, pp 75–95

Jatlow PI: Psychotropic drug disposition during development, in Psychiatric Pharmacosciences of Children and Adolescents. Edited by Popper C. Washington, DC, American Psychiatric Press, 1987, pp 27–44

Joshi PT, Walkup JT, Capozzoli JA, et al: The use of fluoxetine in the treatment of major depressive disorder in children and adolescents. Paper presented at the 36th Annual Meeting of the American Academy of Child and Adolescent Psychiatry, New York, October 1989

Kafantaris V, Campbell M, Padron-Gayol MV, et al: Carbamazepine in hospitalized aggressive conduct disorder children: an open pilot study. Psychopharmacol Bull 28:193–199, 1992

Kemph JP, DeVane CL, Levin GM, et al: Treatment of aggressive children with clonidine: results of an open pilot study. J Am Acad Child Adolesc Psychiatry 32:577–581, 1993

King RA, Riddle MA, Chappell PB, et al: Emergence of self-destructive phenomena in children and adolescents during fluoxetine treatment. J Am Acad Child Adolesc Psychiatry 30:179–186, 1991

Klauber GT: Clinical efficacy and safety of desmopressin in the treatment of nocturnal enuresis. J Pediatr 114:719–722, 1989

Klein RG, Mannuzza S: Hyperactive boys almost grown up, III: methylphenidate effects on ultimate height. Arch Gen Psychiatry 45:1131–1134, 1988

Klein RG, Landa B, Mattes JA, et al: Methylphenidate and growth in hyperactive children. Arch Gen Psychiatry 45:1127–1130, 1988

Klein RG, Koplewicz HS, Kanner A: Imipramine treatment of children with separation anxiety disorder. J Am Acad Child Adolesc Psychiatry 31:21–28, 1992

Klorman R, Brumaghim JT, Fitzpatrick P, et al: Clinical effects of a controlled trial of methylphenidate on adolescents with attention deficit disorder. J Am Acad Child Adolesc Psychiatry 29:702–709, 1990

Klorman R, Brumaghim JT, Salzman LF, et al: Comparative effects of methylphenidate on attention-deficit hyperactivity disorder with and without aggressive/noncompliant features. Psychopharmacol Bull 25:109–113, 1989

Knight MM, Wigder KS, Fortsch MM, et al: Medication education for children: is it worthwhile? Journal of Child Psychiatric Nursing 3:25–28, 1990

Kovacs M: The Children's Depression Inventory (CDI). Psychopharmacol Bull 21:995–998, 1985

Kranzler HR: Use of buspirone in an adolescent with overanxious disorder. J Am Acad Child Adolesc Psychiatry 27:789–790, 1988

Kuperman S, Stewart MA: Use of propranolol to decrease aggressive outbursts in younger patients. Psychosomatics 28:315–319, 1987

Kutcher SP, Reiter S, Gardner DM, et al: The pharmacotherapy of anxiety disorders in children and adolescents. Psychiatr Clin North Am 15:41–67, 1992

Lacouture PG, Gaudreault P, Lovejoy FH: Chronic pain of childhood: a pharmacologic approach. Pediatr Clin North Am 31:1133–1151, 1984

Latz SR, McCracken JT: Neuroleptic malignant syndrome in children and adolescents: two case reports and a warning. Journal of Child and Adolescent Psychopharmacology 2:123–129, 1992

Leckman JF, Ort S, Caruso KA, et al: Rebound phenomena in Tourette's syndrome after abrupt withdrawal of clonidine. Arch Gen Psychiatry 43:1168–1176, 1986

Leckman J, Hardin M, Riddle M, et al: Clonidine treatment of Gilles de la Tourette's syndrome. Arch Gen Psychiatry 48:324–328, 1991

Leonard HL, Swedo SE, Rapoport JL, et al: Treatment of obsessive compulsive disorder with clomipramine and desipramine in children and adolescents. Arch Gen Psychiatry 46:1088–1092, 1989

Leonard HL, Swedo SE, Lenane MC, et al: A double-blind desipramine substitution during long-term clomipramine treatment in children and adolescents with obsessive-compulsive disorder. Arch Gen Psychiatry 48:922–927, 1991

Lewis DW, Pincus JH, Shanok SS, et al: Psychomotor epilepsy and violence in a group of incarcerated adolescent boys. Am J Psychiatry 139:882–887, 1982

Livingston RL, Dykman RA, Ackerman PT: Psychiatric comorbidity and response to two doses of methylphenidate in children with attention deficit disorder. Journal of Child and Adolescent Psychopharmacology 2:115–122, 1992

Mash EJ, Dalby JT: Behavioral interventions in hyperactivity, in Hyperactivity in Children: Etiology, Measurement and Treatment Implications. Edited by Trites RL. Baltimore, MD, University Park Press, 1979, pp 161–216

McBride MC: An individual double-blind crossover trial for assessing methylphenidate response in children with attention deficit disorder. J Pediatr 113:137–145, 1988

McClellan JM, Werry JS: Schizophrenia. Psychiatr Clin North Am 15:131–148, 1992

McDaniel KD: Pharmacologic treatment of psychiatric and neurodevelopmental disorders in children and adolescents (part 1). Clin Pediatr (Phila) 25:65–71, 1986

Menolascino F, Wilson J, Golden C, et al: Medication and treatment of schizophrenia in persons with mental retardation. Ment Retard 24:277–283, 1986

Micheli F, Gatto M, Lekhuniec E, et al: Treatment of Tourette's syndrome with calcium antagonists. Clin Neuropharmacol 13:77–83, 1990

Mikkelsen EJ, Detlor J, Cohen DJ: School avoidance and social phobia triggered by haloperidol in patients with Tourette's disorder. Am J Psychiatry 138:1572–1576, 1981

Munetz MR, Benjamin S: How to examine patients using the Abnormal Involuntary Movement Scale. Hosp Community Psychiatry 39:1172–1177, 1988

Murphy DA, Pelham WE, Lang AR: Aggression in boys with attention deficit-hyperactivity disorder: methylphenidate effects on naturalistically observed aggression, response to provocation, and social information processing. J Abnorm Child Psychol 20:451–466, 1992

Nehra A, Mullick F, Ishak KG, et al: Pemoline-associated hepatic injury. Gastroenterology 99:1517–1519, 1990

Nelles WB, Barlow DH: Do children panic? Clinical Psychology Review 8:359–372, 1988

Nino-Murcia G, Dement WC: Psychophysiological and pharmacological aspects of somnambulism and night terrors in children, in Psychopharmacology: The Third Generation of Progress. Edited by Meltzer HY. New York, Raven, 1987, pp 873–879

Patterson JF: Hepatitis associated with pemoline. South Med J 77:938, 1984

Pauls DL, Leckman JF: The inheritance of Gilles de la Tourette syndrome and associated behaviors: evidence for an autosomal dominant transmission. N

Engl J Med 315:993–997, 1986

Pauls DL, Hurst C, Kruger SD, et al: Evidence against a genetic relationship between Tourette's syndrome and attention deficit disorder. Arch Gen Psychiatry 43:1177–1179, 1986

Pelco LE, Kissel RC, Parrish JM, et al: Behavioral management of oral medication administration difficulties among children: a review of literature with case illustrations. Developmental and Behavioral Pediatrics 8:90–96, 1987

Pelham WE: The effects of stimulant drugs on learning and achievement in hyperactive and learning disabled children, in Psychological and Educational Perspectives on Learning Disabilities. Edited by Torgesen JK, Wong B. New York, Academic Press, 1985, pp 259–295

Pelham WE, Bender ME: Peer relationships in hyperactive children: description and treatment. Advances in Learning and Behavioral Disabilities 1:365–436, 1982

Pelham WE, Murphy HA: Attention deficit and conduct disorders, in Pharmacological and Behavioral Treatment: An Integrative Approach. Edited by Hersen M. New York, Wiley, 1986, pp 108–147

Pelham WE, Schnedler RW, Bologna NC, et al: Behavioral and stimulant treatment of hyperactive children: a therapy study with methylphenidate probes in a within-subject design. J Appl Behav Anal 13:221–236, 1980

Pelham WE, Milich R, Walker JL: Effects of continuous and partial reinforcement and methylphenidate on learning in children with attention deficit disorder. J Abnorm Psychol 95:319–325, 1986

Pelham WE, Sturges J, Hoza J, et al: The effects of sustained release 20 and 10 mg Ritalin b.i.d. on cognitive and social behavior in children with attention deficit disorder. Pediatrics 40:491–501, 1987

Pelham WE, Greenslade KE, Vodde-Hamilton M, et al: Relative efficacy of long-acting stimulants on children with attention deficit-hyperactivity disorder: a comparison of standard methylphenidate, sustained-release methylphenidate, sustained-release dextroamphetamine, and pemoline. Pediatrics 86:226–237, 1990

Pesikoff RB, Davis PC: Treatment of pavor nocturnus and somnambulism in children. Am J Psychiatry 128:778–781, 1971

Petti TA, Law W: Abrupt cessation of high-dose imipramine treatment in children. JAMA 246:768–769, 1981

Pfefferbaum B, Overall JE, Boren HA, et al: Alprazolam in the treatment of anticipatory and acute situational anxiety in children with cancer. J Am Acad Child Adolesc Psychiatry 26:532–535, 1987

Platt JE, Campbell M, Green WH, et al: Cognitive effects of lithium carbonate and haloperidol in treatment-resistant aggressive children. Arch Gen Psychiatry 41:657–662, 1984

Pleak RR, Birmaher B, Gavrilescu A, et al: Mania and neuropsychiatric excitation following carbamazepine. J Am Acad Child Adolesc Psychiatry 27:500–503, 1988

Pliszka SR: Tricyclic antidepressants in the treatment of children with attention deficit disorder. J Am Acad Child Adolesc Psychiatry 26:127–132, 1987

Pliszka SR: Effect of anxiety on cognition, behavior, and stimulant response in ADHD. J Am Acad Child Adolesc Psychiatry 28:882–887, 1989

Popper C: Medical unknowns and ethical consent, in Psychiatric Pharmacosciences of Children and Adolescents. Edited by Popper C. Washington, DC, American Psychiatric Press, 1987, pp 127–161

Poznanski EO, Freeman LN, Mokros HB: Children's Depression Rating Scale-Revised. Psychopharmacol Bull 21:979–989, 1985

Preskorn SH, Weller E, Hughes CW, et al: Depression in prepubertal children: dexamethasone non-suppression predicts differential response to imipramine vs. placebo. Psychopharmacol Bull 23:128–133, 1987

Preskorn SH, Weller E, Jerkovich G, et al: Depression in children: concentration-dependent CNS toxicity of tricyclic antidepressants. Psychopharmacol Bull 24:140–142, 1988

Pynoos RS, Frederick C, Nader K, et al: Life threat and posttraumatic stress in school-age children. Arch Gen Psychiatry 44:1057–1063, 1987

Rapoport JL: Antidepressants in childhood attention deficit disorder and obsessive-compulsive disorder. Psychosomatics 27:30–36, 1986

Rapoport JL, Zametkin A, Donnelly M, et al: New drug trials in attention deficit disorder. Psychopharmacol Bull 21:232–236, 1985

Rapoport JL, Swedo SE, Leonard HL: Childhood obsessive compulsive disorder. J Clin Psychiatry 53 (suppl):11–16, 1992

Rapport MD, Carlson GA, Kelly KL, et al: Methylphenidate and desipramine in hospitalized children, I:

separate and combined effects on cognitive function. J Am Acad Child Adolesc Psychiatry 32:333–342, 1993

Ratey J, Bemporad J, Sorgi P, et al: Brief report: open trial effects of beta-blockers on speech and social behaviors in 8 autistic adults. J Autism Dev Disord 17:439–446, 1987

Ratey J, Sovner R, Parks A, et al: Buspirone treatment of aggression and anxiety in mentally retarded patients: a multiple-baseline, placebo lead-in study. J Clin Psychiatry 52:159–162, 1991

Realmuto GM, Erickson WD, Yellin AM, et al: Clinical comparison of thiothixene and thioridazine in schizophrenic adolescents. Am J Psychiatry 141:440–442, 1984

Regeur L, Pakkenberg B, Fog R, et al: Clinical features and long-term treatment with pimozide in 65 patients with Gilles de la Tourette's syndrome. J Neurol Neurosurg Psychiatry 49:791–795, 1986

Reich W, Welner Z: The Diagnostic Interview for Children and Adolescents-Revised. St. Louis, MO, Washington University, 1988

Reiter S, Kutcher SP: Disinhibition and anger outbursts in adolescents treated with clonazepam. J Clin Psychopharmacol 11:268, 1991

Reiter S, Kutcher S, Gardner D: Anxiety disorders in children and adolescents: clinical and related issues in pharmacological treatment. Can J Psychiatry 37:432–438, 1992

Richardson MA, Haugland G, Craig TJ: Neuroleptic use, parkinsonian symptoms, tardive dyskinesia, and associated factors in child and adolescent psychiatric patients. Am J Psychiatry 148:1322–1328, 1991

Riddle MA, Hardin MT, Cho SC, et al: Desipramine treatment of boys with attention-deficit hyperactivity disorder and tics: preliminary clinical experience. J Am Acad Child Adolesc Psychiatry 27:811–814, 1988

Riddle MA, Hardin MT, King RA, et al: Fluoxetine treatment of children and adolescents with Tourette's and obsessive compulsive disorders: preliminary clinical experience. J Am Acad Child Adolesc Psychiatry 29:45–48, 1990

Riddle MA, King RA, Hardin MT, et al: Behavioral side effects of fluoxetine in children and adolescents. Journal of Child and Adolescent Psychopharmacology 1:193–198, 1990/1991

Riddle MA, Scahill L, King RA, et al: Double-blind, crossover trial of fluoxetine and placebo in children and adolescents with obsessive compulsive disorder. J Am Acad Child Adolesc Psychiatry 31:1062–1069, 1992

Riddle MA, Geller B, Ryan N: Another sudden death in a child treated with desipramine. J Am Acad Child Adolesc Psychiatry 32:792–797, 1993

Rivera-Calimlim L, Griesbach PH, Perlmutter R: Plasma chlorpromazine concentrations in children with behavioral disorders and mental illness. Clin Pharmacol Ther 26:114–121, 1979

Robertson MM, Eapen V: Pharmacologic controversy of CNS stimulants in Gilles de la Tourette's syndrome. Clin Neuropharmacol 15:408–425, 1992

Russo RM, Gururaj VJ, Allen JE: The effectiveness of diphenhydramine HCl in pediatric sleep disorders. J Clin Pharmacol 16:284–288, 1976

Ryan ND: Heterocyclic antidepressants in children and adolescents. Journal of Child and Adolescent Psychopharmacology 1:21–31, 1990

Ryan ND, Puig-Antich J, Cooper T, et al: Imipramine in adolescent major depression: plasma level and clinical response. Acta Psychiatr Scand 73:275–288, 1986

Ryan N, Meyer VA, Dachille S, et al: Lithium antidepressant augmentation in TCA-refractory depression in adolescents. J Am Acad Child Adolesc Psychiatry 27:371–376, 1988a

Ryan ND, Puig-Antich J, Rabinovich H, et al: MAOIs in adolescent major depression unresponsive to tricyclic antidepressants. J Am Acad Child Adolesc Psychiatry 27:755–758, 1988b

Safer DJ: Relative cardiovascular safety of psychostimulants used to treat attention-deficit hyperactivity disorder. Journal of Child and Adolescent Psychopharmacology 2:279–290, 1992

Sallee F, Stiller R, Perel J, et al: Oral pemoline kinetics in hyperactive children. Clin Pharmacol Ther 37:606–609, 1985

Satterfield JH, Satterfield BT, Schell AM: Therapeutic interventions to prevent delinquency in hyperactive boys. J Am Acad Child Adolesc Psychiatry 26:56–64, 1987

Schleifer M, Weiss G, Cohen N, et al: Hyperactivity in preschoolers and the effect of methylphenidate. Am J Orthopsychiatry 45:38–50, 1975

Shapiro AK, Shapiro E: Controlled study of pimozide vs. placebo in Tourette's syndrome. J Am Acad Child Adolesc Psychiatry 23:161–173, 1984

Shapiro E, Shapiro A, Fulop G, et al: Controlled study of haloperidol, pimozide, and placebo for the treatment of Gilles de la Tourette's syndrome. Arch Gen Psychiatry 46:722–730, 1989

Silverstein FS, Boxer L, Johnston MV: Hematological monitoring during therapy with carbamazepine in children. Ann Neurol 13:685–686, 1983

Simeon JG, Ferguson HB: Recent developments in the use of antidepressant and anxiolytic medications. Psychiatr Clin North Am 8:893–907, 1985

Simeon JG, Ferguson HB: Alprazolam effects in children with anxiety disorders. Can J Psychiatry 32:570–574, 1987

Simeon JG, Ferguson HB, Fleet JVW: Bupropion effects in attention deficit and conduct disorders. Can J Psychiatry 31:581–585, 1986

Simeon JG, Thatte S, Wiggins D: Treatment of adolescent obsessive-compulsive disorder with a clomipramine-fluoxetine combination. Psychopharmacol Bull 26:285–290, 1990

Simeon JG, Ferguson HB, Knott V, et al: Clinical, cognitive, and neurophysiological effects of alprazolam in children and adolescents with overanxious and avoidant disorders. J Am Acad Child Adolesc Psychiatry 31:29–33, 1992

Speltz ML, Varley CK, Peterson K, et al: Effects of dextroamphetamine and contingency management on a preschooler with ADHD and oppositional defiant disorder. J Am Acad Child Adolesc Psychiatry 27:175–178, 1987

Spencer T, Biederman J, Steingard R, et al: Bupropion exacerbates tics in children with attention deficit hyperactivity disorder and Tourette's syndrome. J Am Acad Child Adolesc Psychiatry 32:211–214, 1993

Steingard R, Khan A, Gonzalez A, et al: Neuroleptic malignant syndrome: review of experience with children and adolescents. Journal of Child and Adolescent Psychopharmacology 2:183–198, 1992

Strayhorn JM, Rapp N, Donina W, et al: Randomized trial of methylphenidate for an autistic child. J Am Acad Child Adolesc Psychiatry 27:244–247, 1988

Strober M, Morrell W, Lampert C, et al: A family study of bipolar I illness in adolescence: early onset of symptoms linked to increased familial loading and lithium resistance. J Affect Disord 15:255–268, 1988

Strober M, Morrell W, Lampert C, et al: Relapse following discontinuation of lithium maintenance therapy in adolescents with bipolar I illness: a naturalistic study. Am J Psychiatry 147:457–461, 1990

Strober M, Freeman R, Rigali J, et al: The pharmaco-

therapy of depressive illness in adolescence, II: effects of lithium augmentation in nonresponders to imipramine. J Am Acad Child Adolesc Psychiatry 31:16–20, 1992

Sturmey P, Reed J, Corbett J: Psychometric assessment of psychiatric disorders in people with learning difficulties (mental handicap): a review of measures. Psychol Med 21:143–155, 1991

Swanson JM: Measures of cognitive functioning appropriate for use in pediatric psychopharmacological research studies. Psychopharmacol Bull 21:887–890, 1985

Teicher MH, Glod CA: Neuroleptic drugs: indications and guidelines for their rational use in children and adolescents. Journal of Child and Adolescent Psychopharmacology 1:33–56, 1990

Terr LC: Childhood psychic trauma, in Basic Handbook of Child Psychiatry, Vol V. Edited by Call JD, Cohen RL, Harrison SI, et al. New York, Basic Books, 1987, pp 262–272

Thurston LP: Comparison of the effects of parent training and of Ritalin in treating hyperactive children, in Strategic Interventions for Hyperactive Children. Edited by Gittelman M. New York, ME Sharpe, 1981, pp 178–185

Trimble MR: Anticonvulsants in children and adolescents. Journal of Child and Adolescent Psychopharmacology 1:107–124, 1990

Ullmann RK, Sleator EK: Attention deficit disorder children with or without hyperactivity: which behaviors are helped by stimulants? Clin Pediatr (Phila) 24:547–551, 1985

Ullmann RK, Sleator EK: Responders, nonresponders, and placebo responders among children with attention deficit disorder. Clin Pediatr (Phila) 25:594–599, 1986

Varley CK, Trupin EW: Double-blind assessment of stimulant medication for attention deficit disorder: a model for clinical application. Am J Orthopsychiatry 53:542–547, 1983

Venkataraman S, Naylor MW, King CA: Mania associated with fluoxetine treatment in adolescents. J Am Acad Child Adolesc Psychiatry 31:276–281, 1992

Walkup JT, Rosenberg LA, Brown J, et al: The validity of instruments measuring tic severity in Tourette's syndrome. J Am Acad Child Adolesc Psychiatry 31:472–477, 1992

Weller E, Weller R: Neuroendocrine changes in affectively ill children and adolescents. Neurol Clin 6:41–54, 1988

Weller E, Weller R: Depressive disorders in children and adolescents, in Psychiatric Disorders in Children and Adolescents. Edited by Garfinkle BD, Carlson G, Weller EB. Philadelphia, PA, WB Saunders, 1990, pp 3–20

Weller E, Weller R, Fristad M, et al: The dexamethasone suppression test in hospitalized prepubertal depressed children. Am J Psychiatry 141:290–291, 1984

Weller R, Weller E, Tucker S, et al: Mania in prepubertal children: has it been underdiagnosed? J Affect Disord 11:151–154, 1986a

Weller E, Weller R, Fristad M: Lithium dosage guide for prepubertal children: a preliminary report. J Am Acad Child Psychiatry 25:92–95, 1986b

Weller E, Weller R, Fristad M, et al: Dexamethasone suppression test and clinical outcome in prepubertal depressed children. Am J Psychiatry 143:1469–1470, 1986c

Weller E, Weller R, Fristad M, et al: Saliva monitoring in prepubertal children. J Am Acad Child Adolesc Psychiatry 26:173–175, 1987

Whalen CK, Henker B: Therapies for hyperactive children: comparisons, combinations, and compromises. J Consult Clin Psychol 59:126–137, 1991

Whalen CK, Henker B, Castro J, et al: Peer perceptions of hyperactivity and medication effects. Child Dev 58:816–828, 1987

Whalen CK, Henker B, Buhrmester D, et al: Does stimulant medication improve the peer status of hyperactive children? J Consult Clin Psychol 57:545–549, 1989

Whitaker A, Rao U: Neuroleptics in pediatric psychiatry. Psychiatr Clin North Am 15:243–276, 1992

Wilens TE, Biederman J, Geist DE, et al: Nortriptyline in the treatment of ADHD: a chart review of 58 cases. J Am Acad Child Adolesc Psychiatry 32:343–349, 1993

Williams DT, Mehl R, Yudofsky S, et al: The effect of propranolol on uncontrolled rage outbursts in children and adolescents with organic brain dysfunction. J Am Acad Child Psychiatry 21:129–135, 1982

Youngerman J, Canino IA: Lithium carbonate use in children and adolescents. Arch Gen Psychiatry 35:216–224, 1978

Yudofsky SC, Silver JM, Jackson W, et al: The Overt Aggression Scale for the objective rating of verbal and physical aggression. Am J Psychiatry 143:35–39, 1986

Zahn TP, Rapoport, JL, Thompson CL: Autonomic and behavioral effects of dextroamphetamine and placebo in normal and hyperactive prepubertal boys. J Abnorm Child Psychol 8:145–160, 1980

Zametkin AJ, Linnoila M, Karoum F, et al: Pemoline and urinary excretion of catecholamines and indoleamines in children with attention deficit disorder. Am J Psychiatry 143:359–362, 1986

34

Treatment of Substance-Related Disorders

James W. Cornish, M.D., Laura F. McNicholas, M.D., Ph.D., and
Charles P. O'Brien, M.D., Ph.D.

◼ ALCOHOL

Alcoholism is the most prevalent substance use disorder in the United States, affecting approximately 14% of the population at some point in their lives (Robins et al. 1984). The magnitude of this problem is huge, costing 65,000 lives and $136 billion per year (National Institute on Alcohol Abuse and Alcoholism 1990). The natural history of excessive alcohol consumption is known. The amount and pattern of alcohol consumption and the harmful effects of drinking are associated in a predictable manner (Kranzler et al. 1990).

The principal forms of treatment for alcoholism have been self-help or support groups such as Alcoholics Anonymous (see section on self-help groups) or psychosocial treatments in inpatient or outpatient rehabilitation programs or sheltered living situations. There are many 28-day treatment programs that provide group and individual therapy for alcoholic rehabilitation. Unfortunately, psychosocial treatments for alcohol-dependent people have had only limited success in reducing alcohol use (Holder et al. 1991). Although there is ample room for improvement over psychosocial treatment alone, only a few controlled clinical studies have been conducted to test the efficacy of pharmacotherapies in the rehabilitation of

alcohol-dependent patients (Meyer 1989). Pharmacotherapy has been directed at specific indications that often occur during the course of treatment for alcoholism. Studies have been conducted involving alcohol detoxification treatments, alcohol sensitization agents, anticraving agents, and agents to diminish drinking by treating associated psychiatric pathology.

◼ Alcohol Detoxification

Detoxification refers to the clearing of alcohol from the body and the readjustment of all systems to functioning in the absence of alcohol. The alcohol withdrawal syndrome at the mild end may include only headache and irritability, but about 5% of alcoholic individuals have severe withdrawal symptoms (Schuckit 1991) manifested by tremulousness, tachycardia, perspiration, and even seizures ("rum fits"). The presence of malnutrition, electrolyte imbalance, or infection increases the possibility of cardiovascular collapse.

Significant progress has been achieved in establishing safe, effective medications for alcohol withdrawal. Pharmacotherapy with a benzodiazepine is the treatment of choice for the prevention and treatment of the signs and symptoms of alcohol withdrawal (Nutt et al. 1989). Many patients detoxify from alcohol without specific treatment or medications. However, it is difficult to accurately determine which patients require medication for alcohol withdrawal. Patients in good physical condition with uncomplicated, mild to moderate alcohol withdrawal symptoms can usually be treated as outpatients (Hayashida et al. 1989). A typical regimen requires the patient to attend the clinic daily for 5–10 days for clinical evaluations, multiple vitamins, and benzodiazepine pharmacotherapy. A typical medication dosing regimen involves giving enough benzodiazepine on the first day of treatment to relieve withdrawal symptoms— the dose should be adjusted if withdrawal symptoms increase or if the patient complains of excessive sedation. Over the next 5–7 days, the dose of benzodiazepine is tapered to zero. Most clinicians use longer-acting benzodiazepines such as clonazepam, chlordiazepoxide, or diazepam. The usual starting dose of medication on the first day is 25–50 mg of chlordiazepoxide or 10 mg of diazepam given every 6 hours (Schuckit 1991).

The diagnosis of delirium tremens is given to patients who have marked confusion and severe agitation in addition to the usual alcohol withdrawal symptoms (Goodwin 1992). It is important to remember that the risk of mortality is 5% in patients with severe alcohol withdrawal symptoms (Schuckit 1987). Patients who have medically complicated or severe alcoholic withdrawal must be treated in a hospital. Benzodiazepines will usually be sufficient to calm agitated patients; however, some patients may require intravenous barbiturates in order to control extreme agitation (Goodwin 1992).

■ Alcohol Sensitizing Agents

Disulfiram (Antabuse®) is the only medication that has the U.S. Food and Drug Administration (FDA) approval for the treatment of alcohol dependence other than detoxification. Disulfiram inhibits a key enzyme, aldehyde dehydrogenase, involved in breakdown of ethyl alcohol. Following drinking, the alcohol-disulfiram reaction produces excess blood levels of acetaldehyde, which is toxic in that it produces facial flushing, tachycardia, hypotension, nausea and vomiting, and physical discomfort. The usual maintenance dose of disulfiram is 250 mg qd.

There have only been a few randomized controlled trials, and these trials have had mixed results for drug efficacy (Peachy and Naranjo 1984). The most comprehensive trial was the Veterans Administration Cooperative Study of disulfiram treatment of alcoholism. This study was conducted with male veterans and found no differences between disulfiram administered at 250 mg daily and at 1 mg daily (an ineffective dose) and placebo groups in total abstinence, time to first drink, employment, or social stability. Among patients who drank, those in the disulfiram 250-mg dose group reported significantly fewer drinking days (Fuller et al. 1986).

The main problem with disulfiram is that patients frequently stop taking it and relapse to drinking (Goodwin 1992). Disulfiram is most effective when it is used in a clinical setting that emphasizes abstinence and offers a mechanism to ensure that the medication is taken. Drug compliance may be successfully ensured by giving the medication at 3- to 4-day intervals in the physician's office, at the treatment center, or by having a spouse, significant other, or family member administer it.

■ Alcohol Anticraving Agents

According to Volpicelli and colleagues (1992), an ideal pharmacotherapy decreases the craving for alcohol so that there is less motivation to drink and blocks the reinforcing effects of alcohol so that if drinking resumes, there are neither pleasant nor unpleasant effects and few (if any) side effects.

A variety of animal models have implicated the involvement of several neurotransmitter systems in alcohol craving and consumption, including endogenous opioid peptides, catecholamine, serotonin, dopamine, and γ-aminobutyric acid (GABA). The only pharmacological intervention that has thus far shown substantial promise involves the blocking of opioid receptors. There is evidence from animal studies and some human research that alcohol increases endogenous opioid activity. Activation of opioid receptors, therefore, may be involved in the reinforcing properties of alcohol. Opioid antagonists (e.g., naloxone and naltrexone) that block opioid receptors have been found to decrease alcohol consumption in animal models (Altshuler et al. 1980; Myers et al. 1986; Volpicelli et al. 1986). Conversely, rats pretreated with small doses of an opioid agonist such as morphine show increased alcohol drinking (Hubbell et al. 1986), whereas higher doses reduce alcohol drinking. Rats bred for alcohol preference not only have high alcohol consumption but also high endogenous opioid activity, and naltrexone blocks alcohol drinking in these rodents in a dose-related fashion (Froehlich et al. 1990). Collectively, these findings suggest that alcohol consumption is reinforced by an interaction with the endogenous opioid system and that blocking opioid receptors with specific antagonists lessens behavioral reinforcement, which in turn decreases drinking. This hypothesis also explains why higher doses of opioids, which are an external supply of opioid activity, can reduce drinking.

The first human study of the efficacy and safety of naltrexone in the treatment of alcoholism was conducted by Volpicelli and colleagues (1992). This was a 12-week double-blind trial in which 72 subjects were randomly assigned to receive either a 50-mg dose of naltrexone qd or placebo in addition to standard psychosocial treatment. The naltrexone group had lower rates of relapse, fewer drinking days, and less alcohol craving compared with the placebo group. The results indicate that less than half as many naltrexone patients relapsed (23%) as did placebo patients (54.3%). The most striking effects were seen in those who sampled alcohol. Nineteen (95%) of the 20 placebo patients relapsed after they sampled alcohol, compared with only 8 of 16 (50%) of the naltrexone patients. In the other double-blind placebo-controlled study, 97 alcohol-dependent subjects were randomized to receive either naltrexone or placebo and either coping skills/relapse prevention therapy or a supportive therapy (O'Malley et al. 1992). Compared with the placebo group, the naltrexone-treated patients drank on half as many days, drank one-third as much alcohol during occasions of drinking, and had less severe alcohol-related problems. As in the prior study, those randomly assigned to naltrexone had significantly fewer relapses during the 3-month treatment period, and this difference was still present at follow-up 6 months later.

The only FDA-approved indication for naltrexone is in the treatment of opioid dependence. Other studies of naltrexone in alcoholism are under way, and these should help to clarify the role of naltrexone in this disorder. It will be important to determine which patients are most likely to be helped by the opioid antagonist and the optimal amount of psychosocial treatment needed. The evidence so far suggests that naltrexone is most likely to improve relapse rates when combined with a strong psychosocial rehabilitation program.

■ Agents Used to Diminish Drinking by Treating Associated Psychiatric Pathology

Depressed alcoholic patients treated with lithium showed no difference compared with those treated with placebo in a multiple center Veterans Administration study (Dorus et al. 1989). In a study in which desipramine was the pharmacotherapy for alcoholism, the results indicate a trend toward decreased drinking in both depressed and nondepressed subjects (Mason and Kocsis 1991).

McGrath and colleagues (1993) studied alcoholic patients (93% met DSM-III-R [American Psychiatric Association 1987] criteria for dependence) who had an antecedent history of depression (> 90%) or who continued to have depressive symptoms after 6 months of abstinence. Eighty patients were equally randomized to 12 weeks of treatment with either imipramine or placebo. Sixty-five percent of the imipramine-treated patients had a significant reduction in depressive symptoms and alcoholic consumption, compared with 25% for the placebo-treated group.

■ Summary

Benzodiazepines are the pharmacotherapeutic agents of choice for prevention and treatment of the signs and symptoms of alcohol withdrawal. Although disulfiram was no better than placebo when tested in large controlled studies of alcoholism, it is effective when used in clinical settings that stress abstinence and ensure medication compliance. Pharmacotherapy with the opioid antagonist naltrexone appears to markedly decrease relapse rates in abstinent patients who sample alcohol. A recent report indicates that imipramine is beneficial for treating depressed alcoholic patients.

■ BENZODIAZEPINES AND OTHER SEDATIVES

The benzodiazepines have largely replaced older sedative-hypnotic agents, such as barbiturates and meprobamate, in clinical usage. To a great extent, the popularity of the benzodiazepines is because of their safety in overdose situations and because, when first marketed, these agents were thought to have no abuse potential (or almost none). Clinical experience and scientific study have since shown that although the benzodiazepines, as a class of drugs, are certainly safer in isolated overdose situations than the older agents, physiological dependence is certainly possible and occurs with long-term usage, even at therapeutic doses. This has touched off a controversy that has yet to be settled.

Most patients who are in fact physiologically dependent on benzodiazepines do not increase the dose of medication above the physician's prescription or in any other way abuse the prescribed medication. However, if the benzodiazepine were to be abruptly discontinued, the patient would, in all probability, go through a withdrawal abstinence syndrome that could be extremely severe. For instance, abrupt discontinuation of high therapeutic doses of alprazolam has frequently been reported to cause seizures. Thus, any patient treated with a benzodiazepine for a significant length of time (i.e., longer than 3–6 months) should be slowly tapered off medication. This does not preclude the possibility of re-emergence of the patient's symptoms, which may necessitate continued use of the medication. The fact that patients become physiologically dependent on therapeutic doses of benzodiazepines has led some in the field to equate any use of benzodiazepines, in any patient for long-term treatment, with abuse of the drug. This is undoubtedly an overstatement of the abuse of these agents. Significant abuse of benzodiazepines does in fact occur, but it is usually seen in patients also abusing other drugs, *not* in the patient carefully monitored and kept stable on therapeutically indicated benzodiazepines.

Generally speaking, patients who abuse benzodiazepines alone are rare; it is much more common to find benzodiazepine abuse in combination with abuse of other drugs. Alcoholic patients will not infrequently abuse benzodiazepines if the opportunity presents itself, and cocaine- and opioid-abusing patients are also likely to concomitantly use benzodiazepines. Studies of alcoholic patients admitted for detoxification have shown the rate of benzodiazepine use, by urinalysis, to be 28%–41% of the patients (Crane et al. 1988; Ogborne and Kapur 1987; Soyka et al. 1989). Generally, only about one-third of patients with a positive urine test for benzodiazepine admitted to using the drugs.

A variety of studies from Europe have looked at benzodiazepine use in patients using illicit opioids and have found that up to 90% of patients use benzodiazepines to some extent, although most patients deny that they use benzodiazepines or state that they use them for insomnia or anxiety or to reduce withdrawal symptoms. Methadone-maintained patients often use benzodiazepines, but frequently on a sporadic basis. Magura and colleagues (1987) showed that 40% of patients in four methadone programs in New York had urine samples positive for benzodiazepines, whereas studies in England show rates of benzodiazepine-positive urine samples of 54% (Lipsedge and Cook 1987) and 59% (Beary et al. 1987) in methadone patients.

In patients who use benzodiazepines in conjunction with other drugs, the issues of abuse and physiological dependence take on a much different meaning than in the stable patient on long-term prescribed benzodiazepines. If these patients use or abuse more than one substance, the use or abuse of benzodiazepines can seriously interfere with drug abuse treatment for other substances—for example, the patient who is discharged from his or her methadone maintenance program for urine samples consistently positive for illicit benzodiazepines. These patients require detoxification from benzodiazepines, using either a benzodiazepine or phenobarbital taper; evaluation for underlying psychiatric disorders, such as generalized anxiety or panic disorder; and relapse prevention techniques for benzodiazepine abuse.

■ COCAINE

Cocaine abuse in the United States has been an epidemic since the early 1980s. High-purity, low-cost cocaine is widely available. The consequences and byproducts of this epidemic have touched most American communities. The National Household Survey on Drug Abuse (National Institute on Drug Abuse 1991), which is based on a sample of 32,594 people representative of the American population, estimates there are 3 million current cocaine users. When compared with the data for 1985, the current survey shows that weekly (chronic) users have increased from 647,000 to 855,000. Furthermore, the chronic cocaine users are developing a significant number of medical and psychosocial problems. According to data from the Drug Abuse Warning Network, DAWN (Substance Abuse and Mental Health Services Administration 1993), cocaine-related hospital emergencies—especially those for patients age 35 and older—continue to increase (Figure 34–1).

The selection of potential pharmacotherapies have been based on our current understanding of the neurochemical changes that result from chronic stimulant use. Cocaine administration results in increased levels of dopamine in the region of the nucleus accumbens in rats. This is an important part of the brain reward pathways. Cocaine and other abused substances that increase nucleus accumbens dopamine also decreases the threshold for brain-stimulation reward (Kornetsky and Porrino 1992).

Pharmacotherapy of cocaine dependence must be considered separately from pharmacotherapy used to treat complications involved in cocaine abuse, such as depression and psychotic reactions. Although a withdrawal syndrome for cocaine dependence has been proposed (Gawin and Kleber 1986), this withdrawal generally consists simply of tiredness, somnolence, lack of energy, craving for cocaine, and periods of depression. It usually resolves spontaneously over several days, but there is evidence from imaging studies that receptor changes and even brain metabolic effects from chronic cocaine may persist for weeks or months after the last dose of cocaine.

A variety of medications have been used to approach those biochemical changes that are thought to play a role in relapse to compulsive cocaine use.

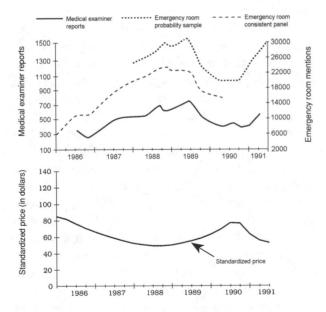

Figure 34–1. Emergency room mentions and medical examiner reports involving cocaine and standardized price of cocaine by quarter, 1986–1991.
Source. Drug Abuse Warning Network and the System to Retrieve Information From Drug Evidence 1986–1991.

Antidepressants have been used based on the theory that they, too, block reuptake of biogenic amines and thus may repair some of the deficit produced by abrupt cocaine withdrawal. The best data have been obtained with desipramine, which is also the medication that has been studied the most. The results from several double-blind studies with desipramine (Arndt et al. 1992; Gawin et al. 1989; Kosten et al. 1992) indicate that it has a modest effect, at best, in inducing abstinence from cocaine. The studies of the Arndt and Kosten research teams both involved methadone maintenance subjects who were abusing cocaine, mainly intravenously. It is possible that patients who only abuse cocaine (not primarily by intravenous administration) may have a better prognosis than cocaine-abusing, methadone-maintained addicts. Further research is needed, particularly among those who abuse nonintravenous drugs, to determine which population of cocaine-addicted individuals benefit most from desipramine pharmacotherapy.

Another approach has been based on animal studies that indicate that cocaine can produce kindling of seizure activity. Kindling is an electrical phenomenon that refers to the increase in seizure activity when a standard subthreshold stimulus is applied repeatedly to certain brain structures, especially the amygdaloid nucleus. Small doses of cocaine applied to the amygdala have also been shown to produce kindling. Thus, the drug carbamazepine, which blocks kindling (Post 1988), might have a role in the treatment of cocaine dependence. Unfortunately, double-blind studies have thus far not shown any benefit from carbamazepine in preventing relapse to cocaine use (Halikas et al. 1992).

■ Summary

There is no medication clearly identified as an effective pharmacotherapy for cocaine-dependent people. Desipramine, which has been studied in several double-blind studies, appears to be moderately effective at inducing abstinence. More research is certainly needed in this important area.

■ OPIOIDS

Pharmacotherapy of opioid dependence has a long history, based no doubt in part because "heroinism" was one of the first recognized drug problems in the United States and therapeutically used congeners of the drug of abuse—heroin—were readily available. Later studies have shown only limited success with nonpharmacological treatment.

■ Detoxification From Opioid Dependence

The classical method of opioid detoxification was, and remains, short-term substitution therapy. The medication traditionally used has been methadone, at a sufficient dose to suppress signs and symptoms of heroin withdrawal abstinence; the methadone is then tapered over a period ranging from 1 week to 6 months. The idea behind a rapid (i.e., 1- or 2-week) detoxification regimen is to quickly achieve total opioid abstinence so that treatment can be continued in a drug-free setting. Detoxification can usually be accomplished in 4–7 days in an inpatient setting, whereas more time is frequently required in the outpatient setting to minimize patient discomfort. Most practitioners considers 21 days sufficient for short-term outpatient detoxification. However, many patients have very chaotic lives when presenting for treatment and require a period of stabilization before they have much hope of maintaining a drug-free lifestyle. As we discuss later in this chapter, the regulations for opioid treatment facilities require that patients be dependent on opioids for most of a year before they may be admitted to methadone maintenance. The 6-month stabilization-detoxification regimen allows these patients to work on the most acute personal and employment problems while stabilized on a relative low dose (30–40 mg qd) of methadone and then to detoxify from methadone to continue treatment in a drug-free setting. More recently, a partial agonist, buprenorphine, has been studied for efficacy in suppressing withdrawal abstinence signs and symptoms. In outpatient trials, Bickel and colleagues (1988) showed buprenorphine to be as effective as methadone in a 10-week double-blind trial (4 weeks on medication taper followed by 6 weeks of placebo). In an open trial, Kosten and Kleber (1988) compared subjects on 3 doses of buprenorphine and found that 4 mg administered sublingually was superior to 2 mg or 8 mg of buprenorphine in suppressing signs and symptoms of withdrawal abstinence, although illicit opiates were present in the urine of patients in both the 2- and 4-mg dose groups

in approximately equal numbers.

There has always been concern about substitution detoxification on the basis that the physician is prolonging the problem by prescribing an addictive medication, even with a tapering regimen. Many of the symptoms of opioid withdrawal abstinence (e.g., diaphoresis, hyperactivity, and irritability) appear to be mediated by overactivity in the sympathetic nervous system. This led Gold and associates (1978, 1980) to attempt to depress this overactivity and thereby ameliorate the withdrawal abstinence syndrome using adrenergic agents that are without abuse potential. Clonidine, an α-adrenergic agonist with inhibitory action primarily at the locus ceruleus, was found to be effective in inpatient populations in decreasing the signs and symptoms of opioid withdrawal abstinence. Outpatient detoxification with clonidine has not been as successful as inpatient treatment. Inpatient studies reported an 80%–90% success rate, whereas outpatient studies have reported success rates as low as 31% in detoxifying patients from methadone and 36% in detoxifying patients from heroin. The problems identified in outpatient clonidine detoxification include access to heroin and other opioids, lethargy, insomnia, dizziness, and oversedation. The last four of these adverse effects were noted in inpatient populations during detoxification with clonidine but were easily managed in the hospital setting.

Clonidine's unacceptable side effects in many patients led researchers to investigate other α-agonists for use in detoxifying opioid-dependent patients. Lofexidine, guanabenz, and guanfacine have all been investigated to varying degrees as detoxification agents. The data thus far indicate that all of these agents have fewer cardiovascular side effects than clonidine. In a double-blind randomized trial comparing methadone, clonidine, and guanfacine in a rapid (12-day) inpatient detoxification program, methadone was significantly better in suppressing signs and symptoms of withdrawal abstinence than either of the α-agonists (San et al. 1990). The authors further concluded that guanfacine was more effective than clonidine in suppressing abstinence and had fewer cardiovascular side effects.

Because clonidine was much less successful for treating outpatients than for inpatients, various approaches—including the above-mentioned alternative α-agonists—were studied in an effort to improve the efficacy of clonidine. One of the major reasons clonidine was less successful in the outpatient setting was the availability of heroin and other opioids to the patient. Naltrexone, a competitive opioid antagonist, was added to the clonidine regimen in efforts to both speed up the time-course of withdrawal and to block the effect of any opioid used illicitly by the patient. As reported by Stine and Kosten (1992), the researchers showed that 82% of patients were successfully detoxified as outpatients in 4–5 days using a single daily dose regimen of clonidine and 12.5 mg of naltrexone. This significantly decreased the time necessary for detoxification. Furthermore, the patients reported few signs or symptoms of withdrawal except for restlessness, insomnia, and muscle aches. This protocol thus not only allowed the patients to detoxify from opioids, but also simultaneously began the patients on naltrexone maintenance (see below).

Loimer and associates (1990, 1991) have conducted work on very rapid opioid detoxification. These methods have involved anesthetizing patients with either methohexital (Loimer et al. 1990) or midazolam (Loimer et al. 1991) and then using naltrexone to precipitate abstinence. These protocols successfully detoxified patients in 48 hours but required major medical intervention (i.e., intubation, mechanical ventilation, and intravenous fluids) and exposed the patients to the risks of general anesthesia.

Two major problems with detoxification (either rapid or slow) have been identified over the years by clinicians and researchers working in this area. The first is that all regimens, regardless of the detoxification agent involved, must be individualized; this eliminates the possibility of standard protocols for opioid detoxification. The second problem is the more serious in terms of patient management—opioid-abusing and -dependent patients in drug-free treatment have an extremely high relapse rate. Maddux and Desmond (1992) reported on six long-term follow-up studies (i.e., 3 years or longer) of drug-free treatment of opiate abuse and dependence. Methadone was used for initial withdrawal, and one study used naltrexone to increase the chances of compliance with a drug-free program. Abstinence rates at follow-up in these studies ranged from 10%–19%; the percentage of patients with unknown status at follow-up ranged from 10%–32%. Because drug-free treatment of opioid users has such high relapse rates, other modalities of treatment have been developed.

■ Maintenance Treatment of Opioid Dependence

Methadone maintenance has been the mainstay of the pharmacotherapy of opioid dependence since its introduction by Dole and Nyswander (1965). Since the 1970s, LAAM (L-α-acetyl-methadol), a long-acting congener of methadone, has been used experimentally for maintenance treatment. It was recently approved by the FDA for this purpose and is available for general use, with Drug Enforcement Agency (DEA) license, in opioid-dependence treatment programs. More recently, buprenorphine has been studied in clinical trials as a maintenance therapy in opioid-dependent patients. It has not yet received FDA approval, but it does have promise as an alternative to methadone maintenance.

■ Methadone

As we discussed, methadone has been used for both short- and long-term detoxification from opioids. However, methadone maintenance is designed to support patients with opioid dependence for months or years while they engage in counseling and other therapy to change their life-styles. Since its introduction, experience with methadone has accumulated in approximately 1.5 million person-years (Gerstein 1992), strongly showing methadone to be safe and effective. Further, this experience has shown that although patients in methadone maintenance show physiological signs of opioid tolerance, there are minimal side effects and the patients' general health and nutritional status improve.

This approach to the treatment of opioid dependence has been controversial from the beginning. Physicians and other treatment professionals who look at opioid dependence using a disease model have little or no problem treating patients with an active drug for long periods of time, especially in light of repeated treatment failures in the absence of active medication therapy. However, many people view methadone maintenance as simply substituting a legal drug for an illegal one, and they refuse to accept any outcome other than total abstinence from all drugs. These people point to long-term follow-up studies of methadone maintenance patients (Maddux and Desmond 1992) that show that 5 years after discharge from the maintenance program, only 10%–20% of the patients are completely abstinent (i.e., not enrolled in methadone maintenance or using illicit opioids). However, long-term follow-up studies on patients discharged from drug-free treatment programs show that only 10%–19% of opioid-dependent patients are abstinent at 3- or 5-year follow-up using the same definition (Maddux and Desmond 1992). In spite of these results on patients discharged from programs, studies on outcome measures other than total abstinence that were done on patients in maintenance treatment consistently show that these patients show marked improvement in various measures.

Investigators have shown up to an 85% decrease in criminal behavior (measured by self-report or arrest records) in patients in treatment, and employment among maintenance patients ranges from 40%–80%. Gerstein (1992) quotes a Swedish study published in 1984 showing the results over 5 years in 34 patients who applied for treatment to the only methadone clinic then in Sweden. The 34 patients were randomly assigned to either methadone maintenance or outpatient drug-free therapy; those patients in drug-free treatment could not apply for methadone for a minimum of 24 months after being accepted into the study. After 2 years, 71% of methadone patients were doing well, compared with 6% of patients admitted to drug-free treatment. After 5 years, 13 of 17 patients remained on methadone and were free of illicit drugs, and 4 of 17 patients had been discharged from treatment for continued drug use. Of the 17 drug-free treatment patients, 9 had subsequently been switched to methadone treatment and were free of illicit drug use and "socially productive." Of the remaining eight patients, five were dead (allegedly from overdose), two were in prison, and one was drug free.

Further, whereas previous generations of individuals who abused drugs had to be concerned about hepatitis B, endocarditis, and other infections, in our own time—when intravenous drug use and concomitant sharing of needles or syringes puts a patient at risk of infection with human immunodeficiency virus (HIV)—the medical consequences of heroin dependence must be taken into account when determining appropriate therapy for a patient. These issues are currently being studied by a variety of methods, but the overall clinical impression of increased general health in patients on methadone maintenance is very strong. Additionally, Metzger and colleagues (1993) have undertaken a study of HIV seroconversion rates in opioid-dependent subjects—152 subjects were in

methadone maintenance treatment and 103 subjects were out of treatment. At baseline, 12% of the subjects were HIV positive—10% of in-treatment and 16% of out-of-treatment subjects. Follow-up of HIV-negative subjects over 18 months showed conversion rates of 3.5% for in-treatment subjects and 22% for those remaining out of treatment. These data suggest that although transmission of HIV still occurs, opioid-abusing intravenous drug users in methadone maintenance programs have a significantly lower likelihood of becoming infected.

Methadone maintenance programs are licensed and regulated by the FDA and the DEA. A program and its physician must be licensed for a methadone maintenance program in order to prescribe or dispense more than a 2-week supply of any opioid to a patient known to be or suspected of being dependent on opioids. Most clinics are ambulatory and are open 6 or 7 days per week, requiring patients to come into the clinic daily to receive medication unless and until patients "earn" privileges (take-home medication) by compliance with the clinic rules and abstinence from illicit substances. For a person to be eligible for methadone maintenance, he or she must be at least age 18 years, physiologically dependent on heroin or other opioids, and must have been dependent on opioids for a period of at least 1 year. The treatment regulations define a 1-year history of addiction to mean that the patient was addicted to an opioid narcotic at some time at least 1 year before admission and was addicted, either continuously or episodically, for most of the year immediately before admission to the methadone maintenance program.

A physician must document evidence of current physiological dependence on opioids before a patient can be admitted to the program; such evidence may be a precipitated abstinence syndrome in response to a naloxone challenge or (more commonly) signs and symptoms of opioid withdrawal, evidence of intravenous injections, or evidence of medical complications of intravenous injections. Exceptions to these requirements are patients who have recently been in penal or chronic care, who have previously been treated, or who are pregnant. In these cases, patients need not show evidence of current physiological dependence, but the physician must justify their enrollment in methadone maintenance. A person under age 18 years must have documented evidence of at least two attempts at short-term detoxification or drug-free treatment (the episodes separated by at least 1 week) and have the consent of his or her parent or legal guardian.

Each clinic sets its own rules within the guidelines set by state and federal agencies. Many clinics are open only 6 days a week, thus giving all patients at least 1 dose of take-home medication weekly; others are open 7 days a week. All clinics must obtain urine toxicologies on patients, but the frequency varies from 2–3 times a week to once a month. Some clinics have set upper limits on the dose of methadone, such that no patient receives more than a dose specified by clinic rules. Certain clinics have dose limits of 30–40 mg, others go as high as 80 mg, and still others have no predetermined dosage limit (although it is rare for a patient to receive more than 100 mg qd). All methadone maintenance clinics must provide counseling for patients, but the amount required is up to the clinic's discretion.

The variability in clinic practice is widespread and (as with the issue of limiting doses) sometimes mandated by state regulators who take a stand with the people advocating total abstinence. These practices continue despite studies showing that doses of at least 60 mg qd were associated with longer retention in treatment, decreased use of illicit drugs, and a lower incidence of HIV infection (Hartel et al. 1988, 1989). Among patients receiving at least 71 mg qd of methadone, no heroin use was detected, whereas patients on doses of 46 mg qd of methadone or lower were five times more likely to use heroin than those receiving higher doses (Ball and Ross 1991). Further, in a comparison of three levels of treatment services in which all patients received at least 60 mg qd methadone, McLellan and colleagues (1993) showed that "enhanced methadone services" patients (i.e., patients receiving methadone plus counseling and on-site medical and psychiatric care, employment, and family therapy) had fewer urine samples positive for illicit substances than did patients in the "standard services" group (methadone plus counseling) or the "minimum services" group (methadone alone). The "standard services" group did significantly better in treatment than did the "minimum services" group. In fact, 69% of the "minimum services" group required transfer to a standard program 12 weeks into the study because of unremitting use of opioids or other illicit drugs.

Yet another issue that has engendered a great deal of controversy is the treatment of opioid-dependent pregnant women. Those who are philo-sophically opposed to methadone treatment would advocate that any woman using illicit opioids (heroin) or enrolled in methadone maintenance who became pregnant should be detoxified. It is currently estimated that up to 2%–3% of babies born each year have had intrauterine exposure to opioids. Because many women with substance abuse problems fear all organizations, including medical ones, they frequently have little or no prenatal care—exposing themselves and their children to the complications of unsupervised pregnancy in the setting of the added severe stressor of maternal addiction.

The complications and treatment of maternal opioid addiction and the effects on the fetus and neonate have been discussed by Finnegan (1991) and Finnegan and Kandall (1992). For our purposes, it should be noted that current evidence shows that pregnant women who wish to be detoxified from opioids (either heroin or methadone) should *not* be detoxified before the 14th week of gestation because of the potential risk of inducing abortion or after the 32nd week of gestation because of possible withdrawal-induced fetal stress (see Finnegan 1991). Most clinicians dealing with pregnant opioid-dependent patients advocate methadone maintenance at a dose of methadone that maintains homeostasis and eliminates opioid craving. This dose must be individualized for each patient and managed in concert with an obstetrician.

◼ LAAM

LAAM is a long-acting opioid agonist recently approved for marketing as a treatment for opioid dependence. Clinical trials conducted in the 1970s showed LAAM to be as effective as methadone in keeping heroin users from using illicit opioids (Jaffe et al. 1970, 1972; Ling et al. 1976). There is extensive literature on the safety and efficacy of LAAM in the treatment of opioid dependence. The major difference between methadone and LAAM is the duration of action of the drugs, which is based on the metabolism of the two drugs. Methadone is slowly metabolized to inactive metabolites; LAAM, on the other hand, is metabolized to two congeners, nor-LAAM and dinor-LAAM, both of which are more potent opioid agonists that LAAM itself. Further, the plasma half-life of methadone is about 35 hours (Gilman et al. 1990), whereas the half-lives for LAAM, nor-LAAM, and dinor-LAAM are estimated to be around 47, 62, and 162 hours, respectively (Finkle et al. 1982). These prolonged half-lives of LAAM and its active metabolites allow for alternate-day dosing or thrice-weekly dosing, without the problem of diverted take-homes that is inherent in methadone maintenance programs that allow take-home medication. It is also crucial to remember that LAAM will not reach steady-state plasma levels for 2–3 weeks after the medication is started or the dose changed. Too rapid an escalation in LAAM dose may result in an unintentional overdose because of drug accumulation; too slow an escalation may result in the patient having withdrawal symptoms and using illicit opioids.

LAAM received FDA approval in 1993 and is available in clinics (regulated by the FDA and the DEA) for the treatment of opioid dependence. In general, a patient who is eligible for methadone maintenance would also be eligible for LAAM maintenance; however, LAAM has not been studied in pregnant women. LAAM would obviously have advantages for the patient who does not want to come to a clinic on a daily basis and who does not require the structure of daily clinic attendance.

■ Buprenorphine

Buprenorphine is a partial agonist of μ-opioid type and is a clinically effective analgesic agent with an estimated potency 25–40 times that of morphine (Cowan et al. 1977). Buprenorphine is currently approved only for use as an analgesic agent, not yet for treatment of opioid dependence. Human pharmacology studies have shown buprenorphine to be 25–30 times as potent as morphine in producing pupillary constriction but less effective in producing morphine-like subjective effects (Jasinski et al. 1978). Further, these studies showed that the physiological and subjective effects of morphine (15–120 mg) were significantly attenuated when morphine was administered 3 hours after buprenorphine in patients maintained on 8 mg qd of buprenorphine. The physiological and subjective effects of 30 mg of morphine were also tested at 29.5 hours after the last dose of chronically administered buprenorphine and were again significantly attenuated.

Studies in opiate-abusing patients have shown that buprenorphine can be administered sublingually (sl) rather than subcutaneously (sc), the route most commonly used for analgesic effect, with only a moderate difference in potency—1.0 mg sc being equal to 1.5 mg sl (Jasinski et al. 1989). In early clinical trials using opioid-dependent patients, it was found that patients would tolerate the sl route and that the dose of buprenorphine could be rapidly escalated to effective doses without significant side effects or toxicity (Johnson et al. 1989). Detoxification from heroin dependence using buprenorphine was as effective as methadone (Bickel et al. 1988) or clonidine (Kosten and Kleber 1988).

Johnson and colleagues (1992) compared buprenorphine (8 mg qd sl) and methadone 20 mg qd or 60 mg qd in a 25-week maintenance study and found that buprenorphine was as effective as 60 mg qd methadone in reducing illicit opioid use and keeping patients in treatment. Both buprenorphine and methadone 60 mg qd were superior to methadone 20 mg qd in this study. It has been shown in both detoxification and maintenance studies that the abrupt discontinuation of buprenorphine in a blind fashion causes only very minor elevations in withdrawal scores on any withdrawal scale (Bickel et al. 1988; Fudala et al. 1990; Jasinski et al. 1978; Johnson et al. 1989; Kosten and Kleber 1988).

Because the issue of take-home medication is likely to arise in any opiate maintenance program, and because methadone take-home medication is likely to be diverted, the option of alternate-day buprenorphine dosing was explored. After 19 heroin-dependent patients were stabilized on buprenorphine (8 mg qd) for 2 weeks, 9 patients continued to receive buprenorphine daily while the other 10 patients, in a blind fashion, received alternate-day buprenorphine doses (8 mg/dose) for 4 weeks. Patients reported some dysphoria on days on which they received placebo. It was also noted that pupils were less constricted on placebo days in the patients on alternate-day therapy, but patients tolerated the 48-hour dosing interval without significant signs or symptoms of opiate withdrawal abstinence (Fudala et al. 1990). This leaves open the possibility of alternate-day medication in the treatment setting, much like dosing regimens using LAAM, eliminating the need for take-home medication. However, unlike LAAM, buprenorphine can be administered on a daily basis until the patient "earns" days away from the clinic.

■ Relapse Prevention

As was noted previously, various methods of detoxifying patients from opioids have been developed—

from substitution and rapidly tapering the dose of opioid to long-term methadone maintenance and a very gradual methadone taper. It was also noted that these methodologies were by and large unsuccessful in achieving permanent opioid abstinence in patients. It has long been thought that both conditioned reactivity to drug-associated cues (Wikler 1973) and protracted withdrawal symptoms (Martin and Jasinski 1969) contribute to the high rate of opioid relapse. The use of a blocking dose of a pure opioid antagonist would allow the patient to extinguish the conditioned responses to opioids by blocking the positive reinforcing effects of the illicit drugs. Naltrexone was shown to be orally effective in blocking the subjective effects of morphine for up to 24 hours (Martin et al. 1973); later studies showed that increasing the dose of naltrexone increased the duration of action.

Patients using naltrexone maintenance for relapse prevention need to be carefully screened, as they must be opioid-free at the start of naltrexone administration. Many practitioners administer a naloxone challenge, which must be negative, before starting naltrexone. Naltrexone is usually administered either daily (50 mg) or thrice-weekly (100 mg, 100 mg, and 150 mg). Although naltrexone is pharmacologically able to block the reinforcing effects of opioids, the patient must take the medication if it is to be effective. Many opioid-addicted patients have very little motivation to remain abstinent. Fram and colleagues (1989) reported that of 300 inner-city patients offered naltrexone, only 15 (5%) agreed to take the medication; 2 months later, only 3 patients remained on naltrexone. However, patients with better identified motivation—among them groups of recovering professionals (physicians, attorneys, etc.) and federal probationers, both of whom face loss of license to practice a profession, or legal consequences—have significantly better success with naltrexone.

■ Summary

There are a variety of well-developed and well-studied treatments—detoxification from opioids, maintenance therapy for dependent patients, and effective (if not well-accepted) relapse prevention pharmacotherapies—available for the opioid-dependent patient. However, even though the area of opioid dependence is probably the most widely studied of the areas of drug abuse, we can currently "cure" only a small percentage of patients coming for help. We must be content with assisting the rest of this patient population to improve their lives and the lives of their families while continuing to deal with the effects of ongoing opioid dependence.

■ SELF-HELP GROUPS

Self-help groups (e.g., Alcoholics Anonymous, Narcotics Anonymous, and Cocaine Anonymous), which are based on a 12-step method of recovery, can be a valuable source of support for the recovering patient. These groups are a fellowship of recovering people interested in helping themselves and each other lead drug-free lives. The groups are very good for reminding people of the adverse consequences of relapse and of the benefits of maintaining abstinence. Many recovering people feel that it is easier and more relevant to hear about some aspects of recovery from another recovering person. Patients can attend meetings as frequently as necessary and can learn more effective management of leisure time. A sponsor—a person in the group with a prolonged time in a drug-free lifestyle—can provide a good role-model for a person in recovery, in addition to providing support and encouragement. Self-help groups are also available to family members and significant others who do not abuse drugs to help them understand the addictive process and how family and interpersonal dynamics can affect the drug-abusing or recovering family member.

■ HALLUCINOGENS

The use and abuse of hallucinogens waxes and wanes much more than the use of some other drugs, such as alcohol and opioids. The major drugs of abuse that fall into this classification are marijuana and related compounds, lysergic acid diethylamide (LSD) and other indolealkylamines (e.g., psilocybin), and phencyclidine (PCP) and its congeners. Marijuana has a relatively constant rate of use, but its use alone almost never causes the user to seek medical attention. The use of LSD and related compounds has changed from the pattern see in the 1960s, when users lived together communally and the life-style of the group frequently revolved around "the psychedelic experience." This is in contrast to the use of hallucinogens today among people in isolated groups, people who engage in polysubstance abuse, adolescents, and young adults who frequent "rave" clubs. Most users of LSD and related compounds are not seen in emergency rooms, but occasionally patients experiencing acute adverse reactions to these drugs are brought in for medical attention. The most frequent adverse effects of LSD and related compounds are acute panic reactions. Most of these reactions—the "bad trips"—do not require any intervention other than a calm atmosphere and reassurance. Occasionally, however, a patient may benefit from a low dose of benzodiazepine to decrease the anxiety associated with the experience. Likewise, patients who are intoxicated with MDMA (methylenedioxymethamphetamine, or "Ecstasy") rarely require more than reassurance or, occasionally, acute benzodiazepine administration—again, to enable patients to deal with the anxiety associated with an adverse experience.

PCP intoxication, however, has serious psychiatric and medical complications. A schizophrenia-like psychotic state can be produced by very low doses of PCP; but behavioral disinhibition (frequently accompanied by anxiety, rage, aggression, and panic), rather than the core psychotic effects, necessitate treatment in most cases where treatment is mandated. There is no convincing evidence of the superiority of either benzodiazepines or neuroleptics in treating a patient with an acute reaction to PCP. Benzodiazepines are frequently used because of their rapid onset of action and because they can be titrated intravenously. If a neuroleptic is required, haloperidol is most commonly used, because many other neuroleptics have significant interaction with the anticholinergic properties of PCP itself. There is a paucity of information on chronic use of PCP and treatment, if indicated, in the chronic user.

■ NICOTINE

According to the U.S. Department of Health and Human Services, there are 51 million smokers in the United States, and tobacco accounts for approximately 400,000 deaths per year (U.S. Department of Health and Human Services 1990). Since the mid-1960s, the incidence of smoking in the United States has progressively decreased by about 1% per year (U.S. Department of Health and Human Services

1989). This remarkable change in tobacco use is a consequence of the realization by many in society that tobacco-related morality and morbidity are entirely preventable. Most of these smokers meet the DSM-III-R criteria for the substance use disorder of nicotine dependence. The behavioral aspects of nicotine dependence are similar to those for alcohol and opiate dependence, as well as the production of tolerance and physical dependence. In about 80% of smokers (Gross and Stitzer 1989), nicotine abstinence leads to well-described withdrawal signs and symptoms (Hughes and Hatsukami 1986).

Pharmacotherapy in the form of nicotine replacement has been a key element in reducing withdrawal symptoms and initiating smoking cessation.

■ Nicotine Replacement

Nicotine polacrilex gum is typically prescribed so that patients have free access to it for periods of up to 4 months. Transdermal nicotine is initially administered in 15- to 21-mg patches for 4–12 weeks, followed by lower-dose patches for up to 8 more weeks. The results from several well-controlled studies confirm that nicotine gum reduces irritability and withdrawal symptoms such as sleep disturbance, difficulty concentrating, and restlessness (Gross and Stitzer 1989; Schneider et al. 1983). Interestingly, nicotine gum does not appear to reduce craving for cigarettes.

Transdermal nicotine also has excellent documentation for its ability to decrease the severity of withdrawal symptoms and also to decrease craving for tobacco (Daughton et al. 1991; Tonnesen et al. 1991).

Neither gum nor transdermal nicotine have any long-term effect on weight gain. Both nicotine preparations provide a significant advantage over placebo in smoking cessation. Stitzer (1991) reviewed seven double-blind, placebo-controlled smoking cessation trials that used nicotine gum. Abstinence rates at 4–6 weeks were 73% for nicotine gum compared with 49% for placebo gum. Most of the transdermal nicotine double-blind studies were reviewed by Palmer and colleagues (1992), who found that quit rates at 4–6 weeks were 39%–71% for nicotine versus 13%–41% for the placebo patches. Beyond the initiation of abstinence, both preparations are associated with a progressive relapse to smoking. After 1 year, abstinence rates are about 25% for the nicotine gum and patch compared with 12% for placebo (Benowitz 1993).

The nasal spray and the inhaler are two new preparations that provide rapid release forms of nicotine. The potential advantage of these rapid-release preparations are that they closely simulate smoking by providing a rapid plasma concentration and oral and sensory stimulation. The results from the initial trials for the nasal spray (Sutherland et al. 1992) and the inhaler (Tonnesen et al. 1993) are similar to those for the gum and patch.

■ Nonnicotine Pharmacotherapies

Propranolol was studied in a double-blind placebo-controlled trial and found to be no better than placebo for smoking cessation (Farebrother et al. 1980).

The antihypertensive agent clonidine is an α_2-adrenergic agonist that has been used for its non-hypertensive effects to treat opiate and alcohol withdrawal symptoms. It has also been studied in the treatment of smokers and found to both decrease nicotine withdrawal symptoms and tobacco craving (Glassman et al. 1984). The researchers reviewed six placebo-controlled trials of clonidine for smoking (Glassman et al. 1990). Five of the trials reported that clonidine-treated patients had significantly better quit rates—4 to 6 weeks—than those treated with placebo. One trial (Franks et al. 1989) reported that clonidine and placebo treatments were equal.

Antidepressant treatment of nicotine dependence has also been investigated. Imipramine was studied in a controlled trial as a treatment for nicotine withdrawal symptoms and smoking cessation but was no better than placebo (Jacobs et al. 1971). Doxepin was compared with placebo in two studies (Edwards et al. 1988, 1989). In both trials, the doxepin-treated subjects performed better; but because these studies contained small numbers of subjects, the investigators consider the findings as preliminary.

■ Psychological Interventions

It is well recognized that smoking is maintained by both behavioral and pharmacological aspects (Jaffe and Kranzler 1979; Leventhal and Cleary 1980). It is not surprising that the combination of nicotine gum replacement and behavioral modification therapy is superior to either treatment alone (Hall et al. 1985; Killen et al. 1984). Hall and Killen (1985) each con-

ducted a controlled combined-treatment trial for smoking cessation. They found that the abstinence rates from these studies, 44% at 12 months and 50% at 10.5 months, were "some of the highest abstinence rates ever reported" (p. 139). To determine the minimum behavioral treatment necessary to optimize abstinence, we need more controlled trials involving combined therapy.

■ Smoking and Psychiatric Disorders

The incidence of smoking among individuals who abuse alcohol, stimulants, and opiates is about 90%; however, alcoholic individuals smoke more cigarettes that do people who abuse other substances (Burling and Ziff 1988).

Many of those who work with psychiatric patients have observed that cigarette smoking is extremely common among schizophrenic patients. Research not only supports this observation but also clearly reveals the extraordinarily high rate of smoking in both schizophrenic inpatients and outpatients. Goff and colleagues (1992) studied schizophrenic outpatients and found that 74% smoked compared to a national average of approximately 30%. About 80%–90% of a group of institutionalized schizophrenic patients were found to smoke (Matherson and O'Shea 1984). There is no known reason for the high rate of nicotine use by schizophrenic individuals. Some have speculated that the dopamine augmenting effect of nicotine may counterbalance a relative dopamine deficiency that exists in individuals with schizophrenia (Glassman 1993). Nicotine-induced changes in other neurotransmitters (e.g., serotonin; Benwell and Balfour 1982) may help to explain why so many people with schizophrenia smoke. Further research is needed to understand nicotine's involvement in the pathophysiology of schizophrenia. It is not unreasonable to expect that future antipsychotics will not only ameliorate psychiatric symptoms but also may decrease nicotine dependence in schizophrenic patients.

Glassman and colleagues (1988) conducted pioneering research establishing the link between major depression and cigarette smoking. Using data from the Epidemiologic Catchment Area (ECA) survey (Regier et al. 1984), they found that 76% of people with a lifetime history of major depression "had ever smoked" compared to 52% of people without a history of depression. Similarly, the incidence of depression was 6.6% in smokers compared with 2.9% in nonsmokers, and smokers with a history of depression had a low rate of cessation. These findings have been replicated by several investigators, and the association between depression and smoking is well supported. Another observation is that depressive symptoms appear during smoking cessation in people with a history of depression (Covey et al. 1990). These researchers also found that alcoholism had the highest association with smoking. Smoking rates among patients with anxiety disorders are at least twice that of people without a psychiatric diagnosis.

It is unclear as to what role smoking plays in psychopathology of these disorders. There is some information supporting smoking in these populations as a maladaptive coping strategy (Revell et al. 1985). Future research on smoking in these targeted populations may indicate the most efficient treatment approaches for patients with both nicotine dependence and a psychiatric disorder.

■ Summary

Nicotine replacement combined with behavior modification therapy is very effective in relieving nicotine withdrawal symptoms and in initiating smoking cessation. We must await the results of future research so as to establish methods of improving long-term nicotine abstinence.

■ REFERENCES

Altshuler HL, Phillips PE, Feinhandler DA: Alteration of ethanol self-administration by naltrexone. Life Sci 26:679–688, 1980

American Psychiatric Association: Diagnostic and Statistical Manual of Mental Disorders, 3rd Edition, Revised. Washington, DC, American Psychiatric Association, 1987

Arndt IO, Dorozynsky L, Woody GE, et al: Desipramine treatment of cocaine dependence in methadone-maintained patients. Arch Gen Psychiatry 49:888–893, 1992

Ball JC, Ross A: The Effectiveness of Methadone Maintenance Treatment. New York, Springer-Verlag, 1991

Beary MD, Christofides J, Fry D, et al: The benzodiazepines as substances of abuse. Practitioner 231:19–20, 1987

Benowitz NL: Nicotine replacement therapy: what has been accomplished—can we do better? Drugs 45:157–170, 1993

Benwell ME, Balfour DJ: The effects of nicotine administration on 5-HT uptake and biosynthesis in rat brain. Eur J Pharmacol 84:71–77, 1982

Bickel WE, Stitzer ML, Bigelow GE, et al: A clinical trial of buprenorphine: comparison with methadone in the detoxification of heroin addicts. Clin Pharmacol Ther 43:72–78, 1988

Burling TA, Ziff DC: Tobacco smoking: a comparison between alcohol and drug abuse in patients. Addict Behav 13:185–190, 1988

Covey LS, Glassman AH, Stetner F: Depression and depressive symptoms in smoking cessation. Compr Psychiatry 31:350–354, 1990

Cowan A, Lewis JW, Macfarlane IR: Agonist and antagonist properties of buprenorphine, a new antinociceptive agent. Br J Pharmacol 60:537–545, 1977

Crane M, Sereny G, Gordis E: Drug use among alcoholism detoxification patients: prevalence and impact on alcoholism treatment. Drug Alcohol Depend 22:33–36, 1988

Daughton DM, Heatley SA, Pendergast JJ, et al: Effect of transdermal nicotine delivery as an adjunct to low-intervention smoking cessation therapy. Arch Intern Med 151:749–752, 1991

Dole VP, Nyswander M: A medical treatment for diacetylmorphine (heroin) addiction: a clinical trial with methadone hydrochloride. JAMA 193:80–84, 1965

Dorus W, Ostrow DG, Anton R, et al: Lithium treatment of depressed and nondepressed alcoholics. JAMA 262:1646–1652, 1989

Edwards NB, Simmons RC, Rosenthal TL, et al: Doxepin in the treatment of nicotine withdrawal. Psychosomatics 29:203–206, 1988

Edwards NB, Murphy JK, Downs AD, et al: Doxepin as an adjunct to smoking cessation. Am J Psychiatry 146:373–376, 1989

Farebrother MJB, Pearce SJ, Turner P, et al: Propranolol and giving up smoking. British Journal of Diseases of the Chest 74:95–96, 1980

Finkle BS, Jennison TA, Chinn DM, et al: Plasma and urine disposition of L-alpha-acetyl-methadol and its principal metabolites in man. J Anal Toxicol 6:100–105, 1982

Finnegan LP: Treatment issues for opioid-dependent women during the perinatal period. J Psychoactive

Drugs 23:191–201, 1991

Finnegan LP, Kandall SR: Maternal and neonatal effects of alcohol and drugs, in Substance Abuse: A Comprehensive Textbook. Edited by Lowinson JH, Ruiz P, Millman RB, et al. Baltimore, MD, Williams & Wilkins, 1992, pp 628–656

Fram DH, Marmo J, Holden R: Naltrexone treatment—the problem of patient acceptance. J Subst Abuse Treat 6:119–122, 1989

Franks P, Harp J, Bell B: Randomized controlled trial of clonidine for smoking cessation in a primary care setting. JAMA 262:3011–3013, 1989

Froehlich JC, Harts J, Lumeng L, et al: Naloxone attenuates voluntary ethanol intake in rats selectively bred for high ethanol preference. Pharmacol Biochem Behav 35:385–390, 1990

Fudala PJ, Jaffe JH, Dax EM, et al: Use of buprenorphine in the treatment of opiate addiction, II: physiologic and behavioral effects of daily and alternate-day administration and abrupt withdrawal. Clin Pharmacol Ther 47:525–534, 1990

Fuller RK, Branchey L, Brightwell DR, et al: Disulfiram treatment of alcoholism: a Veterans Administration cooperative study. JAMA 256:1449–1455, 1986

Gawin FH, Kleber HD: Abstinence symptomatology and psychiatric diagnosis in cocaine abusers. Arch Gen Psychiatry 43:107–113, 1986

Gawin FH, Kleber HD, Byck R, et al: Desipramine facilitation of initial cocaine abstinence. Arch Gen Psychiatry 46:117–121, 1989

Gerstein DR: The effectiveness of drug treatment, in Addictive States, Vol 70. Edited by O'Brien CP, Jaffe JH. New York, Raven, 1992, pp 253–282

Gilman AG, Rall TW, Nies AS, et al (eds): Goodman and Gilman's The Pharmacological Basis of Therapeutics, 8th Edition. New York, Pergamon, 1990

Glassman AH: Cigarette smoking: implications for psychiatric illness. Am J Psychiatry 150:546–553, 1993

Glassman AH, Jackson WK, Walsh BT, et al: Cigarette craving, smoking withdrawal, and clonidine. Science 226:864–866, 1984

Glassman AH, Stetner F, Walsh Raizman PS, et al: Heavy smokers, smoking cessation, and clonidine: results of a double-blind, randomized trial. JAMA 259:2863–2866, 1988

Glassman AH, Helzer JE, Covey LS, et al: Smoking, smoking cessation, and major depression. JAMA 264:1546–1549, 1990

Goff DC, Henderson DC, Amico E: Cigarette smoking in schizophrenia: relationship to psychopathology and medication side effects. Am J Psychiatry 149:1189–1194, 1992

Gold MS, Redmond DE, Kleber HD: Clonidine blocks acute opiate withdrawal symptoms. Lancet 2:599–602, 1978

Gold MS, Pottach AC, Sweeney DR, et al: Opiate withdrawal using clonidine. JAMA 243:343–346, 1980

Goodwin DW: Alcohol: clinical aspects, in Substance Abuse—A Comprehensive Textbook. Edited by Lowinson JH, Ruiz P, Millman RB, et al. Baltimore, MD, Williams & Wilkins, 1992, pp 144–151

Gross J, Stitzer ML: Nicotine replacement: ten-week effects on tobacco withdrawal symptoms. Psychopharmacology (Berl) 93:334–341, 1989

Halikas J, Crosby RD, Graves N: Double-blind carbamazepine enhancement in the treatment of cocaine abuse, in Abstracts: Annual Meeting of the American College of Neuropsychopharmacology. San Juan, Puerto Rico, American College of Neuropsychopharmacology, Abstract 231, 1992

Hall SM, Killen JD: Psychological and pharmacological approaches to smoking relapse prevention. NIDA Res Monogr 53:131–143, 1985

Hall SM, Tunstall C, Rugg D, et al: Nicotine gum and behavioral treatment in smoking cessation. J Consult Clin Psychol 53:256–258, 1985

Hartel D, Selwyn PA, Schoenbaum EE: Methadone maintenance and reduced risk of AIDS and AIDS-specific mortality in intravenous drug users. Fourth International Conference on AIDS, Stockholm, Sweden. Abstract 8526, 1988

Hartel D, Schoenbaum EE, Selwyn PA: Temporal patterns of cocaine use and AIDS in intravenous drug users in methadone maintenance [abstract]. Fifth International Conference on AIDS, Montreal, Canada, 1989

Hayashida M, Alterman AI, McLellan AT, et al: Comparative effectiveness and costs of inpatient and outpatient detoxification of patients with mild-to-moderate alcohol withdrawal syndrome. N Engl J Med 320:358–365, 1989

Holder H, Longabaugh R, Miller W, et al: The cost effectiveness of treatment for alcoholism: a first approximation. J Stud Alcohol 52:517–540, 1991

Hubbell CL, Czirr SA, Hunter GA, et al: Consumption of ethanol solution is potentiated by morphine and attenuated by naloxone persistently across repeated daily administrations. Alcohol 3:39–54, 1986

Hughes JR, Hatsukami D: Signs and symptoms of tobacco withdrawal. Arch Gen Psychiatry 43:289–294, 1986

Jacobs MA, Spilken AA, Norman MM, et al: Interaction of personality and treatment conditions associated with success in a smoking control program. Psychosom Med 33:545–546, 1971

Jaffe JH, Kranzler M: Smoking as an addictive disorder, in NIDA Research Monograph—Cigarette Smoking as a Dependence Process, Vol 23. Edited by Krasnegor NA. Washington, DC, U.S. Government Printing Office, 1979

Jaffe JH, Schuster CR, Smith BB, et al: Comparison of acetylmethadol and methadone in the treatment of long-term heroin users. JAMA 211:1834–1836, 1970

Jaffe JH, Senay EC, Schuster CR, et al: Methadyl acetate vs methadone: a double-blind study in heroin users. JAMA 222:437–442, 1972

Jasinski DR, Pevnick JS, Griffith JD: Human pharmacology and abuse potential of the analgesic buprenorphine. Arch Gen Psychiatry 35:501–516, 1978

Jasinski DR, Fudala PJ, Johnson RE: Sublingual versus subcutaneous buprenorphine in opiate abusers. Clin Pharmacol Ther 45:513–519, 1989

Johnson RE, Cone EJ, Henningfield JE, et al: Use of buprenorphine in the treatment of opiate addiction, I: physiologic and behavioral effects during a rapid dose induction. Clin Pharmacol Ther 46:335–343, 1989

Johnson RE, Jaffe JH, Fudala PJ: A controlled trial of buprenorphine treatment for opioid dependence. JAMA 267:2750–2755, 1992

Killen JD, Maccoby N, Taylor CB: Nicotine gum and self-regulation training in smoking relapse prevention. Behav Res Ther 15:234–248, 1984

Kornetsky C, Porrino LJ: Brain mechanisms of drug-induced reinforcement, in Addictive States, Vol 70. Edited by O'Brien CP, Jaffe JH. New York, Raven, 1992

Kosten TR, Kleber HD: Buprenorphine detoxification from opioid dependence: a pilot study. Life Sci 42:635–641, 1988

Kosten TR, Morgan CM, Falcione J, et al: Pharmacotherapy for cocaine-abusing methadone-maintained patients using amantadine or desipramine. Arch Gen Psychiatry 49:894–898, 1992

Kranzler HR, Babor TF, Laureman RJ: Problems associated with average alcohol consumption and frequency of intoxication in a medical population. Alcohol Clin Exp Res 14:119–126, 1990

Leventhal H, Cleary P: The smoking problem: a review of the research and theory in behavioral risk modification. Psychol Bull 88:370–405, 1980

Ling W, Charuvastra C, Kiam SC, et al: Methadyl acetate and methadone as maintenance treatments for heroin addicts. Arch Gen Psychiatry 33:709–720, 1976

Lipsedge MS, Cook CCH: Prescribing for drug addicts. Lancet 2:451–452, 1987

Loimer N, Schmid R, Lenz K, et al: Acute blocking of naloxone-precipitated opiate withdrawal symptoms by methohexitone. Br J Psychiatry 157:748–752, 1990

Loimer N, Lenz K, Schmid R, et al: Technique for greatly shortening the transition from methadone to naltrexone maintenance of patients addicted to opiates. Am J Psychiatry 148:933–935, 1991

Maddux JF, Desmond DP: Methadone maintenance and recovery form opioid dependence. Am J Drug Alcohol Abuse 18:63–74, 1992

Magura S, Goldsmith D, Casriel C, et al: The validity of methadone clients' self-reported drug use. Int J Addict 22:727–750, 1987

Martin WR, Jasinski DR: Physical parameters of morphine dependence in man: tolerance, early abstinence, protracted abstinence. J Psychiatr Res 7:9–17, 1969

Martin WR, Jasinski D, Mansky P: Naltrexone, an antagonist for the treatment of heroin dependence. Arch Gen Psychiatry 28:784–791, 1973

Mason BJ, Kocsis JH: Desipramine treatment of alcoholism. Psychopharmacol Bull 27:155–161, 1991

Matherson E, O'Shea B: Smoking and malignancy in schizophrenia. Br J Psychiatry 145:429–432, 1984

McGrath PJ, Nunes EV, Delivannides D, et al: Imipramine treatment of depressed alcoholics. Paper presented at the 33rd Annual Meeting of the New Clinical Drug Evaluation Unit Program (NCDEU), Boca Raton, FL, June 1993

McLellan AT, Arndt IO, Metzger DS, et al: The effects of psychosocial services on substance abuse treatment. JAMA 269:1953–1959, 1993

Metzger DS, Woody GE, McLellan AT, et al: Human immunodeficiency virus seroconversion among in- and out-of-treatment intravenous drug users: an 18-month prospective follow-up. J Acquir Immune Defic Syndr 6:1049–1056, 1993

Meyer RE: Prospects for a rational pharmacotherapy of alcoholism. J Clin Psychiatry 50:403–412, 1989

Myers RD, Borg S, Mossberg R: Antagonism by naltrexone of voluntary alcohol selection in the chronically drinking macaque monkey. Alcohol 3:383–388, 1986

National Institute on Alcohol Abuse and Alcoholism: Seventh Special Report to the U.S. Congress on Alcohol and Health. Rockville, MD, U.S. Department of Health and Human Services, 1990

National Institute on Drug Abuse: National Household Survey on Drug Abuse, Population Estimates, 1991 (DHHS Publ No ADM-91-1732). Washington, DC, U.S. Government Printing Office, 1991

Nutt D, Adinoff B, Linnoila M: Benzodiazepines in the treatment of alcoholism, in Recent Developments in Alcoholism, Treatment Research, Vol 7. Edited by Galanter M. New York, Plenum, 1989, pp 283–313

Ogborne AC, Kapur BM: Drug use among a sample of males admitted to an alcohol detoxification center. Alcohol Clin Exp Res 11:183–185, 1987

O'Malley SS, Jaffe AJ, Chang G, et al: Naltrexone and coping skills therapy for alcohol dependence. Arch Gen Psychiatry 49:881–887, 1992

Palmer KJ, Buckley MM, Faulds D: Transdermal nicotine: a review of its pharmacodynamic and pharmacokinetic properties and therapeutic efficacy as an aid to smoking cessation. Drugs 44:498–529, 1992

Peachy JE, Naranjo CA: The role of drugs in the treatment of alcoholism. Drugs 27:171–182, 1984

Post R: Time course of clinical effects of carbamazepine: implications for mechanisms of action. J Clin Psychiatry 49 (suppl 1):35–46, 1988

Regier DA, Myers JK, Kramer M, et al: The NIMH Epidemiologic Catchment Area program: historical context, major objectives, and study population characteristics. Arch Gen Psychiatry 41:934–941, 1984

Revell AD, Warburton DM, Wesnes K: Smoking as a coping strategy. Addict Behav 10:209–224, 1985

Robins LN, Helzer JE, Weissman MM, et al: Lifetime prevalence of specific psychiatric disorders in three sites. Arch Gen Psychiatry 41:949–958, 1984

Substance Abuse and Mental Health Services Administration: Preliminary estimates from the Drug Abuse Warning Network—third quarter 1992 estimates of drug-related emergency room episodes

(Advance Report No 2). Washington, DC, U.S. Government Printing Office, 1993

San L, Cami J, Peri JM, et al: Efficacy of clonidine, guanfacine and methadone in the rapid detoxification of heroin addicts: a controlled clinical trial. British Journal of Addiction 85:141–147, 1990

Schneider NG, Jarvik ME, Forsythe AB, et al: Nicotine gum in smoking cessation: a placebo controlled, double-blind trial. Addict Behav 8:253–261, 1983

Schuckit MA: Alcohol and alcoholism, in Harrison's Principles of Internal Medicine. Edited by Braunwald E, Isselbacher KJ, Petersdorf RG, et al. New York, McGraw-Hill, 1987, pp 2106–2111

Schuckit MA: Alcohol and alcoholism, in Harrison's Principles of Internal Medicine, Vol 2. Edited by Wilson JD, Braunwald E, Isselbacher KJ, et al. New York, McGraw-Hill, 1991, pp 2149–2151

Soyka M, Lutz W, Kauert G, et al: Epileptic seizures and alcohol withdrawal: significance of additional use (and misuse) of drugs and electroencephalographic findings. Epilepsia 2:109–113, 1989

Stine SM, Kosten TR: Use of drug combinations in treatment of opioid withdrawal. J Clin Psychopharmacol 12:203–209, 1992

Stitzer ML: Nicotine-delivery products: demonstrated and desirable effects, in New Developments in Nicotine-Delivery Systems. Edited by Henningfield JE, Stitzer ML. Ossining, NY, Cortland Communications, 1991, pp 35–45

Sutherland G, Stapleton JA, Russell MAH, et al: Randomised controlled trial of nasal nicotine spray in smoking cessation. Lancet 1:324–329, 1992

Tonnesen P, Norrezaard J, Simonsen K, et al: A double-blind trial of a 16-hour transdermal nicotine patch in smoking cessation. N Engl J Med 325:311–315, 1991

Tonnesen P, Norregaard J, Mikkelson K, et al: A double-blind trial of a nicotine inhaler for smoking cessation. JAMA 269:1268–1271, 1993

U.S. Department of Health and Human Services: Reducing the health consequences of smoking: 25 years of progress (a report of the Surgeon General). Washington, DC, U.S. Government Printing Office, 1989

U.S. Department of Health and Human Services: The health benefits of smoking cessation: a report of the Surgeon General. Washington, DC, U.S. Government Printing Office, 1990

Volpicelli JR, Davis MA, Olgin JE: Naltrexone blocks the post-shock increase of ethanol consumption.

Life Sci 38:841–847, 1986

Volpicelli JR, Alterman AI, Hayashida MD, et al: Naltrexone in the treatment of alcohol depen-

dence. Arch Gen Psychiatry 49:886–880, 1992

Wikler A: Dynamics of drug dependence. Arch Gen Psychiatry 28:611–616, 1973

35

Treatment of Eating Disorders

W. Stewart Agras, M.D.

In this chapter, the pharmacological treatment of two classic eating disorders—anorexia nervosa (AN) and bulimia nervosa (BN)—is considered, together with that of binge-eating disorder, which is included as a new entity in DSM-IV (American Psychiatric Association 1994). Of the three disorders, the most is known about the pharmacological treatment of BN, because it is a relatively common problem that has been studied extensively during the past 15 years. Less is known about the pharmacological treatment of anorexia nervosa. Because this is a relatively uncommon disorder, thus militating against controlled research, it is difficult to attain an adequate sample size to evaluate treatment effects.

The treatment of binge-eating disorder has only been formally studied in the past several years. Hence, few studies are available, although it can be argued that much of what we know about the treatment of BN is applicable to binge-eating disorder. Because we know most about the treatment of BN, this disorder will be considered first, followed by the closely related binge-eating disorder, and finally AN.

◼ BULIMIA NERVOSA

BN is a relatively common disorder affecting some 1%–2% of young women (Fairburn and Beglin 1990). The disorder usually has an onset in late adolescence or early adult life, with a prodromal period characterized by dissatisfaction with body shape and a fear of becoming overweight, followed by marked dietary restriction. Sooner or later periods of dietary restriction are followed by episodes of binge-eating experienced as a loss of control over dietary intake, often accompanied by the consumption of large amounts of food. This, in turn, further aggravates both the dissatisfaction with body shape and fears of weight gain. Ultimately, the bulimic person discovers purging, usually in the form of self-induced vomiting, with or without laxative use, or (in rare cases) chewing food and spitting it out.

The DSM-IV diagnosis of BN requires a minimum average of two episodes of binge-eating a week for at least 3 months and allows only self-induced vomiting and laxative use as methods of purging, thus distinguishing BN from diuretic abuse. The diagnosis also requires that the disorder does not occur exclusively during episodes of AN. DSM-IV may distinguish two forms of BN—namely, purging and nonpurging forms, the latter characterized by alternating periods of severe dietary restriction and binge-eating (Task Force on DSM-IV 1993). The implications of this classification for treatment are unknown. Medical complications of BN are relatively rare, the most frequent being potassium depletion and dental caries. Comorbid psychopathology includes major depression, various anxiety disorders including generalized anxiety disorder, social phobia and panic disorder, alcoholism, and personality disorders, particularly those in the Cluster B spectrum. It is now recognized that the natural history of the disorder is frequently one of chronicity (Keller et al. 1992), emphasizing the importance of adequate and early treatment.

Binge-Eating

The form and content of binge-eating episodes have been studied in two ways: in the natural environment by means of self-monitoring, and in the laboratory. Despite reports by bulimic patients that their binges are typically very large, often greater than 5,000 kcal (Johnson et al. 1982), self-monitoring studies of patients with BN revealed a different picture. In the first of these studies, binge-eating episodes averaged 1,459 calories (range 45–5,138 kcal) compared with 321 calories (range 10–1,652 kcal) in nonbinge-eating episodes (Rosen et al. 1986). Sixty-five percent of binge episodes fell within the range of nonbinge episodes. This suggests that when loss of control is made an additional criterion for a binge, there is much variation among and even within individuals in the quantity of food eaten during a binge. In addition, bulimic patients ate more desserts and snacks and less fruits and vegetables in their binge-eating episodes than in nonbinge episodes. Subsequent self-monitoring studies have essentially confirmed the findings of Rosen and colleagues (1986).

Laboratory studies have revealed a somewhat different picture. The average binge is larger than in the self-monitoring studies, varying from a mean of 3,031 kcal to 7,774 kcal across studies, with a range from 83 kcal to 25,755 kcal for binge episodes (Hadigan et al. 1989; Mitchell and Laine 1985). These differences between laboratory and field studies may be partly because of differences in sample selection—many of the participants in laboratory studies were inpatients representing more severe cases. It is also likely that self-monitoring underestimates the caloric content of binges because of deficiencies in recording. One interpretation of the differences between laboratory and field studies is that laboratory studies may overestimate caloric consumption during binge episodes, whereas field studies may underestimate such consumption.

Overall, both field and laboratory studies of the form and content of binge-eating in BN patients suggest the following:

1. The average binge is larger than the average nonbinge episode.

2. There is considerable variation within and between individuals in terms of caloric consumption during a binge.
3. Content (particularly when assessed as food types) may differ between binges and nonbinges.
4. Less certainly, eating rate may be more rapid during binges than during nonbinge episodes.

Etiology of Bulimia Nervosa

Relatively little is known about the etiology of BN. Studies suggest that the disorder is heritable and that familial aggregation is most likely explained by heritability (Kendler et al. 1991). Various neurochemical hypotheses have been suggested, the most frequent being reduction in brain serotonin (5-hydroxytryptamine [5-HT]) synthesis. Recently it has been shown that dietary restriction leads to decreased plasma tryptophan, which in turn would likely reduce 5-HT synthesis. It seems possible that bulimic patients may be particularly sensitive to such changes and become locked in a vicious circle of neurochemical changes once they begin dieting, resulting in an effect on satiety. On the other hand, it must be remembered that food intake is controlled by several neurochemical systems, including norepinephrine and peptide YY, both of which potentiate eating; hence, it may be too early to implicate one particular system. In addition, nutritional state markedly affects these neurochemical systems, making the task of detailing the abnormalities in BN even more complicated.

Social factors are also implicated in BN. During the 1980s, the number of cases of BN seen in clinics around the world increased dramatically (Garner et al. 1985). This increase occurred concurrently with the notion of a thin body shape being portrayed as the ideal for women, despite the fact that few women can meet this social demand without rigorous dieting (Brownell 1991). Such social pressure may have led more women to diet, increasing the risk of binge-eating and purging in the biologically susceptible individual. It is also possible that certain personality types (e.g., those in the Cluster B spectrum) are more affected by such societal changes, perhaps explaining the comorbidity between BN and Cluster B personality disorder.

■ Psychopharmacological Treatment of Bulimia Nervosa

The first controlled pharmacological study of "binge eaters" (a group comprising patients with BN and binge-eating disorder (BED), as purging was not required for entry into the study) compared phenytoin with placebo based on an earlier observation that bulimic patients may have abnormal electroencephalogram (EEG) findings (Wermuth et al. 1977). In this crossover study of relatively brief duration, no evidence was found that phenytoin was effective in reducing binge-eating, nor was there any relationship between EEG abnormalities and reduction in binge-eating. Subsequent studies have focused on the use of antidepressants.

Antidepressant treatment. The use of antidepressants in BN was sparked by the observation that depression is frequently a comorbid feature of the disorder (Pope and Hudson 1982). Disturbances of eating frequently accompany depression, suggesting a linkage between the two disorders. In 1982, two groups of researchers conducted small-scale uncontrolled studies suggesting that both monoamine oxidase inhibitors (MAOIs) and tricyclic antidepressants (TCAs) were useful in reducing binge-eating and purging (Pope and Hudson 1982; Walsh et al. 1982). These observations were followed by a series of double-blind placebo-controlled studies confirming the utility of antidepressants in treating patients with BN, at least in the short term. A wide range of antidepressant agents have been found effective including imipramine (Agras et al. 1987; Mitchell et al. 1990; Pope et al. 1983), desipramine (Agras et al. 1991; Barlow et al. 1988; Blouin et al. 1989; Hughes et al. 1986), phenelzine (Walsh et al. 1984, 1988), trazodone (Pope et al. 1989), bupropion (Horne et al. 1988), and fluoxetine (Fluoxetine Bulimia Nervosa Collaborative Study Group 1992). In these studies, the range of decrease in binge-eating and purging was 30%–91%, with a median of 69%. The range for complete recovery from binge-eating and purging was 10%–60% (median 32%), and the range for dropout from the medication groups was 0%–48% (median 23%). Put another way, of 100 patients with BN, some 77 will persevere with a course of medication treatment, and 25 will be in remission at the end of treatment with a single antidepressant.

Antidepressants are prescribed in the same dosage as used for treating depression—with the exception of fluoxetine, because it has been found that a dosage of 60 mg qd is more effective than one of 20 mg qd in reducing binge-eating and purging (Fluoxetine Bulimia Nervosa Collaborative Study Group 1992). One problem with medication that is given at times other than bedtime is that a significant amount of medication may be purged through subsequent vomiting. Side effects and reasons for dropout from the various medications are similar to those observed in the treatment of depression, with the exception of bupropion, for which a higher than expected proportion of patients with BN had a grand mal seizure (Horne et al. 1988). The authors concluded that bupropion should not be used in BN until the reason for the high proportion of seizures in these patients was established.

In light of the widespread publicity regarding suicidality and fluoxetine, it is reassuring that a large-scale study of the use of fluoxetine in BN found no differences in suicidal thoughts or actions between the subjects on active drug and those on placebo (Wheadon et al. 1992). Only two antidepressants have been found to be no better than placebo: mianserin (Sabine et al. 1983) and amitriptyline (Mitchell and Groat 1984). In the first of these studies, the dosage may have been too low for maximal efficacy. In the second study, a simple form of behavior therapy was used in both groups—perhaps masking the differences between placebo and medication, because both groups showed good and equivalent improvement.

Overall, it appears that most antidepressants are effective in the treatment of BN in the short term, although the effects are limited, with about one-quarter of patients achieving remission on average. Less is known about the long-term effectiveness of antidepressants. In one uncontrolled study (Pope et al. 1985) in which a variety of antidepressants were used over the course of a 2-year follow-up, 50% of patients achieved and maintained remission from binge-eating and purging. The only controlled longer-term follow-up studies have been plagued by sample size problems, with relatively few participants meeting criteria for entry into the follow-up phase of treatment (Pyle et al. 1990; Walsh et al. 1991). Even with continued medication treatment, about one-third of patients in these studies relapsed. There was little evidence that continued treatment with a single antidepressant was more effective than the placebo condition. This raises the question of whether treatment with a different antidepressant of those patients who do not respond initially (or who relapse) would be more effective. One open-label study suggests that about half of such patients will respond to a different antidepressant, with complete remission of symptoms (Mitchell et al. 1989). This would raise the remission rate for the hypothetical cohort of 100 patients to 50. Hence, sequential trials of different antidepressants would seem useful in the treatment of BN.

Combined treatment. Cognitive-behavioral therapy for BN was developed in parallel with the use of antidepressants, and numerous controlled studies suggest that such treatment is effective (Fairburn et al. 1992). Cognitive-behavioral therapy has four distinct phases. First, the extent of the problem is examined by careful history taking and the use of self-monitoring of food intake, binge-eating, and purging. Second, dietary intake is slowly normalized by shaping at least three adequate meals each day. Third, distorted cognitions concerning caloric intake and body shape and weight are corrected. Finally, relapse prevention procedures (e.g., coping with high-risk situations) are practiced. Treatment usually extends over a 6-month period, averaging about 20 sessions. The existence of two different and effective treatments naturally leads to the question of whether the combination of such treatments would be more effective than either one alone. Two studies have examined this question.

The first of these studies used a randomized 2 × 2 design with four experimental groups: imipramine combined with group psychosocial treatment; imipramine with no psychosocial treatment; placebo combined with group psychosocial treatment; and placebo with no psychosocial treatment (Mitchell et al. 1990). Treatment lasted for 10 weeks. The psychosocial treatment was an intensive group variant of cognitive-behavioral therapy, with 5 weekly sessions in the first week and 22 treatment sessions overall. The mean daily dose of imipramine was 217 mg for the psychosocial treatment group and 266 mg for the group receiving medication alone. As might be expected, there was a significantly higher dropout rate for those in the medication groups compared with those on placebo. The results for reductions in binge-eating and purging were quite straightforward. Confirming previous studies, imipramine was found

superior to placebo. However, cognitive-behavioral treatment was found to be superior to imipramine, and there was no additional advantage in reducing binge-eating and purging when the two treatments were combined. The combined treatment was, however, significantly superior to cognitive-behavioral treatment in reducing depression.

In the second study (Agras et al. 1991), participants were randomly allocated to one of three groups: desipramine, cognitive-behavioral treatment, and the combined treatment. Half of the desipramine participants were withdrawn from medication at 16 weeks, and desipramine was discontinued in the remaining half at 24 weeks. Cognitive-behavioral treatment lasted for 24 weeks. Hence, this study examined longer lasting treatments than the 1990 study by Mitchell and colleagues. However, the results were comparable. Eighteen percent of participants stopped taking desipramine by 16 weeks, compared with 4.3% of subjects who stopped cognitive-behavioral treatment. Cognitive-behavioral treatment was significantly superior to desipramine in reducing the frequency of binge-eating and purging, and the combined treatment was no better than cognitive-behavioral treatment alone. At 32 weeks, those withdrawn from desipramine at 16 weeks demonstrated a return to pretreatment levels for binge-eating but not for purging. Those withdrawn at 24 weeks showed no relapse at 32 weeks. Finally, the combined 24-week treatment was more effective in reducing dietary preoccupation and hunger. This study suggests that longer-term antidepressant treatment was better than short-term treatment and that overall, the combined treatment group demonstrated the broadest gains, with 70% of subjects recovered at 32 weeks. Taken together, these studies suggest that the optimal approach to treatment is a combination of cognitive-behavioral treatment and medication.

Predictors of response. Because the use of antidepressants to treat BN was based on the hypothesis that BN is a variant of depression, it was thought that pretreatment level of depression would predict the outcome of antidepressant treatment. In fact, the studies that have examined this proposition have found no evidence that level of depression predicts outcome. Both depressed and nondepressed patients respond equally well to antidepressant treatment (Mitchell and Groat 1984). In addition, different factors predict the antibulimic and antidepressant responses to desipramine in the same group of patients with BN (Blouin et al. 1989). Thus, degree of depression was not a predictor of the antibulimic response, although a higher frequency of purging and a lower bulimia scale on the Eating Disorders Inventory (Garner et al. 1983) did predict a good antibulimic response. On the other hand, those whose depression improved had abnormal dexamethasone suppression tests and were more likely to have a family history of depression. The only other factor to predict outcome is the patient's lowest weight since early adolescence, with those with lower weights (i.e., those who were more anorexic) doing less well (Agras et al. 1987). It should be noted, however, that all studies examining predictors of response have sample sizes too small to accurately determine the characteristics of treatment responders.

Mechanism of action. If the antidepressants do not exert their effect in BN by decreasing depression, then what is the mechanism of action? Two alternative hypotheses have been proposed (Agras and McCann 1987). The first of these hypotheses suggests that although the state of depression does not predict outcome, fluctuant negative moods arising during the day may promote binge-eating. The second hypothesis, based on the finding that desipramine is an anorexic agent in rats, suggests that antidepressants may work by reducing hunger. These hypotheses were tested directly in a study by Rossiter and colleagues (1991). No evidence was found that desipramine reduced fluctuant negative mood. However, desipramine did reduce hunger levels significantly, suggesting that it has an anorexiant effect. This effect was confirmed in a study of BED in which participants on desipramine had significantly greater reductions in hunger than those receiving placebo (McCann and Agras 1990). In addition, it has been found that whereas bulimic patients treated with cognitive-behavioral therapy increase their caloric intake by about 50%, those treated with desipramine stop binge-eating but do not alter their caloric intake (Rossiter et al. 1988)—a finding consistent with desipramine having an anorexiant effect.

Comprehensive treatment of BN. For the most part, patients with BN are best treated as outpatients, unless there are either medical or psychiatric reasons for hospitalization (e.g., an intercurrent physical illness or comorbid psychopathology requiring hospi-

talization, such as a major depression with suicidality). One reason for the usefulness of outpatient treatment is that gains made in the hospital may not carry over to the patient's home, where more complex food stimuli and greater stress are present than in the hospital.

Given the superiority of cognitive-behavioral therapy to medication, it would appear that psychological treatment should be the initial approach in uncomplicated cases of BN. Treatment manuals for this therapy are available (Agras et al. 1991). Should satisfactory progress not be made, antidepressant therapy should be added to the psychological therapy. In cases where there is marked depression accompanying the bulimic symptoms, antidepressant therapy should be combined with cognitive-behavioral therapy, as there is evidence of a superior response of depressive symptoms when antidepressants are used in the treatment of BN. Similarly, where there is marked preoccupation with food and/or hunger, the use of antidepressants should be considered. If the first antidepressant does not lead to therapeutic gains in a reasonable time, the use of alternative antidepressants should be considered.

Other medications. Although there is considerable evidence from controlled trials that most antidepressants are useful in the treatment of BN, few studies of other pharmacological agents exist. Given the possibility that antidepressants act as anorexians in BN, studies of other appetite suppressants are of interest. In one controlled study, it was found that *d*-fenfluramine was significantly more effective in reducing the frequency of binge-eating and purging than was placebo (Russell et al. 1988). However, 40% of patients dropped out of this study. Noncompleters appeared to do better than completers, leading the authors to conclude that *d*-fenfluramine may be useful as an adjunctive treatment for BN, but that further study is needed before definitive conclusions about its efficacy can be reached.

Because opioids are involved in the control of eating, there has been some interest in using opiate antagonists in eating disorders. One study comparing low (50–100 mg qd) and high (200–300 mg qd) doses of naltrexone found that high-dosage patients with BN fared best in reducing binge-eating and purging (Jonas and Gold 1988). However, this was a short-term study, and no data on full recovery were given. Additionally, one patient in the high-dose group demonstrated elevations in liver function tests that normalized after the dose was reduced. The authors suggest that liver function should be monitored at frequent intervals when using high-dose naltrexone. Finally, one relatively large-scale controlled study of lithium in the treatment of BN found no evidence for effectiveness (Hsu et al. 1991). Hence, there is little evidence that medications other than antidepressants are of use in the treatment of BN.

■ BINGE-EATING DISORDER

Although the association between binge-eating and obesity has been noted from time to time in case reports in the literature, it was not until the upsurge of research into the psychopathology and treatment of BN that systematic attention was paid to BED. This entity is included in DSM-IV as a disorder requiring further research attention (Task Force on DSM-IV 1993). The principal features of BED include binge-eating at a frequency of at least twice a week for 6 months, causing marked distress, and not occurring during the course of BN.

A self-monitoring study found that patients with BED consumed some 600 calories during each binge, with high variability among and even within subjects (Rossiter et al. 1992). This suggests that the binges of patients with BED may be smaller than those of patients with BN. Additionally, it was found that patients with BED consumed about 900 kcal less on nonbinge days than on binge days, suggesting that binge-eating alternates with dietary restriction.

About 2% of the general population meet criteria for BED (Bruce and Agras 1992). In clinical populations, in contrast to AN and BN, the ratio of women to men is approximately 3:2. This is the highest rate for men for any eating disorder. Although obesity is not a requirement for the diagnosis of BED, there is a substantial overlap between BED and obesity. Studies have shown that more than one-quarter of the obese subjects meet criteria for BED and that the prevalence of binge-eating increases with increases in Body Mass Index (Marcus et al. 1985; Telch et al. 1988). Because binge-eating appears to precede overweight, binge-eating may be a risk factor for obesity and the multiple health problems associated with overweight. Moreover, the syndrome is associated with comorbid psychopathology similar to that of BN and causes much distress; hence, it is an entity de-

serving of treatment in its own right. In one study, 50% of patients with BED had a history of past major depression, 24% had a history of substance abuse, and a substantial number had had an anxiety disorder (McCann and Agras 1990).

Antidepressant treatment. As noted previously, research into the treatment of BED is in its infancy. Nonetheless, because of the similarity between BN and BED, it has been suggested that treatments effective for BN should also be effective for BED. To date, there has been one double-blind placebo-controlled study of the use of antidepressants in BED (McCann and Agras 1990). In this small-scale study, patients receiving desipramine reduced their binge-eating significantly more than those receiving placebo, and 60% of the desipramine group were abstinent at the end of 12 weeks' treatment. When medication was withdrawn, rapid relapse across all parameters occurred. In addition, hunger was significantly reduced and dietary restraint increased in those assigned to the active drug condition, suggesting that desipramine has an appetite suppressant activity.

Although this study suggests that antidepressants may be useful in the treatment of BED, it should be noted that patients who stopped binge-eating did not lose weight in this study. This finding is in accord with the two controlled psychological treatment studies in this disorder (Telch et al. 1990; Wilfley et al. 1993), neither of which reported significant weight loss in the treated group. Hence, a comprehensive treatment approach would of necessity require combining antidepressants with weight loss therapy. No controlled studies of such a combination or the combination of cognitive-behavioral therapy and antidepressants have appeared in the literature to date.

■ ANOREXIA NERVOSA

AN is a relatively rare disorder characterized by marked weight loss (at least 15% below ideal body weight), an intense fear of gaining weight, disturbance in the experience of body shape (i.e., feeling fat in the face of marked weight loss), and (in females) amenorrhea. The rarity of the disorder militates against the conduct of satisfactory randomized double-blind medication trials, because it is difficult in any one center to acquire an adequate sample size in a reasonable time. Moreover, medication trials should be long enough and use sufficient medication dosage to adequately demonstrate effects in this chronic relapsing disorder. Unfortunately, few of the trials to date meet these criteria, many being of short duration and others using very small doses of medication. Nonetheless, a variety of medications have been evaluated for the treatment of AN, although it is fair to say that none yet appears to have a significant clinical effect.

The first medication to be examined in the treatment of AN was chlorpromazine, given in high doses of up to 1,000 mg daily (Dally and Sargant 1960). Unfortunately, the control group involved a retrospective comparison with patients admitted to the same center several years earlier. It is thus impossible to determine whether the findings were due to cohort or medication effects, particularly as the duration of illness was markedly different between the two cohorts. Moreover, both chlorpromazine and insulin were used together in most patients. Hence, the finding that patients treated with chlorpromazine gained weight more quickly than those not so treated must be viewed with caution. In further studies of antipsychotic agents in the treatment of AN, neither pimozide nor sulpiride (both selective dopamine antagonists) demonstrated clear-cut efficacy (Vandereycken 1984; Vandereycken and Pierloot 1982). There is therefore little evidence for the utility of antipsychotic agents in the treatment of AN.

One of the best studies to date investigated the use of cyproheptadine (up to 32 mg qd) and amitriptyline (up to 160 mg qd) with a placebo control on hospitalized anorexic patients (Halmi et al. 1986). Overall, neither cyproheptadine nor amitriptyline were found to be effective on the rate of weight gain or the number of days required to reach target weight. However, there was an interesting interaction between cyproheptadine and the subtype of AN (bulimic or nonbulimic). In nonbulimic anorexic patients, cyproheptadine was found to significantly decrease the number of days required to reach target weight as compared with amitriptyline. However, in bulimic anorexic patients, cyproheptadine appeared to have a deleterious effect on weight gain. This study suggests that the subtyping of AN into bulimic and nonbulimic variants is valid and that cyproheptadine in doses of 32 mg qd may be of some use in treatment of patients with the nonbulimic subtype. Few side effects of this medication are observed in patients with AN. Other studies of TCA medication, including amitriptyline and clomipramine, have revealed a lack of efficacy in the acute treatment phase, although the dosage of clomipramine was very low (Biederman et al. 1985; Crisp et al. 1987). Similarly, lithium carbonate does not appear effective in promoting weight gain, although the study was only of 4 weeks' duration (Gross et al. 1981).

Two uncontrolled studies suggest that fluoxetine may be useful in the treatment of AN (Gwirtsman et al. 1990; Kaye et al. 1991). The larger of these studies followed 31 patients with AN treated with fluoxetine for about a year following discharge from hospital, finding that 29 patients had maintained their weight at or above 85% of ideal body weight (Gwirtsman et al. 1990). Dosage varied from 20–80 mg, with an average dose for good responders of 26 mg qd. Given the high relapse rate usually found in AN, these findings are highly encouraging and certainly worthy of follow-up in a double-blind placebo-controlled trial.

Overall, apart from the treatment of comorbid psychopathology such as obsessive-compulsive disorder or major depression, there is a limited role for the use of psychopharmacological agents in the treatment of patients with AN. For the nonpurging anorexic patient, cyproheptadine may prove useful in accelerating weight gain during the initial refeeding phase of treatment. In addition, there is tentative evidence that fluoxetine may be of use in the maintenance phase of treatment. This latter finding may assume greater importance if it is confirmed in a controlled study, given the finding that outpatient therapy is as effective as inpatient treatment for AN (Crisp et al. 1991).

CONCLUSION

The place of psychopharmacological agents in the treatment of BN has been well worked out. Adequate treatment using sequential trials of different antidepressants should result in abstinence rates of about 50%. The addition of cognitive-behavioral treatment appears to enhance the effectiveness of the antidepressants. In the case of AN, many clinicians believe that medication does not significantly affect outcome. However, there are encouraging results from the use of fluoxetine in the maintenance phase of treatment of this disabling disorder.

Finally, it is too early to detail the role of pharmacological agents in the treatment of BED. But it might be expected that sequential trials of antidepressants should yield similar results in BED to those in BN. However, the added complication of the need for weight loss among these patients whose treatment is difficult may limit the role of antidepressants in treating this condition.

■ REFERENCES

Agras WS, McCann U: The efficacy and role of antidepressants in the treatment of bulimia nervosa. Annals of Behavioral Medicine 9:18–22, 1987

Agras WS, Dorian B, Kirkley BG, et al: Imipramine in the treatment of bulimia: a double-blind controlled study. International Journal of Eating Disorders 6:29–38, 1987

Agras WS, Rossiter EM, Arnow B, et al: Pharmacologic and cognitive-behavioral treatment for bulimia nervosa: a controlled comparison. Am J Psychiatry 159:325–333, 1991

American Psychiatric Association: Diagnostic and Statistical Manual of Mental Disorders, 4th Edition. Washington, DC, American Psychiatric Association, 1994

Barlow J, Blouin J, Blouin A, et al: Treatment of bulimia with desipramine: a double-blind crossover study. Can J Psychiatry 33:129–133, 1988

Biederman J, Herzog DB, Rivinus TM, et al: Amitriptyline in the treatment of anorexia nervosa: a double-blind, placebo-controlled study. J Clin Psychopharmacol 5:10–16, 1985

Blouin J, Blouin A, Perez E: Bulimia: independence of antibulimic and antidepressant properties of desipramine. Can J Psychiatry 34:24–29, 1989

Brownell KD: Dieting and the search for the perfect body: where physiology and culture collide. Behavior Therapy 22:1–12, 1991

Bruce B, Agras WS: Binge eating in females: a population-based investigation. International Journal of Eating Disorders 12:365–373, 1992

Crisp AH, Lacey JH, Crutchfield M: Clomipramine and "drive" in people with anorexia nervosa: an inpatient study. Br J Psychiatry 150:355–358, 1987

Crisp AH, Norton K, Gowers S, et al: A controlled study of the effects of therapies aimed at adolescent and family psychopathology in anorexia nervosa. Br J Psychiatry 149:82–87, 1991

Dally PJ, Sargant W: A new treatment of anorexia nervosa. British Medical Journal 1:1770–1773, 1960

Fairburn CG, Beglin SJ: Studies of the epidemiology of bulimia nervosa. Am J Psychiatry 147:401–408, 1990

Fairburn CG, Agras WS, Wilson GT: The research on the treatment of bulimia nervosa: practical and theoretical implications, in The Biology of Feast and Famine: Relevance to Eating Disorders. Edited by Anderson GH, Kennedy SH. New York, Academic Press, 1992

Fluoxetine Bulimia Nervosa Collaborative Study Group: Fluoxetine in the treatment of bulimia nervosa. Arch Gen Psychiatry 49:139–147, 1992

Garner DM, Olmsted MP, Polivy J: The eating disorder inventory: a measure of the cognitive-behavioral dimensions of anorexia nervosa and bulimia, in Anorexia Nervosa: Recent Developments. Edited by Darby PL, Garfinkel PE, Garner DM, et al. New York, Alan R Liss, 1983

Garner DM, Olmsted MP, Garfinkel PE: Similarities among bulimic groups selected by weight and weight history. J Psychiatr Res 19:129–134, 1985

Gross HA, Ebert MH, Faden VB, et al: A double-blind controlled trial of lithium carbonate in primary anorexia nervosa. J Clin Psychopharmacol 1:376–381, 1981

Gwirtsman HE, Guze BH, Yager J, et al: Fluoxetine treatment of anorexia nervosa: an open clinical trial. J Clin Psychiatry 51:378–382, 1990

Hadigan C, Kissileff HR, Walsh BT: Patterns of food selection during meals in women with bulimia. Am J Clin Nutr 50:759–766, 1989

Halmi CA, Eckert E, LaDu TJ, et al: Treatment efficacy of cyproheptadine and amitriptyline. Arch Gen Psychiatry 43:177–181, 1986

Horne RL, Ferguson JM, Pope HG, et al: Treatment of bulimia with bupropion: A multicenter controlled trial. J Clin Psychiatry 49:262–266, 1988

Hsu LKG, Clement L, Santhouse R, et al: Treatment of bulimia nervosa with lithium carbonate: a controlled study. J Nerv Ment Dis 179:351–355, 1991

Hughes PL, Wells LA, Cunningham CJ, et al: Treating bulimia with desipramine. Arch Gen Psychiatry 43:182–187, 1986

Johnson WG, Stuckey MK, Lewis LD, et al: Bulimia: a descriptive survey of 316 cases. International Journal of Eating Disorders 2:3–16, 1982

Jonas JM, Gold MS: The use of opiate antagonists in treating bulimia: a study of low-dose versus high-dose naltrexone. Psychiatry Res 24:195–199, 1988

Kaye WH, Weltzin TE, Hsu G, et al: An open trial of

fluoxetine in patients with anorexia nervosa. J Clin Psychiatry 52:464–471, 1991

Keller MB, Herzog DB, Lavori PW, et al: The naturalistic history of bulimia nervosa: extraordinarily high rates of chronicity, relapse, recurrence, and psychosocial morbidity. International Journal of Eating Disorders 12:1–10, 1992

Kendler KS, MacLean C, Neale M, et al: The genetic epidemiology of bulimia nervosa. Am J Psychiatry 148:1627–1637, 1991

Marcus MD, Wing RR, Lamparski DM: Binge Eating and dietary restraint in obese patients. Addict Behav 10:163–168, 1985

McCann UD, Agras WS: Successful treatment of compulsive binge eating with desipramine: a double-blind placebo-controlled study. Am J Psychiatry 147:1509–1513, 1990

Mitchell JE, Groat R: A placebo-controlled, double-blind trial of amitryptiline in bulimia. J Clin Psychopharmacol 4:186–193, 1984

Mitchell JE, Laine DC: Monitored binge-eating behavior in patients with bulimia. International Journal of Eating Disorders 4:177–183, 1985

Mitchell JE, Pyle RL, Eckert ED, et al: Response to alternative antidepressants in imipramine non-responders with bulimia nervosa. J Clin Psychopharmacol 9:291–293, 1989

Mitchell JE, Pyle RL, Eckert ED, et al: A comparison study of antidepressants and structured intensive group psychotherapy in the treatment of bulimia nervosa. Arch Gen Psychiatry 47:149–160, 1990

Pope HG, Hudson JI: Treatment of bulimia with antidepressants. Psychopharmacology (Berl) 78:176–179, 1982

Pope HG, Hudson JI, Jonas JM, et al: Bulimia treated with imipramine: a placebo-controlled double-blind study. Am J Psychiatry 140:554–558, 1983

Pope HG, Hudson JI, Jonas JM, et al: Antidepressant treatment of bulimia: a two-year follow-up study. J Clin Psychopharmacol 5:320–327, 1985

Pope HG, Keck PE, McElroy SL, et al: A placebo-controlled study of trazodone in bulimia nervosa. J Clin Psychopharmacol 9:254–259, 1989

Pyle RL, Mitchell JE, Eckert ED, et al: Maintenance treatment and 6-month outcome for bulimic patients who respond to initial treatment. Am J Psychiatry 147:871–875, 1990

Rosen JC, Leitenberg H, Fisher C, et al: Binge-eating episodes in bulimia nervosa: the amount and type of food consumed. International Journal of Eating Disorders 5:255–267, 1986

Rossiter EM, Agras WS, Losch M, et al: Dietary restraint of bulimic subjects following cognitive-behavioral or pharmacological treatment. Behav Res Ther 26:495–498, 1988

Rossiter EM, Agras WS, McCann U: Are antidepressants appetite suppressants in bulimia nervosa? European Journal of Psychiatry 5:224–231, 1991

Rossiter EM, Agras WS, Telch CF, et al: The eating patterns of non-purging bulimic subjects. International Journal of Eating Disorders 11:111–120, 1992

Russell GFM, Checkley SA, Feldman J, et al: A controlled trial of d-fenfluramine in bulimia nervosa. Clin Neuropharmacol 11 (suppl 1):146–159, 1988

Sabine EJ, Yonace A, Farrington AJ, et al: Bulimia nervosa: a placebo controlled double blind therapeutic trial of mianserin. Br J Clin Pharmacol 15:195–202, 1983

Task Force on DSM-IV: DSM-IV Draft Criteria. American Psychiatric Association, Washington, DC, 1993

Telch CF, Agras WS, Rossiter EM: Binge eating increases with increasing adiposity. International Journal of Eating Disorders 7:115–119, 1988

Telch CF, Agras WS, Rossiter EM, et al: Group cognitive behavioral treatment for the non-purging bulimic: an initial evaluation. J Consult Clin Psychol 58:629–635, 1990

Vandereycken W: Neuroleptics in the short-term treatment of anorexia nervosa: a double-blind placebo-controlled study with sulpiride. Br J Psychiatry 144:288–292, 1984

Vandereycken W, Pierloot R: Pimozide combined with behavior therapy in the short-term treatment of anorexia nervosa: a double-blind placebo-controlled cross over study. Acta Psychiatr Scand 66:445–450, 1982

Walsh BT, Stewart JW, Wright L, et al: Treatment of bulimia with monoamine oxidase inhibitors. Am J Psychiatry 139:1629–1630, 1982

Walsh BT, Stewart JW, Roose SP, et al: Treatment of bulimia with phenelzine: a double-blind, placebo-controlled study. Arch Gen Psychiatry 41:1105–1109, 1984

Walsh BT, Gladis M, Roose SP, et al: Phenelzine vs placebo in 50 patients with bulimia. Arch Gen Psychiatry 45:471–475, 1988

Walsh BT, Hadigan CM, Devlin MJ, et al: Long-term

outcome of antidepressant treatment for bulimia nervosa. Am J Psychiatry 148:1206–1212, 1991

Wermuth BM, Davis KL, Hollister LE, et al: Phenytoin treatment of the binge eating syndrome. Am J Psychiatry 134:1249–1253, 1977

Wheadon DE, Rampey AH, Thompson VL, et al: Lack of association between fluoxetine and suicidality in bulimia nervosa. J Clin Psychiatry 53:235–241, 1992

Wilfley DE, Agras WS, Telch CF, et al: Group cognitive-behavioral therapy and group interpersonal psychotherapy for the non-purging bulimic: a controlled comparison. J Consult Clin Psychol 61:296–305, 1993

36

Treatment of Aggressive Disorders

Stuart C. Yudofsky, M.D., Jonathan M. Silver, M.D., and
Robert E. Hales, M.D.

▦ PREVALENCE AND RELEVANCE OF AGGRESSION IN PSYCHIATRIC AND OTHER MEDICAL PATIENTS

▪ Prevalence

Psychiatrists are frequently called upon to assess and treat patients with aggressive disorders. Approximately 10% of patients with chronic psychiatric disorders admitted to psychiatric services in both the private and not-for-profit sectors exhibited violence toward others just prior to their admissions (Tardiff and Sweillam 1982). Among patients with neuropsychiatric disease—such as patients with posttraumatic brain injury, deliria, and Alzheimer's disease or other dementias—the incidence is much higher. For example, among a sample of outpatients with Alzheimer's disease, Reisberg and colleagues (1987) reported that 48% exhibited agitation, 30% violent behavior, and 24% verbal outbursts, which taken together accounted for the most common of all behavioral symptomatologies in this population. Chandler and Chandler (1988) reported that the most common behavioral problems in a sample of 65 nursing home residents were agitation and aggression, which affected 48% ($n = 32$) of their sample.

Aggression is highly prevalent in both the acute and chronic recovery stages of traumatic brain injury. Rao and colleagues (1985) reported that 96% of 26 patients ($n = 25$) were acutely agitated following traumatic brain injury. But in a prospective study of 100 patients after acute brain injury, Brooke and col-

leagues (1992) documented that 11% were aggressive and agitated and 35% were restless. As with posttraumatic seizure disorders, aggression may occur in patients months or even many years following head injury. Oddy and colleagues (1985) followed 44 patients for 7 years after severe traumatic brain injury, and the researchers determined that agitation occurred in 31% ($n = 14$) of this population. An additional 43% ($n = 19$) had severe irritability, temper outbursts, and aggression.

▪ Relevance

The high prevalence of aggression and violence among psychiatric patients is reflected in reports of assaults by patients against psychiatrists and other physicians. Approximately 40% of psychiatrists report being attacked at least once during their careers, and 48% of psychiatric residents acknowledge that they were assaulted at least once during their residency training programs (New York State Senate Select Committee on Mental and Physical Handicaps 1977; Pardith 1987). In Veterans Administration hospitals nationwide, 12,000 assaultive incidents were reported over a 5-year period (Reid et al. 1985).

Aggression in psychiatric patients exacts an even greater toll on their family members and other primary caregivers than it does on mental health professionals. Rabins and colleagues (1982) studied families and primary caregivers of 55 patients who met DSM-III (American Psychiatric Association 1980) criteria for dementia. Sixty percent ($n = 33$) of the patients had clinical diagnoses of Alzheimer's disease,

18% (n = 10) had multi-infarct dementia, and 22% (n = 12) had other etiologies for their dementia. In response to the first question posed by the Rabins team to the families, "What is the biggest problem you have in caring for the patient?," 22 different problems were isolated. The highest on the list of "most serious" problems faced by the families was aggressive behavior, which 28 of 55 families studied reported to have occurred regularly. When aggression occurred, 75% of the families (n = 41) rated this behavior as the most serious problem with which they were confronted.

In our clinical experience, rageful affects and aggressive behaviors are frequently why elderly patients are referred to psychiatrists for assessment and management. However, a significant percentage of elderly patients with aggression are referred not to psychiatrists, but to nursing home facilities or other restrictive institutional environments such as state hospitals. It is our strong belief that, with appropriate diagnosis and treatment of the medical disorders underlying the aggression (such as delirium secondary to anticholinergic agents) as well as with the enlightened pharmacological management of their aggressive symptoms (such as the use of β-blockers to treat aggression associated with Alzheimer's disease), institutionalization could be avoided for more of these elderly patients. In this chapter, we review nosological, diagnostic, and pathophysiological aspects of aggression and then focus on the pharmacotherapy of aggression in the context of a comprehensive treatment plan.

■ NOSOLOGY OF AGGRESSION

■ Aggression as a Disorder

Largely based on the varying theoretical and clinical approaches of the myriad scientific and professional disciplines studying aggressive behaviors in animal models or in humans, aggression is conceptualized and diagnosed in an unusually broad and disparate fashion. Just as anxiety and depression may be conceptualized either as symptoms or as specific disorders, aggressive behavior may be distinguished as a symptom or as a distinct disorder. The current DSM-IV (American Psychiatric Association 1994) classification of aggressive disorders consists of two diagnoses: intermittent explosive disorder (Table 36–1

[DSM-IV, pp. 609–612]) and organic personality syndrome—explosive type (Table 36–2). Table 36–3 summarizes the DSM-IV diagnostic criteria for personality change due to a general medical condition, aggressive type (Yudofsky et al. 1989). We have expressed disagreement with these diagnostic categorizations and have proposed the specific diagnostic

---

Table 36–1. DSM-IV diagnostic criteria for intermittent explosive disorder

A. Several discrete episodes of failure to resist aggressive impulses that result in serious assaultive acts or destruction of property.

B. The degree of aggressiveness expressed during the episodes is grossly out of proportion to any precipitating psychosocial stressors.

C. The aggressive episodes are not better accounted for by another mental disorder (e.g., antisocial personality disorder, borderline personality disorder, a psychotic disorder, a manic episode, conduct disorder, or attention-deficit/hyperactivity disorder) and are not due to the direct physiological effects of a substance (e.g., a drug of abuse, a medication) or a general medical condition (e.g., head trauma, Alzheimer's disease).

Source. American Psychiatric Association 1994.

Table 36–2. DSM-III-R diagnostic criteria for organic personality syndrome—explosive type

A. Persistent personality disturbance, either life-long or representing a change or accentuation of a previously characteristic trait, involving at least one of the following:

  1. affective instability, e.g., marked shifts from normal mood to depression, irritability, or anxiety
  2. recurrent outbursts of aggression or rage that are grossly out of proportion to any precipitating psychosocial stressors
  3. markedly impaired social judgment, e.g., sexual indiscretion
  4. marked apathy and indifference
  5. suspiciousness or paranoid ideation

B. There is evidence from the history, physical examination, or laboratory tests of a specific organic factor (or factors) judged to be etiologically related to the disturbance.

Specify explosive type if outbursts of aggression or rage are the predominant feature.

Source. American Psychiatric Association 1987.

category of organic aggressive disorder (Table 36–4) to describe the specific condition of dyscontrol or rage and violence secondary to brain lesions (Silver and Yudofsky 1987a; Silver et al. 1992; Yudofsky et al. 1989). We view both organic personality syndrome, explosive type and secondary personality change, aggressive type as "catch basket" diagnoses that are overinclusive and indiscriminate with regard to the number and types of associated symptoms. With entities as disparate as depression, anxiety, impaired social judgment, apathy, and paranoid ide-

---

Table 36–3. DSM-IV diagnostic criteria for personality change due to a general medical condition

A. A persistent personality disturbance that represents a change from the individual's previous characteristic personality pattern. (In children, the disturbance involves a marked deviation from normal development or a significant change in the child's usual behavior patterns lasting at least 1 year.)

B. There is evidence from the history, physical examination, or laboratory findings that the disturbance is the direct physiological consequence of a general medical condition.

C. The disturbance is not better accounted for by another mental disorder (including other medical disorders due to a general medical condition).

D. The disturbance does not occur exclusively during the course of delirium and does not meet criteria for a dementia.

E. The disturbance causes clinically significant distress or impairment in social, occupational, or other important areas of functioning.

Specify type:
    Labile Type: if the predominant feature is affective lability
    Disinhibited Type: if the predominant feature is poor impulse control as evidenced by sexual indiscretions, etc.
    Aggressive Type: if the predominant feature is aggressive behavior
    Apathetic Type: if the predominant feature is marked apathy and indifference
    Paranoid Type: if the predominant feature is suspiciousness or paranoid ideation
    Other Type: if the predominant feature is not one of the above, e.g., personality change associated with a seizure disorder
    Combined Type: if more than one feature predominates in the clinical picture
    Unspecified Type

Source. American Psychiatric Association 1994.

---

ation, these diagnoses have no specificity as they apply to brain loci and pathophysiology that underlie the conditions they purport to describe.

We have seen many patients with brain lesions whose single symptom derivative from the brain impairment is aggressive outbursts that are out of proportion to the precipitating stimulus or provocation. There are animal models in which brain lesions are made in specific brain regions, wherein the animals exhibit increased aggression in response to irritating stimuli but are otherwise quite normal (Eichelman 1971; Leavitt et al. 1989). We also have reservations about whether or not the diagnosis of intermittent explosive disorder actually exists. According to DSM-III-R (American Psychiatric Association 1987), this diagnosis does not apply if the episodes of aggression occur with psychosis, organic mental disorders, antisocial or borderline personality disorder, conduct disorder, or intoxication with a psychoactive substance. These exclusions are so broad that our group, which specializes in the assessment and treatment of aggressive disorders, rarely if ever encounters a patient who meets criteria for this condition.

Our experience is consistent with the report of neurologist Frank Elliott, who also found that 94% of 286 patients ($n = 269$) with histories of recurrent uncontrolled rage attacks that occurred with little or no provocation had objective evidence of developmental or acquired brain deficits (Elliott 1976). We believe that the nosological confusion and imprecision that exist in official diagnostic categorizations have resulted in the pervasive failure of clinicians to diagnose and, consequently, to treat aggressive disorders specifically and effectively in all patient categories.

Table 36–4. Diagnostic criteria for proposed organic aggressive disorder

▼ Persistent or recurrent aggressive outbursts, whether of a verbal or physical nature.

▼ The outbursts are out of proportion to the precipitating stress or provocation.

▼ Evidence from history, physical examination, or laboratory tests of a specific organic factor that is judged to be etiologically related to the disturbance.

▼ The outbursts are not primarily related to the following disorders: paranoia, mania, schizophrenia, narcissistic personality disorder, borderline disorder, conduct disorder, or antisocial personality disorder.

Source. Reprinted from Yudofsky et al. 1989 with permission.

■ Aggression as a Symptom

Rage and aggression most often occur as a consequence of a complexity of experiential and neuropathological conditions. (A review of the brain pathways involved in aggression and the ways in which neuropathology and psychopathology combine to give rise to it can be found in Ovsiew and Yudofsky 1993.) As we discuss later in this chapter, a broad range of conditions and disorders that affect the brain can result in aggressive symptoms. Unfortunately, such symptoms are often not afforded diagnostic primacy and are therefore either not treated at all, or "mistreated" with agents that have do not have antiaggressive properties. In this regard, we have written about "the monosymptomatic mischaracterization of neuropsychiatric disorders" (Yudofsky 1991, pp. 1–4), in which neuropsychiatric conditions with a broad range of symptoms are misconceptualized as being a uniform illness as defined by a singular predominant sign or symptom. An example is the misconceptualization of Alzheimer's disease as a disorder of memory and cognition, without recognition of the agitation, depression, and anxiety that are reported to be among the most disabling aspects of this disorder.

Similarly, Parkinson's disease is conventionally regarded as a movement disorder, but it is well documented that depression, delirium, and dementia are also common concomitants. Schizophrenia is misconceptualized as a psychotic disorder, with the result that a schizophrenic patient's symptoms of depression and aggression often go untreated or mistreated. To focus on the latter example, using antipsychotic agents to treat agitation and aggression that do not stem from psychotic ideation results in oversedated patients. These patients are unnecessarily placed at risk for many other side effects associated with antipsychotic drugs, including irreversible tardive dyskinesia and potentially fatal neuroleptic malignant syndrome (NMS). An overwhelming percentage of patients with schizophrenia whom we have evaluated has included individuals who were prescribed high doses of antipsychotics largely because of their agitated or aggressive behaviors. Uniformly, their psychoses did not change after discontinuation of the antipsychotic drug. In these cases, precise nosology would have helped the clinician arrive at an accurate diagnosis that, in turn, would have led to specific and effective treatment.

■ Distinguishing Between Aggression, Anxiety, and Agitation

As is reviewed in the next section, we developed a rating scale, the Overt Aggression Scale (OAS; Figure 36–1 [Yudofsky et al. 1986]), which encompasses the definition, diagnosis, and operationalization of aggression. Although there are several rating scales used to measure agitation, we believe that, for the purposes of documenting and monitoring the responses of agitation to pharmacological intervention, no existing rating scale is adequate. One major problem is that most rating scales now in use blur the boundaries between anxiety, agitation, and aggression—they depend too heavily on the inferences or idiosyncratic theoretical approaches of the rater.

Figure 36–2 summarizes a new rating scale we developed that is currently undergoing reliability and validity testing. By briefly reviewing this scale, the Overt Agitation Severity Scale (OASS), and comparing it with the OAS, the reader can be helped to differentiate between agitation and aggression. Anxiety and neuropsychiatric syndromes or side effects such as akathisia also require differentiation from aggression. When a clinician confuses akathisia with agitation or aggression, he or she may increase a patient's antipsychotic dose. Apart from the increased sedation from the antipsychotic, the misuse of a neuroleptic in this circumstance ultimately will aggravate the akathisia and result in a vicious cycle of ever-increasing doses of antipsychotic drug and consequent intensification of the akathisia. We advise clinicians to use standardized rating scales such as the OAS and the OASS to help diagnose, document, distinguish, and monitor anxiety, agitation, and aggression.

■ DOCUMENTATION OF AGGRESSION

Accurate documentation of aggressive episodes is critical to record characteristics of aggressive episodes when they occur, to assess effectiveness of interventions in the treatment of violent patients, and to conduct research related to aggressive disorders. To assess the effects of pharmacological agents in the treatment of aggressive behaviors, two of us (S. C. Y. and J. M. S.) developed the one-page OAS to document and measure specific aspects of aggressive behavior based on observable criteria (Figure 36–1

OVERT AGGRESSION SCALE (OAS)

IDENTIFYING DATA

Name of Patient	Name of Rater
Sex of Patient: 1 Male 2 Female	Date / / (month/day/year) Shift: 1 Night 2 Day 3 Evening

☐ No aggressive incidents (verbal or physical) against self, others, or objects during the shift. (check here)

AGGRESSIVE BEHAVIOR (check all that apply)

VERBAL AGGRESSION	PHYSICAL AGGRESSION AGAINST SELF
☐ Makes loud noises, shouts angrily	☐ Picks or scratches skin, hits self, pulls hair (with no or minor injury only)
☐ Yells mild personal insults (e.g., "You're stupid!")	☐ Bangs head, hits fist into objects, throws self onto floor or into objects (hurts self without serious injury)
☐ Curses viciously, uses foul language in anger, makes moderate threats to others or self	☐ Small cuts or bruises, minor burns
☐ Makes clear threats of violence toward others or self (e.g., "I'm going to kill you") or requests to help to control self	☐ Mutilates self, makes deep cuts, bites that bleed, internal injury, fracture, loss of consciousness, loss of teeth

PHYSICAL AGGRESSION AGAINST OBJECTS	PHYSICAL AGGRESSION AGAINST OTHER PEOPLE
☐ Slams door, scatters clothing, makes a mess	☐ Makes threatening gesture, swings at people, grabs at clothes
☐ Throws objects down, kicks furniture without breaking it, marks the wall	☐ Strikes, kicks, pushes, pulls hair (without injury to them)
☐ Breaks objects, smashes windows	☐ Attacks others causing mild to moderate physical injury (bruises, sprains, welts)
☐ Sets fires, throws objects dangerously	☐ Attacks others causing severe physical injury (broken bones, deep lacerations, internal injury)

☐ Time incident began: ____:____ A.M./P.M.	☐ Duration of incident: ____:____ (hours/minutes)

INTERVENTION (check all that apply)

☐ None	☐ Immediate medication given by mouth	☐ Use of restraints
☐ Talking to patient	☐ Immediate medication given by injection	☐ Injury requires immediate medical treatment for patient
☐ Closer observation	☐ Isolation without seclusion (time-out)	☐ Injury requires immediate treatment for other person
☐ Holding patient	☐ Seclusion	

COMMENTS

Figure 36–1. The Overt Aggression Scale.
Source. Reprinted from Yudofsky et al. 1986 with permission.

OVERT AGITATION SEVERITY SCALE (OASS)

Intensity score	Behavior	Not present	Rarely	Some of the time	Most of the time	Always present	Severity score
A.	**Vocalizations and Oral/Facial Movements**						
1 ×	Whimpering, whining, moaning, grunting, crying	0	1	2	3	4	= _____
2 ×	Smacking or licking of lips, chewing, clenching jaw, licking, grimacing, spitting	0	1	2	3	4	= _____
3 ×	Rocking, twisting, banging of head	0	1	2	3	4	= _____
4 ×	Vocal perseverating, screaming, cursing, threatening, wailing	0	1	2	3	4	= _____
B.	**Upper Torso and Upper Extremity Movements**						
1 ×	Tapping fingers, fidgeting, wringing of hands, swinging or flailing arms	0	1	2	3	4	= _____
2 ×	Task perseverating (e.g., opening and closing drawers, folding and unfolding clothes, picking at objects, clothes, or self)	0	1	2	3	4	= _____
3 ×	Rocking (back and forth), bobbing (up and down), twisting or writhing of torso; rubbing or masturbating self	0	1	2	3	4	= _____
4 ×	Slapping, swatting, hitting at objects or others	0	1	2	3	4	= _____
C.	**Lower Extremity Movements**						
1 ×	Tapping or clenching toes; tapping heel; extending, flexing, or twisting foot	0	1	2	3	4	= _____
2 ×	Shaking legs, tapping knees and/or thighs, thrusting pelvis	0	1	2	3	4	= _____
3 ×	Pacing, wandering	0	1	2	3	4	= _____
4 ×	Thrashing legs, kicking at objects or others	0	1	2	3	4	= _____

Total OASS = _____
Subtract baseline OASS = _____
Revised OASS = _____

Instructions for Completing Form

Step one: For each behavior, circle the corresponding frequency.

Step two: For every behavior exhibited, multiply the intensity score by the freqency and record as the Severity Score.

Step three: For the Overt Agitation Severity Score (OASS), total all severity scores and record as Total OASS.

Step four: Does this patient have a neuromuscular disorder (i.e., Parkinson's disease, tardive dyskinesia) affecting

Total OASS? ☐ yes ☐ no

If yes, please establish baseline OASS in nonagitated state and subtract from above Total OASS for Revised OASS.

Comments:

Name of Patient: _____

Sex of Patient: Male (1) Female (2)

Diagnosis: _____

Age: _____ **Race:** _____

Name of Rater: _____

Time of Observation: from _____ am/pm to _____ am/pm

Date: __ __ __ __ __ __
M M D D Y Y

Case ID: _____

Figure 36–2. The Overt Agitation Severity Scale.

Source. Reprinted with permission of Stuart C. Yudofsky, M.D. Copyright © 1994.

[Silver and Yudofsky 1991; Yudofsky et al. 1986]). In the OAS, aggressive behaviors are divided into four categories: verbal aggression, physical aggression against objects, physical aggression against self, and physical aggression against others. Within each category, descriptive statements and numerical scores are provided to define and rate four levels of severity. All behaviors exhibited by a patient during an aggressive episode are checked off by an observer (such as routine hospital staff or a family member). Therapeutic interventions used in response to these aggressive episodes are also listed, rated on the OAS, and checked off by the rater. These interventions are documented, because they may indicate the observer's interpretation of the relative severity of the aggressive behaviors.

Our research, which evaluated more than 5,000 episodes of aggression in chronically hospitalized psychiatric inpatients, demonstrated that hospital records and other official communications and documentations failed to include descriptions of most aggressive behaviors. Using the OAS simultaneously assured that a significantly greater percentage of aggressive episodes and behaviors were documented (Silver and Yudofsky 1987b). We encourage practitioners to use the OAS to establish a baseline score for aggression before beginning psychopharmacological intervention and to use it thereafter to document the efficacy (or lack thereof) of any therapeutic intervention.

The documentation of aggression through the OAS is often essential to *maintaining* a psychopharmacological treatment plan. We are frequently consulted by other physicians or by family members who contend that the psychopharmacological intervention "has stopped working." In these circumstances, professionals and family members are so alarmed by the patient's single episode of violence and its implications that they demand significant revisions in the treatment plan, which often entail abrupt discontinuation of the current pharmacological agent and initiation of another medication. In a significant percentage of these cases, the pharmacological agent has, in fact, been *partially* effective. However, for a variety of reasons (e.g., increased stress, poor compliance, concomitant use of alcohol or illicit substances), the patient's aggression has "broken through" the pharmacological intervention. Documentation of aggressive events using the OAS is highly useful in demonstrating to patients and their families and caregivers when a pharmacological intervention has been partially effective (e.g., the number of aggressive events may have been reduced by 80% and the intensity of the events may have diminished by 94%). These data from the OAS may obviate a potentially deleterious "overreaction" to an aggressive event by caregivers and the discontinuation of an effective pharmacological regimen.

◼ NEUROTRANSMITTERS AND AGGRESSION

Multiple neurotransmitters and neurotransmitter systems are involved in the mediation of aggression, with important roles played by serotonin, norepinephrine, dopamine, acetylcholine, and γ-aminobutyric acid (GABA). In neuropsychiatric disorders, it is the rule rather than the exception that multiple neurotransmitter systems are involved simultaneously in diffuse regions of the brain. Additionally, as we have learned regarding the roles of neurotransmitters in depression, different transmitters may affect one another in influencing aggression. Most frequently, the critical factor relative to the role of neurotransmitters in aggression is the *relationship* between and among the neurotransmitters in both function and dysfunction.

Norepinephrine tracks originate in the locus ceruleus in the lateral tegmental system and course to the forebrain—an area frequently involved in traumatic brain injury and associated with dyscontrol of rage and violent behavior. The β_1-adrenergic receptors have been implicated through their localization in this region (limbic forebrain and cerebral cortex) and are thought to be involved in the mediation of aggressive behavior (Alexander et al. 1979). Animal studies suggest that norepinephrine is involved in many aspects of aggressive behavior, including sham rage, affective aggression, and shock-induced fighting (Eichelman 1987). Higley and associates (1992) documented an association between aggression in free-ranging rhesus monkeys and cerebrospinal fluid (CSF) norepinephrine. Brown and colleagues (1979) reported that humans who exhibit aggressive or impulsive behavior have increased levels of the norepinephrine metabolite 5-hydroxy-3-methoxyphenylglycol (5-MHPG).

Originating in the raphe, located in the pons and

upper brain stem, serotonergic neurons project to the frontal cortex. In a broad variety of studies, lower levels of serotonergic activity have been reported to be associated with increased aggression, including predatory aggression and shock-induced fighting in rats (Eichelman 1987). Clinical studies have implicated lowered serotonin levels in the central nervous system in the expression of aggression and impulsivity in humans, particularly violent self-destructive acts (Kruesi et al. 1992; Linnoila and Virkkunen 1992). Dopamine systems are prominent in both mesolimbic and mesocortical regions of the brain. A variety of indirect evidence indicates that increases in brain dopamine—particularly the release of dopamine after brain lesions—lead to increased aggression in animal models and in humans (Bareggi et al. 1975; Hamill et al. 1987). The profound increases in aggressive behavior after severe traumatic brain injury are thought to be closely associated with subsequent changes of dopaminergic systems (Eichelman et al. 1972).

■ DIFFERENTIAL DIAGNOSIS OF AGGRESSIVE DISORDERS

As with every other symptom or disorder in medicine and psychiatry, the overarching principle is that diagnosis comes before treatment. The history of symptoms in a biopsychosocial context is usually the most critical part of the evaluation. Many psychiatric conditions are associated with aggressive disorders, as summarized in Table 36–5 (Reid and Balis 1987).

As we have noted, organic brain disorders are strongly associated with dyscontrol of rage and violence. Table 36–6 summarizes common etiologies of organically induced aggression, and Table 36–7 lists medications and drugs that are associated with engendering aggression (Yudofsky et al. 1990). Table 36–8 summarizes characteristic features that alert clinicians to the potential presence of organically induced aggression. In soliciting the patient's history of aggression, it is critical to interview family members, teachers, friends, work associates, and others, because patients afflicted by aggressive disorders—as opposed to their families and friends—tend to minimize the disorders' presence and importance (Silver and Yudofsky 1994). In addition, in crafting a multifaceted treatment plan, clinicians should deter-

Table 36–5. DSM-III diagnoses associated with violent behavior

A. Violent Behavior as an Essential Feature
   Intermittent explosive disorder
   Isolated explosive disorder
   Undersocialized conduct disorder, aggressive
   Socialized conduct disorder, aggressive
   Antisocial personality disorder, aggressive
   Borderline personality disorder
   Sexual sadism

B. Violent Behavior as an Associated Feature
   Substance use disorders
   Organic mental disorders
   Mental retardation
   Attention deficit disorder
   Brief reactive psychosis
   Schizophrenic disorder
   Schizoaffective disorder
   Paranoid disorder
   Bipolar disorder
   Posttraumatic stress disorder

C. Violent Behavior as an Infrequent Feature
   Atypical psychosis
   Major depression
   Dysthymic disorder
   Cyclothymic disorder
   Atypical depression
   Paranoid personality disorder
   Histrionic personality disorder
   Schizoid personality disorder
   Schizotypal personality disorder
   Psychogenic fugue
   Adjustment disorder with disturbance of conduct

Source. Reprinted from Reid and Balis 1987, p. 498, with permission.

mine from both patient and observers the context in which the patient's aggression occurs. Information such as the mental status of the patient *prior* to the aggressive event, the nature of the precipitant, the physical and social environment in which aggression occurs, the ways in which the aggressive event is mitigated, and primary and secondary gains related to aggression is essential. If the aggression occurs in the context of a psychiatric disorder, a review of both the individual's and the family's psychiatric history should be emphasized.

For *all* patients with aggression, the clinician must obtain a history of physical illness, make a detailed review of neurological signs and symptoms, and conduct a thorough physical examination. A special focus should be placed on the neurological eval-

Table 36–6. Common etiologies of organically induced aggression

▼ Traumatic brain injury

▼ Stroke and other cerebrovascular disease

▼ Medications, alcohol and other abused substances, over-the-counter drugs

▼ Delirium (e.g., hypoxia, electrolyte imbalance, anesthesia and surgery, uremia)

▼ Alzheimer's disease

▼ Chronic neurological disorders: Huntington's disease, Wilson's disease, Parkinson's disease, multiple sclerosis, systemic lupus erythematosus

▼ Brain tumors

▼ Infectious diseases (encephalitis, meningitis, AIDS)

▼ Epilepsy (ictal, postictal, and interictal)

▼ Metabolic disorders: hyperthyroidism or hypothyroidism, hypoglycemia, vitamin deficiencies, porphyria

Source. Reprinted from Yudofsky et al. 1990. Copyright © 1990, Physicians Postgraduate Press. Used with permission.

Table 36–7. Medications and drugs associated with aggression

▼ Alcohol—intoxication and withdrawal states

▼ Hypnotic and antianxiety agents (e.g., barbiturates, benzodiazepines): intoxication and withdrawal states

▼ Analgesics—opiates and other narcotics—intoxication and withdrawal states

▼ Steroids (prednisone, cortisone, and anabolic steroids)

▼ Antidepressants—especially in initial phases of treatment

▼ Amphetamines and cocaine—aggression associated with manic excitement in early stages of abuse and secondary to paranoid ideation in later stages of use

▼ Antipsychotics—high-potency agents that lead to akathisia

▼ Anticholinergic drugs (including over-the-counter sedatives) associated with delirium and central anticholinergic syndrome

Source. Reprinted from Yudofsky et al. 1990. Copyright © 1990, Physicians Postgraduate Press. Used with permission.

uation and on relevant laboratory testing guided by information from history, physical, and neurological examinations. We find neuropsychological batteries such as the Halsted-Reitan Neuropsychological Battery (Boll 1981) or the Luria-Nebraska Neuropsychological Battery (Golden et al. 1979) more useful than standard psychological scales (e.g., the Minnesota Multiphasic Personality Inventory [MMPI; Hathaway and McKinley 1989]) or projective psycho-

Table 36–8. Characteristic features of organic aggression syndrome

Reactive	Triggered by modest or trivial stimuli
Nonreflective	Usually does not involve premeditation or planning
Nonpurposeful	Aggression serves no obvious long-term aims or goals
Explosive	Buildup is *not* gradual
Periodic	Brief outbursts of rage and aggression; punctuated by long periods of relative calm
Ego-dystonic	After outbursts, patients are upset, concerned, and embarrassed, as opposed to blaming others or justifying behavior

Source. Reprinted from Yudofsky et al. 1990. Copyright © 1990, Physicians Postgraduate Press. Used with permission.

logical tests in evaluating patients with aggressive symptoms and disorders.

■ TREATMENT

■ Overview

Treatment of aggressive symptoms and disorders is guided by the following four "D"s:

1. **D**etermining the etiologies of the psychological and/or organic disorder(s) that may contribute to the aggression
2. **D**elineating the biopsychosocial context in which the aggressive events occur
3. **D**ocumenting and rating the aggression or agitation with the OAS and/or the OASS
4. **D**eveloping a multifaceted treatment plan

Almost without exception, treatment of patients with aggressive disorders requires a multifaceted approach that often combines pharmacological treatments, behavioral treatments, psychodynamically informed psychotherapy, family treatment, and (as indicated) other specific approaches such as spiritual counseling, occupational therapy, or couples treatment. Review of the psychopharmacological management of aggression is the focus of this chapter; therefore, we shall not expand on the other approaches that also have been shown to have efficacy in the treatment of aggression. For a comprehensive review of behavioral treatments of aggression in psychiatric patients, the reader is referred to a review article published in collaboration with us (Corrigan et al. 1993). Table 36–9 summarizes the behavioral treatments of aggression that may be used in combination with pharmacological interventions (Corrigan et al. 1993).

In conceptualizing an approach to the pharmacological treatment of aggression, we differentiate between the acute management of acute aggression (which often constitutes a medical emergency) from the pharmacological treatment of patients with chronic aggression (which often constitutes a prophylactic approach). Currently, no medication for the treatment of aggression has U.S. Food and Drug Administration approval for this indication. Most frequently when medications are used (and often misused), it is their sedating side effects that are sought. Although this may be appropriate in emergency or acute situations, prolonged use of sedation to "cover over" aggressive behaviors has disadvantages. For example, when neuroleptics are used to manage aggression, side effects may emerge, including oversedation, hypotension, confusion, NMS, parkinsonism, akathisia, dystonia, and tardive dyskinesia. When benzodiazepines are used to manage aggression over prolonged periods, side effects such as oversedation, motor disturbances (including poor coordination), mood disturbances, memory impairment, confusion, dependency, overdoses, withdrawal syndromes, and paradoxical violence often complicate treatment (Silver et al. 1992).

■ Pharmacological Management of Acute Aggression and Agitation

Psychiatrists and other physicians most commonly use the sedative side effects of antipsychotics and benzodiazepines in the acute management of aggressive behavior and for acute agitation. However, it must be recognized that these agents are not specific in their capacities to inhibit aggressive behaviors; rather, they "cover over" the respective behaviors and symptoms. As we have stated, sedation may have deleterious effects on arousal and cognitive function. Prolonged use of sedation-producing medications can result in serious disabling side effects such as tardive dyskinesia, or life-threatening drug reactions such as NMS. Therefore, the clinician must establish time limits when prescribing medications for their sedative properties.

Table 36–9. Behavioral treatment of aggression

Strategy	Indications	Special considerations
Token economy	Provides both proactive and reactive strategies for aggressive behaviors	A strict format for implementing contingency management
Aggression replacement		
Differential reinforcement schedules	Replace punishing contingency for previolent behavior	Differential reinforcement of other behaviors is resource intensive; differential reinforcement of incompatible behaviors requires identification of suitable interfering behaviors
Assertiveness training	Effective for patients who become angry when their needs are not met	Patients must work well in skills training groups
Activity programming	Diminishes opportunities for unstructured, frustrating interactions	Activities that patients find reinforcing should be identified
Decelerative techniques		
Social extinction	Effective with previolent patients who respond to social reinforcements	May not work with schizoid patients
Contingent observation	Effective with previolent patients who respond to social reinforcements	Patients must be sufficiently organized to accurately perceive models
Self-controlled time-out	Effective with violent patients immediately after incidents	May diminish risky attempts to seclude or restrain
Overcorrection	Effective with relatively docile patients	Stop if patient struggles with guided practice
Contingent restraint	Effective with violent patients who do not comply with self-controlled time-out and are resistant to guided practice	Decreases inadvertent reinforcement of behaviors that covary with seclusion and restraint

Source. Reprinted from Corrigan et al. 1993. Copyright © 1993, American Psychiatric Association. Used with permission.

Antipsychotic Drugs

Antipsychotics are the most commonly prescribed medications in the treatment of both acute and chronic aggression. Manifestly, these agents are appropriate and effective in treating aggression that derives from psychosis. An example would be to use an antipsychotic drug for a patient who has acute manic psychosis with irritability. This patient had been physically aggressive toward anyone who interfered with his grandiose scheme to redirect the flight plan of a commercial airline on which he was a passenger. A second example of the appropriate use of an antipsychotic medication to treat aggression would be its use for a patient with paranoid schizophrenia who had the delusion that he had to use physical force to protect himself from postal workers, whom he said were "agents who are sent from another planet to kidnap me."

Unfortunately, however, the most common use of antipsychotic medications is in the treatment of patients with chronic aggression associated with organic brain disorders (including schizophrenia). As we have discussed, tolerance develops for the sedative side effects of the neuroleptics, and the ill-advised clinician will increase the dose to maintain the sedation. Often a vicious cycle emerges wherein neuroleptics are increased to "treat" akathisias that are mistaken for increased irritability and agitation of the associated illness. Herrera and colleagues (1988) noted a marked increase in violent behavior among patients with schizophrenia who were treated with haloperidol at doses ranging to 60 mg/day, when compared with violent behaviors that occurred in patients being treated with chlorpromazine at doses to 1,800 mg/day or clozapine at doses ranging to 900 mg/day. We interpret these findings as being the result of haloperidol's increased risk of causing akathisia compared with chlorpromazine or clozapine. These complications and side effects can be avoided by establishing, before initiating neuroleptics to treat acute aggression, a treatment plan that includes 1) operationalized ratings of aggression with the OAS, 2) reduction of neuroleptics when symptoms remit, and 3) specified dates when the antipsychotic agent will be tapered and discontinued.

Unless aggressive behavior is clearly related to psychotic ideation that is responding to treatment with antipsychotic agents, we limit the use of both antipsychotic agents and benzodiazepines for "sedating" aggression to a maximum of 4 weeks. Beyond this time, clinicians must consider whether or not the patient's aggression is chronic and alter the treatment plan accordingly to use medications recommended to treat chronic aggression (see next section).

The essence of managing acute episodes of aggression through sedation by using neuroleptics is to increase the dose of the neuroleptic (often every 1–2 hours) to achieve the lowest dose that will incur the sedation necessary to "control" the violent behaviors. Despite the aforementioned disadvantages of haloperidol in the management of chronic aggression, this medication—because it can be taken orally, intramuscularly, and intravenously, and because of its low level of cardiovascular side effects when compared with other classes of neuroleptics—is most often used. Table 36–10 summarizes guidelines for the use of haloperidol in the acute management of acute aggression.

Benzodiazepines

Benzodiazepines may also be indicated for the acute management of acute agitation and aggression. Intermuscular lorazepam has advantages over other benzodiazepines as an effective medication for the emergency treatment of violent patients (Bick and Hannah 1986). Similar to haloperidol, the advantages of lorazepam in managing acute aggression include its flexible routes of administration (iv, im, or po). In addition, lorazepam has a relatively brief half-life compared with other benzodiazepines such as diazepam or chlordiazepoxide, which can result in the oversedating of the patient through the buildup of too high plasma levels of the respective benzodiaz-

---

Table 36–10. Use of haloperidol in the acute management of aggression

▼ At first, give 1 mg po or 0.5 mg iv or im q 1 hour.

▼ Increase dose by 1 mg q 1 hour until control of aggression is achieved.

▼ Then give haloperidol 2 mg po or 1 mg iv or im q 8 hours.

▼ When the patient is not agitated or violent for a period of 48 hours, taper at rate of 25% of highest daily dose.

▼ If violent behavior reemerges upon tapering drug, reassess etiology and consider changing to a more specific medication to manage chronic aggression.

▼ Do not maintain the patient on haloperidol for more than 6 weeks—except for aggression secondary to psychosis.

Source. Adapted from Yudofsky et al. 1990. Copyright © 1990, Physicians Postgraduate Press. Used with permission.

epine. Table 36–11 summarizes guidelines for the use of lorazepam in the acute management of aggressive behaviors. Other medications such as paraldehyde, chloral hydrate, or diphenhydramine may also be prescribed to sedate patients who exhibit acute aggressive behaviors. But, in general, benzodiazepines and neuroleptics are preferable for reasons of safety and convenience, and because psychiatrists and hospital staff are more familiar with their benefits and risks.

The scientific literature includes many case reports whenever specific pharmacological approaches

are suggested for certain clinical conditions. For example, Gualtieri and colleagues (1989) have reported that amantadine, a dopamine agonist, reduces aggressive behavior in patients recovering from traumatic brain injury; however, our group has not had any experience with this approach. Intensivists who specialize in treating the medical sequelae of trauma may use succinylcholine to achieve a pharmacological paralysis in agitated patients being treated in intensive care units following traumatic brain injury or surgical procedures. Clearly, the application of such interventions is best limited to those professionals who, by virtue of their subspecialty focus, have broad experience and the requisite resources to manage patients safely using these novel approaches.

■ Pharmacological Management of Chronic Aggression and Agitation

When a patient's agitation and aggression persist beyond several weeks, the *prophylaxis* of aggression using specific antiaggressive medications should be considered. We advocate that the decision about the choice of the specific psychopharmacological agent be guided by the determination of the underlying cause of the chronic aggression or by the co-occurrence of other psychiatric symptoms such as anxiety, mania, or depression. Table 36–12 outlines our approach to the pharmacological treatment of chronic aggression.

Antipsychotic Medications

As we have discussed, it is critical to restrict the use of antipsychotic medications to the treatment of ag-

---

Table 36–11. Use of lorazepam in the acute management of aggression

▼ Give lorazepam 1–2 mg po or im.

▼ Repeat every hour until control of aggression is achieved.

▼ If iv dose must be given, push slowly! Do not exceed 2 mg (1 ml) per minute to avoid respiratory depression and laryngospasm; this may be repeated in 30 minutes if required.

▼ Once the patient is no longer violent or agitated, maintain at maximum of 2 mg po or im q 4 hours.

▼ When the patient is not agitated or violent for 48 hours, taper at rate 10% of highest total daily dose.

▼ If violent behavior reemerges upon tapering drug, reassess etiology and consider changing to a more specific medication to manage chronic aggression.

▼ If, after 6 weeks, lorazepam cannot be tapered without reemergence of aggression, reevaluate and revise the treatment plan to include a more specific medication to manage chronic aggression.

Source. Adapted from Yudofsky et al. 1990. Copyright © 1990, Physicians Postgraduate Press. Used with permission.

Table 36–12. Psychopharmacological treatment of chronic aggression

Agent	Indications	Special clinical considerations
Antipsychotics	Psychotic symptoms	Oversedation and multiple side effects
Benzodiazepines	Anxiety symptoms	Paradoxical rage
Carbamazepine (CBZ) Valproic acid (VPA)	Seizure disorder	Bone marrow suppression CBZ and hepatotoxicity (CBZ and VPA)
Lithium	Manic excitement or bipolar disorder	Neurotoxicity and confusion
Buspirone	Persistent underlying anxiety and/or depression	Delayed onset of action
Propranolol (and other β-blockers)	Chronic or recurrent aggression	Latency of 4–6 weeks
Serotonergic antidepressants	Depression or mood lability with irritability	May need usual clinical doses

Source. Adapted from Yudofsky SC et al. 1990. Copyright © 1990, Physicians Postgraduate Press. Used with permission.

gression that is in direct response to psychotic ideation or perception, such as paranoid delusions or command hallucinations. At regular intervals, attempts should be made through tapering of the medication to gauge the efficacy of the antipsychotic agent in treating both the patient's psychosis and the attendant agitation and aggression.

Antianxiety Medications

In various case reports, buspirone, a 5-HT$_{1A}$ agonist, has proven effective in treating patients whose aggression and agitation have been associated with traumatic brain injury (Gualtieri 1991; Ratey et al. 1992a) and in those with dementia (Colenda 1988; Tiller et al. 1988) or who have developmental disabilities and autism (Ratey et al. 1989; Realmuto et al. 1989). Because we have observed that some patients become more aggressive in the initial phases of buspirone treatment, we advocate beginning treatment at low doses (e.g., 5 mg bid) and increasing the dose by 5 mg every 3–5 days. Doses ranging from 45–60 mg/day may be required before treatment, and a latency of 3–6 weeks before therapeutic effects are observed is not uncommon.

Although there have been no double-blind controlled studies of clonazepam in the management of chronic aggression, there are several case reports indicating its benefits in treating agitation in elderly patients (Freinhar and Alvarez 1986) and in a patient who had schizophrenia and seizures (Keats and Mukherjee 1988). We prescribe clonazepam when aggression occurs in patients with pronounced anxiety or when aggression is present with neurologically induced tics and disinhibited motor behavior. Dosages are initiated at 0.5 mg bid and rarely exceed a total daily dose of 6 mg.

Anticonvulsant Medications

Overall, we prioritize the use of anticonvulsant medications (particularly carbamazepine) for the treatment of patients whose chronic aggression is associated with seizure disorders and, as our second choice to β-blockers, in the treatment of chronic aggression related to diffuse neuronal destruction (such as that occurring after traumatic brain injury, middle cerebral arteria stroke, and Alzheimer's disease). The scientific literature is devoid of double-blind placebo-controlled studies measuring the efficacy of carbamazepine in the treatment of aggression. However, several open-label studies indicate that carbamaze-

pine may be effective in reducing aggressive behavior associated with organic brain disorders (Mattes 1988), schizophrenia (Hakoloa and Laulumaa 1982), developmental disabilities (Folks et al. 1982; Yatham and McHale 1988), and dementia (Gleason and Schneider 1990; Leibovici and Tariot 1988). We prescribe carbamazepine in the same doses and with the same blood levels that we use in treating patients with manic-depressive disorder.

Other anticonvulsants have also been suggested to treat patients with aggressive disorders. Second to carbamazepine, the anticonvulsant valproic acid has been used most frequently for this purpose, particularly in patients with organically induced aggression (Giakas et al. 1990; Mattes 1992).

Antimanic Medications

Many researchers suggest lithium's value in treating aggression in patients without bipolar illness but with other specific underlying disorders. Included among this group are patients with mental retardation who exhibit self-directed aggression (Luchins and Dojka 1989) or aggression toward others (Dale 1980), and patients with traumatic brain injury (Haas and Cope 1985). Additionally, aggressive people from special segments of the population, such as children and adolescents (Vetro et al. 1985) or prison inmates (Sheard et al. 1976), have been reported to respond to lithium. The vast majority of the lithium prescribed in treating our patients with aggressive disorders is for those individuals with mania; we prescribe the same dosage of lithium and blood level monitoring as is recommended for patients with bipolar disorder. One caveat, however, is that patients with brain injury have increased sensitivity to the neurotoxic affects of lithium (Hornstein and Seliger 1989; Moskowitz and Altshuler 1991) and must therefore be followed much more closely with neuropsychiatric evaluations and serum lithium levels.

Antidepressant Medications

Although many antidepressants have been suggested for the treatment of aggressive disorders, those agents that act either preferentially or specifically on the serotonergic system of the brain are preferred. Amitriptyline (Jackson et al. 1985; Szlabowicz and Stewart 1990) and trazodone (Pinner and Rich 1988) have been found to be useful in the treatment of aggression; however, most recent reports focus on the use of the selective serotonin reuptake inhibitors

(SSRIs) (Bass and Beltis 1991; Coccaro et al. 1990). We have given fluoxetine and sertraline successfully in treating patients whose aggression is associated with brain lesions. We initiate treatment at relatively low doses (e.g., 10 mg of fluoxetine or 25 mg of sertraline). If antiaggressive effects are not achieved over a period of several weeks, we gradually increase the dose to relatively high ranges (80–100 mg/day of fluoxetine and 200–300 mg/day of sertraline).

Antihypertensive Medications (β-Blockers)

Since 1977, when the first report of the use of β-adrenergic receptor antagonists in the treatment of aggression appeared, more than 25 papers have been published in both the neurological and psychiatric literature that report on the use of β-blockers for this purpose (Yudofsky et al. 1987). The β-blockers that have been investigated in prospective placebo-controlled designs include propranolol (a lipid-soluble nonselective receptor antagonist [Greendyke et al. 1986; Mattes 1988]), nadolol (a water-soluble nonselective receptor antagonist [Alpert et al. 1990; Ratey et al. 1992b]), and pindolol (a lipid-soluble nonselective antagonist with partial sympathomimetic activity [Greendyke and Kanter 1986]). Because a growing body of preliminary evidence suggests that β-adrenergic receptor antagonists are specific and effective agents for the treatment of aggression and violent behaviors in patients with organic brain syndromes, and because of our own extensive experience in treating patients with aggressive neuropsychiatric disorders associated with β-blockers, this approach has become our first line of treatment of organically induced aggression.

Our guidelines for the use of propranolol for this purpose are summarized in Table 36–13. There are several key clinical points related to the use of propranolol. First, the peripheral effects of β blockade (e.g., lowered blood pressure, bradycardia) are frequently saturated when the patient achieves a dose of approximately 280 mg/day. Thereafter, increasing the dose of β-blocker is not usually associated with cardiovascular side effects. Second, because of the long latency of 6–8 weeks before a therapeutic response is achieved, encouragement of the family and other members of the treatment team is an essential component of clinician care. Third, despite reports that depression is commonly associated with use of β-blockers, controlled trials and our own extensive experience indicate that depression is a rare side ef-

Table 36–13.   Clinical use of propranolol

▼ Conduct a thorough medical evaluation.

▼ Exclude patients with the following disorders: bronchial asthma, chronic obstructive pulmonary disease, insulin-dependent diabetes mellitus, congestive heart failure, persistent angina, significant peripheral vascular disease, hyperthyroidism.

▼ Avoid sudden discontinuation of propranolol (particularly in patients with hypertension).

▼ Begin with a single test-dose of 20 mg/day in patients for whom there are clinical concerns with hypotension or bradycardia. Increase dose of propranolol by 20 mg/day every 3 days.

▼ Initiate propranolol on a 20 mg tid schedule for patients without cardiovascular or cardiopulmonary disorder.

▼ Increase the dosage of propranolol by 60 mg/day every 3 days.

▼ Increase medication unless the pulse rate is reduced below 50 bpm, or systolic blood pressure is less than 90 mm Hg.

▼ Do not administer medication if severe dizziness, ataxia, or wheezing occurs. Reduce or discontinue propranolol if such symptoms persist.

▼ Increase dose to 12 mg/kg or until aggressive behavior is under control.

▼ Doses of greater than 800 mg are not usually required to control aggressive behavior.

▼ Maintain the patient on the highest dose of propranolol for at least 8 weeks prior to concluding that the patient is not responding to the medication. Some patients, however, may respond rapidly to propranolol.

▼ Utilize concurrent medications with caution. Monitor plasma levels of all antipsychotic and anticonvulsant medications.

Source. Silver and Yudofsky 1987a. Used with permission of the publisher.

fect of β-blocker use (Yudofsky 1992). Finally, because the use of propranolol is associated with a significant increase in plasma levels of thioridazine, which has an absolute dosage ceiling of 800 mg/day, combining these two medications should be avoided whenever possible (Silver et al. 1986).

■ CONCLUSION

Aggressive disorders are common and have serious and far-reaching consequences for our patients with respect to their functioning at home, at work, and in other social settings. When assessing patients who exhibit aggression, clinicians should focus on careful history taking, a thorough physical examination, and relevant laboratory testing to diagnose any medical condition that could underlie and/or aggravate the aggressive symptom.

Although pharmacological intervention may be highly effective in the treatment of aggression, medications for this purpose should be used in the context of a carefully crafted treatment plan involving the full range of biopsychosocial approaches. When medications are used to treat acute aggression, the sedative side effects of antipsychotic agents or benzodiazepines are commonly required. However, prolonged use of neuroleptics or benzodiazepines frequently lead to disabling side effects; therefore, they should be avoided for the treatment of chronic aggression. A wide range of medications are helpful in the prophylaxis of chronic aggression. The underlying etiology of the patient's aggressive symptomatologies guides the choice of the specific pharmacological agent in the treatment of chronic aggression.

■ REFERENCES

Alexander RW, Davis JN, Lefkowitz RJ: Direct identification and characterization of β-adrenergic receptors in rat brain. Nature 258:437–440, 1979

Alpert M, Allan ER, Citrome L, et al: A double-blind, placebo-controlled study of adjunctive nadolol in the management of violent psychiatric patients. Psychopharmacol Bull 28:367–371, 1990

American Psychiatric Association: Diagnostic and Statistical Manual of Mental Disorders, 3rd Edition. Washington, DC, American Psychiatric Association, 1980

American Psychiatric Association: Diagnostic and Statistical Manual of Mental Disorders, 3rd Edition, Revised. Washington, DC, American Psychiatric Association, 1987

American Psychiatric Association: Diagnostic and Statistical Manual of Mental Disorders, 4th Edition. Washington, DC, American Psychiatric Association, 1994

Bareggi SR, Porta M, Selenati A, et al: Homovanillic acid and 5-hydroxyindole-acetic acid in the CSF of patients after a severe head injury, I: lumbar CSF concentration in chronic brain post-traumatic syndromes. Eur Neurol 13:528–544, 1975

Bass JN, Beltis J: Therapeutic effect of fluoxetine on naltrexone-resistant self-injurious behavior in an adolescent with mental retardation. Journal of Child and Adolescent Psychopharmacology 1:331–340, 1991

Bick PA, Hannah AL: Intramuscular lorazepam to restrain violent patients. Lancet 1:206, 1986

Boll TJ: The Halsted-Reitan Neuropsychological Battery, in Handbook of Clinical Neuropsychology. Edited by Filskov SB, Boll TJ. New York, Wiley, 1981, pp 577–607

Brooke MM, Questad KA, Patterson R, et al: Agitation and restlessness after closed head injury: a prospective study of 100 consecutive admissions. Arch Phys Med Rehabil 73:320–323, 1992

Brown GL, Goodwin FK, Ballenger JC, et al: Aggression in humans correlates with cerebrospinal fluid amine metabolites. Psychiatry Res 1:131–139, 1979

Chandler JD, Chandler JE: The prevalence of neuropsychiatric disorders in a nursing home population. J Geriatr Psychiatry Neurol 1:27, 1988

Coccaro EF, Astill JL, Herbert JL, et al: Fluoxetine treatment of impulsive aggression in DSM-III-R personality disorder patients. J Clin Psychopharmacol 10:373–375, 1990

Colenda CC: Buspirone in treatment of agitated demented patients. Lancet 1:1169, 1988

Corrigan PW, Yudofsky SC, Silver JM: Pharmacological and behavioral treatments for aggressive psychiatric inpatients. Hosp Community Psychiatry 44:125–133, 1993

Dale PG: Lithium therapy in aggressive mentally subnormal patients. Br J Psychiatry 137:469–474, 1980

Eichelman BS: Effect of subcortical lesions on shock-induced aggression in the rat following 6-hydroxydopamine administration. Journal of Comparative and Physiologic Psychology 74:331–339, 1971

Eichelman B: Neurochemical and psychopharmacologic aspects of aggressive behavior, in Psychopharmacology: The Third Generation of Progress. Edited by Meltzer HY. New York, Raven, 1987, pp 697–704

Eichelman B, Thoa NB, Ng KY: Facilitated aggression in the rat following 6-hydroxydopamine administration. Physiol Behav 8:1–3, 1972

Elliott FA: The neurology of explosive rage. Practitioner 217:51–59, 1976

Folks DG, King LD, Dowdy SB, et al: Carbamazepine treatment of selective affectively disordered inpatients. Am J Psychiatry 139:115–117, 1982

Freinhar JP, Alvarez WA: Clonazepam treatment of organic brain syndromes in three elderly patients.

J Clin Psychiatry 47:525–526, 1986

Giakas WJ, Seibyl JP, Mazure CM: Valproate in the treatment of temper outbursts. J Clin Psychiatry 51:525, 1990

Gleason RP, Schneider LS: Carbamazepine treatment of agitation in Alzheimer's outpatients refractory to neuroleptics. J Clin Psychiatry 51:115–118, 1990

Golden CJ, Purisch A, Hammeke TA: The Luria-Nebraska Neuropsychological Battery, A Manual for Clinical and Experimental Uses. Lincoln, NE, University of Nebraska Press, 1979

Greendyke RM, Kanter DR: Therapeutic effects of pindolol on behavioral disturbances associated with organic brain disease: a double-blind study. J Clin Psychiatry 47:423–426, 1986

Greendyke RM, Kanter DR, Schuster DB, et al: Propranolol treatment of assaultive patients with organic brain disease: a double-blind crossover, placebo-controlled study. J Nerv Ment Dis 174:290–294, 1986

Gualtieri CT: Buspirone for the behavior problems of patients with organic brain disorders. J Clin Psychopharmacol 11:280–281, 1991

Gualtieri CT, Chandler M, Coons TB, et al: Amantadine: a new clinical profile for traumatic brain injury. Clin Neuropharmacol 12:258–270, 1989

Haas JF, Cope N: Neuropharmacologic management of behavior sequelae in head injury: a case report. Arch Phys Med Rehabil 66:474–474, 1985

Hakoloa HP, Laulumaa VA: Carbamazepine in treatment of violent schizophrenics. Lancet 1:1358, 1982

Hamill RW, Woolf PD, McDonald JV, et al: Catecholamines predict outcome in traumatic brain injury. Ann Neurol 21:438–443, 1987

Hathaway SR, McKinley JC: Minnesota Multiphasic Personality Inventory—2. Minneapolis, MN, University of Minnesota, 1989

Herrera JN, Sramek JJ, Costa JF, et al: High potency neuroleptics and violence in schizophrenics. J Nerv Ment Dis 176:558–561, 1988

Higley JD, Mehlman PT, Taum DM, et al: Cerebrospinal fluid monoamine and adrenal correlates of aggression in free-ranging rhesus monkeys. Arch Gen Psychiatry 49:436–441, 1992

Hornstein A, Seliger G: Cognitive side effects of lithium in closed head injury [letter]. J Neuropsychiatry Clin Neurosci 1:446–447, 1989

Jackson RD, Corrigan JD, Arnett JA: Amitriptyline for agitation in head injury. Arch Phys Med Rehabil 66:180–181, 1985

Keats MM, Mukherjee S: Antiaggressive effect of adjunctive clonazepam in schizophrenia associated with seizure disorder. J Clin Psychiatry 49:117–118, 1988

Kruesi MJP, Hibbs ED, Zahn TP, et al: A 2-year prospective follow-up study of children and adolescents with disruptive behavior disorders: prediction by cerebrospinal fluid 5-hydroxyindoleacetic acid, homovanillic acid, and autonomic measures? Arch Gen Psychiatry 49:429–435, 1992

Leavitt ML, Yudofsky SC, Maroon JC, et al: Effect of intraventricular nadolol infusion on shock-induced aggression in 6-hydroxydopamine-treated rats. J Neuropsychiatry Clin Neurosci 1:167–172, 1989

Leibovici A, Tariot PN: Carbamazepine treatment of agitation associated with dementia. J Geriatr Psychiatry Neurol 1:110–112, 1988

Linnoila VMI, Virkkunen M: Aggression, suicidality, and serotonin. J Clin Psychiatry 53 (10 suppl):46–51, 1992

Luchins DF, Dojka D: Lithium and propranolol in aggression and self-injurious behavior in the mentally retarded. Psychopharmacol Bull 25:372–375, 1989

Mattes JA: Carbamazepine vs propranolol for rage outbursts. Psychopharmacol Bull 24:179–182, 1988

Mattes JA: Valproic acid for nonaffective aggression in the mentally retarded. J Nerv Ment Dis 180:601–602, 1992

Moskowitz AS, Altshuler L: Increased sensitivity to lithium-induced neurotoxicity after stroke: a case report. J Clin Psychopharmacol 11:272–273, 1991

New York State Senate Select Committee on Mental and Physical Handicaps: Violence revisited: a report on traditional indifference in state mental institutions toward assaultive activity. Albany, NY, New York State Senate (Senator James H. Donovan, Chairman), 1977

Oddy M, Caughlan T, Tyerman A, et al: Social adjustment after closed head injury: a further follow-up seven years after injury. J Neurol Neurosurg Psychiatry 44:564–568, 1985

Ovsiew F, Yudofsky SC: Aggression: a neuropsychiatric perspective, in Rage, Power, and Aggression. Edited by Glick RA, Roose SP. New Haven, CT, Yale University Press, 1993, pp 213–230

Pardith K: Violence and the violent patient [Foreword], in Psychiatry Update: American Psychiatric Association Annual Review, Vol 6. Edited by Hales

RE, Frances AJ. Washington, DC, American Psychiatric Press, 1987, pp 447–450

Pinner E, Rich CL: Effects of trazodone on aggressive behavior in seven patients with organic mental disorders. Am J Psychiatry 145:1295–1296, 1988

Rabins PV, Mace NL, Lucas MJ: The impact of dementia on the family. JAMA 248:333–335, 1982

Rao N, Jellinek HM, Woolson DC: Agitation in closed head injury: haloperidol effects on rehabilitation outcome. Arch Phys Med Rehabil 66:30–34, 1985

Ratey JJ, Sovner R, Mikkelsen E, et al: Buspirone therapy for maladaptive behavior and anxiety in developmentally disabled persons. J Clin Psychiatry 50:382–384, 1989

Ratey JJ, Leveroni CL, Miller AC, et al: Low-dose buspirone to treat agitation and maladaptive behavior in brain-injured patients: two case reports. J Clin Psychopharmacol 12:362–364, 1992a

Ratey JJ, Sorgi P, O'Driscoll GA, et al: Nadolol to treat aggression and psychiatric symptomatology in chronic psychiatric inpatients: a double-blind, placebo-controlled study. J Clin Psychiatry 53:41–46, 1992b

Realmuto FM, August GJ, Garfinkel BD: Clinical effect of buspirone in autistic children. J Clin Psychopharmacol 9:122–124, 1989

Reid WH, Balis GU: Evaluation of the violent patient, in Violence and the Violent Patient, in American Psychiatric Association Annual Review, Vol 6. Edited by Hales RE, Francis AJ. Washington, DC, American Psychiatric Press, 1987, pp 491–509

Reid HW, Bollinger MF, Edwards G: Assaults in hospitals. Bull Am Acad Psychiatry Law 13:1–4, 1985

Reisberg B, Borenstein J, Salob SP, et al: Behavioral symptoms in Alzheimer's disease: phenomenology and treatment. J Clin Psychiatry 48 (5 suppl):27, 1987

Sheard MH, Marini JL, Bridges C, et al: The effects of lithium in impulsive aggressive behavior in man. Am J Psychiatry 133:1409–1413, 1976

Silver JM, Yudofsky SC: Aggressive behavior in patients with neuropsychiatric disorders: the scope of the problem. Psychiatric Annals 17(6):367–370, 1987a

Silver JM, Yudofsky SC: Documentation of aggression in the assessment of the violent patient. Psychiatric Annals 17(6):375–384, 1987b

Silver JM, Yudofsky SC: The Overt Aggression Scale: overview and guiding principles. J Neuropsychiatry Clin Neurosci 3 (suppl 1):S22–S29, 1991

Silver JM, Yudofsky SC: Aggressive disorders, in The Neuropsychiatry of Traumatic Brain Injury. Edited by Silver JM, Yudofsky SC, Hales RE. Washington, DC, American Psychiatric Press, 1994, pp 313–353

Silver JM, Yudofsky SC, Kogan M, et al: Elevation of thioridazine plasma levels by propranolol. Am J Psychiatry 143:1290–1292, 1986

Silver JM, Hales RE, Yudofsky SC: Neuropsychiatric aspects of traumatic brain injury, in American Psychiatric Association Press Textbook of Neuropsychiatry, 2nd Edition. Edited by Hales RE, Yudofsky SC. Washington, DC, American Psychiatric Press, 1992, pp 363–395

Szlabowicz JW, Stewart JT: Amitriptyline treatment of agitation associated with anoxic encephalopathy. Arch Phys Med Rehabil 71:612–613, 1990

Tardiff K, Sweillam A: The occurrence of assaultive behavior among chronic psychiatric inpatients. Am J Psychiatry 139:212–215, 1982

Tiller JWG, Dakis JA, Shaw JM: Short-term buspirone treatment in disinhibition with dementia. Lancet 2:510, 1988

Vetro A, Szentistvanyi L, Pallag M, et al: Therapeutic experience with lithium in childhood aggressivity. Pharmacopsychiatry 14:121–127, 1985

Yatham LN, McHale PA: Carbamazepine in the treatment of aggression: a case report and a review of the literature. Acta Psychiatr Scand 78:188–190, 1988

Yudofsky SC: Psychoanalysis, psychopharmacology and the influence of neuropsychiatry. J Neuropsychiatry Clin Neurosci 3:1–5, 1991

Yudofsky SC: β-Blockers and depression: the clinician's dilemma. JAMA 267:1826–1827, 1992

Yudofsky SC, Silver JM, Jackson M, et al: The Overt Aggression Scale: an operationalized rating scale for verbal and physical aggression. Am J Psychiatry 143:35–39, 1986

Yudofsky SC, Silver JM, Schneider SE: Pharmacologic treatment of aggression. Psychiatric Annals 17:397–407, 1987

Yudofsky SC, Silver J, Yudofsky B: Organic personality disorder, explosive type, in Treatment of Psychiatric Disorders: A Task Force Report of the American Psychiatric Association. Washington, DC, American Psychiatric Press, 1989, pp 839–852

Yudofsky SC, Silver JM, Hales RE: Pharmacologic management of aggression in the elderly. J Clin Psychiatry 51 (10 suppl):22–28, 1990

37

Treatment of Personality Disorders

Robert L. Trestman, Ph.D., M.D., Marie deVegvar, M.D., and
Larry J. Siever, M.D.

Although pharmacotherapy has long been a therapeutic mainstay of the major Axis I syndromes, it is a more recent development that psychopharmacology has gained acceptance as a treatment option for severe personality disorders. This shift reflects the fact that personality disorders have historically been explained in terms of psychodynamic-developmental models, which imply that psychotherapy—whether individual, group, or milieu—would be the major or even sole form of treatment. However, it is increasingly appreciated that biological factors may play an important role in the pathogenesis of personality disorders. Further, the etiology of the disorder may not necessarily determine its treatment. Whether symptoms of anxiety or depression evolved from environmental circumstances or from underlying genetic susceptibilities, they may nonetheless be amenable to psychopharmacological treatment. Thus, the clinician working with patients who have personality disorders will need to be aware of the important role pharmacological treatment may play in these disorders.

Pioneering studies of personality disorder patients demonstrated that pharmacological interventions used in the treatment of affective and schizophrenic disorders might be of benefit (Klein 1968; Klein and Greenberg 1967; Liebowitz and Klein 1981; Rifkin et al. 1972a, 1972b). However, years passed before the field made use of these early findings. More recent studies categorizing patients using DSM-III (American Psychiatric Association 1980) or DSM-III-R (American Psychiatric Association 1987) syndromes, in conjunction with work focused around clinical dimensions, suggest that pharmacological intervention may be beneficial in patients with personality disorder for affective symptoms, including affective instability or transient depression, impulsivity-aggression, psychotic-like symptoms or cognitive-perceptual distortions, and anxiety. These results are complemented by evidence implicating both genetic and biological factors in the pathogenesis of these disorders.

A growing body of studies suggest that genetic factors play an important role in the development of normal personality (Goldsmith 1982; Tellegen et al. 1988). Although the heritability of personality disorders have been less extensively studied, twin studies (Torgersen 1984), adoptive studies (Cloninger et al. 1978), and family studies (Siever et al. 1990; Silverman et al. 1991) suggest that underlying dimensions of personality disorder may be heritable. Developmental studies demonstrate a long-term continuity of behavioral traits such as fearfulness or shyness, which may have specific psychophysiological correlates (Kagan et al. 1988). Comparable studies in primates also suggest behavioral and biological continuity for behavioral dimensions such as aggression or affective sensitivity to separation (Suomi 1991). Biological correlates of personality disorder dimensions in adults are currently under investigation.

In this chapter, we discuss issues of pharmacotherapy for personality disorder patients. Appropriate selection and assessment of patients for pharmacotherapy are initially addressed, as are issues of initiating and maintaining psychopharmacological treatment in this population. Subsequent sections focus on specific syndromes or behavioral dimensions that have received research interest sufficient to tentatively suggest appropriate psychopharmacological intervention. However, many Axis II syndromes do not lend themselves to pharmacological treatment and have not been the focus of controlled treatment studies (e.g., schizoid, narcissistic, histrionic, dependent, and obsessive-compulsive personality disorders); therefore, they are not discussed here.

Further, it is important to note that, although we address the pharmacological treatment of personality disorders, a wide array of psychotherapies exist and are in use. Discussions of the rational selection, use, and efficacy of these therapies, however, are beyond the scope of this chapter.

■ ASSESSMENT FOR TREATMENT

Before considering psychopharmacological treatment of a patient for signs and symptoms of a presumed personality disorder, a formal assessment should be undertaken to evaluate the differential diagnosis and possible complicating medical factors. A proposed sequence for this assessment includes a detailed psychiatric history, substance abuse history, family history, medical history, and physical and laboratory examination. Specific issues of differential diagnosis will be addressed in subsequent sections.

■ Psychiatric History

Now that effective interventions and therapeutics exist for the treatment of many signs and symptoms of psychiatric illness, differential diagnosis becomes increasingly important. Assessment of psychiatric symptomatology, clinical contacts, medication history, and specific response to each of the psychotherapeutic and psychopharmacological interventions are basic to all psychiatric diagnosis and critical to the evaluation of this patient population, many of whom will present with a bewildering array of problems and complaints.

The initial discrimination to be made is usually between Axis I and Axis II diagnoses. In general, Axis I disorders such as schizophrenia, major depression, and bipolar disorder take precedence in the differential diagnosis and treatment priority. For example, if bipolar disorder, Type I, is diagnosed, it is usually the initial target of treatment. When the bipolar disorder is optimally treated, residual personality disorder disturbances may then appropriately be addressed.

In the process of obtaining a detailed past and present psychiatric history, careful attention must be paid not only to the signs and symptoms of psychiatric illness per se, but also to the pattern and timing of their presentation. One explicit example is the presence of impulsive-aggressive behavior, sexual promiscuity, and labile affect. If this symptom cluster is stable over time and has been present since adolescence, Cluster B personality disorders might head the differential list. However, if the symptoms are episodic and associated with increased energy and decreased sleep, Axis I disorders such as bipolar disorder (mania) or organic mental disorder associated with substance intoxication or withdrawal become more likely as primary diagnoses.

Medication history is critical in this assessment. Optimally, for each psychotropic medication taken, the target symptoms, dose, duration, and efficacy should be determined. Given the frequent ambiguity of the behavioral, affective, and cognitive complaints, it is particularly important to operationally define each of the target symptoms assessed.

■ Interviewing of Family Members

Because of the nature of personality disorder diagnoses, it is frequently difficult for this patient population in particular to adequately describe the extent and severity of interpersonal difficulties. It is therefore important to interview family members—with the knowledge and permission of the patient—to improve the data base from which therapeutic interventions will be made. The information to be elicited from the family members is intended to elaborate the nature, extent, and severity of the intra- and interpersonal disturbances experienced by the patient.

■ Substance Abuse and Dependence History

Drug and alcohol use must be carefully assessed and monitored. Before attempting to diagnose and treat personality disorders, substance abuse and/or dependence should be determined and, where found, treated. Symptoms such as affective lability, impulsivity, and aggression that might otherwise be ascribed to personality disorder may remit with the resolution of substance abuse and dependence.

Family History

A thorough family history is of the utmost importance, because it may suggest the existence of biological vulnerabilities to mood disorders, drug and alcohol abuse, and perhaps personality disorders. Even if the patient is unaware of psychiatric illness in the family, it may prove valuable to speak with family members directly (again, with the permission of the patient) to more fully evaluate the potential presence of psychiatric illness in the patient's relatives.

Medical History

There are many medical illnesses that may present as psychiatric illness. Examples include endocrine, neurological, rheumatological, and metabolic disorders that have been reviewed elsewhere (Horvath et al. 1989). Further, medications prescribed for the treatment of other disorders may have cognitive, behavioral, or affective consequences. One common example is the use of steroids in the treatment of severe asthma, chronic obstructive pulmonary disease, or systemic lupus erythematosus. Some of the potential complications arising from the use of high-dose steroids may include agitation, aggressive behavior, and affective lability. Therefore, a careful medical history and review of all medications taken (including nonpsychiatric medications) contributes to the overall accuracy of the diagnostic assessment.

Physical and Laboratory Examinations

A complete physical examination and routine laboratory studies—including blood counts and chemistries, thyroid function tests, serology (for syphilis and human immunodeficiency virus [HIV]), and computed tomography (CT) or magnetic resonance imaging (MRI) of the head, if indicated—should be obtained. Clinical indications should be used to guide the clinician in selecting further tests. If an individual presents with episodic impulsivity and aggression, an electroencephalogram (EEG) might be considered in conjunction with structural imaging of the brain (CT or MRI); antibody testing might also be conducted if autoimmune diseases, such as systemic lupus erythematosus, are a possibility.

If treatment of underlying conditions may not completely correct the disorder, it might at least ameliorate the symptoms. Only when the clinician is convinced that 1) no other treatable physical illness is present and 2) substance abuse and dependence diagnoses are controlled should personality disorder diagnoses be made and pharmacological interventions for them be initiated.

Treatment Initiation and Management of Toxic Effects

When beginning any psychotropic medication in a patient diagnosed with a personality disorder, it is valuable to discuss the treatment in detail with the patient and, where possible, the patient's family. Specific issues to be addressed include 1) clinician-patient agreement about the existence of a problem and the desirability of treating that problem; 2) discussion of the logic of the medication selection, its target symptoms, and potential toxic effects; and 3) an objective procedure for the assessment of treatment progress, or lack thereof.

All medications have predictable dose-dependent toxic effects and idiosyncratic toxic effects. To enhance the probability of a successful medication trial, it is important to attempt to minimize or avoid toxic effects initially. Given the frequent sensitivity to medication side or toxic effects in personality disorder patients and the chronic nature of the disturbances to be treated, a recommended treatment algorithm is to begin with a minimal dose of medication, and incrementally and gradually increase to a therapeutic level. Operationally, the patient might be started with half the dose and half the rate of dosage increase that might be used in an Axis I condition. If toxic effects become manifest, they would then be managed as normal standards of care dictate, with discontinuation, dose reduction, or symptomatic treatment as indicated.

In this chapter, we discuss management of toxicity issues only as they relate specifically to personality disorder patients. General management of toxic effects is beyond the scope of this chapter and is addressed elsewhere in this volume.

■ Assessment of Response

With any patient, it is important to define desired target symptoms and to operationalize the outcome measures. Although this may sound more like a research paradigm than a clinical treatment plan, this approach to the treatment of behavioral, cognitive, anxiety, and/or affective symptoms in personality disorder patients will reduce the risk of inappropriate expectations, ambiguous results, and power struggles between patient and clinician. For example, if the target symptom is reduction of affective instability, a simple 10-cm visual analog scale might be employed: one end might be behaviorally anchored with "most erratic, unstable emotions I have ever experienced," whereas the other might be anchored with "most stable I have ever experienced my emotions to be." The patient would place a mark on this scale to describe his or her experience for the preceding week at baseline and at each subsequent office visit. This provides the clinician with an easy way to objectively chart target symptom change, and the patient with objective criteria to justify either continuation of medication if improvement is noted, or alteration of the medication dose or selection if inadequate progress is seen.

■ Maintenance and Monitoring

Many of the symptoms in personality disorder patients that are a target for pharmacotherapy (such as affective lability or impulsivity) are themselves inconstant. It may then be necessary for the clinician to be willingly to work with the patient to modify the dosing of medications appropriately: increasing selected medications at times of stress, reducing others at times that toxic side effects outweigh benefits.

Monitoring blood levels of medications, where available, may be done to assure appropriate adherence to the medication regimen and to confirm that therapeutic levels are being maintained. As with any medication, where indicated by normal standards of care, periodic monitoring of blood chemistry, electrocardiography, and hematological indices should be performed.

■ Treatment Resistance

Given that, by definition, interpersonal relationships are disturbed in personality disorder patients, it is likely that these disturbances will intrude upon the therapeutic relationship. It is important to realize that these intrusions are by no means limited to psychotherapy. Issues involving adherence to a prescribed medication regimen, consistently and accurately reporting missed doses or side effects, and a willingness to discuss potential problems with medication all may evolve in the psychopharmacological management of any individual patient. It is essential, therefore, for the psychiatrist to be sensitive to these issues and to openly discuss them with the patient. Such discussions should be held at the outset of treatment and at appropriate intervals so that clinician and patient may assure each other of concern on the clinician's part and cooperation and collaboration on the patient's part.

■ SPECIFIC SYNDROMAL TREATMENT

Not all personality disorder syndromes have received psychopharmacological research attention. Indeed, even the most carefully studied of the syndromes is lacking in adequate numbers of well-defined, full-scale, placebo-controlled double-blind studies. What follows are discussions of the psychobiology and psychopharmacological treatment of syndromes that, in our opinion, have received enough attention to support even tentative psychopharmacological treatment recommendations.

■ ECCENTRIC PERSONALITY DISORDERS: SCHIZOTYPAL PERSONALITY DISORDER

A central characteristic of schizotypal personality disorder (SPD) is a dysfunction in perceptual and/or cognitive organization that may be reflected in the impairment of attentional and selective attentional processes. This dysfunction may be expressed in a variety of signs and symptoms, including odd speech; magical thinking; ideas of reference; fleeting perceptual distortions (illusions, transient auditory hallucinations); compromised interpersonal relationships (in which normal motivations of others may be misconstrued); and suspiciousness that may episodically become paranoia (American Psychiatric Association 1987).

Because of these cognitive-perceptual aberrations, patients may experience a great deal of social anxiety. They may be unable to share a common worldview with others and may become "loners," only minimally interacting with those outside of their immediate family. This social isolation may be likened to one of the "negative" or deficit-like symptoms of schizophrenia.

The concept of SPD as a schizophrenia-related disorder or a schizophrenia spectrum disorder is gaining support from several lines of research (Siever and Davis 1991). There is evidence of a genetic association between schizophrenia and SPD (Silverman et al. 1986, 1993; Thaker et al. 1993). In common with schizophrenic patients, SPD patients demonstrate neuropsychological abnormalities, as well as impairment in attention and information processing, in auditory event-related potentials, and in smooth pursuit eye movement (Siever et al. 1990, 1993b). Plasma homovanillic acid (HVA), a peripheral index of dopaminergic activity, is associated with psychosis in patients with schizophrenia (Davidson and Davis 1988; Davis et al. 1985). Preliminary studies with SPD patients show higher concentrations of cerebrospinal fluid (CSF) and plasma HVA in schizotypal patients compared with control subjects (Siever et al. 1991, 1993a), and a correlation between the number of psychotic-like symptoms and the plasma and CSF concentrations of HVA (Siever et al. 1991, 1993a). Furthermore, increases in CSF or plasma HVA might be a predictor of antipsychotic response, a possibility requiring further investigation (Soloff et al. 1994).

■ Differential Diagnoses

Other diagnoses to be considered in the differential include schizophrenia, residual schizophrenia, and the interictal personality sometimes associated with temporal lobe epilepsy (TLE). It is also important to consider the social context of the patient. The patient may come from a culture in which superstitiousness and forms of magical thinking are accepted; if so, it must be determined that the signs and symptoms go beyond that person's cultural norms. Interviews with family members may help in making this distinction.

■ Treatment Selection

Antipsychotics. Low-dose antipsychotic medications have received the most attention in studies con-

ducted over the past two decades with personality disorder patients. In one early open-label study, patients ($N = 120$) with several DSM-II (American Psychiatric Association 1968) personality disorder diagnoses (i.e., borderline, schizoid, paranoid, obsessive-compulsive, hysterical) were treated with an average dose of 3 mg qd of pimozide (Reyntjens 1972). Results demonstrated global improvement in 69% ($n = 83$) of the group (Reyntjens 1972). Similar results were obtained in another early study that used mesoridazine (Barnes 1977). Both studies concluded that antipsychotics were of benefit for the treatment of cognitive disorganization in these patients.

Seventeen SPD patients were treated with haloperidol (maximum 12 mg qd) in a 6-week open-label study (Hymowitz et al. 1986). Mild to moderate improvement in target symptoms of social isolation, odd communication, and ideas of reference were observed in the 50% of patients who remained in the study. This high attrition rate speaks to the intolerance of, and sensitivity to, side effects in this patient population.

Low doses of thiothixene (mean dose 9 mg qd) or haloperidol (mean dose 3 mg qd) were given in a blinded comparison study of 52 patients with histories of recent transient psychotic episodes who met DSM-III-R borderline personality disorder (BPD) or SPD criteria (Serban and Siegel 1984). Eighty-four percent of the patients were noted to be moderately to markedly improved at 3 months follow-up, with decreases in derealization, paranoid ideation, anxiety, and depression.

In a 12-week double-blind placebo-controlled study, 50 BPD or SPD patients were treated with thiothixene (mean dose 8.7 mg qd) (Goldberg et al. 1986). Significant decreases were observed in measures of illusions, psychoticism, phobic anxiety, and ideas of reference; depressive symptoms were unaffected, and there was no improvement noted in measures of global functioning.

Although these results appear promising, it should be kept in mind that all but one of these studies are uncontrolled, and the single double-blind placebo-controlled study (Goldberg et al. 1986) used a heterogeneous sample. Furthermore, there is no evidence that any given agent or class of antipsychotic agent is more effective than another. At this time, medication selection must be made on the basis of expected side-effect profile at the minimum effective dose.

In sum, there is preliminary evidence that low doses of antipsychotic medication (1–2 mg qd of haloperidol equivalent) are effective in at least temporarily reducing or relieving the symptoms of cognitive and perceptual dysfunction in personality disorder patients. Because there are no studies of which we are aware that have looked at long-term chronic use of antipsychotic medications in SPD or related personality disorder patients, no guidelines grounded in research may be proposed. Clinical caution, coupled with concerns for the development of tardive dyskinesia and dystonia, argue that if antipsychotic medications are to be used in this population, they should be administered for short-term use (i.e., months) with subsequent medication withdrawal (if clinically tolerated) and reassessment.

Clinical trials are needed in this area to evaluate 1) efficacy of antipsychotics versus antidepressants versus placebo, 2) optimal dosing, 3) treatment duration, and 4) risk-benefit ratios. Furthermore, with the advent of new antipsychotic medications that are mixed serotonergic and dopamine D_2 antagonists with putatively minimal hematological risk (e.g., risperidone), improved treatment of the deficit-like symptoms and a reduced risk of tardive dyskinesia or dystonia may be possible.

■ Treatment Initiation

It is recommended that antipsychotic medication in this population be started at the level of 1 mg qd or less of haloperidol equivalent. After 1–2 weeks, if no untoward effects emerge, this may be increased to a treatment dose of 2 mg qd of haloperidol equivalent. Before initiating treatment, it is advisable to document any evidence of dyskinesias or dystonias at baseline to determine if any subsequent changes occur.

■ Management of Side Effects

At low antipsychotic doses, minimal side effects are expected. However, akathisia or dystonia and/or dyskinesia are possible. These would be treated as usual. Psychiatrists should periodically assess patients for occurrence of, or change in, dyskinesia or dystonia.

■ Assessment of Response

Beyond global assessment of functioning, target symptoms may be operationalized and followed at each visit to determine treatment efficacy. Although commonly conducted during an unstructured clinical interview, this may also be done with relevant sections of brief standardized instruments (e.g., the Brief Psychiatric Rating Scale [BPRS; Overall and Gorham 1962]) or with patient-specific visual analogue scales as described previously.

■ Treatment Resistance

Some SPD patients are uncomfortable even on low doses of antipsychotic medication, primarily because of behavioral toxicity: dysphoria or a worsening of some of the deficit-like symptoms. If such symptoms arise in the context of otherwise successful pharmacotherapy, the psychiatrist should consider reducing the dose of antipsychotic to the lowest effective level and initiating supportive psychotherapy. If the symptoms persist and the benefit of the antipsychotic argues against discontinuation, a trial with an antidepressant may be considered.

■ IMPULSIVE AND AFFECTIVELY UNSTABLE PERSONALITY DISORDERS: BORDERLINE PERSONALITY DISORDER

The diagnosis of BPD is defined in DSM-III-R as "a pervasive pattern of instability of mood, interpersonal relationships, and self-image," (p. 347) and characterized by criteria that include potentially self-damaging impulsivity, inappropriate or uncontrolled anger, recurrent suicidal threats or gestures, and physically self-damaging acts. Impulsivity-aggression is also characteristic of other personality disorders, although it is expressed somewhat differently in each. For example, in antisocial personality disorder, a disregard for social norms coupled with impulsive aggression may lead to behaviors such as lying, stealing, and destruction of property. Impulsivity-aggression may also play a part in the low frustration tolerance of the histrionic patient and in the rage of the narcissistic patient in response to criticism. This suggests that impulsivity-aggression may be a dimension of behavior that is not restricted to a single psychiatric diagnosis but may occur in both the Cluster B personality disorders and in certain Axis I disorders as well (i.e., intermittent explosive disorder, bipolar disorder—manic type, and conduct disorder).

Serotonin (5-HT) is thought to be a modulatory neurotransmitter with inhibitory effects on a variety of functions that include mood, arousal, cognition, and feeding behavior. There is evidence of an association between increased aggression toward self and/or others and reduced serotonergic function. Support for this relationship comes from a convergence of studies using serotonergic markers, including 5-hydroxyindoleacetic acid (5-HIAA) in CSF (Brown et al. 1982; Linnoila et al. 1983), platelet imipramine binding and receptor sites (Marazziti et al. 1989; Meltzer and Arora 1986), human autopsy studies of metabolites and receptors (Arango et al. 1990; Mann and Arango 1992), and neuroendocrine challenge studies (Coccaro et al. 1988). For example, "net" serotonergic functioning may be measured by the prolactin (PRL) response to fenfluramine, a serotonin-releasing–uptake inhibiting agent. A decreased PRL response to fenfluramine reflects diminished serotonergic function. One study examined 45 patients with personality disorder and/or affective disorder and found that reduced PRL responses to fenfluramine correlated with measures of assault, irritability, and motoric impulsivity in patients with personality disorders, and with suicidal behavior in all patients (Coccaro et al. 1988).

Another key aspect of BPD is affective instability, characterized as rapid, exaggerated shifts in affect in response to emotionally charged environmental stimuli such as criticism, separation from a significant person, or frustration (American Psychiatric Association 1987; Siever and Davis 1991). Affective instability may impair the ability to maintain a stable sense of self and thus disrupt interpersonal relationships. The inability to consistently modulate these mood shifts may also impair learning and the development of cognitive processes, as affective states may influence state-dependent learning (Bartlett and Santruck 1979), and selective memory may be the result of inadequate memory storage and recall. For example, the intense rage of a BPD patient during an argument with a friend may distort the memory of the event to the degree that the patient sees the friend as "all bad" (Kalus and Siever 1993).

To date, there is no definitive biological correlate of affective instability in personality disorders. However, because it is an enduring pattern of behavior, it is likely correlated with a trait abnormality (Siever and Davis 1991). There is evidence of an increased prevalence of affectively labile subjects in the first-degree relatives of BPD patients, suggesting a heritable component to the dimensional characteristic (Silverman et al. 1991). Some of our preliminary studies demonstrate that personality disorder patients with affective instability have a heightened depressive response to the acetylcholinesterase inhibitor physostigmine when compared with personality disorder patients without this dimensional characteristic. These findings suggest that the cholinergic system may play a role in the modulation of affective instability in patients with personality disorder (Steinberg et al. 1994).

The noradrenergic system may also play a part in the regulation of affective instability. One study of compulsive gamblers, for example, observed an increase in noradrenergic function associated with extroversion (Roy et al. 1989). In a preliminary study, we examined 31 patients who met DSM-III criteria for personality disorder and found positive correlations between increased measures of noradrenergic function and measures of irritability and verbal hostility (Trestman et al. 1993). Psychopharmacological interventions might therefore logically target serotonergic or catecholaminergic systems in an attempt to treat BPD patients who are impulsive, aggressive, or affectively labile.

◼ Differential Diagnoses of Impulsivity

Other diagnoses to consider in the differential include the Axis I impulse dyscontrol disorders; bipolar disorder, rapid cycling or mixed subtypes; and organic syndromes secondary to epilepsy, trauma, or substance abuse. Although impulsive aggression associated with TLE is often mentioned in the differential, it is uncommonly the sole presenting symptom and is most often a postictal or interictal phenomenon (Fenwick 1989; Treiman 1991).

◼ Differential Diagnoses of Affective Lability

Clinically, it is important to distinguish affective lability from a major mood disorder such as major depression or rapid-cycling bipolar disorder. The diagnosis of major mood disorder is further complicated by the potential presence of comorbid atypical depression, or of hysteroid dysphoria (Liebowitz and Klein 1981) in personality disorder patients with affective lability.

Atypical depression is not uncommon in personality disorder patients with affective lability and is characterized by dysphoria with prominent mood reactivity, anxiety, rejection hypersensitivity, and markedly decreased energy (sometimes described as "leaden paralysis"). Other features of this disorder include hypersomnia and hyperphagia (especially carbohydrate craving or binge-eating). It is potentially valuable to probe for these symptoms during the initial evaluation, because there is growing evidence of the benefits of monoamine oxidase inhibitors (MAOIs) for atypical depressive features (Liebowitz et al. 1984).

Substance abuse, intoxication, and withdrawal syndromes may also present initially with affective lability, as may connective tissue disorders such as systemic lupus erythematosus, infectious diseases such as HIV-associated encephalopathy, or neurological disorders such as multiple sclerosis or the dementias.

■ Treatment Selection

Serotonin reuptake inhibitors. The serotonin reuptake inhibitor fluoxetine has been used in several studies with BPD patients. Although many of the studies are preliminary, have small sample sizes, or are not double-blind studies, the general results seem to support the efficacy of fluoxetine in BPD patients in a nonspecific manner, or for symptoms of impulsive aggression or affective instability. Twelve patients with BPD were treated in an open-label trial with fluoxetine in doses ranging from 5–40 mg qd (Norden 1989). The patients had a variety of Axis I diagnoses, but none met criteria for a current major depressive episode. Using a clinical global impression rating, 75% of the patients were rated very much improved or much improved and the remaining 25% were rated as moderately improved (Norden et al. 1989). It is interesting to note that, in contrast to the treatment of major depression with an expected response time of 3 weeks or more, patients in this treatment study of impulsive aggression improved within 1 week of treatment. Given the absence of a placebo washout period, it is possible that the results may in part be due to placebo response. Two other small open-label studies have also suggested that fluoxetine may specifically reduce symptoms of impulsivity or aggression in BPD patients (Coccaro et al. 1990; Cornelius et al. 1991).

Twenty-two patients who met DSM-III criteria for BPD and/or SPD were treated in an open-label trial

of fluoxetine (12 weeks duration, 80 mg qd) (Markovitz et al. 1991). There were significant decreases in both affective and impulsive symptoms and the frequency of self-mutilation; self-injurious behavior did not decrease significantly until 9 weeks into the trial. Given the high dosing schedule of 80 mg qd, the delayed response is unlikely attributable to an "underdosing" effect and raises the possibility that the full effects of the drug, regardless of dose, may not be apparent until 9 weeks or longer. In addition, the presence or absence of depression did not appear to influence the outcome with regard to impulsive aggressive behavior, suggesting the possibility of a differential effect of fluoxetine on depression and on impulsive-aggressive behavior.

Twenty-two BPD symptomatic volunteer subjects who did not have a history of suicidal behavior demonstrated significant reductions in impulsive aggressive behavior, irritability, and anger in a 12-week double-blind placebo-controlled study (Salzman et al. 1992) of fluoxetine. An analysis of covariance demonstrated significant decreases in anger that did not correlate with depression scores, a finding consistent with other studies (Coccaro et al. 1990; Markovitz et al. 1991). Further, a preliminary study of patients with BPD suggested that fluoxetine may decrease affective lability per se (Teicher et al. 1989).

Given these findings, there is tentative evidence that fluoxetine may be effective for the treatment of BPD patients, both in terms of reducing severity of global symptomatology and with regard to reducing severity of impulsive aggression and affective instability. More double-blind placebo-controlled studies that are well controlled are needed to confirm these findings and to further investigate optimal dosing strategy, appropriate length of the treatment trial, and potential utility of monitoring fluoxetine serum levels. Overall, fluoxetine would seem a reasonable first choice for the treatment of impulsive aggressive behavior, because it is relatively safe in overdose and may also treat depression and affective lability. Treatment trials have not as yet been conducted with the newer alternative selective serotonin reuptake inhibitors (SSRIs) sertraline and paroxetine. Such trials may prove these agents to be useful alternatives to fluoxetine, given the differing pharmacokinetics and pharmacodynamics of these agents.

Tricyclic antidepressants. Studies conducted with BPD patients on tricyclic antidepressants (TCAs) have generally observed a poor response to treatment (Cole et al. 1984; Soloff et al. 1986a, 1986b, 1989). Coupled with the lethal potential of overdose and the anticholinergic toxicity of these medications, TCAs are not generally recommended for the treatment of BPD patients.

Monoamine oxidase inhibitors. MAOIs are a class of antidepressants that stabilize the noradrenergic system (Cowdry and Gardner 1982; Liebowitz and Klein 1981). One relevant open-label study targeted the treatment of hysteroid dysphoria, a disorder with characteristics of affective lability and rejection sensitivity similar to those seen in BPD patients (Liebowitz and Klein 1981). Three months of open-label treatment with phenelzine was followed with randomization to continued drug or placebo. The results of this preliminary study ($N = 11$) marginally supported the use of MAOIs in this condition: 40% on active medication relapsed, compared with 66% on placebo (Liebowitz and Klein 1981). Consistent with these early findings, a more recent treatment trial of BPD (Cowdry and Gardner 1988) demonstrated that patients on tranylcypromine, even those without current major depression, significantly improved with regard to the target symptoms of impulsivity and affective lability. Furthermore, one study has found that phenylzine may be more effective in the treatment of atypical depression when patients have a comorbid diagnosis of BPD (Parsons et al. 1989).

Given the available (if limited) evidence of MAOI efficacy, one of the practical concerns limiting their more widespread use is the risk of a hypertensive crisis, particularly in patients who may also have difficulties with impulse regulation and therefore be liable to overdose. Reversible inhibitors of MAO-A, which are less likely to induce a hypertensive crisis, may therefore provide an excellent alternative if proven to be as effective as the present nonselective MAOIs for the treatment of affective instability (Liebowitz et al. 1990).

Lithium carbonate. Beyond its role in the treatment of bipolar disorder, lithium may treat affective lability (Van der Kolk 1986), regardless of the syndrome per se. Further, lithium may be effective in decreasing impulsivity in general (Shader et al. 1974), impulsivity associated with affective lability (Rifkin et al. 1972a), and episodic violence, especially in antisocial personality disorder patients (Schiff et al.

1982). Sixty-six impulsive and aggressive prison inmates were treated with lithium carbonate for 3 months in a double-blind placebo-controlled study, and a significant reduction in the number of aggressive acts was observed (Sheard et al. 1976). The anti-aggressive effects of lithium carbonate may be due to its enhancement of serotonergic postsynaptic receptors and/or its possible inhibition of catecholaminergic function (Coccaro et al. 1990), and a decrease in mood lability often associated with impulsivity. More double-blind placebo-controlled studies of patients with a full range of impulsive-aggressive personality disorders would be useful at this time. It may also prove useful to compare the efficacy of fluoxetine and lithium, and (in a controlled study) to assess the efficacy of combination therapy in otherwise treatment refractory patients.

Although clearly documented periods of hypomania or major depressive disorder may not be evident in a given patient, if periods of dysthymia or cyclothymia are noted, a trial of lithium may also be useful (Akiskal 1981; Rifkin et al. 1972b). Lithium carbonate has also been shown to have mood-stabilizing effects in patients with "emotionally unstable personality disorder," a diagnosis characterized by significant affective lability (Rifkin et al. 1972b). An additional indication for the use of lithium may be the presence of bipolar disorder in a first-degree relative of a patient with affective lability.

Anticonvulsants. The presence of mood lability, rage episodes, brief psychotic disturbances, and soft neurological signs in some BPD patients suggested similarities with TLE (despite a normal EEG) and led to trials of anticonvulsants (Gardner and Cowdry 1986a; Klein and Greenberg 1967). One comprehensive double-blind placebo-controlled study conducted over 6 weeks with a crossover design was undertaken to examine the effects of four medications, including carbamazepine, in 16 female patients who met DSM-III-R criteria for BPD (Cowdry and Gardner 1988). Target symptoms included impulsive self-injurious behavior and severe dysphoria. The average dose of carbamazepine was 820 mg qd and those receiving the medication showed a significant decrease in behavioral dyscontrol. Reduction of impulsive aggressive behavior was associated with the capacity to delay action and "reflect." Although the mechanism of action is not yet understood, this study, along with other preliminary trials (Gardner and Cowdry 1986a; Luchins 1984), suggests that carbamazepine may be useful (either alone or as an adjunct to a serotonin reuptake inhibitor) for the control of impulsive aggression.

The anticonvulsant medication carbamazepine may also be effective in stabilizing mood in nonbipolar patients, although its most significant effect has been demonstrated with behavioral dyscontrol (Cowdry and Gardner 1988). Valproic acid—though not specifically studied in this population—is also likely to be similarly effective and may prove to be a viable alternative to carbamezepine in selected BPD patients.

Antipsychotics. A number of studies, both uncontrolled (Brinkley et al. 1979) and placebo-controlled (Cowdry and Garner 1988), have suggested the general benefits of low-dose antipsychotics in individuals with impulsivity, depression, paranoid, and schizotypal features and rejection sensitivity. Five BPD patients with histories of recent transient stress-induced psychotic episodes were treated with minimal doses of high-potency antipsychotics in a preliminary, open-label study. Significant decreases in psychotic-like and affective symptoms were reported (Brinkley et al. 1979).

BPD patients (N = 80) were treated with loxapine (mean 14 mg qd) versus chlorpromazine (mean dose 110 mg qd) in a 6-week double-blind protocol. A decrease in suspiciousness, hostility, and anxiety, as well as improvement in depressed mood, was reported with both agents (Leone 1982). One double-blind placebo-controlled study using a crossover design examined the effects of carbamazepine (mean dose 820 mg qd), tranylcypromine (mean dose 40 mg qd), trifluoperazine (mean dose 7.8 mg qd), and alprazolam (mean dose 4.7 mg qd) on 16 patients who met DSM-III criteria for BPD (Cowdry and Garner 1988). Although trifluoperazine was not well-tolerated, the outcome was moderately favorable: objective ratings noted improvement in suicidality and anxiety.

A significant improvement in hostility, depression, and cognitive-perceptual disturbances was observed in a 12-week thioridazine (mean dose 92 mg qd) open-label study of 11 patients who met DSM-III-R criteria for BPD (Teicher et al. 1989). Six of the 11 patients who completed the study showed decreased symptomatology on the impulse action patterns and psychosis subscales of the Diagnostic

Interview for BPD. In addition, there was improvement in anxiety, interpersonal sensitivity, and paranoid ideation. However, it is interesting to note that, contrary to expectations, the three individuals who met many schizoid and schizotypal criteria became severely depressed and had to discontinue the study. This antipsychotic-induced dysphoria seems, on the basis of clinical experience, to occur more often in patients with SPD or related diagnoses, in contrast to an antidepressant-like effect observed in BPD patients.

Low-dose antipsychotics, in sum, appear potentially useful in the treatment of BPD patients who are more severely impaired, regardless of specific symptoms (Goldberg et al. 1986; Soloff et al. 1986a). It must be kept in mind, however, that these agents have been tested in BPD patients only for relatively short periods (i.e., less than 4 months). Because of the potential for tardive dyskinesia, it may be most prudent to minimize both dose and duration of antipsychotic treatment in BPD patients. Also, because of common antipsychotic side effects, compliance is often a problem. As with most medications, a careful risk-benefit assessment must be made for the specific indication and individual being treated.

Stimulants. One case report using methylphenidate has described improvement of mood lability and impulsivity in an adult diagnosed as having BPD with comorbid attention-deficit disorder (Hooberman and Stern 1984). One finding associated with BPD improvement on tranylcypromine (an MAOI with psychostimulant actions) is a history of childhood attention-deficit hyperactivity disorder (ADHD; Cowdry and Gardner 1988). Furthermore, there is evidence that some patients with antisocial personality disorder have certain electrophysiological responses, such as decreased galvanic skin response and diminished cortical EEG response to novel stimuli (Bloomingdale and Bloomingdale 1988). Electrophysiological findings of a similar nature have been found in ADHD children. This could be a biological correlate of adult residual ADHD, which may be characterized by impulsivity, irritability, mood lability, difficulty focusing, and subtle learning disabilities. Stimulants have proven effective in treating some of these symptoms (Wender et al. 1981).

Although psychostimulants have received only minimal research attention, they may find a useful role in the treatment of impulsive aggression and affective lability. Psychostimulants such as methylphenidate may be considered for the treatment of carefully selected adult BPD patients with well-documented cases of childhood ADHD and with no significant history of drug or alcohol dependence. Carefully controlled studies are needed to evaluate this possibility.

Benzodiazepines. Benzodiazepines have received little controlled attention in the treatment of BPD. One early report with alprazolam in 3 male BPD patients (average dose 2.7 mg qd) suggested a general improvement in overall functioning (Faltus 1984). In a subsequent double-blind placebo-controlled study, 7 of 12 patients (58%) developed serious behavioral dyscontrol (self-mutilation, drug overdoses, aggression) on alprazolam compared with 1 of 12 on placebo (Gardner and Cowdry 1986b). Given the potential dyscontrol problem and the risk of drug dependency, therapy with alprazolam or other benzodiazepines is not indicated at present in this population.

■ Treatment Initiation

Because of the myriad symptoms that BPD patients may present, it is important that the clinician discuss with the patient what symptoms are being targeted with medication. It may also help the patient cooperate fully with treatment if 1) it is specified that only limited success from psychopharmacological intervention is expected, and 2) a logical progression of medication interventions will be made, based on the responses of the individual to treatment.

■ Assessment of Response

Given that several symptoms may be targeted, it will benefit both patient and clinician to objectively define each of the target symptoms with either visual analogue scales or structured instruments (self-report or interview). Each symptom should be assessed for severity at baseline and at each session. It may also be valuable to record a clinical global impression at these same visits, to balance general progress with symptom-specific progress.

■ Treatment Resistance

BPD patients may often resist treatment, intentionally or unintentionally. As many (if not all) of the targeted

symptoms fluctuate, patients may benefit from specific psychoeducation as to the nature of the disturbances and the expected response to treatment. This may help them tolerate the occasional problems without discontinuing treatment.

■ ANXIOUS PERSONALITY DISORDERS: AVOIDANT PERSONALITY DISORDER

Anxiety is an alerting signal that warns of threats to safety, but it can also become maladaptive and interfere with productivity and well-being. It may be reflected in personality characteristics such as shyness, rejection sensitivity, and a diminished ability to perceive and take advantage of positive opportunities. Physiological manifestations include restlessness, wringing of hands, pacing, diaphoresis, palpitations, and gastrointestinal disturbances. Cognitively, anxiety may impair concentration and lead to confusion and perceptual distortion.

One study examined shyness, a trait that appears to be rather stable during childhood development. As youngsters, shy toddlers avoid strangers; as adults, they continued to be uncomfortable and anxious in new situations and social gatherings (Kagan et al. 1988). It would seem that people who have a low set point for physiological arousal in anticipation of threatening consequences might develop avoidant behavior (Kalus and Siever 1993). Although anxiety is a prominent feature of several Axis I disorders (i.e., social phobia, anxiety disorders, obsessive-compulsive disorder [OCD], hyperarousal as a concomitant of a low stimulation threshold) may also contribute to the pathology of the Cluster C diagnoses. Because anxiety may be a prominent feature of many of the personality disorder diagnoses, a target symptom approach may be particularly useful when examining the biological correlates and psychopharmacology of anxiety and inhibition (Siever et al. 1991).

Anxious individuals are characterized by increased tonic levels of sympathetic activity and cortical arousal, slower habituation to new stimuli, and lower sedation thresholds than those of nonanxious individuals (Claridge 1967, 1985; Gray 1982). Studies suggest that the γ-aminobutyric acid (GABA)ergic, serotonergic, and noradrenergic systems each may be involved in the regulation of anxiety and inhibition. Stimulation of the locus ceruleus in primates is associated with responses that closely mimic anxiety in people (Redmond 1987). One hypothesis suggests a role for serotonergic function in harm avoidance, with a positive correlation between serotonin activity and increased avoidance behavior (Cloninger 1987). Consistent with this hypothesis, the postsynaptic serotonin agonist m-chlorophenylpiperazine (m-CPP) increases hormonal release and anxiety in panic disorder patients and increases obsessions in OCD patients (Insel and Zohar 1987; Kahn et al. 1988).

■ Differential Diagnoses

Axis I anxiety disorders constitute the majority of the potentially confounding diagnoses. Most notably, careful assessment of generalized anxiety disorder, panic disorder, OCD, and phobic disorders should be made. Where found, these Axis I disorders may take priority in treatment. Furthermore, avoidant and dependent personality disorders may coexist with, and be secondary to, a major depressive disorder or OCD. Following treatment of the depression or OCD into remission, these apparent personality disorders may also resolve (Ricciardi et al. 1992). Further, when appropriately treated, symptoms of anxiety or excessive inhibition (otherwise attributed to an Axis II disorder) may remit.

■ Treatment Selection

Findings of biological abnormalities in personality disorder patients with anxiety are quite preliminary and do not support the notion of a single neurotransmitter disturbance. By extension to related Axis I disorders, the efficacy of both serotonergic and noradrenergic drugs in panic disorder and the efficacy of serotonin reuptake blockers in OCD may be related to their ability to stabilize these regulatory systems, although their mechanism of action is not yet well understood. Medications such as β-adrenergic receptor antagonists (Gorman et al. 1985), the benzodiazepine alprazolam, and the MAOI phenelzine (Liebowitz et al. 1986) may each be effective in the treatment of some patients with anxiety.

Cowdry and Gardner (1988) found the MAOI tranylcypromine helpful in alleviating anxiety in most patients who had avoidant personality disorder. Alprazolam, used for the treatment of patients with so-cial phobia, was also found to diminish specific symptoms of avoidant personality disorder (e.g., being fearful of saying something foolish, or avoiding social and occupational situations requiring interpersonal contact; Cowdry and Gardner 1988). Case reports have described patients with avoidant personality disorder who were treated with tranylcypromine (30 mg qd), phenelzine (60 mg qd), or fluoxetine (20 mg qd) for 2–3 months (Deltito and Stam 1989). Marked improvement in each case was observed with regard to increased assertiveness, improved occupational and social functioning, and decreased social sensitivity. The improvement in target symptoms was independent of other Axis I diagnoses such as social phobia (Deltito and Stam 1989).

Double-blind placebo-controlled studies are needed to confirm these observations. But there is evidence that MAOIs, SSRIs, β-adrenergic receptor antagonists, and benzodiazepines may each be considered an adjunctive therapy to the overall treatment of patients with personality disorders characterized by anxiety or excessive inhibition.

■ CONCLUSION

Substantial evidence now suggests that there are biological components that contribute to some of the more severe personality disorder syndromes such as SPD and BPD, and to some of the troubling characteristics of personality disorders. These areas include (but may not be limited to) cognitive and perceptual dysfunction, impulsivity and aggression, affective instability, and anxiety or excessive inhibition. Further, there is growing evidence from controlled treatment trials demonstrating the efficacy of psychopharmacological interventions in the treatment of these signs and symptoms.

It is important to emphasize, however, that it may be specific clusters of signs and symptoms that are being treated, and not syndromal personality disorders per se. Although the advantages of categorical syndromal nosologies are clear (including enhanced interrater reliability and operationalized criteria that encourage careful research), the potential pathophysiology may relate more closely to neurobiological dimensions. The observed personality disorders may therefore arise from the patterns of the underlying disturbances acting in concert. Given a growing armamentarium of research tools, the next decade may begin to yield many insights into the pathophysiology that underlies the cognitive, affective, and behavioral disturbances characteristic of the personality disorders.

■ REFERENCES

Akiskal HS: Subaffective disorders: dysthymic, cyclothymic and bipolar II disorders in the "borderline" realm. Psychiatr Clin North Am 4(1):26–46, 1981

American Psychiatric Association: Diagnostic and Statistical Manual of Mental Disorders, 2nd Edition. Washington, DC, American Psychiatric Press, 1968

American Psychiatric Association: Diagnostic and Statistical Manual of Mental Disorders, 3rd Edition. Washington, DC, American Psychiatric Press, 1980

American Psychiatric Association: Diagnostic and Statistical Manual of Mental Disorders, 3rd Edition, Revised. Washington, DC, American Psychiatric Press, 1987

Arango V, Ernsberger P, Marzuk P, et al: Autoradiographic demonstration of increased serotonin 5-HT2 and beta-adrenergic receptor binding sites in the brain of suicide victims. Arch Gen Psychiatry 47:1038–1047, 1990

Barnes RJ: Mesoridazine in personality disorders: a controlled trial in adolescent patients. Diseases of the Nervous System 38:258–264, 1977

Bartlett JC, Santruck JW: Affect-dependent episodic memory in young children. Child Dev 50:513–518, 1979

Bloomingdale LM, Bloomingdale EC: Childhood identification and prophylaxis of antisocial personality disorder. J Forensic Sci 33:187–199, 1988

Brinkley JR, Beitman BD, Freidel RO: Low-dose neuroleptic regimens in the treatment of borderline patients. Arch Gen Psychiatry 3:319–326, 1979

Brown GL, Ebert M, Goyer P, et al: Aggression, suicide and serotonin: relationship to CSF amine metabolites. Am J Psychiatry 139:741–746, 1982

Claridge G: Personality and Arousal. Oxford, England, Pergamon, 1967

Claridge G: Origins of Mental Illness. New York, Blackwell, 1985

Cloninger CR: A systematic method for clinical description and classification of personality variants: a proposal. Arch Gen Psychiatry 44:573–588, 1987

Cloninger CR, Christiansen KO, Reich T, et al: Implications of sex differences in the prevalence of antisocial personality, alcoholism, and criminality for familial transmission. Arch Gen Psychiatry 35:941–951, 1978

Coccaro EF, Siever LJ, Klar H: Serotonergic studies in patients with affective and personality disorders: correlates with suicidal and impulsive aggressive behavior. Arch Gen Psychiatry 45:177–185, 1988

Coccaro EF, Astill JL, Herbert JA, et al: Fluoxetine treatment of impulsive aggression in DSM-III-R personality disorder patients. J Clin Psychopharmacol 10:373–375, 1990

Cole JO, Salomon M, Gunderson J: Drug therapy in borderline patients. Compr Psychiatry 25:249–254, 1984

Cornelius JR, Soloff PH, Perel JM, et al: A preliminary trial of fluoxetine in refractory borderline patients. J Clin Psychopharmacol 11:116–120, 1991

Cowdry RW, Gardner DL: Pharmacology of borderline personality disorder. Arch Gen Psychiatry 139:741–746, 1982

Cowdry RW, Gardner DL: Pharmacotherapy of borderline personality disorder: alprazolam, carbamazepine, trifluoperazine, and tranylcypromine. Arch Gen Psychiatry 45:111–119, 1988

Davidson M, Davis KL: A comparison of plasma homovanillic acid concentrations in schizophrenic patients and normal controls. Arch Gen Psychiatry 45:561–563, 1988

Davis KL, Davidson M, Mohs RC, et al: Plasma homovanillic acid concentration and the severity of schizophrenic illness. Science 227:1601–1602, 1985

Deltito JA, Stam M: Psychopharmacological treatment of avoidant personality disorder. Compr Psychiatry 30:498–504, 1989

Faltus F: The positive effect of alprazolam in the treatment of three patients with borderline personality disorder. Am J Psychiatry 141:802–803, 1984

Fenwick P: The nature and management of aggression in epilepsy. Neuropsychiatric Practice and Opinion 1:418–425, 1989

Gardner DL, Cowdry RW: Positive effects of carbamazepine on behavioral dyscontrol in borderline personality disorder. Am J Psychiatry 143:519–522, 1986a

Gardner DL, Cowdry RW: Alprazolam induced dyscontrol in borderline personality disorder. Am J Psychiatry 142:98–100, 1986b

Goldberg SC, Schulz SC, Schulz PM, et al: Borderline and schizotypal personality disorders treated with low-dose thiothixene versus placebo. Arch Gen Psychiatry 43:680–686, 1986

Goldsmith HH: Genetic influences on personality from infancy to adulthood. Child Dev 54:331–355, 1982

Gorman JM, Liebowitz MR, Fyer AJ, et al: Treatment of social phobia with atenolol. J Clin Psychopharmacol 5:298–301, 1985

Gray JA: The Neuropsychology of Anxiety. Oxford, England, Oxford University Press, 1982

Hooberman D, Stern TA: Treatment of attention deficit and borderline personality disorders with psychostimulants: case report. J Clin Psychiatry 45:441–442, 1984

Horvath TB, Siever LJ, Mohs RC, et al: Organic mental syndromes and disorders. in Comprehensive Textbook of Psychiatry, Vol 5. Edited by Kaplan HI, Sadock BJ. Baltimore, MD, Williams & Wilkins, 1989, pp 599–641

Hymowitz P, Frances A, Jacobsberg LB, et al: Neuroleptic treatment of schizotypal personality disorders. Compr Psychiatry 27:267–271, 1986

Insel TR, Zohar J: Psychopharmacologic approaches to obsessive compulsive disorder, in Psychopharmacology: The Third Generation of Progress. Edited by Meltzer H. New York, Raven, 1987, pp 1205–1209

Kagan J, Reznick S, Snidman N, et al: Childhood derivatives of inhibition and lack of inhibition to the unfamiliar. Child Dev 59:1580–1589, 1988

Kahn RS, Wetzler S, van Praag HM, et al: Behavioral indications for serotonin receptor hypersensitivity in panic disorder. Psychiatry Res 25:101–104, 1988

Kalus O, Siever LJ: The biology of personality disorders, in An Examination of Illness Subtypes: State vs Trait and Comorbid Psychiatric Disorders. Edited by Mann JJ, Kupfer DJ. New York, Plenum, 1993, pp 89–107

Klein DF: Psychiatric diagnosis and a typology of clinical drug effects. Psychopharmacology (Berl) 13:359–386, 1968

Klein DF, Greenberg IM: Behavioral effects of diphenylhydantoin in severe psychiatric disorders. Am J Psychiatry 124:847–849, 1967

Leone NF: Response of borderline patients to loxapine and chlorpromazine. J Clin Psychiatry 43:148–150, 1982

Liebowitz MR, Klein DF: Interrelationship of hysteroid dysphoria and borderline personality disorder. Psychiatr Clin North Am 4:67–87, 1981

Liebowitz MR, Quitkin FM, Steward J, et al: Phenelzine v. imipramine in atypical depression. Arch Gen Psychiatry 41:669–677, 1984

Liebowitz MR, Fyer AJ, Gorman JM, et al: Phenelzine in social phobia. J Clin Psychopharmacol 6:93–98, 1986

Liebowitz MR, Hollander E, Schneier F, et al: Reversible and irreversible monoamine oxidase inhibitors in other psychiatric disorders. Acta Psychiatr Scand Suppl 360:29–34, 1990

Linnoila M, Virkunnen M, Scheinin M, et al: Low cerebrospinal fluid 5-hydroxyindoleacetic acid concentration differentiates impulsive from nonimpulsive violent behavior. Life Sci 33:2609–2614, 1983

Luchins DJ: Carbamazepine in violent non-epileptic schizophrenics. Psychoparmacol Bull 20:569–571, 1984

Mann JJ, Arango V: Integration of neurobiology and psychopathology in a unified model of suicidal behavior. J Clin Psychopharmacol 12 (2, suppl):2S–7S, 1992

Marazziti D, Leo D, Conti L: Further evidence supporting the role of the serotonin system in suicidal behavior: a preliminary study of suicide attempters. Acta Psychiatr Scand 80:322–324, 1989

Markovitz PJ, Calabrese JR, Schulz SC, et al: Fluoxetine in the treatment of borderline and schizotypal personality disorders. Am J Psychiatry 148:1064–1067, 1991

Meltzer HY, Arora RC: Platelet markers of suicidality. Ann N Y Acad Sci 487:271–280, 1986

Norden MJ: Fluoxetine in borderline personality disorder. Prog Neuropsychopharmacol Biol Psychiatry 13:885–893, 1989

Overall JE, Gorham DR: The Brief Psychiatric Rating Scale. Psychol Rep 10:799–812, 1962

Parsons B, Quitkin FM, McGrath PJ: Phenelzine, imipramine, and placebo in borderline patients meeting criteria for atypical depression. Psychopharmacol Bull 25:524–534, 1989

Redmond DE: Studies of the nucleus locus coeruleus in monkeys and hypotheses for neuropsychopharmacology, in Neuropsychopharmacology: The Third Generation of Progress. Edited by Meltzer H. New York, Raven, 1987, pp 967–975

Reyntjens AM: A series of multicentric pilot trials with pimozide in psychiatric practice, I: pimozide in the treatment of personality disorders. Acta Psychiatr

Belg 72:653–661, 1972

Ricciardi JN, Baer L, Jenike MA, et al: Changes in DSM-III-R Axis II diagnoses following treatment of obsessive-compulsive disorder. Am J Psychiatry 149:829–831, 1992

Rifkin A, Levitan SJ, Galewski J, et al: Emotionally unstable personality disorder—a follow-up study. Biol Psychiatry 4:65–79, 1972a

Rifkin A, Quitkin F, Curillo C, et al: Lithium carbonate in emotionally unstable character disorders. Arch Gen Psychiatry 27:519–523, 1972b

Roy A, DeJong J, Linnoila M: Extraversion in pathological gamblers correlates with indices of noradrenergic function. Arch Gen Psychiatry 46:679–681, 1989

Salzman C, Wolfson AN, Miyawaki E, et al: Fluoxetine treatment of anger in Borderline Personality Disorder. Proceedings of the American College of Neuropsychopharmacology, 1992, p 24

Shader RI, Jackson AH, Dodes LM. The anti-aggressive effects of lithium in man. Psychopharmacologia 40:17–24, 1974

Schiff HB, Sabin TD, Geller A, et al: Lithium in aggressive behavior. Am J Psychiatry 139:1346–1348, 1982

Serban G, Siegel S: Response of borderline and schizotypal patients to small doses of thiothixene and haloperidol. Am J Psychiatry 141:1455–1458, 1984

Sheard MH, Marini JL, Bridges DL, et al: The effect of lithium on impulsive aggressive behavior in man. Am J Psychiatry 133:1409–1413, 1976

Siever LJ, Davis KL: A psychobiological perspective on the personality disorders. Am J Psychiatry 148:1647–1658, 1991

Siever LJ, Silverman JM, Horvath T, et al: Increased morbid risk for schizophrenia-related disorders in relatives of schizotypal personality disordered patients. Arch Gen Psychiatry 47:634–640, 1990

Siever LJ, Amin F, Coccaro EF, et al: Plasma homovanillic acid in schizotypal personality disorder. Am J Psychiatry 148:1246–1248, 1991

Siever LJ, Amin F, Coccaro EF, et al: Cerebrospinal fluid homovanillic acid in schizotypal personality disorder. Am J Psychiatry 150:149–151, 1993a

Siever LJ, Kalus OF, Keefe RSE: The boundaries of schizophrenia. Psychiatr Clin North Am 16:217–244, 1993b

Silverman JM, Mohs RC, Siever LJ, et al: Heritability for schizophrenia-spectrum disorder in schizo-

phrenic and schizophrenia related personality disorder patients. Clinical Neuropsychopharmacology 9:271–273, 1986

Silverman JM, Pinkham L, Horvath TB, et al: Affective and impulsive personality disorder traits in the relatives of borderline personality disorder patients. Am J Psychiatry 148:1378–1385, 1991

Silverman JM, Siever LJ, Horvath Coccaro EF, et al: Schizophrenia-related and affective personality disorder traits in relatives of probands with schizophrenia and personality disorders. Am J Psychiatry 150:435–442, 1993

Soloff PH, George A, Nathan RS, et al: Progress in pharmacotherapy of borderline disorders. Arch Gen Psychiatry 43:691–697, 1986a

Soloff PH, George A, Nathan RS, et al: Paradoxical effects of amytriptyline in borderline patients. Am J Psychiatry 143:1603–1605, 1986b

Soloff PH, George A, Nathan RS, et al: Amytriptyline vs haloperidol in borderlines: final outcomes and predictors of response. J Clin Psychopharmacol 9:238–246, 1989

Soloff P, Siever LJ, Cowdry R, et al: Evaluation of pharmacologic treatments in personality disorders, in Clinical Evaluation of Psychotropic Drugs: Principles and Guidelines. Edited by Prien RF, Robinson DS. New York, Raven, 1994, pp 651–673

Steinberg BJ, Trestman RL, Siever LJ: The cholinergic and noradrenergic neurotransmitter systems and affective instability in borderline personality disorder, in Biological and Neurobehavioral Studies of Borderline Personality Disorder. Edited by Silk KR. Washington, DC, American Psychiatric Press, 1994, pp 41–62

Suomi SJ: Primate separation models of affective disorders, in Neurobiology of Learning, Emotion and Affect. Edited by Madden J. New York, Raven, 1991, pp 195–214

Teicher MH, Glod CA, Aaronson ST, et al: Open assessment of the safety and efficacy of thioridazine in the treatment of patients with borderline personality disorder. Psychopharmacol Bull 25:535–549, 1989

Tellegen A, Lykken DT, Bouchard TJ, et al: Personality similarity in twins reared apart and together. J Pers Soc Psychol 54:1031–1039, 1988

Thaker G, Adami H, Moran M, et al: Psychiatric illnesses in families of subjects with schizophrenia-spectrum personality disorders: high morbidity risks for unspecified functional psychoses and schizophrenia. Am J Psychiatry 150:66–71, 1993

Torgersen S: Genetic and nosological aspects of schizotypal and borderline personality disorders. Arch Gen Psychiatry 41:546–554, 1984

Treiman DM: Psychobiology of ictal aggression, in Advances in Neurology. Edited by Smith D, Treiman D, Trimble M. New York, Raven, 1991, pp 341–356

Trestman RL, deVegvar M-L, Coccaro EF, et al: The differential biology of impulsivity, suicide, and aggression in depression and in personality disorders. Biol Psychiatry 33:46A–47A, 1993

Van der Kolk BA: Uses of lithium in patients without major affective illness. Hosp Community Psychiatry 37:675, 1986

Wender PH, Reimherr FW, Wood DR: Attention deficit disorder (minimal brain dysfunction) in adults: a replication study of diagnosis and drug treatment. Arch Gen Psychiatry 38:449–456, 1981

38

Treatment of Psychiatric Emergencies

Michael J. Tueth, M.D., C. Lindsay DeVane, Pharm.D., and Dwight L. Evans, M.D.

Psychiatric emergencies are not found only in the emergency department. They can occur on a medical or surgical floor, in the intensive care unit, on a psychiatric unit, or in an outpatient facility. Regardless of the site of the emergency, the psychiatrist should assess the patient based on subjective complaints and objective findings and then develop a provisional diagnostic impression and a rational treatment plan.

Often the psychiatrist must make decisions based on very limited information. It is usually best to rely heavily on objective findings of the mental status examination. In addition, when only limited data are available, the clinician's treatment plan should be conservative. While choosing the least restrictive environment for the patient, the safety of the patient and others should be foremost in mind. Table 38–1 lists levels of the restrictive environments that may be used, ranging from no hospitalization to physical and chemical restraints.

In this chapter, we discuss the treatment of psychiatric emergencies from the standpoint of requirements for nonpharmacological, limited pharmacological, and primarily pharmacological intervention. Although most psychiatric emergencies require both pharmacological and psychotherapeutic intervention, many also require that legal action or procedures be followed.

■ PSYCHIATRIC EMERGENCIES REQUIRING NONPHARMACOLOGICAL INTERVENTION

Areas of nonpharmacological interventions include decisions regarding admission to the hospital versus discharge to the community, voluntary versus involuntary admission to a psychiatric facility, and legal action requiring involvement or notification of third parties. Although most physicians treat patients who present for treatment voluntarily, emergency physicians and psychiatrists sometimes confine patients to designated psychiatric facilities against the patients' will. All 50 states have statutes requiring physicians to involuntarily detain a patient in a designated psychiatric facility if the patient is judged to be dangerous to self or others. In most states, this concept extends to self-neglect and psychotic conditions. Similarly, all states have statutes that require reporting of suspected child abuse to state and/or county authorities. In addition, some states have included suspected abuse of elderly people as a mandatory reportable situation. Universal statutes also require physicians to contact an intended victim and/or the law enforcement agency in the intended victim's locality if a patient with a psychiatric disorder is judged likely to harm that person in the near future.

Table 38–1. Levels of restrictive environments for psychiatric patients

Out-of-hospital environment
 Out of hospital, alone
 Out of hospital, with family or friends
 Community residence (i.e., halfway house, boarding home, or nursing home)
In-hospital environment
 Medical or surgical floor
 Intensive care unit
 Unlocked psychiatric unit
 Locked psychiatric unit
 Constant one to one observation
 Unlocked seclusion room
 Locked seclusion room
 Leather and chemical restraints in seclusion room

■ Voluntary or Involuntary Admissions

Involuntary confinement in a psychiatric facility necessitates that the patient be judged suicidal or homicidal based on the presence of a mental disorder. Patients who are determined to be dangerous but who are without a mental disorder should be referred to the appropriate law enforcement agency. Any patient who is judged by the clinician to be acutely suicidal, homicidal, or psychotic should be admitted to a psychiatric inpatient unit. In addition, patients who are experiencing self-neglect or deterioration in well-being secondary to a psychiatric disorder should be strongly considered for hospitalization even if they are not actually suicidal, homicidal, or psychotic. Although most of these patients can be voluntarily admitted, a subset of patients who exercise poor judgment and refuse admission secondary to their psychosis or a self-destructive state of mind should be admitted involuntarily.

Suicidal State

Most suicides occur secondary to a mental disorder. The most common mental disorders leading to suicide include major depression, substance abuse, schizophrenia, and severe personality disorders. Various factors have been identified as increasing suicidal risk. These factors include increasing age, history of violence, previous suicidal behavior, male gender, loss of physical health, long duration of depression, and unwillingness to accept help.

Published data have further shown that statistically derived risk factors alone cannot predict suicide.

Although it is not possible to accurately predict suicide among psychiatric patients, the clinician's knowledge and judgment and the patient's communicated intentions remain the most important factors in identifying suicidal risks (Goldstein et al. 1991). Risk factors among alcoholic individuals who commit suicide include continued drinking, major depressive episodes, suicidal communication, poor social support, serious medical illness, unemployment, and living alone (Murphy et al. 1992). Although 2% of patients with panic disorder have been reported to attempt suicide, this percentage increased to 25% in panic disorder patients with a comorbid diagnosis of borderline personality disorder (Friedman et al. 1992). Suicide prevalence in elderly people is at least four times higher than in other adult populations (Spar and LaRue 1990). The second highest prevalence for suicide is in the adolescent population. Comorbidity has been found in most adolescent suicides, including depression, antisocial behavior, and alcohol abuse (Marttunen et al. 1991).

Although self-injurious or self-mutilating behavior is common in patients with borderline personality disorder, Winchel and Stanley (1991) found no predictably useful therapeutic approach for these patients. However, Coccaro and Kavoussi (1991) determined that borderline patients with impulsive-aggressive behavior may respond to serotonergic agents. Recently, the increased prevalence of human immunodeficiency virus (HIV)-positive and acquired immunodeficiency syndrome (AIDS) patients have added another significant risk factor for suicide. Although there is clearly a high risk for suicidal behavior in HIV-positive patients, one study concluded that the risk of completing suicide in AIDS patients is not high but is comparable with suicidality in non-HIV patients (McKegney and O'Dowd 1992). However, another recent study determined that the suicidal risk for persons with AIDS is 7.4-fold higher than for patients who are not HIV positive (Coté et al. 1992).

Homicidal State

Although the vast majority of patients who attempt suicide have a mental disorder, many patients who commit murder or who have homicidal intentions do not have a specific mental disorder. A high correlation exists between sadness and attempted suicide, but there is no correlation between sadness and violence toward others (Apter et al. 1991). The best predictor of violence is a history of violence. However, it has been suggested that clinical decisions regarding dangerousness to others is best determined by the patient's mental state and the need for restraints in the emergency room (Beck et al. 1991).

Self-Neglect and
Nonagitated Psychotic State

Patients who do not take care of their physical needs secondary to a mental disorder and patients who are psychotic but nonviolent may not represent a direct threat to themselves or others. Nevertheless, their condition will sometimes deteriorate without psychiatric intervention. These patients do not usually require involuntary hospitalization, but a decision to commit them involuntarily is occasionally necessary. Rational judgment and consultation with a patient's family is often the best approach in making this decision. Bagby and colleagues (1991) showed that involuntary commitments are generally based on legally mandated factors (e.g., psychosis or dangerousness), but there was some reliance on other factors (e.g., treatability and availability of alternative resources).

Although psychiatric patients who are considered dangerous can be legally detained against their will, they cannot be medicated without their consent unless a court order is obtained. The exception is when the patient is considered an immediate risk to self or others as demonstrated by verbal or behavioral signs. In this situation, a patient can be given medication to control the immediate life-threatening situation, but not after the crisis has passed. Most patients who initially refuse psychiatric medication later voluntarily take medication. Also, patients who are taken to court to determine competency are almost always declared incompetent to make their medication decisions. It has therefore been suggested that the judicial process might be changed—for example, to an in-house clinical review preceding judicial review to make the process more efficient and fair (Hoge et al. 1990; Zito et al. 1991).

■ Notifying Third Parties

Reports of child, elder, and spouse abuse are increasing in our society. Under statute in most states, when a psychiatrist suspects child abuse, it must be reported to the proper county and/or state authorities. Likewise, when a psychiatric patient expresses intentions of harming an individual or individuals, the psychiatrist is required to notify the intended victim(s) and/or notify the appropriate law enforcement agency in the locality of the victim(s). The specifics of this duty to report or warn third parties differ in each state.

■ PSYCHIATRIC EMERGENCIES USUALLY REQUIRING MINIMAL PHARMACOLOGICAL INTERVENTION

Some psychiatric emergency situations should emphasize diagnosis, whereas other clinical presentations are more easily diagnosed. Accurate diagnosis is particularly necessary for first episodes of panic attack, dissociative episodes, catatonia, and mania. Other emergencies require primarily psychotherapeutic intervention. These include patients with adjustment disorders or acute grief reactions, victims of rape and assault, and unstable patients with personality disorders. Use of a benzodiazepine on a short-term basis should be considered together with psychotherapy in these patients. Low to moderate doses of lorazepam or diazepam are recommended (Table 38–2).

Regarding psychiatric emergencies needing crises intervention and outpatient treatment, it was recently reported that patients referred to a multidisciplinary, community-based early intervention team

Table 38–2. Recommended psychopharmacological drug use in psychiatric emergencies

For healthy adult psychiatric patients

For agitation or substance withdrawal
  lorazepam 1–2 mg po, im, or iv every 1–2 hours as needed, or
  diazepam 5–10 mg po, im, or iv every 1–2 hours as needed

For psychotic symptoms
  haloperidol 10–20 mg/day po or im as needed (higher dosages usually are not needed)

For medically ill, delirious, or elderly psychiatric patients

For agitation or substance withdrawal
  lorazepam 0.25–1 mg po, im, or iv every 1–2 hours as needed

For psychotic symptoms
  haloperidol 1–5 mg/day as needed (higher dosages usually are not needed)

who saw the patient at home did much better than patients who were referred to hospital-based psychiatric services (Merson et al. 1992).

Adjustment Disorders

The essential feature of this disorder is a maladaptive reaction to an identifiable psychosocial stressor or stressors occurring within 3 months of the onset of the stressor and has persisted for no longer than 6 months. Symptoms associated with adjustment disorder include anxiety, depression, disturbance of conduct, physical complaints, social withdrawal, and work inhibition (American Psychiatric Association 1987). However, the usual presentation is an adjustment disorder with mixed emotional features. Crisis intervention psychotherapy has proven to be the best treatment for an adjustment disorder. Most crises are self-limited and resolve naturally, but they can definitely be helped by skilled psychotherapeutic intervention. The essential elements of this intervention include establishing rapport with the patient, empathy, listening, obtaining a thorough history, and constructing a plan to deal with the reality of the situation. The therapist helps the patient reestablish his or her defenses, draws on the patient's own resources as well as social support resources, and attempts to increase the patient's confidence and self-esteem (Hyman 1988). It is important to note that hallucinations or delusions are not symptoms of an adjustment disorder but reflect a psychotic disorder. If the initial crisis intervention interview is successful and the patient establishes control of his or her emotions, hospitalization is not usually necessary, but a follow-up outpatient appointment is recommended.

Acute Grief

Although acute grief is an adjustment disorder, it is discussed separately here because of the magnitude of the adjustment. It usually involves the loss of a significant family member or a reaction to an unusual event, such as a natural disaster. Allowing the patient to ventilate his or her feelings is essential. Also, it is imperative that the patient's family or friends be involved in ongoing support of the patient.

Rape and Assault

In addition to necessary medical and surgical evaluation and treatment, the rape or assault victim may need psychiatric intervention and follow-up care. As with the treatment of other acute adjustment disorders, the psychiatrist should follow the lead of the patient in discussing feelings about the assault. It is important for the patient to know that psychological recovery from rape may take months or years and that psychotherapy can be extremely helpful with the recovery process (Hyman 1988).

Borderline Personality Disorder

Patients undergoing acute adjustment disorders who also have a borderline personality disorder usually have much difficulty with recovery. Sometimes they experience intermittent psychotic symptoms, suicidal urges, and loss of emotional control. These patients often need a brief psychiatric admission to prevent further deterioration. Borderline personalities often deteriorate along three lines: affective instability, transient psychotic phenomenon, and impulsive-aggressive behavior. Affective instability has responded to mood stabilizers such as carbamazepine or antidepressants such as tranylcypromine. Transient psychotic symptoms often respond to low-dose neuroleptic medication and impulsive aggressive behavior has responded to serotonergic agents (Coccaro and Kavoussi 1991).

Conditions Requiring Organic Workup

Panic Attack
When for the first time a patient develops signs and symptoms consistent with the diagnosis of panic disorder, he or she should be evaluated medically (by an internist if necessary) to rule out physical causes. The symptoms of a panic attack (including shortness of breath, tachycardia, sweating, and chest pain) are consistent with many medical illnesses, including hypoglycemia, hyperthyroidism, and myocardial infarction or angina. Not until medical conditions have been excluded should a psychiatrist make a diagnosis of panic disorder. Following an initial panic attack, a patient may need a short course of a benzodiazepine to treat the accompanying anxiety and fear before obtaining a medical evaluation.

Dissociative Episodes
Psychogenic amnesia is a relatively rare condition compared with organic amnestic syndrome. Amnesia is a frequent accompaniment of medical-surgical ab-

normalities such as head injury, brain tumor, cardio-vascular incidents, and substance use. Not until organic amnestic disorder has been ruled out should the psychiatrist assume a psychogenic basis for memory loss. Any other dissociative episodes occurring for the first time, such as psychogenic fugue or depersonalization experiences, need an organic evaluation to rule out physical causes.

Dissociative episodes may accompany posttraumatic stress disorder (PTSD). Patients who have experienced extreme traumatic stress can dissociate both at the time of the stressor and intermittently, for years. It was recently reported that Vietnam veterans who had increased levels of combat exposure experienced an increased number of dissociative symptoms years after their combat experiences (Bremner et al. 1992). Although there is no specific emergency treatment for this condition, the patient should be evaluated for possible hospital admission if he or she is in an unstable emotional state. Patients who have experienced an unusual traumatic event such as a natural disaster could in some situations benefit from outpatient treatment to minimize the likelihood of developing PTSD.

Catatonia

Although major depression and schizophrenia (catatonic type) are the most common psychiatric disorders that are associated with catatonia, some medical and neurological conditions also cause this syndrome. Medical causes include hypercalcemia and hepatic encephalopathy. Catatonia may also appear as an adverse drug side effect from neuroleptic medication and phencyclidine (PCP). Neurological causes for catatonia include parkinsonism and encephalitis. Unless the patient has a history of a previous episode of catatonia with an established causative psychiatric diagnosis, he or she should be fully evaluated by medical and/or neurological consultants.

Mania

In patients over age 50, the initial onset of mania is relatively uncommon. Any patient with an initial onset of mania (but especially a patient who is over 50) should be evaluated for organic causes. Various drugs, medical illness, and neurological disease can cause this syndrome. For example, tricyclic antidepressants (TCAs), monoamine oxidase inhibitors (MAOIs), and alprazolam have precipitated hypomania in susceptible patients. Medical illness and neu-

rological disease that can cause the manic syndrome include a hyperthyroid state, multiple sclerosis, and various brain tumors.

Conversion Disorder

A patient with a rather sudden onset of unexplained neurological symptoms should have a full neurological workup before the diagnosis of "conversion hysteria" can be made. Traditionally, the amobarbital (Amytal) interview has been useful for assessment, initial management, and recovery of function in conversion disorders (Perry and Jacobs 1982). It has been reported that intravenous administration of lorazepam accompanied by repeated hypnotic suggestions resulted in full recovery in conversion disorder (Stevens 1990).

■ PSYCHIATRIC EMERGENCIES USUALLY REQUIRING PHARMACOLOGICAL INTERVENTION

Many psychiatric patients require pharmacological intervention as the primary treatment of their condition. These patients include most assaultive or aggressive patients, agitated psychotic patients, substance-intoxicated patients with aggressivity, and patients undergoing substance withdrawal.

■ Assaultive Behavior From Any Cause

On initial presentation it is often impossible to accurately diagnose psychiatrically an assaultive or aggressive individual. Treatment usually precedes a definitive diagnosis. When a patient is assessed to be actively or potentially violent, then quick, decisive, and well-planned action is mandatory. The level of restriction that the psychiatrist chooses for each patient is based on good medical judgment, making use of the least restrictive environment (Table 38–1). However, when a patient is judged to be eminently violent, often a more restrictive environment is needed to minimize potential injury to the patient and others. Every emergency room and psychiatric unit treating potentially violent patients should have a seclusion room with leather restraints available. In implementing the decision to restrain a violent patient, it is essential to act decisively with sufficient manpower to fully control the situation. This usually requires at least five male assistants. Often, when patients see a sufficient show of force, they will voluntarily allow themselves to be restrained.

Most patients who are physically restrained will also require psychopharmacological treatment. Intramuscular or intravenous medication can be used without a patient's consent to treat a life-threatening emergency. The three drugs most often employed in this situation are lorazepam, diazepam, and haloperidol (Table 38–2). Any of these drugs can be given intravenously but are usually given intramuscularly. They are well absorbed if given in a deltoid muscle, but absorption of benzodiazepines may occasionally be erratic (Arana and Hyman 1991). For a healthy adult, the recommended dosage of lorazepam is 1–2 mg every hour as needed; of diazepam, 5–10 mg every hour as needed; and of haloperidol, 5–10 mg bid. Haloperidol is usually only required for patients who are clearly psychotic. However, haloperidol can make certain substance intoxications (e.g., PCP) worse, and it frequently causes acute dystonia early in the course of treatment. Unless the patient is clearly delusional or hallucinating, lorazepam or diazepam is the recommended medication for emergency use.

■ Agitated Psychosis

Psychosis without accompanying behavioral or suicidal problems is not usually considered a psychiatric emergency and can be routinely treated with antipsychotic medication. However, psychosis with agitation, aggression, or violence is probably the most common psychiatric emergency encountered. Again, symptomatic treatment often precedes definitive diagnosis because of the urgency of the situation. Most agitated psychotic patients are diagnosed as having bipolar disorder, schizophrenia, brief reactive psychosis, delirium, or dementia.

Bipolar Disorder

Agitated psychosis can occur in bipolar disorder in two forms: major depression and mania. Electroconvulsive therapy (ECT) is quite effective in the treatment of major depression, especially with catatonia, as well as in severe mania. Moreover, these disorders are more commonly managed psychopharmacologically. Although these disorders have traditionally been treated with neuroleptic medication, more recently, alternative therapies have been suggested.

One study has shown that lithium and valproate were both effective in improving manic symptoms. Valproate was associated with particular effectiveness in treating patients with mixed affective states (Freeman et al. 1992). Pope and colleagues (1991) concluded that valproate was an effective alternative for manic patients who do not tolerate or respond to lithium.

Recent investigations have demonstrated the therapeutic benefits of lorazepam and clonazepam in treating mania. However, one study showed lorazepam to be clearly superior to clonazepam in the treatment of manic symptoms. Sixty-one percent of 13 acutely manic patients ($n = 8$) responded to treatment with lorazepam, with 38.5% ($n = 5$) achieving remission. This compared to an 18.2% response rate ($n = 2$) and 0% remission rate in 11 patients treated with clonazepam (Bradwejn et al. 1990). Lorazepam given orally or intravenously has also been shown to be effective in treating the catatonic syndrome. In one study, 12 of 15 patients responded completely and dramatically (Rosebush et al. 1990).

Schizophrenia

Treatment of schizophrenic exacerbation has changed markedly in the last 5 years. Rapid neuroleptization (tranquilization) using antipsychotics such as haloperidol in 5-mg doses administered every hour as needed has been replaced by using 10–20 mg of haloperidol per day in combination with a benzodiazepine (usually lorazepam) as needed. Several studies have clearly shown that 10–20 mg of haloperidol per day, or the equivalent dose of another antipsychotic, is sufficient as an antipsychotic dose (McEvoy et al. 1991; Rifkin et al. 1991; Van Putten et al. 1990; Volavka et al. 1992). Likewise, benzodiazepine augmentation of neuroleptic medication has been shown to control agitation during exacerbations of schizophrenia (Barbee et al. 1992; Bodkin 1990; Salzman et al. 1991).

Brief Reactive Psychosis

A diagnosis of brief reactive psychosis is common in patients who have a comorbid personality disorder (often borderline personality disorder) and who decompensate under stress. However, it includes any brief psychotic episode not explained by another Axis I disorder. The treatment of agitated psychosis in this disorder is the same as in an exacerbation of schizophrenia, although the neuroleptic drug is usually needed for a shorter period of time.

Delirium

Delirium is defined as an organic mental disorder that develops over a short period of time and fluctuates over the course of a day. Patients show reduced ability to maintain attention, disorganized thinking, and various degrees of reduced level of consciousness, perceptual disturbances, disturbance of the sleep-wake cycle, psychomotor changes, disorientation, and memory impairment (American Psychiatric Association 1987). It is important to always consider delirium as a cause of agitated psychotic behavior, especially in medically ill and elderly patients.

In addition to diagnosing and treating underlying organic causes of delirium and protecting the patient and others from harm while he or she is in a delirious state, medications can help to calm the patient's agitation. Low doses of haloperidol or lorazepam are usually employed. If the delirium is thought to be due to a substance withdrawal state, lorazepam is the drug of choice. It is important to remember that delirium can be accurately diagnosed by electroencephalogram (EEG). An abnormal EEG is virtually always found in delirium (Boutros 1992; Engel and Romano 1959).

Dementia

A patient with dementia can become agitatedly psychotic for various reasons, including delirium, catastrophic reaction, or a reaction to delusions and/or hallucinations. The best treatment for a dementia patient is nonpharmacological, using behavior modification and supportive approaches. However, pharmacotherapy may be indicated; but very low doses of neuroleptics and/or benzodiazepines are recommended, because of the high incidence of side effects including delirium, pseudoparkinsonism, and increased falls. Aggressive behavior in elderly patients with brain damage and dementia can respond to other medications, including serotonin reuptake inhibitors, propranolol, and carbamazepine (Deutsch et al. 1991; Maletta 1990). In addition, buspirone in daily doses of 15–45 mg has been reported to be effective in reducing aggressive behavior in brain-damaged patients (Ratey et al. 1991).

■ Substance Withdrawal

Withdrawal signs and symptoms from alcohol, sedatives and hypnotics, and benzodiazepines are similar. The major signs include tremulousness and autonomic instability (American Psychiatric Association 1987). Also, insomnia and weakness that are not commonly caused by anxiety often do present as symptoms of alcohol or sedative withdrawal. The treatment of withdrawal and prevention of Wernicke-Korsakoff syndrome are important considerations. Alcohol withdrawal is probably best treated with benzodiazepines. Diazepam, due to its relatively long duration of action, has the advantage of providing a smoother tapering period. However, lorazepam is recommended for patients with significant liver disease because its metabolism is less impaired in these patients.

Alcohol withdrawal delirium is a life-threatening illness that usually should be treated in an intensive care unit. It is characterized by delirium developing within a week of the cessation of or reduction of alcohol consumption, accompanied by excessive autonomic activity and usually with fever, perceptual disturbances, and agitation. The presence of a concomitant physical illness predisposes to the syndrome (American Psychiatric Association 1987). Administration of intramuscular thiamine before administration of an intravenous or oral carbohydrate load is necessary in an alcohol-dependent patient to prevent the development of Wernicke-Korsakoff syndrome (Hyman 1988).

■ Substance Intoxication With Violent Behavior

The major substances that lead to violent behavior are cocaine and PCP and, to a lesser extent, amphetamines, hallucinogens, and marijuana. The treatment of psychosis in substance intoxication is similar to the treatment of the agitated psychotic patient (Tables 38–1 and 38–2).

Cocaine

Cocaine use is frequently associated with violence. One study showed transient paranoid states following the use of cocaine in 68% of subjects (Satel et al. 1991). Another study showed 53% of users became psychotic, of which 90% had paranoid delusions and 96% experienced hallucinations, mostly of the auditory type (Brady et al. 1991). Cocaine abuse is common among schizophrenic patients. Compared with those who were abstinent, schizophrenic individuals who used cocaine were hospitalized more frequently, were more likely to be of the paranoid subtype, and were more likely to be depressed during the course of their illness (Brady et al. 1990).

Phencyclidine

The presentation of PCP intoxication can include virtually any combination of psychiatric signs and symptoms. Agitation and violence are particularly common in these patients. Violence can be unprovoked, sudden, and even lethal. Any patient suspected of having PCP intoxication should be treated very cautiously. The person should usually be placed in an isolation room to decrease the amount of external stimuli. If the patient becomes combative, restraints will often be needed. Moderate doses of lorazepam or diazepam (sometimes in combination with haloperidol) are often needed to help calm the patient. Physical restraint may be necessary for a patient intoxicated with phencyclidine if he or she shows aggressive behavior (Hyman 1988).

Other Substance Intoxications

Amphetamines, hallucinogens, and cannabis abuse can cause psychiatric behavioral emergencies, but less often than with the substances already discussed. Any of these substances (including cannabis) can induce psychosis in susceptible individuals. One study found that schizophrenia was 6 times more likely to develop during a 15-year period in heavy cannabis users than in nonusers (Thornicroft 1990).

■ Psychoactive Drug Side Effects

Adverse drug effects necessitating prompt remedial action can occur at any time during pharmacotherapy with psychoactive drugs. One basis for selection of initial therapy is to avoid those drugs producing a high incidence of certain side effect forms (DeVane 1990). Informing patients and family of expected side effects can be comforting. Nevertheless, the clinician can expect patients experiencing an unanticipated and untoward drug reaction to be frightened and to frequently require immediate intervention.

The possible adverse effects from psychoactive drug therapy involve all organ systems. The most urgent side effects requiring attention involve the blood, eyes, and cardiovascular and neurological systems. The prominent drug side effects discussed in the next section may present as psychiatric emergencies. Many less common effects may be equally important and are discussed in standard references.

Antipsychotic Neuroleptics

Because all currently available antipsychotic drugs (with the relative exception of clozapine) block the dopamine D_2-subtype receptor in the nigrostriatal tract, extrapyramidal side effects (EPS) may emerge during therapy (Goetz and Klawans 1981). Symptoms include acute dystonic reactions, akathisias, and parkinsonism (i.e., akinesia, tremor, rigidity). Antipsychotic drug-induced laryngeal and/or pharyngeal dystonia can precipitate cardiac arrhythmias, presumably through vagal reflexes. In addition, akathisia can be distressing and may result in maladaptive reactions, even contributing to suicidal behavior. These reactions require that antipsychotic dosage be kept as low as possible, but EPS are not consistently dose-related. When EPS appear, anticholinergic agents (e.g., benztropine, 0.5–4 mg qd; trihexyphenidyl, 2–10 mg qd; or diphenhydramine, 25–100 mg qd) may be used in treatment. Acute dystonias respond most rapidly to intravenous administration. Caution should be exercised to follow up adequately, as the duration of therapeutic effects following parenteral administration may be brief and acute EPS can reoccur. There is no consistent evidence that one antiparkinsonian drug is consistently superior to another for treatment of EPS.

An increasingly recognized adverse effect of antipsychotic drugs is the neuroleptic malignant syndrome (NMS). This is an acute and potentially lethal reaction manifested by fever, muscular rigidity, central nervous system (CNS) abnormalities, and autonomic dysfunction (Caroff 1980). It may occur at any time during antipsychotic drug treatment, even after the drug has been recently discontinued. The treatment consists of discontinuing the suspected drug and providing supportive treatment and pharmacotherapy. Anticholinergic drugs may act to restore the central balance of dopamine and acetylcholine, one of the purported central mechanisms causing this reaction (Hashimoto et al. 1984). Benztropine (1–2 mg im) or diphenhydramine (25–50 mg im) is recommended. Dopamine agonists have been used orally—either amantadine (200 mg qd) or bromocriptine (15 mg qd) (McCarron et al. 1982; Mueller et al. 1983). Finally, dantrolene sodium (100–300 mg qd) has been successful in relieving skeletal muscle stiffness (May et al. 1983). Treatment may need to be continued for 1–3 weeks.

Antipsychotics produce a variety of cardiovascular effects. In addition to orthostasis, hypotension, and tachycardia, electrocardiogram (ECG) changes are common. The risk of hypotension is increased in elderly patients, with parenteral administration, or when initiating or making large changes in dosage. General recommendations to prevent hypotensive episodes would include making gradual dose increments, instructing patients to stand slowly when they rise from a reclining position, or recommending that elderly patients wear elastic stockings. Many of these patients are voluntarily salt deprived, and salt supplementation of their diet is often very useful. If systolic pressure falls below 90 mm Hg, the dosage should be held or reduced. It may be necessary to position the patient with legs elevated. In cases where shock develops, drug treatment may be necessary. The unopposed β-agonist activity of epinephrine can lead to further decreases in blood pressure, and this drug is therefore not recommended. Preferred pressor treatment would be norepinephrine, phenylephrine, or metaraminol.

ECG changes can include prolongation of Q-T interval; S-T segment depression; blunted, notched, or inverted T waves; or appearance of U waves. The occurrence of serious arrhythmias is rare but can be life threatening. Factors that predispose to ECG changes include hypokalemia, recent food intake, heavy exercise, and alcohol abuse (Nasrallah 1978). Taking a baseline and follow-up ECGs on patients with increased risk factors is recommended. Avoiding the use of strongly anticholinergic phenothiazines, especially in elderly patients, may minimize the risk of causing cardiac effects of antipsychotics (Risch et al. 1982).

Anticholinergic side effects may be prominent with the antipsychotics and can include dry mouth, blurred vision, urinary retention, and constipation. Many of these side effects can be distressing to patients. The avoidance of drugs with high degrees of muscarinic receptor-binding properties is a useful guide in drug selection. A patient with urinary retention may present with overdistension of the bladder, discomfort, or pain. Reducing drug dosage is usually helpful or a trial of bethanechol (10–25 mg tid po) can be considered. Constipation can be accompanied by pain, abdominal rigidity, and vomiting. Mild cases can be treated with diet, increased fluid intake, and exercise. Laxatives should be used in the lowest effective dose. Constipation may be a symptom of paralytic ileus, which (if left untreated) may be fatal. Treatment consists of lowering the drug dose when

possible, correcting fluid and electrolyte balance, and (if necessary) restoring bowel continuity and function by intubation of the gut and relief of abdominal distension and pressure.

The anticholinergic effects of the antipsychotics and antidepressants may aggravate glaucoma, especially the narrow-angle type. Blurred vision from these drugs results from relaxation of the ciliary muscle and loss of accommodation for near vision. Complaints of eye pain, especially in patients over 40, should prompt an ophthalmic examination. It may be necessary to decrease the dose of the offending drug or change to another agent with lower anticholinergic properties. The short-term use of 1% pilocarpine eyedrops may be beneficial for treatment of mydriasis and cycloplegia (Malone et al. 1992).

Drug-induced EEG changes and alteration of the seizure threshold may occur with the antipsychotic drugs (Oliver et al. 1982). A majority of drug-induced seizures are of the generalized tonic-clonic type. The aliphatic phenothiazines and clozapine appear to be the worse offenders, although the occurrence of seizures is considered rare, with less than 1% of patients who receive these drugs being affected. At clozapine doses of 600 mg qd and higher, the risk of seizures appears to increase (Simpson and Cooper 1978). The butyrophenone and piperazine phenothiazines are reported to be associated with a lessor incidence of seizures. Factors that may contribute to the seizure incidence include large or sudden dosage changes, the presence of an organic brain syndrome, or a preexisting seizure disorder or history of head trauma. EEG abnormalities may be present without the occurrence of seizures. In patients already receiving an anticonvulsant regimen to which an antipsychotic is added, plasma concentration of the anticonvulsant should be followed to insure maintenance of a therapeutic level. An adjustment of dosage will be necessary if seizure activity increases.

For terminating status epilepticus, lorazepam has emerged as the agent of first choice at many centers (Treiman 1990). It is as effective as diazepam, with a longer duration of action. Lorazepam can be given intramuscularly or by intravenous infusion (0.05–0.2 mg/kg at 2 mg/min; 8 mg maximal). If lorazepam fails to terminate status epilepticus, then phenytoin is the drug of choice. Attention should be paid to basic life-support measures (i.e., airway and cardiovascular control) and prevention of complications (e.g., rhabdomyolysis, hyperthermia, cerebral edema).

Patients taking clozapine may experience profound hypotension with or without syncope shortly following initiation of therapy, as early as the first or second dose. Although the documented incidence is less than 0.03%, respiratory and/or cardiac arrest has occurred. The most serious reaction to clozapine is agranulocytosis, which can be fatal. Most cases of bone marrow suppression occur between 6 weeks and 6 months after therapy begins, but weekly monitoring of the blood count is justified for the duration of treatment. Prodromal signs of bone marrow suppression include sore throat, low-grade fever, or flu-like symptoms. If the white blood cell (WBC) count is below 3,500, then it should be rechecked biweekly. If the WBC falls below 3,000 or the granulocyte count below 1,500, then the drug should be discontinued. Preventive measures against infection may be necessary, including isolation and antibiotic therapy. Most patients will need hospitalization for close monitoring while bone marrow function returns to normal.

Cyclic Antidepressants

Anticholinergic toxicity (i.e., a delirium or psychosis) can occur from use of any anticholinergic drug, including many of the cyclic antidepressants, antipsychotics, and the antiparkinsonian drugs used to treat EPS. The syndrome results from competitive inhibition of acetylcholine at central and peripheral cholinergic muscarinic receptors. Elderly patients are believed to be especially vulnerable, as well as patients in whom combinations or high doses of anticholinergic agents are used. Recommendations for treatment include discontinuing the offending drug or drugs, conducting a medical and mental status examination to confirm the diagnosis, and restricting the patient's environment (Table 38–1) as necessary to minimize accidental injury. If agitation is present, benzodiazepines may be used (Table 38–2). For severely ill patients, physostigmine (1 mg im) has been useful. This reversible cholinesterase inhibitor results in enhanced central and peripheral cholinergic actions. Cardiac monitoring is recommended when using physostigmine.

The most serious adverse effect of MAOIs is the precipitation of a hypertensive crisis, usually following ingestion of dietary products containing large amounts of tyramine or other substances coadministered with sympathomimetic properties. Management includes discontinuing the MAOI and treating the hypertension. The recommended treatment is intravenous administration of an α-adrenergic blocker. Phentolamine (up to 5 mg iv) has been used. An alternative would be chlorpromazine (25–50 mg im or po), which has the advantage of being routinely available in emergency rooms and psychiatric units. Oral nifedipine has been recommended for patients to carry with them to treat a hypertensive crisis, but it is important to be aware of the potential risk of hypotension following ingestion of nifedipine if the patient is not actually hypertensive (Hesselink 1992).

Priapism may appear in male patients receiving trazodone (often after 1 or 2 weeks of therapy) and, to a much lesser extent, with antipsychotic drugs (Scher et al. 1983). This situation constitutes an emergency, because if left untreated, permanent erectile dysfunction may result. Immediate urological consultation should be sought, as surgical intervention may be necessary. Complaints of unusual erectile activity should be viewed with suspicion as a prodromal symptom of priapism and the drug immediately discontinued.

Epileptogenic effects may occur with the cyclic antidepressants in a similar fashion as with the antipsychotics (Jabbari et al. 1985). Incidence is unknown but may be as high as 3% in patients receiving bupropion at the upper limit of the suggested dose range and higher for patients receiving maprotiline. Patients without a history of a seizure disorder and with a normal EEG are considered to be at low risk. If an isolated seizure occurs, a thorough medical and neurological examination should be performed. The drug dosage should either be lowered or (preferably) the regimen changed to another antidepressant. Prophylactic anticonvulsants are usually not necessary but may be considered for patients who are at high risk for seizure activity (e.g., presence of organicity). Benzodiazepines may be used to terminate seizure activity as described previously for the antipsychotics if seizures continue.

■ SPECIAL PSYCHIATRIC EMERGENCIES

■ Adolescence

Crisis intervention counseling is frequently indicated in the care of adolescent crises. When psychotherapeutic treatment approaches are unsuccessful, neuroleptics, lithium, anticonvulsants, antidepressants, and β-adrenergic blockers have all been recommended for treating violent adolescent behavior. Factors associated with adolescent violence include alcohol and substance use, depression and suicidality, overstimulation, and family issues. Often violence in the adolescent erupts from a strong wish for affectionate contact. The goal of pharmacological treatment is behavior control, whereas the goal of psychotherapy is communication and self-understanding (Marohn 1992).

Geriatrics

Elderly patients are much more likely than younger patients to experience adverse effects of psychotropic medication. Therefore, treating behavioral emergencies in elderly people should be tempered by using a lower initial dosage of medication and slowly raising the total daily dosage (Table 38–2).

Another important statistic is the relatively high suicide rate in elderly people, especially white males over age 75. Whenever an elderly patient talks of suicide ideas or plans or demonstrates suicidal behavior, he or she should be fully evaluated (usually on an inpatient psychiatric unit) for psychopathology.

Psychiatric Drug Overdose

Although it is beyond the scope of this chapter to discuss the specific treatment for each psychotropic drug overdose, several points are of particular importance. It is very problematic to treat an acute overdose patient on a psychiatric unit, unless it is a medical-psychiatric unit equipped to handle medical emergencies. Often what appears to be a simple benzodiazepine overdose on admission, for example, turns out to be a multiple drug ingestion. Patients who have overdosed on a TCA, even those who appear stable, need 24–48 hours of cardiac monitoring—preferably in an intensive care unit, because of the risk of the development of potentially fatal arrhythmias. Sodium bicarbonate is usually considered the first line treatment for serious tricyclic overdosage. Alkalinization of the serum acts to increase the protein binding of the tricyclic, thus decreasing the amount of free drug to block the conducting system in the heart (Jenkins and Loscalzo 1990; Kulig 1992). Although cyclic antidepressants and lithium can be fatal in overdosage, the newer antidepressants (i.e.,

fluoxetine and sertraline) and the benzodiazepines have few if any reported overdose fatalities when taken as sole ingestant (Arana and Hyman 1991). The neuroleptics may produce electrocardiographic changes resembling conduction defects, but the occurrence of serious arrhythmias is rare (Wilson and Weilser 1984).

REFERENCES

American Psychiatric Association: Diagnostic and Statistical Manual of Mental Disorders, 3rd Edition, Revised. Washington, DC, American Psychiatric Association, 1987

Apter A, Kotler M, Sevy S, et al: Correlates of risk of suicide in violent and nonviolent psychiatric patients. Am J Psychiatry 148:833–877, 1991

Arana GW, Hyman SE: Handbook of Psychiatric Drug Therapy, 2nd Edition. Boston, MA, Little, Brown, 1991

Bagby RM, Thompson JS, Dickens SE, et al: Decision making in psychiatric civil commitment: an experimental analysis. Am J Psychiatry 148:28–33, 1991

Barbee JG, Mancuso DM, Freed CR, et al: Alprazolam as a neuroleptic adjunct in the emergency treatment of schizophrenia. Am J Psychiatry 149:506–510, 1992

Beck JC, White KA, Gage B: Emergency psychiatric assessment of violence. Am J Psychiatry 148:1562–1565, 1991

Bodkin JA: Emerging uses for high-potency benzodiazepines in psychotic disorders. J Clin Psychiatry 51 (suppl):41–46, 1990

Boutros NN: A review of indications for routine EEG in clinical psychiatry. Hosp Community Psychiatry 43:716–719, 1992

Bradwejn J, Shriqui C, Koszycki D, et al: Double-blind comparison of the effects of clonazepam and lorazepam in acute mania. J Clin Psychopharmacol 10:403–408, 1990

Brady K, Anton R, Ballenger JC, et al: Cocaine abuse among schizophrenic patients. Am J Psychiatry 147:1164–1169, 1990

Brady KT, Lydiard RB, Malcolm R, et al: Cocaine-induced psychosis. J Clin Psychiatry 52:509–512, 1991

Bremner JD, Southwick S, Brett E, et al: Dissociation in post-traumatic stress disorder in Vietnam combat veterans. Am J Psychiatry 149:328–332, 1992

Caroff SN: The neuroleptic malignant syndrome. J Clin Psychiatry 41:79–82, 1980

Coccaro EF, Kavoussi RJ: Biological and pharmacological aspects of borderline personality disorder. Hosp Community Psychiatry 42:1029–1033, 1991

Coté TR, Biggar RJ, Dannenberg AL: Risk of suicide among persons with AIDS: a national assessment. JAMA 268:2066–2068, 1992

Deutsch LH, Bylsma FW, Rovner BW, et al: Psychosis and physical aggression in probable Alzheimer's disease. Am J Psychiatry 148:1159–1163, 1991

DeVane CL: Fundamentals of Monitoring Psychoactive Drug Therapy. Baltimore, MD, Williams & Wilkins, 1990

Engel GL, Romano J: Delirium: a syndrome of cerebral insufficiency. Journal of Chronic Disease 9:260–277, 1959

Freeman TW, Clothier JL, Pazzaglia P, et al: A double-blind comparison of valproate and lithium in the treatment of acute mania. Am J Psychiatry 149:108–111, 1992

Friedman S, Jones JC, Chernen L, et al: Suicidal ideation and suicide attempts among patients with panic disorder: a survey of two outpatient clinics. Am J Psychiatry 149:680–685, 1992

Goetz CG, Klawans HL: Drug-induced extrapyramidal disorders—a neuropsychiatric interface. J Clin Psychopharmacol 1:297–303, 1981

Goldstein RB, Black DW, Nasrallah A, et al: The prediction of suicide. Arch Gen Psychiatry 48:418–422, 1991

Hashimoto F, Sherman C, Jeffery W: Neuroleptic malignant syndrome and dopaminergic blockade. Arch Intern Med 144:629–630, 1984

Hesselink JMK: Safer use of MAOIs with nifedipine to counteract potential hypertensive crisis. Am J Psychiatry 148:1616, 1992

Hoge SK, Appelbaum PS, Lawlor T, et al: A prospective, multicenter study of patients' refusal of antipsychotic medication. Arch Gen Psychiatry 47:949–956, 1990

Hyman SE: Manual of Psychiatric Emergencies, 2nd Edition. Boston, MA, Little, Brown, 1988

Jabbari B, Bryan GE, Marsh EE, et al: Incidence of seizures with tricyclic and tetracyclic antidepressants. Arch Neurol 42:480–481, 1985

Jenkins JL, Loscalzo J: Manual of Emergency Medicine, Diagnosis and Treatment, 2nd Edition. Boston, MA, Little, Brown, 1990

Kulig K: Initial management of ingestion of toxic substances. N Engl J Med 326:1677–1681, 1992

Maletta GJ: Pharmacologic treatment and management of the aggressive demented patient. Psychiatric Annals 20:446–455, 1990

Malone DA Jr, Camara EG, Krug JH Jr: Ophthalmologic effects of psychotropic medications. Psychosomatics 33:271–277, 1992

Marohn RC: Management of the assaultive adolescent. Hosp Community Psychiatry 43:622–624, 1992

Marttunen MJ, Aro HM, Henriksson MM, et al: Mental disorders in adolescent suicide. Arch Gen Psychiatry 48:834–839, 1991

May DC, Morris SW, Stewart RM, et al: Neuroleptic malignant syndrome: response to dantrolene sodium. Ann Intern Med 98:183–184, 1983

McCarron MM, Boettger ML, Peck JJ: A case of neuroleptic malignant syndrome successfully treated with amantadine. J Clin Psychiatry 43:381–382, 1982

McEvoy JP, Hogarty GE, Steingard S: Optimal dose of neuroleptic in acute schizophrenia: a controlled study of the neuroleptic threshold and higher haloperidol dose. Arch Gen Psychiatry 48:739–745, 1991

McKegney FP, O'Dowd MA: Suicidality and HIV status. Am J Psychiatry 149:396–398, 1992

Merson S, Tyrer P, Onyett S, et al: Early intervention in psychiatric emergencies: a controlled clinical trial. Lancet 339:1311–1314, 1992

Mueller PS, Vester JW, Fermaglich J: Neuroleptic malignant syndrome—successful treatment with bromocriptine. JAMA 249:386–388, 1983

Murphy GE, Wetzel RD, Robins E, et al: Multiple risk factors predict suicide in alcoholism. Arch Gen Psychiatry 49:459–463, 1992

Nasrallah HA: Factors influencing phenothiazine-induced ECG changes. Am J Psychiatry 135:118–199, 1978

Oliver PA, Luchins DJ, Wyall RJ: Neuroleptic-induced seizures. Arch Gen Psychiatry 39:206–209, 1982

Perry JC, Jacobs D: Overview: clinical applications of the amytal interview in psychiatric emergency settings. Am J Psychiatry 139:552–559, 1982

Pope HG, McElroy SL, Keck PE, et al: Valproate in the treatment of acute mania: a placebo-controlled study. Arch Gen Psychiatry 48:62–68, 1991

Ratey J, Sovner R, Parks A, et al: Buspirone treatment of aggression and anxiety in mentally retarded patients: a multiple-baseline, placebo lead-in study.

J Clin Psychiatry 52:159–162, 1991

Rifkin A, Doddi S, Karajgi B, et al: Dosage of haloperidol for schizophrenia. Arch Gen Psychiatry 48:166–170, 1991

Risch SC, Groom GP, Janowsky DS: The effects of psychotropic drugs on the cardiovascular system. J Clin Psychiatry 43(5) (sect 2):16–26, 1982

Rosebush PI, Hildebrand AM, Fulong BG, et al: Catatonic syndrome in a general psychiatric inpatient population: frequency, clinical presentation, and response to lorazepam. J Clin Psychiatry 51:357–362, 1990

Salzman C, Solomon D, Miyawaki E, et al: Parenteral lorazepam versus parenteral haloperidol for the control of psychotic disruptive behavior. J Clin Psychiatry 52:177–180, 1991

Satel SL, Southwick SM, Gawin FH: Clinical features of cocaine-induced paranoia. Am J Psychiatry 148:495–498, 1991

Scher M, Drieger JN, Juergens S: Trazodone and priapism. Am J Psychiatry 140:1362–1363, 1983

Simpson GM, Cooper TA: Clozapine plasma levels and convulsions. Am J Psychiatry 135:99–100, 1978

Spar JE, LaRue A: Geriatric Psychiatry. Washington, DC, American Psychiatric Press, 1990

Stevens CB: Lorazepam in the treatment of acute conversion disorder. Hosp Community Psychiatry 41:1255–1257, 1990

Thornicroft G: Cannabis and psychosis: is there epidemiological evidence for an association? Br J Psychiatry 157:25–33, 1990

Treiman DM: The role of benzodiazepines in the management of status epilepticus. Neurology 40 (suppl 2):32–42, 1990

Van Putten T, Marder SR, Mintz J: A controlled dose comparison of haloperidol in newly admitted schizophrenic patients. Arch Gen Psychiatry 47:754–758, 1990

Volavka J, Cooper T, Czobor P, et al: Haloperidol blood levels and clinical effects. Arch Gen Psychiatry 49:354–361, 1992

Wilson WH, Weilser SJ: Case report of phenothiazine induced torsades de pointes. Am J Psychiatry 141:1265–1266, 1984

Winchel RM, Stanley M: Self-injurious behavior: a review of the behavior in biology of self-mutilation. Am J Psychiatry 148:306–317, 1991

Zito JM, Craig TJ, Wanderling J: New York under the Rivers decision: an epidemiologic study of drug treatment refusal. Am J Psychiatry 48:904–909, 1991

39

Psychopharmacology in the Medically Ill Patient

Alan Stoudemire, M.D., Michael G. Moran, M.D., and
Barry S. Fogel, M.D.

Prescribing psychotropic medications in medically ill patients requires careful risk-benefit assessment. In this chapter, we review the special psychopharmacological considerations that are required in making such risk-benefit assessments for the medical-psychiatric population, including 1) potential interactions between psychotropic medications with drugs used for medical disorders; 2) the effects of impaired renal, hepatic, or gastrointestinal functioning on psychotropic drug metabolism; and 3) side effects of psychotropic drugs that may complicate preexisting medical conditions.

The use of psychotropic drugs in medically ill patients is discussed and recommendations for their use made based on side-effect profiles, drug interactions, and pharmacokinetic properties. Drug interactions of major clinical importance are listed in the tables (Rizos et al. 1988; Sargenti et al. 1988). More extensive critical reviews of the use of psychotropic agents may be found in our more expanded discussions of the area of psychopharmacology (Fogel and Stoudemire 1993; Stoudemire and Fogel 1987; Stoudemire et al. 1991, 1993). The use of psychotropic agents in pregnancy (Cohen et al. 1989, 1991), rapid tranquilization of the agitated medical-surgical patient (Goodman and Charncy 1985), and the use of psychotropic drugs to treat symptoms associated with primary medical disorders (e.g., chronic pain, peptic ulcer disease) are discussed elsewhere (Max et al. 1992).

CARDIAC DISEASE AND CYCLIC ANTIDEPRESSANTS

At therapeutic doses, the cardiovascular risks involved in taking "cyclic" antidepressants (CyADs, or non-monoamine oxidase inhibitor [MAOI] antidepressants) are relatively small in the vast majority of patients (Boston Collaborative Drug Surveillance Program 1972). Although tricyclic antidepressants (TCAs; e.g., imipramine, amitriptyline) have quinidine-like properties that can increase the P-R interval, QRS duration, and QT_c interval and "flatten" the T wave on the electrocardiogram (ECG), these effects are almost never of major clinical significance unless patients have preexisting or latent cardiac conduction defects.

Because of their quinidine-like effects, the TCAs have antiarrhythmic properties and may prolong the refractory period of the action potential of the cardiac conduction system. This quinidine-like effect tends to suppress ectopic pacemakers that cause atrial flutter, atrial fibrillation, ventricular tachycardia, and premature ventricular contractions (PVCs). Thus, if tricyclic agents are used in depressed patients with cardiovascular disease, they may actually suppress PVCs (Bigger et al. 1977).

TCAs may cause ECG changes at therapeutic serum levels in patients with preexisting conduction delays such as atrioventricular (AV) block. Patients with preexisting intraventricular conduction delays (defined as a QRS interval greater than 0.11 seconds), sick sinus syndrome, second-degree heart block, and bifascicular heart block are at higher risk for arrhythmias (Roose et al. 1987). Patients with relatively benign types of heart block such as uncomplicated left bundle branch block, isolated left anterior or left posterior fascicular block, or right bundle branch block are at a relatively lower risk for aggravation of heart block by TCAs (Stoudemire and Atkinson 1988).

A prolonged Q-T interval presents a relative contraindication to CyAD treatment because of the hazard of malignant ventricular arrhythmias (torsades de pointes; an approximate guideline regarding the length of the Q-T for the safe use of TCA is a QT_c interval of no more than 0.440 seconds). Prolonged Q-T intervals may also occur on a congenital basis and present problems in using TCAs. Such patients may not be symptomatic and may only be detected on a routine ECG. In patients without cardiac disease, dangerous prolongations of the QT_c interval (i.e., beyond 0.440 seconds) occur most often in situations involving CyAD overdose (Fricchione and Vlay 1986; Schwartz and Wolf 1978). It should be noted that trazodone, fluoxetine, sertraline, paroxetine, and bupropion have few, if any, quinidine-like side effects compared with TCAs (Fisch 1985; Preskorn and Othmer 1984; Sommi et al. 1987). These drugs are much safer than tricyclic agents in patients with cardiac conduction disease.

Fluoxetine, sertraline, and bupropion have a low affinity for muscarinic, histaminic, and α-adrenergic receptors. They thus have minimal effects on pulse and blood pressure and therefore may offer significant advantages in elderly medically ill patients. There are extremely rare reports of a variety of arrhythmias being attributed to fluoxetine, particularly bradycardia. Reports of arrhythmias associated with fluoxetine have primarily been in patients with concomitant serious medical illness and who are on multiple medications. It has been our experience that cardiac effects with fluoxetine, as with sertraline, are extremely rare; these drugs are to be preferred in patients with a history of cardiac conduction delays, orthostatic hypotension, and congestive heart failure. Bupropion should be considered for such patients as well.

MAOIs, which do not have quinidine-like effects, may also be considered for patients with heart block, as can electroconvulsive therapy (ECT). The use of CyADs in patients with cardiac conduction disease is reviewed in more detail elsewhere (Roose et al. 1987; Stoudemire and Atkinson 1988; Stoudemire and Fogel 1987).

■ CyADs and Myocardial Infarction

It is not known whether a recent myocardial infarction (MI) in itself is a risk factor for cardiotoxicity from CyADs. Secondary complications of MI, such as heart failure, arrhythmias, orthostatic hypotension, and cardiac conduction abnormalities—and the potential influence of CyADs on cardiac rhythm, conduction, blood pressure, and the potential interactions with other drugs—are much more important in assessing the relative safety of CyADs in the post-MI phase (Stoudemire and Fogel 1987). There have been no firm data through prospective study of increased morbidity or mortality associated with the use of CyADs by post-MI patients (Smith et al. 1980). Recent reports from studies of post-MI antiarrhythmic prophylaxis protocols, however, suggest a possible increased risk of morbidity and mortality after MI when drugs with properties similar to those of the tricyclics on cardiac conduction are used. Until more definitive data are available, a conservative approach would be to avoid tricyclics in the post-MI period, if possible, and to treat depression in such patients with selective serotonin reuptake inhibitors (SSRIs) or bupropion.

Cardiac arrhythmias have actually been observed to emerge after TCAs are discontinued, particularly if the withdrawal is rapid (Regan et al. 1989; Van Sweden 1988). Experimental studies involving ligation of the coronary arteries of cats have demonstrated that tricyclics tend to increase retrograde perfusion of the distal component of the occluded artery and decrease the volume of ischemic myocardium (Manoach et al. 1986). Although these observations cannot be generalized to humans, they nevertheless suggest the possibility that TCAs may actually enhance cardiac reperfusion after MI.

The decision to continue or discontinue TCAs after a cardiac event must be evaluated on an individual basis and depends on multiple medical factors, such as the presence of heart block, orthostatic hypotension, and concurrent arrhythmias. Moreover, the complications caused by abrupt tricyclic withdrawal, or exacerbation or relapse of depression in the post-MI period, should also be considered.

Hence, the use of antidepressants in the peri- and post-MI period must always be based on risk-benefit ratio assessment done in consultation with the patient's cardiologist.

■ Orthostatic Hypotension and Congestive Heart Failure

Orthostatic hypotension creates the most problems in medically ill patients treated with traditional tricyclics such as imipramine. Patients with preexisting hypotensive symptoms, impaired left ventricular functioning, or bundle branch block are at increased risk for orthostatic hypotension with tricyclic treatment (Rizos et al. 1988). Although in middle-aged and relatively healthy patients, the use of salt supplements and support hose can partially relieve orthostatic hypotension, these measures are of less benefit in elderly medical patients—and, in the case of salt loading, may be contraindicated in patients with congestive heart failure or hypertension.

Imipramine has little or no effect on cardiac output in most patients, though it may produce orthostatic hypotension, a serious side effect that often prevents its use (Glassman et al. 1983). In patients with normal cardiac output and even in patients with stable or well-compensated congestive heart failure, nortriptyline usually has little or no effect on cardiac output and appears to have significantly less orthostatic hypotensive effects than imipramine (Roose et al. 1981, 1986). At very low levels of cardiac output (20%–25% or less) or in decompensated heart failure, however, tricyclics may exacerbate congestive heart failure.

Bupropion appears to have minimal effects on the cardiovascular system, does not appear to cause orthostatic hypertension, and may actually cause an elevation in blood pressure, particularly in patients with preexisting hypertension. Fluoxetine and sertraline appear to have little or no effect on blood pressure (Cooper 1988). Of the tricyclic agents, nortriptyline has been studied the most extensively in relation to blood pressure changes and has relatively less tendency to cause orthostatic hypotension compared with tertiary tricyclic compounds such as imipramine and amitriptyline. If patients have preexisting symptomatic orthostatic hypotension or develop this condition, drugs such as fluoxetine, sertraline, paroxetine, or bupropion should be used.

■ CyADs AND OTHER MEDICAL CONDITIONS

■ Glaucoma

Narrow-angle glaucoma can be exacerbated by antidepressants with high anticholinergic side effects, but patients with open-angle glaucoma generally can take TCAs with minimal risk. Patients with narrow-angle glaucoma may safely take TCAs if their glaucoma is being treated and monitored (Lieberman and Stoudemire 1987). In general, agents with low or no anticholinergic side effects (e.g., fluoxetine, sertraline, or bupropion) would be preferred in treating this patient population.

■ Urogenital Tract

Patients with known and untreated prostatic hypertrophy are at particular risk for urinary retention from traditional anticholinergic tricyclics. More typically, urinary retention developing with use of a tricyclic often leads to the identification of latent prostatic disease. As with glaucoma, use of drugs with low or no anticholinergic effects would be the preferred choice in patients prone to urinary retention. Trazodone, which has low anticholinergic properties, can cause priapism, although the risk of this complication is low (about 1 in 7,000 males treated) (Falk 1987; Mead Johnson Co., Evansville, IN).

■ Seizure Disorders

Human and animal reports vary in their conclusions as to the effects of CyADs on the seizure threshold (Edwards et al. 1986). Maprotiline, a tetracyclic (in doses above 200 mg qd), as well as bupropion have increased rates of seizures as compared with other CyADs. Among the traditional tricyclic agents, amitriptyline appears most likely to aggravate seizures (Edwards et al. 1986).

When CyADs are given to treated epileptic patients, anticonvulsant levels should be periodically checked and dosages adjusted to maintain the level in the therapeutic range because of possible drug interactions with anticonvulsants (Table 39–1).

Carbamazepine will *lower* tricyclic levels and sodium valproate may *elevate* tricyclic levels. Because bupropion carries greater risk of seizures than other CyADs, it should be avoided in patients with epilepsy

Table 39–1. Reported drug interactions with psychotropic agents: cyclic antidepressants (CyADs)

Medication	Interactive effect
Type I-A antiarrhythmics (quinidine, procainamide)	May prolong cardiac conduction time
Phenothiazines	May prolong Q-T interval and raise CyAD levels
Reserpine Guanethidine Clonidine	May decrease antihypertensive effect
Prazosin and other α-adrenergic blocking agents	Potentiate hypotensive effect
Parenteral sympathomimetic pressor amines (e.g., epinephrine, norepinephrine, phenylephrine)	May cause slight increases in blood pressure
Disulfiram Methylphenidate Cimetidine	Raise CyAD levels
Warfarin	May increase prothrombin time (fluoxetine probably more likely to cause this effect)
Oral contraceptives Ethanol Barbiturates Phenytoin	May lower CyAD levels
Anticholinergic agents	TCA may potentiate side effects
Carbamazepine	Additive cardiotoxicity possible and lower tricyclic levels
Propafenone (Type I-C antiarrhythmic)	May elevate tricyclic levels
Digitoxin	Fluoxetine may displace digitoxin from protein-binding sites and increase bioactive levels of digitoxin; converse is also true
High-fiber diets Cholestyramine	May lower TCA serum levels

as well as in other high-risk patients, such as those with a history of head trauma or patients with abnormal foci on the electroencephalogram, indicating potential enhanced central nervous system (CNS) irritability (Davidson 1989).

■ Pharmacokinetic Considerations

When treating frail, medically ill elderly patients, starting dosages of CyADs should be low (e.g., 10 mg qd of nortriptyline). Dosage should be raised gradually, depending on a patient's toleration of side ef-

fects and response to treatment. Cases have been reported of toxic serum tricyclic levels in elderly patients taking as little as 25 mg qd (Glassman et al. 1985).

Insufficient information exists regarding the effects of medical illness on CyAD metabolism in medically ill patients, but some general observations can be made from limited studies of the use of these drugs in elderly patients (Rockwell et al. 1988). Impaired hepatic protein synthesis (leading to decreased serum albumin) may decrease availability of protein for drug binding, leaving more unbound drug active at receptor sites, and hence more bioactive drug availability at a given dose as compared with patients with normal serum albumin. Plasma levels of the tertiary tricyclics amitriptyline and imipramine also tend to be positively correlated with age (Nies et al. 1977; i.e., increased age equals increased serum level for a given dose). Metabolism of demethylated tricyclics such as nortriptyline and desipramine appears to be less affected by age than imipramine or amitriptyline (Abernethy et al. 1985; Antal et al. 1982; Cutler and Narang 1984; Cutler et al. 1981; Neshkes et al. 1985; Nies et al. 1977).

Elderly and medically ill patients do not always need lower doses of CyADs, and elderly patients may show either great sensitivity or great tolerance to these drugs (Glassman et al. 1985; Rockwell et al. 1988; Stoudemire and Fogel 1987). Primary liver disease and hepatic dysfunction from diseases as well as congestive heart failure may result in slower metabolism of CyADs (and thus a longer half-life) compared with that in healthy patients. A number of drugs may inhibit hepatic enzymes (e.g., antipsychotics, valproate, disulfiram, cimetidine, and methylphenidate) and may thereby increase plasma levels of CyADs (Table 39–1).

It is now well known that fluoxetine (and its principal metabolite norfluoxetine), as well as paroxetine and sertraline, competitively inhibit cytochrome P_{450}/IID6 (Brosen and Skjelbo 1991), an enzyme responsible for the metabolism of tricyclics. Of these three SSRIs, paroxetine is the most potent inhibitor of cytochrome P_{450}/IID6. When any of these drugs are concurrently administered with tricyclics (as well as other psychotropics metabolized via this system such as neuroleptics and carbamazepine), an elevation of serum levels of these concomitantly administered drugs will result. Significant levels of fluoxetine and norfluoxetine may persist for as long as 8 weeks after discontinuation of fluoxetine. Sertraline and paroxetine have elimination half-lives of approximately 24 hours, reach steady state usually within a week, and are eliminated much more rapidly than fluoxetine (usually within 2 weeks) after discontinuation. Introduction of tricyclics following a course of SSRI treatment should start at low doses and be titrated conservatively, with serum levels monitored. Sertraline interacts less with the cytochrome P_{450} system and has less propensity to elevate serum levels of other drugs as compared with paroxetine and fluoxetine (Goff et al. 1991; Grimsley et al. 1991; Pato 1991; Pearson 1990).

Because fluoxetine is tightly bound to plasma protein, the administration of fluoxetine to a patient taking another drug that is tightly bound to protein (e.g., warfarin, digitoxin) could theoretically cause a shift in plasma concentrations resulting in an adverse effect. Conversely, adverse effects may result from displacement of protein-bound fluoxetine by other tightly bound drugs. (These qualities also apply to sertraline and paroxetine, which are also highly protein bound.) Additionally, the protein binding of *digoxin* is approximately 27%; therefore, the binding to plasma protein is relatively low compared with *digotoxin,* which is approximately 90% (Dista Products Company). These effects are primarily theoretical, and there is little evidence to suggest these properties regarding protein binding are of major clinical significance.

■ TRICYCLICS IN PATIENTS WITH RENAL FAILURE AND ON DIALYSIS

The hydroxylated metabolites of tricyclics have been found to be markedly elevated in renal disease and dialysis patients (Dawling et al. 1982; Lieberman et al. 1985) as compared with control subjects. Serum levels of the parent tricyclic compounds (amitriptyline and nortriptyline) also tend to be somewhat higher in dialysis patients as compared with control subjects after oral doses (Lieberman et al. 1985). However, there are no data to indicate the need for routine measurement of the hydroxylated metabolites of TCAs in patients with chronic renal failure or those on dialysis. The fact that these hydroxylated metabolites contribute to side effect hypersensitivity

augers for more conservative titration of doses in this patient population. Table 39–2 summarizes the side-effect profiles of the currently available non-MAOI CyADs.

■ MAOIs IN MEDICALLY ILL PATIENTS

MAOIs may raise special problems in medically ill patients because of their effects on blood pressure and body weight, as well as interactions with medications used in internal medicine. With respect to elderly medically ill patients, the most common effect of MAOIs is orthostatic hypotension. As compared with traditional tricyclics, there is relatively little difference between the orthostatic blood pressure effects of phenelzine compared with that of nortriptyline in patients 55 and older (Georgotas et al. 1987). Effects on blood pressure may be ameliorated by slow, conservative dosing strategies. Divided-dose strategies also will help in minimizing blood pressure effects.

Hypertensive crises may be precipitated by drug interactions with MAOIs. The most consistent offenders are the indirect pressor amines (e.g., ephedrine, pseudoephedrine, and phenylpropanolamine; Table 39–3). Direct pressors (e.g., norepinephrine, epinephrine, and isoproterenol) are relatively safer, and in one well-designed animal study they showed almost no pressor effects (Braverman et al. 1987). Nevertheless, close monitoring of blood pressure would be strongly advisable if these drugs were to be instituted in a patient on MAOIs. Patients receiving bronchodilators are at a higher risk for side effects when on MAOIs; but at least theoretically, they should not have unusual problems as long as indirect sympathomimetics such as ephedrine are clearly avoided. Xanthines and cromolyn would usually be preferable to sympathomimetic drugs in asthmatic patients on MAOIs.

Drug-induced hypertensive episodes would be particularly hazardous in patients with cardiovascular or cerebrovascular disease as well as for patients on oral anticoagulants, because of their greater risk for a cerebral hemorrhage. All patients treated with MAOIs (even those at relatively low risk) should carry 10-mg nifedipine tablets, to be chewed or dissolved under the tongue at the first signs of a hypertensive

Table 39–2.   Side-effect profiles of cyclic antidepressants (CyADs)

	Effect on serotonin reuptake	Effect on norepinephrine reuptake	Sedating effect	Anticholinergic effect	Orthostatic effect	Dose range[d] (mg)
Amitriptyline[a]	++++	++	++++	++++	++++	75–300
Imipramine[a]	++++	++	+++	+++	++++	75–300
Nortriptyline	+++	+++	++	++	+	40–150
Protriptyline	+++	++++	+	+++	+	10–60
Trazodone	+++	±	+++	±[b]	++	200–600
Desipramine	+++	++++	+	+	++	75–300
Amoxapine[c]	++	+++	++	++	++	75–600
Maprotiline	+	++	++	+	++	150–200
Doxepin	+++	++	+++	++	++	75–300
Trimipramine[c]	+	+	++	++	++	50–300
Fluoxetine	++++	–	–	–	–	20–60
Paroxetine	++++	–	–	++	–	20–40
Sertraline	++++	–	–	–	–	50–200
Bupropion	–	–	–	±	–	150–450

Note. Relative potencies (some ratings are approximated) based partly on affinities of these agents for brain receptors in competitive binding studies. – = none, + = slight, ++ = moderate, +++ = marked, ++++ = pronounced, ± = indeterminant.
[a]Available in injectable form.
[b]Most in vivo and clinical studies report the absence of anticholinergic effects (or no difference from placebo). There have been case reports, however, of apparent anticholinergic effects.
[c]Amoxapine and trimipramine have dopamine receptor blocking activity.
[d]Dose ranges are for treatment of major depression. Lower doses may be appropriate for other therapeutic uses.
Source. Reprinted from Richelson 1982 with permission.

reaction (Clary and Schweizer 1987). Nifedipine's hypotensive effect is relatively proportional to the degree of hypertension and has a direct antianginal effect that would be of value for patients with coronary insufficiency. Verapamil has been used for treatment of hypertensive crises, at a dosage of 80 mg po (Merikangas and Merikangas 1988). Drug interactions with MAOIs are summarized in Table 39–3.

All of the MAOIs—but particularly the hydrazides, such as phenelzine and isocarboxazid—are associated with carbohydrate craving and weight gain. Weight gain would be of particular importance in patients with diabetes mellitus and hyperlipidemia. For patients with these and other medical disorders that would be complicated by substantial weight gain, tranylcypromine would typically be the MAOI of choice.

Clinical tradition has usually mandated that MAOIs should always be discontinued prior to anesthesia and surgery. But more recent evidence suggests that surgery or ECT nevertheless can be safely carried out with the concurrent use of MAOIs (El Ganzouri et al. 1985; Stack et al. 1988; Wells and

Bjorksten 1989), providing there is no chance the patient would receive meperidine in the postoperative period.

■ OTHER SPECIAL CONSIDERATIONS

As has been noted earlier, MAOIs do not significantly affect cardiac conduction, although there are few data on the use of these drugs in patients with advanced cardiovascular diseases (McGrath et al. 1987). Phenelzine may slightly reduce heart rate and may actually shorten the Q-T interval (McGrath et al. 1987; Robinson et al. 1982). MAOIs may even have some antiarrhythmic effects; in one animal model of ventricular fibrillation, phenelzine had an antiarrhythmic effect (Verrier 1986).

MAOIs appear less likely than TCAs to aggravate seizures (Edwards 1985), but their pharmacodynamic interactions with some anticonvulsants may create other problems, such as excessive sedation if barbi-

Table 39–3. Reported drug interactions with psychotropic agents: monoamine oxidase inhibitors

Medication	Interactive effect
Meperidine	Fatal reaction
L-Dopa, methyldopa, dopamine, buspirone, guanethidine, cyclic antidepressants, carbamazepine, cyclobenzaprine	Elevation of blood pressure
Direct-acting sympathomimetics Epinephrine, norepinephrine, isoproterenol, methoxamine	Elevation of blood pressure
Indirect-acting sympathomimetics Cocaine, amphetamines, tyramine, methylphenidate, phenethylamine, metaraminol, ephedrine, phenylpropanolamine	Severe hypertension
Direct and indirect-acting sympathomimetics Pseudoephedrine, metaraminol, phenylephrine	Severe hypertension
Serotonergic agents Fluoxetine, tryptophan	"Serotonin syndrome" (ataxia, nystagmus, confusion, fever, tremor)
Caffeine Theophylline Aminophylline	Mild increase in blood pressure
Hypoglycemic agents	Lower blood glucose
Anticoagulants	Prolonged prothrombin time
Succinylcholine	Phenelzine prolongs action
Diuretics Propranolol Prazosin Calcium channel blockers	Increased hypotensive effect

turate anticonvulsants are used. MAOIs, however, may be preferable in many situations to tricyclics in epileptic patients needing antidepressant therapy.

MAOIs may cause a pyridoxine (vitamin B_6) deficiency manifested as peripheral polyneuropathy or as susceptibility to nerve entrapment neuropathy conditions such as carpal tunnel syndrome (Robinson and Kurtz 1987). Pyridoxine deficiency can be treated with 50–100 mg of vitamin B_6 daily. The MAOIs also influence thiamine metabolism (decreasing erythrocyte transketolase [Ali 1985]). In malnourished or alcoholic patients, this effect could theoretically increase the likelihood of clinical symptoms of thiamine deficiency.

BENZODIAZEPINES

Complaints of anxiety and disturbed sleep are the most common indications for use of benzodiazepines among medically ill patients. However, when these complaints arise in medically ill patients who are on a number of medications or in the hospital, care should be exercised in formulating the differential diagnosis. For example, "nervousness" in a pulmonary patient may be due to toxic levels of methylxanthines, excessive use of β-adrenergic inhalers, or high-dose corticosteroids, none of which should be treated with benzodiazepines alone.

Medically Ill Elderly Patients

As with most psychotropics, benzodiazepines present greater risks for elderly patients than for younger ones (Meyer 1982; Thompson et al. 1983). Although there are no benzodiazepines especially safe for elderly medically ill patients, ultrashort-acting agents such as triazolam are more likely to cause confusion, dissociation, and anterograde amnesia (Morris and Estes 1987; Rickels et al. 1988).

Long half-life drugs accumulate and reach steady state slowly, tend to be highly lipophilic, and are cleared slowly after the drug is stopped. These drugs are generally metabolized by oxidation, a hepatic mechanism that decays in efficacy with age and hepatic dysfunction, and for those additional reasons should be used cautiously in elderly patients who are medically ill. For example, adjustments downward in dose, greater time intervals between doses, and close follow-up assessment of cognitive functioning and mood would be indicated. Prototypical benzodiazepines in this group include diazepam, flurazepam, and quazepam.

Shorter-acting drugs are less lipophilic, accumulate less, and clear more rapidly after cessation. Rather than being oxidized, they are conjugated—a metabolic route that loses little effectiveness with aging or hepatic disease. Although the adjustments necessary for medically ill and elderly patients may be proportionately less among this group of drugs than for the longer-acting agents, they are adjustments nonetheless, and close follow-up is indicated (Greenblatt et al. 1983). Drugs with a medium to short half-life include temazepam, oxazepam, and lorazepam.

In patients with hepatic dysfunction due to

cirrhosis, active hepatitis, or metabolic damage, conjugated drugs should be chosen. The hepatic metabolism of lorazepam, oxazepam, and temazepam are less affected by these disorders (Klotz et al. 1975).

Benzodiazepines can induce ventilatory suppression in the setting of certain pulmonary conditions. Those patients who chronically retain CO_2 are at greatest risk, because benzodiazepines reduce the hypoxic response to ventilation—their only remaining ventilatory stimulus (Lakshminarayan et al. 1976; Modeo and Berry 1974). Another high-risk category is that of sleep apnea (the periodic cessation of ventilation during sleep), due either to obstruction or failure of central drive.

■ Other Prescribing Guidelines

Apart from specified high-risk groups, most psychiatrists choose benzodiazepines based on pharmacokinetic properties of the individual drugs. These appear clinically as response time (speed of absorption and lipophilicity), duration of action (functional half-life), and various idiosyncratic adverse effects (e.g., a "high," anterograde amnesia, confusion, and others, often due to lipophilic qualities affecting brain concentration of the drug).

Long-acting benzodiazepines can be used safely even among elderly patients as long as proper dosage and frequency adjustments are made. Intramuscular administration is reliable only with lorazepam and midazolam. The physician should always examine the patient's medication list before prescribing a benzodiazepine or any other sedating medication. Concomitant use of narcotics, barbiturates, or other benzodiazepines may result in untoward sedation or even delirium.

■ Newer Benzodiazepines

Estazolam is a new drug for insomnia. Its elimination half-life increases moderately in elderly patients, to a range of 13–34 hours, from the usual range of 8–24 hours. It is effective in elderly patients at half the usual 2-mg dose for younger patients. There is little rebound insomnia after abrupt cessation (Pierce and Shu 1990). Risk to elderly patients (cognitive impairment) and chronic pulmonary patients (ventilatory suppression) should be considered moderate to high.

Quazepam is a new long-acting benzodiazepine that appears to have preferential BZ1 receptor affinity (Walmsley and Hunt 1991). Because the drug is highly lipophilic and rapidly absorbed, its onset of action is rapid. The duration of action of single doses is brief due to movement to fat stores, but repeated doses will result in accumulation there. The fact that quazepam and flurazepam share a major active metabolite argues for caution in the use of quazepam in elderly medically ill patients, patients with pulmonary disease, and patients with hepatic dysfunction.

When using benzodiazepines as hypnotics or anxiolytics, a thorough differential diagnosis and evaluation of etiology should precede reflexive prescription of a drug. Patients with hepatic or pulmonary disease and elderly patients should probably avoid drugs metabolized by oxidation, and in general, shorter-acting drugs that are conjugated are preferable. Special attention should be given to the patient's need to get up at night because of ataxia and confusion caused by some drugs, such as triazolam. A key strategy for the psychiatrist treating these patients is frequent follow-up in a manner that allows assessment of cognitive functioning, mood, gait, and (when indicated) ventilatory status with blood gases.

■ BUSPIRONE

The use of buspirone, a nonbenzodiazepine anxiolytic, has not been extensively studied in medically ill patients. Buspirone may have advantages in patients with chronic lung disease, because in animal studies it appears to stimulate respiratory drive, as opposed to the general depressant effect on respiration observed with benzodiazepines (Garner et al. 1989; Mendelson et al. 1989). Diazepam may markedly depress ventilatory response to exogenous CO_2 administration, whereas buspirone had no such overall effect (Rapoport 1989; Rapoport et al. 1988). In addition, buspirone does not depress ventilatory response to increasing CO_2 levels. Therefore, buspirone appears to be a potentially safer long-term anxiolytic for treatment of patients with respiratory disease.

Pharmacokinetic studies with buspirone indicate that there are no clinically significant differences between young and elderly patients in standard pharmacokinetic measures with either acute or chronic dosing (Gammans et al. 1989). There appears to be no need to alter the initial doses of buspirone based solely on the patient's age.

■ NEUROLEPTICS

Apart from schizophrenia, delirium is perhaps the most common syndrome treated with neuroleptics among elderly and medically ill patients. The therapeutic efficacy among the various available antipsychotics is essentially the same, and the choice of a particular agent is thus guided by the side-effect profile most likely to be tolerated or to cause the fewest problems in an individual patient. The antipsychotics can be arbitrarily divided into "high-potency" drugs (such as haloperidol and fluphenazine), which are relatively low in sedating and anticholinergic effects and high in extrapyramidal side effects (EPS), and "low-potency" agents, which have opposite characteristics.

The same influences that merge to produce cerebral dysfunction in medically ill patients (i.e., electrolyte disturbances, hypoxemia, volume shifts, systemic infections, medications) make them vulnerable to side effects of any added medication, including neuroleptics. The neuroleptic alone may produce symptomatic improvement in a delirium and thereby induce complacency about the underlying pathogenic cause. Thus, a careful differential diagnosis must be made for the target syndrome (such as delirium) or symptom (such as agitation). Elderly and medically ill patients are generally more sensitive than younger patients to a given oral dose, especially for chlorpromazine. As a result, most psychiatrists use high-potency agents such as haloperidol in the settings described.

■ Cardiac and Pulmonary Disease

Patients with cardiac conduction disease may be susceptible to quinidine-like effects of neuroleptics. The effects on the ECG and on the clinical exam are usually negligible. However, if the patient concurrently takes a Type I antiarrhythmic—including a tricyclic—or has a significant preexisting conduction delay, the effect may be less benign and require close monitoring or even cardiological consultation. If the QT_c interval before starting the neuroleptic is 0.440 seconds or longer, added quinidine-like effects may result in fatal ventricular arrhythmias. Among antipsychotics, thioridazine appears to be the most dangerous drug in this regard (Stoudemire et al. 1993). Drug interactions with neuroleptics are listed in Table 39–4.

The psychiatrist should avoid low-potency agents such as chlorpromazine in patients with symptomatic orthostatic hypotension. These drugs cause a notable degree of α-adrenergic blockade and can worsen blood pressure regulation. High-potency agents are preferred in this setting.

For the patient with an acute MI, the greatest risk again occurs among low-potency drugs, chiefly because of orthostatic hypotension but also because of tachycardia induced by vagolytic anticholinergic ef-

Table 39–4. Reported drug interactions with neuroleptics

Medication	Interactive effect
Type I-A antiarrhythmics	Chlorpromazine or thioridazine may prolong cardiac conduction
Alprazolam Tricyclics β-blockers Chloramphenicol Disulfiram MAOIs Acetaminophen Buspirone Fluoxetine	May increase neuroleptic levels
Barbiturates Hypnotics Rifampin Griseofulvin Phenylbutazone Carbamazepine Phenytoin	Lower neuroleptic levels through induction of hepatic enzymes
Gel-type antacids with Al^{3+} and Mg^{2+}	May interfere with neuroleptic absorption
Narcotics Epinephrine Enflurane Isoflurane	Potentiate hypotensive effects of neuroleptics
α-methyldopa Prazosin ACE-inhibitors (captopril, enalapril)	Increase hypotensive effect
Narcotics Tricyclics Barbiturates	May increase sedative effects of neuroleptics
Iproniazid	May cause encephalopathy and hepatotoxicity when used with neuroleptics
Guanethidine Clonidine	Neuroleptics may decrease blood pressure control
Sodium valproate	Levels of valproate increased by chlorpromazine
Carbamazepine	Clozapine levels lowered by carbamazepine treatment

Note. MAOI = monoamine oxidase inhibitor; ACE = angiotensin-converting enzyme.

fects. High-potency neuroleptics present much less risk for the cardiac patient.

Some asthmatic patients are allergic to salts present in the parenteral solutions of antipsychotics (e.g., sodium bisulfite and sodium sulfite). Susceptible patients should avoid these preparations. The sedation induced by neuroleptics usually presents no ventilatory difficulty for pulmonary patients, even those who chronically retain CO_2.

Other Medical Disorders

The anticholinergic effects of the lower-potency agents may cause or exacerbate cognitive dysfunction in elderly patients and may also lead to increased intraocular pressure in patients with narrow-angle glaucoma. The antimuscarinic effects of these drugs may exacerbate prostatism and contribute to male sexual dysfunction. Thioridazine may induce impotence and retrograde ejaculation (Mitchell and Popkin 1983). Although the higher-potency drugs are less likely to cause these types of anticholinergic problems, they are on the other hand more likely to cause EPS.

Other Side Effects

EPS occur with all neuroleptics except clozapine and occur at a much lower rate with risperidone. The high-potency agents produce these side effects more commonly. Elderly patients are most susceptible to parkinsonian effects and young male patients to dystonias. The hematological effects of clozapine will likely limit its general use, but the Parkinson's disease patient with psychotic symptoms may be an ideal candidate for the drug.

Although all antipsychotics lower the seizure threshold, molindone, fluphenazine (Luchins et al. 1984), thioridazine, and mesoridazine (Edwards et al. 1986) appear to be the least proconvulsant. Reports suggest that chlorpromazine and clozapine are the most problematic in this regard. Combinations of neuroleptics may synergistically lower the seizure threshold. Because neuroleptics may alter the serum levels of anticonvulsant medications, these levels should be monitored during concomitant treatment (Edwards et al. 1986).

Medically debilitated, dehydrated, and neurologically impaired patients appear to be at risk for two potentially catastrophic conditions: neuroleptic ma-

lignant syndrome and neuroleptic-induced catatonia. Delirious patients on antipsychotics thus require close monitoring of fluid status and vital signs (Harpe and Stoudemire 1987; Stoudemire and Luther 1984).

There is increasing evidence for a therapeutic window of efficacy for antipsychotics, making the use of higher doses more likely to cause only more side effects, not bring about greater therapeutic results. Medically ill and elderly patients may respond to doses of haloperidol as low as 0.5–1.0 mg.

Clozapine

Clozapine is a novel antipsychotic with minimal EPS. Problems associated with its use include orthostatic hypotension, lowering of the seizure threshold, anticholinergic toxicity, and significant incidence of agranulocytosis (1%–2%). As a consequence, its indications are restricted to psychosis in Parkinson's disease and refractory schizophrenia. Clozapine may improve the symptoms of that illness (Roberts et al. 1989). The danger of seizure increases with increasing dose. The hematological risk is so grave as to require complete blood counts weekly.

The major side effects of concern for this drug with respect to its use in patients with medical and neurological illness are its high anticholinergic profile, its propensity to cause orthostatic hypertension, its potential to lower the seizure threshold, and the development of clozapine-induced fever and leukopenia. The reported problems with agranulocytosis (1%–2% of patients) require weekly blood monitoring. Of these patients at low doses (below 300 mg qd), 1%–2% are at risk of seizure; this risk increases to 3%–4% for those patients on intermediate doses and to about 5% at higher doses (600–900 mg qd). Nevertheless, clozapine may have advantages in treatment of patients who are prone to EPS and tardive dyskinesia, because it has minimal EPS and has not been reported to cause tardive dyskinesia. The drug may in fact have some beneficial effect in the treatment of tardive dyskinesia caused by traditional neuroleptics.

Clozapine has been used in treating patients with psychosis in Parkinson's disease and has actually been found to improve parkinsonian symptoms (Roberts et al. 1989). Treatment of psychosis in Parkinson's disease should begin with low doses of clozapine—12.5 mg bid (or even lower)—and be titrated upward slowly if needed. Because of clozapine's prominent anticholinergic effects, the extrapyramidal symptoms of Parkinson's disease may actually improve with clozapine treatment.

LITHIUM

Renal Disease

Because the kidney is the route for lithium excretion, renal competence and alterations in intravascular volume status are impediments to the prescription of the drug. Lithium occupies the "sodium space"; thus, any condition altering sodium movement will likely affect the body's handling of lithium. Volume depletion and traditional diuretic use are the most common clinical examples of conditions that raise serum lithium levels. Volume depletion occurs in conditions associated with vomiting, diarrhea, polyuria, and excessive sweating. Physical disability and lessened responsiveness to thirst could also hinder attempts at normal salt and water replacement. The result would be volume contraction and increased renal reabsorption of sodium and of lithium, with higher lithium levels on an unchanged oral dose. Among the diuretics, the thiazides have the most and furosemide the least effect on lithium concentration (Rizos et al. 1988). Potassium-sparing diuretics such as spironolactone may also reduce lithium clearance, but they have been less studied than other diuretics. Drug interactions with lithium are summarized in Table 39–5.

Renal failure patients on dialysis do not eliminate lithium between dialyses, and they therefore require only one dose in this interim. Levels are checked 2–3 hours after the dose, which is given after the dialysis. The dosage range is 300–600 mg qd (Levy 1993).

Advancing age itself generally brings a 30%–40% reduction in glomerular filtration rate and necessitates a proportional reduction in oral dose (Hardy et al. 1987). Older patients and others with CNS disease may show confusion and sedation at levels therapeutic for younger patients (DePaulo 1984). The psychiatrist should closely monitor lithium levels in these groups and aim for the lower end of the therapeutic range.

Almost all patients experience some polyuria on lithium because of its effect in reducing the kidney's ability to concentrate urine. This symptom may be improved by giving the lithium once a day.

Table 39–5. Reported drug interactions with lithium (Li^+)

Medication	Interactive effect
Thiazide diuretics Spironolactone Triamterene Nonsteroidal antiinflammatants (e.g., indomethacin, ibuprofen, phenylbutazone, piroxicam)	Raise Li^+ levels
Acetazolamide Theophylline Aminophylline	Lower Li^+ levels
Calcium channel blockers	May either raise or lower Li^+ levels, effects not clear; verapamil may cause bradycardia when used with Li^+
Metronidazole	May increase lithium levels; may increase chances of nephrotoxicity
Tetracycline	Minor elevation of Li^+ levels
Enalapril and other angiotensin-converting enzyme (ACE) inhibitors	Anecdoctally reported to raise lithium levels; systematic studies show little overall effect

Other Side Effects

Lithium induces hypothyroidism in 2%–15% of patients and goiter in 3%–4%. People with pretreatment elevations of thyroid-stimulating hormone (TSH) are probably at greatest risk for these effects. Monitoring of TSH and free thyroxine (T_4) levels can permit detection of hypothyroidism and prompt appropriate replacement treatment. Lithium cessation is rarely required.

Cardiac effects are generally quite benign, restricted to nonspecific T wave changes in the ECG, and some increased susceptibility to digitalis toxicity (Mittal et al. 1985; Tilkian et al. 1976a, 1976b). Extreme sensitivity to side effects of lithium argues for consideration of alternative treatments for bipolar patients, such as carbamazepine or sodium valproate.

PSYCHOSTIMULANTS

Psychostimulants such as methylphenidate, dextroamphetamine, and pemoline may be used for the treatment of depressed, medically debilitated patients (Kaufmann et al. 1982; Kayton and Raskind 1980; Woods 1986). In addition, methylphenidate has been reported to be effective in the treatment of depression in patients with acquired immunodeficiency syndrome (AIDS) (Fernandez et al. 1988). The dose ranges suggested for methylphenidate vary from 10–40 mg qd and for dextroamphetamine from 10–20 mg qd given in divided doses early in the day. The half-life for methylphenidate is much shorter than dextroamphetamine (2 versus 12 hours).

Psychostimulants, particularly dextroamphetamine, may cause rebound depression, agitation, psychotic reactions, and dependency (Chiarello and Cole 1987). A less controversial indication for their use is in the treatment of pain in cancer patients to counteract the sedation of narcotics (Goldberg and Tull 1984). In this setting, problems with dependency are moot, because most of these patients will have limited life expectancies. Drug interactions are summarized in Table 39–6.

Pemoline is a mild CNS psychostimulant with minimal sympathomimetic activity and a very low abuse potential. Pemoline is primarily used in the treatment of attention-deficit hyperactivity disorder (ADHD) but also has been demonstrated to have antidepressant (Conners and Taylor 1980) and cognitive-enhancing properties (Elizur et al. 1979; Small et al. 1968; Talland et al. 1967). Pemoline has been reported to have antidepressant properties in depressed, debilitated cancer patients similar to the effects of methylphenidate and dextroamphetamine. The usual dose in adults with medical illness is initially 18.75 mg qd or bid, which can be increased over several days to 37.5 mg bid. Side effects that have been reported include agitation, anorexia, and manic behavior. Rare cases of the development or induction of motor tics have been reported in children. Pemoline may also cause a reversible elevation in liver enzymes.

A major advantage of pemoline is that it can be given as a chewable tablet and is reliably absorbed through the buccal mucosa—a route for patients with gastrointestinal motility or absorptive dysfunction (Breitbart and Mermelstein 1992).

■ CARBAMAZEPINE

Carbamazepine's dose-related toxicities include ataxia, diplopia, and sedation. Several additional toxicities are particularly relevant when carbamazepine is used in patients with concurrent medical illness.

Table 39–6. Reported drug interactions with benzodiazepines and psychostimulants

Medication	Interactive effect
Benzodiazepines	
Cimetidine	May elevate serum levels of
Disulfiram	benzodiazepines metab-
Ethanol	olized predominantly by
Isoniazid	oxidation
Estrogens	Tend to lower benzodiaze-
Cigarettes	pine levels
Methylxanthine derivatives	
Rifampin	
Sodium valproate	Enhanced sedative effect of
	benzodiazepines (not
	applicable to lorazepam)
Psychostimulants	
Guanethidine	Decreased antihypertensive effect
Vasopressors	Increased pressor effect
Oral anticoagulants	Increased prothrombin time
Anticonvulsants	Increased levels of pheno-barbital, primidone, phenytoin
Tricyclics	Increased blood levels of cyclic antidepressants
MAOIs	Hypertension

These include hematological toxicity, hepatic toxicity, hyponatremia, quinidine-like cardiac effects, and effects on the pituitary-thyroid axis.

Carbamazepine may produce a transient reduction in white blood count in approximately 10% of patients during the first 4 months of treatment (Rall and Schleifer 1985) and in extremely rare cases produces potentially fatal agranulocytosis and aplastic anemia. The incidence of aplastic anemia has been estimated at 0.5 cases per 100,000 treatment-years (Hart and Easton 1982), but neither the age of the patient nor the duration of treatment predicts the development of aplastic anemia (Pisciotta 1975).

Because of the risk of early neutropenia, weekly or biweekly monitoring of white blood cell (WBC) count is usually advised during the first few months of therapy. Carbamazepine should in most cases be discontinued if the WBC drops below 3,500. However, exceptions may need to be made if the indications for carbamazepine are very strong or if a concurrent medical problem or drug treatment might be contributing to the decreased blood count. In such situations, hematological consultation will assist in determining the appropriate frequency of monitoring and cutoff point for drug discontinuation. Administration of lithium and carbamazepine lowers the risk for neutropenia because lithium stimulates WBC production. Therefore, the lithium-carbamazepine combination might be an option for patients with concurrent medical or hematological problems that suppress the white cell count and who have bipolar disorder unresponsive to lithium alone (Brewerton 1986; Vieweg et al. 1986).

Hepatic toxicity from carbamazepine, like hematological toxicity, comes in benign and relatively benign forms as well as in a rare and malignant form. Mild asymptomatic elevations in serum glutamic-oxaloacetic transaminase (SGOT), serum glutamic-pyruvic transaminase (SGPT), and γ-glutamyl transpeptidase (GGTP) occur in 5%–10% of patients treated with carbamazepine (Jeavons 1983; Pellock 1987). Life-threatening acute hepatitis with liver failure occurs on an allergic basis in less than 1 in 10,000 treated patients (Jeavons 1983). This toxicity most often occurs during the first month of therapy. In patients with preexisting liver disease, carbamazepine would be relatively (but not absolutely) contraindicated. However, frequent monitoring of liver enzymes and prothrombin time (PT) would be a reasonable precaution. In patients without liver disease, elevations of SGOT and SGPT to twice normal levels would generally be acceptable. The upper bounds of transaminase elevation might need to be higher in patients with preexisting hepatic disease who required carbamazepine therapy. Consultation with a gastroenterologist would be indicated to choose both an appropriate schedule for monitoring and criteria for drug discontinuation.

Hyponatremia is a relatively frequent side effect of carbamazepine for which advanced age and higher serum levels are risk factors (Kalff et al. 1984; Lahr 1985; Perucca et al. 1978) and may be aggravated by other conditions predisposing to hyponatremia, such as diuretic use, congestive heart failure, and occult malignancy. Patients with risk factors for hyponatremia should have weekly electrolyte determinations during the first month of carbamazepine therapy. If hyponatremia develops, the clinician's response should depend upon its severity, and sodium levels of less than 125 mEq/L would usually be a reason to discontinue carbamazepine. Lesser degrees of hyponatremia should be considered in relation to the necessity of the drug for the patient. In some cases, drugs aggravating hyponatremia, such as diuretics, can be discontinued instead. Persistent hypo-

natremia after discontinuation of carbamazepine would warrant a full evaluation for inappropriate antidiuretic hormone (ADH) secretion.

Carbamazepine has a tricyclic structure similar to that of TCAs and has quinidine-like cardiac effects. Clinically significant aggravation of heart block has been reported (Beerman and Edhag 1978; Benassi et al. 1987). Patients over 40 or with known cardiac risk factors should have a pretreatment ECG before receiving carbamazepine.

Carbamazepine has been implicated in a large number of drug interactions that are summarized in Table 39–7. Two are particularly deserving of emphasis in the context of psychiatric treatment of medically ill patients. A major effect of carbamazepine is related

Table 39–7. Reported drug interactions with carbamazepine

Medication	Interactive effect
Erythromycin	May raise carbamazepine to toxic levels and precipitate heart block
Antiarrhythmics	May have additive effects on cardiac conduction time
Fluoxetine Cimetidine Diltiazem Verapamil Danazol Propoxyphene	May raise carbamazepine levels to toxic levels
Quinidine Phenytoin Warfarin Tricyclic antidepressants Neuroleptics Propranolol Clonazepam	Serum levels lowered by carbamazepine
Phenobarbital	Decreased serum levels of carbamazepine and increased concentrations of carbamazepine's epoxide metabolite
Valproate	Serum levels of valproate lowered by carbamazepine
Phenytoin	Decreased levels of carbamazepine; phenytoin levels increased when used with carbamazepine
Warfarin	Carbamazepine causes increased metabolism of anticoagulants due to hepatic enzyme induction
Oral contraceptives	Carbamazepine reduces efficacy; loss of contraceptive effect possible

to its potent effect on inducing drug metabolism by the hepatic microsomal system (Perucca and Richens 1989), causing lower serum levels of other drugs metabolized by the liver, including (among many others) TCAs, neuroleptics, propranolol, quinidine, phenytoin, valproic acid, and warfarin. Obtaining levels of drugs metabolized by the hepatic microsomal system should probably be obtained more often in patients taking carbamazepine, and repeated levels of the other medications may be needed if carbamazepine doses are significantly changed.

Because carbamazepine is metabolized by the liver, drugs that inhibit the hepatic metabolic enzymes may raise carbamazepine levels and lead to acute carbamazepine toxicity after a new drug is added. These types of clinically significant interactions have been reported for verapamil (Beattie et al. 1988; MacPhee et al. 1986), diltiazem (Brodie and MacPhee 1986), danazol (Kramer et al. 1986), propoxyphene (Dam et al. 1977), and the antibiotic erythromycin (Wong et al. 1983) and are listed in Table 39–7.

Carbamazepine has two antithyroid effects: it *increases* the peripheral metabolism of thyroid hormone (Aanderud et al. 1981), and it *decreases* TSH secretion by a direct effect on the pituitary (Hein and Jackson 1990). These effects lead to the development of hypothyroidism (Aanderud and Strandjord 1980) or to an increase in the thyroxine requirement for patients already receiving thyroid replacement therapy (DeLuca et al. 1986). Patients receiving combined treatment with lithium and carbamazepine may experience additive antithyroid effects. *TSH levels may not necessarily be elevated even when the patient is hypothyroid because of the effect of carbamazepine on the pituitary.* Patients with thyroid disease should have a complete thyroid function panel after carbamazepine therapy is instituted. Thyroid replacement should be considered if the patient appears hypothyroid, even if the TSH is not elevated (Hein and Jackson 1990).

■ VALPROATE

Sodium valproate is increasingly being applied to patients with bipolar spectrum disorders. The drug's gastrointestinal effects are well known. These problems are markedly reduced by the availability of enteric coated preparations and by patients taking the medications after meals. Although hepatic failure was a major concern with valproate in the past, this problem is encountered almost exclusively in children under age 2 years. The incidence in adults of valproate-related hepatic necrosis is less than 1 in 10,000 (Eadie et al. 1988). In adults, elevations in serum ammonia may occur due to inhibition of urea synthesis, but this is almost always a benign effect and is of concern only in patients with preexisting liver disease. Significant liver disease is a relative contraindication to valproate treatment.

Valproate can increase the PT and decrease fibrinogen levels and the platelet counts, but very rarely do such effects lead to clinically significant bleeding (Stoudemire et al. 1991). Patients should have a coagulation panel (prothrombin time/partial thromboplastin time [PT/PTT]) and a platelet count before having surgery.

With respect to drug interactions, valproate tends to inhibit hepatic enzymes involved in drug metabolism. This effect is in contrast to that of carbamazepine, which is a hepatic enzyme inducer. It should be noted that if carbamazepine and valproate are used together, valproate will raise the concentration of the 10-11-epoxide metabolite of carbamazepine. This metabolite has additional toxicity with carbamazepine and is usually not measured. Hence, the capacity for carbamazepine toxicity is increased when the two drugs are used together. In addition, valproate may displace carbamazepine from serum protein-binding sites, increasing the bioavailable fraction of carbamazepine but without changing the absolute blood level—thus potentially increasing side effects at a given carbamazepine level. With valproate, protein-binding sites are readily saturated. Dose increases beyond this point of saturation may lead to enhanced side effects, even though dose increases are relatively small and absolute serum levels increase only slightly. Drug interactions with valproate are listed in Table 39–8. More detailed discussions of the use of valproate in the medical patient may be found elsewhere (Fogel and Stoudemire 1993; Stoudemire et al. 1991, 1993).

■ ECT IN MEDICALLY ILL PATIENTS

ECT should be considered as a primary treatment for many severely depressed medical patients. In medi-

Table 39–8. Reported drug interactions with valproate

Medication	Interactive effect
Benzodiazepines (except lorazepam)	Sedative effects and serum levels of benzodiazepine increased by valproate
Carbamazepine Phenytoin Phenobarbital	Lower levels of valproate
Phenobarbital	Phenobarbital levels increased by valproate
Phenytoin Carbamazepine	Valproate raises bioavailable phenytoin and carbamazepine by displacing these drugs from serum protein-binding sites
10-11-epoxide metabolite of carbamazepine	Increased levels of this metabolite caused by valproate
Tricyclic antidepressants (TCAs)	TCA levels increased by valproate
Chlorpromazine Cimetidine Salicylates	Increased levels of valproate
Anticoagulants (warfarin)	Increased prothrombin times; valproate also inhibits secondary phase of platelet aggregation

cally debilitated depressed patients and those with advanced cardiovascular disease, appropriate pharmacological management before and during anesthesia can usually attenuate the autonomic responses (i.e., hypertension and tachycardia) that pose the primary risks for elderly patients with cerebrovascular or cardiovascular disease. Advanced technical reviews of the use of ECT and special anesthetic considerations in medically ill patients may be found elsewhere (Knos and Sung 1991; Silver et al. 1986).

■ REFERENCES

Aanderud S, Strandjord RE: Hypothyroidism induced by antiepileptic drugs. Acta Neurol Scand 61:330–332, 1980

Aanderud S, Myking OL, Strandjord RE: The influence of carbamazepine on thyroid hormones and thyroxine-binding globulin in hypothyroid patients substituted with thyroxine. Clin Endocrinol (Oxf) 15:247–252, 1981

Abernethy DR, Greenblatt DJ, Shader RI: Imipramine and desipramine disposition in the elderly. J Phar-

macol Exp Ther 232:183–188, 1985

Ali BH: Effect of some monoamine oxidase inhibitors on the thiamine status of rabbits. Br J Pharmacol 86:869–875, 1985

Antal EJ, Lawson IR, Alderson LM, et al: Estimating steady-state desipramine levels in noninstitutionalized elderly patients using single dose disposition parameters. J Clin Psychopharmacol 2:193–198, 1982

Beattie B, Biller J, Mehlhaus B, et al: Verapamil-induced carbamazepine neurotoxicity: a report of two cases. Eur Neurol 28:104–105, 1988

Beerman B, Edhag O: Depressive effects of carbamazepine on idioventricular rhythm in man. BMJ 2:171–172, 1978

Benassi E, Bo GP, Cociot L, et al: Carbamazepine and cardiac conduction disturbances. Ann Neurol 22:280–281, 1987

Bigger JT, Giardina EGV, Perel JM, et al: Cardiac antiarrhythmic effect of imipramine hydrochloride. N Engl J Med 296:206–208, 1977

Boston Collaborative Drug Surveillance Program Report: Adverse reactions to the tricyclic-antidepressant drugs. Lancet 1:529–531, 1972

Braverman B, McCarthy RJ, Ivankovich AD: Vasopressor challenges during chronic MAOI or TCA treatment in anesthetized dogs. Life Sci 40:2587–2595, 1987

Breitbart W, Mermelstein H: Pemoline: an alternative psychostimulant for the management of depressive disorders in cancer patients. Psychosomatics 33:352–356 1992

Brewerton TD: Lithium counteracts carbamazepine-induced leukopenia while increasing its therapeutic effect. Biol Psychiatry 21:677–685, 1986

Brodie MM, MacPhee GJA: Carbamazepine neurotoxicity precipitated by diltiazem. BMJ 292:1170–1171, 1986

Brosen K, Skjelbo E: Fluoxetine and norfluoxetine are potent inhibitors of $P_{450}IID6$—the source of the sparteine/debrisoquine oxidation polymorphism. Br J Clin Pharmacol 32(1):136–137, 1991

Chiarello RJ, Cole JO: The use of psychostimulants in general psychiatry: a reconsideration. Arch Gen Psychiatry 44:286–295, 1987

Clary C, Schweizer E: Treatment of MAOI hypertensive crisis with sublingual nifedipine. J Clin Psychiatry 48:249–250, 1987

Cohen LS, Heller VL, Rosenbaum JF: Treatment guidelines for psychotropic drug use in pregnancy. Psychosomatics 30:25–33, 1989

Cohen LS, Heller VL, Rosenbaum JF: Psychotropic drug use in pregnancy: an update, in Medical Psychiatric Practice, Vol 1. Edited by Stoudemire A, Fogel BS. Washington, DC, American Psychiatric Press, 1991, pp 615–634

Conners K, Taylor E: Pemoline, methylphenidate and placebo in children with minimal brain dysfunction. Arch Gen Psychiatry 37:923–930, 1980

Cooper GL: The safety of fluoxetine—an update. Br J Psychiatry 153 (suppl 3):77–86, 1988

Cutler NR, Narang PK: Implications of dosing tricyclic antidepressants and benzodiazepines in geriatrics. Psychiatr Clin North Am 7:845–861, 1984

Cutler NR, Zavadil AP III, Eisdorfer C: Concentrations of desipramine in elderly women are not elevated. Am J Psychiatry 138:1235–1237, 1981

Dam M, Kristensen CB, Hensen BS, et al: Interaction between carbamazepine and propoxyphene in man. Acta Neurol Scand 56:603–607, 1977

Davidson J: Seizures and bupropion: a review. J Clin Psychiatry 50:256–261, 1989

Dawling S, Lynn K, Rosser R, et al: Nortriptyline metabolism in chronic renal failure: metabolite elimination. Clin Pharmacol Ther 32:322–329, 1982

DeLuca F, Arrigo T, Pandullo E, et al: Changes in thyroid function tests induced by 2-month carbamazepine treatment in L-thyroxine-substituted hypothyroid children. Eur J Pediatr 145:77–79, 1986

DePaulo JR: Lithium. Psychiatr Clin North Am 7:587–599, 1984

Eadie MJ, Hooper WD, Dickinson RG: Valproate-associated hepatotoxicity and its biochemical mechanisms. Medical Toxicology Adverse Drug Experience 3:85–106, 1988

Edwards JG: Antidepressants and seizures: epidemiological and clinical aspects, in The Psychopharmacology of Epilepsy. Edited by Trimble MR. Chichester, England, Wiley, 1985, pp 119–139

Edwards JG, Long SK, Sedgwick EM, et al: Antidepressants and convulsive seizures: clinical, electroencephalographic, and pharmacological aspects. Clin Neuropharmacol 9:329–360, 1986

El Ganzouri AR, Ivankovich AD, Braverman B, et al: Monoamine inhibitors: should they be discontinued pre-operatively? Anesth Analg 64:592–596, 1985

Elizur A, Wintner I, Davidson S: The clinical and psychological effects of pemoline in depressed

patients: a controlled study. International Pharmacopsychiatry 14:127–134, 1979

Falk WE: Trazodone and priapism. Biological Therapies in Psychiatry 10:9–10, 1987

Fernandez F, Adams F, Levy JK, et al: Cognitive impairment due to AIDS-related complex and its response to psychostimulants. Psychosomatics 29:38–46, 1988

Fisch C: Effect of fluoxetine on the electrocardiogram. J Clin Psychiatry 46:42–44, 1985

Fogel BS, Stoudemire A: New psychotropics in medically ill patients, in Medical-Psychiatric Practice, Vol 2. Edited by Stoudemire A, Fogel BS. Washington, DC, American Psychiatric Press, 1993, pp 69–111

Fricchione GL, Vlay SC: Psychiatric aspects of patients with malignant ventricular arrhythmias. Am J Psychiatry 143:1518–1526, 1986

Gammans RE, Westrick ML, Shea JP, et al: Pharmacokinetics of buspirone in elderly subjects. J Clin Pharmacol 29:72–78, 1989

Garner SJ, Eldridge FL, Wagner PG, et al: Buspirone, an anxiolytic drug that stimulates respiration. Am Rev Respir Dis 139:946–950, 1989

Georgotas A, McCue RE, Friedman E, et al: A placebo-controlled comparison of the effect of nortriptyline and phenelzine on orthostatic hypotension in elderly depressed patients. J Clin Psychopharmacol 7:413–416, 1987

Glassman AH, Johnson LL, Giardina EV, et al: The use of imipramine in depressed patients with congestive heart failure. JAMA 250:1977–2001, 1983

Glassman JN, Dugas JE, Tsuang MT: Idiosyncratic pharmacokinetics complicating treatment of major depression in an elderly woman. J Nerv Ment Dis 173:573–576, 1985

Goff DC, Midha KK, Brotman AW, et al: Elevation of plasma concentrations of haloperidol after the addition of fluoxetine. Am J Psychiatry 148:790–792, 1991

Goldberg RG, Tull RM: Psychosocial Dimensions of Cancer: A Practical Guide for Health Care Providers. New York, Free Press, 1984, pp 111–169

Goodman WK, Charney DS: Therapeutic applications and mechanisms of action of monoamine oxidase inhibitor and heterocyclic antidepressant drugs. J Clin Psychiatry 46:6–22, 1985

Greenblatt DJ, Divoll M, Abernethy DR, et al: Benzodiazepine kinetics: implications for therapeutics and pharmacogeriatrics. Drug Metab Rev

14:251–292, 1983

Grimsley SR, Jann MW, Carter JG, et al: Increased carbamazepine plasma concentrations after fluoxetine coadministration. Clin Pharmacol Ther 50:10–15, 1991

Hardy BG, Shulman KI, MacKenzie SE, et al: Pharmacokinetics of lithium in the elderly. J Clin Psychopharmacol 7:153–158, 1987

Harpe C, Stoudemire A: Aetiology and treatment of the neuroleptic malignant syndrome. Medical Toxicology Adverse Drug Experience 2:166–176, 1987

Hart RG, Easton JD: Carbamazepine and hematological monitoring. Ann Neurol 11:309–312, 1982

Hein MD, Jackson IMD: Thyroid function in psychiatric illness. Gen Hosp Psychiatry 12:232–244, 1990

Jeavons PM: Hepatoxicity in antiepileptic drugs, in Chronic Toxicity of Antiepileptic Drugs. Edited by Oxley J, Janz D, Meinardi H. New York, Raven, 1983, pp 1–46

Kalff R, Houtkooper HA, Meyer JWA, et al: Carbamazepine and sodium levels. Epilepsia 25:390–397, 1984

Kaufmann MW, Murray GB, Cassem NH: Use of psychostimulants in medically ill depressed patients. Psychosomatics 23:817–819, 1982

Kayton W, Raskind M: Treatment of depression in the medically ill elderly with methylphenidate. Am J Psychiatry 137:963–965, 1980

Klotz U, Avant GR, Hoyumpa A, et al: The effects of age and liver disease on the disposition and elimination of diazepam in adult man. J Clin Invest 55:347–359, 1975

Knos GB, Sung YF: Anesthetic management of the high-risk medical patient receiving electroconvulsive therapy, in Medical Psychiatric Practice, Vol 1. Edited by Stoudemire A, Fogel BS. Washington, DC, American Psychiatric Press, 1991, pp 99–144

Kramer G, Theisohn M, von Unruh GE, et al: Carbamazepine-danazol interaction: its mechanism examined by a stable isotope technique. Ther Drug Monit 8:387–392, 1986

Lahr MB: Hyponatremia during carbamazepine therapy. Clin Pharmacol Ther 37:693–696, 1985

Lakshminarayan S, Sahn SA, Hudson LD, et al: Effect of diazepam on ventilatory responses. Clin Pharmacol Ther 20:178–183, 1976

Levy NG: Chronic renal failure, in Psychiatric Care of the Medical Patient. Edited by Stoudemire A, Fogel BS. New York, Oxford University Press, 1993, pp 627–635

Lieberman E, Stoudemire A: Use of tricyclic antidepressants in patients with glaucoma. Psychosomatics 28:145–148, 1987

Lieberman JA, Cooper TB, Suckow RF, et al: Tricyclic antidepressant and metabolite levels in chronic renal failure. Clin Pharmacol Ther 37:301–307, 1985

Luchins DJ, Oliver AP, Wyatt RJ: Seizures with antidepressants: an in vitro technique to assess relative risk. Epilepsia 25:25–32 1984

MacPhee GJ, McInnes GT, Thompson GG, et al: Verapamil potentiates carbamazepine neurotoxicity: a clinically important inhibitory interaction. Lancet 1(8483):700–703, 1986

Manoach M, Netz H, Varon D, Ben-Zeev Z: The effect of tricyclic antidepressants on ventricular fibrillation and collateral blood supply following acute coronary occlusion. Heart Vessels 2:36–40, 1986

Max MB, Lynch SA, Muir J, et al: Effects of desipramine, amitriptyline, and fluoxetine on pain in diabetic neuropathy. N Engl J Med 326:1250–1256, 1992

McGrath PJ, Blood DK, Stewart JW, et al: A comparative study of the electrocardiographic effects of phenelzine, tricyclic antidepressants, mianserin, and placebo. J Clin Psychopharmacol 7:335–339, 1987

Mendelson WB, Martin JV, Rapoport D, et al: Buspirone: stimulation of respiratory rate in freely moving rats [abstract]. Sleep Research 18:62, 1989

Merikangas JR, Merikangas KR: Calcium channel blockers in MAOI-induced hypertensive crisis. Psychopharmacology 96 (suppl):229, 1988

Meyer BR: Benzodiazepines in the elderly. Med Clin North Am 66:1017–1035, 1982

Mitchell J, Popkin M: The pathophysiology of sexual dysfunction associated with antipsychotic drug therapy in males: a review. Arch Sex Behav 12:173–183, 1983

Mittal SR, Mathur AK, Advani GB: Genesis of lithium-induced T wave flattening. Int J Cardiol 7:164–166, 1985

Modeo DG, Berry DJ: Effects of chlordiazepoxide in respiratory failure due to chronic bronchitis. Lancet 2:869–870, 1974

Morris HH, Estes ML: Traveler's amnesia: transient global amnesia secondary to triazolam. JAMA 258:945–946, 1987

Neshkes RE, Gerner R, Jarvik LF, et al: Orthostatic

effect of imipramine and doxepin in depressed geriatric outpatients. J Clin Psychopharmacol 5:102–106, 1985

Nies A, Robinson DS, Friedman MJ, et al: Relationship between age and tricyclic antidepressant plasma levels. Am J Psychiatry 134:790–793, 1977

Pato MT, Murphy DL, DeVane CL: Sustained plasma concentrations of fluoxetine and/or norfluoxetine four and eight weeks after fluoxetine discontinuation [letter to the editor]. J Clin Psychopharmacol 11:224–225, 1991

Pearson HJ: Interaction of fluoxetine with carbamazepine [letter to the editor]. J Clin Psychiatry 51:126, 1990

Pellock JM: Carbamazepine side effects in children and adults. Epilepsia 28 (suppl 3):S64–S70, 1987

Perucca E, Richens A: General principles: biotransformation, in Antiepileptic Drugs, 3rd Edition. Edited by Levy R, Mattson R, Meldrum B, et al. New York, Raven, 1989, pp 23–48

Perucca E, Garratt A, Hebdige S, et al: Water intoxication in epileptic patients receiving carbamazepine. J Neurol Neurosurg Psychiatr 41:713–718, 1978

Pierce MW, Shu VS: Efficacy of estazolam: the United States clinical experience. Am J Med 88 (suppl 3A):6S–11S, 1990

Pisciotta AV: Hematological toxicity of carbamazepine. Adv Neurol 11:355–368, 1975

Preskorn SH, Othmer SC: Evaluation of bupropion hydrochloride: the first of a new class of atypical antidepressants. Pharmacotherapy 4:20–34, 1984

Rall TW, Schleifer LS: Drugs effective in the therapy of the epilepsies, in The Pharmacological Basis of Therapeutics, 7th Edition. Edited by Gilman AG, Goodman LS, Rall TW, et al. New York, Macmillan, 1985, pp 446–472

Rapoport DM: Buspirone: anxiolytic therapy with respiratory implications. Family Practice Recertification 11 (suppl):33–41, 1989

Rapoport DM, Greenberg HE, Goldring RM: Comparison of the effects of buspirone and diazepam on control of breathing [abstract]. Federation of American Societies for Experimental Biology 2:A1507, 1988

Regan WM, Margolin RA, Mathew RJ: Cardiac arrhythmia following rapid imipramine withdrawal. Biol Psychiatry 25:482–484, 1989

Richelson E: Pharmacology of antidepressants in use in the United States. J Clin Psychiatry 43:4–11, 1982

Rickels K, Fox IL, Greenblatt DJ, et al: Clorazepate and lorazepam: clinical improvement and rebound anxiety. Am J Psychiatry 145:312–317, 1988

Rizos AL, Sargenti CJ, Jeste DV: Psychotropic drug interactions in the patient with late-onset depression or psychosis, part 2. Psychiatr Clin North Am 11:253–277, 1988

Roberts HE, Dean RC, Stoudemire A: Clozapine treatment of psychosis in Parkinson's disease. J Neuropsychiatry Clin Neurosci 1:190–192, 1989

Robinson DS, Kurtz NM: Question the experts: what is the degree of risk of hepatotoxicity for depressed patients receiving phenelzine therapy? J Clin Psychopharmacol 7:61–62, 1987

Robinson DS, Nies A, Corcella J, et al: Cardiovascular effects of phenelzine and amitriptyline in depressed outpatients. J Clin Psychiatry 43 (5, part 2):8–15, 1982

Rockwell E, Lam RW, Zisook S: Antidepressant drug studies in the elderly. Psychiatr Clin North Am 11:215–233, 1988

Roose SP, Glassman AH, Siris S, et al: Comparison of imipramine- and nortriptyline-induced orthostatic hypotension: a meaningful difference. J Clin Psychopharmacol 1:316–319, 1981

Roose SP, Glassman AH, Giardina EGV, et al: Nortriptyline in depressed patients with left ventricular impairment. JAMA 256:3253–3257, 1986

Roose SP, Glassman AH, Giardina EGV, et al: Tricyclic antidepressants in depressed patients with cardiac conduction disease. Arch Gen Psychiatry 44:273–275, 1987

Sargenti CJ, Rizos AL, Jeste DV: Psychotropic drug interactions in the patient with late-onset psychosis and mood disorder, part 1. Psychiatr Clin North Am 11:235–252, 1988

Schwartz P, Wolf S: QT interval prolongation as predictor of sudden death in patients with myocardial infarction. Circulation 57:1074–1077, 1978

Silver JM, Yudofsky SC, Kogan M, et al: Elevation of thioridazine plasma levels by propranolol. Am J Psychiatry 143:1290–1292, 1986

Small IF, Sharpley P, Small JG: Influence of Cylert upon memory changes with ECT. Am J Psychiatry 125:837–840, 1968

Smith RC, Chojnacki M, Hu R, et al: Cardiovascular effects of therapeutic doses of tricyclic antidepressants: importance of blood level monitoring. J Clin Psychiatry 41:57–63, 1980

Sommi RW, Crismon ML, Bowden CL, et al: Fluoxetine: a serotonin-specific second-generation antidepressant. Pharmacotherapy 7:1–15, 1987

Stack CG, Rogers P, Linter SPK: Monoamine oxidase inhibitors and anaesthesia. Br J Anaesth 60:222–227, 1988

Stoudemire A, Atkinson P: Use of cyclic antidepressants in patients with cardiac conduction disturbances. Gen Hosp Psychiatry 10:389–397, 1988

Stoudemire A, Fogel BS: Psychopharmacology in the medically ill, in Principles of Medical Psychiatry. Edited by Stoudemire A, Fogel BF. Orlando, FL, Grune & Stratton, 1987, pp 79–112

Stoudemire A, Luther J: Neuroleptic malignant syndrome and neuroleptic-induced catatonia: differential diagnosis and treatment. Int J Psychiatry Med 14:57–63, 1984

Stoudemire A, Fogel BS, Gulley L: Psychopharmacology in the medically ill: an update, in Medical Psychiatric Practice, Vol 1. Edited by Stoudemire A, Fogel BS. Washington, DC, American Psychiatric Press, 1991, pp 29–97

Stoudemire A, Fogel BS, Gulley LR, et al: Psychopharmacology in the medically ill, in Psychiatric Care of the Medical Patient. Edited by Stoudemire A, Fogel BS. New York, Oxford University Press, 1993

Talland GA, Hagen DQ, James M: Performance tests of amnestic patients with Cylert. J Nerv Ment Dis 144:421–429, 1967

Thompson TL II, Moran MG, Nies AS: Psychotropic drug use in the elderly. N Engl J Med 308:134–138 and 194–199, 1983

Tilkian AG, Schroeder JS, Kao JJ, et al: The cardiovascular effects of lithium in man. Am J Med 61:665–670, 1976a

Tilkian JG, Schroeder JS, Kao J, et al: Effect of lithium on cardiovascular performance: a report on extended ambulatory monitoring and exercise testing before and during lithium. Am J Cardiol 38:701–798, 1976b

Van Sweden B: Rebound antidepressant cardiac arrhythmia. Biol Psychiatry 24:360–369, 1988

Verrier RL: Neurochemical approaches to the prevention of ventricular fibrillation. Federation Proceedings 445:2191–2196, 1986

Vieweg WVR, Yank GR, Row WT, et al: Increase in white blood cell count and serum sodium level following the addition of lithium to carbamazepine treatment among three chronically psychotic male patients with disturbed affective states. Psychiatr Q 58:213–217, 1986

Wamsley JK, Hunt ME: Relative affinity of quazepam for type-1 benzodiazepine receptors. J Clin Psychiatry 52 (suppl):15–20, 1991

Wells DG, Bjorksten AR: Monoamine oxidase inhibitors revisited. Can J Anaesth 36:64–74, 1989

Wong YY, Ludden TM, Bell RD: Effect of erythromycin on carbamazepine kinetics. Clin Pharmacol Ther 33:460–464, 1983

Woods SW: Psychostimulant treatment of depressive disorders secondary to medical illness. J Clin Psychiatry 47:12–15, 1986

40

Geriatric Psychopharmacology

Carl Salzman, M.D., Andrew Satlin, M.D., and Adam B. Burrows, M.D.

Psychotropic drugs play an important (but not exclusive) role in the treatment of late-life psychopathology. In this chapter, we review specific uses of psychotropic drugs to treat disorders characterized by disruptive behavior, depression, anxiety, disordered sleep, and impaired cognition.

■ OVERVIEW

There are important differences in the use of psychoactive medications for elderly versus younger adult patients. An appreciation of these differences is essential for optional prescribing of these drugs. Before prescribing, the clinician must consider several processes: 1) physiological changes associated with aging, 2) physiological changes due to disease, 3) the potential influence of concurrent medications, and 4) the social context of illness and treatment.

■ AGING: DEMOGRAPHY AND PHYSIOLOGY

There is considerable variability in the aging process, and the effects of aging and disease may be difficult to distinguish. Yet despite the clinical heterogeneity of the aging population, certain physiological changes are consistently observed. These include changes in nervous system structure and function, such as enhancement of some brain enzymes with aging and increased receptor site sensitivity in several neurotransmitter systems (Morgan et al. 1987; Oreland and Gottfries 1986; Robinson et al. 1977). Age-related changes are also evident in the sensory, respiratory, cardiovascular, gastrointestinal, genitourinary, endocrine, and neuromuscular systems.

A useful generalization often applied to age-related physiological changes is the concept of diminished physiological reserve. In this model, age-related changes in central nervous system (CNS) function may not become clinically apparent until an individual confronts a physiological challenge, such as an acute illness or medical intervention. Under the stress of these circumstances, clinical problems such as disruptive behavior, affective symptoms, and diminished sleep and cognition are revealed through symptoms in a vulnerable system. Thus, illness is typically expressed nonspecifically in elderly patients, and neuropsychiatric symptoms may represent the expression of diverse clinical problems.

■ DISEASE AND DISABILITY

Chronic disease and functional disability characterize the aging population. More than 80% of Americans over age 65 report at least one chronic medical condition, and most have multiple chronic problems (National Center for Health Statistics 1987). Chronic diseases impose functional limitations such that by age 85, half of all Americans have difficulty with at least one daily self-care activity (Dawson et al. 1987). Dementias impose growing challenges on individuals and the health care system. Community-based surveys suggest that 25%–50% of people age 85 and older have dementia, with 40%–70% of dementia cases attributed to Alzheimer's disease (AD) and the remainder primarily to vascular causes (Aronson et al. 1991; Evans et al. 1989; Skoog et al. 1993).

MEDICATIONS AND ELDERLY PATIENTS

Not surprisingly, older individuals consume a disproportionate share of prescription drugs. Although they are 12% of the population, elders over age 65 receive one-third of all prescriptions. Polypharmacy is common; community-dwelling Americans over age 65 fill, on average, 13 prescriptions each year and take twice as many medications as younger Americans (Institute of Medicine 1991; National Center for Health Statistics 1987; Office of Epidemiology and Biostatistics 1987; Stewart et al. 1989). After cardiovascular drugs and analgesics, psychotropic agents are the most frequently prescribed drugs in the treatment of elderly patients.

The risks of medication use in elderly patients are well documented. Adverse drug reactions are more common among elderly people and account for 10%–30% of their hospitalizations (Ancill et al. 1988; Antonijoan et al. 1990; Col et al. 1990; Grymonpre et al. 1988; Institute of Medicine 1991; Ives et al. 1987; Ray et al. 1992). It appears that the risk of adverse drug reactions is not simply due to age-related vulnerability but is instead a function of complex interactions between medical frailty and the prescription of multiple medications (Avorn et al. 1989; Carbonin et al. 1991; Gurwitz and Avorn 1991). Medications requiring monitoring of therapeutic levels, such as antidepressants, may be more likely than other drugs to cause adverse reactions in elderly outpatients (Schneider et al. 1992). Liaison consultation by clinical pharmacists may reduce adverse drug effects (Kroenke and Pinholt 1990; Schneider et al. 1992).

THE SOCIAL CONTEXT OF AGING

How and where will a drug be taken by an elderly patient? Will the cost be an issue? Will the drug be administered by a caregiver? Is the patient in a nurs-

ing home or other long-term care setting?

Approximately 5% of individuals over age 65 and more than 20% of those over age 85 live in nursing homes (National Center for Health Statistics 1987). Many others receive formal and informal care and assistance with daily activities in community settings. As would be expected, nursing home residents have more disability, disease, and dependence than community-dwelling elders. Also, not surprisingly, polypharmacy is commonplace in nursing homes, with reports demonstrating an average of eight medications prescribed per resident (Beers et al. 1988). Psychotropic drugs are among the most frequently prescribed medications in nursing homes. Antipsychotic neuroleptics are ordered for 20%–30% of residents (Avorn et al. 1992; Beardsley et al. 1989; Beers et al. 1988; Garrard et al. 1991).

Unfortunately, medications are commonly prescribed without clear documentation of an appropriate indication (Beardsley et al. 1989; Garrard et al. 1991; Ray et al. 1980; Saban et al. 1982; Zimmer et al. 1986). This problem has been a particular concern with regard to psychotropic medications and was the subject of federal regulation through the Nursing Home Reform Amendments of the Omnibus Budget Reconciliation Act (OBRA) of 1987.

THERAPEUTIC CONSIDERATIONS: PSYCHOTROPIC MEDICATIONS

The Effect of Aging and Disease

Aging and disease contribute to physiological changes that alter the availability and effect of medications. Pharmacodynamic changes describe alterations in the physiological effect produced by a given concentration of drug. Pharmacokinetic changes describe changes in the amount of drug that is made available for clinical effect following a given dose. Aging is associated with both pharmacodynamic and pharmacokinetic changes, and the coexistence of chronic diseases can further alter the body's response to drugs.

Pharmacodynamics. Elderly patients are more sensitive to the therapeutic and toxic effects of psychotropic agents compared with younger patients. For a given concentration of drug, elderly patients usually experience more sedation, anticholinergic toxicity, extrapyramidal side effects (EPS), and orthostatic hypotension. In the setting of degenerative brain diseases such as AD and Parkinson's disease, there may be additional drug sensitivities as the amount of neuronal tissue in key brain areas declines. Patients with AD and acetylcholine deficiency are more sensitive to anticholinergic side effects, whereas patients with Parkinson's disease are more sensitive to dopamine blockade.

Pharmacokinetics. Four pharmacokinetic parameters determine the bioavailability of a drug after administration: absorption, distribution, metabolism, and clearance. Two significant changes occur with aging. First, there is a significant change in distribution. There is an almost universal decrease in lean body mass and a corresponding increase in body fat composition. Fat soluble drugs such as benzodiazepine sedative-hypnotics, neuroleptics, and cyclic antidepressants distribute more widely in the body and will thus take longer to clear. Water-soluble drugs such as lithium distribute through a smaller volume and thus can reach higher tissue concentrations. Second, there are age-related changes in hepatic metabolism of psychotropic drugs. There is an age-related decrement in phase I oxidative biotransformation. This further delays hepatic metabolism and contributes to the prolonged half-lives of many psychotropic drugs, as well as the delayed and prolonged appearance of active intermediate metabolites. The cumulative effect of large volumes of distribution for fat-soluble drugs and delayed hepatic metabolism results in a dramatic prolongation of clinical effect for many agents, especially long-acting benzodiazepines.

Chronic diseases, as well as the aging process, alter the pharmacokinetic patterns of psychotropic drugs. Malnutrition or chronic inflammatory conditions can reduce the synthesis of plasma-binding proteins, resulting in higher free (or bioavailable) drug concentrations. Chronic liver disease or congestion will further delay clearance, leading to higher drug levels for even longer periods. Many though not all older people have reduced glomerular filtration rate. For these individuals, renal clearance of drugs such as lithium will be impaired and higher concentrations will result. Taken as a whole, pharmacological changes associated with aging and disease mean that, for a given dose of most psychoactive drugs, the bioavailable concentration at the target tissue will be higher, and for a given concentration at a CNS site of action, there will be greater physiological effect. These generalizations support the geriatric maxim to start low and go slow when prescribing drugs.

Side effects. In elderly patients, side effects are typically experienced in vulnerable physiological systems. In the cardiovascular system, for example, decreased baroreceptor sensitivity predisposes to orthostatic hypotension, and diminished reserve in the cardiac conduction system predisposes to heart block. Changes in bowel motility predispose to constipation and impaction, whereas bladder weakness and prostatic enlargement predispose to urinary retention. In the CNS, changes in the extrapyramidal and vestibular systems predispose to problems with gait, balance, and posture. Dementia (even early in the course) predisposes to delirium.

■ POLYPHARMACY: ISSUES IN PRESCRIBING PSYCHOACTIVE DRUGS

Given the prevalence of polypharmacy in elderly people, three prescribing problems are common:

1. There is a correlation between the number of medications prescribed and the risk of medication noncompliance.
2. One drug can impair the absorption or metabolism and clearance of another drug or displace it from a protein-binding site.
3. There may also be a confluence of adverse effects. For example, additive effects of vasodilators and antidepressants on blood pressure are common, as are the additive toxic effects from multiple drugs with anticholinergic properties. Monoamine oxidase inhibitors (MAOIs) present special problems with regard to potentially catastrophic interactions with sympathomimetic agents and catecholamine precursors.

■ TREATMENT OF PSYCHOSIS, AGITATION, AND BEHAVIORAL DISRUPTION

Elderly patients who are psychotic or severely ill or who have dementia often manifest behavioral symptoms that require treatment. Prevalence rates of agitation are particularly high in nursing homes (Billig et al. 1991; Cohen-Mansfield et al. 1989; Peabody et al. 1987; Rovner et al. 1986; Wragg and Jeste 1988; Zimmer et al. 1984). Severe agitation, screaming, and assaultiveness are seen frequently in the moderate to severe stages of dementia (particularly AD), as well as with late-life schizophrenia.

■ Treatment Guidelines

Although medications are commonly used to treat severe agitation and psychosis in elderly patients, they are not the only form of treatment. A search for causes of agitation and psychosis should include as possible etiologies drug toxicity, medical illness, pain, frustration, loneliness, reduced sensory input, new environment, diminished nutritional status, and factors in the environment. Treatment approaches include using orienting stimuli, avoiding patient isolation, and using nonpharmacological treatments such as music, exercise, pets, and social contact.

Medications that are commonly used to treat disruptive behavior include neuroleptics, β-blockers, drugs with serotonergic effect, mood stabilizers, and hormones.

■ Neuroleptics

Neuroleptics are the most commonly used drugs to treat severe disruptive behavior in elderly patients (Devanand et al. 1988; Helms 1985; Maletta 1984; Phillipson et al. 1990; Risse and Barnes 1986; Salzman 1987; Schneider et al. 1990a; Small 1988; Wragg and Jeste 1988). These drugs undergo a complicated stepwise hepatic metabolism. The effects of the aging process on this metabolism have not been extensively studied. However, limited data suggest that blood levels of parent compounds and active metabolites are 1½–2 times higher in old patients compared with younger adult control subjects (Aoba et al. 1985; Cohen and Sommer 1988; Forsman and Ohman 1977), although not in all patients.

No data currently suggest that any one neuroleptic is better at controlling agitated behavior or psychotic thinking than any other, given comparable therapeutic doses. Selection of any one neuroleptic (or subclass of neuroleptics) in preference to another is guided by the side-effect profile of each drug or drug class in relation to the patient's history of prior drug response (or lack of response) and the nature of concomitant chronic illness and medication.

Three categories of neuroleptic side effects occur regularly and may be particularly troublesome for older patients. These are sedation, orthostatic hypotension, and EPS. Low-potency neuroleptics such as chlorpromazine and thioridazine commonly cause sedation or orthostatic hypotension. Although sedation may be helpful at bedtime for the disruptive elderly patient, there is often a carryover of sedative effect the next day because of the medications' prolonged elimination half-lives. During the day a sedated elderly person may actually become more agitated and disruptive. For this reason, as well as because of the risk of orthostatic hypotension, low-potency neuroleptics may present a risk in this population. In clinical practice, however, low doses of thioridazine continue to be used for the treatment of agitation with considerable success. As an alternative to low-potency neuroleptics, high-potency medication such as haloperidol and fluphenazine are commonly used because they lack sedating and orthostatic hypotensive properties. Unfortunately, these high-potency compounds are more likely to produce EPS than the low-potency medications. Among the latter, drug-induced Parkinson-like EPS may be associated with a failure to improve behaviorally (Ganzini et al. 1991).

The selection of a neuroleptic to treat behavioral disruption, therefore, requires an appraisal of the risks versus benefits of different neuroleptic compounds. Current clinical practice tends to favor the use of high-potency medications, with an attempt to prevent or minimize EPS by using exceedingly low doses (Devanand et al. 1988, 1989, 1992; Petrie et al. 1982). Clinical experience suggests, for example, that doses of haloperidol in the range of 0.25–1.0 mg one to four times a day may be helpful in diminishing disruptive behavior without producing undue EPS.

In elderly people who have not been previously treated with neuroleptics, tardive dyskinesia develops rapidly and at lower doses than with younger patients (Karson et al. 1990; Lieberman et al. 1984; Saltz et al. 1989; Yassa et al. 1988). Tardive dyskinesia is more common in patients who had evidence of cortical atrophy (Sweet et al. 1992). When neuroleptics are discontinued, there is less improvement in older patients than in younger adults (De Veaugh-Geiss 1988; Smith and Baldessarini 1980; Yassa et al. 1984). However, for some elderly patients with tardive dyskinesia who are maintained on neuroleptics, the symptoms do not increase (Huang 1986; Yassa 1991).

Neuroleptic malignant syndrome may also occur in older patients receiving neuroleptics, more commonly in elderly patients who had either dementia or Parkinson's disease while receiving neuroleptics (Addonizio 1992).

■ Treatment With Nonneuroleptics

A growing body of clinical experience and anecdotal reports (summarized in Salzman 1990a) suggests that drugs such as β-blockers, trazodone, buspirone, serotonergic antidepressants, anticonvulsants, and lithium may aid in managing a variety of agitated behaviors refractory to more conventional treatment.

β-blockers. β-blockers, sometimes modestly helpful in reducing agitated and assaultive behavior in elderly patients, are given in low doses (10–100 mg qd). Not all studies, however, are positive (Risse and Barnes 1986; Weiler et al. 1988). These drugs can be given only to elderly patients who are free of cardiovascular disorder and chronic obstructive pulmonary disease (particularly asthma). Side effects include sedation, orthostatic hypotension, and decreased cardiac output.

Trazodone. The antidepressant drug trazodone has been reported as an effective treatment for agitation and severely disruptive behavior (Greenwald et al. 1986; Pinner and Rich 1988; Simpson and Foster 1986; Tingle 1986). Although no double-blind studies to date compare this drug with placebo or with neuroleptics, clinical experience suggests that it is effective in doses of 50–200 mg qd, with few side effects other than sedation.

Buspirone. This nonbenzodiazepine antianxiety agent has been reported effective in controlling disruptive behavior in older patients in one study (Colenda 1988) but not in another (Strauss 1988). However, oral dyskinesia has been reported in an elderly patient with dementia who received buspirone, and this symptom persisted for at least 4 months after symptom onset (Strauss 1988). As yet, research studies have not compared its effect with that of placebo or other drugs for treating agitation.

The average daily dose range is 20–80 mg in divided doses; side effects are reported to be relatively mild.

Selective serotonin reuptake inhibitors. Current clinical experience suggests that the antidepressant fluoxetine has some antiagitation properties in elderly patients. However, a study (Olafsson et al. 1992) failed to demonstrate effectiveness of fluvoxamine in the treatment of behavioral disruption in elderly dementia patients. However, careful research into the antiagitation properties of the selective serotonin reuptake inhibitors (SSRIs) is essential, because these drugs also tend to be activating and may actually increase agitation in some older patients.

Anticonvulsants and lithium carbonate. In doses of 50–200 mg qd, carbamazepine has also controlled chronic disruptive behavior and agitation in older patients, particularly those with dementia (Leibovici and Tariot 1988). Like carbamazepine, lithium carbonate is sometimes useful in managing disruptive behavior (Holton and George 1985). The therapeutic range is 150–900 mg, in divided doses. Because each of these drugs may produce neurotoxicity characterized by increased agitation, confusion, and disorientation, the lowest possible therapeutic dosage of both is recommended, and each should be discontinued if behavior worsens.

Experience with valproate in managing disruptive behavior is limited but suggests that this drug, like carbamazepine, may be effective in controlling severe agitation.

Estrogen. A single case report (Kyomen et al. 1991) suggests that estrogen (e.g., diethylstilbestrol 1 mg qd or conjugated estrogen 0.625 mg qd) reduces the number of incidents of physical aggression but not of verbal aggression or physical or verbal repetitive behaviors in elderly male patients with dementia.

■ TREATMENT OF DEPRESSION

Depression is the most common psychiatric illness found in the older population (Blazer and Williams 1980). Prevalence rates of depressive disorders in older people reach 20% for major depression and are even higher for milder forms. Suicide rates among depressed elderly people are particularly high (Alexopoulos et al. 1988). Recent research points to the high prevalence of diagnosed major depression in nursing homes and the unusually high mortality (from causes other than suicide) of people diagnosed (Parmelee et al. 1993; Rovner et al. 1991).

Although older people with depressive disorders can present with signs and symptoms similar to those in younger adults, late-life depression is characterized by diagnostic and symptomatic heterogeneity (Alexopoulos 1990). Ascribing diagnostic significance to individual depressive symptoms may be misleading. For example, early morning awakening, appetite disturbance, and low energy (which are characteristic vegetative signs of depression) may each result from the normal aging process, from drugs commonly taken by elderly patients, or from medical conditions more common in elderly people, or some combination of these factors (Salzman et al. 1992).

In addition to heterogeneity of depressive symptom patterns, people over age 65 are remarkably diverse with regard to psychological functioning. Although precise age boundaries are lacking, elderly people are sometimes subdivided into the "young-old" (65 to 75 or 79) and the "old-old" (75 to 80+). Symptomatic presentation of depression may differ between these two categories, although there are considerable similarities and overlap of symptoms. Factors of pharmacokinetic disposition and pharmacodynamic drug sensitivity may be quite different in old-old patients. Response to antidepressant treatment may also be different between these two general categories (Salzman et al. 1993), although, once again, similarities of response also exist and overlap between the two groups is common. Virtually all studies of the pharmacological treatment of late-life depression have focused on the young-old group. A recent review (Salzman et al. 1993) notes that only one controlled study of depressed patients all of whom were over age 75 has been conducted, and the total number of identifiable patients over age 75 who have been studied in *all* antidepressant studies of elderly subjects was 171. Consequently, treatment guidelines for very old patients are based on treatment of young-old or even of young and middle-aged adults and may be misleading.

As a general principle, elderly patients (especially those who are old-old) are more sensitive to the effects of antidepressants than are younger adults, although there is wide interindividual variability. Elderly patients are more likely to experience the side effects of sedation, orthostatic hypotension, and an-

ticholinergic symptoms. Orthostatic hypotension (due to reduced central as well as peripheral controls of blood pressure) may lead to falls and serious fractures. For unclear reasons, pretreatment systolic orthostatic blood pressure may predict clinical response: patients who have large pretreatment systolic orthostatic blood pressure changes in the morning before treatment with antidepressants have a significantly greater response to antidepressant or electroconvulsive therapy (ECT) (Jarvik et al. 1983; Schneider et al. 1986; Stack et al. 1988). In some older patients, sensitivity to anticholinergic side effects of tricyclic antidepressants (TCAs) may limit dosing levels and may cause CNS symptoms of delirium even at therapeutic doses. A review of anticholinergic side effects in elderly patients found that cognitive impairment, which occurs in normal aging, is enhanced and may be associated with behavioral disturbances as well (Meyers 1992). Activation and insomnia resulting from SSRIs may be greater in older patients than in younger patients, although these differences have not been carefully defined by controlled research studies.

Antidepressants, like neuroleptics, undergo complicated hepatic metabolism requiring both phase I reactions (dealkylation, aromatic hydroxylation) and phase II (conjugation). The first set of processes may be affected by the aging process. As a general principle, dealkylation becomes less efficient, leading to higher levels of tertiary tricyclic amines compared with the secondary amine metabolite, and reduced clearance of these compounds, with accumulation and higher blood levels. For these reasons, older patients, on average, need lower doses of antidepressants to achieve therapeutic effect; old-old patients may need even lower doses than young-old patients. Pharmacokinetic data also suggest that for drugs where therapeutic blood level ranges have been established (e.g., nortriptyline and desipramine), older patients respond to the same levels as younger adult counterparts (Cutler et al. 1981; Dawling et al. 1980a, 1980b, 1981; Kanba et al. 1992; Katz et al. 1989; Kitanka et al. 1982; Nelson et al. 1985, 1988). However, the wide range of interindividual variability and limited research data design suggest that the pharmacokinetics of antidepressants in elderly patients have not yet been consistently characterized in this population in comparison with younger patients (von Moltke et al. 1993).

Phase I metabolism of TCAs also produces a

water-soluble hydroxymetabolite whose clearance depends on renal function. This metabolite was previously thought to be inactive; but it is now apparent that, at least in some patients, it may be associated with quinidine-like cardiotoxicity (McCue et al. 1989; Nelson et al. 1988; Schneider et al. 1990b; Young et al. 1984, 1985). Impaired renal function in older patients or in very elderly individuals may lead to higher levels of hydroxymetabolites and the *potential* for cardiotoxicity (Kutcher et al. 1986).

■ Treatment Guidelines

Traditionally, treatment of the depressed elderly patient with antidepressants has followed recommendations for younger and middle-aged adults. ECT or TCAs plus neuroleptics are usually prescribed for delusionally depressed patients (Kroessler and Fogel 1993). TCAs have been the primary treatment for melancholic major depressive disorder, especially on an inpatient service, and MAOIs have been used for less severely depressed patients who do not require hospitalization. The new class of SSRIs has been studied primarily in depressed elderly outpatients and found to be useful for mild to moderately severe patients. These recommendations, however, are based on a small number of studies, with an age sample skewed toward young-old subjects.

Increased clinical experience as well as some more recent studies have suggested that there may not be precise boundaries between these prescribing guidelines, and treatment recommendations for depressed elderly patients may be changing. For example, the combination of fluoxetine and perphenazine has been found effective in the treatment of psychotic depression in a study that included a few patients over age 60 (Rothschild et al., in press). There are many reviews of antidepressant treatment in elderly patients (Alexopoulos 1992; Caine et al. 1993; Dewan et al. 1992; Kim 1988; Koenig and Breitner 1990; Magni et al. 1988; Peabody et al. 1986; Rockwell et al. 1988; Salzman 1990a, 1990b, 1993; Smith and Buckwalter 1992; Weissman et al. 1992).

■ TRICYCLIC ANTIDEPRESSANTS

There have been more than 400 studies of the treatment of serious major depression, nondelusional type, in elderly subjects (Salzman 1994). In general, all TCAs are helpful for elderly patients, although secondary amines are preferred. Regardless of antidepressant used, however, a recent study suggests that elderly patients who have had a serious major depression should be continued on their antidepressant to prevent relapse (Old Age Depression Interest Group 1993).

Although secondary amine TCAs are preferred to tertiary amines because their side effects are usually less intense, the severity of tricyclic-related side effects in elderly patients may be correlated with dose. Because therapeutic blood levels of TCAs in elderly patients may be achieved with lower-than-usual doses, it may be possible to use tertiary amines in elderly patients as long as doses are kept low. A study of low-dose doxepin, for example, showed efficacy without serious side effects (Lakshmanan et al. 1986).

When using TCAs for elderly patients, clinicians are advised to obtain a physical examination and electrocardiogram (ECG) before initiating treatment. Starting doses should be extremely low (e.g., 10–25 mg qd), and dosage increments should be of a similar magnitude. The adage "start low and go slow" is applicable to the use of antidepressants in elderly patients. It must be added, however, that clinicians should try to prescribe the dose of antidepressant that brings about the best therapeutic response with the least amount of side effects, regardless of the final dose. Using the ECG to monitor potential cardiotoxicity will help determine the upper limit of doses.

■ Trazodone

The antidepressant effects of trazodone are unpredictable, making it a less reliable first choice among the various available antidepressants. It is recommended, however, for older patients who have not responded to other compounds, and sometimes it can produce surprising therapeutic effects in the previously treatment-refractory older patient. Although it is sedating and can cause orthostatic hypotension (Gerner et al. 1980), trazodone has minimal anticholinergic properties and does not interfere with memory (Branconnier and Cole 1981).

■ Bupropion

Bupropion has been found effective for elderly subjects in research studies (Branconnier et al. 1983; Halaris 1987). An unusual side effect of falling backward (Szuba and Leuchter 1992) has been reported in a few elderly patients and may be dose related.

Selective Serotonin Reuptake Inhibitors

SSRIs have been prescribed to elderly patients with major depression as well as less serious dysthymic disorders and atypical depressions. The advantages of these drugs is the lack of anticholinergic side effects, cardiotoxicity, and orthostatic hypotension. In research studies, the efficacy of the SSRIs fluoxetine, paroxetine, sertraline, and fluvoxamine is equivalent to that of the TCAs (Dunner et al. 1992; Feighner and Cohn 1985; Feighner et al. 1988; Salzman 1994). In some elderly patients, these drugs cause unacceptable agitation and insomnia. Another report (Brymer and Winograd 1992) also notes that fluoxetine use may be associated with unacceptable weight loss in patients over age 75. Low starting doses and small dosage increments are recommended.

Monoamine Oxidase Inhibitors

MAOIs may be both safe and effective for some older patients with atypical depression characterized by withdrawal, lack of motivation, apathy, and lack of energy (Georgotas et al. 1981, 1983, 1986; Lazarus et al. 1986). Clinical overviews of the use of MAOIs include those of Jenike (1985), Zisook (1985), and Salzman (1992). These drugs are rarely the first-choice antidepressant for major depression. As with TCAs and SSRIs, older patients are likely to experience side effects. Lower doses (e.g., phenelzine 15–20 mg qd, tranylcypromine 10–40 mg qd) than those prescribed for younger adult patients are advised.

MAOIs can be given only to responsible, compliant elderly patients or to those whose medication is carefully supervised. The high risk of toxic drug interactions resulting from the large average number of drugs prescribed for the geriatric population may prevent these drugs from being recommended for many older outpatients.

■ TREATMENT OF MANIA

Elderly bipolar patients who have had many episodes tend to have rapid cycling and severe symptomatology, but bipolar disorder rarely appears for the first time in late life. Several recent studies suggest that first-onset mania in elderly patients is more likely to be associated with neurological impairment than is depression in this age group (Berrios and Bakshi 1991; Shulman et al. 1992; Snowdon 1991) and carries a greater risk for mortality than does depression (Dhingra and Rabins 1991; Shulman et al. 1992). Thus, late-onset mania may represent a different disorder than early-onset mania, or it may be secondary to other conditions.

Treatment Guidelines

Lithium is the primary treatment and prophylaxis for the mania of elderly patients, as it is for younger adults. However, a review (Foster 1992) identified only five studies of antimanic efficacy of lithium in elderly subjects and concluded that the efficacy in elderly bipolar patients is not yet clearly established in the literature. Reviews of lithium effects in older patients include those of Foster (1992), Liptzin (1992), Stone (1989), Jefferson and colleagues (1987), and Glasser and Rabins (1984).

Age-associated reduction of renal clearance of lithium leads to accumulation and increased plasma levels in elders more readily than in younger adults taking the same dosage. This effect is magnified by the reduction in the volume of distribution of lithium in elderly patients, as a result of the relative loss of total body water. Therapeutic plasma levels for older manic patients may need to be only 0.2–0.6 mEq/L. The daily dose necessary to achieve lower blood levels varies among older patients. As a general rule, starting lithium doses are low (e.g., 150–450 mg qd), with dosage increments of 150–300 mg at weekly intervals. However, it is important to recognize that some older manic patients, particularly those with other psychiatric illness, sometimes require doses and blood levels equivalent to those needed by younger patients. One prospective double-blind randomized lithium dose reduction study found that dose reductions of 25%–50% made to achieve serum levels of 0.45 mEq/L resulted in significantly increased affective symptoms in the elderly subjects (Abou-Saleh and Coppen 1989).

Older patients are more sensitive to the therapeutic as well as toxic effects of lithium. The toxic profile of lithium in older people differs in several important aspects from that of younger patients. Tremor and gastrointestinal upset occur in all age groups as side effects. In older patients, however, the first and often the most prominent side effects consist of a spectrum of neurotoxic symptoms, even at low therapeutic levels. In some patients, neurotoxicity may be associated with the presence of underlying neurological disease (Himmelhoch et al. 1980; Kemperman et al. 1989). Subtle but progressive impairment of recent recall (anterograde amnesia), disorientation, aphasia, restlessness, and irritability may appear as the first signs of excessive lithium dosage. This presents a double hazard: overdose and inaccurate interpretation of symptoms of cognitive impairment. Movement disorders also are early signs of toxicity—particularly EPS, dyskinesias, and cerebellar dysfunction, including irregular gait, decreased coordination, and dysarthria. Impaired consciousness also may develop at blood levels therapeutic for younger adults.

Other medical side effects may be common in elderly patients taking lithium. Cardiac effects include altered conduction due to sinus node dysfunction, sinoatrial block, bundle branch block, ventricular irritability, and possible myocardial injury. Lithium may impair urine concentration by the kidneys; this may be more severe in elderly patients who have preexisting deficits in renal concentrating ability. Acute lithium toxicity may result in decreased glomerular filtration rate, and long-term use may be associated with tubular atrophy, glomerular sclerosis, and interstitial fibrosis. Hypothyroidism may be more common in elderly patients taking lithium and can present with more profound consequences, such as myxedema coma.

Alternative medications for the treatment of mania in elderly patients have not been well studied. Neuroleptics are sometimes recommended for elderly patients as adjunctive treatment of severe agitation, insomnia, and potentially harmful behavior in manic patients, particularly in the early stages of treatment before lithium exerts its effect. Anticonvulsants and benzodiazepines have not been studied. There is a single report of seven older patients with mania that demonstrates modest efficacy of valproic acid (McFarland et al. 1990).

TREATMENT OF ANXIETY

In older patients, symptoms of anxiety are common, and the diagnosis of generalized anxiety disorder is not as clearly defined as in younger adults. Clinically significant anxiety symptoms commonly occur in states of depression and dementia, as well as secondary to physical illness or as a result of drug treatment. Panic-phobic anxiety disorder may also occur in older people but is less prevalent than in younger adults and is often associated with physical illness and concomitant psychiatric disorder (Sheikh 1990). Various reviews of the pharmacological treatment of generalized anxiety in elderly patients have been conducted (Allen 1986; Hershey and Kim 1988; Salzman 1990c).

■ Treatment Guidelines

Benzodiazepines, the primary treatment of anxiety, are widely used in the treatment of anxious elderly patients (Beardsley et al. 1989; Beers et al. 1988; Buck 1988; Koepke et al. 1982; Pinsker and Suljaga-Petchel 1984). As a general principle, elderly patients are more sensitive to both the therapeutic and toxic effects of benzodiazepines, or there may be great interindividual variability. Low doses are generally recommended; side effects of sedation, dyscoordination, and cognitive impairment may result from higher doses that are commonly therapeutic for younger adults.

Like other psychotropic drugs, benzodiazepines undergo stepwise hepatic metabolism. The long half-life benzodiazepines that are currently available in the United States undergo both phase I and phase II reactions. Phase I reactions tend to be prolonged in elderly patients, leading to drug accumulation and prolonged half-life. Phase II reactions are unaffected by age. Because short half-life benzodiazepines only require phase II metabolism, they are preferred for older patients (Greenblatt and Shader 1990).

Four types of toxicity occur frequently in older patients: 1) sedation, 2) ataxia and falls (Hale et al. 1988; Rashi and Logan 1986; Ray et al. 1987), 3) psychomotor slowing, and 4) cognitive impairment (Salzman 1990c). The last—an increasing public health concern—is characterized by an anterograde amnesia, diminished short-term recall, increased forgetfulness, and decreased attention. Discontinuing the drug is associated with improved memory and heightened concentration (Salzman et al. 1992).

■ Buspirone

Buspirone is a nonbenzodiazepine anxiolytic that has antianxiety properties in elderly patients. Although research data suggest that it is as effective as benzodiazepines (Napoliello 1986), clinical experience favors benzodiazepines as more rapid and reliable anxiolytics. Because research and clinical experience differ, recommendations for its use remain tentative: buspirone is recommended when benzodiazepines are ineffective or cannot be prescribed.

TREATMENT OF SLEEP DISORDERS

Disordered sleep is a frequent complaint among elderly people (Ancoli-Israel 1989; Pollack and Perlick 1991). Twelve percent of people over age 65 report persistent insomnia, and 1.6% report persistent daytime hypersomnia (Ford and Kamerow 1989). Although only about 12% of Americans are elderly people, they receive 35%–40% of all prescriptions for sedative-hypnotics (Gottlieb 1990).

Treatment Guidelines

Sedative-hypnotic medications are indicated for the short-term treatment of insomnia associated with situational, psychological, psychiatric, or medical conditions that are expected to be time limited or to respond to appropriate therapy. For some elderly patients, long-term use can be justified by the morbidity of chronic sleep deprivation. Regular nightly use, however, may cause significant worsening of cognition, disorientation, confusion, and socially inappropriate behavior in some older people (Regestein 1992). Selection of a particular drug to alleviate sleep problems (like the selection of an antianxiety drug) is guided by the drug's pharmacokinetic properties, its side-effect profile, the patient's medical and emotional health, and the patient's history of prior use of sedative-hypnotics. Reviews of psychotropic drugs to treat sleep disorders in older patients include those of Regestein (1992), Reynolds (1991), and Prinz and colleagues (1990).

Benzodiazepines are the most commonly prescribed sedative-hypnotics. Five are currently marketed for this indication: estazolam, flurazepam, quazepam, temazepam, and triazolam. In general, the benzodiazepines with a long half-life (e.g., flurazepam and, to a lesser extent, quazepam) accumulate and are more likely to produce daytime sedation

in elderly patients. Long-term use can gradually produce a dementia syndrome of cognitive loss, psychomotor retardation, and apathy. Drugs with a shorter half-life cause less daytime sedation and hangover. For example, triazolam, when used in the recommended dose of 0.125 mg, is effective in older patients with sleep fragmentation, daytime sleepiness, and periodic limb movements during sleep (PLMS) (Bonnet and Arand 1991). Withdrawal symptoms and interdose rebound are common. Use of benzodiazepines with an intermediate half-life may be especially useful in elderly patients. Temazepam, which has a half-life of 10–20 hours, has been found to be effective in elderly patients and to cause little hangover, but it has a slow onset of action. The anxiolytic drugs lorazepam and oxazepam are pharmacokinetically similar and are as effective as temazepam for inducing sleep. Estazolam, another benzodiazepine with an intermediate half-life of 12–15 hours, is an effective hypnotic in elderly patients (Vogel and Morris 1992). With intermediate half-life benzodiazepines, daytime performance as well as memory are not adversely affected, and rebound insomnia rarely extends beyond one night following discontinuation.

Other classes of psychotropic drugs are also given to older patients to induce sleep. Sedating neuroleptics such as thioridazine in low doses or antidepressants with sedating side effects such as trazodone and doxepin may be beneficial. Antihistaminic drugs such as diphenhydramine and hydroxyzine also may be helpful in some patients, although these drugs have the potential for anticholinergic, hypotensive, and cardiac side effects. Chloral hydrate is also effective and safe for short-term use. Barbiturates should not be given to elderly patients.

Two new hypnotics that increase delta sleep are now available. Because delta sleep typically decreases with aging, these medications may be of particular benefit to older people. Zolpidem, a clinically effective imidazopyridine hypnotic, does not appear to impair memory (Frattola et al. 1990). Zopiclone, a cyclopyrrolone derivative with a half-life of 5 hours, is as effective as triazolam (Mouret et al. 1990).

TREATMENT OF DEMENTIA

Some degree of memory loss and a slowing of other cognitive processes is common with advancing age. It is called dementia when other cognitive impairments, and impaired social or occupational functioning, accompany the memory loss. Dementia due to neurodegenerative disorders typically follows a slowly progressive course, with worsening attention, orientation, ability to concentrate, visual recognition, and language function in addition to declining short-term and long-term memory. Clinical overviews of the diagnosis and treatment of memory loss include those of Foster and Martin (1990), Crook (1989), and Rosebush and Salzman (1988).

AD is the most common cause of degenerative dementia in elderly people. This idiopathic condition, characterized pathologically by senile plaques and neurofibrillary tangles in the brain, may affect as many as 10% of all people over 65 and nearly 50% of those over 85 (Evans et al. 1989). AD also may cause a variety of psychiatric syndromes, including depression, anxiety, psychosis, and behavioral disturbances such as agitation, sleep-wake cycle disorders, and aggressiveness. At this time there is no known effective treatment to ameliorate or reverse the cognitive impairment caused by AD. Numerous drugs have been studied, based on their presumed effects on those aspects of brain neurochemistry that appear abnormal in AD. Comprehensive reviews of this research include those of Tariot (1992), Miller and colleagues (1992), and Crook and colleagues (1990).

Evidence has suggested that the degree of cognitive impairment in AD patients is correlated with CNS cholinergic deficit (Perry et al. 1978). Restitutive therapies using choline or lecithin as cholinergic precursors have not yielded clinically significant results. Other approaches have used acetylcholinesterase inhibitors to block the enzyme that metabolizes acetylcholine. Three examples are physostigmine, tetrahydroaminoacridine (THA), and velnacrine maleate. Most studies of physostigmine show small improvements in cognition, but the effect is brief (Jenike et al. 1990; Stern et al. 1988). The effects of THA have been both positive and negative. Two trials demonstrated no benefit, but the effect may have been compromised by low doses of the drug (Chatellier and Lacomblez 1990; Gauthier et al. 1990). Three others found improvements that ranged from modest to clinically noticeable by physicians and caregivers (Davis et al. 1992; Eagger et al. 1991; Farlow et al. 1992).

In all of these studies, high rates of liver enzyme elevations—often more than three times normal—have been found. Overall, however, the modest ther-apeutic effects of THA seem to outweigh the possible toxic consequences so that this compound will be available for clinical use in the United States. Other restitutive cholinergic approaches involve the use of muscarinic or nicotinic agonists, or agents that purportedly enhance the potassium-evoked release of acetylcholine (Lavretsky and Jarvik 1992). Acetyl-carnitine may have some direct cholinergic activity, although its mechanism of action is uncertain. Preliminary studies have found some positive effects (Spagnoli et al. 1991), and other studies are in progress.

Restitutive therapies based on known deficits of other neurotransmitters in AD also have been tried. These include attempts to improve

1. Noradrenergic transmission using clonidine or guanfacine
2. Serotonergic function using alaproclate or minaprine
3. γ-aminobutyric acid (GABA)ergic function using tetrahydroisoxazolopyridinol (THIP)
4. Peptide neurotransmission using somatostatin analogues, arginine vasopressin, adrenocorticotropic hormone (ACTH) agonists, thyrotropin-releasing hormone (TRH) analogues, and opiate receptor antagonists

None have been successful in improving cognition, although effects on mood are sometimes seen (Tariot 1992). Studies of selegiline, an MAOI that at low doses appears to be selective for MAO-B, have been encouraging, and additional trials are being conducted.

Evidence suggests that neuronal death in neurodegenerative disorders such as AD may be mediated by a sustained increase in cytosolic free calcium (Branconnier et al. 1992). Increased calcium influx into the cell may be due to changes in the receptor for glutamate, which is part of the N-methyl-D-aspartate (NMDA) receptor complex. Newer therapeutic approaches to AD involve attempts to block calcium channels using antagonists such as nimodipine. One study of nimodipine found significantly less deterioration on some cognitive measures than with placebo, but the short duration of the treatment period limited its clinical relevance (Tollefson 1990). NMDA antagonists, and antagonists at other excitatory amino acid receptors, are in the early stages of development and testing.

Another approach to the treatment of AD involves attempts to enhance CNS cellular metabolism. Hydergine is classified as a metabolic enhancer based on its ability to change cyclic adenosine monophosphate levels. Although hydergine has been studied for more than 20 years, there is evidence that it has only questionable efficacy (Thompson et al. 1990).

The "nootropics" are putative metabolic enhancers that were originally synthesized as GABA derivatives. The first of these was piracetam, and the class now includes oxiracetam, pramiracetam, aniracetam, and vinpocetine. Studies of these drugs indicate variable effects on mood and overall functional status but no clear cognitive effect (Tariot 1992).

Future research on treating the cognitive disorders of AD may be directed at preventing the accumulation of β-amyloid protein fragments, which result from the abnormal processing of the amyloid precursor protein and comprise the core of the senile plaque. Additional research will be directed at targeted drug delivery systems to overcome the problems with drug delivery to the brain caused by peripheral metabolism, poor blood-brain barrier penetration, erratic drug absorption, serum protein binding, systemic adverse effects, and poor patient compliance (Miller et al. 1992).

■ SUMMARY AND CONCLUSION

Psychotropic drugs can benefit the older patient in acute emotional crisis or with chronic recurrent symptoms of severe mental distress that cannot be alleviated solely by other interventions. Regardless of the symptoms being treated or the class of drug used, sound psychotropic treatment may be guided by the following principles:

▼ The elderly patient's current physical illness and medication regimen must be carefully reviewed before beginning treatment.

▼ There is an increased likelihood that concomitant medication for physical illness taken by an older patient may interact adversely with psychotropic drugs.

▼ An older patient is more likely to develop toxic effects from psychotropic drugs, even at doses and blood levels usually considered nontoxic in younger adults.

▼ The average older patient's greater sensitivity to psychotropic drug effects (pharmacodynamics), and the tendency of psychotropic drugs to accumulate and exert greater effect for longer periods (pharmacokinetics), signify the need for low starting doses, low dosage increments, and low therapeutic and maintenance doses to avoid toxicity.

▼ There is great variability in drug response among elderly people. An old-old patient may be even more sensitive to drugs than a young-old patient.

▼ As a corollary, fixed dosing guidelines are not useful when treating an elderly patient. Some older people require doses equal to those prescribed for younger adults.

▼ Close contact and frequent meetings with the older patient under treatment should be routine to assure optimal compliance and to monitor effects and reactions.

■ REFERENCES

Abou-Saleh MT, Coppen A: The efficacy of low-dose lithium: clinical, psychological and biological correlates. J Psychiatr Res 23:157–162, 1989

Addonizio G: Neuroleptic malignant syndrome in the elderly, in Psychopharmacological Treatment Complications in the Elderly. Edited by Shamoian CA. Washington, DC, American Psychiatric Press, 1992, pp 63–70

Alexopoulos GS: Clinical and biological findings in late-onset depression, in American Psychiatric Press Review of Psychiatry, Vol 9. Edited by Tasman A, Goldfinger SM, Kaufmann C. Washington, DC, American Psychiatric Press, 1990, pp 249–262

Alexopoulos GS: Treatment of depression, in Clinical Geriatric Psychopharmacology, 2nd Edition. Edited by Salzman C. Baltimore, MD, Williams & Wilkins, 1992, pp 137–174

Alexopoulos GS, Young RC, Meyers BS, et al: Late-onset depression. Psychiatr Clin North Am 11:101–115, 1988

Allen RM: Tranquilizers and sedative/hypnotics: appropriate use in the elderly. Geriatrics 41:75–88, 1986

Ancill RJ, Embury GD, MacEwan GW, et al: The use and misuse of psychotropic prescribing for elderly psychiatric patients. Can J Psychiatry 33:585–589, 1988

Ancoli-Israel S: Epidemiology of sleep disorders. Clin Geriatr Med 5:347–362, 1989

Antonijoan RM, Barbanoj MJ, Torrent J, et al: Evaluation of psychotropic drug consumption related to psychological distress in the elderly: hospitalized vs. nonhospitalized. Neuropsychobiology 23:25–30, 1990

Aoba A, Kakita Y, Yamaguchi N, et al: Absence of age effect on plasma haloperidol neuroleptic levels in psychiatric patients. J Gerontol 40:303–308, 1985

Aronson MK, Ooi WL, Geva DL, et al: Dementia: age-dependent incidence, prevalence, and mortality in the old-old. Arch Intern Med 151:989–992, 1991

Avorn J, Dreyer P, Connelly K, et al: Use of psychoactive medication and the quality of care in rest homes. N Engl J Med 320:227–232, 1989

Avorn J, Soumerai SB, Everett DE, et al: A randomized controlled trial of a program to reduce the use of psychoactive drugs in nursing homes. N Engl J Med 327:168–173, 1992

Beardsley RS, Larson DB, Burns BJ, et al: Prescribing of psychotropics in elderly nursing home residents. J Am Geriatr Soc 37:327–330, 1989

Beers M, Avorn J, Soumerai SB, et al: Psychoactive medication use in intermediate care facility residents. JAMA 260:3016–3020, 1988

Berrios GE, Bakshi N: Manic and depressive symptoms in the elderly: their relationships to treatment outcome, cognition and motor symptoms. Psychopathology 24:31–38, 1991

Billig N, Cohen-Mansfield J, Lipson S: Pharmacological treatment of agitation in a nursing home. J Am Geriatr Soc 39:1002–1005, 1991

Blazer D, Williams CD: Epidemiology of dysphoria and depression in an elderly population. Am J Psychiatry 137:439–444, 1980

Bonnet MH, Arand DL: Chronic use of triazolam in patients with periodic leg movements, fragmented sleep and daytime sleepiness. Aging 3:313–324, 1991

Branconnier RJ, Cole JO: Effects of acute administration of trazodone and amitriptyline on cognition, cardiovascular function, and salivation in the normal geriatric subject. J Clin Psychopharmacol 1:82S–88S, 1981

Branconnier RJ, Cole JO, Ghazvinian S, et al: Clinical pharmacology of bupropion and imipramine in elderly depressives. J Clin Psychiatry 44:130–133, 1983

Branconnier RJ, Branconnier ME, Walshe TM, et al: Blocking the Ca²⁺-activated cytotoxic mechanisms of cholinergic neuronal death: a novel treatment strategy for Alzheimer's disease. Psychopharmacol Bull 28:175–181, 1992

Brymer C, Winograd CH: Fluoxetine in elderly patients: is there cause for concern? J Am Geriatr Soc 40:902–905, 1992

Buck JA: Psychotropic drug practice in nursing homes. J Am Geriatric Soc 36:409–418, 1988

Caine ED, Lyness JM, King DA: Reconsidering depression in the elderly. American Journal of Geriatric Psychiatry 1:4–20, 1993

Carbonin R, Pahor M, Bernabei R: Is age an independent risk factor for adverse drug reactions in hospitalized medical patients? J Am Geriatr Soc 39:1093–1099, 1991

Chatellier G, Lacomblez L: Tacrine (tetrahydroaminoacridine; THA) and lecithin in senile dementia of the Alzheimer type: a multicentre trial. BMJ 300:495–499, 1990

Cohen BM, Sommer BR: Metabolism of thioridazine in the elderly. J Clin Psychopharmacol 8:336–339, 1988

Cohen-Mansfield J, Marx MS, Rosenthal AS: A description of agitation in a nursing home. J Gerontol 44:77–84, 1989

Col N, Fanale JE, Kronholm P: The role of medication non-compliance and adverse drug reactions in hospitalizations of the elderly. Arch Intern Med 150:841–845, 1990

Colenda CC: Buspirone in treatment of agitated demented patient. Lancet 2:1169, 1988

Crook TH: Diagnosis and treatment of normal and pathologic memory impairment in later life. Semin Neurol 9:20–30, 1989

Crook TH, Johnson BA, Larrabee GJ: Evaluation of drugs in Alzheimer's disease and age-associated memory impairment. Psychopharmacology (Berl) 26:37–55, 1990

Cutler NR, Zavadil AP, Eisdorfer C, et al: Concentrations of desipramine in elderly women. Am J Psychiatry 138:1235–1237, 1981

Davis KL, Thal LJ, Gamzu ER et al: A double-blind, placebo-controlled multicenter study of tacrine for Alzheimer's disease. N Engl J Med 327:1253–1259, 1992

Dawling S, Crome P, Braithwaite RA: Pharmacokinetics of single oral doses of nortriptyline in depressed elderly hospital patients and young healthy volunteers. Clin Pharmacokinet 5:394–401, 1980a

Dawling S, Crome P, Braithwaite RA, et al: Nortriptyline therapy in elderly patients: dosage prediction after single dose pharmacokinetic study. Eur J Clin Pharmacol 18:147–150, 1980b

Dawling S, Crome P, Heyer EJ, et al: Nortriptyline therapy in elderly patients: dosage prediction from plasma concentration at 24 hours after a single 50mg dose. Br J Psychiatry 139:413–416, 1981

Dawson D, Hundershot G, Fulton J: Aging in the eighties: functional limitations of individuals age 65 and over (Advance Data No. 133, June 1987), in Aging America: Trends and Projections, 1986–1987. Washington, DC, U.S. Department of Health and Human Services, 1987

Devanand DP, Sackeim HA, Mayeux R: Psychosis, behavioral disturbance, and the use of neuroleptics in dementia. Compr Psychiatry 29:387–401, 1988

Devanand DP, Sackeim HA, Brown RP, et al: A pilot study of haloperidol treatment of psychosis and behavioral disturbance in Alzheimer's disease. Arch Neurol 46:854–857, 1989

Devanand DP, Cooper T, Sackeim HA, et al: Low dose oral haloperidol and blood levels in Alzheimer's disease: a preliminary study. Psychopharmacol Bull 28:169–173, 1992

De Veaugh-Geiss J: Clinical changes in tardive dyskinesia during long-term follow-up, in Tardive Dyskinesia: Biological Mechanisms and Clinical Aspects. Edited by Wolf ME, Mosnaim AD. Washington, DC, American Psychiatric Press, 1988, pp 89–105

Dewan MJ, Huszonek J, Koss M, et al: The use of antidepressants in the elderly: 1986 and 1989. J Geriatr Psychiatry Neurol 5:40–44, 1992

Dhingra U, Rabins PV: Mania in the elderly: a 5–7 year follow-up. J Am Geriatr Soc 39:581–583, 1991

Dunner DL, Cohn JB, Walshe T III, et al: Two combined, multicenter double-blind studies of paroxetine and doxepin in geriatric patients with major depression. J Clin Psychiatry 53:57–60, 1992

Eagger SA, Levy R, Sahakian BJ: Tacrine in Alzheimer's disease. Lancet 337:989–992, 1991

Evans DA, Funkenstein H, Albert MS, et al: Prevalence of Alzheimer's disease in a community population of older persons. JAMA 262:2551–2556, 1989

Farlow M, Gracon SI, Hershey LA et al: A controlled trial of tacrine in Alzheimer's disease. JAMA 268:2523–2529, 1992

Feighner JP, Cohn JB: Double-blind comparative trials of fluoxetine and doxepin in geriatric patients with major depressive disorder. J Clin Psychiatry 46:20–25, 1985

Feighner JP, Boyer WF, Meredith CH, et al: An overview of fluoxetine in geriatric depression. Br J Psychiatry 153 (suppl 3):105–108, 1988

Ford DE, Kamerow DB: Epidemiological studies of sleep disturbances and psychiatric disorders: an opportunity for prevention? JAMA 262:1479–1484, 1989

Forsman A, Ohman R: Applied pharmacokinetics of haloperidol in man. Current Therapeutic Research 21:396–411, 1977

Foster JR: Use of lithium in elderly psychiatric patients: a review of the literature. Lithium 3:77–93, 1992

Foster JR, Martin CE: Dementia, in Verwoerdt's Clinical Geropsychiatry, 3rd Edition. Edited by Bienenfeld D. Baltimore, MD, Williams & Wilkins, 1990, pp 66–84

Frattola L, Maggioni M, Cesana B, et al: Double blind comparison of zolpidem 20 mg versus flunitrazepam 2 mg in insomniac in-patients. Drugs Exp Clin Res 16:371–376, 1990

Ganzini, L, Heintz R, Hoffman WF, et al: Acute extrapyramidal syndromes in neuroleptic-treated elders: a pilot study. J Geriatr Psychiatry Neurol 4:222–225, 1991

Garrard J, Makris L, Dunham T, et al: Evaluation of neuroleptic drug use under proposed Medicare and Medicaid regulations. JAMA 265:463–467, 1991

Gauthier S, Bouchard R, Lamontagne A, et al: Tetrahydroaminoacridine-lecithin combination treatment in patients with intermediate stage Alzheimer's disease. N Engl J Med 322:1272–1276, 1990

Georgotas A, Mann J, Friedman E: Platelet monoamine oxidase inhibitors as a potential indicator of favorable response to MAOIs in geriatric depression. Biol Psychiatry 16:997–1001, 1981

Georgotas A, Friedman E, McCarthy M, et al: Resistant geriatric depressions and therapeutic response to monoamine oxidase inhibitors. Biol Psychiatry 18:195–205, 1983

Georgotas A, McCue RE, Hapworth W, et al: Comparative efficacy and safety of MAOIs versus TCAs in treating depression in the elderly. Biol Psychiatry

21:1155–1166, 1986

Gerner R, Estabrook W, Steuer J, et al: Treatmemt of depression with trazodone, imipramine, and placebo: a double-blind study. J Clin Psychiatry 41:216–220, 1980

Glasser M, Rabins P: Mania in the elderly. Age Ageing 13:210–213, 1984

Gottlieb GL: Sleep disorders and their management: special considerations in the elderly. Am J Med 88(3A):29S–33S, 1990

Greenblatt DJ, Shader RI: Benzodiazepines in the elderly: pharmacokinetics and drug sensitivity, in Anxiety in the Elderly. Edited by Salzman C, Lebowitz B. New York, Springer, 1990, pp 131–145

Greenwald BS, Marin DB, Silverman SM: Serotoninergic treatment of screaming and banging in dementia [letter]. Lancet 2:1464–1465, 1986

Grymonpre RE, Mitenko PA, Sitar DS, et al: Drug-associated hospital admissions in older medical patients. J Am Geriatr Soc 36:1092–1098, 1988

Gurwitz JH, Avorn J: The ambiguous relationship between aging and adverse drug reactions. Ann Intern Med 114:956–966, 1991

Halaris A: Antidepressant drug therapy in the elderly: enhancing safety and compliance. Int J Psychiatry Med 16:1986–1987, 1986

Hale WE, May FE, Moore MT, et al: Meprobamate use in the elderly. J Am Geriatr Soc 36:1003–1005, 1988

Helms PM: Efficacy of antipsychotics in the treatment of the behavioral complications of dementia: a review of the literature. J Am Geriatr Soc 33:206–209, 1985

Hershey LA, Kim KY: Diagnosis and treatment of anxiety in the elderly. Rational Drug Therapy 22:3–6, 1988

Himmelhoch JM, Neil JF, May F, et al: Age, dementia, dyskinesias, and lithium response. Am J Psychiatry 137:941–945, 1980

Holton A, George K: The use of lithium in severely demented patients with behavioral disturbance. Br J Psychiatry 146:99–104, 1985

Huang CC: Comparison of two groups of tardive dyskinesia patients. Psychiatry Res 19:335–336, 1986

Institute of Medicine: Extending Life, Enhancing Life: A National Research Agenda on Aging. Washington, DC, National Academy Press, 1991

Ives TJ, Bentz EJ, Gwyther RE: Drug-related admissions to a family medicine inpatient service. Arch Intern Med 147:1117–1120, 1987

Jarvik LF, Read SL, Mintz J, et al: Pretreatment ortho-static hypotension in geriatric depression: predictor of response to imipramine and doxepin. J Clin Psychopharmacol 3:368–372, 1983

Jefferson JW, Griest JH, Ackerman DL, et al: Lithium Encyclopedia for Clinical Practice. Washington, DC, American Psychiatric Press, 1987

Jenike MA: The use of monoamine oxidase inhibitors in the treatment of elderly depressed patients. J Am Geriatric Soc 32:571–575, 1985

Jenike MA, Albert M, Heller H, et al: Oral physostigmine treatment for patients with presenile and senile dementia of the Alzheimer's-type: a double-blind, placebo-controlled trial. J Clin Psychiatry 51:3–7, 1990

Kanba S, Matsumoto K, Nibuya M, et al: Nortriptyline response in elderly depressed patients. Prog Neuropsychopharmacol Biol Psychiatry 16:301–309, 1992

Karson CG, Bracha HS, Powell A, et al: Dyskinetic movements, cognitive impairment, and negative symptoms in elderly neuropsychiatric patients. Am J Psychiatry 147:1646–1649, 1990

Katz IR, Simpson GM, Jethanandani V, et al: Steady state pharmacokinetics of nortriptyline in the frail elderly. Neuropsychopharmacology 2:229–236, 1989

Kemperman CJF, Gerdes JH, De Rooij J, et al: Reversible lithium neurotoxicity at normal serum level may refer to intracranial pathology. J Neurol Neurosurg Psychiatry 52:679–680, 1989

Kim KY: Diagnosis and treatment of depression in the elderly. Int J Psychiatry Med 18:211–221, 1988

Kitanka I, Ross RJ, Cutler NR, et al: Altered hydroxydesipramine concentrations in elderly depressed patients. Clin Pharmacol Ther 31:51–55, 1982

Koenig HG, Breitner JCS: Use of antidepressants in medically ill older patients. Psychosomatics 31:22–32, 1990

Koepke HH, Gold RL, Linden ME, et al: Multicenter controlled study of oxazepam in anxious elderly outpatients. Pychosomatics 23:641–645, 1982

Kroenke K, Pinholt EM: Reducing polypharmacy in the elderly: a controlled trial of physician feedback. J Am Geriatr Soc 38:31–36, 1990

Kroessler D, Fogel BS: Electroconvulsive therapy for major depression in the oldest old: effects of medical comorbidity on post-treatment survival. American Journal of Geriatric Psychiatry 1:30–37, 1993

Kutcher SP, Reid K, Dubbin JD, et al: Electrocardiogram changes and therapeutic desipramine and 2-hydroxydesipramine concentrations in elderly depressives. Br J Psychiatry 148:676–679, 1986

Kyomen HH, Nobel KW, Wei JY: The use of estrogen to decrease aggressive physical behavior in elderly men with dementia. J Am Geriatr Soc 39:1110–1112, 1991

Lakshmanan EB, Mion CC, Frengley JD: Effective low dose tricyclic antidepressant treatment for depressed geriatric rehabilitation patients. J Am Geriatr Soc 34:421–426, 1986

Lavretsky EP, Jarvik LF: A group of potassium channel blockers-acetylcholine releasers: new potentials for Alzheimer disease? a review. J Clin Psychopharmacol 12:110–118, 1992

Lazarus LW, Groves L, Gierl B, et al: Efficacy of phenelzine in geriatric depression. Biol Psychiatry 21:699–701, 1986

Leibovici A, Tariot N: Carbamazepine treatment of agitation associated with dementia. J Geriatr Psychiatry Neurol 1:110–112, 1988

Lieberman J, Kane JM, Woerner M, et al: Prevalence of tardive dyskinesia in elderly samples. Psychopharmacol Bull 20:22–26, 1984

Liptzin B: Treatment of mania, in Clinical Geriatric Psychopharmacology, 2nd Edition. Edited by Salzman C. Baltimore, MD, Williams & Wilkins, 1992, pp 175–188

Magni G, Palazzolo O, Bianchin G: The course of depression in elderly outpatients. Can J Psychiatry 33:21–24, 1988

Maletta GS: Use of antipsychotic medications, in Annual Review of Gerontology and Geriatrics, 1984, Vol 4. Edited by Eisdorfer C. New York, Springer, pp 175–220

McCue RE, Georgotas A, Nagachandran N, et al: Plasma levels of nortriptyline and 10-hydroxy-nortriptyline and treatment-related electrocardiographic changes in the elderly depressed. J Psychiatr Res 23:73–79, 1989

McFarland BH, Miller MR, Straumfjord AA: Valproate use in the older manic patient. J Clin Psychiatry 51:479–481, 1990

Meyers BS: Adverse cognitive effects of tricyclic antidepressants in the treatment of geriatric depression: fact or fiction, in Psychopharmacological Treatment Complications in the Elderly. Edited by Shamoian CA. Washington, DC, American Psychiatric Press, 1992, pp 1–16

Miller SW, Mahoney JM, Jann MW: Therapeutic fron-

tiers in Alzheimer's disease. Pharmacotherapy 12:217–231, 1992

Morgan DG, May PC, Finch LE: Dopamine and serotonin systems in human and rodent brain: effects of age and neurodegenerative disease. J Am Geriatr Soc 35:334–345, 1987

Mouret J, Ruel D, Maillard F, et al: Zopiclone versus triazolam in insomniac geriatric patients: a specific increase in delta sleep with zopiclone. Int Clin Psychopharmacol 5 (suppl 2):47–55, 1990

Napoliello MJ: An interim multicentre report on 677 anxious geriatric out-patients treated with buspirone. Br J Clin Pract 40:71–73, 1986

National Center for Health Statistics: Current estimates from the National Health Interview Survey: Vital and Health Statistics 1987, No. 10, in Aging America: Trends and Projections, 1986–1987. Washington, DC, U.S. Government Printing Office, 1987, p 164

Nelson JC, Atillasoy E, Mazure C: Desipramine plasma levels and response in elderly melancholic patients. J Clin Psychopharmacol 5:217–220, 1985

Nelson JC, Atillasoy E, Mazure C, et al: Hydroxy-desipramine in the elderly. J Clin Psychopharmacol 8:428–433, 1988

Office of Epidemiology and Biostatistics, Center for Drug Evaluation and Research: Drug utilization in the United States, 1986. Washington, DC, National Technical Information Service, 1987

Olafsson K, Jorgensen S, Jensen HV, et al: Fluvoxamine in the treatment of demented elderly patients: a double-blind, placebo-controlled study. Acta Psychiatr Scand 85:453–456, 1992

Old Age Depression Interest Group: How long should the elderly take antidepressants? a double-blind placebo-controlled study of continuation/prophylaxis therapy with dothiepin. Br J Psychiatry 162:175–182, 1993

Oreland L, Gottfries CG: Brain monoamine oxidase in aging and in dementia of the Alzheimer type. Prog Neuropsychopharmacol Biol Psychiatry 10:533–540, 1986

Parmelee PA, Katz IR, Lawton MP: Anxiety and association with depression among institutionalized elderly. American Journal of Geriatric Psychiatry 1:46–58, 1993

Peabody CA, Whiteford HA, Hollister LE: Antidepressants and the elderly. J Am Geriatr Soc 34:869–874, 1986

Peabody CA, Warner MD, Whiteford HA, et al: Neuroleptics and the elderly. J Am Geriatr Soc 35:233–238, 1987

Perry E, Tomlinson B, Blessed G, et al: Correlation of cholinergic abnormalities with senile plaques and mental test scores in senile dementia. British Medical Journal 2:1457–1459, 1978

Petrie WM, Ban TA, Berney S, et al: Loxapine in psychogeriatrics: a placebo and standard controlled clinical investigation. J Clin Psychopharmacol 2:122–126, 1982

Phillipson M, Moranville JT, Jeste DV, et al: Antipsychotics. Clin Geriatr Med 6:411–422, 1990

Pinner E, Rich CL: Effects of trazodone on aggressive behavior in seven patients with organic mental disorders. Am J Psychiatry 145:1295–1296, 1988

Pinsker H, Suljaga-Petchel K: Use of benzodiazepines in primary-care geriatric patients. J Am Geriatric Soc 32:595–598, 1984

Pollack CP, Perlick D: Sleep problems and institutionalization of the elderly. J Geriatr Psychiatry Neurol 4:204–210, 1991

Prinz PN, Vitiello MV, Raskind MA, et al: Geriatrics: sleep disorders and aging. N Engl J Med 323:520–526, 1990

Rashi S, Logan RFA: Role of drugs in fractures of the femoral neck. BMJ 292:86, 1986

Ray WA, Federspiel CF, Schaffner W: A study of antipsychotic drug use in nursing homes: epidemiologic evidence suggesting misuse. Am J Public Health 70:485–491, 1980

Ray WA, Griffin MR, Shaffner W, et al: Psychotropic drug use and the risk of hip fracture. N Engl J Med 316:363–369, 1987

Ray WA, Fought RL, Decker MD: Psychoactive drugs and the risk of injurious motor vehicle crashes in elderly drivers. Am J Epidemiol 136:873–883, 1992

Regestein QR: Treatment of insomnia in the elderly, in Clinical Geriatric Psychopharmacology, 2nd Edition. Edited by Salzman C. Baltimore, MD, Williams & Wilkins, 1992, pp 235–253

Reynolds CF: Sleep disorders, in Comprehensive Review of Geriatric Psychiatry. Edited by Sadavoy J, Lazarus LW, Jarvik LF. Washington, DC, American Psychiatric Press, 1991, pp 403–418

Risse SC, Barnes R: Pharmacologic treatment of agitation associated with dementia. J Am Geriatr Soc 34:368–376, 1986

Robinson DS, Sourkes TL, Nies A, et al: Monoamine metabolism in human brain. Arch Gen Psychiatry 34:89–92, 1977

Rockwell E, Lam RW, Zisook S: Antidepressant drug studies in the elderly. Psychiatr Clin North Am 11:215–233, 1988

Rosebush PI, Salzman C: Memory disturbance and cognitive impairment in the elderly, in Handbook of Clinical Psychopharmacology. Edited by Tupin JP, Shader RI, Harnett DS. New York, Jason Aronson, 1988, pp 159–210

Rothschild AJ, Samson AJ, Bessette MP, et al: Efficacy of the combination of fluoxetine and perphenazine in the treatment of psychotic depression (in press)

Rovner B, Kafonek S, Filipp L, et al: Prevalence of mental illness in a nursing home. Am J Psychiatry 143:1146–1149, 1986

Rovner BW, German PS, Brant LJ, et al: Depression and mortality in nursing homes. JAMA 265:993–996, 1991

Saban RJ, Vitug AJ, Mark VH: Are nursing home diagnosis and treatment inadequate? JAMA 243:321–322, 1982

Saltz BL, Kane JM, Woerner MG, et al: Prospective study of tardive dyskinesia in the elderly. Psychopharmacol Bull 25:52–56, 1989

Salzman C: Treatment of agitation in the elderly, in Psychopharmacology: The Third Generation of Progress. Edited by Meltzer HY. New York, Raven, 1987, pp 1167–1176

Salzman C: Recent advances in geriatric psychopharmacology, in American Psychiatric Press Review of Psychiatry, Vol 9. Edited by Tasman A, Goldfinger SM, Kaufmann C. Washington, DC, American Psychiatric Press, 1990a, pp 279–292

Salzman C: The American Psychiatric Association Task Force Report on Benzodiazepine Dependency, Toxicity, and Abuse. J Psychiatr Res 24:35–37, 1990b

Salzman C: Practical considerations of the pharmacologic treatment of depression and anxiety in the elderly. J Clin Psychiatry 51(1) (suppl):40–43, 1990c

Salzman C: Monoamine oxidase inhibitors and atypical antidepressants. Clin Geriatr Med 8:335–348, 1992

Salzman C: Pharmacologic treatment of depression in the elderly. J Clin Psychiatry 54 (suppl):23–28, 1993

Salzman C: Pharmacological treatment of depression in elderly patients, in Diagnosis and Treatment of Depression in Late Life: Results of the NIH Consensus Development Conference. Edited by Schneider LS, Reynolds CF, Lebowitz BD, et al. Washington, DC, American Psychiatric Press, 1994, pp 181–244

Salzman C, Fisher J, Nobel K, et al: Cognitive improvement following benzodiazepine discontinuation in elderly nursing home residents. International Journal of Geriatric Psychiatry 7:89–93, 1992

Salzman C, Schneider LS, Lebowitz BD: Antidepressant treatment of very old patients. American Journal of Geriatric Psychiatry 1:21–29, 1993

Schneider LS, Sloane RB, Staples FR, et al: Pretreatment orthostatic hypotension as a predictor of response to nortriptyline in geriatric depression. J Clin Psychopharmacol 6:172–176, 1986

Schneider LS, Pollock VE, Lyness SA: A metaanalysis of controlled trials of neuroleptic treatment in dementia. J Am Geriatr Soc 38:553–563, 1990a

Schneider LS, Cooper TB, Suckow RF, et al: Relationship of hydroxynortriptyline to nortriptyline concentration and creatinine clearance in depressed elderly outpatients. J Clin Psychopharmacol 10:333–337, 1990b

Schneider JK, Mion LC, Frengley JD: Adverse drug reactions in an elderly outpatient population. Am J Hosp Pharm 49:90–96, 1992

Sheikh JI: Panic disorder, in Anxiety in the Elderly. Edited by Salzman C, Lebowitz B. New York, Springer, 1990, pp 251–266

Shulman KI, Tohen M, Satlin A, et al: Mania compared with unipolar depression in old age. Am J Psychiatry 149:341–345, 1992

Simpson DM, Foster D: Improvement in organically disturbed behavior with trazodone treatment. J Clin Psychiatry 47:191–193, 1986

Skoog I, Nilsson L, Palmertz B, et al: A population-based study of dementia in 85-year-olds. N Engl J Med 328:153–158, 1993

Small GW: Psychopharmacological treatment of elderly demented patients. J Clin Psychiatry 49 (suppl):8–13, 1988

Smith JM, Baldessarini RJ: Changes in prevalence, severity and recovery in tardive dyskinesia with age. Arch Gen Psychiatry 37:1368–1373, 1980

Smith M, Buckwalter KC: Medication management, antidepressant drugs, and the elderly: an overview. Journal of Psychosocial Nursing 30:30–36, 1992

Snowdon J: A retrospective case-note study of bipolar disorder in old age. Br J Psychiatry 158:485–490, 1991

Spagnoli A, Lucca U, Menasce G, et al: Long-term acetyl-L-carnitine treatment in Alzheimer's disease. Neurology 41:1726–1732, 1991

Stack JA, Reynolds CF III, Perel JM, et al: Pretreatment systolic orthostatic blood pressure (PSOP) and treatment response in elderly depressed inpatients. J Clin Psychopharmacol 8:116–120, 1988

Stern Y, Sano M, Mayeux R: Long-term administration of oral physostigmine in Alzheimer's disease. Neurology 38:1837–1841, 1988

Stewart RB, May FE, Moore MY, et al: Changing patterns of psychotropic drug use in the elderly: a five-year update. Annals of Pharmacotherapy 23:610–613, 1989

Stone K: Mania in the elderly. Br J Psychiatry 155:220–229, 1989

Strauss A: Oral dyskinesia associated with buspirone use in an elderly woman. J Clin Psychiatry 49:322–323, 1988

Sweet RA, Benoit H, Mulsant MD, et al: Dyskinesia and neuroleptic exposure in elderly psychiatric inpatients. J Geriatr Psychiatry Neurol 5:156–161, 1992

Szuba MP, Leuchter AF: Falling backward in two elderly patients taking bupropion. J Clin Psychiatry 53:157–159, 1992

Tariot PN: Neurobiology and treatment of dementia, in Clinical Geriatric Psychopharmacology, 2nd Edition. Edited by Salzman C. Baltimore, MD, Williams & Wilkins, 1992, pp 277–299

Thompson TL, Filley CM, Mitchell WD, et al: Lack of efficacy of hydergine in patients with Alzheimer's disease. N Engl J Med 323:445–448, 1990

Tingle D: Trazodone in dementia [letter]. J Clin Psychiatry 47:482, 1986

Tollefson GD: Short-term effects of the calcium channel blocker nimodipine (Bay-e-9736) in the management of primary degenerative dementia. Biol Psychiatry 27:1133–1142, 1990

Vogel GW, Morris D: The effects of estazolam on sleep, performance, and memory: a long-term sleep laboratory study of elderly insomniacs. J Clin Pharmacol 32:647–651, 1992

von Moltke LL, Greenblatt DJ, Shader RI: Clinical pharmacokinetics of antidepressants in the elderly. Clin Pharmacokinet 24:141–160, 1993

Weiler PG, Mungo D, Bernick C: Propranolol for the control of disruptive behavior in senile dementia.

J Geriatr Psychiatry 1:226–230, 1988

Weissman MM, Prusoff B, Sholomskas AJ, et al: A double-blind clinical trial of alprazolam, imipramine, or placebo in the depressed elderly. J Clin Psychopharmacol 12:175–182, 1992

Wragg RE, Jeste DV: Neuroleptics and alternative treatments. Management of behavioral symptoms and psychosis in Alzheimer's disease and related conditions. Psychiatr Clin North Am 11:195–213, 1988

Yassa R: The course of tardive dyskinesia in newly treated psychogeriatric patients. Acta Psychiatr Scand 83:347–349, 1991

Yassa R, Nair V, Schwartz G: Tardive dyskinesia: a two-year follow-up study. Psychosomatics 25:852–855, 1984

Yassa R, Nastase C, Camille Y, et al: Tardive dyskinesia in a psychogeriatric population, in Tardive Dyskinesia: Biological Mechanisms and Clinical Aspects. Edited by Wolf ME, Mosnaim AD. Washington, DC, American Psychiatric Press, 1988, pp 125–133

Young RC, Alexopoulos GS, Shamoian CA, et al: Plasma 10-hydroxynortriptyline in elderly depressed patients. Clin Pharmacol Ther 35:540–544, 1984

Young RC, Alexopoulos GS, Shamoian CA, et al: Plasma 10-hydroxynortriptyline and ECG changes in elderly depressed patients. Am J Psychiatry 142:866–868, 1985

Zimmer JG, Watson N, Trent A: Behavior problems among patients in skilled nursing facilities. Am J Public Health 74:1118–1121, 1984

Zimmer JG, Bentley DW, Valente WM: Systemic antibiotic use in nursing homes: a quality assessment. J Am Geriatr Soc 34:703–710, 1986

Zisook S: A clinical overview of monoamine oxidase inhibitors. Psychosomatics 26:240–246, 1985

41

Psychopharmacology During Pregnancy and Lactation

Zachary N. Stowe, M.D., and Charles B. Nemeroff, M.D., Ph.D.

The management of mental illness during pregnancy and lactation represents a unique and complex clinical situation. Considering the high incidence of mental illness in women of childbearing years and the rise in the number of women that are planning to breast-feed, there is a high probability that the clinician will encounter such situations. The use of psychotropic medications during pregnancy and lactation has been comprehensively reviewed by several groups (Cohen 1989; Cohen et al. 1989; Kerns 1986; Miller 1991, 1994; Robinson et al. 1986; Wisner and Perel 1988). The most common situations encountered include 1) new-onset mental illness or the aggravation of extant symptoms during pregnancy or in the postpartum period; 2) prepregnancy consultation for women with preexisting mental illness and/or currently on psychotropic medications; 3) inadvertent conception during treatment with psychotropic medications; and 4) women at high risk for a postpartum mental illness who are planning to nurse. The literature provides few definitive data to guide the clinician in such situations. However, it is important for the clinician to have all of the available data on potentially toxic effects—somatic and neurobehavioral—of psychotropic medications. As a preamble to expanding on previously suggested treatment guidelines for these clinical conditions (Cohen et al. 1989; Miller 1991), we provide a brief review of the normal physiological changes associated with pregnancy, lactation, and fetal and early infant life. Knowledge of these basic physiolog-

ical alterations may be of some empirical value in selecting medications based on their pharmacokinetic and pharmacodynamic properties in the event that nonpharmacological interventions fail to provide adequate control of symptoms. Further, an important consideration in the selection of psychotropic medication is the available data concerning the possible risks of individual agents from different classes; such information is important for patient education as well as for medical-legal issues. In this chapter, we review the individual classes of medications and discuss potential modifications of previously suggested treatment guidelines.

Review of the extant literature on use of psychotropic medications during pregnancy and lactation reveals a cadre of problems. The most prominent of these are 1) the failure of adequate sample size to establish a significant causal relationship for teratogenic effects of psychotropic medications and 2) the reliance on case reports. Of documented pregnancies 84.5% result in the birth of a viable infant (Kiely 1991; McBride 1972), 2%–4% of whom will have major malformations that impair function and/or require surgical correction, and up to 12% of whom will have minor malformations (Riccardi 1977). The Collaborative Perinatal Project followed a cohort of 50,282 mother-infant pairs from 12 medical centers and found an overall infant malformation rate of 6.5% (Heinonen et al. 1977). Developmental studies have demonstrated that the majority of major malformations occur during the embryonic period (i.e., the 3rd through 8th week of gestation) and that after the 11th week of gestation, most of the organ systems (except for the central nervous system [CNS], teeth, ears, eyes, and external genitalia) are developed (Sadler 1985). Another major issue, noted in previous reviews (Cohen et al. 1989) is that 80% of pregnant women are prescribed medications, and more than one-third of pregnant women may take psychotropic medications at some time during their pregnancy (Doering and Stewart 1978). The majority of previous reports have also failed to control for maternal age, tobacco use, alcohol and drug abuse, potential exposure to environmental toxins, duration and timing of exposure, and extent of prenatal care received. There is also evidence that bias may exist in associating birth defects with psychotropic medications. The association of "in utero" lithium exposure with Ebstein's anomaly of the heart is still virtually considered dogma, yet a comprehensive review of the available data by Cohen and colleagues (1994) places the risk for this malformation at less than 0.1%. Furthermore, any potential relationship between the effect of psychiatric illness itself and the risk of birth defects, as well as of spontaneous miscarriage, has not been studied.

■ PHYSIOLOGY

Physiological alterations during pregnancy and data derived from studies of nonpsychotropic medications support several empirical suggestions for the choice of a psychotropic medication within a given class. One area of growing interest concerns the potential effects of gender differences and the effects of alterations in serum gonadal hormone concentrations on the pharmacokinetics of psychotropic medication (Yonkers et al. 1992). The majority of relevant data concerning the physiological changes associated with pregnancy are derived from therapeutic plasma drug monitoring with nonpsychotropic medications (Boobis and Lewis 1982). Several changes occur during pregnancy that may alter serum concentrations of psychotropic medications, including 1) delayed gastric emptying, resulting in increased exposure to an acidic environment and degradative enzymes; 2) decreased gastrointestinal motility, presumably related to increased progesterone, resulting in potentially more complete absorption of medication; 3) increased volume of distribution (increased body fat,

plasma volume, total body water), resulting in decreased serum concentrations for a given dose; 4) decreased protein binding capacity, resulting in an increase in serum-free drug concentrations (Wood and Hytten 1981); and 5) increased hepatic metabolism, resulting in more rapid degradation of certain medications. However, with the exception of the tricyclic antidepressants, a clear relationship between therapeutic response and serum concentrations has not been established. All of these changes potentially affect the drug concentration to which the fetus may be exposed.

There is no evidence of placental filtering of psychotropic medications; all known psychotropic medications permeate the placental barrier. The mechanism of placental transport is thought to be simple diffusion that is dependent on several properties of the individual medication (molecular size, percentage of protein binding, polarity, lipid solubility), and, of course, duration of exposure (Rayburn and Andresen 1982). The fetus and mother are at equilibrium with respect to circulation. However, the fetus has several distinct physiological attributes: 1) increased cardiac output, 2) increased blood-brain barrier permeability, 3) decreased plasma protein and plasma protein binding affinity, and 4) decreased hepatic enzyme activity. The net effect of these differences is increased fetal CNS exposure to medications and potentially greater CNS drug concentrations.

Following childbirth, the neonate continues to exhibit unique physiological characteristics, including decreased activity of certain hepatic metabolic enzyme systems. Hepatic maturation in the infant appears to occur at a highly variable rate (Warner 1986) and is more delayed in premature infants. Both glucuronidation and oxidation systems are initially immature at birth—as low as 20% of adult levels; the latter system typically matures by 3 months of age (Atkinson et al. 1988). In addition, rates of glomerular filtration and tubular secretion are relatively low in neonates—30%–40% and 20%–30% lower than adult levels, respectively (Welch and Findlay 1981). Hence, the potential for the infant to be exposed to higher serum concentrations of parent compounds and metabolites of any drug needs to be considered.

The excretion of psychotropic medications in breast milk has been reviewed (Buist et al. 1990). The number of women who plan to breast-feed is on the rise, with recent estimates indicating that more than 50% of new mothers leaving the hospital plan to nurse (Briggs et al. 1994a). The information contained in the American Academy of Pediatrics' (1994) recent committee report on the use of medications during breastfeeding is included later in this chapter in our discussion of the classes of medication. The literature is again problematic secondary to differences in the methodology of drug concentration assays, a gradient in breast milk with respect to lipophilic characteristics and protein content (Kauffman et al. 1994; Vorherr 1974). The majority of data have not controlled for which aliquot of breast milk was used for assay. Medications predominantly enter breast milk by passive diffusion of the un-ionized, unbound fraction (J. T. Wilson et al. 1980). The pH gradient between maternal serum and breast milk is a major determinant in the quantity of medication excreted into breast milk. The physicochemical properties of an individual medication appear to be the best predictor of the concentration of drug present in breast milk (see Kacew 1993 for review). These properties include 1) degree of ionization, 2) molecular weight, 3) protein binding, and 4) lipid solubility. Maternal protein binding affects the quantity of drug available for diffusion across the mammillary epithelium, and most drugs have a higher affinity for maternal plasma proteins than for milk proteins (Kacew 1993).

The American Academy of Pediatrics (1994) recently published a committee report on the excretion of drugs and other chemicals into human breast milk. Although admittedly not complete, the report's list of psychotropic medications underscores the need to encourage further collaborative work with pediatricians. The Academy's classification of individual psychotropic medications include 1) drugs that are contraindicated during breastfeeding; 2) drugs whose effects on nursing infants are unknown but may be of concern (i.e., no adverse events have been reported, but the medications are present in human milk and thus conceivably alter CNS development); and 3) maternal medications usually compatible with breastfeeding.

■ ASSESSMENT OF RISK-BENEFIT RATIO

The morbidity and mortality of untreated mental illness during pregnancy and lactation are not well doc-

umented. The majority of pregnant women are not aware of their pregnancy for at least 6 weeks; hence, discontinuation of psychotropic medications may occur after the period of greatest potential risk to the fetus. Such discontinuations may also carry an increased risk of relapse that may result in increased risk to the mother and/or greater exposure to medication. A salient feature of most mental illnesses is impairment of function, as noted in DSM-IV (American Psychiatric Association 1994). Clearly, intervention is warranted if the functional impairment is sufficient to preclude a woman's participation in prenatal care or directly jeopardizes the pregnancy or infant. Another area of concern is the potential negative impact of the neuroendocrine alterations associated with certain mental disorders, such as depression, and stress on pregnancy outcome. Although laboratory animal data have revealed an adverse effect of increased glucocorticoid concentrations on brain development, human studies are based on exposure to exogenous corticosteroids. The impact of maternal mental illness on maternal attachment (Avant 1981) and child development remains controversial (Brazelton 1975; Cradon 1979; Zahn-Waxler et al. 1984).

Cohen and colleagues (1989) considered the risk of psychotropic medication use during pregnancy and lactation to fall into one of five categories: 1) somatic teratogenic risk (see Elia et al. 1987 for review); 2) neurobehavioral teratogenic effects; 3) direct toxic effects to the fetus; 4) drug effects on labor and delivery; and 5) effects on the breast-feeding infant. The category of drug effects on labor and delivery should be expanded to include the entire course of pregnancy. Therefore, obstetric histories—including placental insufficiency, preeclampsia, and urinary or gastrointestinal difficulties—should be closely evaluated to avoid use of any medication that might complicate these conditions. Clearly, potential drug-drug interactions with anesthetic and analgesic medications should also be considered.

To date, the U.S. Food and Drug Administration (FDA) has not approved any psychotropic medication for use during pregnancy or lactation. The current FDA classification system is presented in Table 41–1. One potential confounder of this system is that medications that have been available longer are more likely to have adverse case reports filed. The significance of these adverse case reports is difficult to evaluate.

Table 41–1. U.S. Food and Drug Administration use-in-pregnancy ratings

Category	Interpretation
A	Controlled studies show no risk—Adequate, well-controlled studies in pregnant women have failed to demonstrate risk to the fetus.
B	No evidence of risk in humans—Either animal findings show risk, but human findings do not; or, if no adequate human studies have been done, animal findings are negative.
C	Risk cannot be ruled out—Human studies are lacking, and animal studies are either positive for fetal risk or lacking as well; however, potential benefits may justify potential risk.
D	Positive evidence of risk—Investigational or postmarketing data show risk to the fetus; nevertheless, potential benefits may outweigh risks.
X	Contraindicated in pregnancy—Studies in animals or humans, or investigational or postmarketing reports have shown fetal risks that clearly outweigh any possible benefit to the patient.

Source. Physicians' Desk Reference (1994).

The decision of whether or not to use psychotropic medications during pregnancy and/or lactation not only is a difficult clinical judgment but also carries ethical and potentially legal ramifications regardless of what decision is made. It has been suggested that nonpharmacological interventions be used prior to recommendation of psychotropic agents or electroconvulsive therapy (ECT) (Cohen et al. 1989; Miller 1991). However, in the rapidly changing environment of health care reimbursement and managed health care, nonpharmacological options such as frequent psychotherapy sessions and inpatient hospitalizations may not be readily available.

■ ANTIDEPRESSANTS

Tricyclic antidepressants have been available in the United States since 1963, and their use has extended well beyond treating depression. The development of nontricyclic antidepressants has further broadened the spectrum of clinical utility for antidepressants as a class to include obsessive-compulsive disorder (clomipramine, fluoxetine, paroxetine, sertraline), panic disorder (imipramine, paroxetine, fluoxetine),

pain syndromes (amitriptyline, nortriptyline, doxepin), bulimia (fluoxetine), and premenstrual syndrome (fluoxetine, nortriptyline, clomipramine). Whereas earlier studies (Sim 1963; Zajicek 1981) and clinical lore described pregnancy as a time of psychiatric "well being," recent prospective investigations have found that 10% of women fulfill criteria for a mood disorder (both minor and major) during pregnancy (O'Hara et al. 1990).

Despite the widespread use of antidepressants during pregnancy, no clear association with congenital malformations has been demonstrated (see Table 41–2 for individual medication information). Earlier studies reported an association with various anomalies; the most commonly noted were those affecting the limbs (see Barson 1972, Elia et al. 1987, and McBride 1972 for review). A recent prospective study with a relatively small sample ($N = 18$) demonstrated that there was no increased risk of fetal anomalies and no increased complications during labor and delivery, although short-term withdrawal symptoms were noted in the neonates (Misri and Sivertz 1991). In contrast, there have been reports of fetal tachycardia (Prentice and Brown 1989). The issue of neonatal withdrawal is complicated by the lack of data about maternal dosing during labor. Symptoms reported include tachypnea, tachycardia, cyanosis, irritability, hypertonia, clonus, spasm, and seizure (see Eggermont 1973, Miller 1991, and Webster 1973 for review). Wisner et al. (1993) reported that the tricyclic antidepressant dosage requirement for women with depression during pregnancy may increase over the course of pregnancy to maintain adequate therapeutic serum concentrations and the associated clinical response. Unfortunately, although they did not report any complications, these researchers did not specifically comment on the presence or absence of any neonatal withdrawal phenomena.

There are limited human data on the use of monoamine oxidase inhibitors (MAOIs) during pregnancy and lactation. Although the MAOIs are all FDA category C medications, one prospective study in a small group of patients indicated that in utero tranylcypromine (Parnate) exposure was associated with fetal malformations. Animal studies have demonstrated teratogenic effects associated with the MAOIs (Poulson and Robson 1964). The dietary constraints and potential for hypertensive crisis have precluded much attention being paid to the use of MAOIs during pregnancy (Wisner and Perel 1988).

Table 41–2. Antidepressant medications

Generic name	Trade name	Daily dose (mg/day)[a]	Half-life (hours)[b]	Risk category[c]	American Academy of Pediatrics rating[d]
Tricyclic/heterocyclic antidepressants					
amitriptyline	Elavil, Endep	150–300	10–22	D	Unknown, but of concern
amoxapine	Asendin	150–400	8–20	C_m	Unknown, but of concern
clomipramine	Anafranil	150–250	19–37	C_m	Compatible
desipramine	Norpramin	150–300	12–76	C	Unknown, but of concern
doxepin	Sinequan, Adapin	150–300	11–23	C	Unknown, but of concern
imipramine	Tofranil	150–300	11–25	D	Unknown, but of concern
nortriptyline	Pamelor, Aventyl	75–150	15–93	D	NA
maprotiline	Ludiomil	140–225	21–66	B_m	NA
protriptyline	Vivactil	15–60	54–198	C	NA
Monoamine oxidase inhibitors[e]					
isocarboxazid	Marplan	30–60	NA	C	NA
phenelzine	Nardil	45–90	NA	C	NA
tranylcypromine	Parnate	30–60	NA	C	NA
Selective serotonin reuptake inhibitors					
fluoxetine	Prozac	20–60	24–96	B	Unknown, but of concern
fluvoxamine[f]	Luvox	50–300	17–22	B_m	Unknown, but of concern
paroxetine[f]	Paxil	20–50	24	B_m	NA
sertraline	Zoloft	50–200	26	B	NA
Other antidepressants					
bupropion	Wellbutrin	150–450	8–24	B_m	NA
trazodone	Desyrel	200–300	4–13	C_m	Unknown, but of concern
venlafaxine[f]	Effexor	150–375	5–11	C_m	NA

Note. NA = not applicable.
[a]Dosing strategies adapted from Schatzberg and Cole 1991, Kaplan and Sadock 1993, and, for newer medications, the manufacturer package inserts.
[b]Half-life of elimination is listed for parent compound.
[c]Risk category adapted from Briggs et al. 1994; "m" subscript is for data taken from the manufacturer's package insert.
[d]From American Academy of Pediatrics 1994.
[e]Duration of action is based on irreversible enzyme inhibition; half-life of elimination is not applicable.
[f]Not listed in Briggs et al. 1994; risk category taken from the *Physicians' Desk Reference* (1994).

There are sparse data on the use of the selective serotonin reuptake inhibitors (SSRIs) during pregnancy. A recent study of first-trimester exposure to fluoxetine (mean dose 25.8 mg/day) did not demonstrate an increase in fetal anomalies in 128 women (Pastuszak et al. 1993). In that study, the rate of spontaneous abortion in the subjects was 14.8% compared with 7.8% in the control subjects; however, when subjects were compared with those control subjects exposed to tricyclic antidepressants (n = 74, 12.2% spontaneous abortion rate), no significant increase in spontaneous abortion was associated with in utero fluoxetine exposure. To date, breast milk excretion studies have demonstrated that antidepressants are present in breast milk, with a milk/serum ratio that is typically ≥ 1.0 (Buist et al. 1990). It appears that for amitriptyline (Pittard and O'Neal 1986), desipramine (Stancer and Reed 1986), and trazodone (Verbeeck et al. 1986), there is a peak increase in breast milk concentrations 4–6 hours after an oral dose. Only single case reports are available for fluoxetine (Isenberg 1990) and fluvoxamine (Wright et al. 1991). Our group measured the concentration of sertraline and desmethylsertraline in seven nursing women and found a milk/serum ratio ranging from 0.95–2.35 and 0.80–3.14, respectively (Stowe et al. 1995). Wisner and Perel (1991) reported on seven nursing women treated with nortriptyline: although no infant serum samples had detectable nortriptyline levels ($n = 4$), detectable levels of 10-hydroxynortriptyline were found in two infants. In summary, relatively little is known about antidepressant excretion into breast milk. Furthermore, adjusting both the schedule of dosing of the antidepressant and the infant's feeding schedule may considerably reduce the concentration of the drug to which the infant is exposed.

The majority of investigators recommend using the secondary amine tricyclic antidepressants (nortriptyline and desipramine) (Cohen 1989; Miller 1991). Few data are available concerning the SSRIs, and, as noted above, typically MAOIs are avoided during pregnancy. No human data have been published on novel antidepressants such as bupropion (Wellbutrin) and venlafaxine (Effexor).

■ ANTIPSYCHOTICS

In contrast with other classes of psychotropic medications, antipsychotic agents have a considerably larger database that addresses concerns of neurobehavioral teratogenicity. Additionally, phenothiazines have been widely prescribed to treat pregnancy-associated emesis (typically at lower dose ranges), thereby aiding in separating the effects on pregnancy outcome of having a neuropsychiatric disorder from those of using antipsychotic drugs. Chlorpromazine, haloperidol, and perphenazine have received the greatest scrutiny, and investigators have failed to find a significant association between use of these drugs and major congenital malformations (Goldberg and DiMascio 1978; Hill and Stern 1979; Nurnberg and Prudic 1984). Commonly prescribed antipsychotic medications, as well as agents used to treat their side effects, are listed in Table 41–3.

In a study of 100 women treated with haloperidol (mean dose 1.2 mg/day) for hyperemesis gravidarum, no differences in gestational duration, fetal viability, or birthweight were noted (Van Waes and Van de Velde 1969). In a large prospective study, Milkovich and Van den Berg (1976) followed almost 20,000 women treated for emesis, mostly with phenothiazines. When maternal age, medication, and gestational age of exposure were controlled, the au-

thors found no significant increase in severe anomalies or neonatal survival rates. Similar results have been obtained in several retrospective studies of women treated with trifluoperazine for repeated abortions and emesis (Moriarty and Nance 1963; Rawlings et al. 1963). In contrast, Rumeau-Rouquette and colleagues (1977) reported a significant association of major anomalies with prenatal exposure to phenothiazines with an aliphatic side chain, but not with piperazine- and piperidine-class agents. Reanalysis of the data obtained by Milkovich and Van den Berg did find a significant risk of malformations associated with phenothiazine exposure in the 4th through 10th week of gestation (Edlund and Craig 1976).

Beyond the potential teratogenic risks of these agents is the potential for other side effects of antipsychotic drugs, such as neuroleptic malignant syndrome (NMS) (James 1988) and extrapyramidal side effects (EPS). The symptoms of EPS in the neonate may include increased muscle tone and increased rooting and tendon reflexes that may persist for several months (Cleary 1977; Hill et al. 1966; O'Connor et al. 1981). In addition, in utero exposure to antipsychotics may produce neonatal jaundice (Scokel and Jones 1962) and intestinal obstruction (Falterman and Richardson 1980) postnatally.

Several animal studies have demonstrated that prenatal exposure to antipsychotic medications can cause persistent abnormalities in learning and memory (Hoffeld et al. 1968; Ordy et al. 1966; Robertson et al. 1980). In contrast, Dallemagne and Weiss (1982) did not observe such drug-induced alterations. Human studies have failed to demonstrate significant differences in intelligence quotient (IQ) scores at 4 years of age ($n = 52$ [Kris 1965] and $n = 151$ [Slone et al. 1977]). However, these studies included women exposed to relatively low doses of phenothiazines (Kris 1965).

Antipsychotic drugs, like other psychotropics, are excreted into breast milk (see Buist et al. 1990 for review). The most widely studied is chlorpromazine; seven infants exposed to chlorpromazine did not demonstrate any developmental deficits at 16-month and 5-year follow-ups (Kris and Carmichael 1957). The breast milk concentrations of several other antipsychotics have been measured, including haloperidol (Stewart et al. 1980; Whalley et al. 1981), trifluoperazine and perphenazine (J. T. Wilson et al. 1980), and thioxanthenes (Matheson and Skjaeraasen

Table 41–3. Antipsychotic medications

Generic name	Trade name	Daily dose (mg/day)[a]	Half-life (hours)[b]	Risk category[c]	American Academy of Pediatrics rating[d]
chlorpromazine	Thorazine	200–800	8–35	C	Unknown, but of concern
clozapine	Clozaril	100–800	4–66	B_m	NA
fluphenazine	Prolixin	5–10	14–24	C	NA
haloperidol	Haldol	5–10	12–36	C_m	Unknown, but of concern
loxapine	Loxitane	20–80	4–12	C	NA
mesoridazine	Serentil	100–400	24–48	C	Unknown, but of concern
molindone	Moban	20–80	24–36	C	NA
perphenazine	Trilafon	8–32	8–21	C	Unknown, but of concern
pimozide[e]	Orap	1–10	55	NA	NA
risperidone[e]	Risperdal	1–16	3–20	C	NA
thioridazine	Mellaril	200–600	9–30	C	NA
thiothixene	Navane	10–40	34	C	NA
trifluoperazine	Stelazine	10–40	18–30	C	NA
Medications to treat side effects of antipsychotics					
amantadine	Symmetrel	100–400	15	C_m	NA
benztropine	Cogentin	0.5–6	10–12	C	NA
diphenhydramine	Benadryl	25–150	6–24	C	NA
propranolol	Inderal	20–120	4	C_m	Compatible
trihexyphenidyl	Artane	2–15	10–12	C	NA

Note. NA = not applicable.
[a]Dosing strategies adapted from Schatzberg and Cole 1991, Kaplan and Sadock 1993, and, for newer medications, the manufacturer package inserts.
[b]Half-life of elimination is listed for parent compound.
[c]Risk category adapted from Briggs et al. 1994; "m" subscript is for data taken from the manufacturer's package insert.
[d]From American Academy of Pediatrics 1994.
[e]Not listed in Briggs et al. 1994; risk category taken from the *Physicians' Desk Reference* (1994).

1988). The milk/serum ratio is less than or equal to 1.0. J. T. Wilson et al. (1980) suggested that the physicochemical properties of perphenazine could cause it to become "trapped" in breast milk.

A variety of agents are available for the treatment of EPS. In utero exposure to diphenhydramine (Benadryl) has been the most widely reported. The Collaborative Perinatal Project found an association between first-trimester exposure to diphenhydramine and major and minor anomalies (see Miller 1991 and Wisner and Perel 1988 for review). One study comparing 599 children with oral clefts with 590 control subjects found a significantly higher rate of exposure to diphenhydramine in the children with oral clefts (Saxen 1974). Another group described a possible neonatal withdrawal syndrome associated with diphenhydramine that included tremulousness and diarrhea (Parkin 1974). Case reports of intestinal

obstruction following perinatal exposure to neuroleptics and benztropine (Falterman and Richardson 1980), as well as the potential adverse effects on maternal gastrointestinal motility, warrant cautious use of anticholinergic agents. Animal studies have demonstrated amantadine (Symmetrel) to be a known teratogen (Hirsch and Swartz 1980), yet human reports are lacking.

In summary, antipsychotic medications have been widely used for more than three decades, and the paucity of data linking these agents to either congenital or neurobehavioral deficits would suggest that the risk of these medications are minimal. However, as with all medications, their use should be avoided during the first trimester. Moreover, piperazine phenothiazines (e.g., trifluoperazine, perphenazine) may have less teratogenic potential (Rumeau-Rouquette et al. 1977).

■ ANXIOLYTIC MEDICATIONS

Benzodiazepines and antidepressants are the most commonly used drugs for the treatment of anxiety disorders, and benzodiazepines are the most widely prescribed psychotropic medications. A recent retrospective survey of Medicaid records (1980–1983) of 104,339 pregnant women found that at least 2% had received one or more prescriptions for a benzodiazepine (Bergman et al. 1992). As a class, benzodiazepines readily traverse the placenta, and the presence of benzodiazepines in umbilical cord plasma demonstrates that these drugs accumulate in the fetus after prolonged administration (Mandelli et al. 1975; Shannon et al. 1972); we know that these medications are found in fetal brain, lungs, and heart (Mandelli et al. 1975). The same group (Mandelli et al. 1975) also found that the metabolism of diazepam in fetuses is slower than that in adults, with a fetal $t_{1/2}$ of 31 hours for the parent compound. In contrast to concentrations of other benzodiazepines studied, lorazepam concentrations were lower in cord blood than in maternal serum but were excreted at a slower rate, with excretion of detectable levels 8 days postdelivery (Whitelaw et al. 1981). Earlier studies reported an increased risk of oral clefts following in utero exposure to diazepam (Aarkog 1975; Saxen 1975; Saxen and Saxen 1975); however, later studies failed to demonstrate this association (Entman and Vaughn 1984; Rosenberg et al. 1984; Shiono and Mills 1984). Alprazolam is widely prescribed for a variety of anxiety states, including panic disorder. As of December 1991, the Upjohn voluntary reporting system database on exposure to alprazolam during pregnancy contained the following information: elective abortion, 15%; spontaneous abortion, 7%; and stillborn or neonatal death, 2%—rates comparable to those found in nonmedication-associated pregnancy outcome studies. Congenital anomalies occurred in fewer than 6% of infants who received in utero exposure to alprazolam. Table 41–4 lists benzodiazepine and nonbenzodiazepine anxiolytics and sedative-hypnotics used in the treatment of anxiety disorders and insomnia, respectively.

Long-term, longitudinal follow-up studies are urgently needed. One group has described a "benzodiazepine exposure syndrome" for infants exposed in utero to these drugs that included growth retardation, dysmorphism, and both mental and psychomotor retardation (Laegreid et al. 1987). The same group later reported predominantly neonatal sedation and withdrawal (Laegreid et al. 1989). A second group failed to find an increased incidence of behavioral abnormalities at 8 months of age, and found no difference in IQ scores at 4 years of age, for children exposed to chlordiazepoxide in utero (Hartz et al. 1975). Although the data on the teratogenic effects of fetal exposure to benzodiazepines remain somewhat controversial, the presence of infant withdrawal syndromes has been described by several groups, and symptoms can persist for as long as 3 months (see Miller 1991 for review).

Buist and colleagues (1990) concluded that benzodiazepines at relatively low doses present no contraindications to nursing. In contrast to other classes of psychotropic medications, benzodiazepines appear to have lower milk-to-maternal serum ratios. Wreitland (1987) found a ratio of 0.1 : 0.3 for oxazepam, and estimated that the infant would be exposed to 1/1000th of the maternal dose. The percentage of the maternal dose of lorazepam to which a nursing infant is exposed has been estimated to be 2.2% (Summerfield and Nielsen 1985).

In summary, it is recommended that benzodiazepines not be abruptly withdrawn during pregnancy and that if at all possible, these drugs be tapered sufficiently prior to delivery to limit neonatal withdrawal. Evidence from umbilical cord sampling indicates that lorazepam may not accumulate in the fetus. Lorazepam (Ativan) and oxazepam (Serax) bypass hepatic metabolism and may therefore have less potential for accumulation in the neonate. Finally, as noted in the comprehensive review by Miller (1991), diazepam with sodium benzoate as a preservative may also present some potential difficulties. Clonazepam (Klonopin, FDA category C) appears to have minimal teratogenic risks (Sullivan and McElhatton 1977).

■ MOOD-STABILIZING MEDICATIONS

The management of bipolar disorder during pregnancy has received considerable attention. Unlike depressive, psychotic, and anxiety disorders, the number of clinically efficacious medications for bipolar disorder is more limited (see Table 41–5).

Table 41–4. Anxiolytic and sedative-hypnotic medications

Generic name	Trade name	Daily dose (mg/day)[a]	Half-life (hours)[b]	Risk category[c]	American Academy of Pediatrics rating[d]
Benzodiazepines					
alprazolam	Xanax	0.5–6	12	D_m	NA
chlordiazepoxide	Librium	15–100	< 100	D	NA
clonazepam	Klonopin	0.5–10	34	C	NA
clorazepate	Tranxene	7.5–60	< 100	D	NA
diazepam	Valium	2–60	< 100	D	Unknown, but of concern
halazepam[e]	Paxipam	60–160	< 100	NA	NA
lorazepam	Ativan	2–6	15	D_m	Unknown, but of concern
oxazepam	Serax	30–120	8	D	NA
prazepam[e]	Centrax	20–60	< 100	D	Unknown, but of concern
Benzodiazepines for insomnia					
estazolam[e]	Prosom	1–2	1–2	X	NA
flurazepam	Dalmane	15–30	< 100	X_m	NA
quazepam[f]	Doral	7.5–30	< 100	X_m	Unknown, but of concern
temazepam	Restoril	15–30	11	X_m	Unknown, but of concern
triazolam	Halcion	0.125–0.25	2	X_m	NA
Nonbenzodiazepine anxiolytics and hypnotics					
buspirone[f]	BuSpar	15–60	3–16	B_m	NA
chloral hydrate	Noctec	500–1,500	4–8	C_m	Compatible
zolpidem tartrate[e]	Ambien	5–10	4–6	C	NA

Note. NA = not applicable.
[a]Dosing strategies adapted from Schatzberg and Cole 1991, Kaplan and Sadock 1993, and, for newer medications, the manufacturer package inserts.
[b]Average half-life of elimination for major metabolites; adapted from Kaplan and Sadock 1993, and, for newer medications, the manufacturer package inserts.
[c]Risk category adapted from Briggs et al. 1994; "m" subscript is for data taken from the manufacturer's package insert.
[d]From American Academy of Pediatrics 1994.
[e]Not listed in Briggs et al. 1994b; risk category taken from *Physicians' Desk Reference* (Medical Economics Data 1994).
[f]Briggs et al. 1994b.

Lithium carbonate remains the cornerstone of treatment for bipolar disorder. The Registry of Lithium Babies was established in 1969 for Danish women after case reports of congenital malformations following in utero exposure to lithium (Schou et al. 1973). Further registers were established in Canada and the United States, culminating in the International Register of Lithium Babies. Initial studies suggested a marked increase in cardiovascular malformations, particularly Ebstein's anomaly (Nora et al. 1974; Weinstein and Goldfield 1975). However, as noted previously, Cohen and colleagues (1994) completed an extensive survey of the available information and found an increase in the relative risk of cardiac malformations of 1.2–7.7 and an overall in-

crease in the relative risk for congenital malformations of 1.5–3.0 for in utero lithium exposure. In contrast to animal studies, a 5-year follow-up study failed to find any significant behavioral teratogenic sequelae associated with lithium exposure prenatally (Schou 1976). The recent outcome studies for lithium discontinuation and relapse rates for patients with bipolar disorder (Suppes et al. 1991; Tohen et al. 1990) underscore the need to carefully assess the severity of illness, as outlined by Cohen and colleagues (1994). Briefly, it is recommended that women receive prepregnancy counseling and that for women with a single episode, gradual tapering and an attempt at lithium-free pregnancy are warranted—or, if indicated, reinstitution of lithium after the first trimes-

Table 41–5. Mood-stabilizing medications

Generic name	Trade name	Daily dose (mg/day)[a]	Half-life (hours)[b]	Risk category[c]	American Academy of Pediatrics rating[d]
carbamazepine	Tegretol	400–1,600	12–17	C_m	Compatible
clonazepam	Klonopin	0.5–10	34	C	NA
valproic acid	Depakote (sodium divalproex)	750–2,000	8–10	D	Compatible
lithium carbonate	Eskalith, Lithobid, Lithonate	900–2,400	20	D	Contraindicated

Note. NA = not applicable.
[a]Dosing strategies adapted from Schatzberg and Cole 1991, Kaplan and Sadock 1993, and, for newer medications, the manufacturer package inserts.
[b]Average half-life of elimination for parent compound; taken from the *Physicians' Desk Reference* (1994), Kaplan and Sadock 1993.
[c]Risk category adapted from Briggs et al. 1994; "m" subscript is for data taken from the manufacturer's package insert.
[d]From American Academy of Pediatrics 1994.

ter. It is recommended that the clinician offer a fetal echocardiogram between the 16th and 18th week of gestation for women who were treated with lithium during their first trimester of pregnancy.

The previously noted physiological alterations are of importance in the management of lithium therapy during pregnancy and parturition. The changes in glomerular filtration rate during—and the potential for dehydration at—parturition and the associated rapid fluid status changes warrant close monitoring of lithium levels and a taper/decrease of lithium dosage prior to delivery. In addition, the neonate is at risk for lithium toxicity at serum concentrations lower than maternal concentrations. Symptoms of toxicity include flaccidity, lethargy, and poor suck reflexes that may persist for more than 7 days (Woody et al. 1971). Lithium can also produce reversible changes in thyroid function (Karlsson et al. 1975), cardiac arrhythmias (N. Wilson et al. 1983), hypoglycemia, and diabetes insipidus (Mizrahi et al. 1979).

Several anticonvulsants have also been shown to be effective in the treatment of bipolar disorder. These include carbamazepine, valproic acid, and perhaps clonazepam. The bulk of the literature on the teratogenic risk of these compounds is derived from their use in treating epilepsy during pregnancy. As noted by Cohen and colleagues (1994), these agents have not yet been proven to provide comparable levels of prophylaxis for manic episodes. In utero exposure to both carbamazepine and valproic acid apparently increases the malformation rate in infants of epileptic mothers (Jones et al. 1989; Lindhout and Schimdt 1986). Fetal serum concentrations of carba-

mazepine are approximately 50%–80% of the maternal concentrations (Nau et al. 1982). The risk for spina bifida associated with fetal exposure to carbamazepine is 1% (relative risk is about 13.7%) (Rosa 1991). Similarly, valproic acid is a known human teratogenic drug, with a 1%–2% risk of neural tube defects. As noted by Janz (1982), almost all major and minor malformations associated with mood-stabilizing medications have been reported for infants of epileptic mothers treated with anticonvulsants. Intrauterine growth retardation is one of the most commonly cited potential complications of in utero exposure to valproic acid (see Briggs et al. 1994a for review). Gaily and colleagues (1988) compared the intelligence of 148 children of epileptic mothers (both treated and untreated) and 105 control subjects at 5½ years of age; of the children of epileptic mothers, 4 were considered mentally deficient or of borderline intelligence, whereas none of the control children fulfilled those criteria. Such findings underscore the difficulty in assigning definitive neurobehavioral risk potential to psychotropic medications.

All of the mood-stabilizing medications except for clonazepam appear to carry an increased risk of malformation and a potentially deleterious effect on latter cognitive development. Like other psychotropic medications, mood-stabilizing medications are present in breast milk. Nursing infants can achieve serum lithium concentrations that are 40%–50% of maternal levels (Kirksey and Groziak 1984; Schou and Amdisen 1973). Although there are no reports of toxic effects associated with lithium and nursing, the potential for such toxicity warrants close observation of the infant's hydration status. In contrast, both carbamazepine and valproic acid appear in low concentrations in human milk and both are considered compatible with breastfeeding (American Academy of Pediatrics 1994).

In summary, the management of bipolar disorder during pregnancy requires careful assessment of the disorder and of its severity. If possible, mood-stabilizing medications should be avoided during the first trimester. The guidelines suggested by Cohen et al. (1994) underscore the potentially favorable risk-benefit ratio of lithium use during pregnancy.

■ SUMMARY

There is a paucity of clinical data that support the view that psychotropic medications are teratogenic; in contrast, preclinical laboratory animal studies, which typically used high doses of these agents, reveal definite physical and neurobehavioral teratogenic effects (Elia et al. 1987). Pregnant and nursing women are generally excluded in clinical studies of novel pharmacological agents, and it is doubtful that well-controlled studies will ever be conducted. Although some investigators have suggested that conducting such studies in pregnant and nursing women is unethical (Kerns 1986), one could argue that failure to conduct such studies increases the overall risk to women and infants over time, and may deprive some women of adequate treatment. Several characteristics (route of metabolism, protein binding affinity, lipid partitioning) warrant further study to determine if these physicochemical features affect placental transfer and excretion into breast milk.

Considering the higher prevalence rates of depressive and anxiety disorders in women compared with men, and the particularly high rates of these disorders during childbearing years, it is likely that the clinician will face the complex issues of prescribing psychotropic medications during pregnancy and lactation. In light of the lack of data demonstrating the superior clinical efficacy of a single medication within a given class, we offer the following general treatment recommendations (the assumption is made that the clinician has already exhausted nonpharmacological interventions and that no information involving previous pharmacological response or failure is available):

▼ **Informed consent**—It is not possible to provide a complete list of all risks for any given psychotropic medication. It is important to discuss with the patient the risks of using or not using psychotropic medications and to document that other treatment options have been attempted or considered.

▼ **Choice of medication**—Medications with the following characteristics should be sought:

  ▼ *Greatest documentation of prior use*—Medications that have been available for a longer period of time have a larger database (although predominantly of case reports) in pregnancy and lactation.

  ▼ *Lower FDA risk category (B > C > D)*—The FDA is empirically conservative and has access to the greatest amount of pre- and postmarketing data. Whereas this rating may be controversial for some medications, it is reasonable that medical-legal considerations would support this approach.

  ▼ *Few or no metabolites*—Data from both pregnancy and lactation suggest that drug metabolites, which typically have a longer half-life of elimination, can accumulate. The issue of active versus inactive metabolites is unresolved with respect to teratogenic effects.

  ▼ *Shorter half-life of elimination*—Physiological data indicate that medications may accumulate in the fetus and neonate.

  ▼ *Fewer side effects*—Medications with fewer hypotensive and anticholinergic side effects are preferable. Additionally, the effect on seizure threshold and potential interaction with commonly used obstetric anesthetic and analgesic agents should be minimized.

  ▼ *Concordant data*—Avoid medications with conflicting data; use a clinically comparable alternative if available. This recommendation should also reduce any potential legal liability.

▼ **Dosage**—The goal of treatment during pregnancy and lactation is primarily symptom control, not syndrome resolution. Maintain the minimum effective dose for symptom control and recovery of function. Adjustments may be indicated later in pregnancy as the volume of distribution changes. To minimize the potential for neonatal withdrawal and maternal toxicity after delivery, the dose of medication should be reduced during the 2 weeks prior to delivery.

The number of women choosing to breast-feed is increasing (Briggs et al. 1994a). Adjusting the feeding and dose schedule can reduce the infant's exposure to medication for several agents.

▼ **Communication with pediatrician**—It is highly recommended that the psychiatric clinician discuss medication and potential interactions with the infant's pediatrician. The delay in hepatic maturity may affect the metabolism of psychotropic agents and potentially alter the serum levels of other medications prescribed for the infant.

■ REFERENCES

Aarkog D: Association between maternal intake of diazepam and oral clefts (letter). Lancet 2:921, 1975

American Academy of Pediatrics, Committee on Drugs: The transfer of drugs and other chemicals into human milk. Pediatrics 93:137–150, 1994

American Psychiatric Association: Diagnostic and Statistical Manual of Mental Disorders, 4th Edition. Washington, DC, American Psychiatric Association, 1994

Atkinson HC, Begg EJ, Darlow BA: Drugs in human milk: clinical pharmacokinetic considerations. Clin Pharmacokinet 14:217–240, 1988

Avant K: Anxiety as a potential factor affecting maternal attachment. J Obstet Gynecol Neonatal Nurs 10:416–419, 1981

Barson AJ: Malformed infants. British Medical Journal 2:45, 5804, 1972

Bergman U, Rosa FW, Baum C, et al: Effects of exposure to benzodiazepine during fetal life. Lancet 340:694–696, 1992

Boobis AR, Lewis PJ: Drugs in pregnancy—altered pharmacokinetics. Br J Hosp Med 28:566–573, 1982

Brazelton TB: Mother—infant reciprocity, in Maternal Attachment and Mothering Disorders: A Roundtable. Edited by Klaus MH, Leger T, Trause MA. North Brunswick, NJ, Johnson & Johnson, 1975, pp 49–54

Briggs GG, Freeman RK, Yaffe SJ: Drugs in Pregnancy and Lactation, 4th Edition. Edited by Mitchell CW. Baltimore, MD, Williams & Wilkins, 1994a

Briggs GG, Freeman RK, Yaffe SJ: Drugs in Pregnancy and Lactation, 4th Edition, Vol 7 (Supplement). Edited by Mitchell CW. Baltimore, MD, Williams & Wilkins, 1994b, pp 1–8

Buist A, Norman TR, Dennerstein L: Breastfeeding and the use of psychotropic medication: a review. J Affect Disord 19:197–206, 1990

Cleary MF: Fluphenazine decanoate during pregnancy. Am J Psychiatry 134:815–816, 1977

Cohen LS: Psychotropic drug use in pregnancy. Hosp Community Psychiatry 40:566–567, 1989

Cohen LS, Heller VL, Rosenbaum JF: Treatment guidelines for psychotropic drug use in pregnancy. Psychosomatics 30:1, 25–33, 1989

Cohen LS, Friedman JM, Jefferson JW, et al: A reevaluation of risk of in utero exposures to lithium. JAMA 271:146–150, 1994

Cradon AJ: Maternal anxiety and neonatal wellbeing. J Psychosom Res 23:113–115, 1979

Dallemagne G, Weiss B: Altered behavior of mice following postnatal treatment with haloperidol. Pharmacol Biochem Behav 16:761–767, 1982

Doering JC, Stewart RB: The extent and character of drug consumption during pregnancy. JAMA 239:843–846, 1978

Edlund MJ, Craig TJ: Antipsychotic drug use and birth defects: an epidemiologic reassessment. Compr Psychiatry 25:244–248, 1976

Eggermont E: Withdrawal symptoms in neonates associated with maternal imipramine therapy. Lancet 2(830):680, 1973

Elia J, Katz IR, Simpson GM: Teratogenicity of psychotherapeutic medications. Psychopharmacol Bull 23:531–586, 1987

Entman SS, Vaughn WK: Lack of relation of oral clefts to diazepam use in pregnancy. N Engl J Med 310:1121–1122, 1984

Falterman CG, Richardson CJ: Small left colon syndrome associated with maternal ingestion of psychotropic drugs. J Pediatr 97:308–310, 1980

Gaily E, Kantola-Sorsa E, Granstrom ML: Intelligence of children of epileptic mothers. J Pediatr 113:677–684, 1988

Goldberg HL, DiMascio A: Psychotropic drugs in pregnancy, in Psychopharmacology: A Generation of Progress. Edited by Lipton MA, DiMascio A, Killam KF. New York, Raven, 1978, pp 1047–1055

Hartz SC, Heinonen OP, Shapiro S, et al: Antenatal exposure to meprobamate and chlordiazepoxide in relation to malformations, mental development, and childhood mortality. N Engl J Med 292:726–

728, 1975

Heinonen OP, Stone D, Shapiro S: Birth Defects and Drugs in Pregnancy. Littleton, MA, Publishing Sciences Group, 1977

Hill RM, Stern L: Drugs in pregnancy: effects on the fetus and newborn. Current Therapeutics 20:131–150, 1979

Hill RM, Desmond MM, Kay JL: Extrapyramidal dysfunction in an infant of a schizophrenic mother. J Pediatr 69:589–595, 1966

Hirsch MS, Swartz MN: Antiviral agents. N Engl J Med 302:903–907, 1980

Hoffeld DR, McNew J, Webster RL: Effect of tranquilizing drugs during pregnancy on activity of offspring. Nature 218:357–358, 1968

Isenberg KE: Excretion of fluoxetine in human breast milk. J Clin Psychiatry 51:169, 1990

James ME: Neuroleptic malignant syndrome in pregnancy. Psychosomatics 29:112–119, 1988

Janz D: Antiepileptic drugs and pregnancy: altered utilization patterns and teratogenesis. Epilepsia 23 (suppl 1):S53–S63, 1982

Jones KL, Lacro RV, Johnson KA, et al: Pattern of malformations in the children of women treated with carbamazepine during pregnancy. N Engl J Med 320:1661–1669, 1989

Kacew S: Adverse effects of drugs and chemicals in breast milk on the nursing infant. Journal of Clinical Pharmacology and the Journal of New Drugs 33:213–219, 1993

Kaplan HI, Sadock BJ: Pocket Handbook of Psychiatric Drug Treatment. Baltimore, MD, William & Wilkins, 1993

Kauffman RE, Banner W Jr, Berline CM Jr: The transfer of drugs and other chemicals into human milk. Pediatrics 93:137–150, 1994

Karlsson K, Lindstedt G, Lundberg PA: Transplacental lithium poisoning: reversible inhibition of fetal thyroid (letter). Lancet 1:1295, 1975

Kerns LL: Treatment of mental disorders in pregnancy: a review of psychotropic drug risks and benefits. J Nerv Ment Dis 174:652–659, 1986

Kiely M: Reproductive and Perinatal Epidemiology. Boca Raton, FL, CRC Press, 1991, p 69

Kirksey A, Groziak SM: Maternal drug use: evaluation of risks to breast-fed infants. World Rev Nutr Diet 43:60–79, 1984

Kris EB: Children of mothers maintained on pharmacotherapy during pregnancy and postpartum. Current Therapeutic Research 7:785–789, 1965

Kris E, Carmichael D: Chlorpromazine maintenance therapy during pregnancy and confinement. Psychiatr Q 31:690–695, 1957

Laegreid L, Olegard R, Wahlstrom J, et al: Abnormalities in children exposed to benzodiazepines in utero. Lancet 1:108–109, 1987

Laegreid L, Olegard R, Walstrom J, et al: Teratogenic effects of benzodiazepine use during pregnancy. J Pediatr 114:126–131, 1989

Lindhout D, Schimdt D: In utero exposure to valproate and neural tube defects. Lancet 1:329–333, 1986

Mandelli M, Morselli PL, Nordio S, et al: Placental transfer of diazepam and its disposition in the newborn. Clin Pharmacol Ther 17:564–572, 1975

Matheson I, Skjaeraasen J: Milk concentrations of flupenthixol, nortriptyline and zuclopenthixol and between breast differences in two patients. Eur J Clin Pharmacol 35:217–220, 1988

McBride WG: Limb deformities associated with iminodibenzyl hydrochloride. Med J Aust 1:175–178, 1972

Milkovich L, Van den Berg BJ: An evaluation of the teratogenicity of certain antinauseant drugs. Am J Obstet Gynecol 125:244–248, 1976

Miller LJ: Clinical strategies for the use of psychotropic drugs during pregnancy. Psychiatr Med 9:275–299, 1991

Miller LJ: Psychiatric medication during pregnancy: understanding and minimizing the risks. Psychiatric Annals 24:69–75, 1994

Misri S, Sivertz K: Tricyclic drugs in pregnancy and lactation: a preliminary report. Int J Psychiatry Med 21:157–171, 1991

Mizrahi EM, Hobbs JF, Goldsmith DI: Nephrogenic diabetes insipidus in transplacental lithium intoxication. J Pediatr 94:493–495, 1979

Moriarty AJ, Nance NR: Trifluoperazine and pregnancy. Can Med Assoc J 88:375–376, 1963

Nau H, Kuhnz W, Egger HJ, et al: Anticonvulsants during pregnancy and lactation: transplacental maternal and neonatal pharmacokinetics. Clin Pharmacokinet 7:508–543, 1982

Nora JJ, Nora AH, Toews WH: Lithium, Ebstein's anomaly, and other congenital heart defects. Lancet 2:594–595, 1974

Nurnberg HG, Prudic J: Guidelines for treatment of psychosis during pregnancy. Hosp Community Psychiatry 35:67–71, 1984

O'Connor MO, Johnson GH, James DI: Intrauterine

effect of phenothiazines. Med J Aust 1:416–417, 1981

O'Hara MW, Zekoski EM, Phillips LH, et al: Controlled prospective study of postpartum mood disorders: comparison of childbearing and non-childbearing women. J Abnorm Psychol 99:3–15, 1990

Ordy JM, Samorajski T, Collins RL: Prenatal chlorpromazine effects on liver survival and behavior of mice offspring. J Pharmacol Exp Ther 151:110–125, 1966

Parkin DE: Probable Benadryl withdrawal manifestations in a newborn infant. J Pediatr 85:580, 1974

Pastuszak A, Schick-Boschetto B, Zuber C, et al: Pregnancy outcome following first trimester exposure to fluoxetine (Prozac). JAMA 269:2246–2248, 1993

Physicians' Desk Reference, 48th Edition. Montvale, NJ, Medical Economics Data Production Company, 1994

Pittard WB, O'Neal W: Amitriptyline excretion in human milk. J Clin Psychopharmacol 6:383–384, 1986

Poulson E, Robson JM: Effect of phenelzine and some related compounds in pregnancy. J Endocrinol 30:205–215, 1964

Prentice A, Brown R: Fetal tachyrhythmia and maternal antidepressant treatment. BMJ 298:190, 1989

Rawlings WJ, Ferguson R, Maddison TG: Phenmetrazine and trifluoperazine (letter). Med J Aust 1:370, 1963

Rayburn WF, Andresen BD: Principles of perinatal pharmacology, in Drug Therapy in Obstetrics and Gynecology. Edited by Rayburn WF, Zuspan F. Norwalk, CT, Appleton-Century-Crofts, 1982, pp 1–8

Riccardi VM: The Genetic Approach to Human Disease. New York, Oxford University Press, 1977

Robertson RT, Majka JA, Peter CP, et al: Effects of prenatal exposure to chlorpromazine on postnatal development and behavior of rats. Toxicol Appl Pharmacol 53:541–549, 1980

Robinson HE, Stewart DE, Flak E: The rational use of psychotropic drugs in pregnancy and postpartum. Can J Psychiatry 31:183–190, 1986

Rosa FW: Spina bifida in infants of women treated with carbamazepine during pregnancy. N Engl J Med 324:674–677, 1991

Rosenberg L, Mitchell AA, Parsells JL, et al: Lack of relation of oral clefts to diazepam use during pregnancy. N Engl J Med 309:1281–1285, 1984

Rumeau-Rouquett C, Goujard J, Huel G: Possible teratogenic effect of phenothiazines in human beings. Teratology 15:57–64, 1977

Sadler TW (ed): Langman's Medical Embryology, 5th Edition. Baltimore, MD, Williams & Wilkins, 1985, pp 58–88

Saxen I: Cleft palate and maternal diphenhydramine intake. Lancet 1:407–408, 1974

Saxen I: Association between oral clefts and drugs taken during pregnancy. Int J Epidemiol 4:37–44, 1975

Saxen I, Saxen L: Association between maternal intake of diazepam and oral clefts. Lancet 2(7933): 498, 1975

Schatzberg AF, Cole JO: Manual of Clinical Psychopharmacology. Washington, DC, American Psychiatric Press, 1991, pp 31–242

Schou M: What happened later to the lithium babies?: follow-up study of children born without malformations. Acta Psychiatr Scand 54:193–197, 1976

Schou M, Amdisen A: Lithium and pregnancy, III: lithium ingestion by children breast-fed by women on lithium treatment. British Medical Journal 2:138, 1973

Schou M, Goldfield MD, Weinstein MR, et al: Lithium and pregnancy, I: report from the Registry of Lithium Babies. British Medical Journal 2:135–136, 1973

Scokel PW, Jones WD: Infant jaundice after phenothiazine drugs for labor: an enigma. Obstet Gynecol 20:124–127, 1962

Shannon RW, Fraser GP, Aitken RG, et al: Diazepam in preeclamptic toxaemia with special reference to its effect on the newborn infant. Br J Clin Pract 26:271–275, 1972

Shiono PH, Mills JL: Oral clefts and diazepam use during pregnancy (letter). N Engl J Med 311:919–920, 1984

Sim M: Abortion and the psychiatrist. British Medical Journal 5350:145–148, 1963

Slone D, Siskind V, Heinonen OP, et al: Antenatal exposure to the phenothiazines in relation to congenital malformations, perinatal mortality rate, birth weight, and intelligence quotient score. Am J Obstet Gynecol 128:468–486, 1977

Stancer HC, Reed KL: Desipramine and 2-hydroxy-desipramine in human breast milk and the nursing infant's serum. Am J Psychiatry 143:12, 1597–1600, 1986

Stewart R, Karas B, Springer P: Haloperidol excretion

in human milk. Am J Psychiatry 137:849–850, 1980

Stowe ZN, Kilts C, Ely T, et al: Excretion of sertraline in human breast milk. American Psychosomatic Obstetrics and Gynecology, Abstract, February 1995

Sullivan FM, McElhatton PR: A comparison of the teratogenic activity of the antiepileptic drugs carbamazepine, clonazepam, ethosuximide, phenobarbital, phenytoin, and pyrimidone in mice. Toxicol Appl Pharmacol 40:365–378, 1977

Summerfield RJ, Nielsen MS: Excretion of lorazepam into breast milk. Br J Anaesth 57:1042–1043, 1985

Suppes T, Baldessarini RJ, Faedda GL, et al: Risk of recurrence following discontinuation of lithium treatment in bipolar disorder. Arch Gen Psychiatry 47:1082–1088, 1991

Tohen M, Waternaux CM, Tsuang MT: Outcome in mania: a 4-year prospective follow-up of 75 patients utilizing survival analysis. Arch Gen Psychiatry 47:1106–1111, 1990

Van Waes A, Van de Velde EJ: Safety evaluation of haloperidol in the treatment of hyperemesis gravidarum. J Clin Pharmacol 9:224–227, 1969

Verbeeck RK, Ross SG, McKenna EA: Excretion of trazodone in breast milk. Br J Clin Pharmacol 22:367–370, 1986

Vorherr H: Drug excretion in breast milk. Postgrad Med 56:97–104, 1974

Warner A: Drug use in the neonate: interrelationships of pharmacokinetics, toxicity and biochemical maturity. Clin Chem 32:721–727, 1986

Webster PAC: Withdrawal symptoms in neonates associated with maternal antidepressant therapy. Lancet 2:318–319, 1973

Weinstein MR, Goldfield MD: Cardiovascular malformations with lithium use during pregnancy. Am J Psychiatry 132:529–531, 1975

Welch R, Findlay J: Excretion of drugs in human breast milk. Drug Metab Rev 12:261–277, 1981

Whalley LJ, Blain PG, Prime JK: Haloperidol secreted in breast milk. British Medical Journal 282:1746–1747, 1981

Whitelaw AGL, Cummings AJ, McFadyen IR: Effect of maternal lorazepam on the neonate. British Medical Journal 282:1106–1108, 1981

Wilson JT, Brown RD, Cherek DR, et al: Drug excretion in human breast milk: principles, pharmacokinetics and projected consequences. Clin Pharmacokinet 5:1–66, 1980

Wilson N, Forfar JC, Godman MJ: Atrial flutter in the newborn resulting from maternal lithium ingestion. Arch Dis Child 58:538–549, 1983

Wisner KL, Perel JM: Psychopharmacologic agents and electroconvulsive therapy during pregnancy and the puerperium, in Psychiatric Consultation in Childbirth Settings: Parent- and Child-Oriented Approaches. Edited by Cohen RL. New York, Plenum, 1988, pp 165–206

Wisner KL, Perel JM: Serum nortriptyline levels in nursing mothers and their infants. Am J Psychiatry 148:1234–1236, 1991

Wisner KL, Perel JM, Wheeler SB: Tricyclic dosage requirements across pregnancy. Am J Psychiatry 150:1541–1542, 1993

Wood SM, Hytten FE: The fate of drugs in pregnancy. Clin Obstet Gynecol 8:255–259, 1981

Woody JN, London WL, Wilbanks GD: Lithium toxicity in a newborn. Pediatrics 47:94–96, 1971

Wreitland MA: Excretion of oxazepam in breastmilk. Eur J Clin Pharmacol 33:209–210, 1987

Wright S, Dawling S, Ashford JJ: Excretion of fluvoxamine in breast milk. Br J Clin Pharmacol 31:209, 1991

Yonkers KA, Kando JC, Cole JO, et al: Gender differences in pharmacokinetics and pharmacodynamics of psychotropic medication. Am J Psychiatry 149:587–595, 1992

Zahn-Waxler C, Cummings EM, Ianoff RJ, et al: Young offspring of depressed patients: a population of risk for affective problems and childhood depression, in Childhood Depression. Edited by Cichetti D, Schneider-Rosen K. San Francisco, CA, Jossey-Bass, 1984, pp 81–105

Zajicek E: Psychiatric problems during pregnancy, in Pregnancy: A Psychological and Social Study. Edited by Wolkind S, Zajicek E. London, Academic Press, 1981, pp 57–73

A P P E N D I X   1

Promising Psychopharmacological Agents Available in Europe

Ira D. Glick, M.D., Yves Lecrubier, M.D., Stuart A. Montgomery, M.D., Oldrich Vinar, M.D., D.Sc., and Donald F. Klein, M.D.

In 1991, Vinar and colleagues observed that "U.S. psychiatrists and psychopharmacologists are increasingly aware of the limited armamentarium of medications available for serious mental illness" (p. 201). Since then, at least two new selective serotonin reuptake inhibitors (SSRIs), one mixed serotonin and norepinephrine uptake inhibitor, and one atypical neuroleptic have been added to the available treatments in the United States, but delays in introducing novel agents remain a matter of concern.

In this chapter, we review selected drugs that are available in Europe, but not in the United States, that appear safe and effective and are currently being used in clinical practice, and that are perceived as offering clinically significant advantages over other available medications in the opinion of expert clinical psychopharmacologists.

The reason for discussing these drugs in an American psychopharmacology textbook is that current U.S. Food and Drug Administration (FDA) and customs policy, influenced by pressures from acquired immunodeficiency syndrome (AIDS) patients, allows 3-month supplies of drugs not available in the United States to be imported for use by treatment-resistant patients. It is not clear that any of these drugs are so different and so superior (as was clearly the case with clomipramine in the treatment of obsessive-compulsive disorder [OCD]) as to impel many psychiatrists to arrange to bring one or more of these drugs to the United States to treat their patients; but in special situations this might be worth doing. In addition, our thought was that with the addition of this appendix, *The American Psychiatric Press Textbook of Psychopharmacology* would be more useful for Canadian and European investigators.

■ METHODOLOGY

We collected data from four sources: controlled trials reported in the literature (Gerlach 1991; Hollister 1994; Meltzer 1992; Murphy et al., in press), expert psychopharmacologically oriented clinicians in eight countries, European regulatory agencies, and representatives of the pharmaceutical industry (I. D. Glick, Y. Lecrubier, S. A. Montgomery, D. F. Klein, "Effective and Safe Psychotropics Not Available in the USA," article submitted for publication, 1994). The perception of efficacy and safety of the drugs by the regulatory authorities was assessed by comparing the consistency with which approval had been granted by the authorities in the United Kingdom, France, Denmark, Holland, Sweden, and Canada (Table 1).

Table 1.   Selected foreign regulatory board approvals of medications not available in the United States

Drug	Canada	Denmark	France	Netherland	United Kingdom	Sweden	Total
Clopenthixol		X		X	X		3
Flupentixol	X	X	X	X	X	X	6
Pipamperone			X	X			2
Sulpiride		X	X	X	X		4
Amisulpiride			X				1
Penfluridol		X	X	X			3
Melperone		X		X		X	3
Lofepramine		X			X	X	3
Fluvoxamine	X	X	X	X	X	X	6
Citalopram		X				X	2
Mianserin		X	X	X	X	X	5
Moclobemide	X	X	X	X	X	X	6
Tianeptine			X				1

Chemical structures are listed in Figures 1 and 2; they can be read clockwise starting at 12 o'clock.

■ RESULTS

Our discussions identified a number of drugs that have been found to be effective and are used (sometimes widely) in different parts of Europe. Various clinical features of psychotropic medications not available in the United States are listed in Table 2.

■ Schizophrenia

The key issues are 1) to find drugs that are more effective in treating schizophrenia (particularly in treating its negative symptoms) and to find treatments for patients who are nonresponders to conventional neuroleptics, and 2) to find treatments that are associated with less frequent and less severe extrapyramidal side effects (EPS). Such symptoms are widely perceived as causes of noncompliance.

The conventional treatment in Europe for schizophrenia is still haloperidol, with a change of medication given to patients who are nonresponders after 2–3 weeks. This strategy appears irrational to many U.S. psychopharmacologists—2–3 weeks seems too short a time to give a medication before changing or discontinuing it. In fact, one study has found that schizophrenic patients who had not responded after 6 weeks of a dosage of 30 mg qd of fluphenazine were then continued on the medication for another 6 weeks, by which time two-thirds of them had responded (Quitkin et al. 1975). Clozapine is still used as a first-line treatment in acute episodes by some clinicians, but in most countries this is not permitted.

For this discussion, we divide the drugs into two groups. The first group includes those drugs approved in three or more countries with drug review boards widely perceived to be very rigorous with regard to requirements for approval. The second group includes those drugs with a lesser number of approvals but that we believe to be promising (Table 1).

Clopenthixol, a D_1 and D_2 blocker, has been shown to be equal in efficacy to both haloperidol and fluphenazine. It is widely used, particularly in those countries where depot formulations are used at a dose of 100–300 mg qd. Its principal side effects are sedation and EPS.

Flupentixol, a related drug, is widely used in Europe and is available in Canada. It is well tolerated and has less potential for causing movement disorders than clopenthixol. Opinions on its efficacy vary—from considering it to be an effective drug for negative symptoms to believing that it is less potent than haloperidol. Antipsychotic dosage range is 3–20 mg qd. At lower doses, flupentixol is used as an antidepressant in some countries.

Sulpiride is a D_2 mixed agonist-antagonist that has been available for many years in Europe. It is used in these countries by clinicians who prefer oral to depot formulations and is associated with less EPS than the phenothiazines, but it causes glactorrhea because of its effect on prolactin. Its potency is ques-

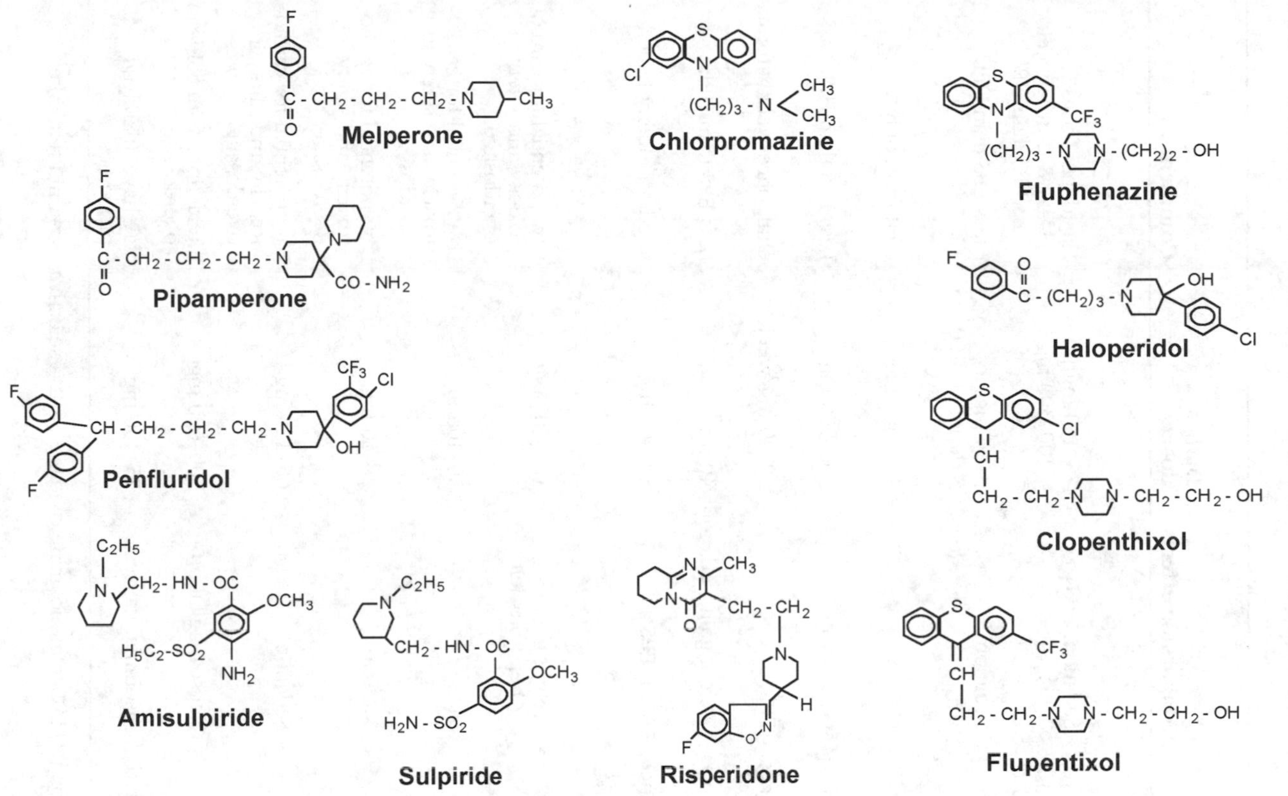

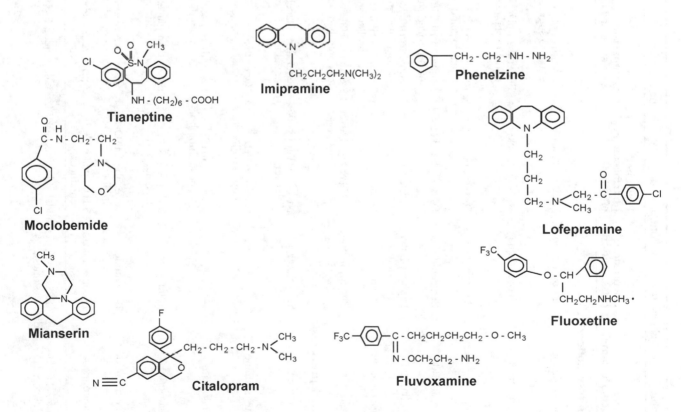

Figure 1. Chemical structures of selected standard and newer antipsychotic drugs.

Figure 2. Chemical structures of selected standard and newer antidepressant drugs.

Table 2. Clinical features of psychotropics not available in the United States

Drug (generic name)	Chemical classification	Presumed pharmacological effects	Comparison with standard drugs	Major side effects	Daily dosage	Comment
Antipsychotics						
Clopenthixol	Thioxanthene	D_1 & D_2 blocker	Better than placebo and equal to standard	Sedation, EPS	75–150 mg po, 100–300 mg im	Has depot forms (2- to 3-day & 2- to 4-week), less EPS than HPL
Flupentixol	Thioxanthene	D_1 & D_2 blocker	Better than placebo and equal to standard	Sedation	3–20 mg po, depot 20–100 mg q 2–4 weeks	? less EPS than HPL
Sulpiride	Benzamide	D_2 blocker	Better than placebo and equal to standard	Galactorrhea, EPS, TD	100–600 mg	Oral form only
Amisulpride	Benzamide	D_2 & D_3 blocker	? equal to HPL in the absence of controlled studies	Galactorrhea	300–900 mg	Less EPS than HPL
Penfluridol	Diphenylbutyl piperidine	D_2 blocker	? equal to HPL in the absence of controlled studies	EPS	20–40 mg/week	Oral, once-weekly form
Pipamperone	Butyrophenone	D_2 blocker	? equal to HPL in the absence of controlled studies	Weight gain, sedation	40 mg	Less EPS than HPL
Melperone	Butyrophenone	$5\text{-}HT_3$ & D_2 blocker	? equal to HPL in the absence of controlled studies	Weak EPS	50–400 mg	Used for elderly patients
Antidepressants						
Lofepramine	Tricyclic	NE & 5-HT reuptake blocker	Better than placebo and equal to standard	Weight gain, ? hepatotoxicity	100–200 mg	Low potential for cardio-toxicity and safety in overdosage
Fluvoxamine	—	Selective 5-HT reuptake inhibitors	Better than placebo and equal to standard	Nausea	50–100 mg	Low potential for cardio-toxicity and safety in overdosage
Citalopram	—	Selective 5-HT reuptake inhibitors	Better than placebo and equal to standard	Nausea	20–60 mg	Low potential for cardio-toxicity and safety in overdosage
Mianserin	Tetracyclic	$5\text{-}HT_{1, 2, 3}$ & α_2 antagonist	Better than placebo and equal to standard	Sedation	60–120 mg	Low potential for cardio-toxicity and safety in overdosage
Moclobemide	Benzamide	Reversible MAO-A inhibitor	Better than placebo and equal to standard	Nausea, agitation	300–600 mg	Interactions with SSRIs in overdosage
Tianeptine	Dibenzothiazine	5-HT uptake enhancer	2 positive placebo-controlled studies	Insomnia, nausea	25–100 mg	May have anxiolytic properties

Note. D = dopamine; EPS = extrapyramidal side effects; HPL = haloperidol; 5-HT = serotonin; MAO = monoamine oxidase; SSRI = selective serotonin reuptake inhibitor; TD = tardive dyskinesia.

tioned by many clinicians, because its bioavailability is poor. Some clinicians have found patient compliance with sulpiride to be good because of its favorable side effect profile; but others have observed that compliance is a problem, as sulpiride is only available in oral form. It is licensed as an antidepressant in France (at low doses), and in many countries it is used to treat schizophrenia with prominent associated depressive (i.e., broadly defined) symptoms.

Amisulpride, a D_2 and D_3 blocker, is also used both as an antidepressant (25–50 mg qd) and as a neuroleptic (300–900 mg qd). It is thought to produce less EPS but has efficacy similar to haloperidol. Amisulpride produces galactorrhea but has no sex-related side effects. It has still not been sufficiently studied to allow for confident assessment, although two placebo-controlled studies suggest improvement in negative symptoms with almost no EPS at a low dosage of 100 mg qd (Boyer et al. 1990; Loo et al. 1993).

Penfluridol, a D_2 blocker, has a fairly high incidence of EPS (about 30%). This drug is inherently long acting, is taken orally once a week, and has been shown to be quite efficacious. Penfluridol has some regulatory problems that have limited its wide use, including an association between its use and the development of pancreatic tumors in beagles. It remains unclear how significant or relevant this finding actually is.

In the opinion of some clinicians, pipamperone, a butyrophenone derivative, seems to be closest in efficacy to clozapine, but with fewer adverse effects. Its side effects include weight gain and sedation.

Melperone, which has 5-HT_3 and D_2 antagonist properties, is available in some countries. It is thought to be as effective as haloperidol, with a lower incidence of EPS.

In addition to the psychotropic drugs listed in Table 2, there are two compounds that may prove useful in the future. Oxyprotipine, a neuroleptic with a decanoate form, is extensively used in the Czech Republic and is thought to have a low incidence of EPS. Pipotiazine, a depot neuroleptic, is used in France. However, the placebo-controlled trial data base is not large enough to draw generalized conclusions on efficacy. It is preliminarily considered to be as effective as fluphenazine but slightly more stimulating.

Remoxipride, a dopamine antagonist, is clearly effective, but it has been withdrawn from the market by its manufacturer.

■ Depression

Clinicians in Europe express two main concerns in the search for drugs that are more effective than conventional antidepressants either for a larger proportion of patients or with a more rapid effect, and in the search for drugs that are better tolerated and safer. European psychiatrists are particularly concerned about potential cardiotoxicity and safety in overdose.

Unlike the U.S. FDA, European regulatory authorities require evidence of antidepressant efficacy in long-term treatment, because depression is recognized as a long-term illness requiring medication over an extended period. Some clinicians in Europe are concerned about finding treatments for other forms of depression, such as dysthymia and recurrent brief depression, but firm recommendations as to which medication to use cannot be made at this time.

The discussions identified a number of drugs not available in the United States that have been found to be effective and are used in different parts of Europe or Canada. Many clinicians considered these drugs to have advantages in terms of side effects and safety over those of other conventional antidepressants.

Lofepramine, a tricyclic antidepressant (TCA), is widely prescribed in the United Kingdom because it has relatively few anticholinergic, sedative, or cardiotoxic effects. It produces some weight gain, and there are reports of an association with hepatotoxicity. Lofepramine is used in particular because of its safety in overdosage.

Two SSRIs are widely used in Europe but are not yet available as antidepressants in the United States.

Fluvoxamine has been widely used in Europe as an antidepressant for many years. It is effective in treating depression and anxiety disorders. In the absence of large fixed-dose studies, clinicians have been uncertain of the optimum therapeutic dose. This is important, because the drug is associated with high levels of nausea, particularly at doses up to 300 mg qd. The widely expressed view was that daily doses as low as 50 mg or 100 mg may be effective (but in a low proportion of patients) and that nausea becomes a more serious problem at doses over 150 mg. Fluvoxamine has been studied in the United States primarily as a treatment for OCD and has recently been recommended for approval by an advisory committee of the FDA.

Citalopram has been available for years in Europe. It is thought to be the most selective SSRI and has a low incidence of side effects and low risk of drug interactions. Many patients respond to doses of 20 mg qd, but higher doses may be needed.

Mianserin has an interesting pharmacological profile. It is an α_2 antagonist as well as a 5-HT$_{1,2}$ and 5-HT$_3$ antagonist. Studies show mianserin's efficacy compared with placebo is similar to that of reference TCAs. Its major advantage is its low potential for cardiotoxicity and its safety in overdose. In some countries, it is widely used to treat geriatric patients, where sedation is considered an advantage. Mianserin's advantages (i.e., that it is noncardiotoxic and not anticholinergic) are counteracted to some extent by concerns about agranulocytosis, which may be seen at a higher rate than with TCAs. It should be noted, however, that this was not borne out in a very large study in England, which showed no evidence of a high degree of agranulocytosis (Inman 1988).

Moclobemide, a reversible monoamine oxidase inhibitor (MAOI), is licensed in most parts of Europe and in Canada. There is a shortage of data on the appropriate dose in the absence of fixed-dose range studies. Moclobemide has been welcomed because of its different mechanism of action (i.e., it is a reversible MAO-A inhibitor, which makes hypertensive crises very rare). It also has a very short half-life of 2 hours. The drug does not appear to interfere with a number of other agents (e.g., tyramine) that produce problems when given with older MAOIs. However, it is advisable to be cautious about co-administering SSRIs and opioids. Even with regard to SSRIs, a paper by Joffe and Bakish (1994) indicates that moclobemide may be combined with fluvoxamine. It has been released in many countries without dietary restrictions and has been shown in Brazilian studies to be useful in treating social phobia. Antidepressant and antianxiety doses are in the range of 300–600 mg qd, but higher doses (e.g., 900 mg qd) have also been tried. In the United States, moclobemide is being studied primarily as an antipanic and antisocial phobic agent.

Tianeptine, a 5-HT uptake enhancer, is licensed as an antidepressant in some parts of Europe. Its efficacy in treating depression has been demonstrated in placebo-controlled studies, and there is also evidence of efficacy for patients with chronic alcoholism. In general, tianeptine appears to be well tolerated, with no anticholineric or cardiovascular effects.

As noted previously, in Europe some clinicians prescribe low doses of neuroleptics as antidepressants. Sulpiride is widely used in low doses as an antidepressant, and amisulpride (dose 25–100 mg) is used in some countries. Amisulpride is licensed for the treatment of dysthymia in Italy. Flupentixol is licensed for use in some countries in Europe as an antidepressant, and there are suggestions of its efficacy in the treatment of depression associated with impulse disorder.

■ Anxiety Disorders

In treating anxiety disorders, there are differences in practice between Europe and the United States. For example, OCD is not regarded as an anxiety disorder in the European diagnostic tradition. Clomipramine has been used in Europe for many years to treat OCD, and the early placebo-controlled trials that demonstrated clomipramine's efficacy were carried out in Europe. In both Europe and the United States, SSRIs have all been widely used in treating OCD and are believed to have advantages, in terms of fewer side effects than clomipramine and better compliance with treatment. Fluoxetine recently was given FDA approval for an indication in OCD, and other SSRIs are currently under FDA review.

Anxiety disorders are considered to be primarily chronic and relapsing. The concern is therefore to find anxiolytics that may be used for long-term treatment. Effective drugs that lack the potential for abuse or dependence would be a major advance. The main choice currently is believed to be between benzodiazepines, which are fast in onset with few side effects but are associated with possible dependence, and antidepressants, which are as effective and lacking in dependence potential but are slower in onset.

Panic disorder is not as widely diagnosed in most of Europe as it is in the United States. Alprazolam is licensed for use in some countries, but there are concerns about possible dependence potential. Clomipramine is widely used in very low doses of 5–15 mg, although there are few controlled data on which to base this practice (Modigh et al. 1992). The SSRIs are increasingly perceived as effective in the treatment of panic disorder. Of this class of drugs, fluvoxamine is the most used and has the best trial data. Dosage is thought to be up to 300 mg qd.

In treating generalized anxiety disorder, the mainstay is benzodiazepines, but there are concerns about dependence. These concerns have led increasingly to off-label use of a variety of antidepressants that are perceived to be as effective although not as rapid acting as benzodiazepines. These antidepressants are thought to be more effective in long-term treatment, but not necessarily safer in view of the toxicity of TCAs in overdose.

Moclobemide has been shown to be efficacious in treating some patients with social phobia. Its efficacy in this indication is in line with the positive results with another reversible MAOI, brofaromine, which has been withdrawn from development. There is insufficient information about appropriate dosage or the population of patients most likely to be responsive to moclobemide.

FDA-APPROVED AND UNAPPROVED DRUGS IN NONAPPROVED CLINICAL CONDITIONS OR COMBINATIONS

Some drugs that are available both in Europe and the United States are used in Europe for indications that are not approved in the United States, particularly for treatment-resistant patients. Newly introduced drugs figure prominently. For example, the SSRIs are prescribed for various addictive behaviors. Fluoxetine is licensed in some countries for the treatment of bulimia and is under review in the United States for this indication.

SSRIs are also being used by some clinicians to treat negative symptoms in schizophrenia. Combinations of haloperidol and antidepressants are sometimes used where there are hypochondriacal symptoms, and combinations of neuroleptics and lorazepam (either intramuscularly or intravenously) are used to treat catatonic stupor in schizophrenia.

DISCUSSION

In this appendix, we have identified 13 drugs that are considered safe, effective, and possibly advantageous over some other drugs. These drugs are used in clinical practice in Europe but are not available in the United States. The drugs that we believe have the most potential are 1) for schizophrenia—flupentixol, clopenthixol, and amisulpride; 2) for depression—lofepramine, fluvoxamine, citalopram, mianserin, tianeptine, and moclobemide; 3) for OCD—fluvoxamine; and 4) for social phobia and panic disorder—moclobemide. In addition, the SSRIs (e.g., sertraline and fluoxetine) have great potential for treating a wide variety of anxiety disorders.

Our interviews with expert clinical psychopharmacologists focused on their frank opinion of the drugs they prescribed in practice and whether these drugs were considered useful and nontoxic. The rationale was that a consistent pattern of opinion and use across countries would be an indicator of those drugs held to be of value. Using clinicians as a data source has the obvious problems of sample bias, bias because of inherent preferences for particular drugs, and lack of systematically collected data and outcome measures. Nevertheless, these clinicians are closer to the relevant information than the independent assessor, and the face value of the data is therefore more powerful.

In conclusion, let us add two caveats. First, expert clinicians tend to be biased toward efficacy over safety. Because they are called upon to treat the most difficult cases and because of their own expert knowledge, they tend to be eager to have new agents available and are less troubled by potential hazards. Regulators tend to be biased in the opposite direction and sometimes (because of economic or liability considerations) so are pharmaceutical manufacturers. On the other hand, we would not want readers to draw the conclusion that many promising drugs are needlessly kept from the U.S. market. A case could also be made that in some other countries, hazardous drugs come to market too quickly. Second, in the world of clinical care, as opposed to clinical trials, clinicians rightly or wrongly select drugs that they believe from their experience show "effectiveness" over time. If European clinicians prefer drugs that really do have a different pharmacological profile than those available in the United States, then we should at least consider the possibility that the Europeans are onto something—witness the story of clomipramine.

REFERENCES

Boyer P, Lecrubier Y, Puech AJ: Treatment of positive and negative symptoms: pharmacologic approaches, in Modern Problems of Pharmacopsychiatry. Edited by Andreasen NC, Ban TA, Freedman AM, et al. Basel, Switzerland, Karger, 1990, 24:152–174

Gerlach J: New antipsychotics: classification, efficacy, and adverse effects. Schizophr Bull 17:289–309, 1991

Hollister LE: New psychotherapeutic drugs. J Clin Psychopharmacol 4:50–63, 1994

Inman WH: Blood disorders and suicide in patients taking mianserin or tricyclics. Lancet 2:90–92, 1988

Joffe RT, Bakish D: Combined SSRI-moclobemide treatment of psychiatric illness. J Clin Psychiatry 55:24–25, 1994

Loo H, Poiruer-Littre MF, Fleurot O, et al: Amisulpride in the long-term treatment of negative schizophrenia: results of a placebo controlled trial. Paper presented at the annual meeting of the Collegium Internationale Neuro-Psychopharmacologicum, Rio de Janeiro, Brazil, June 1993

Meltzer HY (ed): Novel Antipsychotic Drugs. New York, Raven, 1992

Modigh K, Westberg P, Eriksson E: Superiority of clomipramine over imipramine in the treatment of panic disorder: a placebo-controlled trial. J Clin Psychopharmacol 12:251–261, 1992

Murphy LM, Mitchell PB, Potter WZ: Novel pharmacological approaches to the treatment of depression, in Psychopharmacology: The Fourth Generation of Progress. Edited by Bloom FE, Kupfer DJ. New York, Raven (in press)

Quitkin I, Rifkin A, Klein DF: Very high dosage vs. standard dosage fluphenazine in schizophrenia: a double-blind study of nonchronic treatment-refractory patients. Arch Gen Psychiatry 32:1276–1281, 1975

Vinar O, Klein DF, Potter WZ, et al: A survey of psychotropic medications not available in the United States. Neuropsychopharmacology 5:201–217, 1991

Index

*Page numbers printed in **boldface** type refer to tables or figures.*

Abecarnil, 240, 647

Aberrant Behavior Checklist, 696

Abnormal Involuntary Movement Scale (AIMS), 239–240, 284, 684

Acetazolamide
antiepileptic properties of, 369
interaction with carbamazepine, 359
interaction with lithium, **793**

Acetophenazine maleate, **620**

Acetylcholine (ACh), 4, **6,** 10
lithium effects on, 311–312
role in Alzheimer's disease, 391–395, 524
role in depression, 439
role in mood disorders, 457

Acetylcholine precursors, 392, 813

Acetylcholine receptors
muscarinic, 14, 395–396
nicotinic, 12–14, **13,** 395
role in Alzheimer's disease, 395

L-α-Acetyl-methadol (LAAM), 713, 715–716

Achievement testing, 671

Acquired immunodeficiency syndrome (AIDS). *See* Human immunodeficiency virus infection

ACT. *See* α₁ Antichymotripsin

Action potential, 66

Acute phase proteins, 399

Adalat. *See* Nifedipine

Adapin. *See* Doxepin

Adenosine
meprobamate and, 233
in panic disorder, 505

Adenosine triphosphate (ATP), 65

S-Adenosylmethionine, 208

Adenylate cyclase (AC), **18,** 18–19, 21–22, 58
lithium effects on, 315–316
in mood disorders, 458

ADHD. *See* Attention-deficit hyperactivity disorder

Adinazolam, 208

Adjustment disorders, 772

Adolescents. *See* Childhood and adolescent disorders

Adoption studies
of mood disorders, 442
of schizophrenia, 480

β-Adrenergic receptors
β₂-adrenergic receptor, 14, **16,** 18–19
antidepressant effects on, 148–148

Adrenocorticotropic hormone (ACTH)
in Alzheimer's disease, 813
in anorexia nervosa, 561
in bulimia nervosa, 566
in depression, **445,** 445–447
lithium-stimulated secretion of, 318
metyrapone effects on, 546
in panic disorder, 506

Adult attention deficit disorder, 417, 428

Adverse drug effects, 776–778

AF102B, 396

Affective lability, 759–760, 772

Aggression, 735–743
in Alzheimer's disease, 657, 735
associated with mental retardation, 696
in autism, 693
in borderline personality disorder, 758
in children taking fluoxetine, 690
differential diagnosis of, 742–743, **742–743**
documentation of, 738, 741
drug-induced, **743**
emergency treatment for, 773–774
evaluation of patient presenting with, 742–743
5-hydroxyindoleacetic acid level and, 453
as indication for emergency hospitalization, 770–771
neurotransmitters and, 741–742
norepinephrine, 741
serotonin, 439, 742, 759
nosology of, 736–738
aggression as a disorder, 736–737, **736–737**
aggression as a symptom, 738
distinguishing between aggression, anxiety, and agitation, 738, **739–740**
organically induced, 736–737, **736–737, 743**
prevalence of, 735
rating scales for, 738, **739–740**
relevance in psychiatric patients, 735–736
traumatic brain injury and, 735

Aggression treatment, 743–749
  acute, 744–746
    antipsychotics, 745, **745**
    benzodiazepines, 745–746, **746**
    behavioral therapies, 743–744, **744**
  in children and adolescents, 685–687
    assessing treatment response, 686
    assessment for treatment, 685
    β-blockers, 687
    bupropion, 687
    carbamazepine, 686–687
    selecting therapy, 685–686
    trazodone, 687
    treatment resistance, 687
  chronic, **746,** 746–748
    anticonvulsants, 747
    antidepressants, 747–748
    antipsychotics, 746–747
    anxiolytics, 747
    benzodiazepines, 744
    β-blockers, 748, **748**
    lithium, 322, 747
  overview of, 743–744
Agitation
  during alcohol withdrawal, 707, 708
  in Alzheimer's disease, 657
  antipsychotics for, 250
  in autism, 693
  drug-induced
    buspirone, 237
    galanthamine, 394
    selective serotonin reuptake inhibitors, 582
  traumatic brain injury and, 735
  treating in elderly persons, 805–807
Agonists
  benzodiazepine, 130–131, **131,** 220–221
  cholinergic, 395–396
  direct acting versus indirect acting, 9

dopamine, 7–9
  partial vs. full, 12
Agoraphobia, 501, 641. *See also* Panic disorder
  in children and adolescents, 690
Agranulocytosis, drug-induced
  antipsychotics, **627,** 629
  carbamazepine, 358, 608, 611, 794–795
  clozapine, 271–272, 274, 611, 631–633, **632,** 777, 792
  valproate, 365
Akathisia, 251, 255–256, 281–282, 625, **626,** 628, 776. *See also* Extrapyramidal side effects
  amoxapine-induced, 200
  calcium channel blocker–induced, 385
  in children and adolescents, 684
  risperidone-induced, 621
  treatment of, 292
Alaproclate, 813
Alcohol
  amoxapine and, 200
  anxiolytic effects of, 544
  drug interactions with
    antidepressants, 587, **786**
    benzodiazepines, **794**
    trazodone, 198
Alcohol withdrawal, 707–708, 775
  benzodiazepines for, 222, 413–414, 549, 707–709
  protracted, 548–550
  thiamine for, 775
Alcoholics Anonymous, 707, 717
Alcoholism. *See also* Substance dependence disorders
  animal models of, 539–540, 708
  5-hydroxyindoleacetic acid level and, 453
  individual vulnerability and risk of, 538
  low gamma-aminobutyric acid level in, 457

neurobiology of alcohol reinforcement, 543–544
  prevalence of, 707
  treatment of, 707–709
    amphetamine, 418
    benzodiazepines, 222, 413–414, 549, 707–709
    buspirone, 236, 237
    detoxification, 707–708
    disulfiram, 708
    drug therapy of associated psychopathology, 709
    naltrexone, 708–709
    psychosocial therapies, 707
    selective serotonin reuptake inhibitors, 170
  use of benzodiazepines in, 217
Aldehyde dehydrogenase, 708
Allergies, 580
Allosteric modulation, positive, 220
Alpidem, 240
Alprazolam, **130,** 215, 223
  discontinuation of, 128, 129
  drug interactions with
    fluoxetine, **129**
    nefazodone, 207
  half-life of, **218**
  indications for
    avoidant personality disorder, 764
    borderline personality disorder, 762, 763
    children's anxiety in medical setting, 691
    depression, 207, 451
    generalized anxiety disorder, 647
      in children and adolescents, 688
    panic disorder, 215, 218, 222, 223, 643–644
      in children and adolescents, 690
    separation anxiety disorder, 688
    social phobia, 648

plasma concentrations of, **128,** 218
side effects of, 207
use in Europe, 844
use in pregnancy, 830, **831**
Aluminum salts, interaction with β-blockers, 291
Alzheimer's disease (AD), 10, 523–529, 813
  aggression in, 657, 735
  amyloidogenesis in, 525–526
  animal models of, 527–529
    aged nonhuman primates, 527–528
    transgenic mice, 528–529
  brain imaging in, 524
  cholinergic system in, 391, 395
  clinical course of, 524
  clinical features of, 523–524, 657
  cytoskeletal pathology in neurons in, 525
  delusions in, 658–659
  depression in, 664–665
  diagnosis of, 524
  genetics of, 40, 526–527
  incidence of, 657
  neuronal systems vulnerable in, 524–525
  prevalence of, 523
  role of immune system and inflammation in, 399
Alzheimer's disease (AD) treatment, 657–665, 813–814
  antipsychotics, 255, 658–661
  benzodiazepines, 662–663
  buspirone, 662
  carbamazepine, 662
  cognitive enhancers, 391–400, 813–814
    AF102B, 396
    antiinflammatory agents, 399
    arecoline, 395–396
    azaspirodecanes, 396
    bethanechol, 395
    cholinergic-noradrenergic combinations, 397

L-deprenyl, 397
galanthamine, 394
glutamatergic agents, 397–398
HP 029, 393–394
nicotine, 396
oxotremorine, 396
physostigmine, 392
RS-86, 395
tetrahydroaminoacridine, 393
for comorbid depression, 664–665
for disruptive behaviors, 663–664
in long-term care facilities, 658
nimodipine, 378
prevalence of psychotropic drug use, 657–658
selective serotonin reuptake inhibitors, 171
trazodone, 661–662
valproate, 662
Alzheimer's Disease Assessment Scale, 393
Amantadine
  drug interactions with, 289
  history and discovery of, 288
  indications for, 288–289
    extrapyramidal side effects, 256, **284,** 288–289, 627
    neuroleptic malignant syndrome, 776
    protracted cocaine withdrawal, 548
  mechanism of action of, 288
  pharmacokinetics and disposition of, 288
  pharmacological profile of, 288
  side effects and toxicology of, 289
  structure-activity relations for, 288
  use during pregnancy, 829, **829**

Ambien. *See* Zolpidem
Amenorrhea
  in anorexia nervosa, 562–563
  antipsychotic-induced, 629
gamma-Aminobutyric acid (GABA), 4, 10
  drug effects on
    lithium, 313–314, 456
    selective serotonin reuptake inhibitors, 165
    valproate, 362
  effect on extrapyramidal symptoms, 283
  in mood disorders, 456–457
  role in anxiety, 763–764
  role in convulsive disorders, 456
  sites of drug action for, **6**
gamma-Aminobutyric acid (GABA) receptors, 14
  barbiturate actions and, 407
  benzodiazepine actions and, 218–219, 407, 410, **410**
  subtypes of, 456
Aminophosphonopentanoic acid (AP-5), 398
Aminophylline interactions
  with lithium, **793**
  with monoamine oxidase inhibitors, **789**
Amisulpiride, **840–842,** 843, 844
Amitriptyline, 56
  animal studies of
    behavioral effects of olfactory bulb lesions, 86
    chronic mild stress model, 95
    depression of active responding induced by 5-hydroxy-tryptophan, 89
    isolation-induced hyperactivity, 87
    swim test immobility, 89
  biochemical effects of, **144**
  elimination half-life of, **145**

Amitriptyline (continued)
  indications for, **151**
    aggressive behavior, 747
    anorexia nervosa, 731
    enuresis, 151
    panic disorder, 642
    posttraumatic stress
      disorder, 650
  serotonin reuptake inhibition
    by, 141
  structure-activity relationship
    for, 142, **142, 162**
  use in pregnancy, **827**
  weight gain induced by, 153
Amlodipine, **378**
Amnesia. See Memory
  impairment
Amoxapine, 199–200
  avoiding use in Parkinson's
    disease, 579
  biochemical effects of, **144**
  drug interactions with, 200
  elimination half-life of, **145**
  history and discovery of,
    199
  indications for, 199–200
    delusional depression, 150
  mechanism of action of, 199
  metabolite of, 200
  overdose of, 200
  pharmacokinetics and
    disposition of, 199
  pharmacological profile of,
    199
  side effects and toxicology
    of, 200
  structure-activity relationship
    for, **142,** 143, 199, **199**
  use in pregnancy, **827**
Amphetamine, 147, 397. See
  also Dextroamphetamine
  abuse and dependence on,
    419, 430–431
  animal studies of
    blocking tasks, 108
    chronic intoxication,
      110–111
    effects in rats, 85
    isolation-induced
      hyperactivity, 87

    social behavior in
      monkeys, 109–110
  d- and l-isomers of, 420
  historical uses of, 417–419
  interaction with monoamine
    oxidase inhibitors, **789**
  mechanism of action of,
    422–423
  overdose of, 429, 430
  paradoxical quieting effects
    of, 418–419
  pharmacological profile of,
    421, **421**
  side effects and toxicity of,
    429–430
  structure-activity relationships
    for, 419–420
AMPT. See α-Methyl-p-tyrosine
Amygdala lesions, dorsomedial,
  92, **92**
Amyloid precursor protein
  (APP), 399, 525–526,
  528–529
Amyloidogenesis
  in aged monkeys, 528
  in Alzheimer's disease,
    525–526
Amyotrophic lateral sclerosis, 41
Analgesics, interaction with
  antipsychotics, 259
Angiotensin-converting enzyme
  inhibitors, interaction with
  lithium, **793**
Anhedonia, 616
Animal models, 81–113
  of Alzheimer's disease,
    527–529
    aged nonhuman primates,
      527–528
    transgenic mice, 528–529
  of depression, 84–104
    animal assay models, 85–88
    amphetamine
      potentiation, 85
    circadian rhythm
      readjustment, 85–86
    differential operant
      responding for low
      reinforcement,
      86–87

    isolation-induced
      hyperactivity, 87
    kindling, 85
    lesioning of olfactory
      bulbs, 86, 88
    muricide, 85
    summary observations
      of, 87–88
    yohimbine lethality, 85
   homologous models,
    88–104
    chronic mild stress
      model, 94–96
    clonidine withdrawal, 91
    depression of active
      responding
      induced by
      5-hydroxy-
      tryptophan, 89
    exhaustion stress, 94
    isolation/separation-
      induced
      depression in
      monkeys, 92–94,
      93
    lesioning of dorsomedial
      amygdala in dogs,
      92, **92**
    neonatal clomipramine,
      91–92
    reserpine-induced
      reduction of motor
      activity, 88–89
    separation of Siberian
      hamsters, 94
    summary observations
      of, 101–104,
      102–103
    swim test immobility,
      89–91, **90**
    tail suspension test, 91
    uncontrollable shock,
      96–99, **97**
    using selective breeding,
      99–101
   evaluation criteria for, 82–84
    Abramson and Seligman,
      82–83
    McKinney and Bunney, 82
    Willner, 83–84

of neurodegenerative
disorders, 40–41
of schizophrenia, 104–113
animal assay models,
104–105
catalepsy test, 105
conditioned avoidance
responding,
104–105
paw test, 105
self-stimulation
paradigms, 105
homologous models,
105–112
blocking paradigms,
107–108
chronic amphetamine
intoxication,
110–111
high ambient pressure,
111–112
hippocampal damage,
111
latent inhibition
paradigms,
106–107, **107**
prepulse inhibition of
startle reflex,
108–109
rodent interaction, 109
social behavior in
monkeys,
109–110
using selective breeding,
112
summary observations,
112–113
of substance dependence
disorders
alcohol self-administration,
539–540
brain stimulation reward
paradigms, 540–541
conditioned models of
relapse, 544–545
conditioned place
preference
paradigms, 540
drug self-administration,
105, 539

types of, 81–82
animal assay models, 81–82
homologous models, 81–82
Animal studies
of antipsychotics, 250
of benzodiazepines, 216
of buspirone, 235
of lithium effects on
circadian rhythms,
306–307
Aniracetam, 814
Anorexia, drug-induced
amphetamine, 429
fluoxetine, 690
valproate, 365, 680
venlafaxine, 205
Anorexia nervosa (AN), 557–564
bodily changes in, **558,**
558–559
bulimic subtype of, 564–567.
See also Bulimia
nervosa
diagnosis of, 557
metabolic changes in,
558–559, 559–560
neuroendocrine system
adaptations in, 560–561
arginine vasopressin, 564
human growth hormone,
563–564
hypothalamic-pituitary-
adrenal axis, 561–562
hypothalamic-pituitary-
gonadal axis, 562–563
hypothalamic-pituitary-
thyroid axis, 563
melatonin, 564
prolactin, 564
sleep changes in, 560
treatment of, 730–731
antipsychotics, 731
cyproheptadine, 731
fluoxetine, 731
selective serotonin
reuptake inhibitors,
170
tricyclic antidepressants,
731
Anorexiants, 431
Antabuse. *See* Disulfiram

Antacid interactions
with antipsychotics, 259
with benzodiazepines, 224
Anticholinergic drugs
abuse of, 286
animal studies of
chronic mild stress model,
95
tail suspension test, 91
yohimbine lethality, 85
cognitive deficits due to, 391
contraindicated in glaucoma
patients, 153
for extrapyramidal side
effects, 256, **284,**
284–287, 292–294, 627,
776
interaction with
antipsychotics, 258–259
interaction with cyclic
antidepressants, **786**
for neuroleptic malignant
syndrome, 776
use during pregnancy, 829
Anticholinergic effects
of amoxapine, 199, 200
of antipsychotics, **627,** 629,
663, 777, 792
in children and
adolescents, 684
of clomipramine, 690
of clozapine, 273–274
toxicity, 778
of tricyclic antidepressants,
152–153
in elderly persons, 808
of venlafaxine, 205
α_1 Antichymotripsin (ACT), 399
Anticoagulant interactions
with monoamine oxidase
inhibitors, **789**
with stimulants, **794**
with valproate, **797**
Anticonvulsants. *See*
Antiepileptic drugs
Antidepressants
animal studies of, 85–104.
See also Animal models
antihistamine properties of,
580

Antidepressants *(continued)*
  atypical, 195–208, 826
    amoxapine, 199–200
    bupropion, 200–204
    nefazodone, 205–207
    other agents, 207–208
    trazodone, 195–199
    venlafaxine, 204–205
  for children and adolescents,
      681–683
  combinations of, 589–590
    antidepressant and
        stimulant, 589–590
    desipramine and
        fluoxetine, 589
    tricyclic and monoamine
        oxidase inhibitor,
        589
  cost of, 582
  for depressive subtypes, **582,**
      582–585
    atypical depression, 583
    bipolar depression, 584
    delusional depression,
        583–584
    dementia with depression,
        664–665
    depression in
        schizophrenia, 617
    dysthymic disorder, 584
    geriatric depression, 585
    refractory depression, **588,**
        588–589
    unipolar major depression,
        582–583
  discontinuation of, 586
  drug interactions with, 587
  duration of treatment with,
      585–586
  factors influencing choice of,
      580–581
    neurobiological predictors
        of response, 581
    symptomatic predictors of
        response, 580–581
  future development of,
      592–593
  history of, 141–142,
      575–576
  mania induced by, 609

  mechanism of action of, 576
  for medically ill patients,
      576–580, 783–787
    allergies, 580
    cancer, 579–580
    cardiac disease, 577–578,
        579, 783–785
    gastrointestinal disease,
        579, 580
    glaucoma, **579,** 580, 785
    neurological disease,
        578–579, **579,**
        785–786
    renal disease, 787
    urogenital disorders, 785
  monoamine oxidase
      inhibitors, 183–191
  neurotransmitter receptor
      affinity of, 57, 576,
      578
  other drugs used as or with
    alprazolam, 207, 451
    amphetamine, 419
    buspirone, 238, 239
    carbamazepine, 355–357,
        357, 456
    lithium, 321
    stimulants, 417, 423–427
    valproate, 364, 456
  selective serotonin reuptake
      inhibitors, 161–174
  suicide and, 587–588
  tetracyclic, 142, 143. *See also*
      Maprotiline
  therapeutic monitoring of
      blood level of,
      586–587
  use in Europe, 843–844
  use in pregnancy, 826–828,
      827
Antidepressants, tricyclic (TCAs),
    141–154
  animal studies of
    amphetamine potentiation,
        85
    behavioral effects of
        olfactory bulb
        lesions, 86
    chronic mild stress model,
        95

    depression of active
        responding induced
        by 5-hydroxy-
        tryptophan, 89
    differential operant
        responding for low
        reinforcement, 86
    isolation-induced
        hyperactivity, 87
    kindled seizures, 85
    muricide, 85
    reserpine-induced
        reduction of motor
        activity, 89
    swim test immobility, 89
    tail suspension test, 91
    uncontrollable shock
        model, 96
    yohimbine lethality, 85
  biochemical effects of,
      143–145, **144**
  for children and adolescents,
      681–683
    assessing response to, 682
    continuation, maintenance,
        and monitoring of,
        682
    discontinuation of, 683
    initiation of, 682, **682**
    managing side effects of,
        682–683
    resistance to, 683
    selection of, 681
  combined with monoamine
      oxidase inhibitor, 589
  dosage of, 147
    for elderly persons, 808
  drug interactions with,
      153–154, 587, **786**
    antipsychotics, 630
    carbamazepine, 359, 785,
        795
    clozapine, 273
    monoamine oxidase
        inhibitors, 154, 589,
        789
    selective serotonin
        reuptake inhibitors,
        173
    stimulants, **794**

valproate, 366, 785, **797**
duration of treatment with, 585–586
for elderly persons, 146, 153, 585, 786
history and discovery of, 141–142, 576
indications for, 149–151
  anorexia nervosa, 731
  attention-deficit hyperactivity disorder, 673, 677
  atypical depression, 150
  binge-eating disorder, 730
  bipolar depression, 608, 609
  borderline personality disorder, 760–761
  bulimia nervosa, **151,** 727–729
  children's anxiety in medical setting, 691
  delusional depression, 150
  dementia with depression, 664–665
  dysthymic disorder, 584
  enuresis, 150–151, 694
  major depression and melancholia, 149–150
  nicotine dependence, 719
  obsessive-compulsive disorder, 150
  other, 151, **151**
  panic disorder, 151, 641–642, **642**
  posttraumatic stress disorder, 650, 651
  unipolar major depression, 582
lithium augmentation of, 321, 590
mechanism of action of, 147–149, 440, 576
  classical monoamine hypothesis, 147
  receptor sensitivity hypothesis, 147–148
for medically ill patients, 783–787

cardiac disease, 577–578, **579,** 783–785
glaucoma, 580, 785
pharmacokinetic considerations, 786–787
renal failure and dialysis, 787
seizure disorders, 578, **579,** 785–786
urogenital disorders, 785
metabolites of, 145–146
overdose of, 147, 152, 779
pharmacokinetics of, **145,** 145–147, 786–787
in elderly persons, 808–809
receptor affinity of, 133, **144,** 151
side effects and toxicology of, 147, 151–153, **152,** 682–683
  anticholinergic effects, 152–153, 778
  cardiovascular effects, 147, 152, 172, 577–578, 587, 783–785
  in elderly persons, 808–809
  sedation, 153
  weight gain, 153
structure-activity relationships for, **142,** 142–143
therapeutic index of, 147
therapeutic plasma concentration of, 146–147
thyroid hormone augmentation of, 591
use in pregnancy, 826, **827,** 828
Antiepileptic drugs, 351–370, 405
acetazolamide, 369
for aggressive behavior, **746,** 747
amphetamine, 418
barbiturates, 369
benzodiazepines, 366–367, **367**
carbamazepine, 351–359
drug interactions with antidepressants, 587

clozapine, 273
stimulants, **794**
indications for
  agitation in elderly persons, 807
  borderline personality disorder, 761
  dementia, 662
  psychosis, 633–634
meprobamate, 232
oxcarbazepine, 367–368, **368–369**
phenytoin, 368–369
progabide, 369
use in pregnancy, 832, **832**
valproate, 360–366
Antihistamines
animal studies of
  chronic mild stress model, 95
  muricide, 85
  yohimbine lethality, 85
for anxiety, 231
  in children and adolescents, 688, 689
for sedation, 414
for sleep disorders
  in children, 695
  in elderly persons, 812
Antihypertensive agents
depression induced by, **577**
interaction with trazodone, 199
Antiinflammatory agents
for Alzheimer's disease, 399
interaction with lithium, **327,** 329, **793**
Antiparkinsonian drugs
for extrapyramidal side effects, 256, **284,** 284–287, 292
  duration of therapy, 293–294
  prophylaxis, 292
interaction with bupropion, 203
interaction with buspirone, 237
side effects of, 256

Antipsychotic drugs, 247–259, **620**
  animal studies of, 250
  assessing response to, 623–624
  atypical, 263–275. *See also* Clozapine
  behavioral effects of, 250
  in breast milk, 828–829
  buspirone, 234
  for children and adolescents, 683–685
    assessing response to, 683
    continuation, maintenance, and monitoring of, 684
    discontinuation of, 685
    initiation of, 683–684
    managing side effects of, 684–685
    resistance to, 685
  choice of, 619–620
  clozapine, 263–275, 631–634, **632**, 792–793
  discontinuation of, 630–631
  dopamine receptor affinity for, 7, 47, **47**, 57, 619
  dosage of, 248, **249**, 619, **620**, 624–625
  drug interactions with, 258–259, 630, **630**, **791**
    calcium channel blockers, **385**
    carbamazepine, 359, **795**
    lithium, **327**, 328
    selective serotonin reuptake inhibitors, 173
    tricyclic antidepressants, 587
    trihexyphenidyl, 286
    valproate, 366
  effects in animal models of depression
    chronic mild stress model, 95
    isolation-induced hyperactivity, 87
    tail suspension test, 91
    uncontrollable shock model, 96

  effects in animal models of schizophrenia, 104–105
    catalepsy test, 105
    chronic amphetamine intoxication, 110
    conditioned avoidance responding, 104–105, 112
    latent inhibition of conditioned responses, 106, **107**
    paw test, 105
    prepulse inhibition of startle reflex, 108–109
    rat social interaction, 109
    self-stimulation paradigms, 105
    social behavior in monkeys, 110
  effects on gene expression, 35
  for elderly persons, 806–807
  endocrine effects of, 251, 258
  history and discovery of, 247–248
  indications for, 253–255
    aggression
      acute, 745, **745**
      in children and adolescents, 686
      chronic, 746–747
    anorexia nervosa, 731
    autism, 693
    borderline personality disorder, 757, 761–762
    dementia, 255, 658–661
    depot antipsychotics, 255
    depression with psychotic features, 255, 583–584
    mania, 255, 611
      in elderly persons, 811
    obsessive-compulsive disorder, 168, 650
    other conditions, 255
    pregnancy-associated emesis, 828
    rapid neuroleptization, 774
    schizophrenia, 253–254, 615–634

  schizotypal personality disorder, 757–758
  sleep disorders in elderly persons, 812
  symptoms of mental retardation, 255, 696–697
  Tourette's disorder, 691–692
  initiation of, 623
  limitations of, 247
  long-acting depot forms of, 252, 255, 292
  mechanism of action of, 252–253, 283, 618–619
  for medically ill patients, 791–793
    cardiac disease, 791–792
    clozapine, 792–793
    glaucoma, 629, 777, 792
    other medical conditions, 792
    pulmonary disease, 792
    seizure disorders, 258
  motor effects of, 250–251
  pharmacokinetics and disposition of, 251–252
  remoxipride, 621
  resistance to, 631
  risperidone, 620–621
  serotonin antagonist properties of, 490
  side effects and toxicology of, 248, 255–258, 625–630, **626–627**, 684–685, 776–778, 792
    anticholinergic effects, 627, **629**, 663, 777, 792
    cardiovascular effects, 258, 776–777
    in elderly persons, 806–807
    electroencephalographic effects and seizures, 777, 792
    extrapyramidal effects, 250–251, 255–256, 281–294, 625–628, 776, 792
    in neonate, 828
    neuroendocrine effects, 251, 258

neuroleptic malignant
    syndrome, 257, 629,
    776, 792
ocular effects, 258, 629, 777
other effects, 258, 629–630
tardive dyskinesia,
    256–257
structure-activity
    relationships for,
    248–250, **249**
    butyrophenones, 250
    dibenzoxazepines, 250
    diphenylbutylpiperidines,
        250
    phenothiazines, 248
    thioxanthenes, 248
therapeutic plasma levels of,
    624–625, 792
use in Europe, **840–842,**
    840–843
use in pregnancy, 258,
    828–829, **829**
Antithyroid antibodies, 448
Anxiety, drug-induced
    isoproterenol, 505
    nicotine, 396
    oxotremorine, 396
    physostigmine, 392
    venlafaxine, 205
Anxiety disorders. *See also*
    specific disorders
    neurobiology of, 501–513
        obsessive-compulsive
            disorder, 510–513
        panic disorder, 501–507
        posttraumatic stress
            disorder, 509–510
        social phobia, 507–508
    treatment of, 641–651
        in children and
            adolescents, 687–691
        anxiety in medical
            setting, 691
        obsessive-compulsive
            disorder, 689–690
        overanxious disorder
            and generalized
            anxiety disorder,
            688–689
        panic disorder, 690

posttraumatic stress
    disorder, 690–691
separation anxiety
    disorder, 687–688
in elderly persons, 811–812
in Europe, 844–845
generalized anxiety
    disorder, 646–647
obsessive-compulsive
    disorder, 649–650
panic disorder, 641–646
posttraumatic stress
    disorder, 650–651
social phobia, 647–649
Anxiolytics, 641–651
    benzodiazepines, 215–225,
        408–414
    buspirone, 234–241
    for children and adolescents,
        687–691
    effects in animal models of
        depression
        chronic mild stress model,
            95
        isolation-induced
            hyperactivity, 87
        swim test immobility, 89
        tail suspension test, 91
    for elderly persons, 811–812
    for generalized anxiety
        disorder, 646–647
    interaction with
        antipsychotics, 259
    meprobamate, 231–234
    new agents, 240
    for obsessive-compulsive
        disorder, 649–650
    for panic disorder, 641–646
    for posttraumatic stress
        disorder, 650–651
    for social phobia, 647–649
    trazodone, 197
    tricyclic antidepressants, **151**
    use during pregnancy, 830,
        831
    use in Europe, 844–845
Apathy, 616
Apolipoprotein E, 526–527
Apomorphine, 7, **47,** 250, 266,
    449

Arachidonic acid (AA), 3, 17,
    20, **23,** 23–24
Arecoline, 395–396
Arginine vasopressin (AVP)
    for Alzheimer's disease, 813
    in anorexia nervosa, 564
    in obsessive-compulsive
        disorder, 511
Aromatic amino acid
    decarboxylase, 5
Arrhythmias. *See also*
    Cardiovascular effects
    calcium channel blockers for,
        378
    trazodone-induced, 198
    tricyclic antidepressants for
        patients with, 147, 152,
        577–578, 783–785
Artane. *See* Trihexyphenidyl
Asendin. *See* Amoxapine
Aspirin, interaction with
    valproate, 366
Assault victim, 772
Assaultive behavior, 773–774.
    See also Aggression
Assertiveness training, 688
Asthenia, drug-induced
    nefazodone, 207
    venlafaxine, 205
Atarax. *See* Hydroxyzine
Ataraxia, 250
Ataxia, drug-induced
    benzodiazepines, 414
    carbamazepine, 358, 686
    oxcarbazepine, 368
Atenolol
    for extrapyramidal side
        effects, **289**
    for social phobia, 508, 648
Ativan. *See* Lorazepam
Attention-deficit hyperactivity
    disorder (ADHD), 669,
        671–677
    in adults, 417, 428
        borderline personality
            disorder and, 762
        assessing treatment response
            in, 673
        assessment of, 671
        bupropion for, 202, 673

ADHD *(continued)*
  clonidine for, 673, 677
    continuation, maintenance,
      and monitoring of,
      677
    discontinuation of, 677
    initiation of, 677
    managing side effects of,
      677
  differentiating from mania,
    678
  mental retardation and, 696
  placebo response in, 670
  predicting medication
    response in, 672
  selecting treatment for,
    671–672
  stimulants for, 417, 419, 423,
    427–428, 672–677, **675**
    continuation, maintenance,
      and monitoring of, 675
    discontinuation of, 676
    initiation of, 673–675
    managing side effects of,
      675–676, **676**
    resistance to, 676–677
  Tourette's disorder and, 691,
    692
  treating aggression in, 685
  tricyclic antidepressants for,
    673, 677
  urinary incontinence and,
    694
Autistic disorders, 669,
    693–694
  definition of, 693
  placebo response in, 670
  treatment of, 693–694
Autonomic dysfunction, in
    panic disorder, 505–506
Aventyl. *See* Nortriptyline
Avoidant personality disorder
    (APD), 507, 763–764
  anxiety in, 763–764
  differential diagnosis of, 764
  social phobia and, 648
  treatment of, 764
Avolition, 479
Azaspirodecanes, 396
Azaspirones, 235, **236,** 240

B lymphocytes, 461–462
  in depression, 463
Barbital, 405
Barbitone, 406
Barbiturates, 231, 405–408
  contraindications to, 407
  dependence on, 407, 408
  drug interactions with, 408
    antidepressants, 154, 587,
      786
    antipsychotics, 258
    monoamine oxidase
      inhibitors, 189
  history and discovery of,
    405–406
  indications for, 407
    bipolar disorder, 369
  mechanisms of action of,
    406–407
  overdose of, 407, 408
    amphetamine for, 418
  pharmacokinetics and
    disposition of, 406
  pharmacology of, 406–407
  side effects and toxicology
    of, 407–408
  sleep effects of, 406–407,
    412
  structure-activity relations for,
    406, **406**
  tolerance to, 408
  withdrawal from, 407
Barbituric acid, 406, **406**
Barnes Akathisia Rating Scale,
    284
Basal ganglia, 482
  in mood disorders, 461
  in schizophrenia, 482–483,
    483
Beck Depression Inventory,
    681, 682, 696
Bedwetting, 694–695
Behavior modification
  for aggression, 743–744, **744**
  for attention-deficit
    hyperactivity disorder,
    672
  for nicotine dependence, 719
  for obsessive-compulsive
    disorder, 689

  for separation anxiety
    disorder, 688
Beigel-Murphy Scale, 679
Benactyzine, 233
Benadryl. *See* Diphenhydramine
Benzodiazepine agonists,
    130–131, **131,** 220–221, 411,
    411
Benzodiazepine antagonists,
    220, 411, **411**
Benzodiazepine receptors,
    219–220, 219–222
  alcohol effects on, 544
  ligands for, 220–221, 412
  meprobamate actions on,
    233
  nonbenzodiazepine
    hypnotics acting on, 411
  in panic disorder, 505
  peripheral-type, 221–222
  Types I and II, 220
Benzodiazepines, 215–225, 405
  animal studies of, 216
  in breast milk, 830
  dependence on, 414, 709–710
    risk factors for, 645
  discontinuation of, 710
  drug interactions with,
    224–225, **794**
    carbamazepine, 359
    clozapine, 273, 632
    lithium, 327–328
    selective serotonin
      reuptake inhibitors,
      173
    valproate, **797**
  for elderly persons, 217, 644,
    789–790, 811, 812
  electroencephalographic
    effects of, 131–133,
    132–133
  half-lives of, 217–218, **218,**
    409, 789
  history and discovery of, 215,
    408
  indications for, 222–223,
    413–414
    aggressive behavior,
      744–746, **746**
    agitated psychosis, 774

alcohol withdrawal, 222, 413–414, 549, 707–709, 775

avoidant personality disorder, 764

bipolar disorder, 351, 366–367, **367,** 605, 611

borderline personality disorder, 763

dementia, 662–664

extrapyramidal side effects, 291, 628

generalized anxiety disorder, 222–223, 646–647

in children and adolescents, 688–689

in elderly persons, 811

mania, 774

neuroleptic malignant syndrome, 257

panic disorder, 215, 218, 222, 223, **644,** 643–645

phencyclidine intoxication, 718, 776

posttraumatic stress disorder, 222, 223, 651

psychiatric emergencies, 771, **771**

sedation, 408–414

separation anxiety disorder, 688

sleep disorders

in children, 695

in elderly persons, 812

social phobia, 222, 648

symptoms of mental retardation, 697

long-term use of, 224

measuring pharmacodynamic effects of, 131–132

mechanism of action of, 130, **131,** 218–222

benzodiazepine receptors, **219–220,** 219–222

role of gamma-aminobutyric acid, 218–219

for medically ill patients, 789–790

new agents, 790

overdose of, 217, 414, 710, 779

pharmacokinetics and disposition of, 217–218, 409, **409**

in elderly persons, 811

pharmacology of, 217, 409–410, **410**

prescribing guidelines for, 790

shifting to buspirone from, 238

side effects and toxicology of, 130–131, 223–224, 414, 689

in elderly persons, 811

sleep effects of, 412–413, **412–413**

structure-activity relations for, 215–216, **216,** 408–409, **409**

use in pregnancy, 224, 414, 830, **831**

use in sleep apnea patients, 413

withdrawal from, 128–129, 224, 414, 689, 710

rebound anxiety after, 644–645

Benzoic acid, 421, **421**

Benzphetamine, 431

Benztropine

drug interactions with, 287

history and discovery of, 286

indications for, 287

extrapyramidal side effects, 256, **284,** 286–287, 627, 776

in children and adolescents, 684

prophylaxis, 292

neuroleptic malignant syndrome, 776

mechanism of action of, 287

pharmacokinetics and disposition of, 286–287

pharmacological profile of, 286

side effects of, 287

structure-activity relations for, 286

use during pregnancy, 829, **829**

Betaxolol, **289**

Bethanechol, 153, 395

Binge-eating disorder, 725, 730

Biological psychiatry

of Alzheimer's disease, 523–529

of anxiety disorders, 501–513

of eating disorders, 557–567

history of, 439

of mood disorders, 439–464

of schizophrenia, 479–492

of substance dependence disorders, 537–551

Biperiden, **284,** 287

Bipolar disorder. *See also* Depression; Mania; Mood disorders

associated with mental retardation, 696

brain imaging in, 459–461, **460–461**

calcium hyperactivity in, 459

catecholamines in, 451–452

in DSM-IV, 440, 441

genetics of, 444

monoamine oxidase activity in, 456

neuroendocrinology of, 447–448

hypothalamic-pituitary-adrenal axis, **445,** 447

hypothalamic-pituitary-thyroid axis, 448, **449**

rapid cycling, 604–605

secondary, 605

substance abuse and, 605

Bipolar disorder treatment, 603–611

for acute depression, 608–609

for acute mania and hypomania, 606–608

for agitated psychosis, 774

antidepressants, 584

Bipolar disorder treatment
    (continued)
  antiepileptic drugs, 351–370
    acetazolamide, 369
    barbiturates, 369
    benzodiazepines, 351,
        366–367, **367,** 605
    carbamazepine, 351–359,
        584, 606–608
    oxcarbazepine, 367–368,
        368–369
    phenytoin, 368–369
    progabide, 369
    valproate, 360–366, 606,
        607
  bupropion, 202, 583
  calcium channel antagonists,
      378–379, 383–385
  in children and adolescents,
      678–680
  in children and adolescents,
      assessing response to,
      678–679
    assessment for, 678
    lithium, 678–680
    selecting therapy for, 678
    valproic acid, 680
  clozapine, 271, 273
  features of illness affecting,
      603–605, 604
    acute depression, 604
    acute mania and
        hypomania, 603
    comorbid substance abuse,
        605
    secondary bipolar
        disorders, 605
    severity of illness, 604
    subsyndromal variations,
        604–605
      mixed mania, 604
      pure or classical mania,
          604
      rapid cycling, 604–605
  lithium, 303–330, 606–607
  maintenance therapy,
      609–611
    benzodiazepines, 367, 611
    carbamazepine, 352, 357,
        369, 610–611

  clozapine, 611
  lithium, 320–321, 610
  neuroleptics, 611
  oxcarbazepine, 368, **369**
  thyroid hormone, 611
  valproate, 364, 610
during pregnancy, 830–833,
    832
principles of, 605–606
  combining drug therapies,
      605–606
  eliminating mood
      destabilizers, 605
  life charting, 605
  optimizing sleep, 605
  rationale for, 603
  sources of new information
      about, 611
Bizarre behavior, 615, 616
Blessed Dementia Index, 524
Blessed Information-Memory-
    Concentration test, 524
α-Blocker interactions
  with calcium channel
      blockers, 385
  with cyclic antidepressants,
      786
β-Blockers
  discontinuation of, 687
  drug interactions with, 291
    antidepressants, 587
    antipsychotics, 258
    calcium channel blockers,
        385
  history and discovery of, 289
  indications for, 290
    aggression, 748, **748**
      in children and
          adolescents, 686,
          687
    agitation in elderly
        persons, 807
    autism, 694
    avoidant personality
        disorder, 764
    extrapyramidal side effects,
        289, 289–291, 628
    posttraumatic stress
        disorder, 651
    social phobia, 507–508, 648

    symptoms of mental
        retardation, 697
  initiation of, 687
  mechanism of action of, 290
  pharmacokinetics and
      disposition of, 290
  pharmacological profile of,
      290
  side effects and toxicology
      of, 290–291, 687, 807
  structure-activity relations for,
      289–290
Blocking paradigms, 107–108
Blunted affect, 616
Body Mass Index (BMI), 558, 730
Borderline personality disorder
    (BPD), 758–763
  clinical features of, 757–758
  differential diagnosis of,
      759–760
  neurobiology of, 758
  treatment of, 760–763
    anticonvulsants, 761–762
    antipsychotics, 757, 762
    assessing response to, 763
    benzodiazepines, 763
    emergency interventions,
        772
    initiation of, 763
    lithium, 761
    monoamine oxidase
        inhibitors, 761
    resistance to, 763
    selective serotonin
        reuptake inhibitors,
        171, 760
    stimulants, 762–763
    tricyclic antidepressants,
        760–761
Bradykinesia, 255, 627
Brain
  anatomical regions of, 45
  biochemical information
      transfer pathways in,
      3–4
  dopamine and serotonin
      systems in, 9
Brain abnormalities
  in Alzheimer's disease,
      524–526

in anorexia nervosa, 559
in mood disorders, 459–461,
    460–461
in obsessive-compulsive
    disorder, 512–513
in schizophrenia, 112, 459, 486
Brain stimulation reward (BSR)
    paradigms, 540–541, 548
Breast milk. *See also* Pregnancy
    and lactation
    antidepressants in, 827–828
    antipsychotics in, 828–829
    benzodiazepines in, 224, 830
    determinants of drug
        concentration in,
        824–825
    lithium in, 327
Bretazenil, 647
Brief Psychiatric Rating Scale
    (BPRS), 169, 378, 481, 618,
    619, 624, 660
Brofaromine, **184,** 583
Bromide, 405
Bromocriptine
    dopamine receptor affinity
        for, **47**
    for neuroleptic malignant
        syndrome, 257, 629, 776
    for protracted cocaine
        withdrawal, 548
Bronchodilator interactions
    with lithium, **793**
    with monoamine oxidase
        inhibitors, 787, **789**
Bulimia nervosa, 564–567
    age at onset of, 725
    binge-eating episodes in,
        725, 726
    chronicity of, 725–726
    diagnostic criteria for, 725
    etiology of, 726
    medical complications of, 725
    metabolic changes in, **565,**
        565–566
    neuroendocrine changes in,
        566
    physical changes in, 565, **565**
    prevalence of, 725
    psychopathology comorbid
        with, 725

role of serotonin in, 169, 726
sleep changes in, 566
treatment of, 727–730
    antidepressants, **151,**
        169–170, 727–729
    combined with
        cognitive-behavioral
        therapy, 728
    mechanism of action, 729
    predictors of response,
        728–729
    bupropion, 203
    comprehensive therapy, 729
    d-fenfluramine, 729
    lithium, 730
    monoamine oxidase
        inhibitors, 186
    naltrexone, 729–730
    selective serotonin
        reuptake inhibitors,
        169–170
    trazodone, 197–198
Buprenorphine, 712, 716
Bupropion, 200–204, 419
    animal studies of
        chronic mild stress model,
            95
        yohimbine lethality, 85
    drug interactions with,
        203–204
        clozapine, 273
    for elderly persons, 585
    history and discovery of,
        200–201
    indications for, 202–203
        aggression in children and
            adolescents, 686, 687
        attention-deficit
            hyperactivity
            disorder, 202, 673
        bipolar disorder, 202, 583,
            608–609
        bulimia nervosa, 727
        geriatric depression,
            809–810
        unipolar major depression,
            583
    mechanism of action of, 144,
        147, 202
    metabolites of, 201, 202

pharmacokinetics and
    disposition of, 201–202
pharmacological profile of, 201
side effects and toxicology
    of, 203, 583, 687
    seizures, 203, 578, 687,
        778, 785–786
structure-activity relationship
    for, 201, **201**
use in cardiac disease
    patients, 577
use in pregnancy, **827**
BuSpar. *See* Buspirone
Buspirone (BuSpar), 234–241
    abuse liability of, 235
    advantages over
        benzodiazepines, 237
    animal studies of, 235
    dosage of, 237–238
    drug interactions with,
        236–237
        monoamine oxidase
            inhibitors, **789**
        trazodone, 198
    efficacy in panic disorder, 645
    for elderly persons, 236,
        811–812
    history and discovery of,
        234–235
    indications for, 237–240
        aggressive behavior, **746,**
            747, 775
        agitation in elderly
            persons, 807
        anxiety, 237–240, 647
            in children and
                adolescents, 689
            in elderly persons,
                811–812
        autism, 694
        dementia, 662, 664
        depression, 239
        neuropsychiatric disorders,
            239–240
        obsessive-compulsive
            disorder, 168,
            238–239, 650
        social phobia, 238, 648
        symptoms of mental
            retardation, 240, 697

Buspirone *(continued)*
　for medically ill patients, 790
　metabolites of, 236
　neuroendocrine effects of, 236
　pharmacokinetics of, 235–236
　pharmacological profile of,
　　235
　shifting from benzodiazepine
　　to, 238
　side effects of, 237
　structure-activity relationship
　　for, 235, **236**
　use in pregnancy, **831**
Butyrophenones, **249,** 250

Caffeine
　interaction with monoamine
　　oxidase inhibitors, **789**
　role in panic disorder, 505
Calan. *See* Verapamil
Calcitonin, 378
Calcium, in mood disorders,
　458–459
Calcium channel blockers
　(CCBs), 377–385
　binding sites for, 380, **380,**
　　384
　classes of, 378, **378**
　dosage of, 384, **384**
　drug interactions with, 385,
　　385
　　β-blockers, 291
　　lithium, **793**
　　monoamine oxidase
　　　inhibitors, **789**
　history and discovery of,
　　378–379
　indications for, 378, 383–384
　　acute mania, 378–379, 384,
　　　608
　　Alzheimer's disease, 813
　　bipolar disorder, 378–379,
　　　383–385
　lack of familiarity with, 377
　mechanisms of action of,
　　382–383
　pharmacokinetics of,
　　381–382, **382**
　side effects and toxicology
　　of, 384–385

structure-activity
　relationships for,
　379–381, **379–381**
Cancer patients, 579–580
Candidate genes, 443
Cannabis, 717, 776
Carbamazepine, 351–359
　compared with other
　　anticonvulsants, 355
　dosage of, 353, 607, 608
　drug interactions with, 359,
　　795, 795–796
　　antipsychotics, 258, 630
　　calcium channel blockers,
　　　385
　　cyclic antidepressants, **786**
　　lithium, 359, 795
　　monoamine oxidase
　　　inhibitors, **789**
　　oral contraceptives, 359,
　　　607–608
　　selective serotonin
　　　reuptake inhibitors,
　　　173
　　valproate, 366, 606, 796,
　　　797
　history and discovery of,
　　351–352
　indications for, 355–357
　　acute major depression,
　　　355–357, **357,** 456
　　acute mania, 355, **356,**
　　　584, 607–608
　　aggressive behavior, **746,**
　　　747, 775
　　in children and
　　　adolescents,
　　　685–687
　　agitation in elderly
　　　persons, 807
　　bipolar disorder
　　　in children and
　　　　adolescents, 678,
　　　　680
　　prophylaxis, 357, **369,**
　　　610–611
　　borderline personality
　　　disorder, 761–762,
　　　772
　　cocaine abuse, 711

dementia, 662
　posttraumatic stress
　　disorder, 650
　mechanism of action of,
　　354–355
　for medically ill patients,
　　794–796
　metabolites of, 353, **353**
　overdose of, 350, 353
　pharmacokinetics and
　　disposition of, 352–354,
　　353–354, 382
　pharmacological profile of,
　　352
　predictors of response to,
　　357–358
　serum concentration of,
　　353–354
　side effects and toxicology
　　of, 358–359, 607,
　　686–687, 794–796
　slow-release, 352–353
　structure-activity relations for,
　　352, **352**
　use in pregnancy, 359, 687,
　　832, **832**
Cardene. *See* Nicardipine
Cardiac disease patients
　antipsychotics for, 791–792
　cyclic antidepressants for,
　　147, 152, 577–578,
　　783–785
　electroconvulsive therapy for,
　　797
　monoamine oxidase
　　inhibitors for, 787–788
Cardiovascular effects
　of amoxapine, 200
　of amphetamine, 429
　of anorexia nervosa, **558,**
　　558–559
　of antipsychotics, 258, 629,
　　776–777
　of β-blockers, 290–291
　of bulimia nervosa, **565**
　of calcium channel blockers,
　　384–385
　of carbamazepine, 358, 795
　of clomipramine, 690
　of clonidine, 712

of clozapine, 274, **632,** 633
of desipramine in children, 152, 682
of lithium, 326, 793
of physostigmine, 392
of pimozide, 692
of selective serotonin reuptake inhibitors, 172–173
of social phobia, 507–508
of stimulants, 676
of tetrahydroaminoacridine, 393
of trazodone, 198
of tricyclic antidepressants, 147, 152, 577–578, 587, 783–785
of trihexyphenidyl, 285
Cardizem. *See* Diltiazem
Catalepsy
amoxapine and, 199
antipsychotic-induced, 251
buspirone for, 234, 235
Catalepsy test, 105
Catatonia, 773
benzodiazepines for, 351
electroconvulsive therapy for, 621
neuroleptic-induced, 792
Catecholamines, 451. *See also* Dopamine; Epinephrine; Norepinephrine
role in mood disorders, 143, 147, 439, 451
Catechol-O-methyltransferase (COMT), 8, 563
Central nervous system (CNS)
heterogeneity of, 31, 59
integration of, 3
Central nervous system depressants
amoxapine and, 200
interaction with antipsychotics, 259
interaction with diphenhydramine, 288
trazodone and, 198
Central serotonin syndrome (CSS), 172
Centrax. *See* Prazepam

Cerebral blood flow (CBF) studies, 459
in panic disorder, 507
in schizophrenia, 484, 486
Ceretec. *See* [^{99m}Tc]HMPAO
Charcot-Marie-Tooth disease, 41
Chestnut Lodge Longitudinal Study, 616–617
Child Attention Problems (CAP) Rating Scale, 673, **674–675**
Child Behavior Checklist, 671, 673
Child Depression Inventory (CDI), 681, 682, 696
Child Depression Rating Scale Revised (CDRS-R), 681, 682
Childhood and adolescent disorders, 669–697
adolescent crises, 778–779
aggression, 685–687
anxiety disorders, 687–691
anxiety in medical setting, 691
obsessive-compulsive disorder, 689–690
overanxious disorder and generalized anxiety disorder, 688–689
panic disorder, 690
posttraumatic stress disorder, 690–691
separation anxiety disorder, 687–688
attention-deficit hyperactivity disorder, 671–677
autistic disorder, 693–694
developmental toxicology and, 671
drug metabolism and kinetics and, 671
emotional and behavioral symptoms of mental retardation, 696–697
enuresis, 694–695
ethical issues in treatment of, 670
evaluation of, 669
meaning of medication for, 670

measuring treatment outcome in, 670
medication compliance in, 670–671
mood disorders, 678–683
bipolar disorder, 678–680
depression, 680–683
placebo response in, 670
schizophrenia, 683–685
sleep disorders, 695–696
insomnia, 695
sleep terror and sleepwalking, 695–696
Tourette's disorder, 691–693
treatment planning for, 669
Children's Version of the Yale-Brown Obsessive Compulsive Scale, 690
Chlomethiazole, 414
Chloral hydrate, 405, 414
for aggressive behavior, 746
interaction with antidepressants, 587
for sleep disorders
in children, 695
in elderly persons, 812
use in pregnancy, **831**
Chlordiazepoxide, 215, 223
for alcohol withdrawal symptoms, 549, 708
effects on isolation-induced hyperactivity in animals, 87
half-life of, **218**
metabolism of, 217, 409, **409**
use in pregnancy, **831**
p-Chlorophenylalanine, 440
m-Chlorophenylpiperazine (m-CPP), 169, 196, 206, 583, 764
Chlorphentermine, 431
Chlorpromazine, 35, 619
behavioral effects of, 250
in breast milk, 828
cardiovascular effects of, 258
for dementia, 659
dopamine receptor affinity for, 47, **47**

Chlorpromazine (continued)
  dosage of, 248, **249, 620**
  effects on isolation-induced
      hyperactivity in
      animals, 87
  effects on latent inhibition of
      conditioned responses
      in animals, **107**
  history and discovery of,
      141–142, 247–248, 439,
      575
  indications for
    anorexia nervosa, 731
    borderline personality
        disorder, 762
    hypertensive crisis, 778
  interaction with β-blockers,
      291
  interaction with valproate,
      797
  metabolites of, 251
  ocular effects of, 258
  photosensitivity reaction to,
      258
  side effects of, 248
    extrapyramidal side effects
        related to efficacy,
        281
    structure-activity relationship
        for, 248, **249, 840**
  use in pregnancy, 828, **829**
Chlorprothixene, 619, **620**
Cholecystokinin (CCK)
  panic-induced by, 505
  in schizophrenia, 491
Cholestyramine interactions
  with β-blockers, 291
  with cyclic antidepressants,
      786
Choline, 392, 813
Choline acetyltransferase
    (ChAT), 524
Cholinergic agonists, 395–396
  AF102B, 396
  arecoline, 395–396
  azaspirodecanes, 396
  bethanechol, 395
  nicotine, 396
  oxotremorine, 396
  RS-86, 395

Cholinesterase inhibitors,
    392–395
  galanthamine, 394
  HP 029, 393–394
  physostigmine, 392
  tetrahydroaminoacridine,
      393, 813
Chouinard Extrapyramidal
    Rating Scale, 284
Chromosomes, 32
Chronic fatigue syndrome, 203
Ciliary neurotrophic factor
    (CNTF), 41
Cimetidine interactions
  with antipsychotics, 258
  with benzodiazepines, 224,
      794
  with β-blockers, 291
  with carbamazepine, **795**
  with cyclic antidepressants,
      154, **786**
  with moclobemide, 190
  with selective serotonin
      reuptake inhibitors, 173
  with valproate, **797**
  with venlafaxine, 205
Cinnarizine, **378**
Circadian rhythm
  lithium and, 306–307
  mood disorders and, 457
  readjustment in rats, 85–86
  of serotonin release, 9
Citalopram, **840–842**, 843–844
  for alcoholism, 170
  metabolite of, 165–166
  for panic disorder, 169
  pharmacokinetics of,
      165–166, **166**
  sleep effects of, 171
  structure-activity relationship
      for, 162, **162, 841**
Clinical Global Assessment
    Scale, 393, **619**
Clinical Global Impression Scale
    (CGI), 621
Clomipramine (CMI)
  animal studies of
    behavioral effects of
        olfactory bulb
        lesions, 86

differential operant
      responding for low
      reinforcement, 86
  isolation-induced
      hyperactivity, 87
  biochemical effects of, **144**
  dosage of, 150
  effects in neonatal rats,
      91–92
  elimination half-life of, **145**
  indications for, **151**
    anorexia nervosa, 170
    autism, 694
    generalized anxiety
        disorder, 647
    obsessive-compulsive
        disorder, 142, 150,
        168, 649, 839
      associated with
          Tourette's disorder,
          692
    in children and
        adolescents,
        689–690
    panic disorder, 642
  metabolite of, 146, 165, 168
  pharmacokinetics of,
      165–166, **166**
  side effects of, 172
    in children and
        adolescents, 690
    seizures, 150, 578
    sexual dysfunction, 153
  structure-activity relationship
      for, **142**, 143, **162**
  use in Europe, 844
  use in pregnancy, **827**
Clonazepam, 222, 223
  for aggressive behavior, 747
  for alcohol withdrawal
      symptoms, 708
  for bipolar disorder, 366–367,
      367
  interaction with
      carbamazepine, **795**
  interaction with valproate,
      366
  for mania, 774
  for obsessive-compulsive
      disorder, 650

for panic disorder, 643
in children, 690
for social phobia, 648
for treatment-resistant mania,
680
use in pregnancy, 830,
831–832, 832
Clonidine
animal studies of withdrawal
from, 91
discontinuation of, 677
drug interactions with
cyclic antidepressants, 154,
786
trazodone, 198–199
efficacy for mania, 608
growth hormone response to
in depression, 449, 452
in panic disorder, 504
in social phobia, 508
indications for
Alzheimer's disease, 396,
397, 813
attention-deficit
hyperactivity
disorder, 673, 677
autism, 694
nicotine dependence,
719
opioid detoxification,
712–713
posttraumatic stress
disorder, 650
Tourette's disorder,
692–693
treatment-resistant mania,
680
initiation of, 677
side effects of, 677, 712
Clopenthixol, 248, 840,
840–842
Clorazepate, **218,** 223
for generalized anxiety
disorder, 647
indications for, 413
metabolism of, 409, **409**
use in pregnancy, **831**
Clorgiline, 87, 185
Clozapine (Clozaril), 35, 247,
263–275

animal studies of
cocaine self-administration,
105
conditioned avoidance
responding, 105
latent inhibition of
conditioned
responses, **107**
for children and adolescents,
685
compared with typical
antipsychotics, 263,
264
dopamine receptor affinity
for, 47, **47,** 57
dosage of, 272, 273, **620,**
631–632
drug interactions with, 273
benzodiazepines, 273, 632
evaluation before initiation
of, 631
history and discovery of,
271
indications for, 271–273, 792
bipolar disorder
prophylaxis, 611
patients who experienced
neuroleptic malignant
syndrome, 629
psychosis in Parkinson's
disease, 792–793
tardive dyskinesia, 628
treatment-refractory
schizophrenia,
631–634
mechanism of action of,
264–265, 274–275, 283
for medically ill patients,
792–793
metabolites of, 271
neuroleptic augmentation of,
633, **633**
pharmacological profiles of,
265–270, 283
D_2, D_3, and D_4 receptors,
265–267, **266, 268**
D_1 and D_5 receptors,
267–268
serotonin receptors,
268–270

predicting response to, 275
side effects and toxicology
of, 273–274, 631–633,
632, 792
agranulocytosis, 271–272,
274, 611, 631–633,
778
lack of extrapyramidal side
effects, 293, 631
seizures, 273, 777
structure-activity relations for,
250, 271
switching to risperidone
from, 621
use during pregnancy, **829**
use in Europe, 840
Clozaril. *See* Clozapine
CNQX. *See* 6-Cyano-7-
nitroquinoxaline-2,3-dione
Cocaine abuse, 147. *See also*
Stimulants
animal models of, 105, 539
brain imaging in, 548
effect on brain stimulation
reward threshold, 541,
548
effect on synaptic dopamine
level, 8, 9, 56, 711
electroencephalographic
effects of, 548
history of, 417–419
interaction with monoamine
oxidase inhibitors, **789**
kindling of seizure activity
produced by, 711
medical complications of,
710–711, **711**
prevalence of, 710
protracted withdrawal
associated with,
547–548, 711
treatment of, 710–711
carbamazepine, 711
desipramine, 711
intoxication with violent
behavior, 775–776
stimulants for, 429
Cocaine Anonymous, 717
Codeine, **130**
Cogentin. *See* Benztropine

Cognitive enhancers, 391–400, 813–814
  cholinergic agents, 391–396
    acetylcholine precursors, 392, 813
    cholinergic agonists, 395–396
    cholinesterase inhibitors, 392–395
  new approaches, 397–399
    antiinflammatory agents, 399
    glutamatergic agents, 397–398
  other neurotransmitter systems, 396–397
Colestipol, interaction with β-blockers, 291
Complement system, in Alzheimer's disease, 399
Comprehensive Assessment of Symptoms and History (CASH), **618**
Computed tomography (CT)
  in Alzheimer's disease, 524
  in anorexia nervosa, 559
  in mood disorders, 459–460, **460**
  in obsessive-compulsive disorder, 512
  in schizophrenia, 482, 484
COMT. *See* Catechol-O-methyltransferase
Conditioned avoidance responding, 104–105, 112
Conditioned place preference paradigms, 540
Conduct disorder. *See* Aggression treatment, in children and adolescents
Confusion
  antidepressants for patients with, 579
  drug-induced
    amphetamine, 429
    benzodiazepines, 414
    tricyclic antidepressants, 153
Congenital anomalies, 823–824
Congestive heart failure, 785

Conners Parent and Teacher Rating Scales, 678
Constipation, drug-induced, 256
  antipsychotics, 777
  calcium channel blockers, 385
  clozapine, 274
  monoamine oxidase inhibitors, 187
  nefazodone, 207
  tricyclic antidepressants, 153, 682
  trihexyphenidyl, 285
  venlafaxine, 205
Controlled Substances Act, 419, 423
Conversion disorder, 773
Coprolalia, 691
Corgard. *See* Nadolol
Corticosteroids, 440, **577**
Corticosulcal dilatation, 482
Corticotropin-releasing factor (CRF)
  in Alzheimer's disease, 524
  anorexiant effects of, 561
  in mood disorders, 165, **445,** 445–447
  in panic disorder, 506
Cortisol
  in anorexia nervosa, 561–562
  in bulimia nervosa, 566
  in depression, 440, 446, 455, 457
  in posttraumatic stress disorder, 510
Coughing, calcium channel blocker–induced, 385
C-reactive protein, 399
Cushing's disease, 440, 445, 559
Cutaneous effects
  of antipsychotics, 258, 629
  of calcium channel blockers, 384, 385
  of carbamazepine, 686–687
6-Cyano-7-nitroquinoxaline-2,3-dione (CNQX), 398
Cyclic adenosine monophosphate (cAMP), 3, 17–22, **18,** 315, 452

Cyclic guanosine monophosphate (GMP), 20
Cyclobenzaprine, interaction with monoamine oxidase inhibitors, **789**
Cycloplegia, 285
D-Cycloserine, 398
Cyclosporine, **130**
  interaction with buspirone, 237
Cyclothymia, 604
Cylert. *See* Magnesium pemoline
Cyproheptadine, 235
  for anorexia nervosa, 731
  effects on growth hormone, 449
  effects on isolation-induced hyperactivity in animals, 87
Cytochrome P$_{450}$, 129–130, **130,** 173
  P$_{450}$-2D6, 145–146, 173, 587, 786
Cytokines, 461–464
  in Alzheimer's disease, 399

DAG. *See* Diacylglycerol
Dalmane. *See* Flurazepam
Danazol, interaction with carbamazepine, 359, **795**
Dangerousness, 769–771. *See also* Aggression
Dantrolene sodium, 257, 629, 776
DDAVP. *See* Desmopressin
Debrisoquin, 145, 173
Deficit Syndrome Scale, **619**
Delirium, 791
  alcohol withdrawal, 775
  calcium channel blocker–induced, 385
  definition of, 775
  emergency treatment of, 775
  tricyclic antidepressant-induced, 153
Delirium tremens, 708
Delusions, 479, 615, 616
  in Alzheimer's disease, 658–659
  bupropion-induced, 203

Dementia, 523–529, 775, 812–814. *See also* Alzheimer's disease
  treatment of, 391–400, 657–665, 813–814
Demoxepam, **218, 409**
Deoxyribonucleic acid (DNA), 31–38
Depakene; Depakote. *See* Valproate
Depolarization, 66, 304
Depolarization inactivation, 253, 619
L-Deprenyl, 8, 183, **184,** 185
  for Alzheimer's disease, 397
    physostigmine and, 392, 397
  for depression, 190
  drug interactions with, 397
  effects in chronic mild stress model in animals, 95
  history and discovery of, 397
  metabolites of, 397
  for parkinsonian symptoms, 187, 190, 627
  pharmacokinetics and elimination of, 397
  pharmacological profile of, 397
  side effects and toxicity of, 190, 397
  structure of, 397
Depression. *See also* Mood disorders
  in Alzheimer's disease, 664–665
  animal models of, 84–104. *See also* Animal models
  atypical, 150, 186, 583
  bipolar, 584, 604, 608–609
  brain imaging in, 459–461, **460–461**
  catecholamine hypothesis of, 143, 147, 439, 451
  delusional, 583–584
  dexamethasone suppression test for, 440, 446–447, 581
  in children and adolescents, 681

drug-induced, 576, **577**
  β-blockers, 291
  clonidine, 677
  nicotine, 396
  oxotremorine, 396
  reserpine, 439–440
in DSM-IV, 440–441
in elderly persons, 585, 807–810
generalized anxiety disorder and, 646
immune function and, 462–464
medical conditions associated with, 576, **577**
melancholic, 580
menopausal, 449–450, 591–592
mental retardation and, 696
neuroendocrinology of, 440, 445–450
  hypothalamic-growth hormone axis, 448–449, **450**
  hypothalamic-pituitary-adrenal axis, 165, 440, **445,** 445–447
  hypothalamic-pituitary-gonadal axis, 449–450
  hypothalamic-pituitary-thyroid axis, 447–448, **448**
placebo response in child with, 670
poststroke, 578–579
psychotic, 150, 200, 255, 455–456
relapse rate for, 585–586
role of neurotransmitters and receptors in, 144, 450–459
  acetylcholine, 457
  adrenergic receptors, 452–453
  gamma-aminobutyric acid, 456–457
  dopamine and dopamine β-hydroxylase: monoamine oxidase, 455–456

  norepinephrine, **450,** 451–452
  pineal function and circadian rhythm, 457
  second messenger systems, 457–459, **458**
    adenylate cyclase system, 458
    G proteins, 458
    phosphoinositide system and calcium, 458–459
  serotonin, 439–440, 453–455, **454–455**
  schizophrenia and, 617
  smoking and, 719–720
  thyrotropin-releasing hormone stimulation test for, 440
  Tourette's disorder and, 692
  treatment-refractory, 9, **588,** 588–589
  unipolar major, 582–583
Depression treatment, 575–593. *See also* Antidepressants
  for acute depressive episode, 576
  antidepressant combinations for, 589–590
  in children and adolescents, 680–683
    assessing response to, 682
    assessment for, 681
    continuation, maintenance, and monitoring of, 682
    discontinuation of, 683
    initiation of, 682, **682**
    managing side effects of, 682–683
    resistance to, 683
    selecting therapy for, 681
  for depressive subtypes, **582,** 582–585
    alcoholism-associated depression, 709
    atypical depression, 583
    bipolar depression, 584, 608–609

Depression treatment
(continued)
for depressive subtypes
delusional depression,
583–584
dysthymic disorder, 584
geriatric depression, 585
unipolar major depression,
582–583
duration of, 585–586
in elderly persons, 807–810
bupropion, 809–810
monoamine oxidase
inhibitors, 810
selective serotonin reuptake
inhibitors, 810
trazodone, 809
tricyclics, 808, 809
electroconvulsive therapy,
592
estrogen, 591–592
in Europe, 843–844
factors influencing drug
choice for, 580–581
neurobiological predictors
of response, 580–581
symptomatic predictors of
response, 580–581
future of drug therapy for,
592–593
history of, 575–576
lithium augmentation of
antidepressants for,
321, 590–591
medical evaluation prior to,
576–580, **577, 579**
allergies, 580
cancer, 579–580
cardiovascular disease,
577–578
gastrointestinal disease, 580
glaucoma, 580
neurological disease,
578–579
sexual dysfunction, 580
miscellaneous approaches
for, 592
monitoring antidepressant
blood levels during,
586–587

psychiatric evaluation prior
to, 580
for refractory depression,
588, 588–589
changing antidepressant
drug, 588–589
maximizing antidepressant
trial, 588
thyroid hormones and
antidepressants for, 591
Deprol. See
Meprobamate/benactyzine
N-Desalkylflurazepam, 217,
218, 409
Desipramine (DMI), **130**
animal studies of
chronic mild stress model,
95
clonidine withdrawal, 91
differential operant
responding for low
reinforcement, 86
isolation-induced
hyperactivity, 87
muricide, 85
swim test immobility, 89,
91, 101, 104
biochemical effects of,
143–144, **144**
combined with fluoxetine,
129, 589
elimination half-life of, **145**
indications for, **151**
attention-deficit
hyperactivity
disorder, 673, 677
binge-eating disorder, 730
bulimia nervosa, 727
cocaine abuse, 711
panic disorder, 642
posttraumatic stress
disorder, 650
protracted cocaine
withdrawal, 548
methylphenidate potentiation
of, 425
structure-activity relationship
for, 142, **142**
sudden cardiac death in
children on, 152, 682

therapeutic plasma
concentration of, 147,
586–587
use in pregnancy, **827**
Desmethylchlordiazepoxide, **218**
Desmethylcitalopram, 165–166
Desmethylclomipramine, 146,
165, 168
N-Desmethyl-deprenyl, 397
N-Desmethyldiazepam,
217–218, 221, 409, **409**
discontinuation of, 128
plasma concentrations of, **128**
Desmethyl-hydroxynefazodone,
206
Desmethylsertraline, **129,** 165
O-Desmethylvenlafaxine, 204
Desmopressin (DDAVP),
694–695
Desyrel. See Trazodone
Detoxification
from alcohol, 707–708
from benzodiazepines, 710
from opioids, 712–713
Developmental toxicology, 671
Dexamethasone suppression
test (DST), 440, 446–447
in anorexia nervosa, 561–562
in children and adolescents,
681
monoamine oxidase activity
and, 456
Dextroamphetamine (DAMPH,
Dexedrine), 263, 417, 418.
See also Amphetamine
animal studies of
muricide, 85
tail suspension test, 91
clinical use of, **675**
combined with monoamine
oxidase inhibitor, 590
dosage of, 422
indications for
affective disorders, 423
attention-deficit
hyperactivity
disorder, 673–677
potentiation of
antidepressants, 425,
426

prediction of
    antidepressant
    responsiveness, 426
long-acting, 674–675
mechanism of action of, 8, 9,
    423
for medically ill patients,
    793–794
Dextropropoxyphene,
    interaction with
    carbamazepine, 359
Diabetes insipidus,
    nephrogenic, 326
Diabetic neuropathy, 171
Diacylglycerol (DAG), 3, 17, 20,
    22–23, 318, 458
Diagnostic Interview for
    Children and Adolescents
    Revised (DICA-R), 678
Diagnostic Interview Schedule
    (DIS), **618**
Dialysis patients
    cyclic antidepressants for, 787
    lithium for, 793
Diarrhea, drug-induced
    HP 029, 394
    selective serotonin reuptake
        inhibitors, 582
    valproate, 365
Diazepam, 215, 223
    discontinuation of, 128
    drug interactions with, 224
        buspirone, 236
        fluoxetine, **129**
    effects on isolation-induced
        hyperactivity in
        animals, 87
    electroencephalographic
        effects of, 132–133,
        132–133
    half-life of, 217–218, **218,** 409
    indications for, 413, 414
        alcohol withdrawal
            symptoms, 708, 775
        assaultive behavior, 774
        childhood sleep disorders,
            696
        children's anxiety in
            medical setting, 691
        dementia, 663

generalized anxiety
    disorder, 647
    in children and
        adolescents, 688
panic disorder, 643
phencyclidine intoxication,
    776
psychiatric emergencies,
    771, **771**
metabolism of, 217, 409, **409**
plasma concentrations of, **128**
structure of, **409**
use in pregnancy, 830, **831**
Diazepam-binding inhibitor
    (DBI), 221
Dibenzoxazepines, **249,** 250
Diclofenac, interaction with
    lithium, **327,** 329
Diet
    cyclic antidepressants and
        fiber in, **786**
    monoamine oxidase
        inhibitors and tyramine
        in, 187–188, **188,** 190,
        583
Diethylpropion, 419, 431
Diethylstilbestrol, 807
Digoxin interactions
    with benzodiazepines,
        224–225
    with calcium channel
        blockers, 385
    with lithium, **327,** 329
    with nefazodone, 207
    with selective serotonin
        reuptake inhibitors,
        582, **786,** 787
3,4-Dihydrophenylacetic acid
    (DOPAC), 310
2,3-Dihydroxy-6-nitro-7-sulfa-
    moylbenzo(F)quinoxaline
    (NBQX), 398
Diltiazem, **130,** 378, **378**
    antimanic effect of, 379
    dosage of, **384**
    interaction with
        carbamazepine, 359, **795**
    pharmacokinetics of, 382,
        382
    structure of, **379**

6,7-Dinitroquinoxaline-2,3-dione
    (DNQX), 398
Diphenhydramine, 231
    drug interactions with, 288
    history and discovery of, 287
    indications for, 288
        aggressive behavior, 746
        anxiety in children and
            adolescents, 688, 689
        in medical setting, 691
        dementia, 663
        extrapyramidal side effects,
            284, 287–288, 292,
            627, 684, 776
        neuroleptic malignant
            syndrome, 776
        schizophrenia in children,
            683
        sedation, 414
        sleep disorders
            in children, 695
            in elderly persons, 812
    mechanism of action of, 288
    pharmacokinetics and
        disposition of, 287–288
    pharmacological profile of, 287
    side effects and toxicology
        of, 288
    structure-activity relations for,
        287
    use during pregnancy, 829,
        829
Direct acting drugs, 9
Disinhibition, drug-induced
    benzodiazepines, 689, 690
    fluoxetine, 690
Disorientation, benzodiazepine-
    induced, 414
Dissociative episodes, 772–773
Disulfiram
    for alcoholism, 708
    interaction with
        benzodiazepines, 224,
        794
    interaction with cyclic
        antidepressants, **786**
Diuretic interactions
    with lithium, **327,** 329, **793**
    with monoamine oxidase
        inhibitors, **789**

Divalproex sodium, 360–361, 363, 365, 377. *See also* Valproate

Dizziness, drug-induced
amphetamine, 429
benzodiazepines, 414
buspirone, 237
calcium channel blockers, 384
carbamazepine, 358, 686
clomipramine, 690
clonidine, 693
HP 029, 394
monoamine oxidase inhibitors, 187
nefazodone, 207
oxcarbazepine, 368
trazodone, 198
tricyclic antidepressants, 682
venlafaxine, 205

DNA
complementary DNA cloning, 36–37, **36–37**
recombinant DNA technology, 35–38
structure of, 31–32

DNA ligase, 36

DNQX. *See* 6,7-Dinitroquinoxaline-2,3-dione

L-Dopa, 5, 54
interaction with L-deprenyl, 397
interaction with monoamine oxidase inhibitors, **789**
stimulation of growth hormone release by, 449

DOPAC. *See* 3,4-Dihydro-phenylacetic acid

Dopa-decarboxylase, 5

Dopamine agonists, 7–9, 12, **47,** 57
interaction with antipsychotics, 259
for neuroleptic malignant syndrome, 776
partial, 266
psychosis induced by, 263

Dopamine antagonists, 7, **47,** 57
for Tourette's disorder, 691–692

Dopamine (DA), 4, 45–51
comparison of dopamine and serotonin systems in brain, 9
criteria for transmitter role of, 4–5
dopamine receptor affinity for, **47**
dopamine-synthesizing cell groups, **46,** 46–47
effect of chronic opiate administration on, 547
effects of selective serotonin reuptake inhibitors on, 164–165
electrophysiological measures of, 77
interaction with monoamine oxidase inhibitors, **789**
lithium effects on, 309–310
metabolism of, 8
role in depression, 455–456
role in reinforcement of drug-seeking behavior, 545
alcohol, 543–544
opiates, 542
stimulants, 542
role in schizophrenia, 4, 41, 110, 252, 263, 487–489
sites of drug action for, **6**
steps in chemical transmission, 5–9
synaptic regulation of, 54–57, **55**
synthesis, storage, and release of, 5–7
transporters for, 56

Dopamine β-hydroxylase, 456

Dopamine receptors, 5, 7–8, 14, 15, 18, 47–51, 56, 265–268
anatomical distribution of, 47–50, **49, 266**
autoreceptors, 49, 56
colocalization of, 50–51
coupling to G proteins, 58
D_1 receptor, 267–268
D_2 receptor, 265–267
blocking by antipsychotics, 252–253, 263, 265–266, **268**

D_3 receptor, 267
D_4 receptor, 267
D_5 receptor, 268
drug effects on number of, 57
gene structure of, 48
in schizophrenia, 488–489
subtypes of, 47–48

Doral. *See* Quazepam

Down's syndrome, 529

Doxepin
biochemical effects of, **144**
elimination half-life of, **145**
indications for, **151**
for nicotine dependence, 719
structure-activity relationship for, **142,** 143
use in pregnancy, **827**

Doxylamine, 414

Drug Abuse Warning Network (DAWN), 431, 710

Drug efficacy, 12

Drug interactions
with amantadine, 289
with amoxapine, 200
with antidepressants, 587
monoamine oxidase inhibitors, 188–189, **789**
selective serotonin reuptake inhibitors, 129, **129–130,** 173, 582
tricyclics, 153–154, **786**
with antipsychotics, 258–259, 630, **630**
with barbiturates, 408
with benzodiazepines, 224–225, **794**
with β-blockers, 291
with bupropion, 203–204
with buspirone, 236–237
with calcium channel blockers, 385, **385**
with carbamazepine, 359, **795,** 795–796
with clozapine, 273
with L-deprenyl, 397
with diphenhydramine, 288
with lithium, **327,** 327–329, **793**

with moclobemide, 190
with nefazodone, 207
with physostigmine, 392
predictability of, 129–130, **130**
with stimulants, 431–432, **794**
with tetrahydroamino-
acridine, 393
with trazodone, 198–199
with trihexyphenidyl, 286
with valproate, 366, **797**
with venlafaxine, 205
Drugs
active metabolites of, 127
duration of action of, 126
elimination half-life of, 126
interdose fluctuations of, 127,
128
intravenous administration
of, 126
minimum effective
concentration (MEC) of,
126, **126–127**
oral administration of, 127,
127–128
pharmacodynamics of, 125,
130–133
pharmacokinetics of, 125–130
steady-state concentration of,
127–129, **128**
Drug-seeking behavior, 538–540
Dry mouth, drug-induced, 256
amphetamine, 429
antipsychotics, 629, 777
clonidine, 677, 693
clozapine, 273–274
L-deprenyl, 397
monoamine oxidase
inhibitors, 187
nefazodone, 207
selective serotonin reuptake
inhibitors, 172
tricyclic antidepressants, 153,
682
trihexyphenidyl, 285
venlafaxine, 205
Dynorphin, lithium effects on,
313
Dyspepsia, valproate-induced,
365
Dysthymic disorder, 584

Dystonic reactions, acute, 251,
255–256, 282, 625, **626,**
627, 776. *See also*
Extrapyramidal side effects
amoxapine-induced, 200
in children and adolescents, 684
risk factors for, **290,** 292

Eating disorders, 557–567
anorexia nervosa, 557–564,
730–731
binge-eating disorder, 730
bulimia nervosa, 564–567,
725–730
Ebstein's anomaly, 327, 824
"Ecstasy," 420, 718
Edema, peripheral
calcium channel
blocker-induced, 384
monoamine oxidase
inhibitor-induced, 187
Effexor. *See* Venlafaxine
Eicosanoids, 24
Elavil. *See* Amitriptyline
Elderly persons, 803–814
disease and disability among,
803–804
electroconvulsive therapy for,
585
factors affecting psychotropic
drug use in, 804–805
effect of aging and
disease, 804
pharmacodynamics, 804–805
pharmacokinetics, 805
side effects, 805
medication use by, 804
social context of aging
and, 804
physiological changes in, 803
polypharmacy and, 805
psychiatric emergencies in, 779
suicide among, 779
treating anxiety in, 811–812
benzodiazepines, 217, 644,
811
buspirone, 236, 811–812
treating dementia in,
657–665, 812–814. *See*
also Alzheimer's disease

treating depression in, 585,
786, 807–810
bupropion, 585, 809–810
monoamine oxidase
inhibitors, 585, 810
selective serotonin
reuptake inhibitors,
166, 585, 810
trazodone, 197, 585, 809
tricyclics, 146, 153, 585,
809–810
trihexyphenidyl, 286
treating mania in, 810–811
treating psychosis, agitation,
and behavioral
disruption in, 805–807
anticonvulsants, 807
antipsychotics, 806–807
β-blockers, 807
buspirone, 807
estrogen, 807
lithium, 807
selective serotonin
reuptake inhibitors,
807
trazodone, 807
treating sleep disorders in,
812
Electroconvulsive therapy (ECT)
animal studies of
chronic mild stress model,
95
differential operant
responding for low
reinforcement, 86
swim test immobility, 89
uncontrollable shock
model, 96
yohimbine lethality, 85
for elderly persons, 585
indications for
bipolar disorder, 609, 774
major depression, 592
neuroleptic malignant
syndrome, 629
psychosis, 634
schizophrenia, 621
treatment-resistant mania
in adolescents, 680
lithium and, 328–329

ECT *(continued)*
    for medically ill patients,
        796–797
    monoamine oxidase
        inhibitors and, 788
Electroencephalography (EEG),
    67, 69
    antipsychotic effects on, 777,
        792
    benzodiazepine effects on,
        131–133, **132–133**
    in bulimia nervosa, 566
    cocaine effects on, 548
Electrophysiology
    electrochemical gradient,
        65–67, **68–69**
    preparations used in, 73–77
        for invertebrates and lower
            vertebrates, 74
        for recordings from
            dissociated neurons
            and neuronal cell
            cultures, 76–77
        for in vitro recordings from
            brain slices, 75–76, **77**
        for in vivo recordings,
            74–75, **76**
    relationship between
        biochemical and
        electrophysiological
        measures of neuronal
        activity, 77–78
    techniques of, 67–78
        electroencephalographic
            recordings, 67, 69
        field potential recordings,
            69
        intracellular recordings, 70,
            72, **74**
        patch clamp recordings, 73
        single unit extracellular
            recordings, 69–70,
            71–73
Emergency treatment. *See*
    Psychiatric emergencies
Enalapril, interaction with
    lithium, **793**
Endep. *See* Amitriptyline
Endocrine effects. *See also*
    Neuroendocrinology

of antipsychotics, 251, 258,
    629
of buspirone, 236
of carbamazepine, 352, 358
of fenfluramine, 455
of lithium, 325–326
β-Endorphin, 445–446, 464, 546
Enkephalin, 313
Enuresis, 694–695
    causes of, 694
    clozapine-induced, 273
    desmopressin for, 694–695
    lithium-induced, 679
    tricyclic antidepressants for,
        150–151, **151,** 694
Enzymes, 3, 4
Ephedrine, 418
    interaction with monoamine
        oxidase inhibitors, 787,
        789
Epidemiologic Catchment Area
    (ECA) study
    of mood disorders, 442
    of substance abuse, 430
Epinephrine
    effects in social phobia, 508
    interaction with cyclic
        antidepressants, 154, **786**
    interaction with monoamine
        oxidase inhibitors, 787,
        789
    role in posttraumatic stress
        disorder, 509
Epstein-Barr virus, 462
Erythro-hydrobupropion, 201
Erythromycin, interaction with
    carbamazepine, 359, **795**
Eskalith. *See* Lithium
Estazolam, 790, 812
    use in pregnancy, **831**
Estrogen
    for agitation in elderly
        persons, 807
    in anorexia nervosa, 563
    interaction with
        benzodiazepines, 224,
        794
    for menopausal depression,
        591–592
Ethchlorvynol, 414

Ethical issues, 670
Ethyl-β-carboxylate, 221
Ethylpropion, 431
European-approved drugs,
    839–845, **840–842**
    for anxiety disorders, 844–845
    for depression, 843–844
    for schizophrenia, 840, 843
Extrapyramidal side effects
    (EPS), 200, 248, 251,
        255–256, 263, 281–294,
        625–628, **626,** 776, 792
    in children and adolescents,
        684, 692
    effect on treatment outcome,
        281–282
    in elderly persons, 806–807
    etiology of, 282–283
    history of, 281–282
    incidence of, 282
    in neonate, 828
    rating scales for, 283–284
    selective serotonin reuptake
        inhibitor–induced, 172
    serum calcium level and,
        282–283
    types of, 282, 625–628, **626**
Extrapyramidal side effects (EPS)
    treatment, 256, **291,** 291–293
    for acute dystonic reactions,
        627
    for akathisia, 292, 628
    anticholinergic drugs for,
        284, 284–287
        benztropine, 286–287
        biperiden, 287
        procyclidine, 287
        trihexyphenidyl, 284–286
    atypical neuroleptics and, 293
    benzodiazepines for, 291
    buspirone for, 237, 239–240
    depot neuroleptics and, 292
    diphenhydramine for, **284,**
        287–288
    dopaminergic drugs for,
        288–291
        amantadine, 288–289
        β-blockers, **289,** 289–291
    duration of, 293–294
    for parkinsonism, 627

during pregnancy, 829, **829**
prophylactic, 292
for tardive movement
disorders, 292–293, 628

Family studies
of mood disorders, 442
of schizophrenia, 479–480
Family therapy
for attention-deficit
hyperactivity disorder,
672
for obsessive-compulsive
disorder, 689
for panic disorder in
children, 690
for posttraumatic stress
disorder in children, 691
for schizophrenia, 622
for separation anxiety
disorder, 688
Fatigue, 203
drug-induced
carbamazepine, 358
clomipramine, 690
oxcarbazepine, 368
Felodipine, **378**
Fenfluramine, 419, 431
aggression related to prolactin
response to, 759
for autism, 693
for bulimia nervosa, 169, 729
neuroendocrine effects of, 455
for obsessive-compulsive
disorder, 168
Fever, clozapine-induced, 274
Fibrositis, 171
Field potential recordings, 69
Flat affect, 479
Flecainide, interaction with
selective serotonin reuptake
inhibitors, 173
Flunarizine, **378,** 379
Flunitrazepam, **409**
Fluoxetine, 9, 56, 453, 576
animal studies of
depression of active
responding induced
by 5-hydroxy-
tryptophan, 89

differential operant
responding for low
reinforcement, 86
cardiovascular effects of, 784
for children and adolescents,
681
combined with desipramine,
589
drug interactions with, 129,
129–130, 173, 582,
786, 786–787
antipsychotics, 258
bupropion, 203
carbamazepine, **795**
clozapine, 273
monoamine oxidase
inhibitors, **789**
tricyclic antidepressants,
587
valproate, 366
indications for
alcoholism, 170
anorexia nervosa, 731
autism, 694
bipolar depression,
608–609
borderline personality
disorder, 760
bulimia nervosa, 169–170,
727
obesity, 170
obsessive-compulsive
disorder, 649
associated with
Tourette's disorder,
692
in children and
adolescents,
689–690
panic disorder, 168,
642–643, **643**
schizophrenia, 169
social phobia, 648
inhibition of P_{450}-2D6 by, 146
initiating monoamine oxidase
inhibitor after, 166
metabolite of, 128, 165
overdose of, 173–174
pharmacokinetics of,
165–166, **166,** 786–787

side effects in children and
adolescents, 690
sleep effects of, 171
structure-activity relationship
for, **162,** 162–163, **841**
suicidality and, 727
use in cardiac disease
patients, 577, 784
use in pregnancy, 827, **827**
Flupentixol, 105, 248, 840,
840–842, 844
Fluphenazine, 35, 619
for children's anxiety in
medical setting, 691
dosage of, 248, **249, 620**
effects on latent inhibition of
conditioned responses
in animals, **107**
history and discovery of, 248
protein binding of, 252
structure-activity relationship
for, 248, **249, 840**
for Tourette's disorder, 692
use during pregnancy, **829**
Fluphenazine decanoate, 252,
255, **620**
Flurazepam
half-life of, **218,** 409
indications for, 413, 812
metabolism of, 217
structure of, **409**
use in pregnancy, **831**
Fluspirilene, 250
Fluvoxamine, 453, **840–842,**
843
for alcoholism, 170
for autism, 694
drug interactions with, 173
metabolite of, 166
for panic disorder, 169,
642–643, **643**
pharmacokinetics of,
165–166, **166**
structure of, **162, 841**
use in pregnancy, **827**
Follicle stimulating hormone
(FSH)
antipsychotic effects on, 251
in depression, 450
fos gene, 319

Fragile X syndrome, 39–40
Freud, Sigmund, 439

G protein–linked receptors,
14–15, **16**
G protein–linked signal
transduction, 17, **18,** 19
G proteins, 3
effect of chronic opiate
administration on, 547
lithium effects on, 316–317
in mood disorders, 458
Galactorrhea,
antipsychotic-induced, 251,
258, 629
Galanthamine, 394
for Alzheimer's disease, 394
history and discovery of, 394
pharmacokinetics and
disposition of, 394
pharmacological profile of, 394
side effects and toxicity of,
394
structure of, 394
Gallamine, interaction with
diazepam, 224
Gastrointestinal effects
of amphetamine, 429
of anorexia nervosa, **558,** 559
of antidepressants, 580
of antipsychotics, 629
of bulimia nervosa, **565**
of L-deprenyl, 397
of physostigmine, 392
of tetrahydroaminoacridine,
393
of valproate, 365
Geller-Seifter test, 216
Gene expression, 33–38
drug effects on
antipsychotics, 35
cocaine, 548
lithium, 319
opiates, 547
manipulation of, 35–38
complementary DNA
cloning, 36–37, **36–37**
expression of recombinant
genes, 38
genomic cloning, 37

restriction fragment length
polymorphisms, 37,
38
regulation of, **33,** 33–35
variability of, 444
Gene therapy, 41
Generalized anxiety disorder
(GAD), 501
depression and, 646
prevalence of, 646
symptoms of, 646
treatment of, 646–647
antihistamines, 689
benzodiazepines, 222–223,
646–647, 688–689
buspirone, 237–238, 240,
647, 689
in children and
adolescents, 688–689
cognitive-behavioral
therapy, 647
in Europe, 844–845
imipramine, 647
meprobamate, 234
monoamine oxidase
inhibitors, 186
new agents, 647
Genes, 32–33
amplification of, 33
candidate, 443
Genetic code, 32
Genetic engineering, 35
Genetics
degree of penetrance, 444
inheritance patterns, 443
linkage analysis, 443, 444, 480
phenocopies, 444
of psychiatric disorders
Alzheimer's disease, 40,
526–527
mood disorders, 442–445
obsessive-compulsive
disorder, 510–511
panic disorder, 502
personality disorders, 753
schizophrenia, 479–481
Tourette's disorder, 691
restriction fragment length
polymorphisms, 443–444
segregation analysis, 443, 444

single sequence repeat
markers, 444
variable number of tandem
repeats, 444
Genome, 31–33
Genomic cloning, 37
Gepirone, 208, 235, **236**
Geriatrics. *See* Elderly persons
Glaucoma patients, 153, 785
antidepressants for, 580, 785
antipsychotics for, 629, 777,
792
Glucose intolerance, 559, **559**
Glutamate, 4, **6,** 10, 397–398,
549
role in schizophrenia, 489, **490**
Glutamate receptors, 14, 398
alcohol effects on, 549
Glutamatergic agents, 397–398
for Alzheimer's disease,
397–398
glycine site inhibitors, 398
history and background of,
397–398
non-NMDA antagonists, 398
partial agonists, 398
Glutethimide, interaction with
antidepressants, 587
Glycine site inhibitors, 398
Goiter, lithium-induced, 325
Gonadotropin-releasing
hormone (GnRH), 450, 562
Grief, 772
Growth factors, 15, 20
Growth hormone (GH)
in anorexia nervosa, 563–564
in bulimia nervosa, 566
buspirone effects on, 236
response to clonidine
in mood disorders,
448–449, **450**
in panic disorder, 504
in social phobia, 508
Growth hormone–releasing
factor (GRF), 449
Growth retardation,
stimulant-induced, 676
Guanabenz, 712
Guanethidine interactions
with antipsychotics, 259

with cyclic antidepressants, 154, **786**

with monoamine oxidase inhibitors, **789**

with stimulants, **794**

Guanfacine

for Alzheimer's disease, 813

for opioid detoxification, 712

Guanosine diphosphate, 17, **18,** 19

Guanosine triphosphate, 17–19, **18,** 458

Guanylate cyclase, 20

Gynecomastia, antipsychotic-induced, 251

Hair loss, valproate-induced, 365

Halazepam, **218**

use in pregnancy, **831**

Halcion. *See* Triazolam

Haldol. *See* Haloperidol

Hallucinations, 479, 615, 616

in Alzheimer's disease, 657, 658

bupropion-induced, 203

Hallucinogen abuse, 35, 420, 717–718

Haloperidol decanoate, 252, 255

Haloperidol (Haldol), 35, 619

animal studies of

isolation-induced hyperactivity, 87

latent inhibition of conditioned responses, **107**

in breast milk, 828

dopamine receptor affinity for, 47, **47,** 57

dosage of, 248, **249, 620**

drug interactions with

buspirone, 237

fluoxetine, **129**

tricyclic antidepressants, 154

history and discovery of, 248

indications for

aggression, 774

acute, 745, **745**

in children and adolescents, 686

agitation in elderly persons, 806

autism, 693

dementia, 659–661, 663–664

phencyclidine intoxication, 718, 776

psychiatric emergencies, **771**

rapid neuroleptization, 774

schizotypal personality disorder, 757–758

Tourette's disorder, 255, 691–692

treatment-resistant mania, 680

protein binding of, 252

reduced, 251

separation anxiety and school avoidance due to, 687

structure-activity relationship for, **249,** 250, **840**

therapeutic window for, 624

use in Europe, 840

use in pregnancy, 828, **829**

Halstead-Reitan Neuropsychological Battery, 743

Hamilton Rating Scale for Depression (HRS-D), 167, 650, 681

Harm avoidance, 764

Head trauma patients

aggression among, 735

selective serotonin reuptake inhibitors for, 171

Headache

cluster, 322

drug-induced

amphetamine, 429

benzodiazepines, 414

buspirone, 237

calcium channel blockers, 384

HP 029, 394

monoamine oxidase inhibitors, 187

oxcarbazepine, 368

selective serotonin reuptake inhibitors, 582, 690

Hematological effects. *See also* Agranulocytosis

of anorexia nervosa, **558,** 560

of antipsychotics, **627,** 629

of carbamazepine, 358–359, 686, 794–795

of lithium, 322–323

of valproate, 365, 680

"Heroinism," 711–712

Herpes simplex virus

lithium for, 323

mood disorders and, 462

5-HIAA. *See* 5-Hydroxy-indoleacetic acid

Hillside Akathisia Scale, 284

Hippocampus, 111

Hippuric acid, 421, **421**

Homicidal state, 770–771

Homovanillic acid (HVA), 486

antipsychotic effect on, 252–253

bupropion effect on, 202, 203

lithium effect on, 309, 310

predicting response to clozapine by level of, 275

in schizophrenia, 487–488

in schizotypal personality disorder, 757

Hormones. *See* Endocrine effects; Neuroendocrinology

Hospitalization, psychiatric

emergency indications for, 769–771

levels of restrictive environments during, **770**

HP 029, 393–394

for Alzheimer's disease, 394

drug interactions with, 394

history and discovery of, 393–394

pharmacokinetics and disposition of, 394

pharmacological profile of, 394

side effects and toxicity of, 394

structure of, 394

5-HTP. *See* 5-Hydroxytryptophan
Human immunodeficiency virus (HIV) infection
  buspirone for methadone maintenance patients with, 239
  depression in, 462
    stimulants for, 417
  lithium use in, 323
  opioid dependence and, 714
Human leukocyte antigens (HLAs), 480
Huntington's disease (HD), 39
  antipsychotics for, 255
  obsessive-compulsive disorder and, 512
HVA. *See* Homovanillic acid
Hydergine, 814
7-Hydroxyamoxapine, 199
8-Hydroxyamoxapine, 199
Hydroxybupropion, 201, 202
7-Hydroxychlorpromazine, 251
N-Hydroxyethyl-flurazepam, **218**
7-Hydroxyfluphenazine, 251
5-Hydroxyindoleacetic acid (5-HIAA), 144, 168, 486, 581
  lithium effect on, 308
  in obsessive-compulsive disorder, 511
  predicting response to clozapine by level of, 275
  in schizophrenia, 169, 490
  suicidal behavior and, 439, 453
6-Hydroxymelatonin, 202
Hydroxynefazodone, 206
Hydroxynortriptyline, 146
9-Hydroxyrisperidone, 620
5-Hydroxytryptamine. *See* Serotonin
5-Hydroxytryptophan (5-HTP), 9, 54, 89, 449, 455
Hydroxyzine, 231
  for children's anxiety in medical setting, 691
  for sleep disorders
    in children, 695
    in elderly persons, 812

Hyperactivity. *See also* Attention-deficit hyperactivity disorder
  amphetamine for, 419
  in autism, 693
  induced by isolation in rats, 87
Hypercarotenemia, 559
Hypercholesterolemia, 559
Hyperparathyroidism, lithium-induced, 325–326
Hyperpigmentation, antipsychotic-induced, 629
Hypersalivation, drug-induced
  clozapine, 273, **632,** 633
  physostigmine, 392
Hypertension
  amphetamine-induced, 429, 430
  social phobia and, 508
Hypertensive crises, 183, 187–188, 583, 778, 787
  treatment of, 378, 778, 787–788
Hyperventilation, 503
Hypoglycemia
  5-hydroxyindoleacetic acid level and, 453
  lithium-induced, 326
Hypoglycemic agents, interaction with monoamine oxidase inhibitors, **789**
Hypokalemia
  in bulimia nervosa, 565
  lithium-induced, 679
Hypomania, 603, 606–608
Hyponatremia, drug-induced
  carbamazepine, 358, 795
  oxcarbazepine, 368
Hypothalamic-pituitary-adrenal (HPA) axis
  in anorexia nervosa, 561–562
  corticotropin-releasing factor stimulation test of activity of, 446
  immune system and, 464
  in mood disorders, 440, **445,** 445–447
  norepinephrine and, 452
  in panic disorder, 506

  in posttraumatic stress disorder, 510
  in protracted alcohol withdrawal, 549
  serotonin and, 455
  in social phobia, 508
Hypothalamic-pituitary-gonadal (HPG) axis
  in anorexia nervosa, 562–563
  in mood disorders, 449–450
Hypothalamic-pituitary-thyroid (HPT) axis
  in anorexia nervosa, 563
  in mood disorders, 447–448, **448–449**
  in panic disorder, 506
  in social phobia, 508
Hypothyroidism
  carbamazepine-induced, 796
  grading of, 448, **448**
  lithium-induced, 325, 793
  mood disorders and, 445, 447
Hysteresis, counterclockwise, **133**

Ibuprofen, interaction with lithium, **327,** 329, **793**
Idazoxan, 208
[^{123}I]Iofetamine, 459
Iminodibenzyl, 141, 352, **352**
Iminostilbene, **352**
Imipramine (IMI), 56, 453
  animal studies of
    behavioral effects of olfactory bulb lesions, 86
    chronic mild stress model, 95
    circadian rhythm readjustment, 85–86
    depression of active responding induced by 5-hydroxy-tryptophan, 89
    exhaustion stress, 94
    isolation/separation-induced depression in monkeys, 93–94
    muricide, 85
    neonatal clomipramine, 92

reserpine-induced
  reduction of motor
  activity, 89
separation of Siberian
  hamsters, 94
swim test immobility, 89
biochemical effects of, **144**
for children and adolescents,
  682
combined with stimulant,
  424–425, 589–590
drug interactions with
  fluoxetine, **129**
  methylphenidate, 431, 677
  selective serotonin
    reuptake inhibitors,
    173
elimination half-life of, **145**
history and discovery of,
  141–142, 576
indications for, **151**
  alcoholism-associated
    depression, 709
  attention-deficit
    hyperactivity
    disorder, 677
  bipolar disorder, 609
  bulimia nervosa, 727
  childhood sleep disorders,
    696
  dementia with depression,
    664–665
  enuresis, 150–151, 694
  generalized anxiety
    disorder, 647
  nicotine dependence, 719
  panic disorder, 151,
    641–642, **642**
    in children and
      adolescents, 690
  posttraumatic stress
    disorder, 650
  separation anxiety
    disorder, 688
mechanism of action of, 576
metabolic pathways for, **145**
serotonin reuptake inhibition
  by, 141
structure-activity relationship
  for, 142, **142, 841**

therapeutic plasma
  concentration of, 147,
  586–587
thyroid hormone and, 591
use in pregnancy, **827**
Immune system, 461–462
  in Alzheimer's disease, 399
  depression and, 462–464
  glucocorticoids and, 464
  interaction with central
    nervous system,
    462–464
Impulsivity
  in borderline personality
    disorder, 758
  differential diagnosis of, 759
  5-hydroxyindoleacetic acid
    level and, 453
Inappropriate affect, 616
Incertohypothalamic system, 46
Inderal. *See* Propranolol
Indirect acting drugs, 9
Indomethacin
  for Alzheimer's disease, 399
  interaction with lithium, **327,**
    329, **793**
Influenza
  amantadine for, 288
  schizophrenia and, 481
Informed consent
  for drug use during
    pregnancy, 833
  for treatment of minors, 670
Inheritance patterns, 443
Inositol triphosphate (IP$_3$), 3,
  17, 20, 22–23, 458
Interferons, 462
Interleukins, 461–462
  receptors for, 15
  role in Alzheimer's disease,
    399
Intermittent explosive disorder,
  736, **736**
International Statistical
  Classification of Diseases
  and Related Health
  Problems (ICD-10), 441,
  537
Ion-based signal transduction,
  17

Ion channels, 13–14, 65–67,
  68–69, 304
Iprindole
  animal studies of
    chronic mild stress model,
      95
    depression of active
      responding induced
      by 5-hydroxy-
      tryptophan, 89
    differential operant
      responding for low
      reinforcement, 86
    isolation-induced
      hyperactivity, 87
    swim test immobility, 89
    yohimbine lethality, 85
  mechanism of action of, 147
Iproniazid, 9, 183, 440, 575
  animal studies of
    differential operant
      responding for low
      reinforcement, 86
    muricide, 85
    swim test immobility, 89
  for panic disorder, 186
Ipsapirone, 235, **236**
Irritability, drug-induced
  clonidine, 693
  galanthamine, 394
Irritable heart syndrome, 502.
  See also Panic disorder
Isocarboxazid, 183, **184,** 185
  for bulimia nervosa, 186
  for depression, 583
  for panic disorder, 642
  use in pregnancy, **827**
Isoniazid interactions
  with benzodiazepines, 224,
    794
  with carbamazepine, 359
Isoproterenol
  interaction with monoamine
    oxidase inhibitors, 787,
    789
  panic induced by, 505
Isoptin. *See* Verapamil

Jaundice, antipsychotic-induced,
  627

Kennedy's disease (KD), 39
Kerlone. *See* Betaxolol
Kindling, 85
Kinetic-dynamic modeling
procedures, 132–133,
132–134
Klonopin. *See* Clonazepam
Kraepelin, Emil, 439

LAAM. *See* L-α-Acetyl-methadol
Lactation. *See* Breast milk;
Pregnancy and lactation
Laryngeal dystonia, 684, 776
Late luteal phase dysphoric
disorder
monoamine oxidase
inhibitors for, 186
selective serotonin reuptake
inhibitors for, 171
Latent inhibition of conditioned
responses, 106–107, **107**
Laxative abuse, 565
Learned helplessness model,
96–99, **97**
Learning disabilities, 670, 672
Lecithin, 392, 813
Lesch-Nyhan syndrome, 443
Leukopenia, drug-induced
antipsychotics, 629
carbamazepine, 358–359, 686
Leukotrienes, **23,** 24
Leyton Obsessional
Inventory-Child Version, 690
Librium. *See* Chlordiazepoxide
Lidocaine, **130**
Life charting, 605
Ligand-gated ion channels,
13–14, 17
Limbic system, in
schizophrenia, 483–484,
485–486
Linkage analysis, 443, 444
in Alzheimer's disease, 526
in panic disorder, 502
in schizophrenia, 480
β-Lipotropin, 546
Lithium, 303–330, 575, 584
brain distribution of, 324
for children and adolescents,
678–680

continuation, maintenance,
and monitoring of,
679
discontinuation of, 679–680
dosage of, 679
initiation of, 679
managing side effects of,
679
response to, 678
circadian rhythms and,
306–307
combined with monoamine
oxidase inhibitors,
590–591
drug interactions with, **327,**
327–329, **793**
antidepressants, 328
antipsychotics, 328
benzodiazepines, 327–328
bupropion, 203–204
calcium channel blockers,
385
carbamazepine, 359, 795
clozapine, 273
fluoxetine, 173
nonpsychotropic drugs, 329
psychotropic drugs,
327–329
trazodone, 198
effects on neurotransmission,
307–314
acetylcholine, 311–312
gamma-aminobutyric acid
and neuropeptides,
313–314, 456
dopamine, 309–310
norepinephrine, 310–311
serotonin, 307–309
for elderly patients, 793
electroconvulsive therapy
and, 328–329
gene expression and, 319
history and discovery of, 303
indications for, 319–323
acute depression, 321
acute mania, 320, 606–607
in elderly persons,
810–811
affective disorders, 319–320
aggression, 322, **746,** 747

in children and
adolescents, 686
agitation in elderly
persons, 807
antiviral agent, 323
autism, 694
bipolar disorder, 320–321,
610
borderline personality
disorder, 761
bulimia nervosa, 730
cluster headache, 322
hematopoietic disorders,
322–323
obsessive-compulsive
disorder, 168
other psychiatric
conditions, 322
posttraumatic stress
disorder, 650
potentiation of
antidepressant
response, 321, 590
potentiation of clozapine
response, 633
schizophrenia, 321–322
symptoms of mental
retardation, 696, 697
isotopes of, 303–304
mechanism of action of,
306–319, 329–330, 383
for medically ill patients, 793
renal disease, 793
membrane transport and,
304–306
pharmacokinetics and
disposition of, **382**
in elderly persons, 810
physicochemical properties
of, 303–304
side effects and toxicology
of, 323–327, **324,** 679
cardiovascular effects, 326,
793
central nervous system
effects, 324–325
in elderly persons, 810–811
endocrine effects, 325–326
hypoglycemia, 326
hypothyroidism, 793

miscellaneous, 326–327
renal effects, 326
risk factors for, 324
teratogenicity, 327, 831–832
weight gain, 326
signal transduction and,
314–319
adenylyl cyclase, 315–316
G proteins, 316–317
phosphoinositide turnover,
314–315
protein kinase C, 317–319
therapeutic index for, 323–324
time to response to, 607
use in pregnancy, 326,
831–832, **832**
Lithobid, Lithonate. *See* Lithium
Livedo reticularis, 289
Liver disease patients
barbiturates for, 407
benzodiazepines for, 217,
789–790
cyclic antidepressants for, 786
Liver effects
of antipsychotics, 629
of carbamazepine, 795
of HP 029, 394
of magnesium pemoline, 675
of tetrahydroaminoacridine,
393, 813
of valproate, 365, 366, 680
Lofepramine, **840–842,** 843
Lofexidine, 712
Lopressor. *See* Metoprolol
Lorazepam
abuse liability of, 233
biotransformation of, 217
discontinuation of, 128
half-life of, **218**
indications for, 413
aggression, 745–746, **746,**
774
agitated psychosis, 774
alcohol withdrawal, 775
anxiety in children and
adolescents, 688
bipolar disorder, 366–367,
367
conversion disorder, 773
mania, 680, 774

panic disorder, 644
phencyclidine intoxication,
776
psychiatric emergencies,
771, **771**
status epilepticus, 777
intramuscular, 217
use in pregnancy, 830, **831**
Lormetazepam, 217
"Love drug," 420
Loxapine (Loxitane), 143, 150
for borderline personality
disorder, 762
for dementia, 660
dosage of, **249, 620**
structure-activity relationship
for, **249,** 250
use during pregnancy, **829**
Loxitane. *See* Loxapine
Ludiomil. *See* Maprotiline
Luria-Nebraska
Neuropsychological Battery,
743
Luteinizing hormone (LH)
in anorexia nervosa, 562
antipsychotic effects on, 251
in bulimia nervosa, 566
in depression, 450
Luteinizing hormone–releasing
hormone (LHRH), 450
Luvox. *See* Fluvoxamine
Lysergic acid diethylamide
(LSD), 89, 169, 489,
717–718

α_2-Macroglobulin, 399
Magical thinking, 670, 757
Magnesium pemoline, 794
for attention-deficit
hyperactivity disorder,
672–676
clinical use of, **675**
combined with monoamine
oxidase inhibitor, 590
for depression, 423, 425
for medically ill patients,
793–794
Magnetic resonance imaging
(MRI), 304
in Alzheimer's disease, 524

in mood disorders, 459–461,
460
in obsessive-compulsive
disorder, 512
in posttraumatic stress
disorder, 510
in schizophrenia, 112,
482–484, **483, 486**
Magnetic resonance
spectroscopy (MRS), 459, 461
Mania, 603. *See also* Bipolar
disorder; Mood disorders
diagnosis in children and
adolescents, 678
in DSM-IV, 440, 441
drug therapy for, 606–608
antipsychotics, 255
benzodiazepines, 351, 774
calcium channel blockers,
378–379, 383–384
carbamazepine, 355, **356,**
607–608
in elderly persons, 810–811
lithium, 320, 606–607, 774
oxcarbazepine, 368, **368**
phenytoin, 368–369
valproate, **363,** 363–364,
607, 774
verapamil, 608
drug-induced, 609, 773
bupropion, 202
fluoxetine, 690
trazodone, 198
mixed, 604
organic workup for, 773
with psychotic features, 604
pure (classical), 604
role of catecholamines in,
451–452
Mania Rating Scale (MRS), 678
MAOIs. *See* Monoamine oxidase
inhibitors
Maprotiline
biochemical effects of, 144,
144
elimination half-life of, **145**
seizures induced by, 578
structure-activity relationship
for, **142,** 143
use in pregnancy, **827**

Marijuana, 717, 776
Marplan. *See* Isocarboxazid
Mazindol, 431
MDA. *See* 2,3-Methylenedioxy-
    amphetamine
MDMA. *See* Methylenedioxy-
    methamphetamine
Medically ill patients, 783–797
    antidepressants for, 576–580,
        783–787
        allergies, 580
        cancer, 579–580
        cardiac disease, 577–578,
            579, 783–785
        drug interactions, **786**
        gastrointestinal disease,
            579, 580
        glaucoma, **579**, 580, 785
        neurological disease,
            578–579, **579**,
            785–786
        pharmacokinetic
            considerations,
            786–787
        renal failure and dialysis,
            787
        urogenital disorders, 785
    antipsychotics for, 791–793
        cardiac disease, 791–792
        clozapine, 792–793
        drug interactions, **791**
        glaucoma, 629, 777
        other medical conditions,
            792
        pulmonary disease, 792
        seizure disorders, 258
        side effects, 792
    benzodiazepines for,
        789–790
        drug interactions, **794**
    buspirone for, 790
    carbamazepine for, 794–796
        drug interactions, **795**
    electroconvulsive therapy for,
        796–797
    lithium for, 793
        cardiac disease, 793
        drug interactions, **793**
        hypothyroidism, 793
        renal disease, 793

monoamine oxidase
    inhibitors for, 787–789
    cardiac disease, 784, 788
    drug interactions, **789**
    pyridoxine deficiency, 789
    seizure disorders,
        788–789
    stimulants for, 793–794
    drug interactions, **794**
    valproate for, 796
    drug interactions, **797**
Melanocyte-stimulating
    hormone (MSH), 546
Melatonin
    in anorexia nervosa, 564
    in depression, 457
Mellaril. *See* Thioridazine
Melperone, **840–842**, 843
Memory impairment
    drug-induced
        benzodiazepines, 224
        monoamine oxidase
            inhibitors, 187
        tricyclic antidepressants,
            153
        trihexyphenidyl, 285–286
    organic causes of, 773
    psychogenic, 772–773
Menopause, 449–450, 591–592
Mental retardation, 669,
    696–697
    antipsychotics for symptoms
        of, 255, 696–697
    assessment instruments used
        in, 696
    attention-deficit hyperactivity
        disorder and, 696
    buspirone for symptoms of,
        240, 697
    depression and, 696
    schizophrenia and, 696
Meperidine interactions
    with moclobemide, 190
    with monoamine oxidase
        inhibitors, 188–189,
        789
Mephenesin, 231
Meprobamate, 231–234
    abuse liability of, 233
    dosage of, 234

history and discovery of,
    231–232
indications for, 233–234
mechanisms of action of,
    232–233
overdose of, 232
pharmacokinetics and
    disposition of, 232
pharmacological profile of,
    232
structure-activity relationship
    for, 232, **232**
Meprobamate/benactyzine, 233
Mesolimbic system, 46
Mesoridazine, 251, 619
    dosage of, **620**
    effects on latent inhibition of
        conditioned responses
        in animals, **107**
    for schizotypal personality
        disorder, 757
    use during pregnancy, **829**
Metaraminol, interaction with
    monoamine oxidase
    inhibitors, **789**
Metergoline, 512
Methadone detoxification
    regimen, 712–713
Methadone maintenance, 549,
    713–715
    abstinence of patients on,
        713–714
    admittance to programs for,
        714–715
    benzodiazepine use and, 710
    criminal behavior and, 714
    HIV infection and, 239, 714
    interaction with
        carbamazepine, 359
    metyrapone challenge test
        for patients on, 546
    for pregnant women, 715
    regulation of programs for,
        714–715
    for relapse prevention, 717
Methamphetamine, 397, 418, 419
Methohexital, **406**
Methoxamine, interaction with
    monoamine oxidase
    inhibitors, **789**

3-Methoxy-4-hydroxyphenyl-glycol (MHPG), 144, 581
in aggressive persons, 741
buspirone effects on, 236
in mood disorders, 451, 453
in schizophrenia, 491
Methyldopa, interaction with monoamine oxidase inhibitors, **789**
3,4-Methylenedioxyamphetamine, 420
2,3-Methylenedioxyamphetamine (MDA), 420
Methylenedioxymethamphetamine (MDMA), 420, 718
Methylphenidate (MPH), 417
abuse of, 430, 672
clinical use of, **675**
indications for
attention-deficit hyperactivity disorder, 417, 419, 427–428
associated with mental retardation, 696
autism, 693
borderline personality disorder, 762–763
depression, 423–424
imipramine and, 424–425, 589–590
depression in AIDS patients, 794
interaction with cyclic antidepressants, 154, 677, **786**
interaction with monoamine oxidase inhibitors, **789**
mechanism of action of, 8, 9, 422–423
for medically ill patients, 793–794
pharmacological profile of, **421,** 421–422
side effects of, 427
structure-activity relationships for, 420–421
sustained-release, 674
Methylprednisolone, interaction with carbamazepine, 359
α-Methyl-*p*-tyrosine (AMPT), 5, 54

Methysergide, 235, 449
Metoclopramide, **107**
Metoprolol, **130, 289**
Metronidazole, interaction with lithium, **793**
Metyrapone challenge test, 546
Meyer, Adolf, 439
Mianserin, **840–842,** 844
animal studies of
behavioral effects of olfactory bulb lesions, 86
chronic mild stress model, 95
depression of active responding induced by 5-hydroxy-tryptophan, 89
differential operant responding for low reinforcement, 86
isolation-induced hyperactivity, 87
swim test immobility, 89
yohimbine lethality, 85
Microsatellites, 444
Midazolam, **130,** 217
Migraine
selective serotonin reuptake inhibitors for, 171, 579
tricyclic antidepressants for, **151**
Milacemide, 398
Miltown. *See* Meprobamate
Minaprine, 813
Mini-Mental State Examination (MMSE), 393, 524, 664
Minisatellites, 444
Minnesota Multiphasic Personality Inventory (MMPI), 743
MK-212, 166
Moban. *See* Molindone
Moclobemide, 183, **184,** 189–190, **840–842,** 844
for depression, 189, 583
drug interactions with, 190
food interactions with, 190
other psychiatric indications for, 189–190

pharmacokinetics of, 189
side effects of, 190
for social phobia, 189, 845
structure of, **841**
Molecular neurobiology, 31–41
manipulation of gene expression, 35–38
complementary DNA cloning, 36–37, **36–37**
expression of recombinant genes, 38
genomic cloning, 37
restriction fragment length polymorphisms, 37, **38**
molecular components of gene expression, 31–35
DNA structure, 31–32
gene expression and antipsychotic drugs, 35
protein synthesis, 33
regulation of gene expression, 33–35, **34**
RNA synthesis, 32–33
of neurodegenerative disorders, 38–41
animal models, 40–41
cloning target genes, 39–40
gene therapy via fetal implants, 41
Molindone
for aggression in children and adolescents, 686
dosage of, **249, 620**
structure-activity relationship for, **249**
use during pregnancy, **829**
Monoamine oxidase (MAO), 8, 9, 161, 183–184, 440
A and B isoenzymes, 183–184
enzyme kinetics, 184
in mood disorders, 455–456
Monoamine oxidase inhibitors (MAOIs), 56, 57, 183–191, 425–426
animal studies of
amphetamine potentiation, 85
differential operant responding for low reinforcement, 86

MAOIs *(continued)*
  animal studies of
    isolation-induced
        hyperactivity, 87
    muricide, 85
    reserpine-induced
        reduction of motor
        activity, 89
    swim test immobility, 89
    tail suspension test, 91
    uncontrollable shock
        model, 96
    yohimbine lethality, 85
  for children and adolescents,
      683
  classification of, **184**
  combined with lithium,
      590–591
  combined with stimulant, 590
  combined with tricyclic
      antidepressant, 589
  L-deprenyl, 190, 397
  dietary interactions with,
      187–188, **188,** 583
  dosage of, 588
  drug interactions with,
      188–189, 787–788, **789**
    bupropion, 203
    buspirone, 236
    stimulants, **794**
    trazodone, 198
  drug interactions with,
    tricyclic antidepressants,
        154, 589
    venlafaxine, 205
  efficacy of, **185,** 185–186
  for elderly persons, 585
  history and discovery of, 183,
      575–576
  indications for, **185,** 185–187,
      583
    atypical depression, 150,
        583
    avoidant personality
        disorder, 764
    bipolar depression, 608
    borderline personality
        disorder, 761
    bulimia nervosa, 186, 583,
        727

chronic pain, 186–187
    dysthymic disorder, 584
    generalized anxiety
        disorder, 186
    geriatric depression, 810
    obsessive-compulsive
        disorder, 186
    panic disorder, 186, 580,
        583, 642, **642**
    posttraumatic stress
        disorder, 186, 650
    premenstrual dysphoria, 186
    social phobia, 186, 583, 648
    treatment-refractory
        depression, 589
    unipolar major depression,
        185–186, 583
  lithium augmentation of, 321
  mechanism of action of,
      184–185, 440
  for medically ill patients,
      787–789
    cardiac disease, 784, 788
    seizure disorders, 788–789
    surgical patients, 788
  moclobemide, 189–190
  norepinephrine output
      reduced by, 144
  reversible, **184,** 185
  side effects of, 187, 575, 583,
      778
    hypertensive crisis, 183,
        187–188, 583, 778,
        787–788
    pyridoxine deficiency, 789
    weight gain, 788
  stimulant augmentation of,
      426, 431
  use in pregnancy, 826, **827,**
      828
Mood disorders, 439–464. *See
    also* Bipolar disorder;
    Depression; Mania
  brain imaging in, 459–461,
      460–461
  in children and adolescents,
      678–683
  in DSM-IV, 440–441
  epidemiology of, 441–442
  genetics of, 442–445

neuroendocrine and
      neuropeptide
      hypotheses of, 440,
      445–450
    hypothalamic-growth
        hormone axis,
        448–449, **450**
    hypothalamic-pituitary-
        adrenal axis, **445,**
        445–447
    hypothalamic-pituitary-
        gonadal axis, 449–450
    hypothalamic-pituitary-
        thyroid axis, 447–448,
        448–449
    "neuroendocrine window
        strategy," 445
  in pregnancy, 826
  psychoneuroimmunology of,
      461–464
  role of neurotransmitters and
      receptors in, 439, 445,
      450–459
    acetylcholine, 457
    adrenergic receptors,
        452–453
    gamma-aminobutyric acid,
        456–457
    dopamine and dopamine
        β-hydroxylase:
        monoamine oxidase,
        455–456
    norepinephrine, **450,**
        451–452
    pineal function and
        circadian rhythm, 457
    second messenger systems,
        457–459, **458**
      adenylate cyclase
          system, 458
      G proteins, 458
      phosphoinositide system
          and calcium,
          458–459
    serotonin, 453–455,
        454–455
  seasonal, 9
  substance-induced, 441
Motor neuron disease, 41
MPH. *See* Methylphenidate

[⁹⁹ᵐTc]HMPAO, 459
Murder, 770–771
Muscle cramps, carbamazepine-
    induced, 686
Muscle relaxants, 405
Myanesin, 215
Myasthenia gravis, 10
Mydriasis, 285
Myocardial infarction, cyclic
    antidepressants and,
    784–785
Myoclonic jerks, 187, 328
Myotonic dystrophy (MD), 39, 40
Myristoylated alanine-rich C
    kinase substrate (MARCKS),
    318–319

Nadolol
    for aggression in children
        and adolescents, 687
    for extrapyramidal side
        effects, **289**
Naloxone, 232, 366
Naltrexone
    for alcoholism, 708–709
    for autism, 693
    for bulimia nervosa, 729–730
    for opioid dependence
        detoxification, 713
        relapse prevention, 717
Naproxen, interaction with
    lithium, **327,** 329
Narcolepsy
    posttraumatic stress disorder
        and, 509–510
    stimulants for, 417, 418, 423,
        428
    tricyclic antidepressants for,
        151
Narcotics Anonymous, 717
Nardil. *See* Phenelzine
Natural killer cells, 461
    in depression, 463–464
Nausea
    drug-induced
        buspirone, 237
        calcium channel blockers,
            384
        carbamazepine, 358, 686
        clonidine, 677

L-deprenyl, 397
        fluvoxamine, 843
        monoamine oxidase
            inhibitors, 187
        nefazodone, 207
        selective serotonin reuptake
            inhibitors, 582, 690
        tetrahydroaminoacridine,
            393
        valproate, 365, 680
        venlafaxine, 205
    tricyclic antidepressants for,
        151
Navane. *See* Thiothixene
Nefazodone, 205–207, 235
    drug interactions with, 207
    indications for, 206–207
    mechanism of action of, 206
    metabolites of, 206
    overdose of, 207
    pharmacokinetics and
        disposition of, 206
    pharmacological profile of, 206
    side effects and toxicology
        of, 207
    structure-activity relationship
        for, 206, **206**
Nervousness, drug-induced
    buspirone, 237
    selective serotonin reuptake
        inhibitors, 582
    venlafaxine, 205
Neuralgia, tricyclic
    antidepressants for, **151**
Neurodegenerative disorders,
    38–41
    animal models of, 40–41
    cloning target genes for, 39–40
    gene therapy via fetal
        implants for, 41
Neuroendocrinology, 3, 15. *See
    also* Endocrine effects
    of anorexia nervosa, 560–564
    of bulimia nervosa, 566
    of mood disorders, 445–450
    of panic disorder, 506
    of posttraumatic stress
        disorder, 510
    of protracted alcohol
        withdrawal, 549

of social phobia, 508
Neurofibrillary tangles, 524, 525
Neurofibromatosis, 40
Neuroleptic malignant
    syndrome (NMS), 257, 625,
    626, 629, 738, 776, 792
    amoxapine-induced, 200
    in children and adolescents,
        684
    clinical features of, 257, 629
    in elderly persons, 807
    mortality from, 257
    pathophysiology of, 629
    prevention and management
        of, 257, 629, 776
    recurrent, 629
    risk factors for, 629
Neuroleptics. *See* Antipsychotic
    drugs
Neuromodulators, 3
Neurotensin, 35
Neurotransmitters, 3–10, 24,
    45–46
    carbamazepine effects on, 354
    comparison of dopamine and
        serotonin systems in
        brain, 9, 45
    core, 4
    criteria for, 4–5
    lithium effects on, 307–314
    role in aggression, 741–742
    role in mood disorders, 439,
        445, 450–459
    role in schizophrenia,
        487–492
    sites of action in brain, 9–10
    sites of drug action for, 5–9, **6**
    synaptic regulation of, 54–57
        dopaminergic synapse, **55**
        neurotransmitter
            breakdown, 56
        neurotransmitter release, 56
        neurotransmitter reuptake,
            56
        neurotransmitter synthesis,
            54
        postsynaptic mechanisms,
            56–57
        presynaptic mechanisms, 54
        serotonergic synapse, **55**

Neutropenia
  carbamazepine-induced, 794
  lithium for, 323
  valproate-induced, 680
Nialamide, 89
Nicardipine, **378, 384**
Nicotine, 718–720
  for Alzheimer's disease, 396
  changes in tobacco use, 718
  interaction with
      antidepressants, 587
  interaction with
      benzodiazepines, 217,
      224, **794**
  smoking among psychiatric
      patients, 719–720
  substance abuse related to
      use of, 719
  treatment of dependence on,
      718–719
    antidepressants, 719
    clonidine, 719
    nicotine replacement
        therapy, 718–719
    propranolol, 719
    psychological
        interventions, 719
Nifedipine, **130,** 378, **378**
  antimanic effect of, 608
  for depression, 379
  dosage of, **384**
  for hypertensive crisis, 188,
      778, 787–788
  pharmacokinetics of, 382,
      382
  structure of, **381**
Nigrostriatal system, 46
Nikethamide, 418
Nimodipine (Nimotop), 378, **378**
  for Alzheimer's disease, 813
  antimanic effect of, 379, 608
  dosage of, **384**
  structure of, **379, 381**
Nimotop. *See* Nimodipine
Nisoldipine, **378**
Nitrazepam, 409, **409,** 413
Nitrendipine, **378**
Nitric oxide, 17, 20
Noctec. *See* Chloral hydrate
Nomifensine, 85, 89, 207

Nonsteroidal anti-inflammatory
    drugs, interaction with
    lithium, **327,** 329, **793**
Nootropic drugs, 814
Nordazepam, **218**
Norephedrine, 421, **421**
Norepinephrine (NE), 4, 9
  drug effects on
    antidepressants, 143–144,
        144, 154, **786**
    lithium, 310–311
    monoamine oxidase
        inhibitors, 787, **789**
    selective serotonin reuptake
        inhibitors, 164
  growth hormone release
      inhibited by, 449
  role in affective instability,
      759
  role in aggression, 741
  role in anxiety, 763–764
  role in depression, 439, **450,**
      451–452
  role in panic disorder,
      503–504
  role in posttraumatic stress
      disorder, 509
  role in schizophrenia, 491
  role in uncontrollable shock
      model in animals, 97–98
  sites of drug action for, **6**
Norfluoxetine, 128, **129,** 130,
    146, 165, 786
Norpramin. *See* Desipramine
Nortriptyline, **130**
  animal studies of
    differential operant
        responding for low
        reinforcement, 86
    swim test immobility, 89
  biochemical effects of, 144,
      144
  for children and adolescents,
      682
  dosage of, 147
  elimination half-life of, **145**
  indications for, **151**
    attention-deficit
        hyperactivity
        disorder, 673

    enuresis, 151
    panic disorder, 151, 642
  structure-activity relationship
      for, 142, **142**
  therapeutic plasma
      concentration of, 147,
      586–587
  use in pregnancy, **827,** 828
Norverapamil, **378,** 382
NPA. *See* *N*-n-Propylnorapo-
    morphine
Nuclear magnetic resonance
    (NMR) spectroscopy,
    303–304
Nursing Home Reform
    Amendments, 804
Nystagmus, carbamazepine-
    induced, 358

Obesity
  benzodiazepines and, 217
  binge-eating and, 730
  selective serotonin reuptake
      inhibitors for, 170–171
  stimulants for, 417, 419
Obsessive-compulsive disorder
    (OCD), 501, 510–513
  brain imaging in, 512–513
  cerebrospinal fluid studies in,
      511
  heritability of, 510–511
  neuroanatomy of, 512
  prevalence of, 649, 689
  role of serotonin in, 168,
      511–512
    neuropharmacological
        probes of serotonin
        systems, 511–512
    peripheral serotonin
        markers, 511, **511**
  summary of biology of, 513
  Tourette's disorder and, 511,
      512, 691
  treatment of, 649–650
    benzodiazepines, 222
    buspirone, 168, 238–239, 650
    in children and
        adolescents, 689–690
    clomipramine, 142, 150,
        168, 649

clonazepam, 650
duration of, 650
in Europe, 844
monoamine oxidase
inhibitors, 186
neuroleptics, 650
psychotherapy, 650
selective serotonin
reuptake inhibitors,
150, 168, 512, 580,
582, 649
stimulants, 429
trazodone, 197, 650
venlafaxine, 205
Obstetrical complications,
schizophrenia and, 480–481
Obstipation, trihexyphenidyl-
induced, 285
Ohm's law, 70
Olfactory bulb lesioning, 86, 88
Omnibus Budget Reconciliation
Act of 1987, 804
Opioid antagonists
for alcoholism, 708–709
for Alzheimer's disease, 813
for autism, 693
for opioid detoxification, 713
for symptoms of mental
retardation, 697
Opioid dependence, 711–717
L-α-acetyl-methadol (LAAM)
for, 713, 715–716
animal models of, 539
benzodiazepine use and, 710
buprenorphine for, 712, 716
detoxification from, 712–713
medical complications of, 714
methadone maintenance for,
713–715
neurobiology of, 542–543
among pregnant women, 715
preventing relapses of,
716–717
protracted abstinence
syndrome, 546–547
Oral contraceptive interactions
with antidepressants, 587,
786
with carbamazepine, 359,
607–608, **795**

Orap. *See* Pimozide
Organic personality
syndrome—explosive type,
736, **736**
Orthostatic hypotension,
drug-induced
amoxapine, 200
antipsychotics, 258, **627,** 777,
806
clozapine, 274, 792
in elderly persons, 808
monoamine oxidase
inhibitors, 187, 583
nefazodone, 207
risperidone, 621
selective serotonin reuptake
inhibitors, 173
trazodone, 196–198
tricyclic antidepressants, 152,
785, 808
venlafaxine, 205
Overanxious disorder, 688–689
Overdose, 779
of amoxapine, 200
of amphetamine, 429, 430
of barbiturates, 407, 408
of benzodiazepines, 217,
414, 779
of carbamazepine, 350, 353
of nefazodone, 207
of selective serotonin
reuptake inhibitors,
173–174
of trazodone, 198
of tricyclic antidepressants,
147, 152, 779
of valproate, 366
of venlafaxine, 205
Overt Aggression Scale, 738,
739, 741
Overt Agitation Severity Scale
(OASS), 738, **740**
Oxazepam, **218,** 409, **409**
for dementia, 663
indications for, 413
use in pregnancy, 830, **831**
Oxcarbazepine, 351, 367–368,
368–369
for bipolar disorder
prophylaxis, 368, **369**

for mania, 368, **368**
pharmacokinetics of,
367–368
pharmacological profile of,
367
side effects of, 368
Oxiracetam, 814
6-Oxoritalinic acid, 421
Oxotremorine, 396
Oxyprotipine, 843

Pain
carbamazepine for, 351, 352,
355
monoamine oxidase
inhibitors for, 186–187
selective serotonin reuptake
inhibitors for, 171
tricyclic antidepressants for,
151
Pamelor. *See* Nortriptyline
Pancreatitis, valproate-induced,
680
Panic disorder (PD), 223,
501–507
agoraphobia and, 501
autonomic dysfunction in,
505–506
common fears of persons
with, 647
genetics of, 502
neurochemical theories of,
502, 502–505
adenosinergic dysfunction,
505
lactate hypothesis,
502–503
noradrenergic hypothesis,
503–504
respiratory hypotheses,
503
serotonergic dysfunction,
504–505
neuroendocrinology of, 506
hypothalamic-pituitary-
adrenal axis, 506
hypothalamic-pituitary-
thyroid axis, 506
neuroleptic effects in, 645
organic workup for, 772

PD *(continued)*
    other neurobiological models
        of, 505
        benzodiazepine receptor
            sensitivity, 505
        cholecystokinin
            tetrapeptide, 505
        isoproterenol, 505
        positron-emission
            tomography in, 507
    prevalence of, 501, 641
    sleep in, 506–507
    summary of biology of, 507
    symptoms of, 641
Panic disorder (PD) treatment,
        641–646
    antidepressants, 641–643,
        642–643
        monoamine oxidase
            inhibitors, 186, 580,
            583, 642, **642**
        selective serotonin
            reuptake inhibitors,
            168–169, 642–643,
            643
        tricyclics, 151, **151,**
            641–642, **642**
    benzodiazepines, **644,**
        643–645
        alprazolam, 215, 218, 222,
            223, 643–644
    in children and adolescents,
        690
    long-term therapy, 646
    psychotherapy, 645
    short-term acute therapy,
        641–645
    verapamil, 384
Papaverine, 378
Parahydroxyamphetamine, 421,
    421
Parahydroxynorefedron, 421
Parahydroxyritalinic acid, 421
Paraldehyde, 405, 746
Paralytic ileus, 777
Pargyline, 85–86
Parkinsonism, 9, 251, 255–256,
        625, **626,** 627, 663, 776. *See*
        also Extrapyramidal side
        effects

amoxapine-induced, 200
calcium channel
        blocker–induced, 385
    in children and adolescents,
        684
Parkinson's disease (PD), 39,
        738
    amphetamine for, 418
    antidepressants for, 579
    clozapine for, 792–793
    L-deprenyl for, 187, 190, 397
Parnate. *See* Tranylcypromine
Paroxetine, 130, 453, 576
    for children and adolescents,
        681
    drug interactions with, 173,
        582
        tricyclic antidepressants,
            587
    effect on hepatic P_{450}
        enzymes, 146
    metabolite of, 166
    for panic disorder, 642–643,
        643
    pharmacokinetics of,
        165–166, **166,** 786–787
    sleep effects of, 171
    structure-activity relationship
        for, **162,** 162–163
    use in patients with
        cardiovascular disease,
        577
    use in pregnancy, **827**
Pavor nocturnus, 695–696
Paw test, 105
Paxil. *See* Paroxetine
PCP. *See* Phencyclidine
Penfluridol, 250, **840–842,** 843
Pentobarbital, **406**
Peptic ulcer disease,
        antidepressants and, **151,**
        580
Perphenazine
    in breast milk, 828–829
    for children's anxiety in
        medical setting, 691
    dosage of, **249, 620**
    structure-activity relationship
        for, 248, **249**
    use in pregnancy, 828, **829**

Personality change due to
        general medical condition,
        736–737, **737**
Personality disorders treatment,
        753–765. *See also* specific
        personality disorders
    assessing response to, 756
    assessment for, 754–755
        family history, 755
        interviewing family
            members, 754
        medical history, 755
        physical and laboratory
            examinations, 755
        psychiatric history, 754
        substance abuse and
            dependence history,
            754–755
    for avoidant personality
        disorder, 763–764
    for borderline personality
        disorder, 758–763
    initiation of, 755
    maintenance and monitoring
        of, 756
    managing toxic effects of,
        755
    resistance to, 756
    for schizotypal personality
        disorder, 756–758
Pervasive developmental
        disorder, 255
Pharmacodynamics, 130–133
    definition of, 125, 130
    in elderly persons, 804–805
    kinetic-dynamic modeling,
        132–133, **132–134**
    measurement methods,
        130–132
Pharmacokinetics, 125–130
    of amantadine, 288
    of amoxapine, 199
    of antipsychotics, 251–252
    of barbiturates, 406
    of benzodiazepines, 217–218,
        218, 409, **409**
    of benztropine, 286–287
    of β-blockers, 290
    of bupropion, 201–202
    of buspirone, 235–236

of calcium channel blockers, 381–382, **382**

of carbamazepine, 352–354, **353–354**

in children and adolescents, 671

of cyclic antidepressants, **145,** 145–147

in medically ill patients, 786–787

definition of, 125

of L-deprenyl, 397

of diphenhydramine, 287–288

in elderly persons, 805

of galanthamine, 394

of HP 029, 394

implications of two-compartment model, 125–127

intravenous administration, 126, **126–127**

oral administration, 127, **127–128**

of meprobamate, 232

of nefazodone, 206

of oxcarbazepine, 367–368

of physostigmine, 392

predictability of drug interactions, 129–130, **129–130**

of selective serotonin reuptake inhibitors, 165–166, **166**

steady-state condition, 127–129, **128**

of tetrahydroaminoacridine, 393

of trazodone, 196

of trihexyphenidyl, 285

of valproate, **353,** 360–362, 361–362

of venlafaxine, 204

Phencyclidine (PCP), 270, 489, 717–718, 776

Phenelzine, **184,** 185

acetylator type and response to, 185–186

animal studies of differential operant responding for low reinforcement, 86

isolation-induced hyperactivity, 87

indications for

avoidant personality disorder, 764

borderline personality disorder, 761

bulimia nervosa, 186, 727

depression, 185, 583

panic disorder, 186, 642

posttraumatic stress disorder, 186, 650

social phobia, 186, 648

structure of, **841**

use in pregnancy, **827**

Phenmetrazine, 431

Phenobarbital, 405, **406**

drug interactions with

β-blockers, 291

carbamazepine, **795**

valproate, 366, **797**

Phenocopies, 444

Phenothiazines

animal studies of, 89

dosage of, **620**

history and discovery of, 248

interaction with cyclic antidepressants, 154, **786**

metabolism of, 251

structure-activity relationships for, 248, **249**

Phentermine, 431

Phentolamine, 188, 778

Phenylbutazone, interaction with lithium, **327,** 329, **793**

Phenylephrine interactions

with cyclic antidepressants, **786**

with monoamine oxidase inhibitors, **789**

Phenylhydrazine, 183

Phenylisopropylamine. *See* Amphetamine

Phenylketonuria, 39, 443

Phenylpropanolamine, 431

interaction with monoamine oxidase inhibitors, 787, **789**

Phenytoin, 351, 368–369

drug interactions with

β-blockers, 291

carbamazepine, **795**

cyclic antidepressants, 154, **786**

selective serotonin reuptake inhibitors, 582

trazodone, 198

valproate, 366, **797**

for status epilepticus, 777

Phosphoinositide system, 19–20, **20**

lithium effects on, 314–315, 459

in mood disorders, 458–459

Photosensitivity reactions, antipsychotic-induced, 258, 629

Physicians' Desk Reference (PDR), 670

Physostigmine, 392

for Alzheimer's disease, 392, 813

clonidine and, 397

L-deprenyl and, 392, 397

for anticholinergic toxicity, 778

drug interactions with, 392

history and discovery of, 392

mechanism of action of, 392

pharmacokinetics and disposition of, 392

pharmacological profile of, 392

side effects of, 392

structure of, 392

for treatment-resistant mania, 680

Pimozide

for autism, 693

dopamine receptor affinity for, **47**

dosage of, **620**

for schizotypal personality disorder, 757

for Tourette's disorder, 250, 255, 691–692

use during pregnancy, **829**

Pindolol, 455
    for aggression in children
        and adolescents, 687
    for extrapyramidal side
        effects, **289**
Pipamperone, **840–842,** 843
Piquindone, 692
Piracetam, 814
Piroxicam, interaction with
    lithium, **793**
Polymerase chain reaction
    (PCR), 444
Polypharmacy, 805
POMC. *See*
    Pro-opiomelanocortin
Poor metabolizers, 173
Porsolt swim test, 89–91, **90,** 202
Positive and Negative Syndrome
    Scale (PANSS), **619,** 621
Positron-emission tomography
    (PET), 5, 110, 252, 275, 459
    in Alzheimer's disease, 524
    in bulimia nervosa, 566
    of cocaine effects, 548
    in mood disorders, 460–461,
        461
    in obsessive-compulsive
        disorder, 512–513
    in panic disorder, 507
    in schizophrenia, 484, 487
Posttraumatic stress disorder
    (PTSD), 501
    adrenergic dysfunction in, 509
    dissociative episodes and, 773
    neuroendocrinology of, 510
    prevalence of, 650
    psychophysiology of, 509
    sleep studies in, 509–510
    stressors inducing, 509
    symptoms in children,
        690–691
    treatment of, 650–651
        adrenergic inhibitors, 650
        benzodiazepines, 222, 223,
            651
        β-blockers, 651
        carbamazepine, 650
        in children and
            adolescents, 690–691
        lithium, 650

monoamine oxidase
    inhibitors, 186, 650,
    651
selective serotonin
    reuptake inhibitors,
    580, 582
tricyclic antidepressants,
    650, 651
valproate, 650, 651
Potential dependent channels,
    380
Poverty of speech, 616
Pramiracetam, 814
Prazepam, **218, 409**
    use in pregnancy, **831**
Prazosin interactions
    with cyclic antidepressants,
        786
    with monoamine oxidase
        inhibitors, **789**
Prednisone, interaction with
    carbamazepine, 359
Pregnancy and lactation,
    823–834
    drug concentration in breast
        milk, 824–825
    managing mental illness
        during, 823
    physiology of, 824–825
    psychotropic drug use during
        alcohol, 224, 414
        antidepressants, 826–828,
            827
        antipsychotics, 258,
            828–829, **829**
        anxiolytics, 830, **831**
            benzodiazepines, 224,
                414, 830
        assessing risk/benefit ratio
            of, 825–826
        carbamazepine, 359, 832,
            832
        choice of, 833
        communicating with
            pediatrician about,
            834
        dosage of, 833–834
        FDA ratings for, 825, **826,**
            833
        informed consent for, 833

mood stabilizers, 830–833,
    832
    lithium, 326, 831–832
    opioids, 715
    problems in literature on,
        823–824
    valproate, 365, 832, **832**
Premenstrual dysphoric
    disorder, 440
Prenatal risk factors for
    schizophrenia, 480–481
Prepulse inhibition paradigms,
    108–109
Priapism, trazodone-induced,
    198, 687, 778, 785
Procainamide, interaction with
    cyclic antidepressants, **786**
Procardia. *See* Nifedipine
Procyclidine, **284,** 287
Progabide, 369
Prolactin
    in anorexia nervosa, 564
    antipsychotic effects on, 251,
        258, **627,** 629
    buspirone effects on, 236
    serotonin agonist effects on,
        455
Prolixin. *See* Fluphenazine
Prolixin-D. *See* Fluphenazine
    decanoate
Promethazine, 141
Pro-opiomelanocortin (POMC),
    34, 445
    lithium effects on, 313
    opiate effects on, 546–547
Propafenone, **130**
    interaction with cyclic
        antidepressants, **786**
    interaction with selective
        serotonin reuptake
        inhibitors, 173
Propoxyphene, interaction with
    carbamazepine, 359, **795**
Propranolol, **130**
    drug interactions with
        antipsychotics, 259
        carbamazepine, **795**
        monoamine oxidase
            inhibitors, **789**
        thioridazine, 748

indications for
aggregate behavior, 748,
748, 775
in children and
adolescents, 687
extrapyramidal side effects,
256, **289,** 289–291,
628
posttraumatic stress
disorder, 650
in children and
adolescents, 591
social phobia, 507, 648
symptoms of mental
retardation, 697
treatment-resistant mania,
680
side effects of, 687
use during pregnancy, **829**
N-n-Propylnorapomorphine
(NPA), 7
Prosom. *See* Estazolam
Prostaglandins, **23,** 24
Prostatic hypertrophy, 785
Protein kinase C, 22
lithium effects on, 317–319
Protein synthesis, 33
Protracted abstinence
syndrome, 544, 546–550
from alcohol, 548–550
from cocaine, 547–548
from opiates, 546–547
Protriptyline
biochemical effects of, **144**
elimination half-life of, **145**
indications for, **151**
structure-activity relationship
for, **142,** 143
use in pregnancy, **827**
Prozac. *See* Fluoxetine
Pruritus, tricyclic
antidepressants for, **151**
Pseudoephedrine, interaction
with monoamine oxidase
inhibitors, 787, **789**
Pseudoparkinsonism, 282
Psilocybin, 717
Psychiatric emergencies,
769–779
in adolescents, 778–779

conditions requiring organic
workup, 772–773
catatonia, 773
conversion disorder, 773
dissociative episodes,
772–773
mania, 773
panic attack, 772
conditions usually requiring
minimal
pharmacological
intervention, **771,**
771–773
acute grief, 772
adjustment disorders, 772
borderline personality
disorder, 772
rape and assault, 772
conditions usually requiring
pharmacological
intervention, 773–778
agitated psychosis, 774–775
bipolar disorder, 774
brief reactive psychosis,
774
delirium, 775
dementia, 775
schizophrenia, 774
assaultive behavior,
773–774
psychoactive drug side
effects, 776–778
antipsychotics, 776–778
cyclic antidepressants,
778
substance intoxication with
violence, 775–776
cocaine, 775–776
other substances, 776
phencyclidine, 776
substance withdrawal, 775
in elderly persons, 779
nonpharmacological
intervention for,
769–771
notifying third parties, 771
voluntary or involuntary
admissions, 769–771,
770
homicidal state, 770–771

self-neglect and
nonagitated
psychotic state, 771
suicidal state, 770
psychiatric drug overdose,
779
Psychoeducational testing, 671
Psychopathology Instrument for
Mentally Retarded Adults,
696
Psychopharmacology, defined, 3
Psychosis. *See also*
Schizophrenia
brief reactive, 774
drug-induced
amphetamine, 429
bupropion, 203
calcium channel blockers,
385
phencyclidine, 489
emergency treatment of
agitated psychosis, 774–775
nonagitated psychosis, 771
treating in elderly persons,
805–807
Psychotherapies
for alcoholism, 707
for generalized anxiety
disorder, 647
in children and
adolescents, 688
for obsessive-compulsive
disorder, 650, 689
for panic disorder, 645
for posttraumatic stress
disorder in children, 691
for schizophrenia, 253–254,
622
for social phobia, 648–649
Puberty, 562
Pulmonary disease patients
antipsychotics for, 792
benzodiazepines for, 790
buspirone for, 790
monoamine oxidase
inhibitors for, 787
Punished locomotion test, 216
Pyridoxine deficiency, 789
1-Pyrimidinylpiperazine (1-PP),
236

Quality of Life Scale, **619,** 624
Quazepam, 790, 812
  use in pregnancy, **831**
Quinidine, **130**
  drug interactions with
    carbamazepine, **795**
    cyclic antidepressants, **786**
    lithium, **327,** 329
    selective serotonin
      reuptake inhibitors,
      173
Quinpirole, **47**
Quipazine, 166

Raclopride, 47, **47**
Rage. *See* Aggression
Rape, 772
Rapid neuroleptization, 774
Receptor-gated ion channels, 4
Receptors, 3, 4, 10–15, 24–25
  adrenergic
    α_1 receptor, 452
    α_2 receptor, 452
    β_1 receptor, 452–453
    β_2 receptor, 14, **16,** 18–19,
      452–453
    in mood disorders, 452–453
  affinity of antidepressants
    for, 576, **578**
  benzodiazepine, **219–220,**
    219–222
  cholinergic
    muscarinic, 14, 395–396
    nicotinic, 12–14, **13,** 395
    role in Alzheimer's disease,
      395
  classification of, 11
  coupling to G proteins, 58
  definition of, 10–11
  dopamine, 5, 7, 47–51,
    265–268
  drug efficacy and affinity for,
    11–12
  function of, 10
  GABA-A, 14
  glutamate, 14, 398
  growth factor, 15
  interleukin, 15
  molecular structure of, 12,
    13

regulation of number of, 57–58
serotonin, 9, 47, 52–54,
  268–270
superfamilies of, 12–15
  G protein–linked
    receptors, 14–15, **16**
  ligand-gated ion channel
    receptors, 13–14
Remoxipride, 35, 293, 621
Renal disease patients
  cyclic antidepressants for, 787
  lithium for, 793
Renal effects
  of anorexia nervosa, **558,**
    558–559
  of bulimia nervosa, 565, **565**
  of carbamazepine, 358
  of lithium, 326, 793
Repolarization, 66
Reserpine
  animal studies of motor
    activity reduction
    induced by, 88–89
  depression induced by,
    439–440
  effect on synaptic dopamine
    level, 8
  history and discovery of, 248
  interaction with cyclic
    antidepressants, **786**
Respiratory dyskinesia, 282
Resting membrane potential,
  65–66, 304
Restoril. *See* Temazepam
Restraints, 773–774
Restriction fragment length
  polymorphisms (RFLPs), 37,
  38, 443–444
Retinitis pigmentosa, 258, **627,**
  629–630
Ribonucleic acid (RNA), 32–33
Rifampin interactions
  with benzodiazepines, 224,
    794
  with β-blockers, 291
Rigidity, 255, 627, 776
  in children and adolescents,
    684
  in neuroleptic malignant
    syndrome, 257

Risperdal. *See* Risperidone
Risperidone (Risperdal), **249,**
  293, 620–621
  dosage of, 620, **620**
  efficacy studies of, 620–621
  indications for, 621
  mechanism of action of, 620
  metabolite of, 620
  side effects of, 621
  structure of, **840**
  switching from clozapine to,
    621
  use during pregnancy, **829**
Ritalin. *See* Methylphenidate
Ritalinic acid, 421, **421**
Ritanserin, 235
RNA, 32–33
Ro 15-1788, 221
Ro 15-4513, 544
RS-86, 395
"Rum fits," 707

Salbutamol, 87
Salicylates, interaction with
  valproate, **797**
Scale for Assessment of
  Negative Symptoms (SANS),
  619
Scale for Assessment of Positive
  Symptoms (SAPS), **619**
SCH23390, 47
Schedule for Affective Disorders
  and Schizophrenia (SADS),
  618
  for School-Age Children
    (KIDDIE-SADS), 678
Schizoaffective disorders
  antipsychotics for, 253–254
  clozapine for, 273
Schizophrenia, 479–492, 738
  age at onset of, 111
  animal models of, 41,
    104–113. *See also*
    Animal models
  assessment instruments for,
    618, **618–619**
  Bleulerian concept of, 615
  brain abnormalities in, 112,
    459, 481–487
    basal ganglia, 482–483, **483**

cerebellum, 486
limbic system, 483–484, **485–486**
neocortex, 484, 486
soft signs, 481
thalamus and brain stem, 486
ventriculomegaly and corticosulcal dilatation, 459, 482, 616
diagnostic criteria for, 615, **616**
differential diagnosis of, 615
disorganization syndrome in, 616
expressed emotion in family of patient with, 622
genetics of, 479–481
hippocampal changes in, 111
Kraepelinian concept of, 254, 615
mental retardation and, 696
neurochemical abnormalities in, 487–491
dopamine, 4, 41, 110, 252, 263, 487–489
G proteins, 17
glutamate, 489, **490**
norepinephrine, 491
peptides and other neurochemicals, 491
serotonin, 169, 489–491
neuropsychological deficits in, 481
obstetrical complications and, 480–481
psychomotor poverty syndrome in, 616
reality distortion syndrome in, 616
Schneiderian concept of, 615
smoking and, 719
substance abuse and, 617–618
symptoms of
depressive, 617
"first-rank," 615
negative (deficit), 479, 488, 615–617, **617**
positive, 479, 615–617

treatment-refractory, 631–634, **633**
Type I–Type II model of, 615–617
Schizophrenia treatment, 615–634
for agitated psychosis, 774
antipsychotic drugs, 253–254, 618–621, **620**
assessing response to, 623–624, **624**
clozapine, 263–275, 631–634, **632**
continuation, maintenance, and monitoring, 624–625
discontinuation of, 630–631
dosage of, 619, **620,** 624–625
effect on positive and negative symptoms, 616–617
noncompliance with, 625
remoxipride, 621
resistance to, 631
risperidone, 620–621
side effects of, 625–630, **626–627**
assessment for, 615–618
in children and adolescents, 683–685
assessing response to, 683
assessment for, 683
continuation, maintenance, and monitoring of, 684
discontinuation of, 685
initiation of, 683–684
managing side effects of, 684–685
resistance to, 685
selection of, 683
contraindications to drug therapy, 253, 254
electroconvulsive therapy, 621
European-approved drugs for, 840, 843
initiation of, 623
lithium, 321–322

maintenance therapy, 254
psychosocial therapies, 253–254, 621–622
selection of, 618–621
selective serotonin reuptake inhibitors, 169
stimulants, 428–429
Schizotypal personality disorder (SPD), 756–758
antipsychotics for, 757–758
assessing response to, 758
initiation of, 758
managing side effects of, 758
resistance to, 758
clinical features of, 756
differential diagnosis of, 757
relation to schizophrenia, 757
social anxiety in, 757
School avoidance, 687, 692
Seasonal affective disorder (SAD), 9
Second messengers, 3, **4,** 17, 20–25
arachidonic acid pathway, **23,** 23–24
criteria for, 21
cyclic AMP and adenylate cyclase, 21–22
effect of chronic opiate administration on, 547
inositol lipid-based, 22–23
role in mood disorders, 457–459, **458**
Sedation, drug-induced
amoxapine, 200
antipsychotics, **627,** 806
benzodiazepines, 130–131, **131,** 224
clonidine, 677, 692
clozapine, 273, 621, **632,** 633
risperidone, 621
trazodone, 195, 197, 198, 583
tricyclic antidepressants, 153
valproate, 365
venlafaxine, 205
Sedative-hypnotics, 405–415
alcohol-type, 414
antihistamines, 414
barbiturates, 405–408

Sedative-hypnotics (continued)
  benzodiazepines, 408–414
  interaction with
      antipsychotics, 259
  nonbenzodiazepine, 411, **411**
  for sleep disorders in elderly
      persons, 812
  for symptoms of mental
      retardation, 697
  use in pregnancy, 830, **831**
Segregation analysis, 443, 444
Seizures
  alcohol withdrawal, 549, 707
  animal studies of, 85
  antiepileptic drugs for,
      351–370
  drug-induced
    amoxapine, 200
    antipsychotics, **626,** 777,
        792
      in children and
          adolescents, 684
    clozapine, 273, 621,
        632, 633, 777
    bupropion, 203, 578, 687,
        778, 785–786
    clomipramine, 150, 578
    cocaine, 711
    maprotiline, 578
    risperidone, 621
  psychotropic drugs for
      patients with
    antipsychotics, 258, 629
    cyclic antidepressants, 578,
        579, 785–786
    monoamine oxidase
        inhibitors, 788–789
  status epilepticus, 777
Selective serotonin reuptake
    inhibitors (SSRIs), 56, 57,
    141, 161–174, 453
  animal studies of
    behavioral effects of
        olfactory bulb
        lesions, 86
    differential operant
        responding for low
        reinforcement, 86
    uncontrollable shock
        model, 96

  for cardiac disease patients,
      577
  for children and adolescents,
      681
  differentiation from tricyclic
      antidepressants, 149
  dosage of, **166**
  drug interactions with, **129,**
      129–130, 173, 582
    tricyclic antidepressants, 587
  for elderly persons, 585
  history and discovery of, 161,
      576
  indications for, 167–171
    aggressive behavior,
        747–748, 775
    agitation in elderly
        persons, 807
    alcoholism, 170
    atypical depression, 150,
        583
    autism, 694
    avoidant personality
        disorder, 764
    bipolar depression, 608–609
    borderline personality
        disorder, 171, 760
    depression in Parkinson's
        disease, 579
    dysthymic disorder, 584
    eating disorders, 169–170
    generalized anxiety
        disorder, 647
    geriatric depression, 810
    migraine, 171, 579
    miscellaneous, 171
    obesity, 170–171, 580
    obsessive-compulsive
        disorder, 150, 168,
        512, 580, 582, 649
    panic disorder, 168–169,
        642–643, **643**
    poststroke depression, 579
    posttraumatic stress
        disorder, 580, 582
    schizophrenia, 169
    sleep, 171
    suicidality, 171, 587
    treatment-refractory
        depression, 589

  unipolar major depression,
      149, 167–168, 582
  inhibition of cytochrome P_{450}
      subfamilies by, 129–130
  mechanism of action of, 166
  metabolites of, **129,** 165–166
  overdose of, 173–174
  pharmacokinetics and
      disposition of, 165–166,
      166, 786–787
  pharmacological effects of,
      163–165
    corticotropin-releasing
        factor antagonism,
        165
    on dopamine, 164–165
    on gamma-aminobutyric
        acid, 165
    miscellaneous, 165
    on noradrenaline, 164
    on serotonin, **163,** 163–164
  receptor affinity of, 162–163
  side effects and toxicology
      of, 153, 171–173, **172,**
      582, 784
  structure-activity
      relationships for,
      161–163, **162**
  use in Europe, 843–845
  use in pregnancy, 827, **827**
Selegiline. See L-Deprenyl
Self-help groups
  for alcoholism, 707
  for substance dependence,
      717
Self-neglect, 771
Separation anxiety disorder
    (SAD), 687–688
Serax. See Oxazepam
Serentil. See Mesoridazine
Serotonin agonists, 455
Serotonin antagonists, 269–270,
    490
Serotonin (5-HT), 4, 45, 161
  antidepressant effects on,
      143–144, **144**
  circadian rhythm of, 9
  comparison of dopamine and
      serotonin systems in
      brain, 9

effects of lithium on, 307–309
effects of selective serotonin
    reuptake inhibitors on,
    163, 163–164
role in aggression, 439, 741,
    759
role in alcoholism, 170
role in anxiety, 763–764
role in bulimia nervosa, 169,
    726
role in depression, 439,
    453–455, **454–455**
role in obsessive-compulsive
    disorder, 168, **511,**
    511–512
role in panic disorder,
    503–504
role in schizophrenia, 169,
    489–491
role in uncontrollable shock
    model in animals, 98
serotonin-synthesizing cell
    groups, **51,** 51–52
sites of drug action for, **6,**
    162
synaptic regulation of, 54–57,
    55, 454
transporters for, 56
Serotonin receptors, 9, 14, 19,
    47, 52–54, 56, 453–454
anatomical distribution of,
    52–54, **53**
autoreceptors, 53–54
coupling to G proteins, 58
drug effects on, 57
    antidepressants, 148,
        453–454, **578**
    antipsychotics, 268–270
subtypes of, 52, **52,** 163,
    163, 453–454
Serotonin syndrome, 172, 198,
    235, 328
Sertraline, 453, 576
for children and adolescents,
    681
drug interactions with, 582
    tricyclic antidepressants,
        587
metabolite of, **129,** 165
for obesity, 170

for panic disorder, 642–643,
    643
pharmacokinetics of,
    165–166, **166,** 786–787
sleep effects of, 171
structure-activity relationship
    for, **162,** 162–163
use in cardiac disease
    patients, 577
use in pregnancy, 827, **827**
Serzone. *See* Nefazodone
Sexual dysfunction
antidepressants for patients
    with, 580
buspirone for, 237
drug-induced
    antidepressants, 153, 580
    antipsychotics, 251, 258,
        629
    monoamine oxidase
        inhibitors, 187
    selective serotonin
        reuptake inhibitors,
        582
    thioridazine, 792
    trazodone, 198
    venlafaxine, 205
Shyness, 763
Signal transducing proteins, 3
Signal transduction, 15–20, 25
adenylate cyclase–linked, **18,**
    18–19
G protein–linked, 17, **18**
ion-based, 17
lithium effects on, 314–319
other systems for, 20
phosphoinositide-linked,
    19–20, **20**
Simpson-Angus Scale, 284
Simpson/Rockland Scale, 284
Sinequan. *See* Doxepin
Single photon emission
    computed tomography
    (SPECT), 275, 459, 461
in Alzheimer's disease, 524
in obsessive-compulsive
    disorder, 513
in schizophrenia, 484
Single sequence repeat (SSR)
    markers, 444

Site-directed mutagenesis, 15, 35
SKF39383, 47
Sleep disorders
in children, 695–696
    insomnia, 695
    sleep terror and
        sleepwalking,
        695–696
in elderly persons, 812
treating during pregnancy,
    831
Sleep effects
of alcohol, 548
of amphetamine, 429
of antihistamines, 414
of barbiturates, 406–407,
    412
of benzodiazepines, 217,
    412–413, **412–413**
of galanthamine, 394
of meprobamate, 234
of monoamine oxidase
    inhibitors, 187
of selective serotonin
    reuptake inhibitors,
    171, 582, 690
of stimulants, 675
of trazodone, 195, 197
Sleep studies
in anorexia nervosa, 560
in bulimia nervosa, 566
in panic disorder, 506–507
in posttraumatic stress
    disorder, 509–510
to predict antidepressant
    response, 581
Slow hydroxylation, 145–146
Smoking. *See* Nicotine
Social phobia (SP), 501, 507–508
avoidant personality disorder
    and, 648
common fears of persons
    with, 647
generalized and discrete
    forms of, 507
monoaminergic function in,
    508
neuroendocrinology of, 508
prevalence of, 647
summary of biology of, 508

SP (continued)
sympathetic nervous system
function in, 507–508
treatment of, 647–649
benzodiazepines, 222, 648
β-blockers, 507–508, 648
bupropion, 203
buspirone, 238, 648
cognitive-behavioral
therapy, 648–649
moclobemide, 189, 845
monoamine oxidase
inhibitors, 186, 648
Somatostatin, 449
in Alzheimer's disease, 524,
813
in bulimia nervosa, 566
in obsessive-compulsive
disorder, 511
Somnambulism, 695–696
Somnolence, drug-induced
calcium channel blockers, 385
venlafaxine, 205
Sotalol, **289**
Sparteine, 145, 173
Spectamine. See [^{123}I]Iofetamine
Spiperone, 35, **47**
Spironolactone, interaction with
lithium, **793**
SSRIs. See Selective serotonin
reuptake inhibitors
Startle reflex inhibition studies,
108–109
Status epilepticus, 777
Stelazine. See Trifluoperazine
Stevens-Johnson syndrome,
carbamazepine-induced,
358, 608, 687
Stimulants, 8, 417–432
abuse potential of, 417, 672
animal studies of
swim test immobility, 89
tail suspension test, 91
uncontrollable shock
model, 96
classification as controlled
substances, 419, 423
combined with
antidepressants, 589–590
discontinuation of, 676

drug interactions with,
431–432, **794**
monoamine oxidase
inhibitors, **789**
tricyclic antidepressants,
587
history of, 417–419
indications for, 423–429
attention-deficit
hyperactivity
disorder, 417, 419,
423, 427–428, 672–677
associated with
Tourette's disorder,
692
autism, 693
borderline personality
disorder, 762–763
cancer patients, 794
cocaine abuse, 429
depression, 423–424, 427
historical, 417–419
narcolepsy, 417, 418, 423,
428
obsessive-compulsive
disorder, 429
potentiation of
antidepressants,
424–426
prediction of
antidepressant
response, 581
schizophrenia, 428–429
initiation of, 673–675
long-acting, 674–675
mechanism of action of,
422–423
for medically ill patients, 417,
793–794
neurobiology of stimulant
reinforcement, 541–542
pharmacological profile of,
421, 421–422
rebound effects after
withdrawal of, 676
resistance to, 676–677
side effects of, 429–430,
675–676, **676**
structure-activity relationships
for, 419–421

Stroke-related depression,
578–579
Structured Clinical Interview for
DSM-III (SCID), **618**
Substance dependence
disorders, 537–551. See also
Alcoholism
amphetamine abuse and,
430–431
amphetamine for, 418
behavioral neurobiology of
drug-seeking behavior,
538–540
animal models of alcohol
self-administration,
539–540
drug self-administration,
539
biobehavioral theories of
relapse and rapid
reinstatement of
dependence, 544–546
conditioning models,
544–546
homeostatic models, 544
bipolar disorder and, 605
brain stimulation reward
paradigms, 540–541
conditioned place preference
paradigms, 540
definition of, 537
individual vulnerability and
risk of, 538
neurobiology of, 541–544
alcohol reinforcement,
543–544
opiate reinforcement,
542–543
stimulant reinforcement,
541–542
persistent alterations in
homeostasis and risk of
relapse, 546–550
protracted alcohol
abstinence, 548–550
protracted opiate
abstinence, 546–547
protracted withdrawal
phenomena with
cocaine, 547–548

personality disorders and, 754–755

schizophrenia and, 617–618

treatment of, 707–720

alcoholism, 707–709

benzodiazepines and other sedatives, 709–710

cocaine, 710–711, **711**

hallucinogens, 717–718

intoxication with violent behavior, 775–776

nicotine, 718–720

opioids, 711–717

self-help groups, 717

withdrawal, 775

Substance P, 313

Succinylcholine interactions

with gallamine, 224

with monoamine oxidase inhibitors, **789**

Suicidal behavior

adrenal hypertrophy in victims of, 446

α_2 receptor in brain and, 452

antidepressants and, 587–588

in children taking fluoxetine, 690

among elderly persons, 779

emergency hospitalization for, 770

extrapyramidal side effects and, 281

5-hydroxyindoleacetic acid level and, 439, 453

selective serotonin reuptake inhibitors for, 171

Sulfonal, 405

Sulindac, interaction with lithium, **327**

Sulpiride, **47,** 840, **840–842,** 843, 844

Sweating, drug-induced

clomipramine, 690

nefazodone, 207

selective serotonin reuptake inhibitors, 172

venlafaxine, 205

Sydenham's chorea, 512

Symmetrel. *See* Amantadine

Sympathomimetic agents, interaction with monoamine oxidase inhibitors, 188–189

Symptomless autoimmune thyroiditis (SAT), 448

Synaptic effect, 5

Synaptic homeostasis, 7

Synaptic regulation, 54–57

Synaptic resilience, 8, 9

T lymphocytes, 461–462

in depression, 463

Tachykinin, 313

Tandospirone, 235, **236**

Taractan. *See* Chlorprothixene

Tardive dyskinesia (TD), 256–257, 282, 611, 618, 625, **626,** 628. *See also* Extrapyramidal side effects

amoxapine-induced, 200

in children and adolescents, 684

clinical course of, 257

diagnostic criteria for, 256

in elderly persons, 806–807

movements of, 256

pathophysiology of, 628

prevalence of, 256–257

risk factors for, 255, 257, 282, 628

role of gamma-aminobutyric acid in, 283, 628

treatment of, 257, 292–293, 628

buspirone, 239–240

clozapine, 628

verapamil, 384

vitamin E, 628

Tardive dystonia, 282, 628

Targeting of Abnormal Kinetic Effects (TAKE) Scale, 284

TCAs. *See* Antidepressants, tricyclic

Teacher Report Form of Child Behavior Checklist, 671, 673

Tegretol. *See* Carbamazepine

Temazepam

biotransformation of, 217

half-life of, **218**

for sleep disorders in elderly persons, 812

structure of, **409**

use in pregnancy, **831**

Temporal lobe epilepsy, 757

Tenormin. *See* Atenolol

Teratogenicity. *See also* Pregnancy and lactation

of carbamazepine, 359, 687, 832

of lithium, 326, 831–832

of valproate, 365, 832

Terfenadine, **130**

Testosterone

in anorexia nervosa, 563

antipsychotic effects on, **627**

Tetracycline, interaction with lithium, **793**

Tetrahydroaminoacridine (THA), 393

for Alzheimer's disease, 393, 813

dosage of, 394–395

drug interactions with, 393

history and discovery of, 393

mechanism of action of, 393

pharmacokinetics and disposition of, 393

pharmacological profile of, 393

side effects and toxicity of, 393, 813

structure of, 393

Tetrahydroisoxazolopyridinol (THIP), 813

Theophylline interactions

with β-blockers, 291

with carbamazepine, 359

with lithium, **793**

with monoamine oxidase inhibitors, **789**

with tetrahydroamino-acridine, 393

Thiamine, 775

Thiopental, **406**

Thiopentone, 406

Thioridazine, 35, 619

cardiovascular effects of, 258

dosage of, **249,** 258, **620**

effects on latent inhibition of conditioned responses in animals, **107**

Thioridazine *(continued)*
  history and discovery of, 248
  indications for
    aggression in children and
      adolescents, 686
    borderline personality
      disorder, 762
    dementia, 660, 663
    sleep disorders in elderly
      persons, 812
  interaction with propranolol,
    748
  metabolites of, 251
  retinitis pigmentosa induced
    by, 258, **627,** 629–630
  structure-activity relationship
    for, 248, **249**
  use during pregnancy, **829**
Thiothixene
  for dementia, 660
  dosage of, **249, 620**
  effects on latent inhibition of
    conditioned responses
    in animals, **107**
  history and discovery of, 248
  for schizotypal personality
    disorder, 757
  structure-activity relationship
    for, 248, **249**
  use during pregnancy, **829**
Thioxanthenes
  metabolism of, 251
  structure-activity
    relationships for, 248,
    249
THIP. *See* Tetrahydro-
  isoxazolopyridinol
Third-party notification, 771
Thorazine. *See* Chlorpromazine
Thought disorder, 479, 615,
  616
Threo-hydrobupropion, 201,
  202
Thrombocytopenia,
  drug-induced
  carbamazepine, 358–359
  valproate, 365, 680
Thromboxanes, **23,** 24
Thyroid hormones
  in Alzheimer's disease, 813

antidepressants and, 591
for bipolar disorder, 611
for mood disorders, 447
Thyroid-stimulating hormone
  (TSH), 440, 447–448, 563
Thyrotropin-releasing hormone
  (TRH) stimulation test, 440,
  447–448
Tianeptine, **840–842,** 844
Tic douloureux, 223
Tics
  carbamazepine-induced, 686
  in Tourette's disorder,
    691–692
Timolol, **130**
Tindal. *See* Acetophenazine
  maleate
Tofranil. *See* Imipramine
Tolerance, 8
Tourette's disorder, 691–693
  attention-deficit disorders
    and, 691, 692
  depression and, 692
  duration of, 691
  genetics of, 691
  obsessive-compulsive
    disorder and, 511, 512,
    691
  placebo response in, 670
  prevalence of, 691
  treatment of, 691–693
    antipsychotics, 250, 255
    assessing response to, 692
    clonidine, 692–693
    neuroleptics, 692
    selection of, 691–692
Transcription, 33, 34
Tranxene. *See* Clorazepate
Tranylcypromine, 183, **184,** 185,
  397, 419, 440
  animal studies of
    chronic mild stress model,
      95
    differential operant
      responding for low
      reinforcement, 86
  dosage of, 588
  indications for
    avoidant personality
      disorder, 764

borderline personality
    disorder, 761, 762, 772
depression, 185, 583
  bipolar, 608
  treatment-refractory, 589
panic disorder, 642
social phobia, 186
use in pregnancy, 826, **827**
Trazodone, 195–199
  animal studies of
    differential operant
      responding for low
      reinforcement, 86
    isolation-induced
      hyperactivity, 87
  drug interactions with,
    198–199
  efficacy in panic disorder, 642
  for elderly persons, 197, 585
  history and discovery of,
    195–196
  indications for, 197–198
    aggression, 747
      in children and
        adolescents, 687
    agitation in elderly
      persons, 807
    autism, 694
    bulimia nervosa, 727
    dementia, 661–662, 664
    depression, 583
      geriatric, 809
    obsessive-compulsive
      disorder, 168, 650
  mechanism of action of, 196,
    197, 583
  metabolite of, 196, 583
  overdose of, 198
  pharmacokinetics and
    disposition of, 196
  pharmacological profile of,
    196
  serotonin reuptake inhibition
    by, 196, 197, 583
  side effects and toxicology
    of, 198, 583, 687
    priapism, 198, 687, 778, 785
  structure-activity relationship
    for, 196, **196**
  use in pregnancy, **827**

Tremor
    drug-induced
        antipsychotics, 255, 256, 776
        clomipramine, 690
        lithium, 679
        nefazodone, 207
        selective serotonin
            reuptake inhibitors,
            582, 690
        tricyclic antidepressants, 682
        valproate, 365
        venlafaxine, 205
    parkinsonian, 255, 627
Triamterene, interaction with
    lithium, **793**
Triazolam, **130**
    half-life of, **218,** 409
    indications for, 413
    interaction with nefazodone,
        207
    for sleep disorders
        in children, 695
        in elderly persons, 812
    structure of, **409**
    use in pregnancy, **831**
Trichloroethanol, 414
Trifluoperazine
    in breast milk, 828
    dosage of, **249, 620**
    indications for
        autism, 693
        borderline personality
            disorder, 762
        dementia, 660
    structure-activity relationship
        for, 248, **249**
    use during pregnancy, **829**
Triflupromazine, **620**
Trigeminal neuralgia, 351, 352,
    355
Trihexyphenidyl
    abuse of, 286
    drug interactions with, 286
    history and discovery of,
        284–285
    indications for, 285
        extrapyramidal side effects,
            256, **284,** 284–286,
            292, 776
    mechanism of action of, 285

pharmacokinetics and
        disposition of, 285
    pharmacological profile of, 285
    side effects and toxicology
        of, 285–286
    structure-activity relations for,
        285
    use during pregnancy, **829**
Trilafon. *See* Perphenazine
Trimipramine, **142,** 143,
    144–145
Tryptophan
    growth hormone release
        stimulated by, 449
    interaction with monoamine
        oxidase inhibitors, **789**
    for obsessive-compulsive
        disorder, 168
    serum level as predictor of
        antidepressant
        response, 581
Tuberoinfundibular system, 46
Tumor necrosis factor (TNF), 462
    in Alzheimer's disease, 399
Twin studies
    of mood disorders, 442, 444
    of panic disorder, 502
    of schizophrenia, 479–481
Two-compartment model,
    125–127, **126–128**
Tyramine, dietary
    moclobemide and, 190
    monoamine oxidase inhibitors
        and, 187–188, **789**
Tyrosine, 5, 54
Tyrosine hydroxylase, 5, 7, 54,
    563

Uncontrollable shock model of
        depression, 96–99, **97**
Urethan, 405
Urinary retention, drug-induced,
    256
    antipsychotics, 629, 777
    clozapine, 274
    monoamine oxidase
        inhibitors, 187
    tricyclic antidepressants, 153,
        785
    trihexyphenidyl, 285

Urticaria
    antipsychotic-induced, 629
    tricyclic antidepressants for,
        151

Valium. *See* Diazepam
Valproate, 351, 360–366
    dosage of, 361–362, 607, 608
    drug interactions with, 366,
        796, **797**
        benzodiazepines, **794**
        carbamazepine, 359, 606,
            795, 796
        clozapine, 273
        fluoxetine, **129**
    history and discovery of, 360
    indications for, 363–364
        acute major depression,
            364, 456
        aggressive behavior, **746,**
            747
        bipolar disorder, 364, 610
        in children and
            adolescents, 680
        dementia, 662
        mania, **363,** 363–364, 607,
            774
        in elderly persons, 811
        posttraumatic stress
            disorder, 650, 651
        seizures, 363
    initiation of, 680
    mechanism of action of,
        362–363
    for medically ill patients, 796
    metabolites of, 361
    overdose of, 366
    pharmacokinetics of, **353,**
        360–362, **361–362, 382**
    pharmacological profile of,
        360
    predictors of response to,
        364–365
    resistance to, 680
    side effects and toxicology
        of, 365–366, 680
    structure-activity relations for,
        360, **360**
    use in pregnancy, 365, 832,
        832

Valpromide, 360
Variable number of tandem
     repeats (VNTRs), 444
Velnacrine maleate, 813
Venlafaxine, 204–205
     drug interactions with, 205
     history and discovery of, 204,
          576
     indications for, 204–205
     mechanism of action of, 204
     metabolite of, 205
     overdose of, 205
     pharmacokinetics and
          disposition of, 204
     pharmacological profile of,
          204
     side effects and toxicology
          of, 205
     structure-activity relationship
          for, 204, **204**
     use in pregnancy, **827**
Ventricular brain ratio, 460, 461
Ventriculomegaly
     in mood disorders, 460
     in schizophrenia, 459, 481,
          482, 616
Verapamil, **378**
     antidepressant effect of, 379
     antimanic effect of, 378–379,
          384, 608, 680
     dosage of, **384**
     history and discovery of, 378
     interaction with
          carbamazepine, 359,
          795
     metabolites of, 382
     pharmacokinetics of, 382, **382**

structure of, **379**
Vesprin. *See* Triflupromazine
Vietnam combat exposure, 773
Viloxazine, 86
Vinpocetine, 814
Violence. *See* Aggression
Viqualine, 170
Visken. *See* Pindolol
Vistaril. *See* Hydroxyzine
Visual disturbances,
     drug-induced, 256
     antipsychotics, 258, 629,
          777
     carbamazepine, 358, 686
     clozapine, 274
     monoamine oxidase
          inhibitors, 187
     tricyclic antidepressants, 153
     trihexyphenidyl, 285
     venlafaxine, 205
Vitamin E, for tardive
     dyskinesia, 628
Vivactil. *See* Protriptyline
Vogel punished drinking test,
     216
Vomiting
     drug-induced
          carbamazepine, 686
          fluoxetine, 690
          valproate, 365, 680
          venlafaxine, 205
     self-induced, 725
Von Economo's encephalitis, 512

Warfarin interactions
     with carbamazepine, 359,
          795

with selective serotonin
     reuptake inhibitors,
     173, 582, 787
with tricyclic antidepressants,
     154
with valproate, **797**
Weight changes, drug-induced
     antipsychotics, **627**
     in children and
          adolescents, 684
     clozapine, **632,** 633
     lithium, 326, 679
     monoamine oxidase
          inhibitors, 187, 583
     risperidone, 621
     selective serotonin reuptake
          inhibitors, 172, 690
     tricyclic antidepressants, 153
     valproate, 365
Wellbutrin. *See* Bupropion
Wernicke-Korsakoff syndrome,
     775

Xanax. *See* Alprazolam
"XTC," 420, 718

Yohimbine, 85

Zidovudine, 323
Zimeldine
     for alcoholism, 170
     animal studies of, 86
Zoloft. *See* Sertraline
Zolpidem, 411, **411,** 812
     use in pregnancy, **831**
Zopiclone, 220, 411, **411,** 812